Physiological Bases of Human Performance During Work and Exercise

For Elsevier:

Commissioning Editor: Claire Wilson
Development Editor: Catherine Jackson
Production Manager: Kerrie-Anne Jarvis
Designer: Sarah Russell
Illustrator: Cactus
Illustration Manager: Kirsteen Wright

Physiological Bases of Human Performance During Work and Exercise

Edited by

Nigel A.S. Taylor PhD
Human Performance Laboratories, School of Health Sciences, University of Wollongong, Wollongong, Australia

Herbert Groeller PhD
Human Performance Laboratories, School of Health Sciences, University of Wollongong, Wollongong, Australia

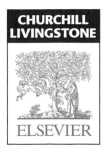

CHURCHILL LIVINGSTONE

ELSEVIER

EDINBURGH   LONDON   NEW YORK   OXFORD   PHILADELPHIA   ST LOUIS   SYDNEY   TORONTO   2008

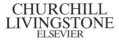

CHURCHILL
LIVINGSTONE
ELSEVIER

© 2008, Elsevier Limited. All rights reserved.
First published 2008

ISBN: 978 0 443 10271 4

British Library Cataloguing in Publication Data
A catalogue record for this book is available from the British Library.

Library of Congress Cataloging in Publication Data
A catalog record for this book is available from the Library of Congress.

Notice
Knowledge and best practice in this field are constantly changing. As new research and experience broaden our knowledge, changes in practice, treatment and drug therapy may become necessary or appropriate. Readers are advised to check the most current information provided (i) on procedures featured or (ii) by the manufacturer of each product to be administered, to verify the recommended dose or formula, the method and duration of administration, and contraindications. It is the responsibility of the practitioner, relying on their own experience and knowledge of the patient, to make diagnoses, to determine dosages and the best treatment for each individual patient, and to take all appropriate safety precautions. To the fullest extent of the law, neither the Publisher nor the Editors assume any liability for any injury and/or damage to persons or property arising out or related to any use of the material contained in this book.

The Publisher

Contents

Contributors

David G Allen MBBS PhD
Professor of Physiology, School of Medical Sciences, University of Sydney, Sydney, NSW, Australia

Markus Amann PhD
Senior Scientist, Institute of Physiology, ETH Zurich and University of Zurich, Zurich, Switzerland

Tuula-Maria Asikainen DMedSci
Director, Occupational Health Service, Health Centre of Pori, Pori, Finland

Adrian E Bauman PhD
Professor of Public Health, Centre for Physical Activity and Health, School of Public Health, University of Sydney, Sydney, NSW, Australia

Louise M Burke PhD
Professor, Head of Department of Sports Nutrition, Australian Institute of Sport, Belconnen, ACT, Australia

Paolo Cerretelli MD
Professor of Physiology, Dipartimento di Scienze e Tecnologie Biomediche, Università degli Studi di Milano, Milan, Italy

Manu V Chakravarthy MD PhD
Instructor in Medicine, Washington University School of Medicine, St Louis, Missouri, USA

Samuel N Cheuvront PhD RD
Research Physiologist, US Army Research Institute of Environmental Medicine, Thermal and Mountain Medicine Division, Natick, Massachusetts, USA

John R Clarke PhD
Scientific Director, Navy Experimental Diving Unit, Panama City, Florida, USA

Jerome A Dempsey PhD
Professor, John Rankin Laboratory of Pulmonary Medicine, University of Wisconsin School of Medicine, Madison, Wisconsin, USA

Pietro E di Prampero MD
Professor in Human Physiology, Sezione di Fisiologia Umana, Dipartimento di Scienze e Tecnologie Biomediche, Udine, Italy

Ola Eiken MD PhD
Director of Research, Swedish Defence Research Agency, Karolinska Institutet, Stockholm, Sweden

Björn Ekblom MD PhD
Professor, Åstrand Laboratory of Work Physiology, Swedish School of Sport and Health Sciences and Department of Physiology and Pharmacology, Karolinska Institet, Stockholm, Sweden

Patricia C Fehling PhD FACSM
Associate Professor, Department of Exercise Science, Skidmore College, Saratoga Springs, New York, USA

Keith George PhD
Professor of Exercise and Cardiovascular Physiology, Research Institute for Sport and Exercise Sciences, School of Exercise and Sports Sciences, Liverpool John Moores University, Liverpool, UK

Geoffrey Goldspink PhD ScD FRSC
Emeritus Professor of Anatomy and Developmental Biology, Department of Surgery, University College, London, UK

José González-Alonso PhD
Professor of Sports and Exercise Physiology, Centre for Sports Medicine and Human Performance, Brunel University, Middlesex, UK

Daniel J Green PhD
Professor of Cardiovascular Physiology, Research Institute for Sport and Exercise Sciences, School of Exercise and Sports Sciences, Liverpool John Moores University, Liverpool, UK

Herbert Groeller PhD
Lecturer, Human Performance Laboratories, School of Health Sciences, University of Wollongong, Wollongong, NSW, Australia

Shona L Halson PhD
Senior Recovery Scientist, Department of Physiology, Australian Institute of Sport, Belconnen, ACT, Australia

Mark Hargreaves PhD
Professor, Department of Physiology, University of Melbourne, Melbourne, Victoria, Australia

Helmut Hinghofer-Szalkay MD
Chair, Institute of Physiology, Medical University Graz, and Director and Founder, Institute of Adaptive and Spaceflight Physiology, Graz, Austria

Sue L Hooper PhD
Director, Centre of Excellence for Applied Sport Science Research, Queensland Academy of Sport, Sunnybank, Queensland, Australia

Arthur B Jenkins PhD
Associate Professor, School of Health Sciences, University of Wollongong, Wollongong, Australia

Asker E Jeukendrup MSc PhD
Professor of Exercise Metabolism, School of Sport and Exercise Sciences, University of Birmingham, Birmingham, UK

Michael J Joyner MD
Professor of Anesthesiology and Physiology, Deputy Director for Research and Associate Dean, Department of Anesthesiology, Mayo Clinic, Rochester, Minnesota, USA

Keisho Katayama PhD
Visiting Assistant Professor, John Rankin Laboratory of Pulmonary Medicine, University of Wisconsin School of Medicine, Madison, Wisconsin, USA, and Associate Professor, Research Center of Health, Physical Fitness and Sports, Nagoya University, Nagoya, Japan

W Larry Kenney PhD
Professor of Physiology and Kinesiology, Pennsylvania State University, Pennsylvania, USA

Bente Kiens PhD DSc
Department of Human Physiology, Copenhagen Muscle Research Centre, Institute of Exercise and Sports Sciences, University of Copenhagen, Copenhagen, Denmark

Paavo V Komi PhD
Research Director, Neuromuscular Research Centre, Department of Biology of Physical Activity, University of Jyväskylä, Jyväskylä, Finland

Narihiko Kondo PhD
Associate Professor, Department of Human Performance and Expression, Kobe University, Kobe, Japan

John A Krasney PhD
Professor, Department of Physiology and Biophysics, University at Buffalo, School of Medicine and Biomedical Sciences, Buffalo, New York, USA

Katriina Kukkonen-Harjula DMedSci
Senior Researcher, UKK Institute for Health Promotion Research, Tampere, Finland

Graham D Lamb MSc PhD
Senior Principal Research Fellow of the NHMRC, Department of Zoology, LaTrobe University, Melbourne, Victoria, Australia

Benjamin D Levine MD
Professor, University of Texas Southwestern Medical Center at Dallas, Institute for Exercise and Environmental Medicine, S Finley Ewing Jr Chair for Wellness at Presbyterian Hospital of Dallas and Harry S Moss Heart Chair for Cardiovascular Research, Dallas, Texas, USA

Michael L Lindinger PhD
Associate Professor, Department of Human Health and Nutritional Sciences, University of Guelph, Ontario, Canada

Carsten Lundby PhD
Assistant Professor, Centre for Idraet, Århus Universitet, Copenhagen, Denmark

Laurel T Mackinnon PhD
Adjunct Associate Professor, School of Human Movement Studies, University of Queensland, Brisbane, Queensland, Australia

Peter L McLennan PhD
Associate Professor, Graduate School of Medicine, University of Wollongong, Wollongong, NSW, Australia

Claudio Marconi MD
Associate Professor of Physiology, Istituto di Bioimmagini e Fisiologia Molecolare Consiglio Nazionale delle Ricerche, Milan, Italy

Igor B Mekjavic PhD
Professor and Scientific Counsellor, Department of Automatics, Biocybernetics and Robotics, Jozef Stefan Institute, Ljubljana, Slovenia

Andy Miah PhD
Reader in New Media and Bioethics, School of Media, Language and Music, University of the West of Scotland, Ayr, Scotland

Scott J Montain PhD
Research Physiologist, US Army Research Institute of Environmental Medicine, Military Nutrition Division, Natick, Massachusetts, USA

James B Morrison PhD
Professor Emeritus, School of Kinesiology, Simon Fraser University, Burnaby, British Columbia, Canada

Michelle F Mottola PhD FACSM
Director, R Samuel McLaughlin Foundation, Exercise and Pregnancy Laboratory, and Associate Professor, School of Kinesiology, University of Western Ontario, London, Ontario, Canada

Marco V Narici MSc PhD
Professor in Physiology of Ageing, Institute for Biomedical Research into Human Movement and Health, Manchester Metropolitan University, Manchester, UK

Louise H Naylor PhD
Postdoctoral Research Fellow, School of Sports Science, Exercise and Health, Royal Perth Hospital, Perth, WA, Australia

Alan M Nevill PhD
Professor of Biostatistics, Research Institute of Healthcare Sciences, University of Wolverhampton, Walsall, UK

Caroline Nicol PhD
Assistant Professor, Institut des Sciences du Mouvement, UMR 6233, Faculté des Sciences du Sport, Marseille, France

Timothy D Noakes MB ChB MD DSc FACSM
Professor of the Discovery Health Chair of Exercise and Sports Science, MRC/UCT Research Unit for Exercise Science and Sports Medicine, Department of Human Biology, University of Cape Town and Sports Science Institute of South Africa, Cape Town, South Africa

Hiroshi Nose MD PhD
Department of Sports Medical Sciences, Shinshu University Graduate School of Medicine, Asahi Matsumoto, Japan

Sarah A Nunneley MD MS
Research Scientist (Retired), Air Force Research Laboratory, and Editor-in-Chief, Aviation, Space and Environmental Medicine, Lexington, Virginia, USA

Lars Nybo PhD
Associate Professor, Department of Human Physiology, Institute of Exercise and Sport Sciences, University of Copenhagen, Copenhagen, Denmark

Kent B Pandolf PhD MPH
Senior Scientist (Retired), US Army Research Institute of Environmental Medicine, Natick, Massachusetts, USA

David R Pendergast EdD
Professor, Department of Physiology and Biophysics, University at Buffalo, School of Medicine and Biomedical Sciences, Buffalo, New York, USA

Guy Plasqui PhD
Assistant Professor, University of Maastricht, Maastricht, The Netherlands

David N Proctor PhD
Associate Professor of Kinesiology, Physiology and Medicine, Noll Laboratory, Pennsylvania State University, Pennsylvania, USA

Kyra E Pyke PhD
Assistant Professor, School of Kinesiology and Health Studies, Queen's University, Kingston, Ontario, Canada

Thomas W Rowland MD
Pediatric Cardiologist, Baystate Medical Center, Springfield, Massachusetts, USA

Michael N Sawka PhD
Chief, Thermal and Mountain Medicine Division, US Army Research Institute of Environmental Medicine, Natick, Massachusetts, USA

Niels H Secher MD PhD
Professor of Anaesthesiology, Department of Anaesthesiology, Rigshospitalet, Copenhagen, Denmark

Jeffrey O Segrave PhD
Professor and David H Porter Endowed Chair, Skidmore College, Saratoga Springs, New York, USA

Roy J Shephard MD PhD DPE
Professor Emeritus of Applied Physiology, Faculty of Physical Education and Health and Department of Public Health Sciences, Faculty of Medicine, University of Toronto, Toronto, Canada

Denise L Smith PhD FACSM
Professor and Class of 1961 Term Chair, Department of Exercise Science, Skidmore College, Saratoga Springs, New York, USA

Claire E Stewart PhD
Professor in Molecular and Cellular Biology, Institute for Biomedical Research into Human Movement and Health, Manchester Metropolitan University, Manchester, UK

Michael K Stickland PhD
Assistant Professor, Division of Pulmonary Medicine, Department of Medicine, University of Alberta, Edmonton, Alberta, Canada

Janet L Taylor MBBS MBiomedE MD
Senior Research Fellow, Prince of Wales Medical Research Institute, Randwick, NSW, Australia

Nigel AS Taylor PhD
Associate Professor, Human Performance Laboratories, School of Health Sciences, University of Wollongong, Wollongong, NSW, Australia

Kevin D Tipton PhD
School of Sport and Exercise Sciences, University of Birmingham, Birmingham, UK

Michael J Tipton PhD
Professor of Human and Applied Physiology, Institute of Biomedical and Biomolecular Science, Department of Sport and Exercise Science, University of Portsmouth, Portsmouth, UK

Michael E Tschakovsky PhD
Associate Professor, School of Kinesiology and Health Studies, Queen's University, Kingston, Ontario, Canada

Hidde P van der Ploeg PhD
Academic Research Fellow, Centre for Physical Activity and Health, School of Public Health, University of Sydney, Sydney, NSW, Australia

Cristiana P Velloso PhD
Honorary Lecturer and Research Fellow, Division of Applied Biomedical Research, King's College, London, UK

Peter D Wagner MD
Professor of Medicine and Bioengineering, Division of Physiology, Department of Medicine, University of California, San Diego, California, USA

Jürgen Werner PhD
Professor, Institute of Biomedical Engineering, Ruhr University, Bochum, Germany

Håkan Westerblad MD PhD
Professor of Physiology, Department of Physiology and Pharmacology, Karolinska Instituet, Stockholm, Sweden

Brian J Whipp PhD DSc
Visiting Professor, Institute of Membrane and Systems Biology, Faculty of Biological Sciences, University of Leeds, Leeds, UK

Matthew D White PhD
Assistant Professor, Laboratory for Exercise and Environmental Physiology, School of Kinesiology, Simon Fraser University, Burnaby, British Columbia, Canada

Ronald J White PhD
Senior Fellow, Universities Space Research Association, Center for Advanced Space Studies, Houston, Texas, USA

Greg P Whyte PhD
Professor, Research Institute for Exercise and Sports Sciences, Liverpool John Moores University, Liverpool, UK

Preface

Human performance extremes co-exist with the possibility of a failure to adequately regulate the internal environment (*milieu intérieur*; Bernard 1865), impending fatigue and physiological catastrophe. People of all ages regularly approach these points. The principal focus of this book is the physiology of acute human stress and adaptation, as experienced during work and recreational activities. These topics will first be explored within temperate, sea-level conditions and then across a wide range of hostile environments from the cold of Antarctica to the heat of Death Valley (USA), and from depths of Challenger Deep (Mariana Trench) through the mountains and into space.

A wide selection of monographs are available that deal with the physiological challenges that confront workers, adventurers, athletes and those who pursue exercise as a form of recreation. Most of these publications target undergraduate university students or the lay reader. With an increased level of sophistication and scientific depth in many human and applied physiology programmes across the world, it became evident that a text was required for more advanced and postgraduate students, for recent university graduates engaged as scientists, and for experienced scientists and practitioners seeking a distillation of current knowledge and critical thinking concerning physiological function during work and exercise. This book represents the first iteration of our attempt to provide such a work.

In striving to achieve our goal, we enlisted 80 authors from Africa, Asia, Australia, Europe and North America. These authors represent a balance of highly experienced senior scientists as well as the next generation of scientists. We asked each author to provide a critical assessment of the scientific literature within their field, aiming to produce material at a level approximating that of a peer-reviewed, scientific review published within the mainstream physiology journals. In presenting this material, many authors have stimulated thought, discussion and debate on topics for which there is not yet a consensus.

In keeping with our desire to encourage critical thinking in student readers, we have deliberately sought focused discussion on topics that are often hotly debated within the scientific literature or at international conferences. Our aim within these Topical Debates and Discussions was to stimulate readers to question assumed facts, and what better way to learn how to question than to see how the main protagonists engage in this process? Many scientists differ in their interpretation of experimental data, some quite dramatically. However, whilst a consensus is often not obtained, few would deny the right of the scientist to apply his or her own interpretation to experimental observations. Future generations of scientists must continue to embrace this principle. Consider the thoughts of Isaac Asimov (1996, p. 226) on this matter:

> . . . when people thought the Earth was flat, they were wrong. When people thought the Earth was spherical they were wrong. But if you think that thinking the Earth is spherical is just as wrong as thinking the Earth is flat, then your view is wronger than both of them put together.

The topics covered within this book have, for pragmatic reasons, been grouped within six sections. However, as readers will discover, there is extensive overlap among chapters. Many chapter titles refer to human performance, although this is not to imply any one form of performance, but to embrace all forms of physical endeavour across a breadth of stressful conditions. We have tried, within the confines of such work, to allocate space for authors to explore performance limits in men and women, from adolescents to the aged. While the bulk of this text focuses upon those in good health, one section is dedicated to the interaction of disease and exercise, both as a causal agent, in the case of our increasingly more sedentary lifestyles, and a therapeutic modality. Finally, performance optimisation is discussed with regard to hydration and the use of dietary and other supplements.

References

Asimov I 1996 The relativity of wrong. Kensington Books, New York
Bernard C 1865 Introduction à l'étude de la medicine experimentale. Baillière et Fils, Paris

SECTION 1

Limitations and adaptations

SECTION CONTENTS

Section introduction: Processes of human adaptation
Roy J. Shephard

Throughout life, the human body seeks to maintain the constancy of what Claude Bernard (1878) has termed the *milieu intérieur*: the bloodstream, body fluids and tissue spaces. This requires an appropriate sequence of both behavioural and biological responses when the body is faced by internal or external stresses that threaten the stability of the internal environment. For example, the stress posed by the separate or combined challenges of performing intense cardiorespiratory or neuromuscular exercise (Chapters 1–7), and life in adverse environments that are marked by extremes of temperature, decreases in barometric pressure or the absence of normal gravitational stimuli (Chapters 9, 19–29).

If stress exposure is prolonged, as when performing a bout of endurance exercise, some behavioural and physiological adjustments may occur during a single exposure. But more typically, the body's response develops progressively, as a given stimulus is repeated over several days, weeks or even months. In the case of exercise, the process is described as training, but for most other stresses, whether considered alone or in combination with exercise, the process is described as acclimation or acclimatisation (Shephard 1982; Chapters 21 and 25). A distinction is sometimes drawn between acclimation (exposure to a unique challenge, for example, repeated sessions of heat or cold exposure in a climatic chamber) and acclimatisation (exposure to a total environment, for example, residence in a tropical city or an arctic settlement).

There is also a theoretical possibility that the body will show or develop a genetic adaptation (Shephard 1978). This implies the emergence of a genetic variant, either by chance or as a consequence of gene doping (Miah 2004; Chapter 8), that confers a substantial competitive margin when an individual performs a particular type of exercise or faces a given environmental challenge. A person's advantage could be immediate, but it could also include a faster than normal rate of acclimation to a given situation or there might be a larger ultimate biological response. In earlier times, such a genotype could well facilitate survival in a hostile habitat, so that over a number of generations a population might emerge showing an inherent adaptation to a specific habitat, an ability to adjust rapidly to a specific stress or a favourable ultimate response.

The immediate biological adjustment to a given stress comprises three main elements: habituation, learning and physiological training or acclimation (Shephard 1969). Habituation is essentially a subconscious psychological process whereby a person becomes accustomed to a given stress. For instance, over the course of a few days, a given intensity of exercise seems less difficult to perform or a given environmental temperature becomes less stressful. In consequence, the immediate physiological reactions of the body, such as an increase in heart rate, become smaller.

Learning, in contrast, involves cognitive and cerebellar processes. For example, a cyclist may discover that a given amount of external work can be performed more efficiently if the thrust of the leg is exerted through a larger fraction of a pedal movement. Likewise, the cerebellum stores information on more efficient movement patterns, and an individual who moves to a cold mid-western city in the United States discovers the advantages of walking on the sunny side of the street during a winter stroll. As a consequence of such learning, the physiological responses to a given rate of work or a given environmental challenge are again reduced.

Training involves a more coordinated response of the body. Initially, adjustments of the autonomic nervous system increase the central blood volume, allowing a given cardiac output to be maintained at a lower heart rate (Chapters 3 and 21), and an enhanced coordination of neuromuscular firing yields a greater force for the activation of a given muscle mass. Subsequently, changes in protein synthesis increase cardiac and muscle masses. Thus, an increase of left ventricular mass allows for a more efficient oxygen delivery to exercising muscles, and a given muscle force can be developed at a smaller fraction of maximal muscle force; both changes further reduce physiological strain (e.g. lower heart rate response) when undertaking a given task.

For each of these elements (habituation, learning, training), multiple regression analysis suggests that the pattern of adjustment is determined by the intensity of the stimulus relative to the individual's initial status, the frequency and the duration of the stimulus, in that order of importance (Shephard 1968; Chapter 21). When comparing studies, it is thus vital to have details concerning the previous experience of the subjects concerned, and also the nature of the forcing function used to induced adaptation.

The major thrust of the Human Adaptability Project of the International Biological Programme was to explore influences of the more fundamental process of genetic adaptation upon current phenotypes. The project organisers suggested studying the characteristics of various indigenous peoples with minimal exposure to modern civilisation, and who were thought to be exercising extremely hard in order to meet the basic demands of life in adverse habitats. The hope of the investigators was to demonstrate regional differences of genome that had developed in consequence of challenges to survival, such as those found in the circumpolar regions (Milan 1980). In fact, the programme observed relatively few unique patterns of adaptation in the isolated human communities that were studied (Shephard & Rode 1996; Chapter 21).

Several possible reasons for the lack of genotypic adaptation were advanced. First, many indigenous populations tend to exploit the junction of several differing ecosystems, because access to a number of environments offers them the resource of a wide range of animal and plant foods. Thus, any genetic adaptations that developed to help survival in one particular ecosystem would be disadvantageous when hunting or cultivating in other adjacent ecosystems. Second, although some environments, such as the circumpolar regions, do make heavy demands on physiological systems, in other regions of the globe, indigenous peoples seem to live with a relatively low daily energy expenditure (Shephard 1978). Furthermore, studies of the human genome, as yet, have identified few gene combinations that make more than a minor impact upon human performance (Wolfarth et al. 2005). Moreover, the survival of humans in a challenging environment depends more upon the learning of appropriate skills than on brute strength; there may indeed be a genotype that facilitates such learning of skills, but the processes of cerebral adaptation are much more difficult to study than a mere listing of advantageous changes in physique. Humans also learn behavioural techniques of insulating themselves from many environmental challenges by appropriate choices of clothing (the Inuit parka) and home design (the igloo). Finally, the norms of most societies dictate the help of those in need, rather than a competitive struggle for survival, so that adaptive pressures are much less than those encountered by some animal species.

Favourable changes in genotype are unlikely to be lost. However, the competitive advantages of training and acclimation disappear within a few weeks, whether this be the loss of exercise training through a period of bed rest or space travel (Chapters 9 and 26) or the return of an athlete to sea level following a period of living high and training low (Levine & Stray-Gundersen 1997; Chapter 25). The progressive loss of the impressive cardiorespiratory fitness of the circumpolar Inuit over 20 years' exposure to modern urban living (Shephard & Rode 1996) is perhaps the most convincing argument against significant environmental adaptation of the human genome, at least in recent years.

References

Bernard C 1878 Leçons sur les phenomènes de la vie. Baillière, Paris

Levine BD, Stray-Gundersen J 1997 'Living high, training low': effect of moderate altitude acclimatization with low altitude training on performance. Journal of Applied Physiology 83:102–112

Miah A 2004 Genetically modified athletes. Biomedical ethics, gene doping and sport. Taylor and Francis, Boca Raton, FL

Milan FA 1980 The human biology of circumpolar populations. Cambridge University Press, London

Shephard RJ 1968 Intensity, duration and frequency of exercise as determinants of the response to a training regimen. Internationale Zeitschrift für Angewandte Physiologie 26:272–278

Shephard RJ 1969 Learning, habituation and training. Internationale Zeitschrift für Angewandte Physiologie 25:13–24

Shephard RJ 1978 Human physiological work capacity. Cambridge University Press, London

Shephard RJ 1982 Physiology and biochemistry of exercise. Praeger, New York

Shephard RJ, Rode A 1996 The health consequences of 'modernization'. Cambridge University Press, London

Wolfarth B, Bray MS, Hagberg JM, Pérusse L, Rauramaa R, Rivera MA, Roth SM, Rankinen T, Bouchard C 2005 The human gene map for performance and health-related fitness phenotypes: the 2004 update. Medicine and Science in Sports and Exercise 37:881–903

Chapter 1

Cardiovascular responses to exercise and limitations to human performance

Michael E. Tschakovsky Kyra E. Pyke

1 INTRODUCTION: CHARACTERISTICS OF HUMAN ACTIVITY AND PERFORMANCE LIMITATIONS

Human activity in work and exercise takes on many forms. It can vary in terms of the muscle mass used, and span the range from very short, high-intensity power output requirements (e.g. sprinting, power lifting), through to ultra-long sustained power outputs (e.g. iron man triathlon, Kalahari bushmen spending 2–3 days of constant pursuit in a hunt). Human performance is ultimately a reflection of muscle power output, which depends upon muscle metabolic and contractile function.

A true performance limit may be defined as the point at which the exercising muscles are unable to maintain the required power output for a given exercise intensity (fatigue). This is illustrated in Figure 1.1A for sustained cycling exercise efforts, with the mechanisms resulting in this exponential power decay described in Chapters 5 and 6. Figures 1.1B and C show that the power requirement for steady-state exercise intensities (B: solid lines), or for progressively

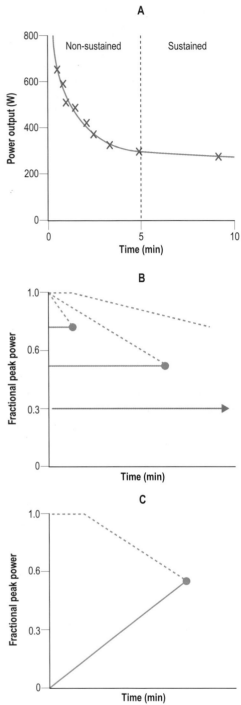

increasing work rates (C), can no longer be met when the power fatigue curve (dashed line) declines to intersect with the power curve. Thus, while power outputs at ~30–40% of peak power can be sustained for prolonged periods, fatigue occurs more rapidly at higher work intensities.

In this chapter, we focus on the cardiovascular limits to human performance during whole-body exercise challenges, during short through to extended duration maximum sustainable power outputs (Figure 1.1B), and during progressive increases in power output to exhaustion. The emphasis is on developing a conceptual understanding of: (1) how the cardiovascular system regulates exercising muscle oxygenation and arterial blood pressure; (2) how oxygenation affects muscle metabolism and contractile function; and (3) how this may explain human performance limitations.

1.1 Defining the role of the cardiovascular system in human performance

Homeostasis (Chapter 18) is a foundation principle defining the role the cardiovascular system plays in determining human performance. The regulated variables of systemic interest are mean arterial pressure, blood gases and blood acidity (pH), regulated by the cardiovascular and respiratory control mechanisms. However, there are intramuscular variables that also appear to be regulated during exercise.

1.1.1 The challenge to homeostasis during exercise and the role of the cardiovascular system

Exercise challenges equilibrium at the contracting muscle, elevating the demand for adenosine triphosphate (ATP) to fuel force production. This demand is met by various metabolic pathways (Chapters 6 and 7), but since intramuscular ATP concentration (ATP) changes very little during exercise (Chapters 6 and 10.3), it is clear that it must also be a key regulated variable. The immediate ATP demand is met via phosphocreatine breakdown and rapid increases in glycolysis, resulting in the accumulation of inorganic phosphate, adenosine diphosphate, lactate and hydrogen ions. These metabolites affect muscle contractile and metabolic function (Chapter 6), and must be stabilised at levels that allow sustained muscle power output (Conley et al. 2001, Westerblad & Allen 2003).

For this stabilisation to occur, ATP must be provided primarily via aerobic metabolism. This necessitates adjustment of not only physiological processes inside exercising muscle fibres (Tschakovsky & Hughson 1999), but also pulmonary (Chapter 2) and cardiovascular processes that maintain muscle oxygenation at a level to support the required metabolic rate. Oxygen transport from the alveoli to the mitochondria is the result of a series of alternating convective (oxygen delivery) and diffusive (flux) processes (Figure 1.2). These two steps are the responsibility of the cardiovascular system and determine the rate at which oxygen enters and is used by exercising muscle fibres, as well as the intramuscular oxygen content for a given diffu-

Figure 1.1 (A) The duration that a given power output can be maintained during cycling. From Conley (2001) with permission. (B) Fractional peak power output during sustainable, time-dependent maximal efforts (solid lines) and theoretical fatigue curves (dashed lines) that intersect earlier at higher work intensities. These intersections indicate failure to sustain required power output. (C) Similar to B but with power output progressively increased (ramp forcing function).

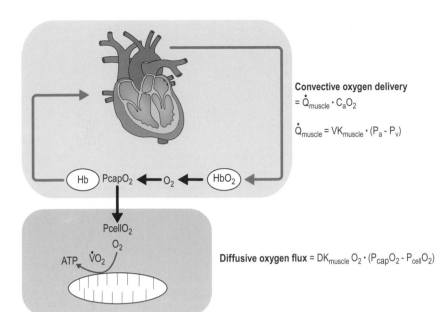

Figure 1.2 The cascade of oxygen delivery. Convective oxygen delivery is a function of total muscle blood flow ($\dot{Q}$), which is a function of muscle vascular conductance (K_{muscle}) and the arterial to venous pressure gradient (P_a–P_v), and arterial oxygen content (C_aO_2). Diffusive oxygen delivery (flux) is a function of the diffusive (diffusion) capacity of the muscle for oxygen ($D_{muscleO2}$) and an oxygen pressure gradient from the capillary to the cytosol ($P_{cap}O_2$–$P_{cell}O_2$), thus affecting oxygen uptake ($\dot{V}_{O_2}$).

Convective oxygen delivery
$= \dot{Q}_{muscle} \cdot C_aO_2$

$\dot{Q}_{muscle} = VK_{muscle} \cdot (P_a - P_v)$

Diffusive oxygen flux $= DK_{muscle}O_2 \cdot (P_{cap}O_2 - P_{cell}O_2)$

sive oxygen flux. During steady-state exercise, the diffusive flux is equal to the rate of oxygen uptake ($\dot{V}_{O_2}$). However, changes in the balance between the convective oxygen delivery and oxygen uptake can result in changes in the capillary and cytosolic oxygen pressure. Thus, in the context of homeostasis, we can identify muscle oxygenation as a key regulated variable guiding the cardiovascular response to exercise, although it is still not clear which aspect of muscle oxygenation is sensed (Jagger et al. 2001).

Oxygenation of essential organs must be maintained, and this is achieved through the regulation of mean arterial blood pressure, ensuring a reliable driving force for tissue perfusion. In this environment, adjustments to organ vascular conductance, through localised vasodilatation or vasoconstriction, can then control organ blood flow and thereby allow regulation of tissue oxygenation.

2 MODELS FOR UNDERSTANDING THE DETERMINANTS OF EXERCISING MUSCLE OXYGENATION AND ARTERIAL BLOOD PRESSURE

Models that provide background concerning the principles governing mass flow, compartment pressures and the nature of physiological control systems are now discussed (see Chapter 18 for a detailed discussion of control theory concepts). These models are useful tools with which to explore and develop a conceptual understanding of integrated pulmonary, cardiovascular, muscle contractile and metabolic responses to exercise.

2.1 Convective and diffusive movement: the mass flow model

Figure 1.3A identifies the key structural and functional characteristics of the cardiovascular system that dictate mass flow. In this chapter, the focus is on the flow of blood and oxygen molecules. Mass flow requires an energy gradient. In the case of blood (mass) flow, this is in the form of

a pressure gradient between upstream and downstream segments of the vascular tree, necessary to overcome inherent flow resistances. The inverse of resistance is conductance, which describes the degree to which flow is permitted rather than resisted, and it is this term that will be used throughout this chapter. For the diffusion (mass flow) of oxygen from the blood into the muscle fibres (diffusive flux), the energy gradient is a concentration (partial pressure) gradient for oxygen in solution between these sites.

From this model, several key points may be derived that are essential to understanding the sections that follow. First, the same flow can be achieved if equal and opposite adjustments in energy gradient and conductance occur. Second, the downstream energy can be maintained at a higher level for the same flow if the conductance is elevated. Third, for a given conductance, an increase in flow can only be achieved if there is an increase in the energy gradient.

2.2 Blood volume and oxygen concentration in a defined compartment: conservation of mass model

Figure 1.3B illustrates the determinants of mass volume and pressure within a compartment. Arterial blood volume and pressure result from the balance between inflow (cardiac output; $\dot{Q}$) and outflow (systemic vascular conductance and the pressure gradient). When vascular conductance increases but cardiac output does not, arterial blood pressure drops. This will eventually reduce outflow as the pressure gradient decreases, until inflow again matches outflow, but at a reduced arterial volume and pressure. The central veins, the large arteries and the peripheral veins are also compartments of relevance to understanding dynamic changes in, and the stabilisation of, arterial blood flow and blood pressure. Similarly, for diffusive oxygen flux and partial pressure, the compartments of primary interest are the capillary plasma space and the cytosolic space in the active muscle fibres.

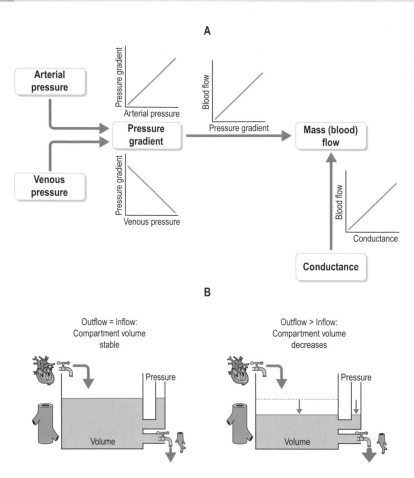

Figure 1.3 (A) The mass flow model, illustrating how blood flow is proportionally linked to the blood pressure gradient via arterial and venous pressure relationships, and to vascular conductance through vasomotor tone. (B) The conservation of mass model, describing how arterial blood volume and pressure result from the balance between cardiac output and systemic vascular conductance and the pressure gradient.

Some key points are essential to understanding the sections that follow. First, flows into and out of the compartment are determined by the mass flow model (Figure 1.3A). Second, changes in volume (concentration) can only occur if there is an imbalance between inflow and outflow (turnover). Third, increased inflow, relative to outflow, will increase compartment volume (concentration) and the pressure gradient for outflow. Thus, outflow will increase to eventually equal inflow but at a new, stable elevated compartment volume (concentration); the inverse is also true. Fourth, when outflow is fixed, increasing inflow elevates compartment volume (concentration) and pressure. This reduces the energy gradient for inflow, so that it returns to the original level, but at a higher compartment volume (concentration).

2.3 Physiological control strategies: integrated control model

The principles of physiological regulation (control systems) are discussed in detail in Chapter 18. Below are summarised the actions and interactions of feedback and feedforward (related disturbance loop, central command), as they relate to minimising the effects of disturbances to the regulated cardiovascular variables (Figure 1.4).

2.3.1 Feedback control
Feedback control utilises a closed loop (afferent flow) for continuous control or modulation of critical physiologi-

cal functions (e.g. cardiac output, total peripheral resistance). Changes in the regulated variable (e.g. mean arterial pressure) are continuously monitored, and this information is used to guide adjustments in the controlled system and thereby correct errors in the regulated variable to restore homeostasis (Chapter 18). For example, high-pressure baroreceptors (carotid sinus and aortic arch) continuously sense local blood pressure, with an elevation causing stretch-induced feedback. This occurs during exercise. Such feedback results in cardiac output and total peripheral vascular conductance adjustments, via the (efferent) autonomic nervous system, enabling blood pressure restoration. Historically, physiologists have used engineering models to describe regulation, assuming the presence of either reference or error signals, and, in some cases, the presence of set-points. Contemporary modellers challenge the need for these concepts (Chapter 18).

However, it must be remembered that if homeostasis is not disturbed, there will be no change in afferent flow received by the control system. Therefore, feedback is an essential control system component and the magnitude by which the change in the regulated variable is reduced (attenuated) is termed the gain (sensitivity) of feedback control (Chapter 18). It appears that physiological control systems have relatively modest gains in order to promote adequate stability (Houk 1988).

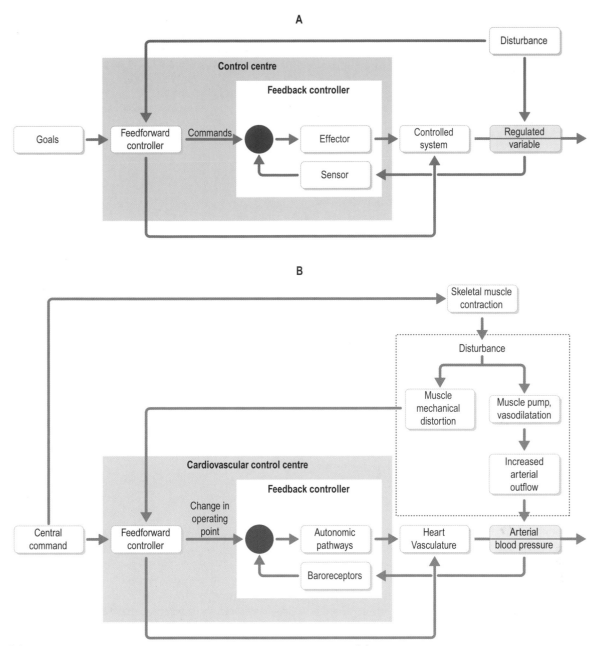

Figure 1.4 (A) A schematic representation of feedforward and feedback control. (B) Arterial blood pressure regulation showing parallel central command (feedforward) to activate the muscle, and cardiovascular feedforward. Skeletal muscle activation affects blood pressure, with arterial baroreceptors providing feedback. After Houk (1988) with permission.

2.3.2 Feedforward control

Feedforward control (related disturbance loop, central command) generates commands to the controlled system without using feedback information about the regulated variable. However, it can be directed by initial sensory information about a disturbance that will eventually alter the regulated variable. This means that the moment-to-moment regulation is under open-loop control (Chapter 18) and without feedback, so the accuracy of the initial response cannot be evaluated. In essence, we can view the feedforward commands as a best guess at the appropriate physiological response to prevent a disruption of the regulated variable. The better its best guess, the smaller the homeostatic disturbance.

3 THE CARDIOVASCULAR RESPONSE TO EXERCISE: REGULATING MUSCLE OXYGENATION

Exercise increases the metabolic demand for oxygen, requiring cardiovascular adjustments that elevate muscle blood flow: increased muscle vascular conductance and cardiac output, and decreased vascular conductance in resting tissues (redistribution; Figures 1.3A and 1.3B). Since muscle blood flow increases many-fold with exercise but arterial blood pressure changes relatively little, it is the change in vascular conductance that primarily determines muscle blood flow. Cardiac output increases and vasoconstriction in the non-exercising tissues facilitate maintenance of mean arterial pressure (Figure 1.3B); these variables are controlled to regulate mean arterial pressure. This section explores what is known about regulation of oxygen delivery to exercising muscles.

3.1 The relationship between oxygen delivery and metabolic demand

Considerable evidence supports the notion that oxygen delivery is adjusted in proportion (tightly regulated) to metabolic demand in exercise. This requires negative feedback control, with supporting evidence coming from the linear relationship between muscle blood flow and work rate or oxygen uptake ($\dot{V}_{O_2}$; Saltin et al. 1998). Depending on the oxygen-carrying capacity of blood and oxygen extraction at the exercising muscle, muscle blood flow would need to increase by ~5.5–7.0 $L \cdot min^{-1}$ for every 1 $L \cdot min^{-1}$ increase in oxygen uptake. Typically, muscle blood flow increases linearly until exhaustion in a progressive exercise test (Saltin et al. 1998; Figure 1.5).

Further support comes from studies in which the oxygen-carrying capacity of blood has been manipulated. If oxygen delivery is regulated, then an altered oxygen-carrying capacity should result in an opposite change in muscle blood flow, for a given steady-state exercise intensity. This often (Calbet et al. 2006, Koskolou et al. 1997), though not always (Richardson et al. 1995b), appears to be the case. When it is the case, the changes in blood flow tend to completely offset the changes in oxygen content so that oxygen delivery is preserved. However, it is not known whether these restorations in oxygen delivery preserve intracellular oxygen partial pressure. This is a critical question to answer and will be addressed in section 7.4.2.

However, this seemingly tight feedback regulation of oxygen delivery to metabolic demand does not occur when oxygen delivery is manipulated by arterial pressure-induced changes in muscle blood flow. Experiments demonstrating this have simply examined the exercising limb blood flow response when the limb is in different positions relative to heart level: altered hydrostatic pressure. Regardless of whether the position of the exercising muscle group, relative to the heart, is different at the onset of exercise or changed during steady-state submaximal exercise, muscle blood flow adapts to a higher level if arterial pressure at the muscle is higher (Shoemaker et al. 1998). However, within any limb position, the relationship between metabolic demand and oxygen delivery remains linear with progressive increases in exercise intensity, indicating a proportional adjustment in oxygen delivery with metabolic demand (Figure 1.5).

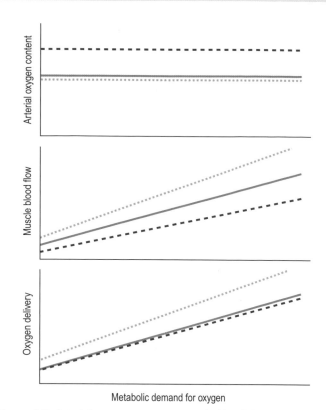

Figure 1.5 Arterial oxygen content, muscle blood flow and oxygen delivery in normal conditions (solid line), elevated arterial oxygen content (dashed line) and elevated local exercising muscle blood pressure (dotted line), each as a function of exercise intensity.

3.2 Oxygen delivery and the metabolic demand for oxygen

With a step increase (forcing function) in exercise intensity, oxygen delivery (muscle blood flow) must increase to meet the new metabolic demand for oxygen. The adjustment to a new steady state is called the dynamic response, which occurs in an exponential fashion, with different components of the cardiovascular and respiratory systems displaying different time constants. These time constants provide insight into the characteristics of the control mechanisms (feedforward or feedback) that modulate these adjustments and in this section, we examine the characteristics of the dynamic cardiovascular response to step increases in exercise intensity.

3.2.1 Dynamic response characteristics of muscle oxygen delivery (muscle blood flow)

There are currently no techniques with which to measure the dynamic response of exercising muscle blood flow during whole-body exercise, and the information we do have regarding blood flow changes during a step forcing function comes primarily from exercise involving smaller muscle groups (forearm and knee extension/flexion;

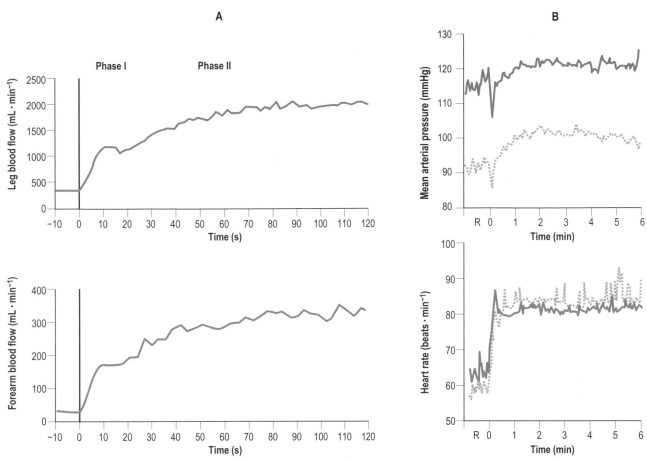

Figure 1.6 (A) Leg blood flow during rhythmic two-legged knee extension/flexion exercise and forearm handgrip exercise, in response to a step increase (forcing function) from rest to moderate-exercise intensity. From Tschakovsky (2004) with permission. (B) Mean arterial blood pressure at the level of the exercising leg, and heart rate in upright (solid line) and supine (dotted line) positions in response to a step increase from rest to moderate-exercise intensity. Modified from MacDonald et al. (1998) with permission.

MacDonald et al. 1998, Saunders et al. 2005). Data from these experimental models are extrapolated here to represent the response to whole-body exercise, and are characterised by an immediate but incomplete initial increase that plateaus at about 5–7 s (Figure 1.6A).

This blood flow is maintained until a second slower increase (Phase II) occurs, beginning at approximately 20 s. In low- to moderate-intensity exercise, muscle blood flow reaches a steady state during this phase (MacDonald et al. 1998, Saunders et al. 2005). At higher intensity exercise, a third and very slow increase in blood flow (Phase III) is observed, commencing ~1.5–2 min after the start of exercise (Saunders et al. 2005). The magnitude of the initial increase (Phase I) is proportional to the exercise intensity, as is the ultimate steady-state blood flow. Since arterial blood pressure changes are relatively small compared to muscle blood flow, it is not surprising that changes in muscle vascular conductance essentially mirror muscle blood flow responses (Saunders et al. 2005).

Important questions to ask here are: What type of control system might be involved in the Phase I and II increases in blood flow? Since both phases are proportional to exercise intensity, what sort of vasodilatory signals arise from the muscle and in proportion to the exercise intensity? What are the implications of this type of control system, and what is its contribution to the steady-state response, for cardiovascular limitations to human performance?

3.3 Oxygen delivery to exercising muscle: feedforward control

The immediate increase in muscle blood flow (Figure 1.5) is consistent with a feedforward control system, which can involve sensing disturbances that are related to the disruption of a regulated variable (Figure 1.4A). Two types of mechanisms are thought to contribute to the initial exercise hyperaemia response: muscle pumping and rapid vasodilatation. The latter are more related to neuromuscular activation and mechanical events of muscle activation rather than to muscle metabolism. Conclusions regarding the relative contribution of these mechanisms depend on the experimental model and type of exercise (Tschakovsky & Sheriff 2004).

However, the current view is that, in humans, the rapid exercise hyperaemia always has a vasodilatory component, and can be accompanied by a muscle pump effect when venous pressure is high prior to the onset of contractions.

3.3.1 The muscle pump

Muscle activation compresses the arteries and veins within the active muscle. Due to the presence of one-way valves in the venous side, activation expels blood towards the heart, with no backflow upon relaxation, leaving intramuscular veins empty during muscle relaxation. Eliminating the venous volume, and therefore venous pressure, is thought to result in an immediate increase in the arteriovenous pressure gradient upon relaxation (Figure 1.3A), and may contribute to the immediate exercise hyperaemia (Tschakovsky & Sheriff 2004). It has also been proposed that muscle relaxation may result in a negative venous pressure, with the veins being actively pulled open upon relaxation, since they are tethered to the surrounding muscle tissue. This could effectively suck blood through the vascular bed into the veins (Laughlin 1987).

The muscle pump effect should be maximised when exercise begins under conditions of high venous pressures, as would be the case with the limbs below the heart. This is because the larger the starting venous pressure, the greater the increase in arteriovenous pressure gradient when the veins are emptied and their pressure drops. For example, Tschakovsky et al. (1996) found that rhythmic squeezing of the resting forearm with an inflatable cuff, designed to mimic the mechanical venous emptying effect of contraction, increased forearm blood flow when the forearm was below heart level (dependent) and when there was an initial venous volume and pressure available to be reduced. In contrast, when the forearm was above heart level, forearm venous pressure was already at zero, and forearm cuff inflation did not increase forearm blood flow.

Muscle activation also compresses blood vessels, temporarily impeding muscle blood flow; a negative effect. So, muscle pumping is associated with an enhancement effect and an impedance effect. What is the net effect on muscle blood flow?

It has recently been demonstrated, in exercising human quadriceps muscles, that the muscle pump enhancement of blood flow more than offsets contraction-induced reduction in blood flow at low-intensity exercise, resulting in a blood flow response beyond that due to vasodilatation (Lutjemeier et al. 2005). However, as the exercise intensity increases, the contraction-induced impairment begins to outweigh the enhancement effect, such that the muscle pump no longer improves blood flow beyond the effect of vasodilatation alone, and at high intensities, muscle activation actually impairs muscle blood flow.

3.3.2 Rapid vasodilatation: neuromuscular activation

The presence of a rapid vasodilatation at the onset of exercise has been demonstrated repeatedly (Hamann et al. 2004a, Shoemaker et al. 1998, Tschakovsky et al. 1996, 2004, VanTeeffelen & Segal 2006). However, the mechanism(s) responsible for this immediate vasodilatation have proven difficult to isolate. It has been demonstrated in humans that the peak blood flow response (indicative of vasodilatation) following a single forearm activation is proportional to contraction intensity (Hamann et al. 2004b, Tschakovsky et al. 2004). Acetylcholine is released by the motor neurons to stimulate muscle activation; it is also a vasodilator. In humans and dogs, it appears fairly clear that acetylcholine does not contribute to this rapid vasodilatation. Supporting evidence comes from experiments in which the ability of the muscle to contract was blocked (paralysed) and then the motor nerves were either maximally activated voluntarily (Dyke et al. 1998) or via motor nerve electrical stimulation (Naik et al. 1999). In both cases, despite maximal motor nerve acetylcholine release, there was absolutely no change in muscle blood flow.

Potassium is released from muscle fibres as part of the fibre membrane potential pattern. It appears that the increase in potassium in the interstitial space of the muscle is in proportion to activation intensity (Hnik et al. 1976) and duration (Green et al. 2000), and occurs very rapidly (Hnik et al. 1976). However, it still has not been determined exactly how potassium causes vasodilatation and, as a result, compelling evidence for a role of potassium in exercise hyperaemia has yet to be found.

3.3.3 Rapid vasodilatation: mechanical events of contraction

As an alternative to muscle activation factors, there is a potential for vasodilatation when resistance vessels are mechanically distorted during muscle activity (Tschakovsky & Sheriff 2004). This effect has recently been identified in isolated rodent vessels (Clifford et al. 2006). In that study, blood vessels were subjected to external pressures at different durations and frequencies, resulting in an immediate increase in vessel diameter, following a brief compression. This effect has since been demonstrated at very low compression pressures and it seems to be increased by the frequency of compressions.

3.3.4 Summary of rapidly acting feedforward mechanisms

The reduction in venous pressure, the release of factors involved in muscle activation and the mechanical distortion of resistance vessels can each be viewed as disturbances occurring in the muscle and associated with the onset of increased oxygen demand. However, these factors do not provide information concerning the matching of oxygen delivery and metabolic demand. Therefore, they act to initiate a feedforward vascular control response that adjusts oxygen delivery rapidly, but somewhat inadequately (Figure 1.4). Accordingly, there is a mismatch between the response of oxygen delivery relative to demand, and that requires correction to ensure adequate muscle oxygenation.

3.4 Regulating oxygen delivery to exercising muscle: feedback control

The Phase II oxygen delivery response (Figure 1.6) is thought to largely reflect feedback control (Figure 1.4), since its onset is delayed, local adjustments are slower and a steady state is ultimately reached in this phase (Hughson 2003). One might expect that, if the purpose of vasodilatation is to ensure adequate oxygenation to support aerobic metabolism, there would be an oxygen-sensing system that controlled vascular conductance in response to sensed changes in muscle oxygenation (Harder et al. 1996). To date, no such system, originating within the muscle fibre, has been found. Instead, feedback control relies upon the production of factors related to metabolic rate and the balance between oxygen offered to the muscle and oxygen extracted from the blood. In addition, there is a need for mechanisms that can communicate muscle demand for blood flow upstream to blood vessels that are not in the muscle, but which contribute a considerable amount to vascular conductance for flow through the muscle. Ultimately, feedback control is characterised as requiring a supply–demand mismatch and the magnitude of the mismatch determines the magnitude of the physiological response.

3.4.1 Metabolic hypothesis

Due to the close relationship between muscle metabolism and blood flow it has been hypothesised that some substance released from the contracting muscle, in proportion to metabolic rate, may cause vasodilatation (Shepherd 1983). The conservation of mass model shows that an exercise-induced mismatch between muscle production (and release) of vasodilatory metabolites into the interstitial space (metabolite inflow), and metabolite removal (metabolite outflow) will elicit a local metabolite accumulation (turnover). This accumulation indicates the extent of the mismatch between blood flow and metabolism; it causes vasodilatation and it elevates interstitial metabolite removal. Blood flow eventually increases to the point where a balance between metabolite production and removal is reached at a stable but elevated concentration of metabolites.

Although the metabolic hypothesis's simplicity and apparent logic make it attractive, it has proven difficult to isolate the specific muscle metabolite(s) that explain the increase in blood flow. Attempts to identify the proportional contribution of a number of known vasodilators that are released in exercising muscle have often met with failure. For example, lactate (Shepherd 1983) and hydrogen ions (Shepherd 1983, Street et al. 2001), inorganic phosphate (Shepherd 1983), carbon dioxide (Clifford & Hellsten 2004), adenosine (Radegran & Hellsten 2000) and ATP (Clifford & Hellsten 2004) are all metabolites that reveal increased production and release during muscle activation, and which can cause vasodilatation. However, blockade of the effect of any single vasodilator rarely affects steady-state blood flow. An exception may be adenosine. Infusion of an antagonist of the adenosine receptor in humans blocks the effect of adenosine. This approach has demonstrated a 20% reduction in exercising muscle blood flow (Radegran & Calbet 2001). However, these experimental approaches are inappropriate for systems in which there may be redundancy. The current opinion is that the elimination of one vasodilator mechanism is likely to result in the compensatory increase of another. Thus, advancement in understanding blood flow control in exercise awaits new experimental approaches that can identify this redundancy.

When considered in the context of human performance and the role of the cardiovascular system in meeting metabolic oxygen demand, this type of feedback may have negative implications. Let us consider the following: metabolite concentrations increase with exercise intensity, indicating that a greater mismatch is required to evoke increases in oxygen delivery as metabolic demand increases. Furthermore, this type of feedback is an indirect indication of the matching between oxygen delivery and metabolic demand. Therefore, while such feedback control might result in a linear increase in blood flow with muscle metabolism, muscle fibre oxygenation may be increasingly compromised with increased exercise intensity in order for an adequate mismatch to exist and increase muscle blood flow.

3.4.2 The red blood cell as an oxygen sensor

The observation that oxygen delivery via blood flow is tightly regulated to oxygen demand also suggests there may be an oxygen sensor responding to the metabolic demand for oxygen (Ellsworth et al. 1995). The red blood cell transports oxygen, with haemoglobin saturation in muscle capillaries reflecting the balance between the flow and use of oxygen (Figures 1.2 and 1.3B). If red cell oxygen content could be communicated to the vascular smooth muscle, such that reduced content resulted in vasodilatation, it could serve to correct a mismatch between oxygen demand and supply.

It is now clear that red blood cells release ATP in response to desaturation (González-Alonso et al. 2002, Jagger et al. 2001). ATP binds to endothelial cell receptors, triggering a conducted vasodilatation (Crawford et al. 2006). This means that a progressive vasodilatation travels upstream to the resistance vessels that determine flow to regions where oxygen demand has increased relative to its supply.

3.4.3 Upstream communication of metabolic demand: cell–to–cell conducted vasodilatation

Examination of the architecture of the vascular bed has led to the conclusion that, in addition to direct local mechanisms for vasodilatation in exercising muscle, mechanisms that communicate metabolic demand to upstream resistance vessels are necessary to fully explain the magnitude of the blood flow increase observed during exercise (Segal 2000). Capillaries and terminal arterioles are embedded between the contracting muscle fibres, and are therefore exposed to the metabolic and mechanical environment of the muscle. However, larger upstream resistance vessels, both within and external to the muscle, must also dilate for a full expression of exercise hyperaemia. Therefore, local vascular control requires mechanisms that can communicate the downstream muscle metabolic demand to these upstream resistance vessels.

Cell-to-cell conduction of vasodilatation from distal vessels to proximal (upstream) vessels is now known to be one such mechanism, and it occurs via ion channels (gap junctions) between endothelial cells or smooth muscle cells (Emerson et al. 2002, Segal & Jacobs 2001). Evidence comes from the following observations. First, when muscle fibres in contact with a capillary bed are stimulated, flow through the capillaries increases due to vasodilatation of upstream arterioles that are not in contact with the muscle fibres of the capillary bed (Berg et al. 1997). This upstream vaso-dilatation does not occur when gap junction blockade is employed. In addition, Segal & Jacobs (2001) found that rhythmic muscle contractions resulted in feed artery dilation, but not when conduction was prevented via interruption of the endothelial cells.

3.4.4 Upstream communication of metabolic demand: flow-mediated vasodilatation

Flow-mediated vasodilatation results from local flow elevations that increase friction of the red blood cells against the endothelial cells lining the blood vessel (shear stress), leading to the release of the vasodilators nitric oxide and prostaglandins (Busse et al. 2002, Koller et al. 1995, Pohl et al. 1986, Smiesko et al. 1985). Thus, increases in downstream conductance or pressure gradient would increase flow through upstream vessels. This would increase shear stress and induce vasodilatation, thereby helping to coordinate the dilation of remote vessels with that of vessels closer to the site of metabolic activity.

However, the contribution of nitric oxide and prostaglandins to exercise hyperaemia in humans appears to be minimal at best. Numerous studies have failed to affect exercising muscle blood flow by the blockade of nitric oxide or prostaglandins alone (Radegran & Hellsten 2000, Shoemaker et al. 1996). Nitric oxide appears to have no role in hyperaemia when blockade is achieved before exercise (Shoemaker et al. 1997), but recent results have demonstrated about 20% reduction in hyperaemia when blockade was initiated after steady-state exercising muscle blood flow was established (Schrage et al. 2004). Finally, Segal & Jacobs (2001) found that when conducted vasodilatation in response to muscle activation was interrupted, no flow-mediated dilatation occurred at the upstream site, despite a significant increase in shear stress. Thus, the role for a flow-mediated mechanism of ascending vasodilatation remains unclear.

3.4.5 Summary of feedback vascular control mechanisms: implication for muscle oxygenation

Metabolic vasodilatation and cell-to-cell conduction of vasodilatation a short distance up the vascular tree are likely to ensure that blood flow is precisely targeted and quickly directed to areas of increased metabolism. The question arises as to whether the demand/supply mismatch results in a vascular response that regulates oxygenation to the point where no change of consequence to muscle contractile and metabolic function occurs. Stated another way, oxygenation can have an impact on muscle contractile and metabolic function. Oxygenation is ultimately regulated to a steady-state level by feedback mechanisms. Feedback regulation relies upon detecting a mismatch. However, is this mismatch large enough to eventually compromise muscle metabolic and contractile function?

An answer to this question can be found, in part, by examining the effect of altering muscle oxygenation during exercise. This is the focus of the second part of this chapter. First, however, we will turn our attention to the regulation of arterial blood pressure during exercise. What will become clear from this examination is that arterial blood pressure regulation competes with local oxygenation regulation.

4 THE CARDIOVASCULAR RESPONSE TO EXERCISE: REGULATING ARTERIAL BLOOD PRESSURE

Arterial blood pressure provides the driving force for blood flow. Therefore, the regulation of arterial blood pressure is essential for adequate tissue perfusion. The maintenance of arterial blood pressure requires that arterial inflow (cardiac output) balances with arterial outflow (peripheral tissue perfusion) at the desired arterial pressure (Figure 1.3B). Since exercise results in immediate and substantial increases in peripheral outflow at the exercising muscle, blood pressure regulation during exercise requires an elevated cardiac output. This may also require reductions in arterial outflow to non-exercising tissue, and potential restraining of arterial outflow in exercising muscle (Figure 18.9). The latter response has important implications for muscle oxygenation.

4.1 The relationship between arterial blood pressure and metabolic demand

A hallmark of steady-state arterial blood pressure during exercise is that it increases with increasing exercise intensity. It is now established that this results from an apparent resetting of the operating point of blood pressure (the pressure the cardiovascular system is trying to maintain; see Chapter 18, sections 2.2.3 and 2.3). It is the baroreflex negative feedback loop that is primarily responsible for this, with additional effects due to the muscle metaboreflex.

4.2 Arterial pressure changes with a step increase in metabolic demand

The dynamic response of arterial blood pressure to a step change in exercise intensity is shown in Figure 1.6B as an immediate pressure drop. This can be explained by applying the conservation of mass model (Figure 1.3B), where cardiac output determines arterial inflow and total vascular conductance determines arterial outflow. A pressure drop indicates that increases in total vascular conductance exceed the rise in cardiac output. However, since heart rate increases immediately (feedforward; Figure 1.3B), cardiac output is also instantaneously increased. Therefore, the change in vascular conductance is very large and the arterial circulation begins to empty, and pressure is reduced. At ~12 s into exercise (Toska & Eriksen 1994), arterial blood pressure begins to increase, indicating now that cardiac output is exceeding arterial outflow. This is thought to represent the onset of baroreflex-mediated sympathetic vasoconstriction (Toska & Eriksen 1994). This increase in blood pressure then progresses to a new steady state over the next 1–2 min. During this time, exercising muscle vascular conductance is still increasing, but it is apparent that cardiac output must be increasing to a greater extent in order for arterial blood pressure to increase.

4.2.1 Arterial blood pressure regulation during exercise: rapid, initial feedforward cardiovascular control

Let us return to our control model of the circulation (Figures 1.4A,B). We can consider arterial blood pressure regulation in much the same way as the local vascular control mechanisms in the exercising muscle. Thus, we have disturbances that are sensed and can translate into immediate feedforward commands to the controlled system (heart and vasculature) to anticipate the coming disturbance of blood pressure.

4.2.1.1 Central command

Central command (Chapter 18) is hypothesised to be a parallel neural signal to the feedforward controller (Figure 1.4B). This parallel signal ultimately causes immediate increases in heart rate, a resetting of the negative feedback baroreflex for arterial blood pressure and vasoconstriction in many vascular beds (e.g. skin and viscera). In this way, the impact of exercise on arterial outflow (vasodilatation), via immediate effects on cardiac output, is anticipated. It also sets in motion the process of feedback control by disturbing mean arterial pressure from its regulated steady state. Thus, central command occurs in parallel to motor command, which is the initiator of physiological disturbances that would result in a drop in arterial blood pressure if no compensatory response (increasing cardiac output) occurs.

Central command was identified by observing increases in cardiac output and arterial blood pressure in response to attempted contractions of paralysed muscle (Mitchell & Victor 1996). It appears to be proportional to the motor command (Ogoh et al. 2002), which would be reflective of the mass of muscle activated and exercise intensity. This fits with the view that central command is a best guess at the cardiovascular response necessary to regulate blood pressure in the face of increased muscle demand for oxygen.

4.2.1.2 Muscle pump: translocation of peripheral blood volume to the heart

Muscle activation expels blood from the muscle vascular bed towards the heart, increasing central venous pressure (Sheriff et al. 1993) and stroke volume, via the Frank–Starling mechanism. That is, a greater central venous pressure increases atrial and ventricular filling during diastole, preloading (stretching) the heart to a more optimal force generating length. Thus, there is a compensatory increase in cardiac output that helps offset the impact of increased muscle vascular conductance on arterial pressure.

4.2.1.3 Muscle mechanoreflexes

In skeletal muscle, type III afferent nerve endings sense mechanical events in the muscle (Leshnower et al. 2001), with muscle activation stimulating these mechanosensitive afferents. This is the equivalent of sensing muscle activation, with the magnitude of the afferent response appearing to be proportional to the activated muscle mass and activation intensity (Williamson et al. 1994). However, the response evoked by this reflex is a resetting of the baroreflex, which, in this instance, does not evoke increases in cardiac output, but rather peripheral vasoconstriction (Gallagher et al. 2001, Yamamoto et al. 2004), in the attempt to regulate arterial blood pressure.

It is important to understand that all feedforward responses occur simultaneously with exercise onset. Since arterial pressure drops at this point (Figure 1.6B), it is clear that the effect of feedforward regulation of muscle oxygenation (vascular conductance) exceeds the effect of feedforward regulation of arterial blood pressure.

4.2.2 Arterial blood pressure regulation during exercise: slower feedback cardiovascular control

The delayed, slower corrective increase in arterial blood pressure (Phase 2) is primarily the result of feedback regulation, as is the continued regulation of arterial blood pressure during exercise.

4.2.2.1 Arterial baroreflex

The arterial baroreflex is a negative feedback reflex, with sensors in the aortic arch and carotid arch vessel walls being activated by pressure-induced vessel stretching. Increased afferent flow from these baroreceptors inhibits sympathetic flow to the heart and blood vessels, and increases parasympathetic flow to the heart. Blood pressure reductions elicit the opposite responses. This reflex has a modest gain (1.7–7.0), with recent human research indicating a maximal gain of ~3 (Chapter 18). This means that the arterial blood pressure disturbance is only ~30% of that which may have occurred without the baroreflex-initiated cardiovascular adjustments (Ogoh et al. 2006).

The baroreflex-mediated increase in sympathetic nerve traffic to peripheral resistance vessels appears to be directed at both exercising and resting skeletal muscle (Keller et al. 2004). So, there is an increase in sympathetic vasoconstrictor influence in exercising muscle. In the context of cardiovascular limits to human performance, the question arises as to whether this might interfere with muscle oxygenation by restricting muscle blood flow in exercise below that which local vascular feedforward and feedback mechanisms are attempting to accomplish.

4.2.2.2 Muscle metaboreflex

Feedback also comes from muscle metaboreceptors that are sensitive to metabolites related to oxygenation and therefore signal local metabolic strain through type IV afferent nerve endings (Vissing et al. 1998). It is thought that a metabolite build-up beyond a certain threshold indicates that oxygenation of the muscle is inadequate (Rowell & O'Leary 1990). This reflex is not involved in arterial pressure regulation during mild exercise, as indicated by a lack of change in blood pressure when exercising muscle blood flow is reduced. However, it is active in more intense exercise. This is demonstrated by the observation that increases in muscle oxygenation reduce blood pressure during heavy exercise (Strange et al. 1990). This is an important first clue regarding the adequacy of muscle oxygenation in submaximal exercise.

Since the reflex sensors are actually detecting muscle metabolic stress and not arterial blood pressure, it is likely that this feedback reflex causes a blood pressure elevation as a means of improving muscle blood flow (mass flow model; Figure 1.3A), thus improving muscle oxygenation. The metaboreflex elevates arterial pressure by increasing cardiac output and peripheral vasoconstriction (Rowell & O'Leary 1990; Chapter 19). Like the baroreflex, its sympathetic vasoconstrictor outflow is directed to all muscles. This again raises the question: Is there a cardiovascular limit to performance that is associated with this peripheral vasoconstriction?

5 THE INTERACTION OF MUSCLE OXYGEN DELIVERY REGULATION AND ARTERIAL BLOOD PRESSURE REGULATION

The previous section has identified that the two regulated variables, exercising muscle oxygenation (blood flow) and arterial blood pressure, may have competitive influences on the exercising muscle vascular conductance. This leads us to ask the question: How do sympathetic vasoconstriction and exercising muscle vasodilatory control interact?

5.1 Sympathetic restraint: defending arterial blood pressure

During single-leg quadriceps exercise, peak muscle vascular conductance can be upwards of 3 L·min^{-1}·kg^{-1} of muscle tissue (Richardson et al. 1995a). If a 74 kg person has ~35 kg of muscle, with a conservative estimate of 15 kg of active muscle during running or cycling, this means that, if all that muscle was maximally vasodilated, these muscles could accept ~45 L·min^{-1} of flow. Maximal cardiac output of an average fit, healthy person is ~20–25 L·min^{-1}. Thus, peak arterial outflow capacity is much greater than peak arterial inflow capacity and, if allowed, would result in a drastic drop in arterial blood pressure (Figure 1.3B).

So how is this prevented? Recall that the arterial baroreflex maintains blood pressure at progressively higher levels with increases in exercise intensity, primarily through sympathetic vasoconstriction (Ogoh et al. 2003), which is sent to resting and exercising muscle (Hansen et al. 1994). In addition, in heavy exercise (>80%) most of the cardiac output is directed to the exercising muscles, and most of the resting tissue is already substantially vasoconstricted (Rowell 1997). This means that only in exercising muscle is there enough vascular conductance available to change blood pressure. So, is there sympathetic vasoconstriction in exercising muscle?

There are two experimental models that have been used to investigate this question. In the first approach, sympathetic blockade of vasoconstriction in dogs (Buckwalter et al. 1997, O'Leary et al. 1997) and humans (Shoemaker et al. 1997) has demonstrated that exercising muscle blood flow increases considerably following blockade. Interestingly, this occurs with only a small reduction in arterial blood pressure (O'Leary et al. 1997), as an increase in heart rate (O'Leary et al. 1997) or vasoconstriction of other vascular beds (Buckwalter et al. 1997) appears to partially compensate for elevated exercising muscle vascular conductance.

The second model uses patients with autonomic failure, who lack the ability to sympathetically vasoconstrict any vascular beds, and who demonstrate marked reductions in arterial pressure with the onset of exercise. Some of this is because of an unrestrained exercising muscle vasodilatation (Puvi-Rajasingham et al. 1997). Again, it is interesting to note that exercising muscle blood flow is higher in these persons despite reduced arterial pressure. This indicates that the net result of compromising arterial blood pressure regulation, and allowing full expression of muscle vasodilatation, is enhanced muscle oxygenation!

5.2 Functional sympatholysis: optimising exercising muscle oxygen delivery

While sympathetic restraint clearly exists in exercising muscle, it is now well established that the responsiveness of resistance vessels in exercising muscle to a given sympathetic vasoconstrictor influence is blunted (Fadel et al. 2001, Tschakovsky et al. 2002). Furthermore, this blunting effect increases with exercise intensity. This means that a given increase in sympathetic nerve traffic results in less vasoconstriction in exercising muscle than in resting muscle, even if that resting muscle received a vasodilator to elicit the same blood flow that would occur during exercise (Tschakovsky et al. 2002). Nevertheless, arterial blood pressure regulation is not compromised (Fadel et al. 2001).

6 SUMMARY OF CARDIOVASCULAR REGULATION DURING EXERCISE AND IMPLICATIONS FOR HUMAN PERFORMANCE

The cardiovascular system is charged with the role of adequate oxygenation of exercising muscle to support function. Feedback mechanisms are responsible for regulating oxygenation to meet these demands. In any feedback control system, exercise displaces regulated variables away from a monotonic steady state, and this homeostatic disturbance is never completely abolished. Accordingly, feedback control predicts that oxygenation is not optimal.

However, the issue does not end here. We have just seen that the regulation of arterial blood pressure, while perhaps not necessitating sympathetic restraint of exercising muscle blood flow at submaximal exercise intensities, nevertheless does so. We have also seen that removal of arterial baroreflex-mediated sympathetic vasoconstrictor influence in exercising muscle results in significant increases in muscle blood flow during submaximal exercise, with minimal compromise to arterial blood pressure when the cardiovascular system is able to compensate (Buckwalter et al. 1997, O'Leary et al. 1997).

Several questions arise: Is the vascular conductance and resulting blood flow, in the absence of sympathetic restraint, the true target of local vascular feedback control? Is the local feedback regulation of muscle oxygenation compromised by the overriding influence of arterial blood pressure regulation? Insight into these questions could come from determining the impact on human performance in submaximal exercise (sustainable power output or time trial), when exercising muscle sympathetic restraint is eliminated. While these specific conditions have not been properly investigated, the effect of manipulating oxygenation by other means has been extensively investigated, so that we do have some concrete understanding of whether the normal cardiovascular support of muscle metabolic and contractile function is limiting to human performance.

7 CARDIOVASCULAR LIMITATIONS TO HUMAN PERFORMANCE: IMPACT OF OXYGENATION ON MUSCLE METABOLIC AND CONTRACTILE FUNCTION

The first half of this chapter introduced the concept that limitations to muscle power output could occur if cardiovascular responses to exercise did not maintain adequate muscle oxygenation. The competition between sympathetic vasoconstriction, for the purpose of arterial blood pressure regulation, and local vasodilatation, for the purpose of muscle oxygenation, appears to be a central issue requiring further investigation of true performance limitations. Indeed, this topic is also discussed, although for a different purpose, with respect to exercise in the heat (Chapter 19).

We will now examine in more detail exactly how oxygenation can impact upon metabolic and contractile func-

tion, and whether the normal state of oxygenation may not be optimal, meaning that cardiovascular limitations to human performance do exist. To do so, we will answer the following questions: How does muscle oxygenation affect muscle power output? Does convective oxygen delivery limit oxygenation required to support peak aerobic power output? Does diffusive oxygen transport into muscle fibres limit oxygenation? How do convective and diffusive oxygen transport mechanisms interact to determine muscle oxygenation? Is peak sustainable (submaximal) muscle power output limited by cardiovascular determinants of muscle oxygenation, and if so, how?

7.1 Muscle oxygenation and muscle power output

The muscle contractile apparatus and associated ion pumps are the source of the ATP demand, which is satisfied through several metabolic pathways. Intramuscular ATP concentration (ATP) remains very stable, at least until phosphocreatine is exhausted, even at volitional exhaustion, so the ATP demand and supply systems are almost always in balance. Oxygen availability can determine the demand for ATP, and intracellular metabolite concentrations from phosphocreatine breakdown and glycolysis affect muscle force production and power (Chapter 6).

7.1.1 The oxygen dependence of mitochondrial respiration and muscle power output

Figure 1.7 shows how mitochondrial respiration interacts with phosphocreatine metabolism and glycolysis to buffer ATP. Changes in phosphate energy state regulate mitochondrial ATP production, since it reflects muscle ATP demand, and oxygen and redox state can modulate mitochondrial ATP production. The rate of mitochondrial respiration can be independently determined by each of these factors, and it can be affected by their combined influence. For example, at a fixed redox state and intracellular oxygen content, an increase in phosphate energy state will increase mitochondrial ATP production (Wilson & Rumsey 1988). In addition, the effect on mitochondrial ATP production of a change in one of these variables can be compensated by opposite changes in any (or all) of the other factors. For instance, if intracellular oxygen content decreases, phosphate energy state can increase, and redox state can increase to maintain mitochondrial ATP production (Wilson 1994, Wilson et al. 1983).

These interactions occur at intracellular oxygen concentrations found in exercising human muscle, with oxygen, redox and phosphate energy states providing a net drive for ATP production. The implications of this net drive of mitochondrial respiration on intracellular metabolites, muscle force production and motor drive are illustrated in Figure 1.8B, which is the key to understanding how oxygen can affect muscle power output, as addressed within the next four sections.

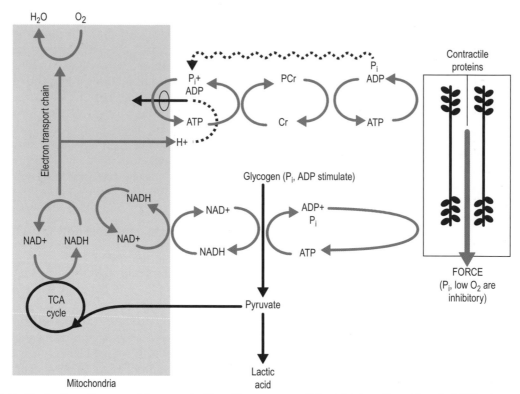

Figure 1.7 Schematic illustration of an exercising muscle fibre. The enzymes of the tricarboxylic acid cycle (TCA), electron transport chain and ATP synthase requires oxygen, adenosine diphosphate (ADP), inorganic phosphate (Pi) and reduced nicotinamide adenine dinucleotide (NADH) as substrates to produce ATP. Contractile proteins use ATP, with immediate needs being met by phosphocreatine (PCr) breakdown, liberating Pi and creatine (Cr). Glycogen is metabolised to supply pyruvate for the oxygen-dependent mitochondrial ATP production, with some becoming lactic acid. The build-up of Pi and ADP serves as a controller for mitochondrial metabolism, communicating ATP demand. Pi and ADP increase glycolysis in excess of mitochondrial pyruvate use, with lactic acid production increasing. High Pi and a low oxygen levels directly reduce force production (Chapter 6). The overall reaction for mitochondrial respiration (metabolism) is:

$$NADH + 1/2\ O_2 + H^+ + 3ADP + 3Pi \rightarrow 3ATP + NAD^+ + H_2O$$

7.1.2 Interaction of ATP supply systems

Sustaining a match between ATP supply and demand requires predominantly mitochondrial respiration. Intracellular energy systems are tightly integrated (Figure 1.7), influencing the rate of substrate production and consumption across systems. Of greatest importance, however, is the adjustment of mitochondrial ATP supply, which requires a disruption to cellular homeostasis of the redox and phosphate energy states. The concept of net drive explains how the magnitude of this disruption is sensitive to oxygen availability.

7.1.3 Oxygen availability affects muscle metabolic and contractile function: insight from stimulated muscle activations

The concept that aerobic ATP supply adjusts to meet ATP demand is a familiar one, describing the response at the onset of exercise. However, the reverse can also occur. For example, experiments using a dog hindlimb model (with isolated circulation) have shown that, when oxygen delivery is reduced (i.e. muscle blood flow or oxygen content)

from its normal steady-state exercise level while motor drive (stimulation) remains constant, muscle power output decreases (Hogan et al. 1992; Figure 1.8B), as does oxygen uptake. This response of skeletal muscle power output (ATP demand) adjusting to oxygen availability has been termed the oxygen conformer response (Hochachka 1988, Hogan et al. 1998, 1992).

There is also evidence to support a beneficial effect of an increased muscle oxygen delivery (blood flow) on force production and metabolism. For instance, increasing oxygen supply above normal during a constant electrical stimulation of dog (Brechue et al. 1993, Vrabas et al. 2002) and human (thumb) muscle (Wright et al. 2000) has been shown to increase muscle oxygen uptake and force production. However, we know little about the mechanisms involved.

Motor nerve stimulation is not voluntary exercise and we are concerned here with limits to human performance. So, what might happen when the same changes in oxygen availability are imposed during voluntary human exercise?

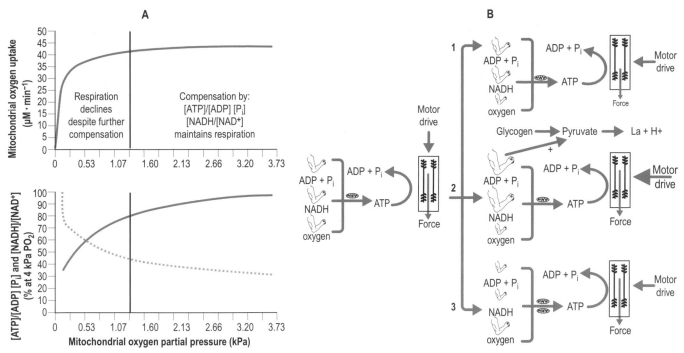

Figure 1.8 (A) Mitochondria oxygen uptake (upper graph), and phosphorylation (solid line) and redox states (dashed line; lower graph) as a function of mitochondrial oxygen partial pressure in isolated cells. After Wilson (1983) with permission. As oxygen tension is reduced, oxygen uptake is maintained by adjusting phosphate energy and redox states, with the vertical dotted line indicating the oxygen tension below which compensations cannot sustain oxygen uptake. (B) The net drive concept: three scenarios. During steady-state exercise, there is a given motor drive and ATP production, due to the combined drive of oxygen, redox and phosphate energy state. Scenario 1: reduced oxygen at the same motor drive reduces force production and ATP demand. Scenario 2: reduced oxygen requires increased motor drive to maintain force output and ATP demand, but drive from phosphate energy and redox states must increase to maintain ATP production. Scenario 3: increased oxygen allows normal force production at a lower motor drive and lower phosphate energy and redox states.

7.1.4 Oxygen availability affects muscle metabolic and contractile function: insight from voluntary exercise

The oxygen conformer response of stimulated skeletal muscle to reduced oxygen delivery can be compensated by increasing motor drive, thus restoring force production and aerobic ATP production (Figure 1.8B). However, the net drive hypothesis predicts that, to maintain oxygen uptake when oxygen is reduced, one would require compensatory changes in redox or phosphate energy states. The observations of Haseler et al. (1998) and Hogan et al. (1999) in exercising human calf muscle are consistent with this hypothesis. In both studies, inspired oxygen was changed between hypoxic (10% oxygen), normoxic (21% oxygen) and hyperoxic states (100% oxygen) during steady-state, submaximal exercise. These conditions change the partial pressure of oxygen in the exercising muscle (Richardson et al. 1995c, 2006).

Haseler et al. (1998) changed the gas composition during steady-state conditions, resulting in the expected compensatory changes in inorganic phosphate; moving from hypoxia to hyperoxia decreased inorganic phosphate concentration. In the second study, it was observed that the more oxygen that was available, the less evident was the depletion of phosphocreatine at a given level of submaximal exercise

intensity, when exercise intensity increased progressively until exhaustion (ramp function). An important observation, with regard to human performance, was that, for all gas mixtures, exhaustion occurred at the same level of phosphocreatine depletion (Chapter 6), but this happened at increasing power outputs with increasing inspired oxygen.

Recently, Amann et al. (2006a) have examined how arterial oxygenation might affect the central motor output and subsequent muscle power output chosen by trained cyclists during a 5 km time trial. Physiologically, athletes were faced with finding the highest continuous muscle power output that can be sustained just long enough to complete 5 km. The results clearly showed that a greater central motor output (power output) was chosen under conditions of greater arterial and muscle oxygenation. This is entirely consistent with muscle oxygenation affecting the metabolic and contractile function of muscle at submaximal work rates.

7.1.5 Oxygen availability affects muscle metabolic and contractile function: impact of oxygen on lactic acid

Lactic acid accumulation is the consequence of a mismatch between glycolytic flux to pyruvate and the flux of pyruvate into the mitochondria (Spriet et al. 2000). Can oxygen availability contribute to this mismatch?

In the past, it was argued that a steep increase in blood lactate concentration during a progressive (ramp) increase in exercise intensity indicated an inadequate oxygen supply for aerobic ATP supply (Davis et al. 1982, Wasserman 1984): the anaerobic threshold (Wasserman 1984). The concept was that glycolysis was increased to make up the aerobic deficit; this view is no longer universally accepted (Chapters 6 and 10.3).

We now know that lactic acid production can occur in fully aerobic conditions (Connett et al. 1990), even at rest (Richardson et al. 2006). Recently, it has been proposed that changes in lactic acid production are due to changes in circulating levels of epinephrine (Richardson 2000), a potent stimulator of glycolysis. So epinephrine could increase glycolytic flux to exceed mitochondrial pyruvate uptake. Observations that have led to this hypothesis include: (1) the onset and magnitude of blood lactate accumulation coinciding with the onset and magnitude of arterial epinephrine (Schneider et al. 2000, Turner et al. 1995); (2) this happens whether there is normal, increased or reduced oxygen availability (Richardson 2000); and (3) blood lactate increases with exercise intensities above ~50% peak work rate, even when intracellular oxygen tension does not change (Richardson 2000, Richardson et al. 2001).

Remember that greater changes in the phosphate energy state are required to maintain mitochondrial respiration rate at a lower intracellular oxygen tension, and less oxygen means more inorganic phosphate and adenosine diphosphate, both of which are potent stimulators of glycolysis (Spriet et al. 2000). So, do we see an effect of oxygen availability on lactic acid when there is no change in epinephrine in a contracting muscle? The answer is yes. Muscle lactate concentration at the same submaximal oxygen uptake is ~50% greater when oxygen delivery is reduced by ~30% in an isolated contracting dog muscle, where no systemic epinephrine response occurs (Hogan et al. 1992). There are also substantially elevated intramuscular inorganic phosphate and adenosine diphosphate concentrations. This supports a role for oxygen availability in influencing lactic acid production, but it is not due to a lack of ATP supply via aerobic metabolism.

Why is an impact of oxygen on lactic acid important for human performance? It has been observed that, when cycling under hypoxic conditions, the blood lactate increase begins at a lower work rate (Hughson et al. 1995). Conversely, in the hyperoxic state, the onset of blood lactate accumulation occurs at a higher work rate (Knight et al. 1996, Mateika & Duffin 1994). It is clearly established that the peak power output that can be sustained for prolonged periods (e.g. marathon racing pace) is just below that which results in the onset of blood lactate accumulation (Coyle 1995, Fohrenbach et al. 1987, Stellingwerff et al. 2006). Therefore, this increase in lactate is indicative of processes that can impair muscle contractile function, and is a

believed to be a key signpost of a human performance limit (Coyle 1995). However, Chapter 6 will present evidence that acidosis does not necessarily contribute to muscle fatigue. This leaves the unanswered question of what performance-limiting processes are occurring with the onset of blood lactate accumulation.

7.1.6 Summarising the critical concepts
Five summary points need to be recalled. (1) When motor nerve stimulation is constant, muscle force production and oxygen uptake changes follow intracellular oxygen content. (2) To maintain force production and oxygen uptake in voluntary exercise, motor nerve activation must change to compensate for changes in intracellular oxygen content. (3) The phosphate energy and redox states required to achieve a given mitochondrial respiration rate are affected by intracellular oxygen content. (4) Lactic acid production can be affected by intracellular oxygen content because of changes in inorganic phosphate and adenosine diphosphate concentrations. (5) Blood lactate accumulation is a marker of the peak sustainable power output.

A key take-home message here is that intracellular oxygen content is a critical determinant of muscle metabolism and power output. It warrants equal, if not greater consideration than maximal oxygen flux to properly understand the cardiovascular limitations to human performance.

7.2 Diffusive oxygen flux and intracellular oxygen partial pressure: dependence on the cardiovascular system

The oxygen cascade illustrated in Figure 1.2 provides a visual frame of reference for identifying structural and functional limitations of the cardiovascular system that impact upon diffusive oxygen flux and intracellular oxygen partial pressure in exercising muscles. It also provides critical equations that define the interaction of factors determining oxygen movement from the lungs to the mitochondria.

7.2.1 Equations for exploring cardiovascular limitations
1. Convective transport of oxygen to the exercising muscle is the product of muscle blood flow and the arterial oxygen content.

2. Muscle blood flow is the product of vascular conductance and the arteriovenous pressure gradient. Vascular conductance is determined by the interaction of local vasodilator and sympathetic neural vasoconstrictor influences, while arterial pressure is determined by the interaction of cardiac output and total vascular conductance.

3. The diffusive transport of oxygen to the mitochondria of exercising muscle (oxygen uptake: $\dot{V}_{O_2}$) is described by Fick's Law of Diffusion, and is the product of intra-

muscular oxygen diffusive conductance and the oxygen partial pressure gradient from the capillary to the cell. It is in this last step that the determinants of oxygen flux and intracellular oxygen tension are represented. From Fick's Law of Diffusion, two conclusions become evident: (a) intracellular oxygen tension, for a given oxygen uptake, can be higher if oxygen diffusion or capillary oxygen tension is increased; (b) limitations to oxygen diffusion or capillary oxygen tension determine both peak diffusive oxygen flux and intracellular oxygen in exercising muscles.

7.3 Does convective oxygen delivery to the exercising muscle limit the muscle oxygenation required to support peak aerobic power output?

To answer this question, researchers have created experimental conditions where only convective oxygen transport to the muscle was manipulated during whole-body, upright exercise. In animal models, it is possible to increase peak muscle blood flow by increasing peak cardiac output by cutting the rigid pericardium surrounding the heart, thereby permitting greater preloading of myocardial cells (Hammond et al. 1992, Stray-Gundersen et al. 1986).

7.3.1 Evidence for convective oxygen transport limitations to peak aerobic power output

Peak aerobic ATP production in exercising muscle depends upon the number of functional mitochondria, if oxygen is at saturating levels. If that were the case during upright whole-body exercise, then we would not expect an increase in muscle oxygenation to cause an increase in peak oxygen uptake ($\dot{V}_{O_2peak}$). This is the basis for the experimental approach used to determine whether oxygen transport limits muscle aerobic power output.

Increasing the maximal delivery of oxygen to exercising muscle in humans has been accomplished in a number of ways. One method uses autologous reinfusion (blood doping), where blood is withdrawn and frozen and reinfused after the original blood volume has been restored. If whole blood is reinfused, there is an increase in total blood volume and total haemoglobin, but not the arterial oxygen content per litre of blood. In this case, peak cardiac output is increased, indicating the importance of blood volume in determining cardiac function. The assumption is that an elevated peak cardiac output increases exercising muscle blood flow and convective oxygen delivery to the muscle. If only red blood cells are reinfused, there is an increase in haemoglobin concentration, but peak cardiac output is not increased. Thus, an elevated peak convective oxygen delivery to the exercising muscles is due to a greater arterial oxygen content. Both procedures generally increase peak oxygen uptake during upright, whole-body exercise (Sawka et al. 1987, Spriet et al. 1986).

Breathing hyperoxic air primarily elevates dissolved arterial oxygen content, as haemoglobin is 97–98% saturated under normoxic conditions (Knight et al. 1993). In such studies, it has also been consistently observed that an increase in arterial oxygen content leads to an increase in peak oxygen uptake. However, the increase is only ~5–8%, since the solubility of oxygen dictates that only a relatively small volume can be dissolved in plasma.

A particularly clever approach has been the comparison of single-leg knee extensor exercise with upright cycling. This takes advantage of the fact that the baroreflex-initiated vasoconstriction of exercising muscle must occur in order to maintain blood pressure during whole-body exercise, since the pumping capacity of the heart cannot match the vasodilatory capacity of exercising muscle (Andersen & Saltin 1985, Rowell 1992). The degree of sympathetic restraint of the exercising muscle blood flow is much less during single-leg knee extensions, involving only a muscle mass of ~2–4 kg, since peak exercising muscle blood flow does not threaten blood pressure. So here is a model with which to compare peak oxygen uptake of the quadriceps during upright cycling, relative to a state when its peak blood flow is allowed to be far greater.

If we examine the data presented in Figure 1.9 in combination with the discussion regarding the regulation of muscle blood flow and arterial blood pressure, a number of conclusions can be drawn concerning how and why convective oxygen delivery during whole-body exercise limits peak aerobic power. During cycling, the quadriceps of one leg form part of a much larger exercising muscle mass and peak oxygen delivery, per unit muscle mass, is substantially less during cycling than knee extension exercise (Figure 1.9A). In addition, the normalised peak oxygen uptake is greater for knee extension exercise. In other words, if peak convective oxygen delivery is increased, the quadriceps muscle is able to use this extra oxygen. This demonstrates that, during cycling, muscle metabolic and contractile functions are limited by the peak convective oxygen delivery, since blood pressure regulation dictates that muscle blood flow will be restrained when both legs are exercised.

In addition, Figure 1.9B shows that increases in the capillary oxygen tension, accompanying increases in inspired oxygen, further increase peak oxygen uptake during knee extension exercise. Peak muscle blood flow is not elevated in hyperoxic relative to normoxic knee extension exercise, but peak convective oxygen delivery is increased, as hyperoxia increases the arterial oxygen content. Thus, convective oxygen delivery is a determinant of the capillary oxygen tension driving oxygen diffusion into the muscle. Increasing convective oxygen delivery will increase the diffusion of oxygen from the blood into muscle fibres. As is evident from Figure 1.9C, it also can elevate intracellular oxygen tension. Recall that a given oxygen uptake requires a smaller change in phosphate energy and redox states at a higher intracellular oxygen partial pressure. Therefore, we expect that a higher oxygen uptake can be reached before the

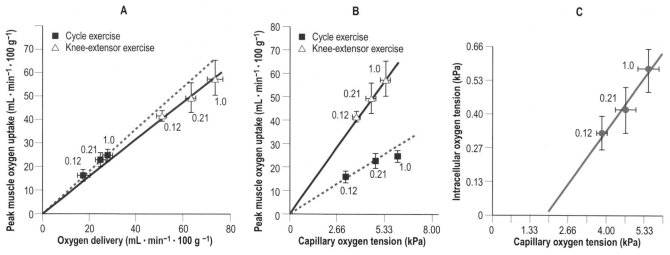

Figure 1.9 Cycling and single-leg knee extensor exercise breathing hypoxic (12% oxygen: 0.12), normoxic (21% oxygen: 0.21) and hyperoxic (100% oxygen: 1.0) gas mixtures. (A, B) Peak muscle (leg) oxygen uptake normalised to the active muscle mass as a function of maximal oxygen delivery at peak exercise (A) and mean capillary partial pressure of oxygen (B). (C) Intracellular partial pressure of oxygen in the exercising quadriceps as a function of mean capillary partial pressure of oxygen. Adapted from Richardson (2000) and Richardson et al. (1999) with permission.

maximal change in phosphate energy and redox state occurs.

One final key observation: the slope of the relationship between capillary oxygen tension and oxygen uptake represents the diffusive conductance for oxygen into the muscle. The higher the conductance, the greater the absolute change in oxygen flow for a given change in pressure. Thus, when the oxygen partial pressure gradient increases from hypoxia to hyperoxia, there is a greater change in the diffusive oxygen flux (reflected by oxygen uptake) into the muscle fibres. The steeper slope for knee extension exercise means there is an enhanced diffusive conductance. Therefore, if we apply Fick's Law of Diffusion to compare the quadriceps during knee extension and cycling, we find that the higher diffusive conductance at the same capillary oxygen tension and oxygen uptake would predict a higher intracellular oxygen partial pressure during knee extension exercise than cycling.

7.3.1.1 Summary

Limitations to convective oxygen delivery in upright cycling stem from the need to restrain exercising muscle blood flow to defend arterial blood pressure, in the face of an insufficient peak cardiac output. Increasing peak convective oxygen delivery above that observed during upright cycling increases muscle oxygenation and peak oxygen uptake. Increases in peak convective oxygen delivery increase the capillary oxygen partial pressure and thereby intracellular oxygen tension. This allows a higher work rate to be attained before maximal tolerated changes in the phosphate energy and redox states occur.

7.4 Does the diffusive transport of oxygen from the blood into the muscle fibre limit the muscle oxygenation required to support peak oxygen uptake?

An important observation in Figure 1.9 is that the increase in peak oxygen uptake is not proportional to the increase in convective oxygen delivery. That is, the amount of oxygen left in the blood draining from the exercising muscle increases with increasing inspired oxygen conditions; the arteriovenous oxygen difference decreases. This indicates there is a limitation to the rate of oxygen diffusion from the blood into the muscle fibres. To investigate this, researchers have created experimental conditions where the capillary-to-cell oxygen partial pressure gradient is increased, independently of convective oxygen delivery, by modifying the haemoglobin affinity for oxygen.

7.4.1 Evidence for diffusive oxygen transport limitations to peak muscle aerobic power output

When convective oxygen delivery to exercising muscle is maintained under conditions where capillary oxygen tension is manipulated, peak oxygen uptake tracks changes in oxygen tension (Hogan et al. 1989, 1990, 1991b). For example, Hogan et al. (1989) studied two conditions with the same convective oxygen delivery (~14.5 mL·100 g⁻¹·min⁻¹), but with different combinations of muscle blood flow and oxygen content: low blood flow (73 mL·100 g⁻¹·min⁻¹) with high oxygen content (20.5 mL·100 mL⁻¹); and high blood flow (115 mL·100 g⁻¹·min⁻¹) with low oxygen content (13 mL·100 mL⁻¹). The venous oxygen tension for the first condition (~3.33 kPa) was higher than condition two (~2.66 kPa), resulting in a higher peak oxygen uptake (10.4 versus 9.1 mL·100 g^{-1}·min^{-1}).

These data, combined with the observation that peak oxygen uptake does not increase proportionately with increases in peak convective oxygen delivery, demonstrate that the intramuscular oxygen diffusion sets the peak diffusive oxygen flux and therefore the peak oxygen uptake. Intramuscular oxygen diffusion depends primarily on the ratio of the capillary to muscle fibre surface areas (Mathieu-Costello & Hepple 2002) and the spatial matching of tissue perfusion to regions of elevated metabolic demand. The former represents the available surface area for diffusion, whilst the latter describes the relative homogeneity of blood flow to metabolic demand. Indeed, this flow-to-metabolism heterogeneity contributes to limiting how much of the oxygen delivered to the muscle can actually enter the exercising muscle fibres – diffusive flux (Calbet et al. 2005, Saltin et al. 1986).

7.4.2 How do convective and diffusive oxygen transport interact to determine muscle oxygenation?

It is now generally appreciated that it is inappropriate to ask: What is the limiting factor for peak oxygen uptake?

Instead, it is clear that factors determining convective oxygen delivery and diffusive transport of oxygen (and muscle metabolic characteristics) interact to determine peak oxygen uptake. Essentially, convective delivery determines the capillary oxygen tension, and intramuscular oxygen diffusion sets the maximal diffusive oxygen flux for that particular capillary oxygen partial pressure (Wagner 1992). Muscle metabolic aerobic capacity determines the change in phosphorylation and redox state required for a given oxygen uptake at a given oxygenation level.

Figure 1.10 describes the interrelationship between the limits to diffusive oxygen flux (Fick's Law of Diffusion) and convective oxygen delivery (Fick Principle), and how these dictate peak oxygen uptake. Imagine that one could control the oxygen tension of blood and that the intramuscular mitochondrial capacity to use oxygen was not limited. Manipulating the oxygen tension would cause a proportional change in mass flow (diffusive oxygen flux) and oxygen uptake (Figure 1.10A; see also Chapter 10.1).

However, in vivo, there needs to be a source of oxygen that can maintain the oxygen tension of the blood. This is where convective oxygen delivery plays a role. In Figure 1.10B, a line representing convective oxygen delivery has been added (Fick Principle). Where this line intercepts the

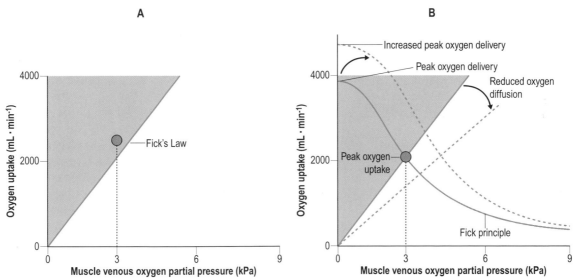

Figure 1.10 (A) The relationship between peak oxygen uptake and the driving pressure for oxygen diffusion into muscle fibres, as defined by Fick's Law of Diffusion: oxygen uptake = oxygen diffusive conductance • mixed venous oxygen partial pressure ($\dot{V}_{O_2} = D_{muscle}O_2 \cdot P_vO_2$). The estimate of driving pressure is venous oxygen tension, which is linearly related to capillary oxygen partial pressure. The slope of solid line (Fick's Law) is determined by the ease with which oxygen diffuses from the blood into the muscle fibres (diffusive conductance), and defines the upper limit for the diffusive flux of oxygen at a given driving pressure (dotted line). Thus, oxygen uptakes in the shaded area cannot be supported, due to a diffusion limitation. (B) A solid curve describing the Fick Principle has been added: oxygen uptake = cardiac output • arteriovenous oxygen difference ($\dot{V}_{O_2} = \dot{Q} \cdot [C_aO_2 - C_vO_2]$). Its shape is a function of the oxygen dissociation curve and it shows peak oxygen delivery to the muscle ($\dot{Q} \cdot C_aO_2$) as the intercept with the ordinate. The intersection of the lines describing Fick's Law and the Fick Principle indicates the peak oxygen uptake possible for the given peak oxygen delivery. Increasing peak oxygen delivery (Fick Principle dashed line) increases peak oxygen uptake through an increase in the driving pressure for diffusive oxygen flux (the intercept moves up the Fick Law line). Reducing diffusive oxygen conductance (Fick Law dashed line) reduces peak oxygen uptake at a given peak oxygen delivery, because it requires a higher driving pressure for a given diffusive oxygen flux. Adapted from Wagner (1992) with permission.

abscissa, there is no blood flow (oxygen delivery) to the muscle and no oxygen is consumed. The intercept with the ordinate represents the theoretical maximal oxygen delivery to the mitochondria, if all of the oxygen was extracted from the blood as it passed through the exercising muscle. Of course, this would mean that the capillary oxygen tension would essentially be zero. But Fick's Law of Diffusion shows there can be no diffusive oxygen flux into the muscle fibres in this state. Therefore, the line describing Fick's Law of Diffusion defines the limit to which we can follow the Fick Principle line from the x-axis intercept (no oxygen delivered to the mitochondria) to the y-axis intercept (all the oxygen sent to the muscle is taken up by the muscle). Indeed, the intersection of the lines describing these two relationships sets the limit for peak oxygen uptake (see Chapter 10.1). The dashed lines for these relationships illustrate how manipulating convective oxygen delivery capacity (e.g. muscle blood flow) or intramuscular oxygen diffusion (e.g. capillary-to-fibre contact surface area) changes peak oxygen uptake.

In light of the points discussed in section 7.3.1, a critical outcome concerning the interaction between convective oxygen delivery and diffusive conductance for oxygen becomes evident. That is, under conditions of improved peak convective oxygen delivery, we not only have a higher capillary oxygen tension but also a higher intracellular tension (Richardson et al. 1995c, 1999). This results in a smaller change in the phosphate energy and redox states for a given oxygen uptake, less motor drive to produce a given muscle power output, and therefore a higher oxygen uptake can be achieved before these variables reach a level that limits muscle contractile function.

7.4.3 How is peak sustainable muscle power output limited by cardiovascular determinants of muscle oxygenation?

Submaximal performance can be assessed using three indices: time to exhaustion at a set power output; peak sustainable power output over fixed distance (time trial); and peak power output over a given time (Figure 1.1A). Each of these indices can be improved by increasing arterial oxygen content, by manipulating haemoglobin concentration or oxygen content of the inspired air (Amann et al. 2006a,b, Buick et al. 1980, Eiken & Tesch 1984, Eiken et al. 1987, Gledhill et al. 1999) or by elevating exercising muscle blood flow (Wright et al. 1999, 2000). In the former case, section 3.1 (regulation of muscle oxygenation) demonstrated that the majority of the evidence indicates that convective oxygen delivery is tightly regulated, such that any

increase in arterial oxygen content imposed by investigators is offset by a reduction in submaximal exercising muscle blood flow (Calbet 2000, Saltin et al. 1986). But how is performance affected?

There are two possible explanations, and these are based on the impact of intracellular oxygen tension on muscle metabolic and contractile function (section 7.1). There is evidence that increases in arterial oxygen content, at the same convective oxygen delivery, result in increased capillary oxygen tension at a given submaximal oxygen uptake (Hogan et al. 1989), or possibly improvements in intramuscular oxygen diffusion (Hogan et al. 1991a). Fick's Law of Diffusion predicts this would result in a higher intracellular oxygen tension. Alternatively, increased arterial oxygen content is not completely offset by decreased submaximal muscle blood flow (Richardson et al. 1995b), and this also would similarly elevate intracellular oxygen tension, with resulting consequences to muscle metabolic and contractile function.

7.4.3.1 Regulation of muscle oxygenation: a paradox?

We have established that increases in muscle oxygenation imposed under experimental conditions can clearly improve muscle metabolic and contractile function. The result is that human performance in work and exercise can be improved above the 'normal' condition. So why does the integrated response of the cardiovascular system to exercise result in an apparent underoxygenation as far as muscle performance is concerned?

This remains an unanswered question. Evidence from experiments where sympathetic restraint of muscle blood flow has been removed, resulting in an elevated submaximal muscle blood flow, would indicate that part of the reason may be the competing regulation of arterial pressure, and the characteristics of the control mechanisms involved in that regulation. Another possibility might be that the nature of local muscle feedback control of vasodilatation requires an error signal and therefore muscle oxygenation will be compromised. Finally, an important consideration is that the human body is a complex integrated physiological system with a multitude of different functions and structures necessary to sustain life. These range from being at the level of organ systems to cells through to molecular interactions. It may be that optimising muscle oxygenation purely for the outcome of acute muscle performance may have associated with it negative consequences for other aspects of physiological function. Therefore, oxygenation is regulated to a level that minimises these potentially negative consequences.

References

Amann M, Eldridge MW, Lovering AT, Stickland MK, Pegelow DF, Dempsey JA 2006a Arterial oxygenation influences central motor output and exercise aperformance via effects on peripheral locomotor muscle fatigue. Journal of Physiology 575(Pt 3):937–952

Amann M, Romer LM, Pegelow DF, Jacques AJ, Hess CJ, Dempsey JA 2006b The effects of arterial oxygen content upon peripheral locomotor muscle fatigue. Journal of Applied Physiology 101(1):119–127

Andersen P, Saltin B 1985 Maximal perfusion of skeletal muscle in man. Journal of Physiology 366:233–249

Berg BR, Cohen KD, Sarelius IH 1997 Direct coupling between blood flow and metabolism at the capillary level in striated muscle. American Journal of Physiology 272(6 Pt 2):H2693–H2700

Brechue WF, Ameredes BT, Andrew GM, Stainsby WN 1993 Blood flow elevation increases VO_2 maximum during repetitive tetanic contractions of dog muscle in situ. Journal of Applied Physiology 74(4):1499–1503

Buckwalter JB, Mueller PJ, Clifford PS 1997 Sympathetic vasoconstriction in active skeletal muscles during dynamic exercise. Journal of Applied Physiology 83(5):1575–1580

Buick FJ, Gledhill N, Froese AB, Spriet L, Meyers EC 1980 Effect of induced erythrocythemia on aerobic work capacity. Journal of Applied Physiology 48(4):636–642

Busse R, Edwards G, Félétou M, Fleming I, Vanhoutte PM, Weston AH 2002 EDHF: bringing the concepts together. Trends in Pharmacological Sciences 23(8):374–380

Calbet JA 2000 Oxygen tension and content in the regulation of limb blood flow. Acta Physiologica Scandinavica 168(4):465–472

Calbet JA, Holmberg HC, Rosdahl H, van Hall G, Jensen-Urstad M, Saltin B 2005 Why do arms extract less oxygen than legs during exercise? American Journal of Physiology. Regulatory, Integrative and Comparative Physiology 289(5):R1448–R1458

Calbet JA, Lundby C, Koskolou M, Boushel R 2006 Importance of hemoglobin concentration to exercise: acute manipulations. Respiratory Physiology and Neurobiology 151(2–3):132–140

Clifford PS, Hellsten Y 2004 Vasodilatory mechanisms in contracting skeletal muscle. Journal of Applied Physiology 97(1):393–403

Clifford PS, Kluess HA, Hamann JJ, Buckwalter JB, Jasperse JL 2006 Mechanical compression elicits vasodilatation in rat skeletal muscle feed arteries. Journal of Physiology 572(Pt 2):561–567

Conley KE, Kemper WF, Crowther GJ 2001 Limits to sustainable muscle performance: interaction between glycolysis and oxidative phosphorylation. Journal of Experimental Biology 204(Pt 18):3189–3194

Connett RJ, Honig CR, Gayeski TE, Brooks GA 1990 Defining hypoxia: a systems view of VO_2, glycolysis, energetics and intracellular PO_2. Journal of Applied Physiology 68(3):833–842

Coyle EF 1995 Integration of the physiological factors determining endurance performance ability. Exercise and Sports Sciences Reviews 23:25–63

Crawford JH, Isbell TS, Huang Z, Shiva S, Chacko BK, Schechter AN, Darley-Usmar VM, Kerby JD, Lang JD Jr, Kraus D, Ho C, Gladwin MT, Patel RP 2006 Hypoxia, red blood cells and nitrite regulate NO-dependent hypoxic vasodilation. Blood 107(2):566–574

Davis JA, Whipp BJ, Lamarra N, Huntsman DJ, Frank MH, Wasserman K 1982 Effect of ramp slope on determination of aerobic parameters from the ramp exercise test. Medicine and Science in Sports and Exercise 14(5):339–343

Dyke CK, Dietz NM, Lennon RL, Warner DO, Joyner MJ 1998 Forearm blood flow responses to handgripping after local neuromuscular blockade. Journal of Applied Physiology 84(2):754–758

Eiken O, Tesch PA 1984 Effects of hyperoxia and hypoxia on dynamic and sustained static performance of the human quadriceps muscle. Acta Physiological Scandinavica 122(4):629–633

Eiken O, Hesser CM, Lind F, Thorsson A, Tesch PA 1987 Human skeletal muscle function and metabolism during intense exercise at high O_2 and N_2 pressures. Journal of Applied Physiology 63(2):571–575

Ellsworth ML, Forrester T, Ellis CG, Dietrich HH 1995 The erythrocyte as a regulator of vascular tone. American Journal of Physiology 269(6 Pt 2):H2155–H2161

Emerson GG, Neild TO, Segal SS 2002 Conduction of hyperpolarization along hamster feed arteries: augmentation by acetylcholine. American Journal of Physiology. Heart and Circulation Physiology 283(1):H102–H109

Fadel PJ, Ogoh S, Watenpaugh DE, Wasmund W, Olivencia-Yurvati A, Smith ML, Raven PB 2001 Carotid baroreflex regulation of sympathetic nerve activity during dynamic exercise in humans. American Journal of Physiology. Heart and Circulation Physiology 280(3):H1383–H1390

Fohrenbach R, Mader A, Hollmann W 1987 Determination of endurance capacity and prediction of exercise intensities for training and competition in marathon runners. International Journal of Sports Medicine 8(1):11–18

Gallagher KM, Fadel PJ, Smith SA, Norton KH, Querry RG, Olivencia-Yurvati A, Raven PB 2001 Increases in intramuscular pressure raise arterial blood pressure during dynamic exercise. Journal of Applied Physiology 91(5):2351–2358

Gledhill N, Warburton D, Jamnik V 1999 Haemoglobin, blood volume, cardiac function and aerobic power. Canadian Journal of Applied Physiology 24(1):54–65

González-Alonso J, Olsen DB, Saltin B 2002 Erythrocyte and the regulation of human skeletal muscle blood flow and oxygen delivery: role of circulating ATP. Circulation Research 91(11):1046–1055

Green S, Langberg H, Skovgaard D, Bulow J, Kjaer M 2000 Interstitial and arterial-venous $[K^+]$ in human calf muscle during dynamic exercise: effect of ischaemia and relation to muscle pain. Journal of Physiology 529(Pt 3):849–861

Hamann JJ, Buckwalter JB, Clifford PS 2004a Vasodilatation is obligatory for contraction-induced hyperaemia in canine skeletal muscle. Journal of Physiology 557(Pt 3):1013–1020

Hamann JJ, Buckwalter JB, Clifford PS, Shoemaker JK 2004b Is the blood flow response to a single contraction determined by work performed? Journal of Applied Physiology 96(6):2146–2152

Hammond HK, White FC, Bhargava V, Shabetai R 1992 Heart size and maximal cardiac output are limited by the pericardium. American Journal of Physiology 263(6 Pt 2):H1675–H1681

Hansen J, Thomas GD, Jacobsen TN, Victor RG 1994 Muscle metaboreflex triggers parallel sympathetic activation in exercising and resting human skeletal muscle. American Journal of Physiology 266:H2508–H2514

Harder DR, Narayanan J, Birks EK, Liard JF, Imig JD, Lombard JH, Lange AR, Roman RJ 1996 Identification of a putative microvascular oxygen sensor. Circulation Research 79(1):54–61

Haseler LJ, Richardson RS, Videen JS, Hogan MC 1998 Phosphocreatine hydrolysis during submaximal exercise: the effect of FIO_2. Journal of Applied Physiology 85(4):1457–1463

Hník P, Holas M, Krekule I, Křiz N, Mejsnar J, Smiesko V, Ujec E, Vyskocil F 1976 Work-induced potassium changes in skeletal muscle and effluent venous blood assessed by liquid ion–exchanger microelectrodes. Pflugers Archiv 362(1):85–94

Hochachka PW 1988 Patterns of O_2-dependence of metabolism. Advances in Experimental Medicine and Biology 222:143–151

Hogan MC, Roca J, West JB, Wagner PD 1989 Dissociation of maximal O_2 uptake from O_2 delivery in canine gastrocnemius in situ. Journal of Applied Physiology 66(3):1219–1226

Hogan MC, Bebout DE, Gray AT, Wagner PD, West JB, Haab PE 1990 Muscle maximal O_2 uptake at constant O_2 delivery with and without CO in the blood. Journal of Applied Physiology 69(3):830–836

Hogan MC, Bebout DE, Wagner PD 1991a Effect of hemoglobin concentration on maximal O_2 uptake in canine gastrocnemius muscle in situ. Journal of Applied Physiology 70(3):1105–1112

Hogan MC, Bebout DE, Wagner PD 1991b Effect of increased Hb–O_2 affinity on VO_2max at constant O_2 delivery in dog muscle in situ. Journal of Applied Physiology 70(6):2656–2662

Hogan MC, Arthur PG, Bebout DE, Hochachka PW, Wagner PD 1992 Role of O_2 in regulating tissue respiration in dog muscle working in situ. Journal of Applied Physiology 73(2):728–736

Hogan MC, Gladden LB, Grassi B, Stary CM, Samaja M 1998 Bioenergetics of contracting skeletal muscle after partial reduction of blood flow. Journal of Applied Physiology 84(6): 1882–1888

Hogan MC, Richardson RS, Haseler LJ 1999 Human muscle performance and PCr hydrolysis with varied inspired oxygen fractions: a ^{31}P-MRS study. Journal of Applied Physiology 86(4):1367–1373

Houk JC 1988 Control strategies in physiological systems. FASEB Journal 2(2):97–107

Hughson RL 2003 Regulation of blood flow at the onset of exercise by feed forward and feedback mechanisms. Canadian Journal of Applied Physiology 28(5):774–787

Hughson RL, Green HJ, Sharratt MT 1995 Gas exchange, blood lactate and plasma catecholamines during incremental exercise in hypoxia and normoxia. Journal of Applied Physiology 79(4): 1134–1141

Jagger JE, Bateman RM, Ellsworth ML, Ellis CG 2001 Role of erythrocyte in regulating local O_2 delivery mediated by hemoglobin oxygenation. American Journal of Physiology. Heart and Circulation Physiology 280(6):H2833–H2839

Keller DM, Fadel PJ, Ogoh S, Brothers RM, Hawkins M, Olivencia-Yurvati A, Raven PB 2004 Carotid baroreflex control of leg vasculature in exercising and non-exercising skeletal muscle in humans. Journal of Physiology 561(Pt 1):283–293

Knight DR, Schaffartzik W, Poole DC, Hogan MC, Bebout DE, Wagner PD 1993 Effects of hyperoxia on maximal leg O_2 supply and utilization in men. Journal of Applied Physiology 75(6): 2586–2594

Knight DR, Poole DC, Hogan MC, Bebout DE, Wagner PD 1996 Effect of inspired O_2 concentration on leg lactate release during incremental exercise. Journal of Applied Physiology 81(1):246–251

Koller A, Huang A, Sun D, Kaley G 1995 Exercise training augments flow-dependent dilation in rat skeletal muscle arterioles. Role of endothelial nitric oxide and prostaglandins. Circulation Research 76(4):544–550

Koskolou MD, Roach RC, Calbet JA, Rådegran G, Saltin B 1997 Cardiovascular responses to dynamic exercise with acute anemia in humans. American Journal of Physiology 273(4 Pt 2): H1787–H1793

Laughlin MH 1987 Skeletal muscle blood flow capacity: role of muscle pump in exercise hyperemia. American Journal of Physiology 253(5 Pt 2):H993–H1004

Leshnower BG, Potts JT, Garry MG, Mitchell JH 2001 Reflex cardiovascular responses evoked by selective activation of skeletal muscle ergoreceptors. Journal of Applied Physiology 90(1): 308–316

Lutjemeier BJ, Miura A, Scheuermann BW, Koga S, Townsend DK, Barstow TJ 2005 Muscle contraction–blood flow interactions during upright knee extension exercise in humans. Journal of Applied Physiology 98(4):1575–1583

MacDonald MJ, Shoemaker JK, Tschakovsky ME, Hughson RL 1998 Alveolar oxygen uptake and femoral artery blood flow dynamics in upright and supine leg exercise in humans. Journal of Applied Physiology 85(5):1622–1628

Mateika JH, Duffin J 1994 The ventilation, lactate and electromyographic thresholds during incremental exercise tests in normoxia, hypoxia and hyperoxia. European Journal of Applied Physiology. Occupational Physiology 69(2):110–118

Mathieu-Costello O, Hepple RT 2002 Muscle structural capacity for oxygen flux from capillary to fiber mitochondria. Exercise and Sports Science Reviews 30(2):80–84

Mitchell JH, Victor RG 1996 Neural control of the cardiovascular system: insights from muscle sympathetic nerve recordings in humans. Medicine and Science in Sports and Exercise 28(10 Suppl): S60–S69

Naik JS, Valic Z, Buckwalter JB, Clifford PS 1999 Rapid vasodilation in response to a brief tetanic muscle contraction. Journal of Applied Physiology 87(5):1741–1746

Ogoh S, Wasmund WL, Keller DM, O-Yurvati A, Gallagher KM, Mitchell JH, Raven PB 2002 Role of central command in carotid baroreflex resetting in humans during static exercise. Journal of Physiology 543(Pt 1):349–364

Ogoh S, Fadel PJ, Nissen P, Jans Ø, Selmer C, Secher NH, Raven PB 2003 Baroreflex-mediated changes in cardiac output and vascular conductance in response to alterations in carotid sinus pressure during exercise in humans. Journal of Physiology 550(Pt 1): 317–324

Ogoh S, Brothers RM, Barnes Q, Eubank WL, Hawkins MN, Purkayastha S, O-Yurvati A, Raven PB 2006 Effects of changes in central blood volume on carotid–vasomotor baroreflex sensitivity at rest and during exercise. Journal of Applied Physiology 101(1):68–75

O'Leary DS, Robinson ED, Butler JL 1997 Is active skeletal muscle functionally vasoconstricted during dynamic exercise in conscious dogs? American Journal of Physiology 272:R386–R391

Pohl U, Holtz J, Busse R, Bassenge E 1986 Crucial role of endothelium in the vasodilator response to increased flow in vivo. Hypertension 8(1):37–44

Puvi-Rajasingham S, Smith GD, Akinola A, Mathias CJ 1997 Abnormal regional blood flow responses during and after exercise in human sympathetic denervation. Journal of Physiology 505(Pt 3):841–849

Radegran G, Calbet JA 2001 Role of adenosine in exercise–induced human skeletal muscle vasodilatation. Acta Physiologica Scandinavica 171(2):177–185

Radegran G, Hellsten Y 2000 Adenosine and nitric oxide in exercise-induced human skeletal muscle vasodilatation. Acta Physiologica Scandinavia 168(4):575–591

Richardson RS 2000 What governs skeletal muscle VO$_2$max? New evidence. Medicine and Science in Sports and Exercise 32(1): 100–107

Richardson RS, Kennedy B, Knight DR, Wagner PD 1995a High muscle blood flows are not attenuated by recruitment of additional muscle mass. American Journal of Physiology 269(5 Pt 2):H1545–H1552

Richardson RS, Knight DR, Poole DC, Kurdak SS, Hogan MC, Grassi B, Wagner PD 1995b Determinants of maximal exercise VO$_2$ during single leg knee-extensor exercise in humans. American Journal of Physiology 268(4 Pt 2):H1453–H1461

Richardson RS, Noyszewski EA, Kendrick KF, Leigh JS, Wagner PD 1995c Myoglobin O$_2$ desaturation during exercise. Evidence of limited O$_2$ transport. Journal of Clinical Investigation 96(4):1916–1926

Richardson RS, Grassi B, Gavin TP, Haseler LJ, Tagore K, Roca J, Wagner PD 1999 Evidence of O2 supply-dependent VO2max in the exercise-trained human quadriceps. Journal of Applied Physiology 86(3):1048–1053

Richardson RS, Newcomer SC, Noyszewski EA 2001 Skeletal muscle intracellular PO$_2$ assessed by myoglobin desaturation: response to graded exercise. Journal of Applied Physiology 91(6):2679–2685

Richardson RS, Duteil S, Wary C, Wray DW, Hoff J, Carlier PG 2006 Human skeletal muscle intracellular oxygenation: the impact of ambient oxygen availability. Journal of Physiology 571(Pt 2):415–424

Rowell LB 1992 Reflex control of the circulation during exercise. International Journal of Sports Medicine 13(Suppl 1):S25–S27

Rowell LB 1997 Neural control of muscle blood flow: importance during dynamic exercise. Clinical and Experimental Pharmacology and Physiology 24(2):117–125

Rowell LB, O'Leary DS 1990 Reflex control of the circulation during exercise: chemoreflexes and mechanoreflexes Journal of Applied Physiology 69(2):407–418

Saltin B, Kiens B, Savard G, Pedersen PK 1986 Role of hemoglobin and capillarization for oxygen delivery and extraction in muscular exercise. Acta Physiological Scandinavia 556(Suppl):21–32

Saltin B, Rådegran G, Koskolou MD, Roach RC 1998 Skeletal muscle blood flow in humans and its regulation during exercise. Acta Physiologica Scandinavica 162(3):421–436

Saunders NR, Pyke KE, Tschakovsky ME 2005 Dynamic response characteristics of local muscle blood flow regulatory mechanisms in human forearm exercise. Journal of Applied Physiology 98(4):1286–1296

Sawka MN, Young AJ, Muza SR, Gonzalez RR, Pandolf KB 1987 Erythrocyte reinfusion and maximal aerobic power. An examination of modifying factors. Journal of the American Medical Association 257(11):1496–1499

Schneider DA, McLellan TM, Gass GC 2000 Plasma catecholamine and blood lactate responses to incremental arm and leg exercise. Medicine and Science in Sports and Exercise 32(3):608–613

Schrage WG, Joyner MJ, Dinenno FA 2004 Local inhibition of nitric oxide and prostaglandins independently reduces forearm exercise hyperaemia in humans. Journal of Physiology 557(Pt 2):599–611

Segal SS 2000 Integration of blood flow control to skeletal muscle: key role of feed arteries. Acta Physiologica Scandinavica 168(4):511–518

Segal SS, Jacobs TL 2001 Role for endothelial cell conduction in ascending vasodilatation and exercise hyperaemia in hamster skeletal muscle. Journal of Physiology 536(Pt 3):937–946

Shepherd JT 1983 Circulation to skeletal muscle. In: Shepherd JT, Abboud FM, Geiger SR (eds) Handbook of physiology. The cardiovascular system: peripheral circulation and organ blood flow. American Physiological Society, Bethesda, MD

Sheriff DD, Zhou XP, Scher AM, Rowell LB 1993 Dependence of cardiac filling pressure on cardiac output during rest and dynamic exercise in dogs. American Journal of Physiology 265(1 Pt 2): H316–H322

Shoemaker JK, Naylor HL, Pozeg ZI, Hughson RL 1996 Failure of prostaglandins to modulate the time course of blood flow during dynamic forearm exercise in humans. Journal of Applied Physiology 81:1516–1521

Shoemaker JK, Halliwill JR, Hughson RL, Joyner MJ 1997 Contributions of acetylcholine and nitric oxide to forearm blood flow at exercise onset and recovery. American Journal of Physiology 273(5 Pt 2):H2388–H2395

Shoemaker JK, Tschakovsky ME, Hughson RL 1998 Vasodilation contributes to the rapid hyperemia with rhythmic contractions in humans. Canadian Journal of Physiology and Pharmacology 76(4):418–427

Smiesko V, Kozik J, Dolezel S 1985 Role of endothelium in the control of arterial diameter by blood flow. Blood Vessels 22(5):247–251

Spriet LL, Gledhill N, Froese AB, Wilkes DL 1986 Effect of graded erythrocythemia on cardiovascular and metabolic responses to exercise. Journal of Applied Physiology 61(5):1942–1948

Spriet LL, Howlett RA, Heigenhauser GJ 2000 An enzymatic approach to lactate production in human skeletal muscle during exercise. Medicine and Science in Sports and Exercise 32(4):756–763

Stellingwerff T, Leblanc PJ, Hollidge MG, Heigenhauser GJ, Spriet LL 2006 Hyperoxia decreases muscle glycogenolysis, lactate production and lactate efflux during steady-state exercise. American Journal of Physiology. Endocrinology and Metabolism 290(6):E1180–E1190

Strange S, Rowell LB, Christensen NJ, Saltin B 1990 Cardiovascular responses to carotid sinus baroreceptor stimulation during moderate to severe exercise in man. Acta Physiologica Scandinavica 138(2):145–153

Stray-Gundersen J, Musch TI, Haidet GC, Swain DP, Ordway GA, Mitchell JH 1986 The effect of pericardiectomy on maximal oxygen consumption and maximal cardiac output in untrained dogs. Circulation Research 58(4):523–530

Street D, Bangsbo J, Juel C 2001 Interstitial pH in human skeletal muscle during and after dynamic graded exercise. Journal of Physiology 537(Pt 3):993–998

Toska K, Eriksen M 1994 Peripheral vasoconstriction shortly after onset of moderate exercise in humans. Journal of Applied Physiology 77(3):1519–1525

Tschakovsky ME, Hughson RL 1999 Interaction of factors determining oxygen uptake at the onset of exercise. Journal of Applied Physiology 86(4):1101–1113

Tschakovsky ME, Sheriff DD 2004 Immediate exercise hyperemia: contributions of the muscle pump vs. rapid vasodilation Journal of Applied Physiology 97(2):739–747

Tschakovsky ME, Shoemaker JK, Hughson RL 1996 Vasodilation and muscle pump contribution to immediate exercise hyperemia. American Journal of Physiology 271(4 Pt 2):H1697–H1701

Tschakovsky ME, Sujirattanawimol K, Ruble SB, Valic Z, Joyner MJ 2002 Is sympathetic neural vasoconstriction blunted in the vascular bed of exercising human muscle? Journal of Physiology 541(2):623–635

Tschakovsky ME, Rogers AM, Pyke KE, Saunders NR, Glenn N, Lee SJ, Weissgerber T, Dwyer EM 2004 Immediate exercise hyperemia in humans is contraction intensity dependent: evidence for rapid vasodilation. Journal of Applied Physiology 96(2):639–644

Turner MJ, Howley ET, Tanaka H, Ashraf M, Bassett DR Jr, Keefer DJ 1995 Effect of graded epinephrine infusion on blood lactate response to exercise. Journal of Applied Physiology 79(4):1206–1211

VanTeeffelen JW, Segal SS 2006 Rapid dilation of arterioles with single contraction of hamster skeletal muscle. American Journal of Physiology. Heart and Circulation Physiology 290(1):H119–H127

Vissing J, Vissing SF, MacLean DA, Saltin B, Quistorff B, Haller RG 1998 Sympathetic activation in exercise is not dependent on muscle acidosis. Direct evidence from studies in metabolic myopathies. Journal of Clinical Investigation 101(8):1654–1660

Vrabas IS, Dodd SL, Crawford MP 2002 Interaction of blood flow and oxygen delivery affects peak VO$_2$ and fatigue in canine muscle in situ. European Journal of Applied Physiology 86(3):273–279

Wagner PD 1992 Gas exchange and peripheral diffusion limitation. Medicine and Science in Sports and Exercise 24(1):54–58

Wasserman K 1984 The anaerobic threshold measurement in exercise testing. Clinics in Chest Medicine 5(1):77–88

Westerblad H, Allen DG 2003 Cellular mechanisms of skeletal muscle fatigue. Advances in Experimental Medicine and Biology 538:563–570

Williamson JW, Mitchell JH, Olesen HL, Raven PB, Secher NH 1994 Reflex increase in blood pressure induced by leg compression in man. Journal of Physiology 475(2):351–357

Wilson DF 1994 Factors affecting the rate and energetics of mitochondrial oxidative phosphorylation. Medicine and Science in Sports and Exercise 26(1):37–43

Wilson DF, Rumsey WL 1988 Factors modulating the oxygen dependence of mitochondrial oxidative phosphorylation. Advances in Experimental Medicine and Biology 222:121–131

Wilson DF, Erecinska M, Silver IA 1983 Metabolic effects of lowering oxygen tension in vivo. Advances in Experimental Medicine and Biology 159:293–301

Wright JR, McCloskey DI, Fitzpatrick RC 1999 Effects of muscle perfusion pressure on fatigue and systemic arterial pressure in human subjects. Journal of Applied Physiology 86(3):845–851

Wright JR, McCloskey DI, Fitzpatrick RC 2000 Effects of systemic arterial blood pressure on the contractile force of a human hand muscle. Journal of Applied Physiology 88(4):1390–1396

Yamamoto K, Kawada T, Kamiya A, Takaki H, Miyamoto T, Sugimachi M, Sunagawa K 2004 Muscle mechanoreflex induces the pressor response by resetting the arterial baroreflex neural arc. American Journal of Physiology. Heart and Circulation Physiology 286(4):H1382–H1388

Chapter 2

Pulmonary responses to exercise and limitations to human performance

Michael K. Stickland Markus Amann Keisho Katayama
Jerome A. Dempsey

1 INTRODUCTION

The respiratory system is responsible for the first two steps in the convective (oxygen delivery) and diffusive (flux) oxygen transport processes (Chapter 1; Figure 1.2) from the inspired air to muscle mitochondria. These steps include: the difference in oxygen partial pressure (PO_2) from inspired air to alveolar gas, which is determined by the matching of alveolar ventilation to metabolic rate, and the transfer of oxygen from alveolar gas to pulmonary capillaries. The respiratory system simultaneously regulates carbon dioxide levels in the body by providing adequate alveolar ventilation, and thus avoiding the rise in arterial carbon dioxide (respiratory acidosis). Importantly, arterial blood gas homeostasis should be maintained at a minimum energy expense, in terms of metabolic cost to the organism. In addition, pulmonary vascular resistance and vascular pressures must remain low to limit the load on the right heart, and prevent hydrostatic oedema or damage to the delicate alveolar–capillary interface.

From rest to moderate exercise, blood gas homeostasis is well maintained in the healthy human (Table 2.1). However, during high-intensity exercise, impairments in pulmonary gas exchange can develop, which negatively impact arterial oxygen content (and thus systemic oxygen delivery) and, as a consequence, locomotor muscle fatigue and athletic performance. At the same time, the considerable ventilatory requirement needed at high metabolic rates in highly trained athletes can result in additional blood flow to the respiratory muscles at a cost of reduced blood flow to locomotor muscle. Consequently, the increased work of breathing during high-intensity exercise can also contribute to a reduction in oxygen delivery, and therefore muscle fatigue and impaired performance. This chapter will examine the

Table 2.1 Ventilation, pulmonary gas exchange and pulmonary circulation responses during incremental exercise (ramp function) in a healthy, untrained young adult (70 kg; maximal oxygen uptake ($\dot{V}O_{2max}$) = 40–45 mL·kg^{-1}·min^{-1}) and peak exercise values for two highly trained young adults (body mass 70 kg; $\dot{V}O_{2max}$ = 60–65 mL·kg^{-1}·min^{-1})

	Untrained								Trained A	Trained B
	Relative exercise intensity (% maximal oxygen uptake)									
	Rest	15	30	45	60	75	90	100	100	100
$\dot{V}O_2$ (L·min^{-1})	0.24	0.45	0.90	1.35	1.80	2.25	2.70	3.00	5.25	5.25
$\dot{V}CO_2$ (L·min^{-1})	0.19	0.40	0.77	1.21	1.71	2.31	3.00	3.30	6.04	6.04
$\dot{V}E$ (L·min^{-1})	6	14	22	35	51	75	100	115	183	168
$\dot{V}A$ (L·min^{-1})	4	9	18	28	41	60	81	94	150	138
V_T (L)	0.6	0.9	1.2	1.6	2.2	2.5	2.6	2.6	3.1	2.9
f_R (breaths·min^{-1})	10	15	18	22	23	30	38	44	59	58
V_D/V_T	0.35	0.28	0.21	0.20	0.19	0.18	0.18	0.18	0.18	0.18
EELV (% TLC)	0.50	0.49	0.46	0.45	0.44	0.43	0.42	0.42	0.48	0.48
Gas exchange										
PaO_2 (kPa)	12.7	12.7	12.4	12.4	12.3	12.5	12.5	12.5	12.0	9.3
PAO_2 (kPa)	13.5	13.5	13.5	13.5	14.3	14.9	15.2	15.6	15.6	14.9
$PaCO_2$ (kPa)	5.5	5.5	5.5	5.5	5.2	4.7	4.4	4.1	4.1	5.1
A–aDO$_2$ (kPa)	0.8	0.8	1.1	1.1	2.0	2.4	2.7	3.1	3.6	5.6
pH	7.40	7.40	7.38	7.36	7.34	7.30	7.29	7.28	7.25	7.25
S_aO_2 (%)	97	97	97	97	96	96	95	95	93	86
$\dot{V}A/\dot{Q}$	0.8	1.3	2.0	2.5	2.9	3.5	4.1	4.5	4.7	4.3
Pulmonary circulation										
$\dot{Q}$ (L·min^{-1})	5	7	9	11	14	17	20	21	32	32
PCBV (mL)	83	95	107	119	137	155	173	180	180	180
Transit time (s)	1.00	0.81	0.71	0.65	0.59	0.55	0.52	0.51	0.33	0.33
PAP (mmHg)	13	15	17	20	23	27	29	32	30	30
PAWP (mmHg)	8	9	10	12	13	15	17	21	14	14
PVR (kPa·min^{-1}·s^{-1})	8.00	6.86	6.22	5.82	5.71	5.65	4.80	4.19	4.00	4.00

$\dot{V}O_2$, oxygen uptake; $\dot{V}CO_2$, expired carbon dioxide; $\dot{V}E$, minute ventilation; $\dot{V}A$, alveolar ventilation; V_T, tidal volume; f_R, breathing frequency; V_D/V_T, dead space to tidal volume ratio; EELV (% TLC), end-expiratory lung (expiratory reserve volume) volume as a percentage of total lung capacity; P_aO_2, arterial PO$_2$; P_AO_2, alveolar PO$_2$; P_aCO_2, arterial PCO$_2$; A–aDO$_2$, alveolar to arterial oxygen partial pressure difference; S_aO_2, arterial oxyhaemoglobin saturation; $\dot{V}A/\dot{Q}$, global ventilation to perfusion ratio; $\dot{Q}$, cardiac output; PCBV, pulmonary capillary blood volume; Transit time, mean pulmonary capillary transit time; PAP, mean pulmonary artery pressure; PAWP, pulmonary artery wedge pressure; PVR, pulmonary vascular resistance.
Units conversion: 1 mmHg = 0.133 kPa.

acute respiratory responses to exercise, as well as how the respiratory system may limit exercise performance in both normal and highly trained subjects.

2 EXERCISE HYPERPNOEA

In healthy humans, breathing in all physiological states is remarkably well controlled. Accordingly, the arterial partial pressures of oxygen and carbon dioxide, along with its acidity, are regulated precisely throughout mild to moderate exercise (Dempsey et al. 1995, Kaufman & Forster 1996, Waldrop et al. 1996, Ward 1994).

These relationships are shown in the following alveolar gas equations, where alveolar gas partial pressures are approximately equal to the ratio of the metabolic requirement to alveolar ventilation.

Equation 1: $P_ACO_2 = [\dot{V}_{CO_2} \div \dot{V}_A] \cdot K$

Equation 2: $P_AO_2 = P_IO_2 - [\dot{V}_{O_2} \div \dot{V}_A] \cdot K$

where:

P_ACO_2 and P_AO_2 = alveolar carbon dioxide and oxygen partial pressures (it is assumed $P_ACO_2 \approx$ arterial PCO$_2$)
$\dot{V}_{CO_2}$ and $\dot{V}_{O_2}$ = volumes of carbon dioxide expired and oxygen consumed
$\dot{V}_A$ = alveolar ventilation
P_IO_2 = inspired partial pressure of oxygen
K = constant (0.863).

Table 2.1 illustrates the interrelation of these variables, as one goes from rest to exercise. With exercise, there is an increased metabolic rate, with alveolar ventilation increasing to regulate arterial blood gases at resting levels (Figure

18.9). This is accomplished by increasing both tidal volume and breathing frequency. Thus, ventilation is controlled to facilitate the regulation of blood gas partial pressures. If ventilation does not meet the metabolic demand, arterial carbon dioxide partial pressure (P_aCO_2) would increase, impacting acid–base regulation, while alveolar oxygen partial pressure (P_AO_2) would decrease, negatively impacting upon oxygen delivery. As illustrated in Table 2.1, the body tightly regulates P_AO_2 and P_aCO_2 up to moderate-intensity exercise. However, once past ~60% of maximal oxygen uptake (peak aerobic power; $\dot{V}_{O_{2max}}$) in

an untrained subject, alveolar ventilation increases disproportionately relative to metabolic demand, resulting in an increase in P_AO_2 and a reduction in P_aCO_2 (Chapter 10.3). Exactly how the body is able to tightly control ventilation with the increased metabolic rate of exercise is discussed in the following section.

2.1 Control of breathing

Several mechanisms have been proposed to explain exercise-induced hyperpnoea (Figure 2.1), including feed-

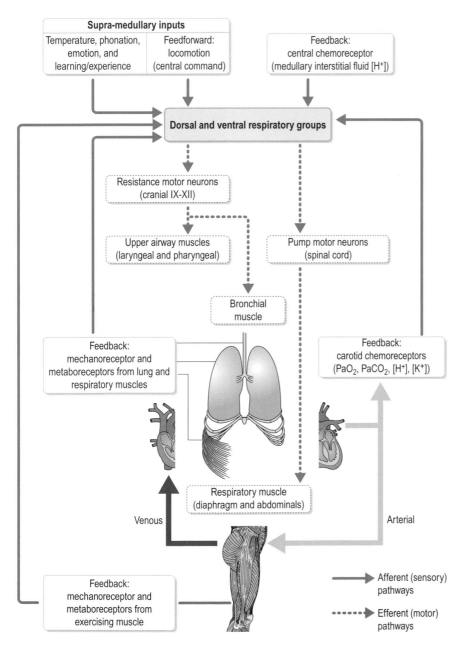

Figure 2.1 Schematic overview of proposed mechanisms for the control of breathing during exercise. Efferent (motor) pathways: motor output carried in cranial and spinal nerves, and innervating muscles of the upper airway, bronchial muscle and respiratory muscles. Afferent pathways: inputs to the dorsal and ventral respiratory groups (medulla oblongata) originating from central (supramedullary regions, central chemoreceptors) and peripheral sites (working muscles, lung, respiratory muscles, carotid chemoreceptors). Also see control models in Chapters 1 and 18.

forward from central command, proportional to skeletal muscle activation, and feedback to the dorsal and ventral respiratory groups that is triggered by stimuli associated with physical activity, and may involve afferents of central and peripheral origin, including chemoreceptor (P_aO_2, P_aCO_2, pH), metaboreceptor (lactate, potassium ions) and mechanoreceptor activity (muscles, airways, lungs, blood vessels), carbon dioxide flow to the lung and short-term potentiation (after-effects). In this section, we focus upon feedforward (central command), carbon dioxide flow to the lung, receptors in working locomotor muscles and the carotid body. In addition, we discuss the mechanisms of exercise hyperpnoea during heavy, dynamic exercise.

2.1.1 Central command

The central feedforward mechanism has been hypothesised to have a primary role in exercise hyperpnoea (Waldrop et al. 1996). This hypothesis was first introduced by Krogh & Lindhard (1913) and referred to as cortical irradiation, with both animal and human studies supporting the hypothesis (Waldrop et al. 2006). In animal studies it has been shown that descending drive from the supraspinal area, that provides the neural drive for locomotion, can elicit an increase in cardiorespiratory function, even in the absence of contracting muscle (Eldridge et al. 1985, Waldrop et al. 1996). The locomotor areas that provide descending drive to the spinal locomotor circuits are located in discrete regions of the hypothalamus, the diencephalons of the midbrain and in the premotor cortex (Eldridge et al. 1981, Waldrop et al. 1996, 2006). These areas project to the medullary cardiorespiratory neurons and directly to the cervical and lumbar spinal motor neurons.

Recent human studies have provided circumstantial evidence favouring a role for central command in exercise hyperpnoea. It has been reported that a greater ventilatory response to exercise appeared after partial muscle nerve paralysis. That is, central neural drive must have been higher compared with that during exercise without paralysis (Innes et al. 1992). In another study (Thornton et al. 2001), subjects under hypnosis were asked to imagine exercise and hyperventilation occurred (i.e. ventilation beyond metabolic demand, reducing P_aCO_2). At the same time, positron emission tomography was used to image the brain and increased brain activity in motor areas was found (Thornton et al. 2001). Furthermore, neuroimaging techniques measuring brain blood flow distribution have also shown that several motor cortical areas were activated using exercise imagery (Williamson et al. 2002).

Based on these findings, it is generally accepted that feedforward contributes directly to hyperpnoea during dynamic exercise. Since it is simultaneous, parallel excitation of the neural circuits containing locomotor and cardiorespiratory neurons, hyperpnoea associated with feedforward will occur much faster than any feedback mechanism could operate. Therefore, feedforward is likely to be the major contributor to the immediate hyperpnoea during the first 20 s following exercise onset.

2.1.2 Carbon dioxide flow to the lung

Increases in alveolar ventilation are well correlated with an enhanced metabolic rate, during steady-state exercise. For example, Casaburi et al. (1977), using sinusoidal exercise in varying time domains, showed a strong correlation in the time constants of minute ventilation and carbon dioxide production. In addition, a strong linear relationship between ventilation and carbon dioxide production was found during exercise induced by electrical stimulation in paraplegic subjects with complete lesions of the spinal cord, removing both feedforward and feedback pathways (Brice et al. 1988). These results support the hypothesis that exercise hyperpnoea is linked to metabolism via carbon dioxide production. This hypothesis is also supported by animal studies; when carbon dioxide flow to the lung was removed via extracorporeal circulation, reductions in ventilation occurred in proportion to decreased carbon dioxide production (Phillipson et al. 1981).

Judging from the above, there is little doubt that carbon dioxide flow does affect the control of ventilation. Carbon dioxide-sensitive receptors in the lung have been identified in anaesthetised animals (Green & Schmidt 1984). However, these receptors may not be sufficiently sensitive to produce the five- to ten-fold increase in ventilation observed during light to moderate intensity exercise, but they may be important to the drive to breathe at rest.

2.1.3 Receptors in working locomotor muscles

It is well established that various receptors in the limb skeletal muscle and tendons are sensitive to mechanical events (stretch, pressure, tension), to metabolic changes produced by contracting limb skeletal muscle (lactic acid and bradykinin; Kaufman & Forster 1996) and to the venous vascular distension caused by increasing muscle blood flow (Haouzi et al. 2004). The most important afferent nerve fibres in muscle are classified as type III (primary mechanical) and type IV (primary metabolic; Kaufman & Forster 1996). When these fibres are stimulated, electrically, pharmacologically or via perfusion of acid or other metabolites into their arterial blood supply, increases in phrenic nerve activity and breathing frequency occur (Kaufman & Forster 1996). When muscle contraction was caused by direct electrical stimulation in an animal, and the venous effluent blood from the working muscle directed to a second resting animal via cross-circulation, thereby eliminating the carbon dioxide flow stimulus, hyperpnoea was still apparent in the stimulated animal (Kao 1963). In humans, it has been reported that abrupt increases in ventilation can be achieved at the onset of passive exercise, performed either while awake or asleep (Ishida et al. 1993, Miyamura et al. 1997). In addition, it has been recently considered that type III and IV fibres within the adventitia of the venous vasculature in the muscle respond to the mechanical changes associated with venous distension (Haouzi et al. 2004).

These results in both animals and humans indicate that the reflex arose from the stimulation of mechanoreceptors in the exercising muscle. Overall, these data show the existence of ventilatory responses to stimuli originating in the locomotor skeletal muscle, and suggest that feedback mechanisms from receptors in the working muscle contribute to the exercise hyperpnoea.

2.1.4 Carotid chemoreceptors

The carotid chemoreceptors are small bilateral organs located near the bifurcations of the common carotid arteries, and are fast-responding receptors for changes in the partial pressures of oxygen and carbon dioxide and hydrogen ion concentration of the arterial blood (Lumb & Nunn 2000). Furthermore, carotid chemoreceptors also respond to changes in the concentrations of potassium, catecholamines and adenosine, as well as blood temperature and osmolality (Lumb & Nunn 2000). However, since arterial blood gases and acidity remain constant and other factors (catecholamines) that can stimulate carotid chemoreceptors do not increase during light to moderate exercise, it is assumed that the contribution of the carotid bodies to the control of ventilation during light and moderate exercise at sea level may be relatively minor (Kaufman & Forster 1996).

How do carotid chemoreceptors contribute during moderate exercise? Ventilation during exercise in humans decreases quickly when breathing an oxygen-enriched gas mixture. Thus, the carotid chemoreceptors are likely to play an important role as 'error detectors' by fine tuning the ventilatory response to ensure sufficient and precise isocapnic hyperpnoea during light to moderate exercise (Dempsey et al. 1995, Kaufman & Forster 1996).

2.1.5 Short-term potentiation

When respiratory feedback stimuli are abruptly terminated, central respiratory motor output will still continue. This has been termed short-term potentiation (after-effect). This response was shown following electrical simulation of the carotid sinus nerve in the anaesthetised animal (Eldridge & Gill-Kumar 1978), and also following brief hypoxic ventilatory simulation in humans (Badr et al. 1992). These after-effects of respiratory motor output also occur in response to a wide variety of sensory stimuli. It is considered that short-term potentiation acts as a smoothing or stabilising effect on the ventilatory response to prevent overshoots and undershoots in ventilation during periods of transition between increases and decreases in ventilatory stimuli (Dempsey et al. 2006). Therefore, it is conceivable that this after-effect contributes to the hyperventilatory response not only after cessation of exercise but also following changing exercise intensities, or even to the slow (secondary) increase in ventilation during completion of a single workload, although direct supporting evidence is lacking.

2.1.6 The hyperventilation during heavy exercise

Once exercise intensity increases beyond ~60% of maximal oxygen uptake in untrained subjects, ventilation increases disproportionately to the metabolic demand, resulting in an increase in P_AO_2 and a reduction in P_aCO_2. The degree of hyperventilation can be substantial, driving P_aCO_2 1–2 kPa (8–15 mmHg) below resting values at maximal exercise (Table 2.1). What causes this extra drive to breathe?

Current candidates include disproportionate increases in feedback mechanisms of carotid chemoreceptors responding to arterial hydrogen ion concentration or receptors in locomotor working muscle, and disproportionate increases in feedforward mechanism in the presence of locomotor muscle fatigue. During heavy exercise, increases in hydrogen ion concentration occur and the carotid chemoreceptors must contribute something to the hyperventilatory response. In humans, there is a good correlation between plasma hydrogen ion concentration and exercise-induced hyperventilation, and this correlation provides much of the basis for the theory that heavy exercise hyperventilation is mediated by increased hydrogen ions stimulating carotid chemoreceptors (Kaufman & Forster 1996). However, to our knowledge, the definitive experiments to test the role of carotid chemoreceptors have not yet been carried out. Previous studies have used carotid body denervation experiments (asthmatics with denervated carotid bodies) to clarify the relative importance during heavy exercise (Wasserman et al. 1975). However, it has been postulated that these denervated patients are not an appropriate model for examining the role of the carotid chemoreceptors in exercise hyperpnoea, because of the potential confounding mechanical limitations to airflow in these patients due to their asthmatic condition. Furthermore, carotid body denervation is accompanied by significant changes in key elements of the remainder of the central (Liu et al. 2003) and peripheral (Serra et al. 2002) respiratory control systems (Forster 2003).

There are some reports that neither metabolic acidosis nor the carotid bodies were shown to be required for the hyperventilation to heavy exercise. Patients with McArdle's syndrome are incapable of producing lactic acid, but hyperventilation appears during heavy exercise (Hagberg et al. 1982). This finding is often cited as evidence against the hypothesis that metabolic acidosis and carotid chemoreceptor stimulation are related to hyperpnoea during heavy exercise (Chapter 10.3). However, patients with McArdle's syndrome hyperventilate even during submaximal exercise. Thus, other factors that are not present in normal subjects are likely to be present in such patients. Therefore, this model may also be inappropriate to evaluate the mechanisms for hyperpnoea during heavy exercise in typical humans (Kaufman & Forster 1996).

When dietary-induced glycogen depletion was used to prevent almost all of the exercise-induced increase in lactic acid, a normal hyperventilatory response remained (Busse et al. 1991). In addition, there is a report that dopamine, an inhibitory neurotransmitter in the carotid body, diminished the hypoxic ventilatory response, while it had no effect on the ventilatory response during incremental exercise (Henson et al. 1992). Furthermore, when exercising animals were studied before and after carotid body denervation, ventilatory response to heavy exercise was slightly greater following carotid body denervation, while levels of metabolic acidosis were the same (Kaufman & Forster 1996). Thus, it may be that hypocapnia during heavy exercise inhibits carotid chemoreceptor activity (Dempsey & Smith 1994). From these data, it is evident that neither metabolic acidosis nor the carotid bodies are required for the hyperventilation during heavy exercise (Chapter 10.3).

How do we interpret these inconsistent data? Undoubtedly, hydrogen ions increase during heavy exercise, and thus it is safe to state that the carotid chemoreceptors are involved to a significant extent in the hyperventilation during heavy exercise. Furthermore, potassium, catecholamines and adenosine concentrations all increase during heavy exercise and these stimulate carotid chemoreceptors. However, increased carotid chemoreceptors feedback alone is unlikely to be sufficient to explain the 20–30% hyperventilation observed during heavy exercise.

Although there is no direct evidence, feedback from pulmonary receptors sensitive to carbon dioxide flow, and the receptors in working locomotor muscle could be enhanced during heavy exercise (Kaufman & Forster 1996). It has been reported that somatic afferents from limb muscle receptors are sensitive to venous distension via increases in blood flow (Haouzi et al. 2004), and feedback from these receptors, due to increased muscle blood flow, may be enhanced during heavy exercise. Additionally, since limb muscle fatigue occurs during heavy exercise, additional central neural drive (motor unit recruitment) could be needed to maintain locomotor muscle force (Chapter 5). Limb muscle electromyography has shown a marked increase in activity, indicating increased feedforward and coincident changes in electromyographic activity and ventilation appeared (Mateika & Duffin 1994). Therefore, an additional mechanism for hyperventilation during heavy exercise may be increased feedforward (Kaufman & Forster 1996).

In summary, as compared with isocapnic hyperpnoea of light to moderate exercise, the concentration of known carotid chemoreceptor stimuli increase in the arterial blood during heavy exercise. Thus, we can be fairly certain that carotid chemoreceptors contribute to some extent to the hyperventilation during heavy exercise. As well, the additional strong descending output from feedforward and the ascending input from locomotor muscle are likely to contribute to the hyperventilatory response to heavy exercise.

2.2 Exercise hyperpnoea – conclusion

Based on studies regarding hyperpnoea during exercise, there are two candidates in the locomotor-linked stimuli:

central feedforward and feedback from muscles receptors (Figure 2.1). When either of these mechanisms is removed, the ventilatory response to exercise remains nearly normal (Waldrop et al. 1986). Consequently, neither input is required for normal exercise hyperpnoea, although both inputs are clearly capable of producing a sufficiently strong ventilatory response. Therefore, we propose that these two major stimuli act together to provide the primary stimulus to exercise hyperpnoea. Additional short-term potentiation, together with carotid chemoreceptor input, provides fine tuning of the ventilatory response to ensure precise normocapnic hyperpnoea (Dempsey et al. 2006).

3 BREATHING PATTERN

The precise matching of alveolar ventilation with metabolic rate during exercise is achieved by increasing minute ventilation. This increase is accomplished by increases in both tidal volume and breathing frequency (Table 2.1, Figure 2.2). The increased tidal volume slightly increases airway dead space, due to tethering effects of the lung parenchyma on airway lumen size. However, the relative tidal volume increase exceeds this effect, and the dead space to tidal volume ratio decreases during exercise from resting values of ~0.35 to ~0.20, translating into more efficient alveolar ventilation. During low to moderate intensity exercise, both tidal volume and breathing frequency increase roughly in proportion to exercise intensity, whereas at higher intensities, tidal volume reaches a plateau, and further increases in ventilation are accomplished by increases in breathing frequency alone.

Increases in breathing frequency are accomplished by reducing both the inspiratory (T_I) and expiratory times (T_E). However, the ratio of inspiratory time to total breath cycle duration (T_{TOT}), the duty cycle (T_I/T_{TOT}), increases only slightly during exercise (~0.40 at rest to ~0.50 during high-intensity exercise). The fact that the inspiratory duty cycle remains low is important and beneficial, because prolonged diaphragmatic activations hinder blood flow to this muscle, possibly precipitating diaphragmatic fatigue (Bellemare & Grassino 1982).

The increase in tidal volume is achieved by reducing the end-expiratory lung volume below the functional residual capacity (achieved by activating expiratory muscles) and increasing the end-inspiratory lung volume (Figure 2.2). At lower exercise intensities, increases in ventilation are adequately achieved through tidal volume changes, rather than just increasing breathing frequency, which would increase dead space ventilation, and compromise effective alveolar ventilation. To minimise the work of breathing during heavier exercise, tidal volume increases only to ~70% of the vital capacity, a lung volume beyond which lung compliance decreases markedly and the respiratory pressure production required for a given change in volume is very large.

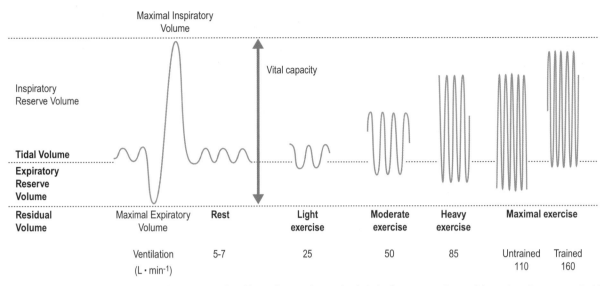

Figure 2.2 Changes in breathing pattern during exercise. The spirograph on the left is from a resting subject showing normal tidal volume, maximum expiration to residual lung volume, then maximal inspiration to total lung capacity. With light to heavy exercise (in both untrained and highly trained subjects) the increase in ventilation is achieved by increasing breathing frequency and tidal volume. Tidal volume increases by encroaching on the expiratory and inspiratory reserve volumes. The reduced end-expiratory lung volume is maintained at maximal exercise in the normally fit subject (maximal oxygen uptake ($\dot{V}_{O_{2max}}$) 45 mL·kg^{-1}L·min^{-1}). In the trained subject ($\dot{V}_{O_{2max}}$ = 75 mL·kg^{-1}L·min^{-1}), ventilation, breathing frequency and tidal volume are all higher, and at maximal exercise end-expiratory lung volume is increased to near resting values due to expiratory flow limitations.

4 TIDAL FLOW–VOLUME LOOP

Tidal exercise flow–volume curves, plotted within the maximal volitional flow–volume envelope, provide a simple and useful method for assessing flow limitation and its consequences during exercise. In the normal, healthy human, the maximal attainable flow at any given lung volume is usually much greater than the spontaneous flows reached during exercise of any intensity. Thus, there is usually a large reserve for increasing ventilation, even at maximal exercise. However, endurance-trained individuals, with high maximal exercise ventilation, may intersect the boundary of the expiratory portion of the maximal flow–volume envelope, and thus become flow limited (Figure 2.3). This may also occur in untrained individuals with abnormally small airways, or in those with compromised lung elastic recoil and ability to produce high airflows, due to dynamic airway collapse, as observed in obstructive lung disease (e.g. asthma). Furthermore, expiratory flow limitation during exercise appears to occur more often in women, primarily because of smaller airways and lower maximal expiratory flow rates, than in age- and height-matched men (McClaran et al. 1998). Importantly, a flow–volume limitation that develops with exercise can inhibit the ventilatory response to exercise, reducing P_AO_2 and negatively affecting arterial blood gas status (see section 9).

5 AIRWAY RESPONSES DURING EXERCISE

5.1 Upper airway

The upper airway comprises the nose, mouth, pharynx and larynx and provides the majority of resistance to airflow at rest and during exercise, although flow resistance within the bronchial tree is greatest in the medium-sized bronchi, prior to the seventh generation. Additionally, each region has the potential to independently contribute to alterations in airway resistance during exercise. Thus, the work required to produce the airflow necessary during exercise would become excessively large during even low-intensity exercise, if several mechanisms were not in place to reduce airway resistance in the upper airway. First, the route of airflow switches from predominantly nasal to oronasal breathing when ventilation reaches approximately 30 L·min^{-1} (Dempsey et al. 1996). Second, nasal resistance decreases during exercise in an intensity- and duration-dependant manner, secondary to sympathetically mediated vasoconstriction of the nasal mucosal vasculature (Forsyth et al. 1983). Finally, the nasal dilatory muscles, and presumably the skeletal muscles of pharyngeal and laryngeal regions, contract in phase with, but slightly preceding, inspiratory muscle recruitment, and this drive to the upper airway muscles is increased with increasing ventilation, resulting in decreased resistance and a less collapsible airway (Forsyth et al. 1983). Therefore, the work required to overcome flow

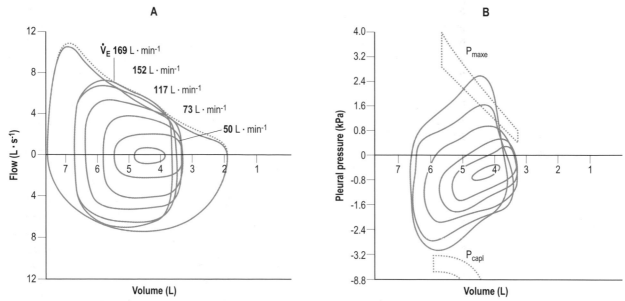

Figure 2.3 Flow–volume and pressure–volume relationships in a young healthy adult, at rest and during exercise. The maximal (outer envelope) flow–volume relationship is obtained via maximal volitional inspiratory and expiratory efforts, before (solid line) and immediately following exercise (broken line). For the pressure–volume relationships, only tidal breaths from rest through to maximal exercise are shown. In addition, the maximum inspiratory pleural pressures (P_{capl}) are shown at the specific peak volume and flows achieved during tidal breathing in heavy exercise. For minute ventilations up to 115 L·min^{-1}, approximating peak exercise in an untrained adult (Table 2.1), the inspiratory muscles are activated at only ~40–50% of capacity. The more highly trained subject is shown achieving ventilations >150 L·min^{-1} at higher metabolic rates. Under these conditions, the tidal flow–volume loop encroaches on the maximum flow–volume envelope, end-expiratory lung volume rises and the inspiratory muscles approach 90% of their dynamic capacity for force output and shortening velocity. The broken area on the expiratory side indicates an expiratory pressure for any given lung volume (P_{maxe}), beyond which extra expiratory muscle effort will not produce a higher flow. In almost all instances up to ventilations of ~150 L·min^{-1}, this critical expiratory pressure is not exceeded, but it is exceeded slightly in the highly trained athlete at maximum exercise.

resistance during exercise is minimised by adjustments occurring in the upper airway that decrease flow resistance.

5.2 Bronchial diameter

Bronchial dilatation during exercise is well documented in healthy humans. Furthermore, bronchodilator influence is very powerful, as evidenced by the prevention of an increase in pulmonary resistance during exercise after histamine inhalation in asthmatic subjects, who exhibit large increases in resistance during histamine inhalation at rest. Additionally, the forced expiratory volume in 1 s (FEV$_1$) is increased immediately after exercise, in both normal and asthmatic individuals. There are several potential mechanisms contributing to this bronchodilator effect. A primary component of the exercise-induced increase in airway calibre is withdrawal of vagal parasympathetic tone to the airways, which occurs at the onset of exercise (Bowes et al. 1984, Kaufman et al. 1985, Warren et al. 1984). Mechanical influences may also play a substantial role in increasing airway calibre. Since the airways are tethered open by the lung parenchyma, increasing end-inspiratory lung volume and

operating lung volumes during exercise enlarge airway diameter. Finally, local release of chemical mediators from airway resident and non-resident cells might affect bronchial airway calibre during exercise. Airway mast cells, macrophages, neutrophils, eosinophils, epithelial cells and smooth muscle cells have the potential to release a variety of chemical mediators that may alter airway calibre. Consequently, the release of such bronchodilator mediators could help explain increased airway calibre during exercise (Beck 1999).

6 ENERGY COST OF THE WORK OF BREATHING DURING EXERCISE

The work performed by the respiratory muscles per litre of ventilation increases fairly linearly from rest to maximal exercise, from approximately 0.5 J·L^{-1} up to >4 J·L^{-1} in normal, healthy humans. Given a resting ventilation of 6 L·min^{-1} and a peak exercise ventilation >150 L·min^{-1} in endurance-trained athletes, this translates into a 200-fold increase in the work of breathing, from 3 J·min^{-1} at rest to >600 J·min^{-1} at peak exercise. The oxygen cost of the work of breathing (when normalised to ventilation) also increases linearly with ventilation, to a maximum of ~2.85 mL $O_2 \cdot L^{-1}$ (Aaron et al. 1992). However, when the work is expressed per unit time ($J \cdot min^{-1}$), respiratory muscle work increases non-linearly with ventilation. Thus, respiratory muscle oxygen uptake can reach ~15% of the total oxygen uptake during maximal exercise in trained athletes and, in turn, ~15% of total cardiac output must be directed to the respiratory muscles (Aaron et al. 1992). In the untrained young adult working maximally, about 10% of the oxygen uptake and cardiac output is directed to the respiratory muscles. To ensure this proportion of blood flow is diverted to the respiratory muscles (to maintain adequate perfusion), autonomic reflexes originating from the respiratory muscles are thought to be enacted (Harms et al. 1997; section 10.2).

7 PULMONARY CIRCULATION

The lungs are unique in that they are the only organ that receives all the blood pumped from the heart and thus, the lungs must accommodate the entire increase in cardiac output during exercise. The pulmonary circulation is under limited adrenergic (Kane et al. 1994) or endothelial (Duncker et al. 2000, Kane et al. 1994, Lindenfeld et al. 1983, Manohar & Goetz 1998, Merkus et al. 2004, Newman et al. 1986) control during exercise, and therefore, because of its unique in-series relationship, the pulmonary circulation is tightly coupled to left (downstream) ventricular function. At the same time, the pulmonary microcirculation has been engineered to maximise gas exchange efficiency, and as a result, vessel walls are very thin and distensible. Correspondingly, pulmonary vascular resistance and perfusion pressures are about one-fifth of those observed in the systemic circulation at rest.

With upright exercise, there is an increase in venous return to the heart, causing a central shift of blood volume into the thorax (Flamm et al. 1990). This increases both right and left ventricular filling pressures (Reeves et al. 1990), helping to maintain, or increase, both end-diastolic volume and stroke volume, despite reductions in filling time secondary to exercise-induced tachycardia. Pulmonary venous pressure can be predicted from pulmonary artery wedge pressure, which is said to reflect left-ventricular end-diastolic pressure (Thadani & Parker 1978). Importantly, Reeves & Taylor (1996) have shown that ~80% of the variance in mean pulmonary artery pressure is due to pulmonary arterial wedge pressure, and therefore the dominant determinant of pulmonary artery pressure during exercise is left ventricular filling pressure.

The rise in both pulmonary arterial and pulmonary arterial wedge pressures with exercise recruits previously unperfused pulmonary capillaries, increasing capillary blood volume, and the area for gas diffusion and diffusion capacity (Johnson et al. 1960). The augmented pulmonary vascular pressures with exercise also act to distend pulmonary vessels (Reeves et al. 2005) and this increase in diameter, combined with capillary recruitment, results in reduced pulmonary vascular resistance with incremental exercise (Stickland et al. 2004b, Wagner et al. 1986). In addition, capillary recruitment helps to maintain the red blood cell capillary transit time necessary for complete gas exchange (>0.25 s). Mean pulmonary capillary transit time (s) is equal to the ratio of pulmonary capillary blood volume and blood flow (cardiac output). Using resting data from Table 2.1, resting capillary transit time is slightly <1.0 s: pulmonary capillary blood volume ~83 mL and cardiac output ~5000 mL·min⁻¹. At peak exercise in untrained subjects, despite the fourfold increase in pulmonary flow (cardiac output) from rest, capillary transit time is reduced only to ~0.51 s, due to a doubling of the pulmonary capillary blood volume. Thus, capillary recruitment during exercise is an important response as it serves to increase diffusion and reduce pulmonary vascular resistance, while limiting the reduction in capillary transit time.

8 LUNG FLUID HOMEOSTASIS

Fluid homeostasis within the lung microcirculation is governed by the Starling forces, which include the hydrostatic pressure gradient from the vessel lumen to the interstitial space. This gradient pushes fluid out of the venous ends of capillaries and into the interstitial space (pulmonary oedema), and is counteracted by the osmotic pressure of the plasma proteins, which promotes fluid reabsorption into the capillary, and the permeability of the blood–gas barrier. This relationship can be expressed in the following equation:

Equation 3: $Q_{VC} = L_P A[(P_C - P_{TIF}) - \sigma(\pi_C - \pi_T)]$

where:

Q_{VC} = fluid filtration
L_P = filtration constant per unit area (index of permeability)
A = membrane area available for filtration
P_C = hydrostatic pressure within the lumen
P_{TIF} = hydrostatic pressure of the interstitial fluid surrounding the vessel
σ = reflection coefficient for proteins
π_C = plasma oncotic pressure
π_T = tissue fluid oncotic pressures.

It is important for the lung to remain relatively dry for gas exchange. At rest, there is a small outward flow of plasma fluid (~10–20 mL·h⁻¹) from the capillaries into the interstitial space of the alveolar wall. The fluid passes into the perivascular and peribronchiolar spaces of the lung, with the lymphatic system transporting this fluid to the hilar lymph nodes. With exercise, lymph flow increases substantially, due to augmented pulmonary capillary pressures and capillary surface area (Coates et al. 1984). In addition, the augmented ventilation with exercise increases lymph flow, acting as a safety mechanism to oppose oedema formation in the alveoli or interstitial space (Koizumi et al. 2001). Thus, the lymphatic system is vitally important in preventing the exudation of fluid into the alveoli during exercise. In spite of this, the considerable increase in pulmonary capillary wall stress with exercise greatly increases the risk for exercise-induced hydrostatic pulmonary oedema, or even stress failure (West 2000, West & Mathieu-Costello 1995). Indeed, evidence suggests that pulmonary oedema, or vascular damage, does develop with exercise in fit subjects (Caillaud et al. 1995, Hanel & Mortensen 2003, Hopkins et al. 1997, McKenzie et al. 2005, Young et al. 1987). However, this typically occurs only following very severe exercise.

Some would propose that athletes would have greater pulmonary artery pressures during exercise because of their elevated cardiac output, and therefore would be more likely to develop oedema during exercise than less trained subjects. Recently, Stickland et al. (2006b) showed that trained subjects have better left ventricular compliance at peak exercise compared with untrained, as pulmonary artery wedge pressure was lower at peak exercise, despite a markedly greater cardiac output. Pulmonary vascular resistance and pulmonary artery pressure were not different between trained and untrained at peak exercise, which indicates that, to achieve greater pulmonary blood flows, fitter subjects accomplish the increased driving pressure not through higher pulmonary artery pressures, but by having better cardiac compliance and therefore lower pulmonary venous pressures (Table 2.1). While exercise increases pulmonary capillary wall stress, which may lead to oedema or damage, the enhanced cardiac compliance in trained subjects limits the increase in pulmonary artery pressure during exercise. Therefore, trained athletes may not be at any greater risk of oedema formation during exercise. The prevalence and mechanism(s) for exercise-induced pulmonary oedema and damage remain unclear, and require further investigation.

9 PULMONARY GAS EXCHANGE

The ability of the lungs to oxygenate the blood has not traditionally been considered as a limitation in oxygen delivery during exercise (Saltin et al. 1968; section 10 and Chapter 10.1). However, Dempsey et al. (1984) observed that many highly trained athletes (maximal oxygen uptake = 72 mL·kg^{-1}·min^{-1}), exercising at high workloads, exhibited significant arterial hypoxaemia. It is now accepted that most humans develop an impairment of pulmonary gas exchange with exercise, as demonstrated by a widening of the alveolar–arterial oxygen partial pressure difference (P$_A$O$_2$–P$_a$O$_2$). The magnitude of this gas exchange impairment appears to be primarily determined by metabolic rate, as steady-state exercise does not show a time-dependent increase in this gradient (Stickland et al. 2004a, Wetter et al. 2001), and highly trained athletes, who are able to exercise at higher metabolic rates, are most likely to demonstrate an exaggerated alveolar–arterial partial pressure difference (section 9.1). While most healthy humans develop a widened

pressure gradient during exercise, the hyperventilatory response (and increased P$_A$O$_2$) compensates for this, resulting in little change in P$_a$O$_2$ from rest (Table 2.1).

Exercise-induced arterial hypoxaemia is defined as a significant fall in P$_a$O$_2$ (>1.4 kPa) and haemoglobin saturation (S$_a$O$_2$, >5%) from rest (Dempsey & Wagner 1999). This typically occurs during exercise in some, but not all, trained subjects, and is due to a substantial widening of the alveolar–arterial oxygen partial pressure difference, combined with a blunted hyperventilatory response, resulting in a decreased P$_a$O$_2$, S$_a$O$_2$ and total arterial oxygen content relative to rest (Figure 2.4; Dempsey & Wagner 1999, Powers et al. 1988). Arterial hypoxaemia occurs in susceptible individuals during brief, high-intensity endurance exercise (>90% maximal effort; Dempsey & Smith 1984, Harms et al. 1998a, Powers et al. 1992, Wetter et al. 2001), and some subjects develop hypoxaemia at submaximal exercise, which worsens as work rate is further increased (Rice et al. 1999a).

The mechanisms for the widened alveolar–arterial oxygen partial pressure gradient with exercise are discussed

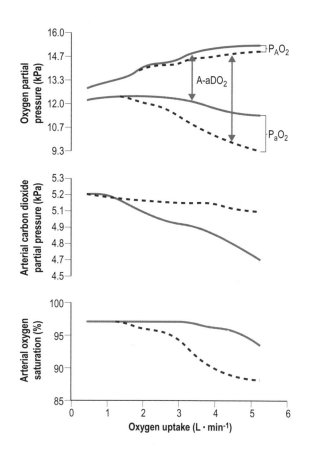

Figure 2.4 Gas exchange in a highly trained subject who does not develop exercise-induced arterial hypoxaemia during incremental exercise (ramp function), compared with a subject who experiences arterial hypoxaemia.

in a later section. However, it is important to emphasise that subjects displaying hypoxaemia typically demonstrate a minimal hyperventilatory response to heavy exercise, such that it is insufficient to raise P_AO_2 enough to compensate for the widened gradient, and prevent P_aO_2 from falling. Mechanical limitations to inspiratory and expiratory flows are the main cause of the constrained hyperventilatory response (Dempsey & Wagner 1999). Much of the mechanical constraints on ventilation appear to be imposed by the airways that have an upper limit to flow, especially during expiration, as defined by the maximum flow–volume envelope (section 4).

The fall in arterial oxygen saturation (S_aO_2) and total oxygen content (C_aO_2) can have an important effect on oxygen delivery and exercise (section 10; Chapters 1 and 10.1). Arterial oxygen content follows arterial saturation, but will be modified by haemoglobin concentration, which generally increases slightly from rest to heavy exercise, due to a 5–10% shift of fluid from the plasma to the interstitial space of the active muscles (Maw et al. 1998; haemoconcentration) at the start of exercise (Chapter 19).

Conceptually, it is important to differentiate between the decrease in saturation due to a shift in the oxyhaemoglobin dissociation curve, and a fall secondary to a drop in P_aO_2 (Dempsey & Wagner 1999). Table 2.1 and Figure 2.4 highlight this by illustrating the exercise response in two highly trained athletes. The subject who does not experience arterial hypoxaemia (A) develops impaired gas exchange, as demonstrated by a widening of the alveolar–arterial oxygen partial pressure difference at peak exercise. However, the hyperventilatory response to exercise (increased P_AO_2, decreased P_aCO_2) compensates for most of this, with little change in P_aO_2 relative to resting values. Thus, the decrease in saturation, from 97% at rest to 93% at peak exercise, is due entirely to a temperature- and pH-induced shift in the oxyhaemoglobin dissociation curve. The subject experiencing arterial hypoxaemia (B) develops a greater gas exchange impairment, as demonstrated by a much greater increase in the alveolar–arterial oxygen pressure gradient at peak exercise, and also experiences a blunted hyperventilatory response, resulting in a drop in P_aO_2 to ~9.3 kPa at peak exercise. In this subject, the drop in P_aO_2 combined with the temperature and pH effects on the oxyhaemoglobin dissociation curve result in a substantial drop in arterial oxygen saturation from rest (97%) to peak exercise (86%). Thus, while nearly all subjects develop an increase in the alveolar–arterial oxygen partial pressure difference with exercise, fewer (mostly highly trained) subjects develop arterial hypoxaemia, secondary to an exaggerated alveolar–arterial oxygen gradient and a blunted hyperventilatory response.

During prolonged moderate-intensity exercise (<80% maximal), arterial hypoxaemia is lessened with exercise duration because of the time-dependent increase in ventilation and P_aO_2, while arterial pH remains near normal, or even shifts in an alkaline direction over time (Hanson et al.

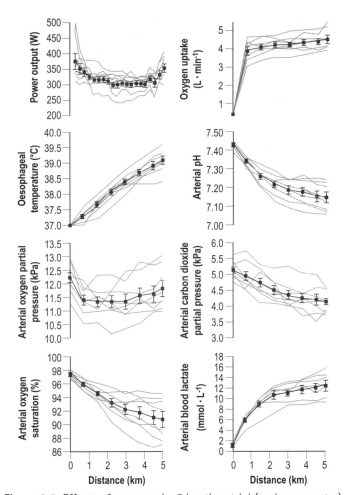

Figure 2.5 Effects of a normoxic, 5 km time trial (cycle ergometer) on the physiological responses of trained cyclists. Thin lines are individual data ($N = 8$), with thick lines showing mean responses. Mean time was 483.4 ± 7.5 s (range 437.5–478.4 s). Haemoglobin concentration was 14.4 ± 0.5 g·L^{-1} and arterial oxygen content was 19.8 ± 0.8 mL O$_2$·100 mL^{-1} at rest and 16.4 ± 0.7 mL O$_2$·100 mL^{-1}/ 20.9 ± 1.0 mL O$_2$·100 mL^{-1} at kilometre 5. Note the progressive reduction in arterial haemoglobin saturation, due to a reduced P_aO_2 in the early stage of exercise, and then a progressive metabolic acidosis and increasing blood temperature. Modified after Amann et al. (2006a), with permission.

1982, Stickland et al. 2004a). During high-intensity sustained exercise (>80% maximal) involving either constant workload or race conditions, arterial hypoxaemia will continue to develop, primarily because of a progressive metabolic acidosis, and an increased core temperature (Amann et al. 2006a, Wetter et al. 2001). Figure 2.5 highlights the gas exchange response during a 5 km cycling time trial. Within the first kilometre, P_aO_2 decreases from rest, reducing saturation ~2%. Arterial oxygen partial pressure begins to increase during the latter half of the time trial, due to the time-dependent increase in ventilation. Despite this, saturation continues to drop because of reduced arterial pH and increased core temperature. This example further highlights the independent effects of the oxyhaemoglobin dissociation curve and P_aO_2 on arterial saturation.

9.1 Determinants of pulmonary gas exchange

The alveolar–arterial oxygen partial pressure difference is determined by ventilation–perfusion matching, diffusion limitations, extrapulmonary shunting (e.g. thebesian drainage and bronchial circulation) and intracardiac and intrapulmonary shunts. Much of our understanding of pulmonary gas exchange and exercise has been obtained from the multiple inert gas elimination technique, which is the best gas exchange-dependent technique available to functionally evaluate ventilation–perfusion matching (Wagner et al. 1986). With this technique, arterial and exhaled levels of six intravenously infused inert gases, encompassing a wide range of solubility in blood, are used to calculate ventilation–perfusion mismatching and diffusion limitations (i.e. the amount of alveolar–arterial oxygen tension gradient not explained by ventilation–perfusion heterogeneity).

9.1.1 Extrapulmonary shunt

Deoxygenated blood returning from the bronchial and thebesian veins is dumped directly into the left atrium (venous admixture), mixing with the newly oxygenated blood from the pulmonary circulation, decreasing oxygen tension within the left atrium. The deoxygenated blood bypasses the pulmonary circulation entirely; an extrapulmonary shunt. The multiple inert gas elimination technique does not allow for the calculation of an extrapulmonary shunt. However, breathing 100% oxygen and examining the change in P_aO_2 relative to room air provides an estimate of the combined intra- and extrapulmonary shunt. Using the 100% oxygen technique, pulmonary shunting has been estimated to be <1% during exercise (Wagner et al. 1986), and thus unlikely to be a major contributor to the widened alveolar–arterial oxygen gradient with exercise.

9.1.2 Intrapulmonary shunt

Blood that passes through the pulmonary circulation but does not take part in gas exchange is defined as right-to-left shunt, or an intrapulmonary shunt. In addition, intracardiac shunts (e.g. patent foramen ovale) also allow blood to bypass the lungs, increasing the alveolar–arterial oxygen difference. Healthy subjects do not demonstrate an intrapulmonary shunt, either at rest or during exercise, as evaluated by gas exchange-dependent techniques (Dempsey & Wagner 1999). Therefore, right-to-left shunting has not been considered an important contributor to the widened alveolar–arterial oxygen difference during exercise. However, recent work using non-gas exchange-dependent techniques suggests that large-diameter arteriovenous shunt vessels

are recruited during exercise (Eldridge et al. 2004, Stickland et al. 2004b, 2006a, Whyte et al. 1992). It has been proposed that these vessels may not be detected using traditional techniques (e.g. multiple inert gas elimination) because partial gas exchange may occur either before or within these vessels, and thus these vessels may not shunt pure mixed venous blood, but may contribute to the widened alveolar–arterial oxygen gradient during exercise (Stickland & Lovering 2006). The recruitment of these vessels during exercise appears related to this gradient (Stickland et al. 2004b). However, these findings are contrary to the multiple inert gas elimination technique and oxygen breathing data, and require further work to determine shunt size and magnitude.

9.1.3 Ventilation–perfusion matching

During exercise, ventilation increases more than cardiac output, and therefore the global ventilation–perfusion ratio increases with exercise (Table 2.1). Despite this, regional ventilation–perfusion matching within the lung deteriorates with incremental exercise, widening the alveolar–arterial oxygen gradient. It has been estimated that regional ventilation–perfusion mismatching accounts for virtually all of this increase from rest to moderate-intensity exercise (Wagner et al. 1986), and with further increases in exercise intensity, the ventilation–perfusion mismatch increases (Hopkins et al. 1994) or remains constant (Rice et al. 1999b, Wagner et al. 1986). Therefore, regional ventilation–perfusion mismatches are said to contribute from ~30% to up to ~60% of the alveolar–arterial oxygen gradient during severe to maximal exercise. However, it is important to again highlight that a rise in the global ventilation–perfusion ratio acts to increase P_AO_2 and therefore, despite greater regional ventilation–perfusion heterogeneity and a widened alveolar–arterial oxygen difference, P_aO_2 is maintained close to resting levels in most subjects.

9.1.4 Diffusion limitation

The multiple inert gas elimination technique allows for calculation of a diffusion limitation, based upon the alveolar–arterial oxygen gradient not accounted for by the ventilation–perfusion mismatch. A diffusion limitation is not found in healthy humans at rest. However, during more strenuous exercise (oxygen uptake >2.5 L·min^{-1}) a diffusion limitation typically begins to develop (Hammond et al. 1986, Hopkins et al. 1994, Rice et al. 1999b, Wagner et al. 1986). At peak exercise, the widened alveolar–arterial oxygen gradient is therefore said to be due to a combination of a diffusion limitation and a ventilation–perfusion mismatch.

9.2 Mechanism for ventilation–perfusion mismatch and diffusion limitation during exercise

West (2000) and West & Mathieu-Costello (1995) have described how hydrostatic oedema or even stress failure may develop with exercise due to high pulmonary vascular pressures. Wagner et al. (1986) demonstrated a strong correlation between mean pulmonary artery pressure and a ventilation–perfusion mismatch during exercise. These findings have led to the suggestion that pulmonary oedema explains the ventilation–perfusion mismatch, diffusion limitation and the corresponding widened alveolar–arterial oxygen gradient during exercise. While substantial evidence exists indicating that interstitial oedema or damage develops with severe exercise (Caillaud et al. 1995, Hanel & Mortensen 2003, Hopkins et al. 1997, McKenzie et al. 2005, Young et al. 1987), direct links between oedema and the exercising alveolar–arterial oxygen difference have not been found (Edwards et al. 2000, Zavorsky et al. 2006). Moreover, acute increases in pulmonary vascular pressures do not further widen this gradient during exercise (Stickland et al. 2006a). These results indicate that, while oedema or stress failure may develop during exercise, the link to the impairment in gas exchange observed with exercise remains unclear.

Dempsey et al. (1984) proposed that a diffusion limitation may develop during high-intensity exercise due to an inadequate time for oxygen equilibration with haemoglobin, across the blood–gas barrier. As noted above, capillary recruitment during exercise helps maintain capillary transit time. However, the capillary blood volume will plateau at an oxygen uptake of ~3.5 $L \cdot min^{-1}$ (Warren et al. 1991). In athletes who can exercise above 4.5 $L \cdot min^{-1}$, and with a cardiac output >32 $L \cdot min^{-1}$ (Table 2.1), pulmonary capillary transit time drops to <0.33 s and could infringe upon equilibration time. Data obtained from the multiple inert gas elimination technique would tend to support this hypothesis, as a diffusion limitation typically develops at oxygen uptake >2.5 $L \cdot min^{-1}$ (Hammond et al. 1986, Hopkins et al. 1994, Rice et al. 1999b, Wagner et al. 1986). However, isolated lung studies that have attempted to replicate exercise by reducing capillary transit time to 0.18 s, while maintaining a near homogenous ventilation–perfusion distribution, and a mixed venous oxygen tension of ~2.9 kPa, have not shown any effect of red cell transit time on the alveolar–arterial oxygen difference (Ayappa et al. 1996).

9.3 Gas exchange – conclusion

Despite the well-documented impairment of gas exchange observed in healthy humans with exercise, considerable debate remains as to its mechanism. Data exist that support the popular theories of oedema development and reduced red cell transit time, and there is even recent work suggesting the recruitment of large-diameter arteriovenous vessels. Unfortunately, determining whether these potential mechanisms contribute to the widened alveolar–arterial oxygen gradient during exercise is difficult, due to the many problems associated with accurate measurement during whole-body exercise.

10 PULMONARY LIMITATIONS TO EXERCISE

10.1 Healthy sedentary versus highly trained individuals

The respiratory system of normal healthy, young individuals (maximal oxygen uptake ≤55 $mL \cdot kg^{-1} \cdot min^{-1}$) is generally overengineered, ensuring effective pulmonary gas exchange, even in the face of maximal whole-body endurance exercise (Figure 2.6). This statement is substantiated by a variety of observations obtained during maximal systemic exercise (Rodman et al. 2002). First, as documented in Table 2.1, despite a substantial increase in alveolar–arterial oxygen gradient, P_aO_2 is maintained near to resting levels, due to increased alveolar ventilation, which effectively raises P_AO_2 and arterial oxygen saturation drops ≤3%. Second, airway resistance and lung compliance are maintained near resting levels, and in untrained subjects, the oxygen cost of breathing is ≤10% of maximum oxygen uptake and cardiac output, and intrathoracic pressure changes developed by the respiratory muscles approximate only 40–60% of their maximal capacity. Accordingly, objective measures of force output by the diaphragm, before and after exercise, show that the diaphragm does not fatigue as a result of incremental exercise to exhaustion. Finally, since the tidal flow–volume loop remains well within the maximal flow–volume envelope (Figure 2.3), expiratory flow limitations are not a limiting factor during maximum exercise, and alveolar ventilation increases unrestricted and out of proportion to carbon dioxide production as P_aCO_2 is reduced to ≥1.33 kPa below resting levels.

10.2 What are the weaknesses in the respiratory system that compromise oxygen delivery?

Despite these near-perfect and highly efficient respiratory responses to exercise, there are two circumstances in which the healthy respiratory system presents a significant limitation to oxygen delivery and exercise performance. The first threat to the convective oxygen delivery to the working locomotor muscles is an exercise-induced reduction in arterial oxygen content (hypoxaemia). This can develop during either progressive incremental exercise, or over time during high-intensity sustained exercise. It occurs due to reduced P_aO_2 (in a minority of subjects) and more commonly as a result of a rightward shift in the oxyhaemoglobin dissociation curve, mediated by metabolic acidosis and hyperthermia.

A second threat to oxygen delivery is the hyperventilation of heavy sustained exercise (>90% maximal) causing substantial increases in both inspiratory and expiratory muscle work, leading to diaphragm and expiratory muscle fatigue (Babcock et al. 1995, 2002, Taylor et al. 2006). Whereas arterial hypoxaemia might impose a reduction to limb oxygen delivery only in a subpopulation of highly trained athletes, this second threat is an important limitation to

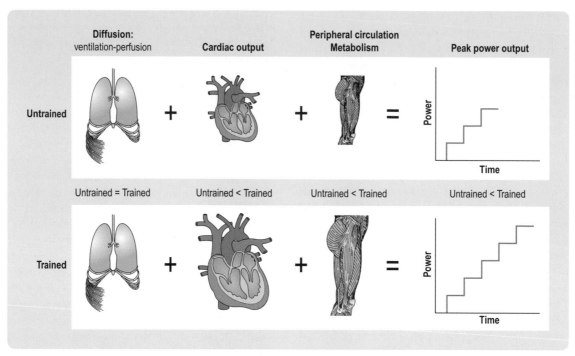

Figure 2.6 Schematic representation of the oxygen delivery chain, comparing an untrained person and an endurance-trained athlete.

performance across the range of fitness levels in healthy individuals.

Diaphragmatic fatigue is determined objectively by stimulating the phrenic nerves supramaximally and measuring transdiaphragmatic pressure (oeosophageal versus gastric pressure), before and immediately following exercise. Significant diaphragm fatigue does not occur during incremental exercise to fatigue; rather, it is induced by sustained heavy-intensity exercise. Even though diaphragm force during tidal breathing falls during the latter stages of sustained heavy exercise, alveolar ventilation is not compromised, presumably due to accessory muscle recruitment. However, fatiguing contractions and accumulation of metabolites in the inspiratory and expiratory muscles activate unmylenated group IV phrenic afferents (Hussain et al. 1991, Pickar et al. 1994) which, in turn, increase sympathetic vasoconstrictor activity in the working limb via a supraspinal reflex (St Croix et al. 2000). The result is a reduction in blood flow to the working locomotor muscles and (presumably) an increase in blood flow to the respiratory muscles, indicating a competitive relationship for a limited cardiac output (Harms et al. 1997, Manohar 1986; Figure 2.7). At maximal exercise (>90% maximal) in the highly trained subject, the respiratory muscles now require up to 15–16% of the maximal oxygen uptake and cardiac output (Harms et al. 1998b). Thus, in contrast to arterial hypoxaemia, the work of breathing induced by heavy, sustained exercise has no effect on arterial oxygen content, but the reduction in oxygen delivery is caused by reduced limb blood flow, in favour of the respiratory muscles. For example, increasing respiratory muscle work reduces blood

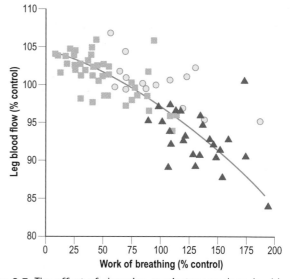

Figure 2.7 The effect of changing respiratory work on leg blood flow during peak cycling exercise. Modified from Harms et al. (1997), with permission. The circles are during normal breathing, squares are for inspiratory unloading and the triangles represent inspiratory loading.

flow to the legs, while reducing the work of breathing increases leg blood flow (Figure 2.7).

It should be noted that a threat to convective oxygen delivery to the working muscle via arterial hypoxaemia is experienced only by a subgroup of highly trained endurance athletes, and can develop even at submaximal exercise intensities. However, the threat to oxygen delivery via diaphragm and expiratory muscle fatigue, and the subsequent reduction in blood flow to the working locomotor muscles occurs in healthy untrained and trained subjects, but only at sustained, high-intensity endurance exercise (>85% maximal).

10.3 What are the consequences of a reduced convective oxygen delivery on peripheral locomotor muscle fatigue?

Fatigue is defined as any exercise-induced reduction in the ability to exert muscle force or power (Bigland-Ritchie & Woods 1984), and can be divided into a peripheral and a central component (Chapter 5). Central fatigue is defined as a progressive reduction in neural drive to the working muscle, whereas peripheral fatigue represents force reductions due to changes at or distal to the neuromuscular junction (Chapter 6). Peripheral muscle fatigue of the quadriceps can be revealed by comparing quadriceps force output evoked by supramaximal stimulation of the femoral nerve before and immediately following exercise (Polkey et al. 1996).

Amann et al. (2006b) and Romer et al. (2006a) have recently shown that changes in convective oxygen delivery to the working muscle significantly affected exercise-induced peripheral fatigue. Thus, a blunted systemic oxygen delivery exaggerates the rate of peripheral fatigue development and, in contrast, an augmentation in oxygen delivery (increased arterial oxygen content) attenuates the rate of fatigue during prolonged high-intensity, whole-body exercise.

Arterial hypoxaemia is characterised by a 5–8% reduction in oxygen saturation, from rest to high-intensity exercise (Figure 2.4). Yet even this relatively small reduction and the associated limb oxygen delivery have been demonstrated to significantly affect the magnitude of peripheral fatigue induced via high-intensity endurance exercise (≥90% maximal; Romer et al. 2006a). During two cycling exercise sessions at an identical power output and duration, arterial hypoxaemia was allowed to develop in the first trial and prevented during the second trial, via increasing the fractional concentration of inspired oxygen (0.24–0.30). In the latter trial, end-exercise peripheral muscle fatigue (quadriceps) was reduced by more than 50% compared to that measured after the first trial. These changes were accompanied by reductions in the rate of rise of blood lactate concentration, and perceptions of dyspnoea and limb discomfort during exercise.

The work of breathing required during high-intensity exercise has also been shown to affect end-exercise locomotor muscle fatigue (Romer et al. 2006b). To quantify these effects, a mechanical ventilator, capable of reducing the force required by the inspiratory muscles during breathing by 50–60%, was used during strenuous cycling exercise to significantly attenuate the work of breathing. Exercise-induced peripheral fatigue, measured as described above, was reduced by about one-third compared to the control trial (no breathing assistance). In contrast, enhancing inspiratory muscle work (resistive loading) by ~80% greater than the control trial almost doubled end-exercise muscle fatigue. This effect has been attributed to increased sympathetic vasoconstrictor activity in the working limb (Figure 2.7) which, in turn, reduces quadriceps oxygen delivery and increases exercise-induced peripheral muscle fatigue.

10.4 To what extent is endurance exercise performance affected by the limits of the respiratory system?

Impairments in pulmonary gas exchange and redistribution of the locomotor muscle blood flow (reduced oxygen delivery) have deleterious effects on endurance performance.

10.4.1 Performance loss imposed by exercise–induced arterial hypoxemia

The consequences of hypoxaemia on exercise performance may be revealed by adding just sufficient oxygen to the inspired air to prevent the fall in haemoglobin saturation during exercise. The measurable threshold of hypoxaemia-induced limitations to peak aerobic power occurs at a saturation reduction of ~3–4% (Harms et al. 2000a). Beyond this threshold, a linear association between the changes in saturation and maximal oxygen uptake is observed, such that each further 1% reduction in saturation (or oxygen content) causes a 1–2% reduction in peak aerobic power. By preventing arterial haemoglobin desaturation, the plateau of oxygen uptake, relative to work rate, is delayed until a higher work rate is reached. These observations also confirm that convective oxygen delivery to the working muscle, as determined by blood flow, arterial oxygen content and oxygen extraction, is the important limiting factor to maximal oxygen uptake in healthy subjects, as opposed to the metabolic capacity of the muscle mitochondria (Chapter 10.1).

Similarly, Amann et al. (2006a) have recently demonstrated a significant limiting effect of hypoxaemia on 5 km cycling time trial performance (Figure 2.5). Arterial oxygen content and thus oxygen delivery were increased by ~8% when the exercise-induced fall in oxygen saturation was prevented by increasing oxygen content of the inspired air. This resulted in a 2–5% reduction in the time to completion, and up to a 5% increase in mean power output.

10.4.2 Performance loss imposed by the work of breathing

The effects of the work of breathing on exercise performance (time to exhaustion) have been revealed by reducing the work of the respiratory muscles, using ventilatory assistance during constant-workload cycling at 90% of maximal aerobic power. A 60% reduction in work of breathing resulted in a 4% increase in leg blood flow (oxygen delivery) and a 3% elevation in leg oxygen uptake. The time to the limit of exhaustion was increased by ~14% when the work of breathing was reduced by ~50% (Harms et al. 2000b). This significant effect on exercise performance has indirectly been confirmed by increasing the work of the respiratory muscles by about 28%, resulting in ~15% reduction in time to exhaustion. When combined, these experiments emphasise the significant effect of respiratory muscle work on performance, during strenuous exercise.

It also needs to be mentioned that performance alterations occurred coincidentally with changes in the rate of rise in perceived exertion, both for limb discomfort (fatigue) and dyspnoea. It is thought that an increased effort perception affects the higher central nervous system such that it reduces motor output, thereby limiting exercise performance. While the specific peripheral sources of either reflex inhibition of central motor output or of heightened perceptions of effort or discomfort have not been conclusively identified (Gandevia 2001), it is likely that mechanoreceptor and metaboreceptors in the fatiguing limb (and respiratory) muscles are an important source of the heightened sensory feedback (Chapter 5).

10.4.3 Fatigue development and exercise performance

The effects of muscle oxygen delivery on peripheral muscle fatigue development have recently been postulated to determine exercise (race) performance. Increases in convective oxygen delivery, via increases in inspired oxygen or haemoglobin concentration, are known to reduce end-exercise effort perception, and the rate of peripheral fatigue development. Amann et al. (2006a) recently hypothesised that peripheral fatigue development, as affected by arterial oxygen content, is a significant determinant of central motor output during exercise, thereby preventing peripheral fatigue development beyond a critical threshold or sensory tolerance limit. Thus, acting via inhibitory feedback to higher motor areas, peripheral fatigue influences central motor drive and exercise performance. In summary, the rate of peripheral muscle fatigue development, which is sensitive to arterial oxygen content and delivery, might operate as a (dose-dependent) trigger of central fatigue (reduced central motor drive), which in turn influences exercise performance.

This theory should not be interpreted as meaning that fatigue (reduced performance) is solely based on peripheral feedback from the working muscles, especially not in conditions of severe hypoxia. Various investigators suggest that hypoxia-sensitive sources of central motor output inhibition exist outside influences related to peripheral muscle fatigue and its associated afferent feedback, even at sea level. For example, metabolic turnover of neurotransmitters in cerebral tissue is sensitive to hypoxia and even to intense exercise (at sea level), and may influence the brain's perception of effort, triggering the onset of central fatigue during exercise (Davis & Bailey 1997).

10.5 Pulmonary limitations to exercise – relative importance

We need to clarify that while the lung, airways and respiratory muscles present a significant limitation to both peak and endurance exercise performance in healthy subjects exercising at sea level, these limitations occur only in a subpopulation of endurance-trained athletes (arterial hypoxaemia), only under conditions of high-intensity, sustained exercise (respiratory muscle fatigue), and their influence is limited to a maximum effect of ~15% on either maximal oxygen uptake or endurance performance time. As emphasised earlier, the lung, airways and chest wall are structurally overbuilt for most demands imposed by peak or low-intensity endurance exercise. When combined with a multicomponent, highly sensitive neurochemical ventilatory control system, the healthy respiratory system's response to most types of exercise is nearly perfect, in terms of the efficiency and precision with which arterial blood gases are regulated. Under these conditions, the primary weak links in the delivery and utilisation of oxygen lie within the cardiovascular (Chapter 1) and muscle metabolic systems (Chapter 6). However, when exercising underwater and at high attitudes, pulmonary function can be limiting (Chapters 23 and 24).

11 EXPOSURE TO ALTITUDE

Additional respiratory limits to exercise performance, at or near sea level, occur during acute or chronic exposure to altitude (Chapter 24). Hypoxia aggravates the proposed threats to limb oxygen delivery in two ways. First, the alveolar–capillary diffusion limitation becomes more pronounced, due to a decreased P_AO_2 (driving pressure) at any given alveolar ventilation. Consequently, arterial hypoxaemia is exaggerated in the highly trained subject, even at mild elevations (1500–2000 m), imposing a further reduction in convective oxygen delivery. Second, acute but especially chronic hypoxic exposures potentiate the hyperventilatory response to exercise, markedly increasing ventilatory work (Thoden et al. 1969). Thus, the work of breathing and exercise-induced diaphragmatic fatigue would be expected to play a more significant role in determining limb blood flow and oxygen delivery. These effects might be offset to some extent if the endurance capacity and fatigue resistance of the respiratory muscles are enhanced during acclimatisation to hypoxia. On the other hand, the potential positive effects of acclimatisation (Chapter 25) will be opposed by the greater exercise hyperventilation and increased work of breathing.

12 GENDER DIFFERENCES IN PULMONARY FUNCTION

Recent work has examined whether gender affects the pulmonary responses and limitations to exercise. The menstrual cycle can modulate the ventilatory response to exercise through changes in circulating progesterone and oestrogen. Progesterone administration results in hyperventilation at rest and exercise, as well as increasing the resting ventilatory response to hypoxia and hypercapnia (Moore et al. 1987, Schoene et al. 1981). Oestrogen affects fluid retention and blood volume. Resting diffusion capacity is lower during the early follicular phase of the menstrual cycle, when circulating oestrogen and progesterone are lowest (Sansores et al. 1995). However, no studies have associated exercise pulmonary function with menstrual phase.

Relative to men of the same height, women have smaller diameter airways (Mead 1980), lung volumes and diffusion surfaces (Schwartz et al. 1988, Thurlbeck 1982). Smaller airway diameters mean women would be more likely to develop mechanical limits to expiratory flow. Indeed, tidal volume and minute ventilation are mechanically constrained during maximal exercise in many fit women, because the demand for high expiratory flows encroaches on the maximum flow–volume envelope (McClaran et al. 1998). The increased expiratory flow limitation increases the likelihood of respiratory muscle fatigue (Harms 2006), although this has not been examined. The smaller diffusion surface, combined with this flow limitation, could also negatively impact pulmonary gas exchange and hypoxaemia. Recent support for this was given by Hopkins & Harms (2004) who showed that, when data from several studies were compiled, females had a greater alveolar–arterial oxygen gradient and a lower P_aO_2 at the same relative oxygen uptake (Chapter 11).

13 EFFECTS OF AGEING ON PULMONARY FUNCTION

Normal ageing causes reductions in lung elastic recoil, vital capacity, diffusion surface area and chest wall compliance (Chapter 16). Importantly, longitudinal studies have shown that habitual physical activity does not slow the normal age-related decrease in lung function (McClaran et al. 1995). As a result, a significant expiratory flow limitation with the accompanying increase in end-expiratory lung volume is observed in fit elderly individuals, even during submaximal exercise (Johnson et al. 1991). The reduced surface area for diffusion with ageing, which is secondary to an increase in alveolar size, combined with a reduction in alveoli number (Janssens et al. 1999), could negatively impact upon exercise gas exchange. Prefaut et al. (1994) found that older athletes typically had a wider alveolar–arterial oxygen gradient and a correspondingly lower P_aO_2 than younger athletes during exercise, although others have failed to find a greater prevalence of arterial hypoxaemia in older, fit athletes (Johnson et al. 1994, Miller & Dempsey 2004). Normal ageing reduces cardiac compliance in untrained subjects, increasing pulmonary venous and arterial pressures (Arbab-Zadeh et al. 2004), and increasing the likelihood of exercise-induced pulmonary oedema or damage. Importantly, cross-sectional data have shown that master athletes have improved cardiac compliance (Arbab-Zadeh et al. 2004), suggesting that master athletes are less likely to develop exercise-induced oedema or lung damage, when compared to their age-matched sedentary counterparts.

14 SUMMARY

The respiratory system has the potential to limit exercise in several ways. First, exercise-induced arterial hypoxemia, whether due to impaired gas exchange, a blunted ventilatory response to exercise or a shift in the oxyhaemoglobin dissociation curve, will reduce arterial oxygen saturation and convective oxygen delivery. Second, the considerable ventilatory requirement during high-intensity exercise can cause a redistribution of blood flow to the respiratory muscles, reducing oxygen delivery to the locomotor muscles. Third, exercise performance may be curtailed via the striking effect of dyspnoea (secondary to respiratory muscle fatigue) and perceptions of limb discomfort (secondary to locomotor muscle fatigue) on the central nervous system, which could consciously or subconsciously determine effort. These respiratory limitations are relatively minor contributions in the young, untrained person during brief exercise bouts at sea level, but gain in importance in the highly trained subject, during high-intensity endurance exercise, with ageing or at high altitudes.

References

Aaron EA, Seow KC, Johnson BD, Dempsey JA 1992 Oxygen cost of exercise hyperpnea: implications for performance. Journal of Applied Physiology 72(5):1818–1825

Amann M, Eldridge MW, Lovering AT, Stickland MK, Pegelow DF, Dempsey JA 2006a Arterial oxygenation influences central motor output and exercise performance via effects on peripheral locomotor muscle fatigue. Journal of Physiology 575(3): 688–689

Amann M, Romer LM, Pegelow DF, Jacques AJ, Hess CJ, Dempsey JA 2006b Effects of arterial oxygen content on peripheral locomotor muscle fatigue. Journal of Applied Physiology 101(1):119–127

Arbab-Zadeh A, Dijk E, Prasad A, Fu Q, Torres P, Zhang R, Thomas JD, Palmer D, Levine BD 2004 Effect of aging and physical activity on left ventricular compliance. Circulation 110(13):1799–1805

Ayappa I, Brown LV, Wang PM, Katzman N, Houtz P, Bruce EN, Lai-Fook SJ 1996 Effect of blood flow on capillary transit time and oxygenation in excised rabbit lung. Respiratory Physiology 105(3):203–216

Babcock MA, Pegelow DF, McClaran SR, Suman OR, Dempsey JA 1995 Contribution of diaphragmatic power output to exercise-induced diaphragm fatigue. Journal of Applied Physiology 78(5): 1710–1719

Babcock MA, Pegelow DF, Harms CA, Dempsey JA 2002 Effects of respiratory muscle unloading on exercise-induced diaphragm fatigue. Journal of Applied Physiology 93(1):201–206

Badr MS, Skatrud JB, Dempsey JA 1992 Determinants of poststimulus potentiation in humans during NREM sleep. Journal of Applied Physiology 73(5):1958–1971

Beck KC 1999 Control of airway function during and after exercise in asthmatics. Medicine and Science in Sports and Exercise 31(1 Suppl):S4–11

Bellemare F, Grassino A 1982 Effect of pressure and timing of contraction on human diaphragm fatigue. Journal of Applied Physiology 53(5):1190–1195

Bigland-Ritchie B, Woods JJ 1984 Changes in muscle contractile properties and neural control during human muscular fatigue. Muscle Nerve 7(9):691–699

Bowes G, Shakin EJ, Phillipson EA, Zamel N 1984 An efferent pathway mediating reflex tracheal dilation in awake dogs. Journal of Applied Physiology 57(2):413–418

Brice AG, Forster HV, Pan LG, Funahashi A, Hoffman MD, Murphy CL, Lowry TF 1988 Is the hyperpnea of muscular contractions critically dependent on spinal afferents? Journal of Applied Physiology 64(1):226–233

Busse MW, Maassen N, Konrad H 1991 Relation between plasma K+ and ventilation during incremental exercise after glycogen depletion and repletion in man. Journal of Physiology 443: 469–476

Caillaud C, Serre-Cousine C, Anselme F, Capdevilla X, Prefaut C 1995 Computerized tomography and pulmonary diffusing capacity in highly trained athletes after performing a triathlon. Journal of Applied Physiology 79(4):1226–1232

Casaburi R, Whipp BJ, Wasserman K, Beaver WL, Koyal SN 1977 Ventilatory and gas exchange dynamics in response to sinusoidal work. Journal of Applied Physiology 42(2):300–311

Coates G, O'Brodovich H, Jefferies AL, Gray GW 1984 Effects of exercise on lung lymph flow in sheep and goats during normoxia and hypoxia. Journal of Clinical Investigation 74(1):133–141

Davis JM, Bailey SP 1997 Possible mechanisms of central nervous system fatigue during exercise. Medicine and Science in Sports and Exercise 29(1):45–57

Dempsey JA, Smith CA 1994 Do carotid chemoreceptors inhibit the hyperventilatory response to heavy exercise? Canadian Journal of Applied Physiology 19(3):350–359

Dempsey JA, Wagner PD 1999 Exercise-induced arterial hypoxemia. Journal of Applied Physiology 87(6):1997–2006

Dempsey JA, Hanson PG, Henderson KS 1984 Exercise-induced arterial hypoxaemia in healthy human subjects at sea level. Journal of Physiology 355:161–175

Dempsey JA, Forster HV, Ainsworth DM 1995 The regulation of hyperpnea, hyperventilation and respiratory muscle recruitment during exercise. In: Dempsey JA, Pack AI (eds) The regulation of breathing. Marcel Dekker, New York, 1065–1134

Dempsey JA, Adams L, Ainsworth DM 1996 Airway, lung and respiratory muscle function during exercise. In: Rowell LB, Shepard JT (eds) Handbook of physiology section 12, exercise: regulation and integration of multiple systems. Oxford University Press, New York

Dempsey JA, Miller JD, Romer LM 2006 The respiratory system. ACSM's advanced physiology. Lippincott, Williams and Wilkins, Philadelphia, 246–299

Duncker DJ, Stubenitsky R, Tonino PA, Verdouw PD 2000 Nitric oxide contributes to the regulation of vasomotor tone but does not modulate O(2)-consumption in exercising swine. Cardiovascular Research 47(4):738–748

Edwards MR, Hunte GS, Belzberg AS, Sheel AW, Worsley DF, McKenzie DC 2000 Alveolar epithelial integrity in athletes with exercise-induced hypoxemia. Journal of Applied Physiology 89(4):1537–1542

Eldridge FL, Gill-Kumar P 1978 Lack of effect of vagal afferent input on central neural respiratory after discharge. Journal of Applied Physiology 45(3):339–344

Eldridge FL, Millhorn DE, Waldrop TG 1981 Exercise hyperpnea and locomotion: parallel activation from the hypothalamus. Science 211(4484):844–846

Eldridge FL, Millhorn DE, Kiley JP, Waldrop TG 1985 Stimulation by central command of locomotion, respiration and circulation during exercise. Respiratory Physiology 59(3):313–337

Eldridge MW, Dempsey JA, Haverkamp HC, Lovering AT, Hokanson JS 2004 Exercise-induced intrapulmonary arteriovenous shunting in healthy humans. Journal of Applied Physiology 97(3):797–805

Flamm SD, Taki J, Moore R, Lewis SF, Keech F, Maltais F, Ahmad M, Callahan R, Dragotakes S, Alpert N 1990 Redistribution of regional and organ blood volume and effect on cardiac function in relation to upright exercise intensity in healthy human subjects. Circulation 81(5):1550–1559

Forster HV 2003 Plasticity in the control of breathing following sensory denervation. Journal of Applied Physiology 94(2):784–794

Forsyth RD, Cole P, Shephard RJ 1983 Exercise and nasal patency. Journal of Applied Physiology 55(3):860–865

Gandevia SC 2001 Spinal and supraspinal factors in human muscle fatigue. Physiological Reviews 81(4):1725–1789

Green JF, Schmidt ND 1984 Mechanism of hyperpnea induced by changes in pulmonary blood flow. Journal of Applied Physiology 56(5):1418–1422

Hagberg JM, Coyle EF, Carroll JE, Miller JM, Martin WH, Brooke MH 1982 Exercise hyperventilation in patients with McArdle's disease. Journal of Applied Physiology 52(4):991–994

Hammond MD, Gale GE, Kapitan KS, Ries A, Wagner PD 1986 Pulmonary gas exchange in humans during exercise at sea level. Journal of Applied Physiology 60(5):1590–1598

Hanel B, Law I, Mortensen J 2003 Maximal rowing has an acute effect on the blood-gas barrier in elite athletes. Journal of Applied Physiology 25:25

Hanson P, Claremont A, Dempsey J, Reddan W 1982 Determinants and consequences of ventilatory responses to competitive endurance running. Journal of Applied Physiology 52(3):615–623

Haouzi P, Chenuel B, Huszczuk A 2004 Sensing vascular distension in skeletal muscle by slow conducting afferent fibers: neurophysiological basis and implication for respiratory control. Journal of Applied Physiology 96(2):407–418

Harms CA 2006 Does gender affect pulmonary function and exercise capacity? Respiratory Physiology and Neurobiology 151(2–3):124–131

Harms CA, Babcock MA, McClaran SR, Pegelow DF, Nickele GA, Nelson WB, Dempsey JA 1997 Respiratory muscle work compromises leg blood flow during maximal exercise. Journal of Applied Physiology 82(5):1573–1583

Harms CA, McClaran SR, Nickele GA, Pegelow DF, Nelson WB, Dempsey JA 1998a Exercise-induced arterial hypoxaemia in healthy young women. Journal of Physiology 507(Pt 2):619–628

Harms CA, Wetter TJ, McClaran SR, Pegelow DF, Nickele GA, Nelson WB, Hanson P, Dempsey JA 1998b Effects of respiratory muscle work on cardiac output and its distribution during maximal exercise. Journal of Applied Physiology 85(2):609–618

Harms CA, McClaran SR, Nickele GA, Pegelow DF, Nelson WB, Dempsey JA 2000a Effect of exercise-induced arterial O2 desaturation on VO2max in women. Medicine and Science in Sports and Exercise 32(6):1101–1118

Harms CA, Wetter TJ, St Croix CM, Pegelow DF, Dempsey JA 2000b Effects of respiratory muscle work on exercise performance. Journal of Applied Physiology 89(1):131–138

Henson LC, Ward DS, Whipp BJ 1992 Effect of dopamine on ventilatory response to incremental exercise in man. Respiratory Physiology 89(2):209–224

Hopkins SR, Harms CA 2004 Gender and pulmonary gas exchange during exercise. Exercise and Sport Sciences Reviews 32(2): 50–56

Hopkins SR, McKenzie DC, Schoene RB, Glenny RW, Robertson HT 1994 Pulmonary gas exchange during exercise in athletes. I. Ventilation-perfusion mismatch and diffusion limitation. Journal of Applied Physiology 77(2):912–917

Hopkins SR, Schoene RB, Henderson WR, Spragg RG, Martin TR, West JB 1997 Intense exercise impairs the integrity of the pulmonary blood-gas barrier in elite athletes. American Journal of Respiratory and Critical Care Medicine 155(3):1090–1094

Hussain SN, Chatillon A, Comtois A, Roussos C, Magder S 1991 Chemical activation of thin-fiber phrenic afferents. 2. Cardiovascular responses. Journal of Applied Physiology 70(1):77–86

Innes JA, De Cort SC, Evans PJ, Guz A 1992 Central command influences cardiorespiratory response to dynamic exercise in humans with unilateral weakness. Journal of Physiology 448:551–563

Ishida K, Yasuda Y, Miyamura M 1993 Cardiorespiratory response at the onset of passive leg movements during sleep in humans. European Journal of Applied Physiology. Occupational Physiology 66(6):507–513

Janssens JP, Pache JC, Nicod LP 1999 Physiological changes in respiratory function associated with ageing. European Respiratory Journal 13(1):197–205

Johnson RL Jr, Spicer WS, Bishop JM, Forster RE 1960 Pulmonary capillary blood volume, flow and diffusing capacity during exercise. Journal of Applied Physiology 15:893–902

Johnson BD, Reddan WG, Seow KC, Dempsey JA 1991 Mechanical constraints on exercise hyperpnea in a fit aging population. American Review of Respiratory Diseases 143(5 Pt 1):968–977

Johnson BD, Badr MS, Dempsey JA 1994 Impact of the aging pulmonary system on the response to exercise. Clinics in Chest Medicine 15(2):229–246

Kane DW, Tesauro T, Koizumi T, Gupta R, Newman JH 1994 Exercise-induced pulmonary vasoconstriction during combined blockade of nitric oxide synthase and beta adrenergic receptors. Journal of Clinical Investigation 93(2):677–683

Kao F 1963 An experimental study of the pathways involved in exercise hyperpnea employing cross-circulation techniques. In: Cunningham D, Lloyd B (eds) The regulation of human respiration. Oxford University Press, London, 461–502

Kaufman MP, Forster HV 1996 Reflexes controlling circulatory, ventilatory and airway responses to exercise. In: Rowell LB, Shepard JT (eds) Handbook of physiology section 12, exercise: regulation and integration of multiple systems. Oxford University Press, New York, 381–447

Kaufman MP, Rybicki KJ, Mitchell JH 1985 Hindlimb muscular contraction reflexly decreases total pulmonary resistance in dogs. Journal of Applied Physiology 59(5):1521–1526

Koizumi T, Roselli RJ, Parker RE, Hermo-Weiler CI, Banerjee M, Newman JH 2001 Clearance of filtered fluid from the lung during exercise: role of hyperpnea. American Journal of Respiratory and Critical Care Medicine 163(3 Pt 1):614–618

Krogh A, Lindhard J 1913 The regulation of respiration and circulation during the initial stages of muscular work. Journal of Physiology 47:112–136

Lindenfeld J, Reeves JT, Horwitz LD 1983 Low exercise pulmonary resistance is not dependent on vasodilator prostaglandins. Journal of Applied Physiology 55(2):558–561

Liu Q, Kim J, Cinotte J, Homolka P, Wong-Riley MT 2003 Carotid body denervation effect on cytochrome oxidase activity in pre-Botzinger complex of developing rats. Journal of Applied Physiology 94(3):1115–1121

Lumb A, Nunn JF 2000 Nunn's applied respiratory physiology. Butterworth-Heinemann, Oxford

McClaran SR, Babcock MA, Pegelow DF, Reddan WG, Dempsey JA 1995 Longitudinal effects of aging on lung function at rest and exercise in healthy active fit elderly adults. Journal of Applied Physiology 78(5):1957–1968

McClaran SR, Harms CA, Pegelow DF, Dempsey JA 1998 Smaller lungs in women affect exercise hyperpnea. Journal of Applied Physiology 84(6):1872–1881

McKenzie DC, O'Hare T, Mayo J 2005 The effect of sustained heavy exercise on the development of pulmonary edema in trained male cyclists. Respiratory Physiology and Neurobiology 145(2–3):209–218

Manohar M 1986 Blood flow to the respiratory and limb muscles and to abdominal organs during maximal exertion in ponies. Journal of Physiology 377:25–35

Manohar M, Goetz TE 1998 L-NAME does not affect exercise-induced pulmonary hypertension in thoroughbred horses. Journal of Applied Physiology 84(6):1902–1908

Mateika JH, Duffin J 1994 Coincidental changes in ventilation and electromyographic activity during consecutive incremental exercise tests. European Journal of Applied Physiology. Occupational Physiology 68(1):54–61

Maw GJ, Mackenzie IL, Taylor NAS 1998 Human body-fluid distribution during exercise in hot, temperate and cool environments. Acta Physiologica Scandinavica 163(3):297–304

Mead J 1980 Dysanapsis in normal lungs assessed by the relationship between maximal flow, static recoil and vital capacity. American Review of Respiratory Diseases 121(2):339–342

Merkus D, Houweling B, Zarbanoui A, Duncker DJ 2004 Interaction between prostanoids and nitric oxide in regulation of systemic, pulmonary and coronary vascular tone in exercising swine. American Journal of Physiology. Heart and Circulation Physiology 286(3):H1114–H1123

Miller JD, Dempsey JA 2004 Pulmonary limitations to exercise performance: the effects of healthy aging and COPD. In: Massaro DJ, DeCarlo Massaro G, Chambon P (eds) Lung development and regeneration. Marcel Dekker, New York, 483–524

Miyamura M, Ishida, K Hashimoto I, Yuza N 1997 Ventilatory response at the onset of voluntary exercise and passive movement in endurance runners. European Journal of Applied Physiology. Occupational Physiology 76(3):221–229

Moore LG, McCullough RE, Weil JV 1987 Increased HVR in pregnancy: relationship to hormonal and metabolic changes. Journal of Applied Physiology 62(1):158–163

Newman JH, Butka BJ, Brigham KL 1986 Thromboxane A2 and prostacyclin do not modulate pulmonary hemodynamics during exercise in sheep. Journal of Applied Physiology 61(5):1706–1711

Phillipson EA, Duffin J, Cooper JD 1981 Critical dependence of respiratory rhythmicity on metabolic CO2 load. Journal of Applied Physiology 50(1):45–54

Pickar JG, Hill JM, Kaufman MP 1994 Dynamic exercise stimulates group III muscle afferents. Journal of Neurophysiology 71(2):753–760

Polkey MI, Kyroussis D, Hamnegard CH, Mills GH, Green M, Moxham J 1996 Quadriceps strength and fatigue assessed by magnetic stimulation of the femoral nerve in man. Muscle and Nerve 19(5):549–555

Powers SK, Dodd S, Lawler J, Landry G, Kirtley M, McKnight T, Grinton S 1988 Incidence of exercise induced hypoxemia in elite endurance athletes at sea level. European Journal of Applied Physiology. Occupational Physiology 58(3):298–302

Powers SK, Martin D, Cicale M, Collop N, Huang D, Criswell D 1992 Exercise-induced hypoxemia in athletes: role of inadequate hyperventilation. European Journal of Applied Physiology. Occupational Physiology 65(1):37–42

Prefaut C, Anselme F, Caillaud C, Masse-Biron J 1994 Exercise-induced hypoxemia in older athletes. Journal of Applied Physiology 76(1):120–126

Reeves JT, Taylor AE 1996 Pulmonary hemodynamics and fluid exchange in lungs during exercise. In: Rowell LB, Shepard JT (eds) Handbook of physiology section 12, exercise: regulation and integration of multiple systems. Oxford University Press, New York, 585–613

Reeves JT, Groves BM, Cymerman A, Sutton JR, Wagner PD, Turkevich D, Houston CS 1990 Operation Everest II: cardiac filling pressures during cycle exercise at sea level. Respiratory Physiology 80(2–3):147–154

Reeves JT, Linehan JH, Stenmark KR 2005 Distensibility of the normal human lung circulation during exercise. American Journal of Physiology. Lung Cellular and Molecular Physiology 288(3): L419–425

Rice AJ, Scroop GC, Gore CJ, Thornton AT, Chapman MA, Greville HW, Holmes MD, Scicchitano R 1999a Exercise-induced hypoxaemia in highly trained cyclists at 40% peak oxygen uptake. European Journal of Applied Physiology. Occupational Physiology 79(4):353–359

Rice AJ, Thornton AT, Gore CJ, Scroop GC, Greville HW, Wagner H, Wagner PD, Hopkins SR 1999b Pulmonary gas exchange during exercise in highly trained cyclists with arterial hypoxemia. Journal of Applied Physiology 87(5):1802–1812

Rodman JR, Haverkamp HC, Gordon SM, Dempsey JA 2002 Cardiovascular and respiratory system responses and limitations to exercise. In: Weisman RJ, Zeballos RJ (eds) Clinical exercise testing. Karger, New York, 1–17

Romer LM, Haverkamp HC, Lovering AT, Pegelow DF, Dempsey JA 2006a Effect of exercise-induced arterial hypoxemia on quadriceps muscle fatigue in healthy humans. American Journal of Physiology. Regulatory, Integrative and Comparative Physiology 290(2): R365–375

Romer LM, Lovering AT, Haverkamp HC, Pegelow DF, Dempsey JA 2006b Effect of inspiratory muscle work on peripheral fatigue of locomotor muscles in healthy humans. Journal of Physiology 571(Pt 2):425–439

St Croix CM, Morgan BJ, Wetter TJ, Dempsey JA 2000 Fatiguing inspiratory muscle work causes reflex sympathetic activation in humans. Journal of Physiology 529(Pt 2):493–504

Saltin B, Blomqvist G, Mitchell JH 1968 Response to exercise after bed rest and after training. Circulation 38(5 Suppl):VII1–78

Sansores RH, Abboud RT, Kennell C, Haynes N 1995 The effect of menstruation on the pulmonary carbon monoxide diffusing capacity. American Journal of Respiratory and Critical Care Medicine 152(1):381–384

Schoene RB, Robertson HT, Pierson DJ, Peterson AP 1981 Respiratory drives and exercise in menstrual cycles of athletic and nonathletic women. Journal of Applied Physiology 50(6):1300–1305

Schwartz J, Katz SA, Fegley RW, Tockman MS 1988 Sex and race differences in the development of lung function. American Review of Respiratory Diseases 138(6):1415–1421

Serra A, Brozoski D, Hodges M, Roethle S, Franciosi R, Forster HV 2002 Effects of carotid and aortic chemoreceptor denervation in newborn piglets. Journal of Applied Physiology 92(3):893–900

Stickland MK, Lovering AT 2006 Exercise-induced intrapulmonary arteriovenous shunting and pulmonary gas exchange. Exercise and Sport Sciences Reviews 34(3):99–106

Stickland MK, Anderson WD, Haykowsky MJ, Welsh RC, Petersen SR, Jones RL 2004a Effects of prolonged exercise to exhaustion on left-ventricular function and pulmonary gas exchange. Respiratory Physiology and Neurobiology 142(2–3):197–209

Stickland MK, Welsh RC, Haykowsky MJ, Petersen SR, Anderson WD, Taylor DA, Bouffard M, Jones RL 2004b Intra-pulmonary shunt and pulmonary gas exchange during exercise in humans. Journal of Physiology 561(Pt 1):321–329

Stickland MK, Welsh RC, Haykowsky MJ, Petersen SR, Anderson WD, Taylor DA, Bouffard M, Jones RL 2006a Effect of acute increases in pulmonary vascular pressures on exercise pulmonary gas exchange. Journal of Applied Physiology 100(6):1910–1917

Stickland MK, Welsh RC, Petersen SR 2006b Does fitness level modulate the cardiovascular hemodynamic response to exercise? Journal of Applied Physiology 100(6):1895–1901

Taylor BJ, How SC, Romer LM 2006 Exercise-induced abdominal muscle fatigue in healthy humans. Journal of Applied Physiology 100(5):1554–1562

Thadani U, Parker JO 1978 Hemodynamics at rest and during supine and sitting bicycle exercise in normal subjects. American Journal of Cardiology 41(1):52–59

Thoden JS, Dempsey JA, Reddan WG, Birnbaum ML, Forster HV, Grover RF, Rankin J 1969 Ventilatory work during steady-state response to exercise. Federal Proceedings 28(3):1316–1321

Thornton JM, Guz A, Murphy K, Griffith AR, Pedersen DL, Kardos A, Leff A, Adams L, Casadei B, Paterson DJ 2001 Identification of higher brain centres that may encode the cardiorespiratory response to exercise in humans. Journal of Physiology 533(Pt 3):823–836

Thurlbeck WM 1982 Postnatal human lung growth. Thorax 37(8):564–571

Wagner PD, Gale GE, Moon RE 1986 Pulmonary gas exchange in humans exercising at sea level and simulated altitude. Journal of Applied Physiology 61(1):260–270

Waldrop TG, Iwamoto GA 2006 Point: supraspinal locomotor centers do contribute significantly to the hyperpnea of dynamic exercise. Journal of Applied Physiology 100(3):1077–1079

Waldrop TG, Mullins DC, Millhorn DE 1986 Control of respiration by the hypothalamus and by feedback from contracting muscles in cats. Respiratory Physiology 64(3):317–328

Waldrop TG, Eldridge FL, Iwamoto GA, Mitchell JH 1996 Central neural control of respiration and circulation during exercise. In: Rowell LB, Shepard JT (eds) Handbook of physiology section 12, exercise: regulation and integration of multiple systems. Oxford University Press, New York, 333–380

Ward SA 1994 Peripheral and central chemoreceptor control of ventilation during exercise in humans. Canadian Journal of Applied Physiology 19(3):305–333

Warren JB, Jennings SJ, Clark TJ 1984 Effect of adrenergic and vagal blockade on the normal human airway response to exercise. Clinical Science (London) 66(1):79–85

Warren GL, Cureton KJ, Middendorf WF, Ray CA, Warren JA 1991 Red blood cell pulmonary capillary transit time during exercise in athletes. Medicine and Science in Sports and Exercise 23(12): 1353–1361

Wasserman K, Whipp BJ, Koyal SN, Cleary MG 1975 Effect of carotid body resection on ventilatory and acid-base control during exercise. Journal of Applied Physiology 39(3):354–358

West JB 2000 Invited review: pulmonary capillary stress failure. Journal of Applied Physiology 89(6):2483–2489; discussion 2497

West JB, Mathieu-Costello O 1995 Stress failure of pulmonary capillaries as a limiting factor for maximal exercise. European Journal of Applied Physiology. Occupational Physiology 70(2):99–108

Wetter TJ, St Croix CM, Pegelow DF, Sonetti DA, Dempsey JA 2001 Effects of exhaustive endurance exercise on pulmonary gas exchange and airway function in women. Journal of Applied Physiology 91(2):847–858

Whyte MK, Peters AM, Hughes JM, Henderson BL, Bellingan GJ, Jackson JE, Chilvers ER 1992 Quantification of right to left shunt at rest and during exercise in patients with pulmonary arteriovenous malformations. Thorax 47(10):790–796

Williamson JW, McColl R, Mathews D 2002 Brain activation by central command during actual and imagined handgrip under hypnosis. Journal of Applied Physiology 92(3):1317–1324

Young M, Sciurba F, Rinaldo J 1987 Delirium and pulmonary edema after completing a marathon. American Review of Respiratory Diseases 136(3):737–739

Zavorsky GS, Saul L, Murias JM, Ruiz P 2006 Pulmonary gas exchange does not worsen during repeat exercise in women. Respiratory Physiology and Neurobiology 153(3):226–236

Chapter 3

Cardiovascular and pulmonary adaptations to endurance training

Daniel J. Green   Louise H. Naylor   Keith George
Jerome A. Dempsey   Michael K. Stickland   Keisho Katayama

1 CARDIAC AND VASCULAR ADAPTATIONS TO ENDURANCE TRAINING
Keith George   Daniel Green   Louise Naylor

Endurance training is a unique cardiovascular stimulus in humans. No other lifestyle or pharmacological intervention causes comparable functional adaptation or structural remodelling of the heart or vasculature. With the possible exception of severe, prolonged endurance exercise (Green et al. 2006), cardiac adaptations to endurance training are entirely beneficial in terms of human health (Lee et al. 1999, Myers et al. 2002, Tanasescu et al. 2002). Indeed, the importance of such habitual exercise for health is that it may normalise the level of physical conditioning expected of humans from an evolutionary perspective (Booth et al. 2002; Chapter 28).

1.1 Exercise and cardiovascular adaptations: definitions

The elements of an exercise prescription are multidimensional, encompassing modality, intensity, duration, frequency (volume) and progression, all of which conceivably impact on the outcome. To reduce this complexity, the effect of training has often been delimited to the impact of aerobic or endurance exercise; repetitive dynamic (low–moderate intensity) activation of large muscle groups. This has an historical rationale, since most studies of the past century used such exercise as an intervention strategy, providing considerable adaptation data. This section adheres to this convention, although examples are highlighted where adaptation to other intensities or modes of exercise are described.

The Fick Principle provides a valuable first-principles roadmap for considering the physiological adaptations to exercise (Chapter 1). It states that oxygen uptake ($\dot{V}_{O_2}$) is dependent upon central oxygen delivery and peripheral tissue extraction. Delivery is principally a function of heart rate and stroke volume, with the latter being the difference between end-diastolic and end-systolic volumes. End-diastolic volume is determined by factors affecting preload, which relates to the extent to which ventricular myocytes are stretched prior to contracting, and is simply comprehended in terms of the length–tension curve of muscle. Preload is dependent upon ventricular filling time and atrioventricular filling pressure gradient. End-systolic volume is determined by preload (due to the Frank–Starling effect), cardiomyocyte contractility (inotropic status) and afterload (the pressure the ventricle must produce to eject blood into the aorta).

1.2 Effect of an acute bout of exercise: the Fick Principle

It is axiomatic that physiological adaptation occurs in a manner that enhances the capacity of an organism to respond to subsequent presentation of the same stimulus (Chapter 21). The effects of exercise training are therefore best understood if first placed in the context of the impact of acute bouts of endurance exercise on the cardiovascular system.

1.2.1 Fick and the acute exercise response

In response to endurance exercise, cardiac output can increase by as much as eightfold (Ekblom & Hermansen 1968), whilst heart rate rises by two- to fourfold, accounting for ~60% of the rise in cardiac output (Ekblom & Hermansen 1968). However, when the heart is paced in resting subjects to levels achieved during exercise, no substantive increase in cardiac output occurs (Bevegard et al. 1967), reinforcing the importance of the concomitant rise in stroke volume during exercise, which may either plateau at ~60% of maximal aerobic power ($\dot{V}_{O_{2max}}$) (Crawford et al. 1985, Ehsani et al. 1991, Higginbotham et al. 1986a, Janicki et al. 1996, Younis et al. 1990) or increase continually to near maximal effort (Gledhill et al. 1994, Mortensen et al. 2005, Spina et al. 1992); the difference in these studies perhaps relates to endurance training status (Figure 3.1).

1.2.1.1 Afterload

Afterload has conventionally been related to the level of systemic arterial pressure in humans. Mean arterial pressure (a valid index of mean aortic pressure (Rowell et al. 1968)) increases during dynamic exercise. Aortic pressure changes from rest (~112/68 mmHg) to peak exercise (~154/70 mmHg), increasing ejection pressure from approximately 103 to 137 mmHg (Janicki et al. 1996). If preload and contractility were constant, this afterload increase might decrease stroke volume by ~10 mL. Clearly, preload and myocardial contractility drive stroke volume during upright exercise, in spite of an increased afterload.

1.2.1.2 Contractility

Most studies have observed a progressive decrease in end-systolic volume during dynamic exercise (Figure 3.1;

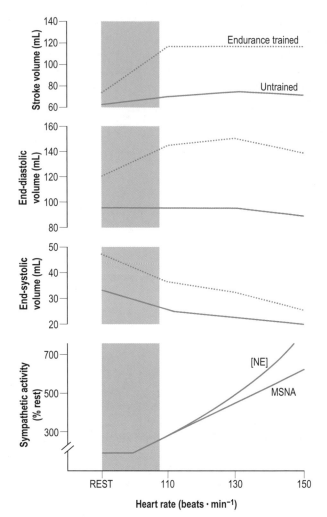

Figure 3.1 Cardiovascular responses to exercise in endurance-trained (dashed lines) and untrained subjects. The lower panel shows indices of sympathetic activity: muscle sympathetic nerve activity (MSNA) and plasma norepinephrine concentration (NE). Endurance training increases stroke volume at rest and throughout exercise, due to increased end-diastolic volume, which accompanies ventricular remodelling, enhanced ventricular compliance and the release of pericardial constraint (Figure 3.2). The enhanced stroke volume cannot be attributed to decreases in end-systolic volume with training, as this is higher in trained subjects. Figures reproduced from Schairer et al. (1992), Rowell et al. (1996) with permission.

Janicki et al. 1996, Schairer et al. 1992) which, in the presence of increasing systemic arterial pressure, ejection pressure and afterload, can be taken as evidence of enhanced myocardial contractility. The average decline in end-systolic volume during exercise is estimated at ~18 mL (Janicki et al. 1996). Along with an increase in end-diastolic volume, this could account for stroke volume changes during exercise, despite the impact of increased afterload.

Sympathetic activity does not begin to increase until heart rate exceeds ~100 beats·min^{-1} (Rowell 1993, Rowell & O'Leary 1990), whereas much of the stroke volume elevation occurs at low–moderate intensities (Figure 3.1). It seems reasonable to infer, therefore, that the inotropic effects of catecholamines are predominantly effective at moderate–high exercise intensities. This emphasises the importance of preload on stroke volume at low–moderate intensities, and implies that decreases in end-systolic volume, which contribute to the risc in stroke volume at these exercise intensities, are a likely secondary consequence of venous return (preload) and the Frank–Starling effect.

1.2.1.3 Preload

Most studies indicate that end-diastolic volume is either increased or maintained during progressive intensity exercise (Janicki et al. 1996); the difference in these studies may relate to training status (Figure 3.1; Schairer et al. 1992). Due to variations in the precision of measurement techniques and postural control, many studies have probably underestimated the rise in end-diastolic volume during the transition from rest to exercise. This is because data were frequently collected in the supine posture, minimising gravitational effects on venous return (Higginbotham et al. 1986b). For example, moving from a seated to supine posture (rest) increases stroke volume to within 20% of its peak (Thadani & Parker 1978). It has been estimated that the increase in left ventricular end-diastolic volume during upright submaximal cycling, from seated rest, is ~24 mL (Crawford et al. 1985). This would increase stroke volume by a similar magnitude, assuming constant contractility and afterload (Janicki et al. 1996).

Given that diastolic filling time decreases during incremental exercise, from ~0.55 s at 70 beats·min^{-1} to ~0.12 s at 195 beats·min^{-1} (Rowell 1993), a maintenance or increase in end-diastolic volume must result from an increased pressure gradient across the atrioventricular valves during diastole. An important concept here is that enhanced ventricular filling may result from increased atrial filling pressure, as estimated from central venous pressure and pulmonary artery wedge pressure, but it may also be related to reduced ventricular pressures, which would aid filling via suction.

Venous return increases during exercise, as a consequence of the skeletal muscle, respiratory and counter-current pumps, and also due to a redistribution of blood from the inactive to the active muscles. Thus, most of the increase in cardiac output goes to tissues that can rapidly and efficiently pump it back to the heart (Rowell 1993). At heart rates <100 beats·min^{-1}, this redistribution predominantly occurs as a consequent of non-autonomic adjustments. The muscle pump probably increases blood flow through the active muscles (Sheriff 2005), and further redistribution occurs due to vasodilator metabolites released from active muscle (section 2.1.1.3). Progressive increases in sympathetically mediated vasoconstrictor flow to inactive regions assists venous return at higher intensities (>100 beats·min^{-1}), redistributing blood away from compliant beds and towards the active skeletal muscle.

Evidence in humans indicates that indices of ventricular filling pressure (pulmonary artery wedge and central venous pressures) increase rapidly at the onset of exercise, and continue to rise until exhaustion (Higginbotham et al. 1986b, Reeves et al. 1990, Sheriff et al. 1993). As there is little evidence for a decline in ventricular filling pressures during dynamic exercise (Janicki et al. 1996), it has been suggested that the efficiency of the venous return pumps must at least match that of the heart itself (Libonati 1999, Rowell 1993). Indeed, the 'stroke volume' of the muscle and respiratory pumps must exceed that of the heart during intense exercise, given that the frequency of skeletal muscle and diaphragmatic contractions is substantially lower than heart rate.

End-diastolic and stroke volumes during exercise may also rise due to enhanced diastolic suction into the ventricles. Ventricular end-systolic volume progressively decreases during incremental exercise, whilst end-diastolic volume increases, before exhibiting a plateau in untrained subjects (Figure 3.1). The return of the left ventricle to a similar or larger volume at the end of diastole, from a smaller volume at end-systole, might involve a greater rebound suction. Recent studies have reported that the velocity at which the ventricular wall moves increases with exercise intensity, during incremental exercise (Quintana et al. 2004).

Interestingly, many studies indicate that end-diastolic volume increases during low–moderate exercise (40–70% maximal), beyond which there is a plateau (Janicki et al. 1996). Thus, a greater proportion of this increase occurs during the transition from light to moderate exercise. This raises the possibility that, at higher heart rates, filling time may begin to compromise the capacity of an increased filling pressure gradient to sustain the increase in end-diastolic volume, a suggestion supported by data from dogs which indicates that, at heart rates >170 beats·min^{-1}, ventricular contractions begin before the full resolution of diastole (Weisfeldt et al. 1978). An alternative explanation is that the continued rise in end-diastolic volume is circumscribed by pericardial constraint or ventricular stiffening (section 2.1.3). Evidence for pericardial restraint during exercise exists in animals (Hammond et al. 1992, Stray-Gundersen et al. 1986) and humans (Janicki 1990, Reeves et al. 1990). In dogs and pigs, surgical removal of the pericardium increased stroke volume (~17%), cardiac output (~20%) and oxygen uptake (~7%) during maximal exercise (Stray-Gundersen et al. 1986), primarily due to increased left ventricular end-diastolic volume (~33%; Hammond et al. 1992; Figure 3.2). In humans, removal of pericardial constraint transformed the plateau in stroke volume at higher exercise stages to a continual rise (Janicki 1990).

The similarity between the degree to which stroke volume is increased following pericardial section and endurance training (Figure 3.2) has prompted the suggestion that the pericardium plays an important role in limiting end-diastolic volume and stroke volume in untrained subjects

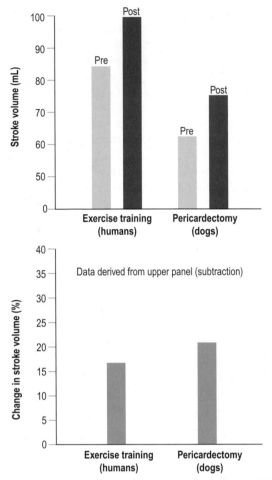

Figure 3.2 Similarity in changes in stroke volume induced by endurance training (left) and pericardiectomy (right). Figure based on data derived from DeMaria et al. (1978) and Stray-Gundersen et al. (1986). Also see Chapters 10.1 and 10.2.

(Chapter 10.2). However, regardless of whether the end-diastolic volume plateau in untrained subjects results from compromised filling time or ventricular stiffness and pericardial constraint, it remains that if end-diastolic volume and preload do indeed plateau during moderate–intense exercise, in the context of increasing afterload, further increases in stroke volume at higher exercise intensities would necessarily be dependent upon enhanced contractility and decreases in end-systolic volume.

1.2.2 Fick and the acute exercise response: summary

It seems clear that enhanced stroke volume during acute bouts of endurance exercise occurs despite an increase in afterload. A progressive decrease in end-systolic volume provides some evidence that contractility increases during exercise, although it might also be due to a Frank–Starling effect driven by enhanced preload. If contractility is an important determinant of stroke volume, it is probably mostly at higher exercise intensities and is sympathetically driven (Figure 3.1).

The increase in preload with acute exercise occurs despite decreased filling time, and is a result of increased venous return and ventricular suction. The increase in preload is likely to be a particularly important determinant of the stroke volume increase during light–moderate exercise, before any increase in sympathetic drive occurs. Thus, it appears that the venous return pumps prime the performance of the heart during dynamic exercise in upright humans. Contractility-driven decreases in end-systolic volume are likely to become important at higher intensities, where there is evidence that the rise in end-diastolic volume is attenuated as a consequence of compromised filling time or ventricular stiffening and pericardial constraint. The relative importance of these factors differs with training status (section 2.1.3).

2 ENDURANCE TRAINING AND CARDIAC OUTPUT

Resting cardiac output does not appreciably change after endurance training (Pluim et al. 1998, Zandrino et al. 2000). This belies the changes in heart rate and stroke volume; resting heart rate can decrease by ~50%, with stroke volume compensating to maintain cardiac output at a level commensurate with resting metabolic demand. Endurance training effects are manifest at matched absolute workloads,

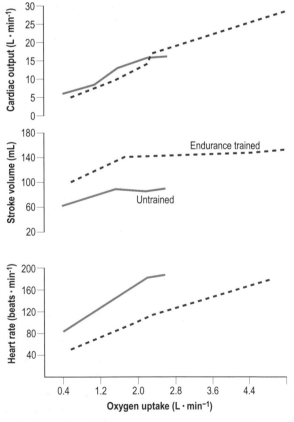

Figure 3.3 Central cardiac changes during incremental exercise in trained (dashed lines) and untrained subjects. Figure reproduced with permission from Saltin (1969).

where oxygen delivery is achieved at a lower heart rate and higher stroke volume (Figure 3.3). This relative bradycardia expands the range over which heart rate can rise (heart rate reserve). Maximal heart rate does not change appreciably with training (section 2.2), and the training-induced increase in maximal cardiac output (~10–30%) is, in this sense, entirely due to an increase in maximal stroke volume (Ekblom & Hermansen 1968). In healthy sedentary subjects, the increase in maximal cardiac output accounts for around 50% of the increase in maximal aerobic power associated with endurance training. In trained athletes, in whom tissue-based adaptations to enhance oxygen extraction are optimised, the small improvements in aerobic power with training are predominantly due to enhanced stroke volume (Clausen 1977, Rowell 1974, Saltin et al. 1968).

2.1 Stroke volume and exercise training

Most of the increase in stroke volume occurs during the transition from rest to moderate exercise (Figure 3.1, 3.3), and this holds for trained and untrained subjects, although the absolute workload at which trained subjects reach any given heart rate increases. Maximal stroke volume generally occurs between 40–50% of maximal aerobic power (~110–120 beats·min^{-1}) in untrained subjects. Following endurance training, stroke volume may not exhibit this plateau or may plateau later (Gledhill et al. 1994, Mortensen et al. 2005, Spina et al. 1992).

Recently, Mortensen et al. (2005) reported a rise in stroke volume to ~80% of maximal work rate in young trained individuals, with a subsequent decline at higher intensities, associated with decreased cardiac output and vascular conductance. They concluded that oxygen delivery to the exercising muscles limits aerobic power in trained subjects (Chapters 10.1 and 10.2). The reason for this plateau in stroke volume at higher exercise intensities in trained subjects is not related to decreased central venous pressure or pulmonary artery wedge pressure, and there is no evidence that it is due to an increased afterload. This has led to speculation that, as in dogs (Weisfeldt et al. 1978), decreased filling time may compromise stroke volume in trained individuals at higher heart rates (section 1.2.1.3). In untrained subjects, pericardial constraint may be more important for the plateau in end-diastolic volume and stroke volume, because these occur at lower relative exercise intensities and heart rates, where diastolic filling time should be adequate. The impact of endurance training on the determinants of the stroke volume response is considered in detail below.

2.1.1 Does endurance training modulate afterload?

Despite the marked increase in maximal cardiac output following endurance training, mean aortic pressure at maximal exercise (~140 mmHg) does not differ between the trained and untrained subjects (Ekblom 1969, Rowell 1993). Given that arterial pressure is the product of cardiac output and systemic vascular resistance, this indicates that vascular conductance must increase with training to accommodate the increased cardiac output. This is reinforced by the observation that, at matched absolute exercise intensities, arterial pressure is lower, despite similar cardiac outputs (Fisman et al. 1990, Fleg et al. 1994, Gledhill et al. 1994). The conductance elevation must occur predominantly within active muscles, since these tissues are the major site of blood flow redistribution during exercise (Rowell 1993). Such increases in vascular conductance must result from changes in the structure or function of the vasculature; evidence for both possibilities is presented below.

2.1.1.1 Consideration of functional elements of the vascular tree

Adaptations to the resistance vessels (arteries and arterioles) have been a primary research focus since they control the distribution of blood (Krogh 1912), and have the greatest impact upon systemic vascular conductance and arterial pressure. Large, more elastic arteries absorb the impact of systolic ejection, so that adaptation that favours increased elasticity will moderate systolic arterial pressure, an important adaptation given the enhanced ejection volumes resulting from endurance training. Conduit arteries are those principally involved in catastrophic ischaemic events in humans, and the impact of training on their structure and function is therefore of great clinical relevance. Finally, training-induced microvascular angiogenesis in terminal arterioles and capillaries (Brown 2003) represents an important training effect that enhances the capacity for tissue oxygen extraction.

In general terms, enhanced vascular conductance in the trained state might result from increases in vessel structure (arteriogenesis), enhanced functional vasodilatation or reduced vasoconstriction. As is the case with cardiac adaptations, training effects on the vasculature might best be considered in the context of the nature of the acute exercise stimulus. To this end, mechanisms responsible for the exercise hyperaemic response to dynamic exercise are briefly considered.

2.1.1.2 Vascular responses to an acute bout of endurance exercise

It has been known for several decades that numerous by-products of metabolism induce vasodilatation of resistance vessels when infused intraarterially (Laughlin et al. 1996, Shepherd 1983, Whelan 1967). This has encouraged a largely fruitless search for a sole agent that could explain exercise hyperaemia, an endeavour further complicated by the recent suggestion that vasodilator by-products of metabolism exhibit redundancy, whereby inhibition of one pathway during exercise results in upregulation of another (Boushel & Kjaer 2004, Green et al. 2004, Schrage et al. 2004). Whilst metabolic dilatation cannot explain the rapid rise in muscle blood flow following the onset of exercise, an increase that some ascribe to the perfusion impact of the muscle pump (Sheriff 2005), it is clear that some combination of vasodilator metabolites is important to the steady-state exercise hyperaemia in humans.

Recently, some interesting alternative explanations for exercise hyperaemia have been proposed, relating local vasodilatation to haemoglobin dissociation. In one such model, the binding of oxygen to haemoglobin in the lungs also facilitates the binding of nitric oxide to haemoglobin, and its bound transport in the blood as S-nitrosohaemoglobin. Subsequent dissociation of oxygen from haemoglobin in metabolically active tissues reverses S-nitrosohaemoglobin binding, thereby offloading nitric oxide in close proximity to the active skeletal muscle fibres, causing vasodilatation of the surrounding microvessels (Gow & Stamler 1998, Stamler et al. 1997). A recent variation to this schema proposes that adenosine triphosphate (ATP) is released from haemoglobin in hypoxic regions, such as metabolically active tissue, leading to vasodilatation of local arterioles by stimulating endothelial nitric oxide release, with a similar result to that described above (González-Alonso et al. 2002).

These explanations provide elegant hypotheses for the observation of a tight coupling between oxygen demand and delivery, and preferential vasodilatation in regions that are most metabolically active (González-Alonso et al. 2006).

Whichever combination of vasodilator mechanisms is activated during exercise, it is important to note that the interstitial fluid into which these substances are released bathes smaller arterioles and microvessels, whereas the primary sites of the control of perfusion and blood flow distribution in skeletal muscle lie upstream in the larger arteries and arterioles (Green et al. 1996b, Segal 1992). Thus, unless some counter-current exchange of vasodilator metabolites into the arterial vessels occurs as they are washed out through the veins (Green et al. 1996b), the explanation for a post-training enhancement in vasodilatation is unlikely to be directly attributable to the repeated effects of metabolic vasodilator agents during repeated exercise bouts.

One hypothetical explanation for the vasodilatation of the upstream resistance vessels, or feed arteries, relates to the control of vascular shear stress across the endothelium. Shear stress is proportional to blood velocity and inversely related to arterial diameter, and it transduces signals that release vasodilator agents, in particular nitric oxide from the vascular endothelium (Furchgott & Zawadzki 1980). This local paracrine mechanism acts to homeostatically regulate local shear forces by modulating arterial diameter (Dimmeler & Zeiher 2003, Hutcheson & Griffith 1991, Koller & Kaley 1991, Neibauer & Cooke 1996), with the inherent capacity for nitric oxide production being dependent upon the magnitude of changes in local shear experienced at different levels of the vascular tree (Laughlin et al. 2003a, b). During exercise, increased arterial pressure combines with the decrease in downstream microvessel resistance caused by accumulating metabolites (Green et al. 1996b) and the perfusion effects of the muscle pump (Laughlin 1987, Sheriff

2005). This increased perfusion gradient may increase shear stress across the arterioles that control muscle blood flow and its distribution (Segal 1992). This, in turn, causes local endothelium-dependent vasodilatation. In this way, blood is preferentially distributed with the aid of localised 'steal effects' to the metabolically active regions within a muscle (Segal 1992).

Animal data support the existence of this 'ascending' vasodilatation (Green et al. 1996b), and some human studies have reported nitric oxide release from resistance and conduit arteries during acute bouts of exercise (Duffy et al. 1999a,b, Dyke et al. 1995, Gilligan et al. 1994, Hickner et al. 1997). The impact of exercise on other paracrine agents, such as prostacyclin, has been less well studied but may also contribute to shear stress-mediated resistance and feed artery dilatation (Duffy et al. 1999a, Green et al. 1996b).

In summary, the best current explanation for the control of the vasculature during incremental exercise appears to involve a combination of microvessel dilation, as a consequence of localised metabolite build-up and nitric oxide, as well as ATP off-loading from haemoglobin. As a consequence, ascending vasodilatation of larger, upstream resistance vessels occurs. These mechanisms combine to cause feed and resistance artery dilatation that is specific to the metabolically active muscle. The coupling of microvessel and shear stress-mediated resistance vessel vasodilatation satisfies the observed temporal, spatial and quantal aspects of exercise hyperaemia, although much work remains to confirm the existence of this schema in humans.

2.1.1.3 Endurance training and vasculature function: evidence for enhanced vasodilatation

Several reviews have focused on evidence regarding changes in endothelial function resulting from endurance training (Jasperse & Laughlin 2006, Maiorana et al. 2003). A summary of these is provided below.

Studies using endurance training in small muscle groups in healthy adults indicate that this form of training does not consistently improve vasodilator function (Green et al. 1994, 1996a), possibly due to an inadequate active muscle mass, or the lack of substantive haemodynamic changes that might induce shear stress-mediated adaptations (Green et al. 2004). Studies have, however, observed evidence of increased resistance and conduit vessel cross-sectional area following the training of small muscle groups (Dinenno et al. 2001, Green et al. 1996a, Schmidt-Trucksass et al. 2000, Sinoway et al. 1986), suggesting structural remodelling or arteriogenic change (section 2.1.1.5). This vascular remodelling may normalise shear stress and negate the requirement for functional adaptations (Green et al. 2004).

Exercise involving large muscle groups produces shear stress changes not always apparent with localised training (Green et al. 2005). In one study, basal resistance vessel endothelial function was enhanced in response to 4 weeks of endurance cycling (Kingwell et al. 1997), whilst relatively intense exercise improved conduit artery endothelial

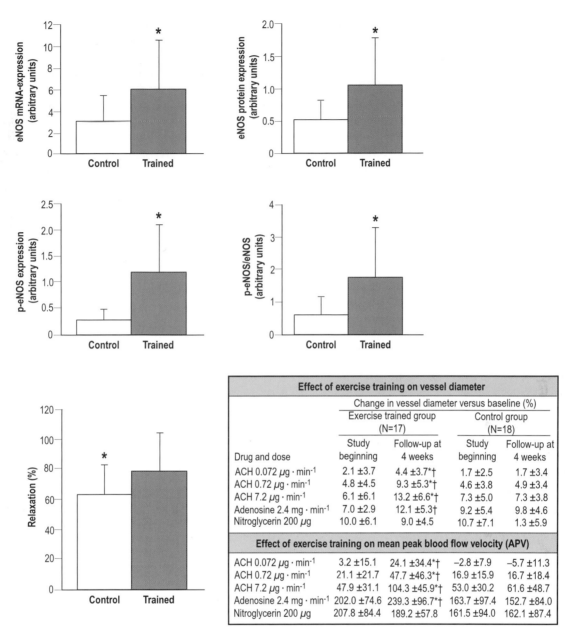

Figure 3.4 Summary of the findings of Hambrecht et al. (2003, with permission). Four weeks of exercise training in coronary disease patients was associated with increased mRNA and protein expression of eNOS and phosphorylated eNOS in samples of the left internal mammary artery of exercise-trained subjects, harvested at the time of the bypass surgery. In vitro relaxation responses (%) to the endothelium-dependent and nitric oxide-mediated vasodilator, acetylcholine, were also enhanced, along with in vivo endothelium-dependent responses (tabluated).

function in healthy young subjects (Clarkson et al. 1999). Other endurance-training studies, performed in patients with endothelial dysfunction, have consistently observed improvement in conduit and resistance vessel endothelial function (Maiorana et al. 2003). Taken together, these studies indicate that endurance training of large muscle groups improves vasodilator function, with these beneficial effects being generalised, since lower limb training improves upper limb conduit and resistance vessel function (Green et al. 2004, Linke et al. 2001, Maiorana et al. 2001, 2003).

In terms of the putative mechanisms responsible for enhanced active vasodilator function following training, the role of shear stress was recently confirmed in a study involving assessment of internal mammary artery function in patients with coronary artery disease (Hambrecht et al. 2003). Four weeks of endurance cycling increased endothelium-dependent vasodilatation of this artery, with no change evident in non-trained controls. During coronary bypass surgery that followed the training programme, a section of the artery was harvested. Enhanced in vitro vasodilator function, and significantly higher nitric oxide synthase mRNA and protein expression were confirmed in the arteries of trained subjects, along with higher phosphorylation of the shear stress transducing elements of this enzyme

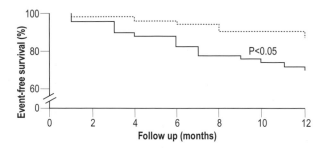

	Endurance training group (N=43)		Stent group (N=37)		
	Baseline	12 months	**Baseline**	After surgery	12 months
Minimal lumen diameter (mm)	0.66±0.06	0.69±0.08	0.53±0.04	2.57±0.05†	1.91±0.07*†
Relative stenosis diameter (%)	77.9±1.7	76.5±2.4	80.7±1.5	11.8±0.9†	31.3±2.0*†

* P<0.001 versus after surgery
† P<0.001 training versus stent group

Figure 3.5 Event-free survival in patients randomised to undergo endurance training (dashed line) and percutaneous coronary intervention with stenting. The inset table shows changes in lumen and stenosis diameters in each group at entry and after 12 months. Stenting significantly increased lumen diameter and decreased relative stenosis diameter of target lesions, but there was significantly higher event-free survival in the training group. Coronary intervention treats a short segment of the diseased coronary tree, whereas endurance training exerts beneficial effects throughout the entire arterial bed. Redrawn from Hambrecht et al. (2004) with permission.

which correlated with the in vivo improvement in vasodilator function (Figure 3.4). These unique and convincing human data are consistent with a shear-stress mechanism for enhanced endothelial function with training. An alternative explanation, which is not mutually exclusive, is that degradation of endothelium-derived vasodilators by free radicals during acute exercise (Adams et al. 2002, Fukai et al. 2000) is attenuated with endurance training (Ennezat et al. 2001).

Whilst vascular tone is a balance between the interplay of dilator and constrictor influences, the studies summarised above provide strong evidence for enhanced active vasodilator function following endurance training in humans. Improvement in conduit endothelial function may have important implications for atherothrombotic risk in humans (Green et al. 2004, Hambrecht et al. 2004; Figure 3.5), whereas improvement in the intrinsic vasodilator capacity of resistance vessels may contribute to the enhanced vascular conductance, and the decrease in resting and submaximal blood pressures observed following such conditioning. Indeed, enhanced vasodilator function may be particularly

relevant at low-to-moderate exercise intensities (<100 beats·min^{-1}), because there is little evidence for a marked contribution of sympathetic outflow and vasoconstrictor restraint at these intensities (Figure 3.1).

2.1.1.4 Endurance training and vasculature function: evidence for decreased vasoconstriction

Indirect evidence of reduced sympathetic vasoconstriction following endurance training comes from the suggestion that, at given absolute workloads, plasma norepinephrine (noradrenaline) spill-over from vasomotor nerves is lower following training (Galbo 1983, Rowell 1993).

The relevance of changes in vasoconstrictor tone following training is better appreciated if one considers the importance of vasoconstriction of active skeletal muscle beds during endurance exercise. This was classically demonstrated by training studies that confined the training stimulus to one leg, and demonstrated that blood flow and oxygen uptake increased during maximal one-legged exercise of the trained limb, whereas during two-legged exercise, blood flow and maximal aerobic power were attenuated (Davies & Sargeant 1975, Gleser 1973, Klausen et al. 1982, Saltin et al. 1976). This indicates that, during single leg exercise, the training-induced increase in cardiac output (stroke volume) was directed to the trained limb, increasing its oxygen delivery and aerobic power. Adding the untrained leg, with the attendant increase in total vascular conductance, was associated with relative vasoconstriction, presumably to regulate blood pressure (Rowell 1993). In this context, it was recently estimated that if trained subjects were able to use the combined vascular conductance of all the leg and arm muscles during maximal exercise, maximal aerobic power should be ~20% higher than that actually observed (Calbet et al. 2004).

Such studies imply that training-induced changes in vascular structure and vasodilator function can increase vascular conductance to the extent that it exceeds the capacity of the cardiovascular system to regulate blood pressure. Since pressure regulation is critical (Chapters 1 and 18), vasoconstriction in active muscles must occur (Rowell 1993). Such vasoconstriction probably begins at moderate–high intensity exercise and results from a combination of a central command-mediated resetting of the baroreflex and muscle chemoreflex activation (Rowell et al. 1996). Evidence for a sympathetically induced increase in vasoconstrictor tone at lower intensities (<100 beats·min^{-1}) is scant.

2.1.1.5 Endurance training and vascular structure

The prevailing evidence indicates that endurance training induces changes in arterial calibre (arterial remodelling or arteriogenesis). Autopsy and angiographic studies have revealed enlarged coronary arteries in athletes (Currens & White 1961, Pelliccia et al. 1990) and physically fit individuals (Hildick-Smith et al. 2000, Mann et al. 1972, Rose et al. 1967), whilst cross-sectional studies have consistently reported larger skeletal muscle conduit (Dinenno et al. 2001,

Schmidt-Trucksass et al. 2000) and resistance (Green et al. 1996a, Sinoway et al. 1986) vessels in athletes. Longitudinal training studies also provide evidence for increased vessel diameter in resistance (Green et al. 1994, Sinoway et al. 1987) and conduit vessels (Dinenno et al. 2001, Miyachi et al. 1998, Naylor et al. 2006). These observations are supported by animal studies (Brown 2003), and the plasticity of arterial adaptation was recently demonstrated when significant increases in conduit diameters were observed in highly trained athletes following the resumption of their training regimen after a brief lay-off period (Naylor et al. 2006).

The mechanisms responsible for arteriogenic changes may be linked to a shear stress stimulus on the endothelium, during repeated exercise. This is supported by a classic study in which carotid arteries (rabbit) were unilaterally ligated to induce chronic decreases in blood flow (Langille & O'Donnell 1986). The flow reduction significantly reduced the size of the ligated vessel, an adaptation that was dependent upon the presence of the endothelium. Similar studies confirm that shear stress is autoregulated and provides an endothelium-dependent stimulus to arterial remodelling (Kamiya & Togawa 1980), which enlarge to homeostatically regulate wall shear (Tronc et al. 1996, Tuttle et al. 2001).

It is concluded that endurance training induces structural enlargement in the resistance and conduit vessels. This acts to mitigate the increases in transmural pressure and wall stress that accompanies repeated endurance exercise (Prior et al. 2004, Tronc et al. 1996).

2.1.1.6 Summary: vascular adaptation and the contribution of afterload to enhanced stroke volume

Increased vascular conductance following endurance training is associated with a lower arterial blood pressure at matched submaximal workloads, and a reduced afterload may therefore help increase stroke volume during submaximal exercise. Evidence presented above strongly indicates that training increases the lumenal area of conduit and resistance vessels, and the capacity for producing paracrine vasodilators. Exercise training also decreases vasoconstrictor outflow at matched absolute workloads and oxygen uptakes. Such adaptations impact on the potential vasodilator reserve of active muscles during exercise. Given that the major increase in stroke volume occurs in the transition from low to moderate intensities, before sympathetic activity markedly increases, it can be inferred that increased active vasodilator capacity or structural vascular enlargement, rather than reduced tonic vasoconstriction, plays a more dominant role in the decreased afterload, which may assist stroke volume to rise following training. During maximal exercise, arterial pressure is similar before and after training, but cardiac output is higher. Whilst this is consistent with increased vascular conductance with training, it provides limited evidence for a contribution of reduced afterload to the rise in maximal stroke volume.

2.1.2 Does endurance training alter cardiac contractility?

The relationship between end-systolic volume and arterial pressure can provide some insight into training-induced changes in contractility, as can the concentrations of catecholamines during exercise and changes in β-adrenoceptor density. Studies comparing athletes with controls, or using longitudinal endurance training designs, typically report increases in resting end-systolic volume (Brandou et al. 1993, Crouse et al. 1992, Fisman et al. 1990, Rubal et al. 1986, Seals et al. 1994). Hence, at rest, even though arterial pressure is similar or slightly decreased after training, there appears to be no evidence for a lower end-systolic volume. The increase in resting stroke volume must therefore primarily be the result of ventricular remodelling, favouring enhanced end-diastolic volume (section 2.1.3.1). This, in turn, is likely to result from repetitive increases in preload, as a consequence of enhanced venous return during repeated bouts of exercise. This view is consistent with the reasoning presented above (section 1.2.1.2) regarding the importance of venous return preload, and the Frank–Starling effect for achieving the major proportion of the increases in stroke volume which occurs at exercise intensities below ~100 beats·min^{-1}.

The question of whether training modifies cardiac contractility during exercise is difficult to discern, due to the absence of reliable end-systolic volume data during exercise, and also because simultaneous changes occur in loading conditions which can affect end-systolic volume. Nonetheless, Schairer et al. (1992) reported higher end-systolic volumes at all matched submaximal heart rates following training, including rates well above 100 beats·min^{-1}, where sympathetic activity should be apparent (Figure 3.1). As previously stated, catecholamine concentrations are similar at matched relative exercise intensities, and lower at matched absolute workloads following training (Galbo 1983, Rowell 1993). Furthermore, longitudinal studies have consistently demonstrated that muscle sympathetic nerve activity responses to dynamic exercise are attenuated after training (Ray & Hume 1998), and recent evidence suggests that endurance training is associated with no change, or a decline, in β-adrenoceptor density (Barbier et al. 2006).

Thus, even though arterial pressures (and ejection pressures) are decreased at submaximal exercise workloads following training, the available evidence implies that end-systolic volume is increased (one possible exception involved elderly men; Ehsani et al. 1991). This evidence, together with the lack of evidence for higher catecholamine concentrations or β-adrenoceptor density (Barbier et al. 2006), suggests that changes in stroke volume accompanying endurance training are not due to enhanced cardiac contractility. Possibly, ejection fraction is already so high during intensive exercise in unconditioned individuals (~85%) that any scope for further training-induced changes is small, and would contribute little to enhanced cardiac performance after training (Rowell 1993).

Sport	LVID$_d$ (mm)	Sport	Wall thickness (mm)
(1) Endurance cycling	5.91	Rowing	2.13
(2) Cross-country skiing	5.41	Endurance cycling	2.02
(3) Swimming	4.90	Swimming	1.71
(4) Pentathlon	4.35	Canoeing	1.70
(5) Canoeing	4.23	Long-distance track	1.49
(6) Sprint cycling	3.97	Water polo	1.38
(7) Rowing	3.87	Sprint cycling	1.35
(8) Long-distant track	3.47	Weightlifting	1.23
(9) Soccer	3.11	Wrestling/judo	1.21
(10) Team handball	2.87	Tennis	1.00
(11) Tennis	2.69	Pentathlon	0.98
(12) Roller hockey	2.41	Cross-country skiing	0.98
(13) Boxing	2.25	Boxing	0.94
(14) Alpine skiing	2.13	Roller skating	0.88
(15) Fencing	2.09	Soccer	0.76
(16) Taekowando	2.07	Roller hockey	0.69
(17) Water polo	2.02	Fencing	0.63
(18) Diving	1.70	Sprint track	0.54
(19) Roller skating	1.68	Volleyball	0.39
(20) Volleyball	1.43	Diving	0.38
(21) Bobsledding	1.35	Alpine skiing	0.29
(22) Weightlifting	1.32	Field weight events	0.25
(23) Wrestling/judo	1.25	Taekwondo	0.23
(24) Equestrian	0.43	Team handling	0.19
(25) Field weight events	0.18	Equestrian	0.13
(26) Yachting	0.10	Bobsledding	0.07
(27) Sprint track	0.00	Yachting	0.00

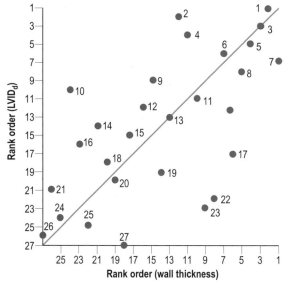

Figure 3.6 The relationship between left ventricular cavity dimensions (i.e. internal ventricular diameter at the end of diastole (LVID$_d$) and wall thickness in athletes from different sports. Numbers on the graph correspond to those in the table in parenthesis. Redrawn from Spirito et al. (1994) with permission.

2.1.3 Does endurance training alter preload?

Human data consistently indicate that end-diastolic volume increases with endurance training, both at rest and during exercise (Brandou et al. 1993, Morganroth et al. 1975, Pelliccia et al. 1999, Rerych et al. 1980, Schairer et al. 1992; Figure 3.6). In untrained subjects, end-diastolic volume will plateau (it may not rise) at low heart rates (Janicki et al. 1996). This implies that pericardial constraint and ventricular stiffness are more important limiting factors than diastolic filling time. This is reinforced by the observation that cutting of the pericardium acutely increases stroke volume (Barnard 1898, Hammond et al. 1992, Stray-Gundersen et al. 1986; Figure 3.2), suggesting that humans operate on the steep portion of the Frank–Starling curve, and that filling pressure, even at rest, is high enough to increase stroke volume if the restraint is removed.

In endurance athletes, the rise in stroke volume and end-diastolic volume may continue beyond 40–50% of maximal exercise capacity and heart rate (Gledhill et al. 1994, Mortensen et al. 2005, Schairer et al. 1992, Spina et al. 1992). The reasons for this improvement could conceivably include ventricular enlargement (remodelling), enhanced filling pressure (perhaps associated with enhanced blood volume), enhanced ventricular compliance or reduced pericardial constraint. These factors are inter-related and are considered below (also consult the discussion within Chapter 10.2).

2.1.3.1 Endurance training and cardiac remodelling

Morphological cardiac adaptations can be understood in the context of the Law of La Place, the implication of which is that cardiac muscle hypertrophies to match the workload imposed on the ventricle, such as to maintain a constant relationship between chamber pressure and the ratio of wall thickness to ventricular radius. This allows wall tension to be homeostatically maintained.

This schema has been used to explain early observations that two forms of athlete's heart develop as a consequence of differing training programmes (Morganroth et al. 1975). It was proposed that endurance athletes were subjected to repetitive increases in cardiac preload, resulting in eccentric left ventricular hypertrophy, characterised by increased left ventricular cavity dimensions (end-diastolic volume), and a proportional increase in left ventricular wall thickness to normalise myocardial strain and end-diastolic wall stress. In contrast, resistance athletes experience repetitive increases in cardiac afterload, resulting in concentric left ventricular hypertrophy. This manifests as an increased wall thickness to normalise the increased wall tension associated with the rise in arterial pressure, but with little or no effect on cavity size (end-diastolic volume).

There is some evidence supporting the La Place-based schema relating pressure or volume overload and training-induced ventricular remodelling. In animals the degree of ventricular wall thickening occurs in direct proportion to the duration of static training and the amount of isometric work (Muntz et al. 1981), and there is a general consensus that in humans, end-diastolic volume and left ventricular mass are increased in athletic populations (Brandou et al. 1993, Morganroth et al. 1975, Pelliccia et al. 1999, Pluim et al. 1999, Schairer et al. 1992, Scharhag et al. 2002), and with training (Abergel et al. 2004, DeMaria et al. 1978, Naylor et al. 2005, Shapiro & Smith 1983, Stein et al. 1980, Wieling et al. 1981). Detraining is associated with rapid reversal of these effects (Ehsani et al. 1978), and echocardiographic findings are now being endorsed by data from more sensitive cardiac magnetic resonance imaging techniques.

Whilst there is general acceptance of the impact of endurance training on left ventricular mass and end-diastolic volume, it is notable that two meta-analyses were unable to conclusively demonstrate differences in cardiac adaptations between resistance and endurance training modalities (Fagard 2003, Pluim et al. 1999). Nonetheless, substantial differences are evident between groups of athletes, with endurance athletes generally displaying greater adaptation than strength athletes (see Figure 3.6) (Pelliccia et al. 1999, Spirito et al. 1994, Urhausen & Kindermann 1989, Wernstedt et al. 2002).

2.1.3.2 Endurance training and ventricular compliance

The impact of training-induced hypertrophy on ventricular compliance is a topic of considerable interest because of the important negative relationship between pathological hypertrophy (e.g. hypertension, diabetes) and ventricular diastolic function (Bella et al. 2002, Fischer et al. 2003, Schillaci et al. 2002, Wang et al. 2003). However, evidence from cross-sectional comparisons indicates that, even when physiological ventricular hypertrophy is observed with training, there is no evidence for detrimental effects on diastolic function in elite endurance-trained (Caso et al. 2000, Fagard 2003, Libonati 1999, Pela et al. 2004, Pluim et al. 1999) or strength-trained athletes (Colan et al. 1985, MacFarlane et al. 1991, Yeater et al. 1996). Indeed, there is evidence from transmitral blood velocity (Di Bello et al. 1996) and myocardial tissue velocity (Pela et al. 2004) that diastolic function at rest is improved in athletes. What is difficult to determine from such studies is whether these changes simply reflect a lower resting heart rate, improved preload or a combination of these, rather than enhanced intrinsic relaxation properties.

Some insight is available from two studies, performed at rest, using the rapid infusion of saline and lower-body negative pressure to modulate ventricular filling pressure, in combination with stroke volume measurement (Arbab-Zadeh et al. 2004, Levine et al. 1991). Both young and old endurance-trained athletes exhibited Frank–Starling curves that were shifted upwards and to the left relative to controls. That is, for the same pulmonary artery wedge pressure, athletes had greater stroke volume. It was concluded

that endurance training improved ventricular compliance. These observations were recently extended by Stickland et al. (2006) using estimates of pulmonary artery wedge pressure and stroke volume during exercise in matched trained and untrained subjects. Left ventricular filling pressures were lower at similar submaximal stroke volume in the trained subjects. Filling pressures remained lower in these subjects, even at maximal exercise, when stroke volume and end-diastolic volume were significantly higher. They concluded that trained subjects possessed superior diastolic function and compliance during both submaximal and maximal exercise.

Conceivably, ventricular compliance might increase as a result of training due to enhanced ventricular suction, intrinsic myocardial changes that occur in concert with ventricular remodelling (Libonati 1999, Moore & Korzick 1995) or decreased ventricular wall stiffness, related to the possible removal of pericardial constraint. The increased systolic contraction force during dynamic exercise, largely due to enhanced preload and the Frank–Starling effect, results in augmented systolic fibre shortening, a smaller end-systolic volume, and a consequent increase in diastolic elastic recoil (Libonati 1999), thereby enhancing the gradient for left ventricular filling (Stickland et al. 2006). Although training is associated with increased end-systolic volume, end-diastolic volume also increases such that the possibility for enhanced recoil and ventricular suction after training remains feasible. From a cellular perspective, exercise training may enhance compliance by altering calcium uptake (sarcoplasmic reticulum) and cardiomyocyte relaxation, or other so-called active relaxation metabolic processes (Moore & Korzick 1995, Naylor et al. 2008, Tate et al. 1990).

2.1.3.3 Endurance training and pericardial remodelling

Several lines of evidence are consistent with the possibility that the pericardium plays an important role in limiting the increase in end-diastolic volume during exercise in untrained subjects. This evidence includes the fact that cutting of the pericardium increases end-diastolic volume and stroke volume (Barnard 1898, Hammond et al. 1992, Stray-Gundersen et al. 1986), indicating that if this apparent impediment is removed, then the ventricular filling pressure gradient is capable of enhancing end-diastolic volume, preload and stroke volume. There is a similarity between the degree to which stroke volume is increased following pericardial section and the magnitude of training-induced adaptation (Figure 3.2; Stray-Gundersen et al. 1986). The observation that end-diastolic volume either fails to increase during exercise in untrained subjects or attains a plateau at low workloads (Ahmad & Dubiel 1990, Crawford et al. 1985, Ehsani et al. 1991, Higginbotham et al. 1986a, Janicki et al. 1996, Younis et al. 1990), despite continuous increases in filling pressures (central venous pressure, pulmonary artery wedge pressure), also implies that an impediment to diastolic filling, rather than compromised filling time or pressure, is responsible (Warburton et al. 2002). Indeed, acute blood volume expansion increases filling pressure during exercise, but not stroke volume (Robinson et al. 1966b).

A further line of evidence for the importance of the constraining effects of the pericardium comes from studies of diastolic ventricular interaction; that is, the transient impact of acute changes in right ventricular volume on left ventricular end-diastolic volume (Wiliams & Frennaux 2006). These studies indicate that a reduction in right ventricular volume paradoxically, and transiently, increases left ventricular end-diastolic volume (Atherton et al. 1997, Guazzi et al. 1995), as a consequence of a rightward septal shift. Collectively, these studies imply that the acute reduction in right ventricular volume enhances the compliance of the left ventricle by relieving the constraining effect of the pericardium.

In summary, the possibility that endurance training stimulates pericardial remodelling, as a consequence of repetitive increases in venous return and ventricular filling pressure, seems reasonable on several grounds. First, an acute increase in filling pressures in resting subjects induces a larger stroke volume in athletes than controls (Arbab-Zadeh et al. 2004, Levine et al. 1991), indicating enhanced compliance, possibly as a result of reduced constraint. Second, pericardial plasticity is supported by studies in which ventricular filling pressures were chronically elevated, increasing pericardial size (Freeman & LeWinter 1984). Third, repetitive exercise stimulates increases in ventricular filling pressures. Pericardial adaptation, in response to increased ventricular pressure, results in both a geometric enlargement (Freeman et al. 1984) and a reduced intrinsic pericardial stiffness (Lee et al. 1985).

2.1.3.4 Endurance training and blood volume
It has long been believed that blood volume expansion partially explains enhanced cardiovascular performance following endurance training (Sawka et al. 2000; Chapter 27.3). Elevated blood volume, via increased plasma or red cell volumes, has the theoretical potential to increase preload by increasing central blood volume and filling pressure.

Endurance athletes appear to have a larger blood volume than non-athletes (Chapter 27.3), even after adjustment for body size. Some training studies occasionally report no change in blood volume, but on average, endurance training induces ~10% increase in blood volume (Sawka et al. 2000). Changes of this magnitude result from a rapid plasma volume expansion (1–2 d), with a slower (2–3 wk) increase in red cell volume, although evidence for this is limited. Interestingly, it seems that training duration has little effect on blood volume changes, with nearly all the volume expansion occurring within the first 2–3 weeks of training (Sawka et al. 2000).

The impact of these changes on cardiac preload, stroke volume and maximal aerobic power is more controversial.

Studies have reported correlation coefficients for blood volume expansion and increases in maximal oxygen uptake, between 0.52 and 0.92 (Sawka et al. 2000). Whilst these data indicate that blood volume expansion may be one of a number of mechanisms by which stroke volume is enhanced with training, such simplistic statistical associations may overplay the role of blood volume. The time-course of blood volume adaptation to training may not match that of stroke volume and may only be of importance in the initial or early adaptation (i.e. <2–3 wk). Furthermore, the assumed impact of enhanced blood volume on central venous pressure, end-diastolic volume and preload may be an oversimplification, since exercise alters cardiac output and its distribution in ways that affect central venous pressure, irrespective of blood volume changes (Rowell 1993).

2.1.3.5 Summary: endurance training and preload
The evidence presented throughout this chapter indicates an important role for increases in preload as a stimulus for endurance training-induced changes in cardiac structure and function, and, therefore, functional capacity. Preload increases during dynamic exercise, as reflected in an elevated end-diastolic volume at low to moderate exercise intensities. This increase is associated with enhanced venous return and filling pressure, in concert with increased ventricular suction.

As exercise intensity increases, end-diastolic volume exhibits a plateau in untrained subjects, which appears to be due to ventricular stiffness and pericardial constraint. Hence, volume loading of the left ventricle and pericardium at end-diastole represents a major stimulus for adaptation with endurance training, with eccentric ventricular hypertrophy occurring. This cardiac remodelling, possibly assisted by an enlarged blood volume, enables end-diastolic volume to increase to a greater degree during exercise in trained individuals. At the same time, pericardial remodelling releases the restraint on end-diastolic volume. The result is that end-diastolic volume increases more in trained than untrained individuals, such that filling time may ultimately limit continued increases in end-diastolic volume and stroke volume at higher exercise intensities.

2.1.4 Summary: endurance training effects on stroke volume
An increased stroke volume is the single largest endurance training adaptation affecting cardiac output, oxygen delivery and oxygen uptake in humans.

Whether individuals are trained or untrained, most of the stroke volume increase occurs in the transition from rest to moderate-intensity exercise. The pattern of this increase differs following training, with a plateau occurring later in the trained state. Training effects on contractility are likely to be of marginal significance given the high ejection fraction evident even before training occurs. Hence, increased contractility during exercise is not a major contributor to training-induced increases in stroke volume.

Endurance training increases vascular conductance and, at matched submaximal workloads, this is associated with decreased afterload. Structural vascular remodelling and improved vasodilator function following training are likely contributors to this decrease in afterload.

Increases in preload during exercise provide a potent physiological stimulus to cardiac and pericardial remodelling, and increased ventricular compliance. Consequently, endurance training is associated with a higher end-diastolic volume, an adaptation that largely accounts for the higher stroke volume and cardiac output following training. Ventricular and pericardial remodelling, and enhanced chamber compliance, mean that a smaller rise in filling pressure is required to increase stroke volume following training (Janicki et al. 1996, Rowell 1993).

2.2 Endurance training and heart rate

Physical conditioning is associated with increased parasympathetic drive, which is largely responsible for the bradycardia evident in the trained state. Regardless of training status, however, increases in heart rate below ~100 beats·min^{-1} are driven by withdrawal of parasympathetic inhibition (Ekblom et al. 1972, Maciel et al. 1986, Robinson et al. 1966a). By decreasing heart rate at rest and during submaximal exercise, endurance training increases the range across which heart rate increases before sympathetic recruitment occurs. Thus, although the relationship between heart rate and absolute oxygen uptake (or workload) is modified by endurance training, the relationship between heart rate and indices of sympathetic activity remains unaltered (Clausen 1977, Rowell 1974, 1986).

Training-induced rate reductions suggest increased cardiac filling time at given absolute work rates. In this way, the relative bradycardia contributes to the increase in preload which, in turn, induces adaptations in ventricular and pericardial remodelling which enhance stroke volume (section 2.1.3).

A final consideration is that increases in maximal aerobic power following endurance training cannot be attributed to increases in heart rate. Maximal heart rate is, if anything, slightly lower (~5 beats·min^{-1}) in trained athletes than matched controls (Whyte et al. 2008). Teleologically, this can be seen as advantageous, since the increase in end-diastolic volume in the trained state means that diastolic filling time becomes a more important issue in trained than untrained individuals. The mechanisms responsible for this slight decrease in maximal heart rate are unknown but structural adaptation in the conducting system accompanying ventricular remodelling seems unlikely, since both endurance and resistance athletes, in whom the stimulus and nature of ventricular remodelling differ, exhibit similar decreases in peak heart rate (Whyte et al. 2008). Residual parasympathetic drive also seems unlikely, since at such high exercise intensities sympathetic control dominates. Perhaps a decrease in sympathetic drive (Ray & Hume 1998) or β-adrenoceptor density play a role (Barbier et al. 2006).

3 CONCLUSION: CARDIOVASCULAR ADAPTATIONS

Dynamic contraction of large muscle groups is associated with rapid increases in venous return. Hence, preload and the Frank–Starling mechanism are responsible for enhanced stroke volume and cardiac output during exercise, with increased contractility perhaps playing a role as exercise becomes intense and sympathetic outflow increases. Repeated increases in venous return and increased diastolic filling time coupled with the relative bradycardia following training represent a potent preload training stimulus for ventricular and pericardial remodelling. Afterload is lower following endurance training, and there is evidence for resistance and conduit arteriogenesis, as well as increases in active vasodilator capacity and decreases in tonic vasoconstrictor outflow. At maximal exercise intensities, vascular conductance is increased to accommodate the increase in maximal cardiac output.

In keeping with the importance of exercise in an evolutionary setting, the human cardiovascular system adapts rapidly and precisely to support increased exercise loads. Repetitive acute cardiovascular responses to endurance exercise lead to chronic adaptations that improve health and promote more efficient responses to exercise. Given that diseases of cardiovascular aetiology are the predominant causes of death and disability in the developed world, and that these are exacerbated by physical inactivity (Chapters 17.1 and 28), exercise training may be the nearest approximation to a public health panacea available in the 21st century.

4 RESPIRATORY SYSTEM ADAPTATIONS TO TRAINING
Jerome Dempsey   Michael Stickland   Keisho Katayama

The heart, systemic circulation and skeletal muscle adapt structurally and functionally to chronic exercise training by increasing their capacity for oxygen delivery and utilisation, resulting in increased peak metabolic rate and work capacity. In normal, healthy untrained humans, the lungs are overbuilt, easily meeting requirements for ventilation and gas exchange during even maximal exercise (Chapter 2). However, with chronic endurance training, increased peak and sustainable metabolic rates place a greater demand on the lungs and respiratory muscles for ventilation and gas exchange, and there are instances of arterial hypoxaemia, ventilatory inadequacies and diaphragm fatigue in some highly trained subjects. This implies that the lung and chest wall do not always experience appropriate adaptations in parallel with changing metabolic requirements. We will now discuss the capabilities of the lung and the respiratory muscles to adapt to various types of chronic exercise stress.

4.1 Evidence for pulmonary system adaptability to stress

Lung structure, lung volumes and the alveolar–capillary diffusion surface area show substantial plasticity in response to specific stresses. Pneumonectomy (partial lung resection) promotes a relatively rapid and almost complete restoration to normal lung volume and diffusion capability, achieved by increasing protein synthesis, and the addition of alveolar and capillary number and volume in the remaining lung tissue. While these postpneumonectomy adaptations are almost complete in the maturing lung during a phase of somatic growth, remarkably, even the mature adult lung shows significant recovery of diffusion capacity following partial pneumonectomy (Takeda et al. 1999). Increased and decreased caloric intake also prompts adaptations in lung structure. For example, increasing caloric intake in rodents causes an increased rate of cell division, leading to increased alveolar size and number, and increased lung elastic recoil pressure; similar adaptations in the opposite direction occur with caloric restriction (Massaro et al. 2004).

Finally, adaptations to chronic hypoxia are manifested in the human natives of high altitude, and even in the sea-level natives with long-term residency at high altitudes (>3000 m) who show an extraordinarily large pulmonary diffusion capacity at rest and exercise (Dempsey et al. 1971, Wagner et al. 2002; Chapter 25). That this adaptation may be acquired upon exposure to chronic hypoxia in the sea-level native is shown in the increased lung diffusion capacity and alveolar–capillary diffusion surface in canines exposed to high altitude during maturation. Similar responses of gas exchange surfaces to chronic hypoxia are also observed in the gills of fish, the skin of frogs and the tracheal systems of tetrapods.

In humans, the high diffusion capacity is combined with enlargement of the carotid chemoreceptors and a greatly blunted ventilatory response to hypoxia at rest, and especially during exercise in the human. This combination results in a highly efficient response to exercise in hypoxia, whereby the long-term resident of high altitude achieves a level of arterial oxygenation during exercise which is comparable to that in the sea-level native sojourning at high altitude. However, because of the high diffusion capacity and narrowed alveolar to arterial oxygen partial pressure difference, the high-altitude resident does not require the extreme levels of hyperventilation (and increased work of breathing and its sequelae) experienced by the sojourner. The stimuli that induce lung structures to adapt to pneumonectomy, caloric imbalances and chronic hypoxia have not been specifically identified, although accompanying changes in oxygen uptake or mechanical manipulation of the lung are not thought to be required perturbations for such adaptive lung growth.

Inspiratory and expiratory muscles also show quite remarkable adaptation to increased loads. Recent studies employing muscle biopsies in humans showed that the chronic lung overloading, through increased airway resistance, hyperinflation and elastic loads in chronic obstructive pulmonary disease patients, resulted in a shift toward a more oxidative phenotype in the diaphragm and accessory muscles during disease development (Levine et al. 2001). These structures also show increases in the proportion of slow-twitch oxidative (type I) fibres. An even more remarkable adaptation occurs in response to the hyperinflation developed in emphysema (Farkas & Roussos 1982). As lung elastic recoil is lost, airways close on expiration, gas is trapped and volumes increase, and the diaphragm is forced to operate at shorter lengths and flatter geometric configurations. To improve force production in these circumstances, sarcomeres are progressively lost in the diaphragm's myofibrils. Thus, the remaining sarcomeres operate at near optimal length, thereby greatly improving force production. Finally, to sustain resting ventilation, we use only a small fraction of the maximum capacity of the diaphragm for force generation; nevertheless there are substantial effects of removing this phasic respiratory muscle activity. For example, inducing complete electrical silence of the diaphragm in a rodent (via mechanical ventilation) for only 3 days results in significant myofibril damage, and a 50% loss of force production (Powers et al. 2002).

4.2 Absence of positive adaptations of endurance training on the airways and gas exchange surface area

Slightly larger lung volumes, higher maximum flow–volume envelopes and lung diffusion capacities are often, but not always, present in highly trained endurance athletes, especially swimmers, when compared to their untrained contemporaries of similar stature. These superior characteristics of lung function are especially obvious in young female swimmers (Andrew et al. 1972, Mostyn et al. 1963) and in elderly (60–80 y) male long-distance runners (Johnson et al. 1991). On the other hand, it is unlikely that the training process per se caused these characteristics. This lack of a cause–effect relationship is evidenced from longitudinal studies in rodents and humans. In rats and mice, high-intensity daily training, carried out throughout maturation, had no significant effect on lung morphology (Ross & Thurlbeck 1992). Even so-called waltzing mice, who are in constant motion throughout life because of a genetic vestibular defect, showed no differences from their normally active litter mates. In humans, most longitudinal training studies are of only a few weeks to months duration, and show no effects on lung diffusion capacity at rest or exercise (Reuschlein et al. 1968).

In humans, Andrew et al. (1972) carried out repeated measures of lung function and diffusion at rest and exercise over several years in a group of prepubescent competitive swimmers. McClaran et al. (1995) conducted a similar longitudinal study over 7 years in a group of elderly, competitive long-distance runners (63–78 y), all of whom had over 20 years of habitual training, and who continued high-mileage programmes throughout the study. In both studies, lung volumes, maximal flows and diffusion capacity were consistently greater in the athletes compared to age-, height- and mass-matched sedentary counterparts. However, neither the rate of rise in diffusion and lung volumes with increasing age during maturation in the younger age groups, nor the rate of decline in diffusion capacity and maximal flow–volume envelopes throughout the 7-year period in the ageing elderly athletes, were different between the athletic and non-athletic controls.

An obvious conclusion from these studies is that superior lung function, at any age, is a selected characteristic that is brought to the athlete's endeavours, rather than being caused by the habitual training. The other broader scientific lesson to be learned from this contrast of cross-sectional and longitudinal comparisons is that the correlative data obtained in the former type of study do not confer cause–effect!

If the lung is indeed malleable to specific chronic stimuli, why does endurance training not elicit these kinds of adaptations in the lung parenchyma and airways? One explanation is that dynamic exercise is not sufficiently stressful to the lung to warrant positive adaptive morphological responses (Chapter 21). However, there is ample evidence that the limits of lung function and structure are being challenged during high-intensity endurance exercise in trained humans, as shown by the occasional development of arterial hypoxaemia, expiratory flow limitation, even stress failure of the blood–gas barrier, and significant release of inflammatory mediators in the airways and pulmonary vasculature (Chapter 2).

4.3 Negative adaptations to training

While the repeated physiological stresses associated with daily endurance training do not elicit positive structural adaptations in the lung and airways, some indirect evidence indicates that these repeated stresses might elicit negative consequences, especially when training is carried out in the presence of cold, dry air or urban pollutants, and at high, sustained intensities.

Lung biopsy studies in cross-country skiers show increased collagen deposition and remodelling in the bronchiolar airway walls (Karjalainen et al. 2000), which are likely to reflect the effects of repeated inflammatory mediator release (Figure 3.7). One wonders whether the high prevalence of asthma-like symptoms reported in many populations of endurance athletes may be attributed in part to these training-induced structural changes. Furthermore, the finding that the widened alveolar to arterial oxygen partial pressure difference and hypoxaemia in some habitually active athletes (Chapter 2) occurs not only at extremely high peak work rates, but also during moderate submaximal exercise intensity, implies an abnormal gas exchange function in these selected athletes. It has also been suggested that structural elements of the blood–gas barrier

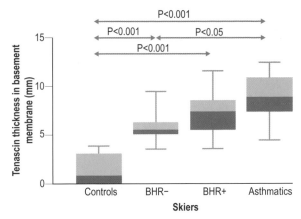

Figure 3.7 Thickness of tenascin immunoreactive band in subepithelial basement membrane zone in controls, in cross-country skiers with and without bronchial hyperresponsiveness (BHR), and in asthmatic subjects. The basement membrane thickness is increased in all skiers relative to control subjects, indicating airway remodelling from chronic exercise training. In addition, skiers with asthma-like airway hyperresponsiveness tended to have a greater degree of remodelling. Redrawn from Karjaleinen et al. (2000) with permission.

may undergo remodelling in response to the repeated stress accompanying heavy dynamic exercise. For example, patients with mitral stenosis have chronically elevated pulmonary vascular pressures and demonstrate thickening within the basement membrane of the blood–gas barrier (Kay & Edwards 1973). Is it possible, then, that elevations of pulmonary vascular pressures that occur repeatedly with heavy exercise in highly trained endurance athletes may also serve as a stimulus to thicken the basement membrane? We present these as untested possibilities. Adequate testing of these hypotheses will require detailed, invasive longitudinal studies of the lungs and airways throughout different types of training regimens.

4.4 Respiratory adaptations across species

There are additional instructive examples from comparative physiology, illustrating how organ system adaptability might differ markedly in the face of the very large alterations in maximal metabolic requirements experienced among sedentary and athletic species of similar body mass. For example, when comparing the cow with the horse, or the dog with a goat, the more athletic animal has an almost twofold higher maximal aerobic power and comparable heart and limb muscle mitochondrial volumes and capillary densities, but only a 20–30% increase exists in the athlete's alveolar–capillary diffusion surface (Weibel et al. 1992).

Thoroughbred horses have a maximal aerobic power that is four times that of sedentary humans and twice that of the fittest humans, but consistently show exercise-induced arterial hypoxaemia, carbon dioxide retention, pulmonary hypertension and haemorrhaging of the lung parenchyma during even submaximal exercise (Bayly et al. 1989). This equine product of genetic engineering is an extreme example of an underbuilt lung that has been left way behind the capacity of the cardiovascular and metabolic systems, especially with regard to the capability of the pulmonary vasculature to accept the extraordinarily high cardiac outputs achieved during exercise.

On the other hand, there are extremely fit animals, such as the pronged horned antelope, that are capable of producing five- to sixfold increases in maximal oxygen uptake above the fittest humans. These animals show an upregulation of structure in the diffusion surface of the lung which is proportional to their extraordinary maximal aerobic power.

4.5 Training–induced alterations in the ventilatory response to exercise

Endurance training generally reduces ventilation during both moderate and high-intensity exercise (Casaburi et al. 1987). Training also reduces circulating blood lactate, potassium, norepinephrine and temperature, all of which are important peripheral chemoreceptor stimuli. Accordingly, a significant relationship exists between training-induced increases in blood-borne metabolites and ventilation. Several claims have also been made that carotid chemoreceptor sensitivity may be reduced in the highly trained. However, while ventilatory chemoresponsiveness does vary widely among healthy humans, the results are conflicting concerning a consistent change in ventilatory responsiveness to chemoreceptor stimuli, as a result of physical training. In fact, recent direct recordings of carotid sinus nerve activity (healthy rabbits) showed no effect of endurance training on carotid chemoreceptor responsiveness to acute hypoxia (Zucker et al. 2004). Accordingly, it is most likely that the reduced ventilatory response following endurance training (or in highly trained athletes) is attributable to reduced chemoreceptor stimuli, which in turn are closely linked with the training effect on metabolite production in the active muscles.

4.6 Pulmonary vascular adaptations to training

Cross-sectional data indicate that pulmonary vascular resistance is not different between trained and untrained subjects at peak exercise (Stickland et al. 2006). There has been concern that, to obtain high blood flows (i.e. cardiac output) during exercise in athletes, extremely high pulmonary artery (driving) pressures are required. Chronic endurance improves diastolic function (Levy et al. 1993, Nixon et al. 1991), which is likely to explain the improved cardiac compliance both at rest (Arbab-Zadeh et al. 2004, Levine et al. 1991) and during exercise (Stickland et al. 2006). This has

the effect of reducing mean left atrial pressure at any given stroke volume. Indeed, Stickland et al. (2006) found that trained subjects actually have lower mean left atrial (pulmonary venous) pressures at peak exercise compared with untrained, and that these subjects accomplish the higher pulmonary driving pressure not through elevations in pulmonary artery pressure, but by having better cardiac compliance and therefore lower pulmonary venous pressures compared with less fit subjects. These results indicate that, while no change is observed in pulmonary vascular resistance from chronic exercise, cardiac adaptations from endurance training play an important role in limiting potentially damaging increases in pulmonary artery pressure during exercise.

Despite no apparent change in pulmonary vascular resistance, exercise training (<8 wk) has been shown to improve endothelial-dependent relaxation of the pulmonary arteries in animals, through increased nitric oxide bioavailability (Chen & Li 1993, Johnson et al. 2001). Surprisingly, however, when animals were trained for 16 weeks, no differences were observed between trained and sedentary animals (Johnson & Laughlin 2000). Interestingly, when pulmonary blood flow was chronically elevated, but without increases in pulmonary vascular pressures, no change in nitric oxide bioavailability was observed, suggesting that the combination of both elevated blood flow and pressure is required for pulmonary endothelial adaptation (Everett et al. 1998). Indeed, it has been suggested that increasing left atrial and pulmonary venous and arterial pressures accentuates radial stretch, providing a greater stimulus for endothelial adaptation (Johnson & Laughlin 2000). Endurance training improves cardiac compliance, both at rest and during exercise, and this would reduce pulmonary artery and venous pressures during exercise, as well as vessel wall stress, and the stimulus for endothelial adaptation. Therefore, it is possible that favourable adaptations in cardiac function result in reduced pulmonary blood vessel strain and a plateau, or even a reversal of training-induced pulmonary endothelial function.

4.7 Respiratory muscle adaptations to training

Respiratory muscle stimuli that accompany chronic endurance training are, unlike stimuli for the lung and airways, apparently sufficient to positively affect respiratory muscle structure and function. However, the training regimen must be substantial in both intensity and duration.

Studies in rodents show that some moderate-intensity training regimens that are capable of producing significant increases in the metabolic capacity of active muscles and maximal oxygen uptake have little or no effect on the structure or function of the diaphragm (Fregosi et al. 1987). However, with heavier intensity and longer duration training, 20–30% increases in mitochondrial enzyme activity occur in inspiratory and expiratory muscles, along with an increased antioxidant capacity that protects against fatigue development. Phenotypic adaptations also occur in fibre type in the fast myosin heavy chain isoforms in the diaphragm, and similar training-induced changes have even been reported in selective dilator muscles of the upper airway (Vincent et al. 2002). So, given the significance of these adaptive changes in structure and function, the overload stimulus of the respiratory muscles during exercise training appears to parallel that of the limb locomotor muscles. However, training-induced upregulation of oxidative capacity of the limb versus that of respiratory muscle (when comparisons are made between muscles of similar fibre type) is always substantially greater in the former.

Cross-sectional human data support data obtained in rodents, in that the respiratory muscles do adapt to chronic endurance exercise, and thereby reduce their fatigability. Babcock et al. (1996) examined the effects of high-intensity sustained exercise on diaphragm fatigue, as determined from exercise-induced changes in the force output of the diaphragm in response to supramaximal electrical stimulation of the phrenic nerves. Both highly fit and normal subjects developed similar diaphragmatic fatigue following exercise. However, the fit subjects exercised at a higher absolute workload, which required higher carbon dioxide production, greater ventilation, and thus greater diaphragm force production throughout exercise. These comparisons indicate that the respiratory muscles are adaptable to training, enabling greater ventilatory work for a given amount of fatigue. Nevertheless, even in highly trained endurance athletes, sustained high-intensity exercise causes significant fatigue in the diaphragm and expiratory muscles, and potentially elicits reflexes from these muscles with wide-ranging cardiovascular effects (Chapters 1 and 2).

4.8 Respiratory muscle training

Several studies have tested the hypothesis that specific respiratory muscle training enhances exercise performance. The rationale for this may reside in the cardiovascular consequences of respiratory muscle work during heavy exercise (Chapter 2). The logic is that respiratory muscle training would increase the endurance of inspiratory and expiratory muscles, rendering them more fatigue resistant, and perhaps even more mechanically efficient during whole-body, dynamic exercise. In turn, the more efficient, fatigue-resistant, trained respiratory muscles would not require as large a fraction of the cardiac output or accumulate metabolites as readily as in the untrained state, thereby preventing potential reflex vasoconstrictive effects within the locomotor muscles. If locomotor and respiratory muscles are more fatigue resistant, this might also mean less sensory feedback from the muscles, resulting in a reduced intensity of perception of locomotor and respiratory effort (perceived exertion) at given work rates or exercise durations.

Several studies reported little effect of respiratory muscle training on endurance performance, while others have claimed large effects. However, these studies rarely employed objective, reliable tests of exercise performance and did not include a placebo control group, the latter being an absolute necessity in studies where the endpoint involves a performance test that is determined by maximal volitional effort.

Some recent studies have used reliable and valid measures, such as simulated time-trial performances, in combination with a placebo control, and most of these observations indicate that respiratory muscle training has a very small, but possibly significant effect on endurance performance in healthy fit subjects. Furthermore, biopsy studies using patients with chronic obstructive pulmonary disease attest to the plasticity of the diaphragm in response to specific chronic overload (respiratory muscle training). These studies showed significant increases in the proportion of type I fibres and the size of type II fibres in the external intercostals (Ramirez-Sarmiento et al. 2002). Unfortunately, most studies have not focused on why respiratory muscle training might show beneficial effects on whole-body exercise performance. For example, mechanisms such as improved respiratory muscle efficiency, reduced exercise-induced respiratory or limb muscle fatigue, or altered blood flow distribution during exercise may account for these changes.

4.9 Summary

The current evidence demonstrates that the lung, airway and respiratory muscles are indeed malleable structures that show many positive adaptations to a variety of chronic stresses. This plasticity occurs during maturation and even in the mature respiratory system, and is evident in both animals and humans. Similarly, endurance training, especially that of high intensity and long duration, stimulates the further development of high oxidative, fatigue-resistant respiratory muscles. However, the structures of the developing, mature or even ageing lung and airways appear resistant to the training stimulus. Limited data even indicate that the delicate airway epithelium, capillary endothelium and alveolar–capillary interface may be negatively impacted by the repeated shear stresses and inflammatory mediatory release accompanying high-intensity exercise. Despite the presence (or absence) of respiratory system adaptations to chronic endurance training, we need to recall that the lung and respiratory muscles in the untrained have substantial structural reserves, and that even in the highly trained, exercise-induced mechanical constraints to ventilation and arterial hypoxaemia occur rarely, and respiratory muscle fatigue with its attendant cardiovascular consequences occurs only when exercise is of very high intensity, and sustained to or near exhaustion.

References

Abergel E, Chatellier G, Hagege AA, Oblak A, Linhart A, Ducardonnet AJM 2004 Serial left ventricular adaptations in world-class professional cyclists. Implications for disease screening and follow-up. Journal of the American College of Cardiology 44:144–149

Adams V, Hambrecht R, Erbs S 2002 Impact of physical exercise training on the expression of NAD(P)H-oxidase and angiotensin-II receptors in the left mammary artery of patients with coronary artery disease. Circulation 106:II–354

Ahmad M, Dubiel JP 1990 Left ventricular response to exercise in regular runners and controls. Clinical Nuclear Medicine 15:630–635

Andrew GM, Becklake MR, Guleria JS, Bates DV 1972 Heart and lung functions in swimmers and nonathletes during growth. Journal of Applied Physiology 32:245–251

Arbab-Zadeh A, Dijk E, Prasad A, Fu Q, Torres P, Zhang R, Thomas JD, Palmer D, Levine BD 2004 Effect of aging and physical activity on left ventricular compliance. Circulation 110:1799–1805

Atherton JJ, Moore TD, Lele SS, Thomson HL, Galbraith AJ, Belenkie I, Tyberg JV, Frenneaux MP 1997 Diastolic ventricular interaction in chronic heart failure. Lancet 349:1720–1724

Babcock MA, Pegelow DF, Johnson BD, Dempsey JA 1996 Aerobic fitness effects on exercise-induced low-frequency diaphragm fatigue. Journal of Applied Physiology 81:2156–2164

Barbier J, Reland S, Ville N, Rannou-Bekono F, Wong S, Carré F 2006 The effects of exercise training on myocardial adrenergic and muscarinic receptors. Clinical Autonomic Research 16:61–65

Barnard H 1898 The functions of the pericardium. Journal of Physiology (London) 22:43–48

Bayly WM, Hodgson DR, Schulz DA, Dempsey JA, Gollnick PD 1989 Exercise-induced hypercapnia in the horse. Journal of Applied Physiology 67:1958–1966

Bella JN, Palmieri V, Roman MJ, Liu JE, Welty TK, Lee ET, Fabsitz RR, Howard BV, Devereux RB 2002 Mitral ratio of peak early to late diastolic filling velocity as a predictor of mortality in middle-aged and elderly adults. The Strong Heart Study. Circulation 105:1928–1933

Bevegard S, Jonsson B, Karlof I, Lagergren H, Sowton E 1967 Effect of changes in ventricular rate on cardiac output and central venous pressures at rest and during exercise in patients with artificial pacemakers. Cardiovascular Research 1:21–33

Booth FW, Chakravarthy MV, Spangenburg EE 2002 Exercise and gene expression: physiological regulation of the human genome through physical activity. Journal of Physiology (London) 543:399–411

Boushel R, Kjaer M 2004 Redundancy reflects versatility of blood flow regulation mechanisms. Journal of Physiology (London) 557:346

Brandou MUP, Wagngarten M, Rondon E, Giorgi MCP, Hironaka F, Negrao CE 1993 Left ventricular function during dynamic exercise in untrained and moderately trained subjects. Journal of Applied Physiology 75:1989–1995

Brown MD 2003 Exercise and coronary vascular remodelling in the healthy heart. Experimental Biology and Medicine 88:645–658

Calbet JA, Jensen-Urstad M, Van Hall G, Holmberg HC, Rosdahl H, Saltin B 2004 Maximal muscular vascular conductances during whole body upright exercise in humans. Journal of Physiology (London) 558:319–331

Casaburi R, Storer TW, Wasserman K 1987 Mediation of reduced ventilatory response to exercise after endurance training. Journal of Applied Physiology 63:1533–1538

Caso P, D'Andrea A, Galderisi M, Liccardo B, Severino S, De Simone L, Izzo A, D'Andrea L, Mininni N 2000 Pulsed Doppler tissue imaging in endurance athletes: relation between left ventricular preload and myocardial regional diastolic function. American Journal of Cardiology 85:1131–1136

Chen H, Li H-T 1993 Physical conditioning can modulate endothelium-dependent vasorelaxation in rabbits. Arteriosclerosis and Thrombosis 13:852–856

Clarkson P, Montgomery HE, Mullen MJ, Donald AE, Powe AJ, Bull T, Jubb M, World M, Deanfield JE 1999 Exercise training enhances endothelial function in young men. Journal of the American College of Cardiology 33:1379–1385

Clausen J-P 1977 Effect of physical training on cardiovascular adjustments to exercise in man. Physiological Reviews 57:779–815

Colan SD, Sanders SP, MacPheraon D, Borow KM 1985 Left ventricular diastolic function in elite athletes with physiologic cardiac hypertrophy. Journal of the American College of Cardiology 6:545–549

Crawford MH, Petru MA, Rabinowitz C 1985 Effect of isotonic exercise training on left ventricular volume during upright exercise. Circulation 72:1237–1243

Crouse SF, Rohack JJ, Jacobsen DJ 1992 Cardiac structure and function in women basketball athletes: seasonal variation and comparisons with nonathletic controls. Research Quarterly in Exercise and Sport 63:393–401

Currens JH, White PD 1961 Half century of running: clinical, physiological and autopsy findings in the case of Clarence De Mar, 'Mr. Marathoner.' New England Journal of Medicine 265:988–993

Davies CTM, Sargeant AJ 1975 Effects of training on the physiological responses to one- and two-leg work. Journal of Applied Physiology 38:377–381

DeMaria A, Neumann A, Lee G, Fowler W, Mason DT 1978 Alterations in ventricular mass and performance induced by exercise training in man evaluated by echocardiography. Circulation 57:237–244

Dempsey JA, Reddan WG, Birnbaum ML, Forster HV, Thoden JS, Grover RF, Rankin J 1971 Effects of acute through life-long hypoxic exposure on exercise pulmonary gas exchange. Respiratory Physiology 13:62–89

Di Bello V, Santoro G, Talarico L, Di Muro C, Caputo MT, Giorgi D, Bertini A, Bianchi M, Giusti C 1996 Left ventricular function during exercise in athletes and sedentary men. Medicine and Science in Sports Exercise 28:190–196

Dimmeler S, Zeiher AM 2003 Exercise and cardiovascular health. Get active to AKTivate your endothelial nitric oxide synthase. Circulation (Editorial) 107:3118–3120

Dinenno FA, Tanaka H, Monahan KD, Clevenger CM, Eskurza I, DeSouza CA, Seals DR 2001 Regular endurance exercise induces expansive arterial remodelling in the trained limbs of healthy men. Journal of Physiology (London) 534:287–295

Duffy SJ, Castle SF, Harper RW, Meredith IT 1999a Contribution of vasodilator prostanoids and nitric oxide to resting flow, metabolic vasodilation and flow-mediated dilation in human coronary circulation. Circulation 100:1951–1957

Duffy SJ, New G, Tran BT, Harper RW, Meredith IT 1999b Relative contribution of vasodilator prostanoids and NO to metabolic vasodilation in the human forearm. American Journal of Physiology 276:H663–H670

Dyke CK, Proctor DN, Deitz NM, Joyner MJ 1995 Role of nitric oxide during prolonged rhythmic handgripping in humans. Journal of Physiology (London) 448:259–265

Ehsani A, Hagberg J, Hickson R 1978 Rapid changes in left ventricular dimensions and mass in response to physical conditioning and deconditioning. American Journal of Cardiology 42:52–56

Ehsani AA, Ogawa T, Miller TR, Spina RJ, Jilka SM 1991 Exercise training improves left ventricular systolic function in older men. Circulation 83:96–103

Ekblom B 1969 Effect of physical training on oxygen transport system in man. Acta Physiologica Scandinavica 328(Suppl):1045

Ekblom B, Hermansen L 1968 Cardiac output in athletes. Journal of Applied Physiology 25:619–625

Ekblom B, Goldbarg AN, Kilblom ASA, Astrand P-O 1972 Effects of atropine and propranolol on the oxygen transport system during exercise in man. Scandinavian Journal of Clinical Laboratory Investigation 30:35–42

Ennezat PV, Malendowicz SL, Testa M, Colombo PC, Cohen-Solal A, Evans T, LeJemtel TH 2001 Physical training in patients with chronic heart failure enhances the expression of genes encoding antioxidative enzymes. Journal of the American College of Cardiology 38:194–198

Everett AD, Le Cras TD, Xue C, Johns RA 1998 eNOS expression is not altered in pulmonary vascular remodeling due to increased pulmonary blood flow. American Journal of Physiology 274: L1058–L1065

Fagard R 2003 Athlete's heart. Heart 89:1445–1461

Farkas GA, Roussos C 1982 Adaptability of the hamster diaphragm to exercise and/or emphysema. Journal of Applied Physiology 53:1263–1272

Fischer M, Baessler A, Hense HW, Hengstenberg C, Muscholl M, Holmer S, Döring A, Broeckel U, Riegger G, Schunkert H 2003 Prevalence of left ventricular diastolic dysfunction in the community. Results from a Doppler echocardiographic-based survey of a population sample. European Heart Journal 24:320–328

Fisman EZ, Frank AG, Ben-Ari E, Kessler G, Pines A, Drory Y, Kellermann JJ 1990 Altered left ventricular volume and ejection fraction responses to supine dynamic exercise in athletes. Journal of the American College of Cardiology 15:582–588

Fleg JL, Schulman SP, O'Connor FC, Gerstenblith G, Becker LC, Fortney S, Goldberg AP, Lakatta EG 1994 Cardiovascular responses to exhaustive upright cycle exercise in highly trained older men. Journal of Applied Physiology 77:1500–1506

Freeman GL, LeWinter MM 1984 Pericardial adaptations during chronic dilation in dogs. Circulation Research 54:294–300

Fregosi RF, Sanjak M, Paulson DJ 1987 Endurance training does not affect diaphragm mitochondrial respiration. Respiratory Physiology 67:225–237

Fukai T, Siegfried MR, Ushio-Fukai M, Cheng Y, Kojda G, Harrison DG 2000 Regulation of the vascular extracellular superoxide dismutase by nitric oxide and exercise training. Journal of Clinical Investigation 105:1631–1639

Furchgott RF, Zawadzki JV 1980 The obligatory role of endothelial cells in the relaxation of arterial smooth muscle by acetylcholine. Nature (London) 288:373–376

Galbo H 1983 Hormonal and metabolic adaptation to exercise. Thieme-Stratton, New York

Gilligan DM, Panza JA, Kilcoyne CM, Waclawiw MA, Casino PR, Quyyumi AA 1994 Contribution of endothelium-derived nitric oxide to exercise-induced vasodilation. Circulation 90:2853–2858

Gledhill N, Cox D, Jamnik R 1994 Endurance athletes' stroke volume does not plateau: major advantage is diastolic function. Medicine and Science in Sports and Exercise 26:1116–1121

Gleser MA 1973 Effects of hypoxia and physical training on hemodynamic adjustments to one-legged exercise. Journal of Applied Physiology 34:655–659

González-Alonso J, Olsen B, Saltin B 2002 Erythrocytes and the regulation of human skeletal muscle at onset of intense dynamic exercise. Circulation Research 91:1046–1055

González-Alonso J, Mortensen SP, Dawson EA, Secher NH, Damsgaard R 2006 Erythrocytes and the regulation of human skeletal muscle blood flow and oxygen delivery: role of erythrocyte count and oxygenation state of haemoglobin. Journal of Physiology (London) 572:295–305

Gow A, Stamler J 1998 Reactions between nitric oxide and haemoglobin under physiological conditions. Nature 391:169–173

Green DJ, Cable NT, Fox C, Rankin JM, Taylor RR 1994 Modification of forearm resistance vessels by exercise training in young men. Journal of Applied Physiology 77:1829–1833

Green DJ, Fowler DT, O'Driscoll JG, Blanksby BA, Taylor RR 1996a Endothelium-derived nitric oxide activity in forearm vessels of tennis players. Journal of Applied Physiology 81:943–948

Green DJ, O'Driscoll JG, Blanksby BA, Taylor RR 1996b Control of skeletal muscle blood flow during dynamic exercise. Sports Medicine 21:119–146

Green DJ, Maiorana AJ, O'Driscoll G, Taylor R 2004 Topical review: effects of exercise training on vascular endothelial nitric oxide function in humans. Journal of Physiology (London) 561:1–25

Green DJ, Bilsborough W, Naylor LH, Reed C, Wright J, O'Driscoll G, Walsh JH 2005 Comparison of forearm blood flow responses to incremental handgrip and cycle ergometer exercise: relative contribution of nitric oxide. Journal of Physiology (London) 562:617–628

Green DJ, Naylor LH, George K 2006 Cardiac and vascular adaptations to exercise. Current Opinion in Clinical Nutrition and Metabolic Care 9(6):677–684

Guazzi M, Pepi M, Maltagliati A, Celeste F, Muratori M, Tamborini G 1995 How the two sides of the heart adapt to graded impedance to venous return with head-up tilting. Journal of the American College of Cardiology 26:1732–1740

Hambrecht R, Adams V, Erbs S, Linke A, Kränkel N, Shu Y, Baither Y, Gielen S, Thiele H, Gummert JF, Mohr FW, Schuler G 2003 Regular physical activity improves endothelial function in patients with coronary artery disease by increasing phosphorylation of endothelial nitric oxide synthase. Circulation 107:3152–3158

Hambrecht R, Walther C, Möbius-Winkler S, Gielen S, Linke A, Conradi K, Erbs S, Kluge R, Kendziorra K, Sabri O, Sick P, Schuler G 2004 Percutaneous coronary angioplasty compared with exercise training in patients with stable coronary artery disease: a randomized trial. Circulation 109:1371–1378

Hammond HK, White FC, Bhargava V, Shabetai R 1992 Heart size and maximal cardiac output are limited by the pericardium. American Journal of Physiology 263:1675–1681

Hickner RC, Fisher JS, Ehsani AA, Kohrt WM 1997 Role of nitric oxide in skeletal muscle blood flow at rest and during dynamic exercise. American Journal of Physiology 273:H405–H410

Higginbotham MB, Morris KG, Williams RS, Coleman RE, Cobb FR 1986a Physiological basis for the age-related decline in aerobic work capacity. American Journal of Cardiology 57:1374–1379

Higginbotham MB, Morris KG, Williams RS, McHale PA, Coleman RE, Cobb FR 1986b Regulation of stroke volume during submaximal and maximal upright exercise in normal man. Circulation Research 58:281–291

Hildick-Smith DJ, Johnson PJ, Wisbey CR, Winter EM, Shapiro LM 2000 Coronary flow reserve is supranormal in endurance athletes: an adenosine transthoracic echocardiographic study. Heart 84:383–390

Hutcheson IR, Griffith TM 1991 Release of endothelium-derived relaxing factor is modulated both by frequency and amplitude of pulsatile flow. American Journal of Physiology 261: H257–H262

Janicki JS 1990 Influence of the pericardium and ventricular interdependence on left ventricular diastolic and systolic function in patients with heart failure. Circulation 81:15–20

Janicki JS, Sheriff DD, Robotham JL, Wise RA 1996 Cardiac output during exercise: contributions of the cardiac, circulatory and respiratory systems. In: Rowell LB, Shepherd JT (eds) Handbook of physiology. Section 12: exercise: regulation and integration of multiple systems. Oxford University Press, Oxford

Jasperse JL, Laughlin MH 2006 Endothelial function and exercise training: evidence from studies using animal models. Medicine and Science in Sports and Exercise 38:445–454

Johnson BD, Reddan WG, Seow KC, Dempsey JA 1991 Mechanical constraints on exercise hyperpnea in a fit aging population. American Review of Respiratory Disease 143:968–977

Johnson LR, Laughlin MH 2000 Chronic exercise training does not alter pulmonary vasorelaxation in normal pigs. Journal of Applied Physiology 88:2008–2014

Johnson LR, Rush JW, Turk JR, Price EM, Laughlin MH 2001 Short-term exercise training increases ACh-induced relaxation and eNOS protein in porcine pulmonary arteries. Journal of Applied Physiology 90:1102–1110

Kamiya A, Togawa T 1980 Adaptive regulation of wall shear stress to flow change in the canine carotid artery. American Journal of Physiology 239:H14–H21

Karjalainen EM, Laitinen A, Sue-Chu M, Altraja A, Bjermer L, Laitinen LA 2000 Evidence of airway inflammation and remodeling in ski athletes with and without bronchial hyperresponsiveness to methacholine. American Journal of Respiratory and Critical Care Medicine 161:2086–2091

Kay JM, Edwards FR 1973 Ultrastructure of the alveolar-capillary wall in mitral stenosis. Journal of Pathology 111:239–245

Kingwell BA, Sherrard B, Jennings GL, Dart AM 1997 Four weeks of cycle training increases basal production of nitric oxide from the forearm. American Journal of Physiology 272:H1070–H1077

Klausen K, Secher NH, Clausen JP, Hartling O, Trap-Jensen J 1982 Central and regional circulatory adaptations to one-legged training. Journal of Applied Physiology 52:976–983

Koller A, Kaley G 1991 Endothelial regulation of wall shear stress and blood flow in skeletal muscle microcirculation. American Journal of Physiology 260:H862–H868

Krogh A 1912 Regulation of the supply of blood to the right heart (with a description of a new criculation model). Scandinavian Archives of Physiology 27:227–248

Langille BL, O'Donnell F 1986 Reductions in arterial diameter produced by chronic decreases in blood flow are endothelium-dependent. Nature 231:405–407

Laughlin MH 1987 Skeletal muscle blood flow capacity: role of muscle pump in exercise hyperemia. American Journal of Physiology 253:H993–H1004

Laughlin MH, Korthuis RJ, Duncker DJ, Bache RJ 1996 Control of blood flow to cardiac and skeletal muscle during exercise In: Rowell LB, Shepherd JT (eds) Handbook of physiology. Section 12: exercise: regulation and integration of multiple systems. Oxford University Press, Oxford

Laughlin MH, Rubin LJ, Rush JW, Price EM, Schrage WG, Woodman CR 2003a Short-term training enhances endothelium-dependent dilation of coronary arteries, not arterioles. Journal of Applied Physiology 94:234–244

Laughlin MH, Turk JR, Schrage WG, Woodman CR, Price EM 2003b Influence of coronary artery diameter on eNOS protein content. American Journal of Physiology 284:H1307–1312

Lee M-C, LeWinter MM, Freeman G, Shabetai R, Fung YC 1985 Biaxial mechanical properties of the pericardium in normal and volume overloaded dogs. American Journal of Physiology 249:222–230

Lee CD, Blair SN, Jackson AS 1999 Cardiorespiratory fitness, body composition and all-cause and cardiovascular disease mortality in men. American Journal of Clinical Nutrition 69:373–380

Levine B, Lane L, Buckey J, Friedman D, Blomqvist C 1991 Left ventricular pressure-volume and Frank–Starling relations in endurance athletes. Implications for orthostatic tolerance and exercise performance. Circulation 84:1016–1023

Levine S, Nguyen T, Shrager J, Kaiser L, Camasamudram V, Rubinstein N 2001 Diaphragm adaptations elicited by severe chronic obstructive pulmonary disease: lessons for sports science. Exercise and Sports Science Reviews 29:71–75

Levy WC, Cerqueira MD, Abrass IB, Schwartz RS, Stratton JR 1993 Endurance exercise training augments diastolic filling at rest and during exercise in healthy young and older men. Circulation 88:116–126

Libonati JR 1999 Myocardial diastolic function and exercise. Medicine and Science in Sports and Exercise 31:1741–1747

Linke A, Schoene N, Gielen S, Hofer J, Erbs S, Schuler G, Hambrecht R 2001 Endothelial dysfunction in patients with chronic heart failure:

systemic effects of lower-limb exercise training. Journal of the American College of Cardiology 37:392–397

McClaran SR, Babcock MA, Pegelow DF, Reddan WG, Dempsey JA 1995 Longitudinal effects of aging on lung function at rest and exercise in healthy active fit elderly adults. Journal of Applied Physiology 78:1957–1968

MacFarlane N, Northbridge DB, Wright AR, Grant S, Dargie HJ 1991 A comparative study of left ventricular structure and function in elite athletes. British Journal of Sports Medicine 25:45–48

Maciel BC, Gallo L, Marin Neto JA, Lima Filho EC, Martins LEB 1986 Autonomic nervous control of the heart rate during dynamic exercise in normal man. Clinical Science (London) 71:457–467

Maiorana A, O'Driscoll G, Dembo L, Cheetham C, Goodman C, Taylor R, Green D 2000 Effect of aerobic and resistance exercise training on vascular function in heart failure. American Journal of Physiology 279:H1999–H2005

Maiorana A, O'Driscoll G, Cheetham C, Dembo L, Stanton K, Goodman C, Taylor R, Green D 2001 The effect of combined aerobic and resistance exercise training on vascular function in type 2 diabetes. Journal of the American College of Cardiology 38:860–866

Maiorana A, O'Driscoll GJ, Taylor RR, Green DJ 2003 Exercise and the nitric oxide vasodilator system. Sports Medicine 33:1013–1035

Mann GV, Spoerry A, Gray M, Jarashow D 1972 Atherosclerosis in the Masai. American Journal of Epidemiology 95:26–37

Massaro D, Massaro GD, Baras A, Hoffman EP, Clerch LB 2004 Calorie-related rapid onset of alveolar loss, regeneration and changes in mouse lung gene expression. American Journal of Physiology. Lung Cellular and Molecular Physiology 286:L896–906

Miyachi M, Iemitsu M, Okutsu M, Onodera S 1998 Effects of endurance training on the size and blood flow of the arterial conductance vessels in humans. Acta Physiologica Scandinavica 163:13–16

Moore RL, Korzick DH 1995 Cellular adaptations of the myocardium to chronic exercise. Progress in Cardiovascular Diseases 37:371–396

Morganroth J, Maron B, Henry W, Epstein S 1975 Comparative left ventricular dimensions in trained athletes. Annals of Internal Medicine 82:521–524

Mortensen SP, Dawson EA, Yoshiga CC, Dalsgaard MK, Damsgaard R, Secher NH, González-Alonso J 2005 Limitations to systemic and locomotor limb muscle oxygen delivery and uptake during maximal exercise in humans. Journal of Physiology (London) 566:273–285

Mostyn EM, Helle S, Gee JB, Bentivoglio LG, Bates DV 1963 Pulmonary diffusing capacity of athletes. Journal of Applied Physiology 18:687–695

Muntz K, Gonyea W, Mitchell J 1981 Cardiac hypertrophy in response to an isometric training program in the cat. Circulation Research 49:1092–1101

Myers J, Prakash M, Froelicher V, Partington S, Atwood JE 2002 Exercise capacity and mortality among men referred for exercise testing. New England Journal of Medicine 346:793–801

Naylor L, Arnolda L, Deague J, Playford D, O'Driscoll G, Green DJ 2005 Reduced diastolic function in elite athletes is augmented with the resumption of exercise training. Journal of Physiology (London) 563:957–963

Naylor L, O'Driscoll G, Fitzsimons M, Arnolda L, Green DJ 2006 Effects of training resumption on conduit arterial diameter in elite rowers. Medicine and Science in Sports and Exercise 38:86–92

Naylor LH, George K, O'Driscoll G, Green DJ 2008 The athlete's heart: A contemporary appraisal of the "Morganroth hypothesis." Sports Medicine 38:69–90

Neibauer J, Cooke JP 1996 Cardiovascular effects of exercise: role of endothelial shear stress. Journal of the American College of Cardiology 28:1652–1660

Nixon JV, Wright AR, Porter TR, Roy V, Arrowood JA 1991 Effects of exercise on left ventricular diastolic performance in trained athletes. American Journal of Cardiology 68:945–949

Pela G, Bruschi G, Montagna L, Manara M, Manca C 2004 Left and right ventricular adaptation assessed by Doppler tissue echocardiography in athletes. Journal of the American Society of Echocardiography 17:205–211

Pelliccia A, Spataro A, Granata J, Biffi A, Caselli G, Alabiso A 1990 Coronary arteries in physiological hypertrophy: echocardiographic evidence of increased proximal size in elite athletes. International Journal of Sports Medicine 11:120–126

Pelliccia A, Culasso F, Di Paolo F, Maron B 1999 Physiologic left ventricular cavity dilatation in elite athletes. Annals of Internal Medicine 130:23–31

Pluim BM, Lamb HJ, Kayser HW, Leujes F, Beyerbacht HP, Zwinderman AH, van der Laarse A, Vliegen HW, de Roos A, van der Wall EE 1998 Functional and metabolic evaluation of the athlete's heart by magnetic resonance imaging and dobutamine stress magnetic resonance spectroscopy. Circulation 97:666–672

Pluim BM, Zwinderman AH, van der Laarse A, van der Wall EE 1999 The athlete's heart. A meta-analysis of cardiac structure and function. Circulation 100:336–344

Powers SK, Shanely RA, Coombes JS, Koesterer TJ, McKenzie M, Van Gammeren D, Cicale M, Dodd SL 2002 Mechanical ventilation results in progressive contractile dysfunction in the diaphragm. Journal of Applied Physiology 92:1851–1858

Prior BM, Yang HT, Terjung RL 2004 What makes vessels grow with exercise training? Journal of Applied Physiology 97:1119–1128

Quintana M, Saha SK, Rohani M, Del Furia F, Bjernby J, Lind B, Brodin LA 2004 Assessment of the longitudinal and circumferential left ventricular function at rest and during exercise in health elderly individuals by tissue-Doppler echocardiography: relationship with heart rate. Clinical Science 106:451–457

Ramirez-Sarmiento A, Orozco-Levi M, Guell R, Barreiro E, Hernandez N, Mota S, Sangenis M, Broquetas JM, Casan P, Gea J 2002 Inspiratory muscle training in patients with chronic obstructive pulmonary disease: structural adaptation and physiologic outcomes. American Journal of Respiratory and Critical Care Medicine 166:1491–1497

Ray CA, Hume KM 1998 Sympathetic neural adaptations to exercise training in humans: insights from microneurography. Medicine and Science in Sports and Exercise 30:387–391

Reeves JT, Groves BM, Cymerman A, Sutton JR, Wagner PD, Turkevich D, Houston CS 1990 Operation Everest II: cardiac filling pressures during cycle exercise at sea level. Respiration Physiology 80:147–154

Rerych SK, Scholz PM, Sabiston DC, Jones RH 1980 Effects of exercise training on left ventricular function in normal subjects: a longitudinal study by radionuclide angiography. American Journal of Cardiology 45:244–252

Reuschlein PS, Reddan WG, Burpee J, Gee JB, Rankin J 1968 Effect of physical training on the pulmonary diffusing capacity during submaximal work. Journal of Applied Physiology 24:152–158

Robinson BR, Epstein SE, Beiser GD, Braunwald E 1966a Control of heart rate by the autonomic nervous system: studies in man on the interrelation between baroreceptor mechanisms and exercise. Circulation Research 19:400–411

Robinson BR, Epstein SE, Kahler RL, Braunwald E 1966b Circulatory effects of acute expansion of blood volume: studies during maximal exercise and at rest. Circulation Research 19:26–32

Rose G, Prineas RJ, Mitchell JRA 1967 Myocardial infarction and the intrinsic calibre of coronary arteries. British Heart Journal 29:548–552

Ross KA, Thurlbeck WM 1992 Lung growth in newborn guinea pigs: effects of endurance exercise. Respiratory Physiology 89:353–364

Rowell LB 1974 Human cardiovascular adjustments to exercise and thermal stress. Physiological Reviews 54:75–159

Rowell LB 1986 Human circulation: regulation during physical stress. Oxford University Press, New York

Rowell LB 1993 Human cardiovascular control. Oxford University Press, New York

Rowell LB, O'Leary DS 1990 Reflex control of the circulation during exercise: chemoreflexes and mechanoreflexes. Journal of Applied Physiology 69:407–418

Rowell LB, Brengelmann GL, Blackmon JR, Bruce RA, Murray JA 1968 Disparities between aortic and peripheral pulse pressures induced by upright exercise and vasomotor changes in man. Circulation 37:954–964

Rowell LB, O'Leary DS, Kellogg DL 1996 Integration of cardiovascular control systems in dynamic exercise. In: Rowell LB, Shepherd JT (eds) Handbook of physiology. Section 12: exercise: regulation and integration of multiple systems. Oxford University Press, Oxford

Rubal BJ, Moody JM, Damore S, Bunker SR, Diaz NM 1986 Left ventricular performance of the athletic heart during upright exercise: a heart rate controlled study. American Journal of Physiology 262:1361–1364

Saltin B 1969 Physiological effects of physical conditioning. Medicine and Science in Sport 1:50–56

Saltin B, Blomqvist G, Mitchell JH, Johnson RLJ, Wildenthal K, Chapman CB 1968 Response to exercise after bed rest and after training. Circulation 38(Suppl 7):1–78

Saltin B, Nazar K, Costill DL, Stein E, Jansson E, Essen B, Gollnick PD 1976 The nature of the training response: peripheral and central adaptations to one-legged exercise. Acta Physiologica Scandinavica 96:289–305

Sawka MN, Convertino VA, Eichner ER, Schneider SM, Young AJ 2000 Blood volume: importance and adaptations to exercise training, environmental stresses and trauma/sickness. Medicine and Science in Sports and Exercise 32:332–348

Schairer JR, Stein PD, Keteyian S, Fedel F, Ehrman J, Alam M, Henry JW, Shaw T 1992 Left ventricular response to submaximal exercise in endurance-trained athletes and sedentary adults. American Journal of Cardiology 70:930–933

Scharhag J, Schneider G, Urhausen A, Rochette V, Kramann B, Kindermann W 2002 Athlete's heart. Right and left ventricular mass and function in male endurance athletes and untrained individuals determined by magnetic resonance imaging. Journal of the American College of Cardiology 40:1856–1863

Schillaci G, Pasqualini L, Verdecchia P, Vaudo G, Marchesi S, Porcellati C, de Simone G, Mannarino E 2002 Prognostic significance of left ventricular diastolic dysfunction in essential hypertension. Journal of the American College of Cardiology 39:2005–2011

Schmidt-Trucksäss A, Schmid A, Brunner C, Scherer N, Zäch G, Keul J, Huonker M 2000 Arterial properties of the carotid and femoral artery in endurance-trained and paraplegic subjects. Journal of Applied Physiology 89:1956–1963

Schrage WG, Joyner MJ, Dinenno FA 2004 Local inhibition of nitric oxide and prostaglandins independently reduces forearm exercise hyperaemia in humans. Journal of Physiology (London) 557:599–611

Seals DR, Hagberg JM, Spina RJ, Rogers MA, Schechtman KB, Ehsani AA 1994 Enhanced left ventricular performance in endurance trained older men. Circulation 89:198–205

Segal SS 1992 Communication among endothelial and smooth muscle cells coordinates blood flow control during exercise. News in the Physiological Sciences 7:152–156

Shapiro L, Smith R 1983 Effect of training on left ventricular structure and function. An echocardiographic study. British Heart Journal 50:534–539

Shepherd JT 1983 Circulation to skeletal muscle In: Shepherd JT, Abboud FM, Geiger SR (eds) Handbook of physiology. The cardiovascular system: peripheral circulation and organ blood flow. American Physiological Society, Bethesda, MD, 319–370

Sheriff D 2005 The muscle pump raises muscle blood flow during locomotion. Journal of Applied Physiology 99:371–375

Sheriff DD, Zhou XP, Scher AM, Rowell LB 1993 Dependence of cardiac filling pressure on cardiac output during rest and dynamic exercise in dogs. American Journal of Physiology 265:316–322

Sinoway LI, Musch TI, Minotti JR, Zelis R 1986 Enhanced maximal metabolic vasodilation in the dominant forearms of tennis players. Journal of Applied Physiology 61:673–678

Sinoway LI, Shenberger J, Wilson J, McLaughlin D, Musch TI, Zelis R 1987 A 30-day forearm work protocol increases maximal forearm blood flow. Journal of Applied Physiology 62:1063–1067

Spina RJ, Ogawa T, Martin WH, Coggan AR, Holloszy JO, Ehsani AA 1992 Exercise training prevents decline in stroke volume during exercise in young healthy subjects. Journal of Applied Physiology 72:2458–2462

Spirito P, Pelliccia A, Proschan MA, Granata M, Spataro A, Bellone P, Caselli G, Biffi A, Vecchio C, Maron BJ 1994 Morphology of the 'athlete's heart' assessed by echocardiography in 947 elite athletes representing 27 sports. American Journal of Cardiology 74:802–806

Stamler JS, Jia L, Eu JP, McMahon TJ, Demchenko IT, Bonaventura J, Gernert K, Piantadosi CA 1997 Blood flow regulation by S-nitrosohemoglobin in the physiological oxygen gradient. Science 276:2034–2037

Stein R, Michiellie D, Diamond J, Horwitz B, Kransnow N 1980 The cardiac response to exercise training: echocardiographic analysis at rest and during exercise. American Journal of Cardiology 46:219–225

Stickland MK, Welsh RC, Petersen SR, Tyberg JV, Anderson WD, Jones RL, Taylor DA, Bouffard M, Haykowsky MJ 2006 Does fitness level modulate the cardiovascular hemodynamic response to exercise? Journal of Applied Physiology 100:1910–1917

Stray-Gundersen J, Musch TI, Haidet GC, Swain DP, Ordway GA, Mitchell JH 1986 The effect of pericardectomy on maximal oxygen consumption and maximal cardiac output in untrained dogs. Circulation Research 58:523–530

Takeda S, Hsia CC, Wagner E, Ramanathan M, Estrera AS, Weibel ER 1999 Compensatory alveolar growth normalizes gas-exchange function in immature dogs after pneumonectomy. Journal of Applied Physiology 86:1301–1310

Tanasescu M, Leitzmann MF, Rimm EB, Willett WC, Stampfer MJ, Hu FB 2002 Exercise type and intensity in relation to coronary heart disease in men. Journal of the American Medical Association 288:1994–2000

Tate CA, Taffet GE, Hudson SL, Blaylock RP, McBride RP, Micheal LH 1990 Enhanced calcium uptake of cardiac sarcoplasmic reticulum in exercise-trained rats. American Journal of Physiology 258:H431–H435

Thadani U, Parker JO 1978 Hemodynamics at rest and during supine and sitting bicycle exercise in normal subjects. American Journal of Cardiology 41:52–59

Tronc F, Wassef M, Esposito B, Henrion D, Glagov S, Tedgui A 1996 Role of NO in flow-induced remodeling of rabbit common carotid artery. Arteriosclerosis Thrombosis and Vascular Biology 16:1256–1262

Tuttle JL, Nachreiner RD, Bhuller AS, Condict KW, Connors BA, Herring BP, Dalsing MC, Unthank JL 2001 Shear level influences artery remodelling, wall dimension, cell density and eNOS expression. American Journal of Physiology 281:H1380–H1389

Urhausen A, Kindermann W 1989 One- and two-dimensional echocardiography in body builders and endurance-trained subjects. International Journal of Sports Medicine 10:139–144

Vincent HK, Shanely RA, Stewart DJ, Demirel HA, Hamilton KL, Ray AD, Michlin C, Farkas GA, Powers SK 2002 Adaptation of upper airway muscles to chronic endurance exercise. American Journal of Respiratory and Critical Care Medicine 166:287–293

Wagner PD, Araoz M, Boushel R, Calbet JA, Jessen B, Rådegran G, Spielvogel H, Søndegaard H, Wagner H, Saltin B 2002 Pulmonary gas exchange and acid-base state at 5,260 m in high-altitude Bolivians and acclimatized lowlanders. Journal of Applied Physiology 92:1393–1400

Wang M, Yip GW, Wang AY, Zhang Y, Ho PY, Tse MK, Lam PK, Sanderson JE 2003 Peak early diastolic mitral annulus velocity by tissue Doppler imaging adds independent and incremental prognostic value. Journal of the American College of Cardiology 41:820–826

Warburton DE, Haykowsky MJ, Quinney HA, Blackmore D, Teo KK, Human DP 2002 Myocardial response to incremental exercise in endurance-trained athletes: influence of heart rate, contractility and the Frank–Starling effect. Experimental Physiology 87:613–622

Weibel ER, Taylor CR, Hoppeler H 1992 Variations in function and design: testing symmorphosis in the respiratory system. Respiratory Physiology 87:325–348

Weisfeldt ML, Frederiksen JW, Yin FCP, Weiss JL 1978 Evidence of incomplete left ventricular relaxation in the dog: prediction from time constant for isovolumic pressure fall. Journal of Clinical Investigation 62:1296–1302

Wernstedt P, Sjostedt C, Ekman I, Thuomas K-A, Areskog NH, Nylander AE 2002 Adaptation of cardiac morphology and function to endurance and strength training. A comparative study using MR imaging and echocardiography in males and females. Scandinavian Journal of Medicine and Science in Sports 12:17–25

Whelan RF 1967 Control of the peripheral circulation in man. Charles C Thomas, Illinois

Whyte GP, George K, Shave R, Middleton N, Nevill AM 2008 Training induced changes in maximum heart rate. International Journal of Sports Medicine, Epub ahead of print

Wieling W, Borghols E, Hollander A, Danner S, Dunning A 1981 Echocardiographic dimensions and maximal oxygen uptake in oarsmen during training. British Heart Journal 46:190–195

Williams L, Frenneaux M 2006 Diastolic ventricular interaction: from physiology to clinical practice. Nature Clinical Practice and Cardiovascular Medicine 3:368–376

Yeater R, Reed C, Ullrich I, Morise A, Borsch M 1996 Resistance trained athletes using or not using anabolic steroids compared to runners: effects on cardiorespiratory variables, body composition and plasma lipids. British Journal of Sports Medicine 30:11–14

Younis LT, Melin JA, Robert AR, Detry JMR 1990 Influence of age and sex on left ventricular volumes and ejection fraction during upright exercise in normal subjects. European Heart Journal 11:916–924

Zandrino F, Molinari G, Smeraldi A, Odaglia G, Masperone M, Sardanelli F 2000 Magnetic resonance imaging of athlete's heart: myocardial mass, left ventricular function and cross-sectional area of the coronary arteries. European Radiology 10:319–325

Zucker IH, Patel KP, Schultz HD, Li YF, Wang W, Pliquett RU 2004 Exercise training and sympathetic regulation in experimental heart failure. Exercise and Sports Science Reviews 32:107–111

Chapter 4

Neuromuscular adaptations to exercise

Paavo V. Komi Caroline Nicol

CHAPTER CONTENTS

1 INTRODUCTION

The functional adaptations that occur with strength (resistance) and power training are typically interpreted within the context of a two-component model, consisting of a neural component, that accounts for training-induced changes in motor unit activation (Duchateau et al. 2006, Enoka 1997, Sale 2003), and a muscle–tendon component, that describes changes occurring at the muscle (Goldspink 1983, MacDougall 2003) and extracellular matrix levels (Kjaer 2004).

The concept of neural adaptation arises from three major observations (Sale 2003): an almost immediate increase in strength at the onset of training, a strength increase that could only partly be accounted for by muscle hypertrophy, and the cross-training effects, wherein training of one limb increases strength in the contralateral, untrained limb. The time course and magnitude of contributions made by neural and muscular adaptations will, in any case, be affected by the neuromuscular challenge posed by the training stimulus. The present chapter focuses primarily on the neural and mechanical factors associated with resistance training adaptations, and gives less emphasis to metabolic and hypertrophic factors. However, both neural and mechanical components interact, and adaptations often occur in parallel.

Skeletal muscle is one of the most adaptive structures in the body and each of its structural aspect may be expected to change, given the appropriate stimulus. Structural plasticity involves both quantitative (hypertrophy) and qualitative (isoform or phenotype of protein) changes of the different cellular components, with training-induced adaptation being a multidimensional phenomenon that has been recently shown to affect gene transcription and protein translation rates, via mechanical signalling pathways. Recent evidence shows that the first training session, which induces muscle damage, stimulates protein synthesis and degradation (Phillips 2000), with adaptation (hypertrophy) commencing earlier than previously thought. It remains uncertain how quickly this process leads to hypertrophy and strength increases, but this evidence questions the validity of the belief that the neural adaptations take place first, then trigger hypertrophic adaptation (Komi 1986, Moritani & deVries 1979, Sale 2003). The mechanisms behind mechanical loading resulting in altered gene expression and gene protein content have not so far been clearly identified (Goldspink & Harridge 2003).

In skeletal muscles, up to 10% of the cytoskeleton is collagen tissue. New evidence indicates there is close coupling between myogenesis and development of the intramuscular extracellular matrix (Collinsworth et al. 2000, Schmalbruch & Lewis 2000). The extracellular matrix within tendon tissue, as well as peri- and intramuscular tissue, is recognised as a functional link between skeletal muscle cells and bone. Thus, in addition to the force transmission that occurs in muscle–tendon (in-series) structures, elements of the cytoskeleton are thought to transfer a substantial amount of force in the lateral direction (Huijing 1992, Street 1983, Trotter & Purslow 1992). Apart from connecting muscles to bones and improving the functional movement range of the muscle–tendon complex, tendon structures are important as shock absorbers during high-impact motions, and contribute to the efficiency of locomotion and explosive movements (Alexander 1991, Komi 2000, Komi & Ishikawa 2006). This is due to tendon compliance, which allows storage and recycling (recoil) of elastic energy, but it is also due to the fact that tendon recoil takes up some of the length of the muscle–tendon unit. Tendons and extracellular connective tissue are dynamic structures that adapt to mechanical loading, expressing both structural and functional adaptations (Kjaer 2004).

The major focus of this chapter is upon the neuromechanical adaptations to strength and power training, which include training-induced structural and functional changes, and these are examined from the points of view of the traditional force–length (length–tension), force-velocity and power–velocity relationships.

2 MUSCLE–TENDON MECHANICS

2.1 From isolated actions to true muscle function

To help understand the way that skeletal muscle functions in normal locomotion, the relation between stimulus and response needs to be examined in more isolated muscle actions: isometric, concentric and eccentric. The most frequently studied muscle action is the isometric form of exercise, which refers to activation while the muscle–tendon unit length remains somewhat constant. Isometric action in locomotion is not, however, meaningless, since it plays a very important role in the process of preactivation of muscle before the other actions take place. Concentric action refers to muscle shortening while it is active, and eccentric action means lengthening of the active muscle. From these two dynamic forms, eccentric action plays perhaps a more important role in locomotion. When the active muscle–tendon unit is lengthening, following preactivation, it forms a basis for the stretch–shortening (eccentric–concentric

muscle actions) cycle, which is the natural form of muscle function in most daily activities involving joint movement.

2.2 Force–time characteristics

All joint movements involve a time delay, calculated from initiating the first intentional motor command (or reflex; e.g. proprioceptive feedback) and consisting of neuronal conduction delays (e.g. synaptic transmission), events of excitation–contraction coupling and mechanical characteristics of muscle fibres. In this regard, the isometric action is a very convenient way in which to describe the stimulus-response characteristics of skeletal muscle.

Figure 4.1 illustrates how the first principle of muscle mechanics, the force–time relation, varies as a function of stimulus strength, and between muscles and species (Figure 4.1A). The size of a single twitch response depends on the stimulus strength: a single shock, if strong enough, produces only a small twitch; two repetitive shocks add to the force of the first stimulus, when applied before complete recovery from the first stimulus (Figure 4.1C). Imagine a real movement situation, in which a load is fixed to the muscle, with the load not moving until the stimulus strength reaches (or exceeds) that necessary to overcome the total load (Figure 4.1B). When stimulus frequency is increased, force gradually reaches the state of a tetanus, which describes the maximum force–time characteristic of a muscle in an isometric action (Figure 4.1C).

The most fundamental feature for human locomotion is the difference between the fast (glycolytic) type II and endurance (oxidative) type I muscles fibres. Muscles consisting of mainly fast-twitch fibres (innervated more heavily by fast conducting α-motoneurons) have a faster rate of force development (Komi 1984, McComas 1996).

The present discussion has relevance due to the possibility for training modifying the force–time curve of a specific muscle or muscle group. In sport, the time to develop force is crucial, because total action times for a specific muscle may vary by <1 s. Thus, if the leg extensors achieve peak force >1000 ms after initiation, this implies that, for some activities, movement would already be over before peak forces were reached. Consequently, strength and power training studies have recently concentrated on examining the force–time curve during its early rise, with several methods being used to assess the rate of force development. Mirkov et al. (2004) found most of these methods could be considered to be fairly reliable, but their (external) validity for evaluating the ability to perform rapid movements was questionable. The force–time curve reveals that, if the movement begins at the point of zero electromyographic activity (force is also zero), then the practical consequences would be catastrophic. Nature corrects this by appropriately preactivating muscles before movement begins. Preactivation is preprogrammed (Mevill-Jones & Watt 1971), and is designed to take up the tension before movement initiation,

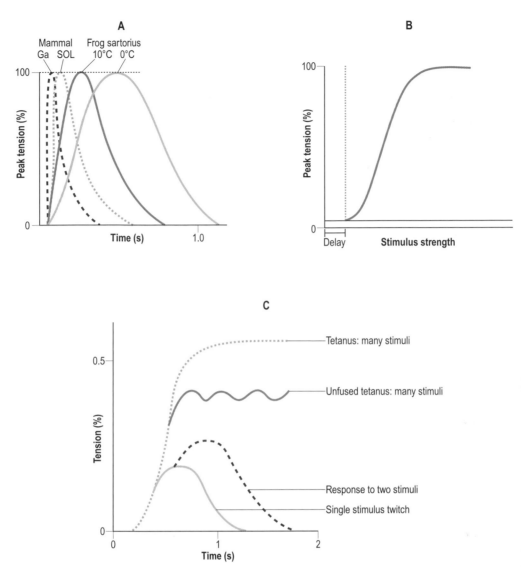

Figure 4.1 (A) The mechanical response (twitch) of mammalian muscle (GA, gastrocnemius; SOL, soleus) and frog (sartorius) muscle. In the frog, the twitch was measured at two incubation temperatures. Force is normalised to its peak (100%) for all conditions. (B) The relationship between stimulus strength and size of the twitch response. There is a delay before tension starts to rise. In normal locomotion, this delay is taken away by preprogrammed muscle action, such as occurs before contact with the ground during running. (C) When the stimulus is repeated the force begins to summate, eventually reaching a state of tetanus. Modified from Wilkie (1968) with permission.

and corresponds usually, but not always, to the isometric phase of the muscle action. Its electromyographic magnitude is a function of an expected static load or an impact load to be received (e.g. running; Komi et al. 1987). This preactivity corresponds to the initial stimulation, and is included in the measurement of concentric and isometric actions (Edman et al. 1978, Hill 1938).

2.3 Force–length relationship

Resting muscle–tendon structures are elastic and resist stretching forces. However, as it stretches, the muscle becomes less extensible. That is, its passive force–length curve becomes steeper (Figure 4.2), and this is largely determined by connective tissue structures (endomysium, perimysium, epimysium, tendon).

The active curve in Figure 4.2 constitutes the contractile component, whose form represents the contribution of the contractile material (fascicle or muscle fibres) to the total force curve, which is the sum of the active and passive forces at given muscle lengths. However, the active curve is not a continuous curve, but represents discrete data points, observed when the muscle is stimulated maximally from different lengths. The total force–length relationship

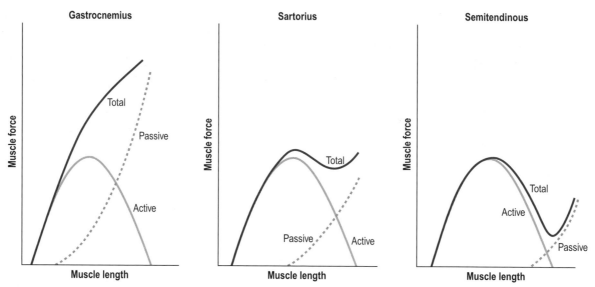

Figure 4.2 Active and passive force–length relationships of three frog muscles. The total muscle force curve is the sum of these curves. Note that the passive curve adds to the total force at different regions of the active curves, but always at some length greater than maximal force development. Modified from Wilkie (1968) with permission.

differs among muscles. Thus, no single relationship can be described that would be applicable for all skeletal muscles. From these curves, it is the active component that has received more attention; it resembles the force–length curve of individual sarcomeres, and the form of this curve comes from the number of cross-bridges that are being formed at different sarcomere lengths. It is unfortunate that conclusive and direct evidence of training-induced changes in sarcomere length is lacking, especially in humans. However, sarcomere numbers have been examined both in immobilisation and physical activity, and evidence shows these are not fixed, even in adults, but can increase and decrease.

For the muscle–tendon complex, however, exhaustive fatigue has been shown to shift the total force–length and force–angle curves to the right (Komi & Rusko 1974, Whitehead et al. 2001), and, in severe eccentric type exercise, this shift has been considered to reliably indicate the degree of muscle damage (Jones et al. 1997; Chapter 5).

2.4 Force–velocity relationship

Hill's classical paper (Hill 1938) describes the force–velocity relationship of an isolated muscle preparation (Figure 4.3), obtained using a constant electrical stimulation against different mechanical loads. The muscle was clamped at a fixed length and maximally stimulated. When the isometric force–time curve reached its maximum, the muscle was released, and its (concentric) shortening speed determined. These measurements can be extended to eccentric muscle action by allowing the muscle to actively resist an imposed

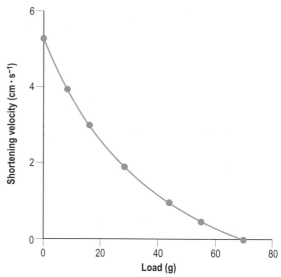

Figure 4.3 The classic force–velocity curve for the frog sartorius muscle at 0°C. The line is not continuous, but represents a discrete relationship of distinct data points. Redrawn from Hill (1938) with permission.

stretch that begins after the maximal (isometric) force has been reached. When human experiments have followed the methods applied to isolated muscles (Edman et al. 1978, Hill 1938), the voluntary concentric and eccentric force–velocity relationships were similar to those observed in isolated preparations (Komi 1973, Wilkie 1950). This includes the finding of similar maximal electromyographic activities in all contraction modes (eccentric, isometric and concentric) and velocities (Komi 1973). The observation that the voluntary eccentric force can sometimes be less than the isometric force (Westing et al. 1991) may be explained by differences between experiments, especially when the pre-activation was not maximal before recording the concentric and eccentric forces at different velocities of shortening and stretch, respectively. It may also be due to the inhibition of electromyographic activity.

Although the Hill curve was never designed to describe the instantaneous force–velocity relationship (stretch–shortening cycle), it has been used successfully to follow training adaptations in human skeletal muscle. These adaptations deal with power training, especially for sport activities requiring high levels of force and speed. From the Hill curve, it can be calculated that mechanical power (force times velocity) peaks under conditions when speed and force represent 30–50% along the force–velocity curve. Peak power is very sensitive to differences in muscle fibre composition. For instance, Faulkner (1986) demonstrated that human muscle peak power output for fast-twitch fibres was fourfold that of slow-twitch fibres, due to their greater shortening velocity for a given afterload. In the mixed muscle, the fast-twitch fibres may contribute 2.5 times more than the slow-twitch fibres to total power production.

In human experiments, it is difficult to use concentric and eccentric velocities that can adequately load the muscles across the range of physiological speeds (as described above). The maximum speed of most of the commercially available instruments can cover only ~20–30% of the different physiological maxima. As Goldspink (1978) has demonstrated, the peak efficiencies of isolated fast- and slow-twitch fibres occur at completely different contraction speeds. Therefore, it is possible that in measurements of the force–velocity curve in humans, when the maximum angular velocity reaches 3–4 rad·s^{-1}, only the contraction speeds of slow-twitch fibres will be studied. The peak power of the fast-twitch fibre may occur at angular velocities more than three times greater than our present measurement systems allow. Notwithstanding this, Tihanyi and collaborators (1982) were able to show a clear difference in force–velocity and power–velocity curves in leg extension movement between subject groups who differed in the fibre composition of vastus lateralis.

What happens to the fascicle length (magnitude and change of length) during different muscle actions? In our recent studies, we were able to demonstrate that during pure concentric action the fascicles show normal shortening (Finni et al. 2003), the magnitude of which may be intensity dependent (Reeves et al. 2003). In pure eccentric actions, fascicle lengthening (active resistance to stretch) should be expected, and has been demonstrated by Finni and collaborators (2003) for vastus lateralis. However, Reeves and collaborators (2003) reported for tibialis anterior that the

fascicles may operate at greater lengths at higher velocities of shortening (4 rad·s^{-1}), as compared to slower concentric action speeds. The fascicle lengths during eccentric action remained constant at all isokinetic speeds, but they were also shorter than those measured at higher concentric velocities. Although the latter finding does not directly imply the magnitude or even direction of shortening/lengthening, it may stress an important point: the fascicle length change may be dependent on the muscle and also on the specific movement. This notion becomes even more important when the fascicle–tendon interaction is studied under conditions of different intensity stretch–shortening cycle exercise.

3 STRETCH–SHORTENING CYCLE OF MUSCLE FUNCTION

3.1 Definition of the stretch–shortening cycle

The stretch–shortening cycle is illustrated in Figure 4.4 for the leg extensor muscle during the ground contact phase of running. The preactivated muscle begins its eccentric action upon first contacting the ground, when the muscle–tendon unit lengthens. This active eccentric (braking) phase is followed, without delay, by the shortening (concentric) action which, depending upon the intensity of effort, can take place in many cases as a recoil phenomenon, with relatively low electromyographic activity. Consequently, the stretch–shortening cycle is important for locomotion, since it takes up the unnecessary delays in the force–time relationship by bringing the preactivated force up to the level necessary to meet the expected eccentric loading. It also helps the concentric action (push-off) to produce peak power (maximal

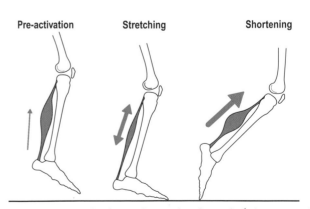

Figure 4.4 The stretch–shortening cycle of muscle (triceps surae) muscle during running. The cycle begins with the preprogrammed preactivity before toe contact with the ground. During contact, the activated muscle is first stretched (eccentric action), followed by shortening (concentric) muscle action. Adapted from Komi (2000) with permission.

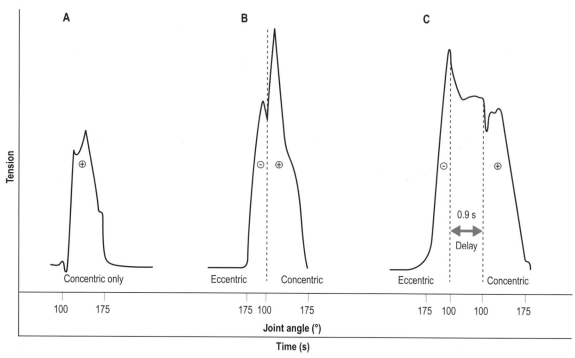

Figure 4.5 Three force-time traces for knee extension (100–175°), all performed with maximal voluntary activation. (A) A pure maximal concentric action. (B) Concentric muscle action is preceded by an eccentric (stretching) action, but no delay is allowed between these actions; note the force enhancement. (C) An identical action, but with a time delay between stretching and shortening; concentric force potentiation is reduced. Adapted from Komi (1983) with permission.

efforts) or generate force more economically (submaximal efforts).

Cavagna and colleagues were among the first to describe the mechanisms of this performance potentiation in experiments on isolated frog sartorius muscle (Cavagna et al. 1965), and later in human forearm flexors (Cavagna et al. 1968). Figure 4.5 illustrates knee extensor action (Komi 1983), and shows that the time delay (coupling time) between stretch (eccentric) and shortening (concentric) has influences on force and power output in the concentric phase of the cycle. That is, a short coupling time enhances performance. In addition, a shorter coupling time also improves economy (Aura & Komi 1986). The mechanisms of this potentiation will involve the entire muscle–tendon unit: fascicles and tendinous tissue.

Until recently, it was very difficult to measure much more than the force–angle relationship in situ, forcing the estimation of force–length changes. Accurate tensile force calculations have now been performed in vivo, by applying devices directly to tendons (buckle transducer (Komi 1990), optic fibre method (Komi et al. 1996)). With the development of real-time ultrasonography, it is now possible to non-invasively examine the in vivo behaviour of fascicles and tendinous tissues (aponeuroses and tendon in series) during exercise. Such measurements have been performed

at rest (Kawakami et al. 1993), but also in isometric actions (Fukunaga et al. 1997, Maganaris et al. 1998, Narici et al. 1996), showing that the muscle–tendon architecture undergoes remarkable changes. Some studies have succeeded in exploring these changes during activities with different intensity of the stretch–shortening cycle: walking (Fukunaga et al. 2001, Ishikawa et al. 2005a), running (Ishikawa et al. 2007) and jumping (Ishikawa & Komi 2004, Ishikawa et al. 2003, 2005b, Kawakami et al. 2002). The complexity of the interaction between fascicular and tendinous tissues is discussed below.

3.2 The instantaneous force–velocity relationship during the stretch–shortening cycle

The direct application of the force–velocity relationship of isolated muscle to natural locomotion, such as the stretch–shortening cycle, is difficult, since isolated preparations use constant electrical stimulation. Instead, it is necessary to measure the instantaneous force–velocity relationship in humans, using the buckle transducer or fine optic fibre. Both techniques are very sensitive to small variations in tensile force during normal activities. For example, the buckle transducer method revealed (surprisingly) that gastrocnemius and soleus demonstrated a small but meaning-

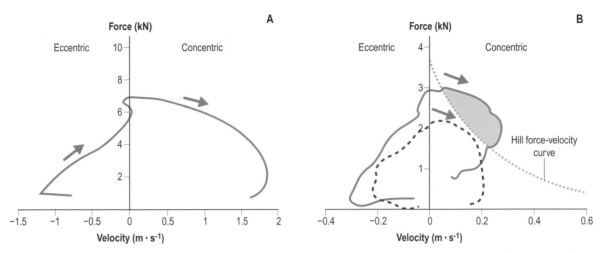

Figure 4.6 Instantaneous force–velocity curves, measured with a buckle transducer on the Achilles tendon during running (A: 9 m·s^{-1}), and with an optic fibre for the Achilles (solid) and patellar tendons (dashed) during hopping (B). Note the force potentiation during the concentric phase of the stretch–shortening cycle (shaded area). Adapted from Komi (1992; A) and Finni et al. (1998; B) with permission.

ful stretch–shortening cycle action during cycling (Gregor et al. 1991). Traditionally, cycling was considered an almost pure form of positive (concentric) work.

A characteristic of these instantaneous force–velocity curves is the considerable force potentiation, as seen during the push-off (concentric) phase of running (Figure 4.6A). Furthermore, force–velocity measurements during the contact phase of running revealed a curve that was completely different from the classic Hill relationship (Figure 4.3). Figure 4.6B, obtained simultaneously for the patella and Achilles tendons (optic fibre technique), demonstrates two important aspects of human skeletal muscle function. First, in short-contact hopping actions, triceps surae behaves like a bouncing ball. Second, when the hopping intensity is increased or changed to another type of movement, the contribution of the patella tendon force increases, and that of the Achilles may decrease (Finni et al. 2001). The Hill curve, obtained during a constant maximal (concentric) action, is superimposed, and the shaded area denotes remarkable performance potentiation, even though the hopping effort was submaximal. Animal experiments have obtained similar results (Gregor et al. 1988).

Such a difference between the instantaneous and classical curves is partly due to differences in muscle action between the two conditions. Isolated preparations primarily quantify the shortening properties of the contractile elements, whilst natural locomotion uses the whole stretch–shortening cycle, and involves the controlled release of elastic forces from the muscle–tendon unit that were generated during the eccentric phase. Some of energy recovery occurs during the shortening phase, resulting in performance potentiation. Thus, natural locomotion may produce more efficient muscle function that differs markedly from that observed in isolated preparations. In addition, during

stretch–shortening cycle activity performed without fatigue, electromyographic activity usually peaks before the eccentric phase ends, thereby confirming the importance of the eccentric phase.

3.3 Role of stretch reflexes in stretch–shortening cycle exercise

A characteristic of this performance enhancement phenomenon, at a given shortening velocity, is a very low electromyographic activity during the concentric phase, but a very pronounced contribution of the short-latency, stretch reflex component. This reflex contributes significantly to electromyographic activity and force generation during the transition phase from eccentric to concentric muscle action (Figure 4.7). This has been convincingly shown for soleus and gastrocnemius muscles, although the ultrasound measurements of Fukunaga et al. (2001) have demonstrated a continuous shortening of the fascicles during ground contact when walking. This finding did not support muscle spindle stretching and sensitisation of the Ia afferent fibres. However, our recent ultrasound measurements, performed at a higher sampling frequency, showed a very short-lived but clear fascicle stretch of gastrocnemius, immediately after ground contact (Ishikawa et al. 2007). Earlier evidence for the short-latency, stretch reflex component in gastrocnemius comes from the studies of Fellows et al. (1993), who used the ischaemic blocking method to isolate the Ia afferent information acting on spinal pathways during fast running. The control (non-ischaemic) runs demonstrated that gastrocnemius had a clear stretch reflex component during the contact phase, with the average electromyographic activity being twice that of maximal voluntary isometric plantarflexion. During ischaemic blocking, gastrocnemius electromyographic

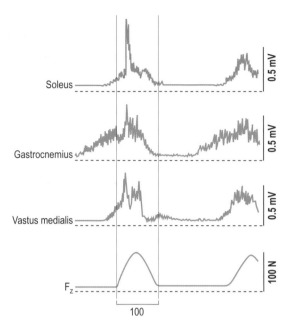

Figure 4.7 The short-latency, stretch reflex component in the drop jump. Records are average, rectified electromyographic traces and force (bottom trace). The two vertical lines denote the beginning and the end of contact on the ground, respectively. Note the sharp reflex peaks in the early contact phase. Adapted from Komi & Gollhofer (1997) with permission.

activity (during contact) was dramatically reduced but there was no change in preactivation. These results emphasise the importance of Ia afferents in the stretch–shortening cycle activities and may help explain performance potentiation.

4 TRAINING INFLUENCES ON THE MUSCLE–TENDON UNIT STRUCTURE AND FUNCTION

4.1 Adaptation of muscle fibre cross–sectional area

It is well accepted that postnatal muscle growth occurs by hypertrophy of individual fibres rather than the appearance of new fibres (Goldspink et al. 1983). Muscle fibre cross-sectional area follows a steady increase before puberty and, for boys, a rapid increase during and, for a while, after puberty. This precedes a progressive loss of muscle mass starting as early as 30 years and becoming significant at ~40 years. Training-induced hypertrophy of skeletal muscle is known to be associated with increased myofibrillar content of individual fibres. This may lead to an increased number of fibres (hyperplasia). In humans, however, there seems to be no evidence for muscle fibre splitting. The superiority of eccentric actions for stimulating hypertrophy has been reported in animal studies, but it is less clear for human studies.

It is generally accepted, however, that hypertrophy is more pronounced in fast muscle fibres (Thorstensson 1976).

This has been attributed to the relatively greater loading of those motor units during heavy load training, relative to daily activities. There is also ample evidence that muscle cells continue to adapt if the period of training is extended. Indeed, muscle fibre size and adaptation are determined by the nature of the adaptation stimulus (type of training; Chapter 21). Similarly, endurance training specifically influences the size of slow fibres, and can ultimately lead to smaller fibre cross-sectional areas, a trend that optimises oxygen uptake dynamics by reducing diffusion distances, thus allowing the muscle to sustain oxidative metabolism longer. This trend may be counteracted by combined resistance and endurance training (Kraemer et al. 2001).

What are the mechanisms of hypertrophy? Although biochemical events are not the major focus in this chapter, some answers to this question can be found at the molecular level. There are two ways in which proteins are accumulated. First, there may be an increased rate of protein synthesis. Second, there can be a reduced rate of protein breakdown. Since protein turnover is the balance between synthesis and breakdown, then total protein content reflects changes in either process. Recent data indicate that eccentric and concentric resistance exercise can increase net (intramuscular) protein balance, being detectable within 3 h of exercise (Phillips et al. 1997). Importantly, the limited human data indicate there is no difference in protein turnover between fibre types (Rennie & Tipton 2000).

However, clear evidence exists for a selective response which depends upon the type of training. This is in line with a recent hypothesis that muscle fibre phenotype is determined by stretch and force generation, and controlled at the gene transcription level (Chapter 8). More precisely, the regulation of growth is thought to be limited by the rate of translation of the message into protein. Goldspink (1977) reported increases in protein synthesis in stretched and immobilised rat skeletal muscle. The subsequent observations of a positive effect of stretch in both innervated and denervated muscle give support to a passive myogenic response, rather than an active component triggered by sensory receptors within the stretched muscle (Goldspink et al. 1974). This could give support to the possible beneficial use of high-load eccentric training to induce both hypertrophy, and increased force and power production. Recently, Shepstone and collaborators (2005) shed light on this problem, presenting evidence that higher-velocity eccentric actions can lead to greater hypertrophy and strength gains than eccentric training with slower stretch velocities.

4.2 Adaptation of muscle cross-sectional area

Investigators comparing differences in strength and muscle size between young and elderly individuals (Chapter 16) have related force (or torque) to the anatomical cross-sectional area of muscles (at 90° to the muscle belly) or total muscle volume (magnetic resonance imaging, computed tomography scanning). A general observation concerning strength training is that disproportionate changes take place between the anatomical cross-sectional and muscle fibre cross-sectional areas, with the former increasing to a greater extent (Aagaard et al. 2002). One explanation is that training changes fibre pennation angle rather than modifying the contractile and non-contractile material. Likewise, a greater increase in anatomical cross-sectional area has been observed in most (Higbie & Cureton 1996, Seger et al. 1998) but not all studies (Jones & Rutherford 1987). Finally, the hypertrophic response to eccentric training is reported to be longer lasting than the concentric adaptation (Hather et al. 1991). The reader is referred to Aagaard & Thorstensson (2003), Roy and collaborators (2003) and, for adaptations related to the sedentary lifestyle and ageing, to Chapters 9, 16 and 28.

With regard to the muscle length adaptation, there is a considerable increase during postnatal development, resulting from the serial addition of sarcomeres (Williams & Goldspink 1971). This has a major influence on the total force-length curve, since the force is dependent on the number of cross-bridges that can be engaged. Eccentric exercise shifts the length-tension relation so that the optimum length moves towards longer muscle lengths. This has now been demonstrated for both animals and humans (Brockett et al. 2001, Jones et al. 1997), and the size of this shift has been shown to correlate with previous exercise-induced muscle damage.

It has been proposed that the adaptation process, following the first bout of eccentric exercise, involves the repair of the damaged fibres, and the incorporation of additional sarcomeres in series (Morgan 1990). This mechanism has been proposed as providing protection against subsequent muscle damage (Brockett et al. 2001, Lynn & Morgan 1994). However, this hypothesis has been challenged by Koh & Herzog (1998), who did not observe a change in sarcomere number following eccentric type training. On the other hand, evidence exists that muscle adapts in the opposite direction after a regular programme of concentric exercise, and may become more vulnerable to damage from subsequent eccentric exercise (Whitehead et al. 1998).

4.3 Possibilities of stretch–shortening cycle training

The stretch–shortening cycle is the natural form of muscle action, and loads the neuromuscular system in a very complex way. It uses high-load eccentric (impacts) and combinations of eccentric and concentric muscle actions. The whole muscle–tendon unit is involved in these cycles. When repeated until exhaustion, such exercise causes considerable muscle damage, and is associated with an overall muscle performance reduction, as well as reduced stretch reflex function and maximal activation. Recovery from such fatigue is a long-term process and follows a bimodal fashion (Chapter 5).

The training benefits of exploiting stretch–shortening cycle activities (e.g. plyometrics) are not well known, despite the fact that such training is commonly used. However, Malisoux and collaborators (2006) undertook a breakthrough experiment (humans), revealing the training effects of a short-term (8 wk), maximal-effort stretch–shortening cycle exercise protocol (drop jumping). Their results showed remarkable performance enhancement in strength and power tests, but also, more importantly, in the mechanical performance of single muscle fibres. At the single-fibre level, the fibre diameter, peak force and shortening velocity increased, leading to enhanced fibre power. These effects were found for all fibre types.

On a whole-muscle electromyographic level, it is known that stretch–shortening cycle training enhances maximal electromyographic activity (Kyröläinen et al. 2004), but the sites of this adaptation are unknown. It is anticipated that future studies will reveal the mechanism of trainability with the neural components of the stretch–shortening cycle, especially the facilitatory and inhibitory influences within the nervous system.

5 NEUROMECHANICAL ADAPTATIONS

It is well known that almost any exercise that utilises force levels beyond those encountered in daily activities will lead to strength adaptation. A second important aspect of muscle function is the force–velocity principle. Figure 4.8 summarises how these factors result in strength adaptation.

In the overload principle, force development is crucial, and eccentric actions, if performed with full preactivation, could be useful for strength training. Eccentric training can indeed be beneficial for increasing maximal electromyographic activity and force (Häkkinen et al. 1981, Komi & Buskirk 1972), provided training is progressive, and excessive muscle soreness is avoided.

The force–velocity principle emphasises the specificity of training. That is, the effects of training are usually more pronounced when the performance is measured under the conditions of the training load, angular position and movement velocity. The effects of strength and power training, for example, can be both of muscular and neural origin. However, it is the neural adaptations that take place first, and present the conditions for muscular hypertrophy to participate in the process of performance improvement (Komi 1986, Moritani & deVries 1979).

It is quite remarkable that the literature is mostly composed of investigations that have concentrated on the training-induced changes in strength, determined as improvement in muscle force (maximal voluntary contraction). In many activities, however, the ability to develop force within the initial 100–200 ms of contraction (explosive muscle power) is equally, or even more important than maximal force itself. To generate the greatest possible force or power in a short time, and in the intended direction of movement, the nervous system faces at least four challenges: (1) full activation of

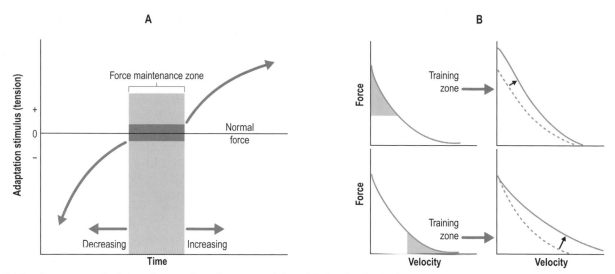

Figure 4.8 Two important principles of strength and power training: (A) Overload principle: the affect of the adaptation stimulus is a function of the force generated, relative to the tension experienced in daily activities and the duration of the stimulus. (B) Force–velocity principle: strength adaptation is a function of the load (upper left) and movement velocity (lower left) chosen for training, with the resultant adaptations affecting the shape of the force–velocity curve (right). Both A and B adapted from Komi (1975) with permission.

the agonist muscle(s); (2) appropriate activation of the synergistic muscle(s); (3) suitable input from the antagonist muscles; and (4) proper utilisation of sensory feedback in preparation to, and execution of the movement.

The mechanical response (performance) occurs in parallel with the neural input (activation), and individuals who demonstrate a slow rate of electromyographic development will usually have a slow force development. Thus, one purpose of training is to change the electromyographic-time and force–time curves. However, the locus of these changes depends upon the type of training employed.

The requirement of complete activation of the prime mover (agonist) muscles is naturally the most important of these challenges. This can be performed by a more consistent recruitment of the highest threshold motor units, and by increasing motor unit firing rate, with special attention for the occurrence of doublets and triplets. The second and third requirements make the agonist action easier by the appropriate activation of synergists and antagonists that oppose the primary action.

5.1 Neural adaptation to resistance and power training: influence on the force–time relationship

Studies using classical strength or power training programmes have concentrated on the first two challenges. The major observation of studies using high-intensity training loads is the improvement in maximum force output. Increases in strength are reported to occur along with increased neural drive, over the entire duration of muscle action. These findings are not dramatically new. However, selective adaptations of the rate of force development and

maximum force capacity have been reported for specific training regimens. For instance, resistance (strength) training primarily leads to an enhanced maximum force, whereas explosive (power) training results in adaptations related to the rate of force development (Aagaard et al. 2002, Häkkinen & Komi 1986). The following is an attempt to separate these two classic training methods (high-load versus high-speed), and their neural adaptations. New data have shown that cross-education (contralateral) is possible, and that unilateral, voluntary muscle training has contralateral effects at both the cortical and segmental levels (Hortobagyi et al. 2003). In addition, eccentric training at fast velocities may have a greater cross-education effect than slow-velocity training (Farthing & Chilibeck 2003).

High-load strength training is believed to result in a neural adaptation of the agonist (increased activation), synergist (more appropriate activation) and antagonist muscles (decreased activation). Increased maximal electromyographic activity (agonist) is thought to be due to the central command for skeletal muscle having some activation reserve that is not fully used in the untrained state. In general, neural adaptation reduces antagonist activity, and increases the net force produced by the agonist-antagonist groups. However, in some circumstances, it may be desirable to increase antagonist coactivation so that joint stiffness can be increased; for example, during high-impact load situations.

Muscle coactivity is the concurrent activation of agonist and antagonist muscles surrounding a joint, and it may arise from reduced reciprocal inhibition, mediated segmentally by the Ia inhibitory interneuron, or from an elevated central activation impinging on the antagonistic motoneurons, or from some combination of these mechanisms (Humphrey & Reed 1983). The most commonly ascribed role of this coactivity is to increase joint stiffness and limb stability (Baratta et al. 1988, Hortobagyi & De Vita 2000). In sequential movements, increased coactivity is expected to result in shorter time delays (Enoka 1983) and reduced effort (Hazan 1986). Challenging and high-precision tasks are typically associated with strong coactivation (Pearson 1958). However, it is also well known that exercise training and skill acquisition tend to decrease coactivity (Amiridis et al. 1996).

High-speed (explosive, ballistic) training has a different objective. The aim is not to increase strength per se, but to increase the speed with which loaded actions can be performed. For instance, it is known from electrical stimulation studies that an increase in initial firing rate (e.g. from 60 to 100 Hz) may not increase the peak isometric force, but it does allow for an increased rate of force development, which occurs in the early part of the force–time curve. The experiments in this regard are very encouraging and have dramatically changed the concept of force and power production, and their adaptation in sports activities (Komi 1986) in young as well as in elderly subjects (Kamen & Knight 2004).

The most conclusive evidence for modification of the force–time curve comes from Duchateau's group (Van Cutsem et al. 1998), observing that explosive training of human tibialis anterior resulted in greater discharge rates of both single motor units (Figure 4.9) and the entire motor unit pool. Instantaneous firing rate has increased, twitch contraction is shorter and there is a simultaneous increase in the rate of force development. Two other observations need to be mentioned. First, explosive training caused the instantaneous discharge rates of the motor unit firing very early during activation, reaching values >200 Hz (Figure 4.9A). Second, it increased the number of doublet motor unit discharges during the early phase of maximal activation. Doublet firing refers to the repetitive firing of a single motor unit at an interspike interval ≤5 ms. The functional significance of doublets is their contribution to the rate of force development. Thus, strong evidence has been presented that explosive training causes motor units to be activated earlier, to fire in a doublet pattern and to increase their overall firing rate.

The possible contribution of increased motor unit synchronisation to rate of force development is more debatable. Some strongly favour that increased synchronisation plays an important role in enhancing the rate of force development (Semmler 2002). Others, although agreeing that synchronised firing of motor units may increase due to explosive training, feel that its contribution to the rate of force development is not very meaningful (Duchateau et al. 2006).

These adaptations to explosive training (increased motor unit firing rate, doublet discharge and synchronisation) may contribute to an increased voluntary movement speed, and an enhanced rate of force production during subse-quent muscle activation. These are fundamental attributes of skeletal muscle function during many sporting activities. Of course, there is the possibility that cross-over effects may exist between high-load and explosive training. For example, depending on the initial training status, it is quite possible that, with a very low starting performance, either form of training will result in performance increases, even when tests to measure performance were intended for use with the other training protocol. Indeed, a significant force enhancement is known to result from the addition of only one high-frequency extraneural pulse (Burke et al. 1970).

5.2 Neural adaptation and the force–velocity principle

As introduced above, the classical force-velocity curve (Hill 1938) can be used to quantify training influences. In addition, the training load and velocity can be prescribed from this curve to target specific adaptations. Although the mechanisms regarding neural adaptations are similar to those already discussed, the adaptations to force–velocity training are so important that they warrant special attention.

From the force–velocity curve and its sensitivity to muscle fibre composition, one would expect that training adaptations of this curve, or the power–velocity curve had been exhaustively explored. The situation is unfortunately the opposite. Although the specificity of strength and power training has been well explored with regard to neural and mechanical adaptations (Komi 1986, Moritani & Yoshitake 1998, Sale 2003), Kaneko (Kaneko 1970, 1974, Kaneko et al. 1983) and Duchateau & Hainaut (1984) can be considered pioneers in research involving the power curve and human skeletal muscle training.

For example, Kaneko (1974) followed the time course of changes in the force–velocity characteristics and maximal power output, to training loads applied at discrete points along that curve (0%, 30%, 60%, 100% of maximal contraction force) over a 20-week period. His major finding was that mechanical power was improved most at the point on the force–velocity curve that corresponded to the training load. This specificity of explosive power training was later confirmed by Kaneko and collaborators (1983), who showed that training with maximal actions and zero load was most effective for the training of maximal velocity. High-load (100%) training resulted in the greatest improvement for maximal strength. From these studies it was concluded that the force–velocity curve adaptation is very specific, and could be used to follow adaptations in the mechanical properties of muscle to different training modes. It is important to note that when the training load was selected to correspond to maximal power, the outcome was the greatest improvement in overall maximal power.

Moritani & Muro (1987) extended these studies to examine neural activation in the course of maximal training, using biceps brachii (human) loaded to 30% of its maximal isometric force. They showed a dramatic increase

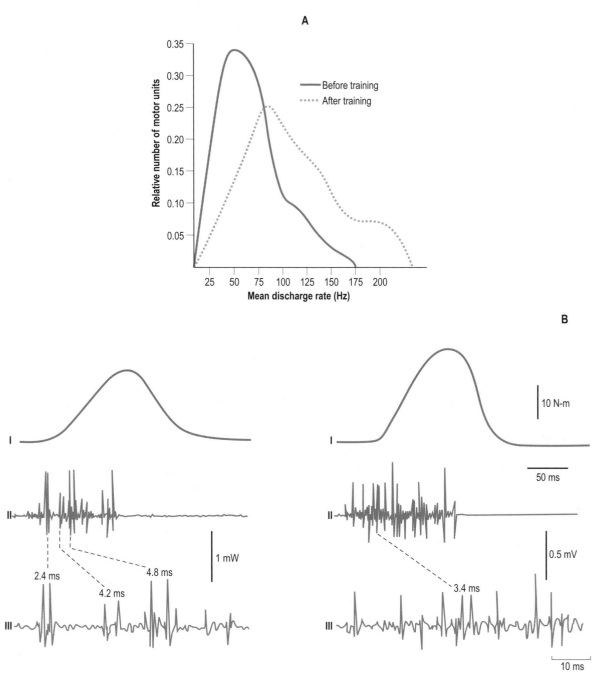

Figure 4.9 (A) The impact of explosive training (12 wk) on motor unit discharge (tibialis anterior). Note the rightward shift in the distribution of maximum firing rates. (B) Mechanograms (I) and electromyographic records at normal (II) and slower (III) chart speeds, showing doublet discharges after explosive training. Left: motor units firing at 2.4, 4.2 and 4.8 ms during activation. Right: one motor unit firing 14, 12.5 and 6 ms, then a doublet discharge of 3.4 ms. Note how quickly the motor unit activity finishes relative to the mechanical record. Adapted from Van Cutsem et al. (1998) with permission.

in muscle activation, and suggested that the short-term training-induced shifts in the force–velocity relationship, and that mechanical power might have been brought about by a neural adaptation expressed as increased muscle activation and more synchronous motor unit activation patterns (Moritani 2003). Consequently, results from studies that have used discrete parts of the force–velocity curve as adaptation stimuli are in line with the principle of training adaptation specificity (Chapter 21), and also with the adaptation mechanisms described above for explosive training.

5.3 Neural adaptation to sensorimotor training

The metabolic changes in skeletal muscle, following strength and explosive training, are also very specific to the training protocol used, and these principles also apply to the metabolic and atrophic changes due to ageing (Chapter 16). However, less is known about how exercise and training affect the metabolic and morphological properties of the motoneurons. Consequently, information regarding training adaptation of neuronal pathways is based on human studies that have examined the electrophysiological properties of motor units, including their recruitment and firing rates.

Stimulation techniques, such as H-, M- and V-wave recordings and interpolation twitch techniques, have been used to follow the possible neural adaptations, and sites where these could occur. Despite many attempts and publications, it still remains uncertain where the sites of these adaptations might be located; they could be at any point from the central command to the propagation of an action potential.

The sensorimotor system incorporates all the afferent, efferent and central integration, and processing for the maintenance of joint stability. This concept extends from Sherrington's definition of the proprioceptive system to include a more complex connection between sensory pathways and motor pathways, than the simple reflex arc (Lephart et al. 2000). Sensory information arises in this case from the peripheral mechanoreceptors (skin, joints, ligaments, tendons, muscles) as well as from visual and vestibular receptors. It is still debated as to how this sensory information is transmitted (Lephart et al. 2000), the relative importance (weighting) of these afferent signals (Bergenheim et al. 2000, Ribot-Ciscar et al. 2003, Roll et al. 2000), and the mechanisms by which the sensory information mediates motor control: feedback versus feedforward control (Lam et al. 2006, Lephart et al. 2000; Chapter 18). These questions are important for our comprehension of neural adaptation induced by sensorimotor training.

In terms of training adaptation, the target of sensorimotor training has mostly been defined as improving the functional stability or postural stabilisation in a rehabilitative or injury prevention sense. Proprioception has mostly been examined in patients ranging from vestibular deficits (Lacour et al. 1997) to chronic ankle instability (Tropp 1986). The role of somatosensory (prioceptive and tactile) information has also been demonstrated by altering or limiting somatosensory input through the use of anaesthetic blockade (Konradsen et al. 1993), or platform translations under different visual and surface conditions (Horak et al. 1990). More recently, a few studies have demonstrated (Gollhofer 2003, Granacher et al. 2006, Gruber & Gollhofer 2004) that proprioceptive training (using unstable platforms, ankle pads and uneven surfaces) generally improves afferent responses. From these studies it also appears that 4 weeks of sensorimotor training has positive effects on the rate of force

development during maximal voluntary contraction, especially in its early phase (Gollhofer 2003, Gruber & Gollhofer 2004). In accordance with the effects of explosive training (Aagaard et al. 2002), sensorimotor training increases the rate of force development without enhancing maximum strength, and the early gain in force development occurs along with an increased mean voluntary activity.

The improvements in postural stability are associated with an increased reflex activation in young (Gollhofer et al. 2000, Gruber & Gollhofer 2004), as well as in elderly men (Granacher et al. 2006). The gain in muscle activation is attributed to an enhanced reflex contribution acting at the spinal level and induced by the sensorimotor training itself. Finally, Bruhn and collaborators (2006) examined the neuromuscular effects of combined sensorimotor and resistance training. Both training regimens had positive effects on the rate of force development, as well as maximal strength. However, improvements caused by sensorimotor training could only be achieved when it was performed first. It was suggested that the sensorimotor training can have preconditioning effects on strength training.

At present, knowledge concerning the most appropriate modes for sensorimotor training is still rudimentary. The challenge is to develop techniques that may help locate the sites in the neuromuscular system (including supraspinal sites), where these changes take place.

5.3.1 Vibration training

Vibration training refers to the use of mechanical oscillatory movements, either whole-body or at specific joints or muscles, for the purpose of enhancing performance (force and power output). Similar to sensorimotor training, the mechanisms related to vibration training are largely unknown. However, several overviews have been recently published on this topic (Cardinale & Bosco 2003, Mester et al. 2003, Nordlund & Thorstensson 2007, Rehn et al. 2007) and should be consulted.

Vibration training is not new but this method of strength training has attracted more attention in the last two decades. First, as safety considerations are particularly important in vibration techniques, it is worth noting that clear recommendations have been recently defined (Mester et al. 2006). When vibration training is properly designed, this method may be considered effective for improving maximal strength, power and flexibility. Importantly, its evaluation is facing the common time delay of the loading-induced adaptation process that includes a decreasing (fatigue) period, followed by a progressive recovery, and finally an overcompensation phase (Mester et al. 2003). Similar to resistance training, a threshold load appears necessary to obtain significant positive effects, but the literature is still lacking precision on the proper range of frequencies, amplitudes and exposure duration of the vibration. In terms of mechanisms, the increase in strength has frequently been attributed to the so-called tonic vibration reflex induced by the activation of Ia afferents of the muscle spindles with the potential contribution of skin and type II afferents (Park & Martin 1993, Romaiguère et al. 1991). Further research is needed, however, to define the exact underlying physiological processes.

6 FASCICLE–TENDON INTERACTIONS IN NATURAL HUMAN MOVEMENT

During natural muscle function, in which muscles are actively stretched and subsequently shortened (stretch–shortening cycle), the descriptions above refer to the entire muscle–tendon unit. However, this may not apply to the individual compartments of the muscle–tendon unit, such as contractile tissue, aponeurosis or tendon. Several studies have reported that the muscle fibres shorten during the braking phase, even if the muscle–tendon unit is stretching (Biewener & Corning 2001, Griffiths 1991, Roberts et al. 1997). Others have demonstrated that the fascicle behaves almost isometrically during stretch–shortening cycles. In addition, our recent measurements with extremely high-impact, loaded drop jumps show that the fascicles could stretch and shorten similar to those of the muscle–tendon unit (Ishikawa & Komi 2004, Ishikawa et al. 2003). These observations have been made with the same muscle group, but during different tasks. We must therefore consider how the stretch–shortening cycle behaviour inside a single muscle–tendon unit may differ across different types of stretch–shortening cycle exercise, and also across different muscles. Can these mechanical behaviours be generalised (modelled) across different situations?

6.1 Muscle specificity

The literature indicates that fascicles either maintain a constant length, shorten or lengthen during the early phase of stretch–shortening cycle exercises. However, we believe that the mechanical behaviour of muscle and tendon may be specific to a given muscle–tendon unit. Consequently, the fascicle behaviour of two different muscles (medial gastrocnemius and soleus) was measured simultaneously during walking. The soleus fascicles were lengthened with increasing muscle activation, but the medial gastrocnemius fascicles kept at a constant length during the single support phase of walking. These different fascicle behaviours can be observed in other stretch–shortening cycle movements as well (drop jumps, hopping, running; Ishikawa et al. 2005a, b, 2007). Consequently, the fascicles in a biarticular muscle do not show the same stretch–shortening cycle behaviour as a monoarticular muscle. Differences in fascicle behaviour between these two muscles support the concept of previous studies (Elftman 1939, Alexander 1974), which suggested that biarticular muscle (e.g. medial gastrocnemius) could play a greater energy conservation role during human locomotion, relative to monoarticular muscle (e.g. soleus).

Furthermore, our results show that leg muscles (human), which are commonly accepted as being synergists, do not have similar mechanical behaviour within the fascicles during locomotion. Although one may conclude that such muscle specificity exists, particularly for comparisons between mono- and biarticular muscles, some caution should be used. Although it is clear that fascicle stretching during ground contact is much greater in soleus than medial gastrocnemius, one should not assume that medial gastrocnemius fascicles do not undergo stretching. When we increased (ultrasound) sampling frequency from 50 to 96 Hz, we observed a very short but clear stretching of medial gastrocnemius fascicles during the early breaking phase of contact in jogging (Ishikawa et al. 2007). This can be taken as an important observation, and proof that there is enough fascicle stretching to activate the stretch reflex component in the medial gastrocnemius. As discussed earlier, stretch reflexes play an important role in potentiating performance in the stretch–shortening cycle.

6.2 Movement specificity

Fascicle–tendinous tissues interaction may also display movement specifity. It is well known that muscle elasticity plays an important role in muscle function and performance potentiation (Cavagna et al. 1968). It is also known that the resonant frequency of the elastic component of human ankle extensors varies considerably (2.6–4.3 Hz; Bach et al. 1983, Cavagna et al. 1997). Consequently, the utilisation of this elasticity may occur in the same way during the contact phase of all stretch–shortening cycle exercises. For example, running and hopping have short contact phases, whilst walking and counter movement jumps have long contact phases. Ishikawa et al. (2007) have shown that medial gastrocnemius behaviour (muscle-tendon unit, fascicle and tendinous tissues) during the contact phase of running and walking is different from that of soleus. Although the muscle–tendon unit and tendinous tissues were lengthened during the braking phase in both conditions, the medial gastrocnemius fascicles behaved differently. Except for the early quick lengthening, as discussed above, the usual pattern was overall shortening during ground contact of running. In walking, they lengthened slightly during the single support phase. In jumping (Souza et al. 2007), the gastrocnemius fascicle length was found to be either constant, shortened or initially lengthened before shortening, even though the muscle–tendon units were lengthened in each condition. These results can indicate the existence of movement-specific fascicle behaviour.

6.3 Intensity specificity within the movement

If the muscle–tendon interaction is subject to muscle and movement specificity, one may also wonder whether the intensity of effort modifies the interaction during stretch–shortening cycle exercises. For example, a common finding of many drop jump studies is that, as the height of the drop preceding the rebound is increased, performance can initially improve (Asmussen & Bonde-Petersen 1974, Bosco & Komi 1981) but eventually will decrease (Komi & Bosco 1978, Walshe & Wilson 1997). Consequently, the fascicle–tendinous tissues interaction could be modified by the pre-stretch and rebound intensity efforts.

Experimental results confirm this assumption (Ishikawa & Komi 2004, Ishikawa et al. 2005b). For example, when high-intensity stretch–shortening cycle exercises were performed on the sledge apparatus, vastus lateralis fascicles and tendinous tissues behaved similarly to the muscle–tendon unit, according to the stretch–shortening cycle concept. However, the length changes of the fascicles and tendinous tissues were unequally distributed along the muscle–tendon unit. In addition, the stretching and shortening amplitudes of tendinous tissues increased with increasing rebound intensities. Greater recoil in tendinous tissues at higher rebound intensities was clearly seen at the end of the push-off phase. These results imply that, during stretch–shortening cycle exercises, not only the stretch intensity, but also the rebound intensity can have considerable influence on elastic energy storage and subsequent recoil during the push-off phase, via fascicle length modification. This is under the influence of the activation pattern, with its modulation depending upon the jumping task.

It is worth noting that, for a specific muscle, there may be critical prestretch intensities that can be tolerated, in the sense that if this stretch speed is exceeded (e.g. very high drop jump), the fascicles may lose their ability to resist the stretch. Consequently, the attached cross-bridges will be broken, and the subsequent rebound height in the concentric push-off phase is decreased (Ishikawa et al. 2003). This phenomenon may explain why, after a certain drop height, jumping performance decreases (Asmussen & Bonde-Petersen 1974, Komi & Bosco 1978). Thus, we conclude that, depending upon the intensity of the prestretch and rebound phases, the elastic potentiation of subsequent muscle action will also vary.

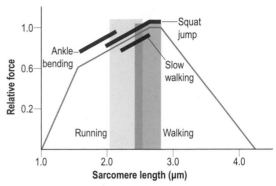

Figure 4.10 A proposed scheme for human medial gastrocnemius muscles to utilise various parts of the sarcomere force–length relation during different activities. The shaded areas indicate the range of the sarcomere lengths for the contact phases of walking and running. Note that the working length of sarcomeres shifts to the ascending (left) limb when the activity changes from walking to running. Adapted from Fukunaga et al. (2002) and Ishikawa et al. (2007) with permission.

6.4 Fascicle–tendon interactions: concluding remarks

Although studies relating to the fascicle–tendon interaction are still in their developmental stage, several important conclusions can be noted. No generalised pattern of fascicle–tendinous tissues interaction is available for universal application across muscles, actions or intensities. This is because these interactions are muscle, movement and intensity specific. A great challenge for future research is to find out how and why training and ageing modify these interactions. We may also suggest, based on current knowledge, that the sarcomere force–length curve is equally problematic, and may face a list of difficulties similar to those encountered when investigating fascicle–tendon interactions. However, in Figure 4.10, we illustrate our current thinking concerning how the ascending and descending limbs of the sarcomere length–tension relationship may be used during different physical activities.

References

Aagaard P, Simonsen EB, Andersen JL, Magnusson P, Dyhre-Poulsen P 2002 Increased rate of force development and neural drive of human skeletal muscle following resistance training. Journal of Applied Physiology 93:1318–1326

Aagaard P, Thorstensson A 2003 Neuromuscular aspects of exercise-adaptive responses evoked by strength training. In: Kjaer M, Krogsgaard M, Magnusson P, Engebretsen L, Roos H, Takala T, Woo S (eds) Textbook of sports medicine. Blackwell Science, Oxford, 70–106

Alexander RM 1974 The mechanics of jumping by a dog. Journal of Zoology (London) 173:549–573

Alexander RM 1991 Energy–saving mechanisms in walking and running. Journal of Experimental Biology 160: 55–69

Amiridis IG, Martin A, Morlon B, Martin L, Cometti G, Pousson M, van Hoecke J 1996 Co–activation and tension–regulating phenomena during isokinetic knee extension in sedentary and highly skilled humans. European Journal of Applied Physiology and Occupational Physiology 73:149–156

Asmussen E, Bonde–Petersen F 1974 Apparent efficiency and storage of elastic energy in human muscles during exercise. Acta Physiologica Scandinavica 92:537–545

Aura O, Komi PV 1986 Effects of prestretch intensity on mechanical efficiency of positive work and on elastic behavior of skeletal muscle in stretch–shortening cycle exercise. International Journal of Sports Medicine 7:137–143

Bach TM, Chapman AE, Calvert TW 1983 Mechanical resonance of the human body during voluntary oscillations about the ankle. Journal of Biomechanics 16(1):85–90

Baratta R, Solomonow M, Zhou BH, Letson D, Chuinard R, D'Ambrosia R 1988 Muscular coactivation. The role of the antagonist musculature in maintaining knee stability. American Journal of Sports Medicine 16:113–122

Bergenheim M, Ribot–Ciscar E, Roll JP 2000 Proprioceptive population coding of two–dimensional limb movements in humans. I. Muscle spindle feedback during spatially oriented movements. Experimental Brain Research 134:301–310

Biewener AA, Corning WR 2001 Dynamics of mallard (Anas platyrynchos) gastrocnemius function during swimming versus terrestrial locomotion. Journal of Experimental Biology 204:1745–1756

Bosco C, Komi PV 1981 Prestretch potentiation of human skeletal muscle during ballistic movement. Acta Physiologica Scandinavica 111:135–140

Brockett CL, Morgan DL, Proske U 2001 Human hamstring muscles adapt to eccentric exercise by changing optimum length. Medicine and Science in Sports and Exercise 33:783–790

Bruhn S, Kullmann N, Gollhofer A 2006 Combinatory effects of high intensity strength training and sensorimotor training on muscle strength. International Journal of Sports Medicine 27(5):401–406

Burke RE, Rudomin P, Zajac FE 1970 Catch property in single mammalian motor units. Science 168:122–124

Cardinale M, Bosco C 2003 The use of vibration as an exercise intervention. Exercise and Sport Sciences Reviews 31(1):3–7

Cavagna GA, Dusman B, Margaria R 1968 Positive work done by a previously stretched muscle. Journal of Applied Physiology 24:21–32

Cavagna GA, Mantovani M, Willems PA, Musch G 1997 The resonant step frequency in human running. Pfügers Arch 434(6):678–684

Cavagna GA, Saibene FP, Margaria R 1965 Effect of negative work on the amount of positive work performed by an isolated muscle. Journal of Applied Physiology 20:157–158

Collinsworth AM, Torgan CE, Nagda SN, Rajalingam RJ, Kraus WE, Truskey GA 2000 Orientation and length of mammalian skeletal myocytes in response to unidirectional stretch. Cell and Tissue Research 302:243–251

Duchateau J, Hainaut K 1984 Isometric or dynamic training: differential effects on mechanical properties of a human muscle. Journal of Applied Physiology 56:296–301

Duchateau J, Semmler JG, Enoka R 2006 Training adaptations in the behaviour of human movement units. Journal of Applied Physiology 101:1766–1775

Edman KAP, Elzinga G, Noble MIM 1978 Enhancement of mechanical performance by stretch during tetanic contractions of vertebrate skeletal muscle fibres. Journal of Physiology (London) 281:139–155

Elftman H 1939 The function of muscles in locomotion. American Journal of Physiology 125:339–356

Enoka RM 1983 Muscular control of a learned movement: the speed control system hypothesis. Experimental Brain Research 51(1):135–145

Enoka RM 1997 Neural adaptations with chronic physical activity. Journal of Biomechanics 30(5):447–455

Farthing JP, Chilibeck PD 2003 The effect of eccentric training at different velocities on cross–education. European Journal of Applied Physiology 89:570–577

Faulkner JA 1986 Power output of the human diaphragm. American Review of Respiratory Disease 134(5):1081–1083

Fellows SJ, Dömges F, Töpper R, Thilmann AF, Noth J 1993 Changes in the short and long latency stretch–reflex components of the triceps surae muscle during ischaemia in man. Journal of Physiology 472:737–748

Finni T, Komi PV, Lepola V 2001 In vivo muscle mechanics during natural locomotion is dependent on movement amplitude and contraction intensity. European Journal of Applied Physiology 85:170–176

Finni T, Ikegawa S, Lepola V, Komi PV 2003 Comparison of force–velocity relationships of vastus lateralis muscle in isokinetic and in stretch–shortening cycle exercises. Acta Physiologica Scandinavica 177:483–491

Fukunaga T, Ichinose Y, Ito M, Kawakami Y, Fukashiro S 1997 Determination of fascicle length and pennation in a contracting human muscle in vivo. Journal of Applied Physiology 82:354–358

Fukunaga T, Kawakami Y, Kubo K, Kanehisa H 2002 Muscle and tendon interaction during human movements. Exercise and Sport Sciences Reviews 30(3):106–10

Fukunaga T, Kubo K, Kawakami Y, Fukashiro S, Kanehisa H, Maganaris CN 2001 In vivo behaviour of human muscle tendon during walking. Proceedings of the Biological Sciences/Royal Society 268(1464):229–233

Goldspink DF 1977 The influence of activity on muscle size and protein turnover. Journal of Physiology 264:283–296

Goldspink DF, Garlic PJ, McNurlan MA 1983 Protein turnover measured in vivo and in vitro in muscles undergoing compensatory growth and subsequent denervation atrophy. Biochemical Journal 210(1):89–98

Goldspink G 1978 Energy turnover during contraction of different types of muscles. In: Asmussen E, Joergensen K (eds) Biomechanics VI/A. University Park Press, Baltimore, 27–29

Goldspink G 1983 Alterations in myofibril size and structure during growth, exercise and changes in environmental temperature. In: Peachey LD (ed) Handbook of physiology. American Physiology Society, Baltimore, 539–554

Goldspink G, Harridge S 2003 Cellular and molecular aspects of adaptation in skeletal muscle. In: Komi PV (ed) Strength and power in sport, 2nd edn. Blackwell, Oxford, 231–251

Goldspink G, Tabary C, Tabary JC, Tardieu C, Tardieu G 1974 Effect of denervation on the adaptation of sarcomere number and muscle extensibility of the functional length of the muscle. Journal of Physiology (London) 236:733–742

Gollhofer A 2003 Proprioceptive training: considerations for strength and power production. In: Komi PV (ed) Strength and power in sport, 2nd edn. Blackwell, Oxford, 331–342

Gollhofer A, Alt W, Lohrer H 2000 Active joint control–importance of proprioceptive activation on functional neuro–muscular properties. In: Schmidt R, Benesch S, Lipke K (eds) Chronic ankle instability. Libri Verlag, Ulm, Germany, 317–325

Granacher U, Gollhofer A, Strass D 2006 Training induced adaptations in characteristics of postural reflexes in elderly men. Gait and Posture 24(4):459–466

Gregor RJ, Komi PV, Browning RC, Järvinen M 1991 A comparison of the triceps surae and residual muscle moments at the ankle during cycling. Journal of Biomechanics 24:287–297

Gregor RJ, Roy RR, Whiting WC, Lovely RG, Hodgson JA, Edgerton VR 1988 Mechanical output of the cat soleus during treadmill locomotion in vivo vs. in situ characteristics. Journal of Biomechanics 21(9):721–732

Griffiths RI 1991 Shortening of muscle fibers during stretch of the active cat medial gastrocnemius muscle: the role of tendon compliance. Journal of Physiology 436:219–236

Gruber M, Gollhofer A 2004 Impact of sensorimotor training on the rate of force development and neural activation. European Journal of Applied Physiology 92:98–105

Häkkinen K, Komi PV 1986 Training–induced changes in neuromuscular performance under voluntary and reflex conditions. European Journal of Applied Physiology 55(2):147–155

Häkkinen K, Komi PV, Tesch P 1981 Effect of combined concentric and eccentric strength training and detraining on force–time, muscle fiber and metabolic characteristics of leg extensor muscles. Scandinavian Journal of Sports Sciences 3(2):50–58

Hather BM, Tesch PA, Buchanan P, Dudley GA 1991 Influence of eccentric actions on skeletal muscle adaptations to resistance training. Acta Physiologica Scandinavica 143:177–185

Hazan Z 1986 Optimized movement trajectory and joint stiffness in unperturbed, inertially loaded movements. Biological Cybernetics 53:373–382

Higbie EJ, Cureton KJ 1996 Effect of concentric and eccentric training on muscle strength, cross–sectional area and neural activation. Journal of Applied Physiology 81(5):2173–2181

Hill AV 1938 The heat and shortening of the dynamic constant of muscle. Proceedings of the Royal Society of London Series B 126:136–195

Horak FB, Nashner LM, Diener HC 1990 Postural strategies associated with somatosensory and vestibular loss. Experimental Brain Research 82(1):167–177

Hortobagyi T, De Vita P 2000 Muscle pre– and coactivity during downward stepping are associated with leg stiffness in aging. Journal of Electromyography and Kinesiology 10:117–126

Hortobágyi T, Taylor JL, Petersen NT, Russell G, Gandevia SC 2003 Changes in segmental and motor cortical output with contralateral muscle contractions and altered sensory inputs in humans. Journal of Neurophysiology 90:2451–2459

Huijing PA 1992 Elastic potential of muscle. In Komi PV (ed) Strength and power in sport. Blackwell Scientific Publications, Oxford, 151–168

Humphrey DR, Reed DJ 1983 Separate cortical systems for control of joint movement and joint stiffness: reciprocal activation and coactivation of antagonist muscles. In: Desmedt JE (ed) Motor control mechanisms in health and disease. Raven Press, New York, 347–372

Ishikawa M, Finni T, Komi PV 2003 Behaviour of vastus lateralis muscle–tendon during high intensity SSC exercises in vivo. Acta Physiologica Scandinavica 178:205–213

Ishikawa M, Komi PV 2004 Effects of different dropping intensities on fascicle and tendinous tissue behavior during stretch–shortening cycle exercise. Journal of Applied Physiology 96:848–852

Ishikawa M, Komi PV, Grey MJ, Lepola V, Bruggemann GP 2005a Muscle–tendon interaction and elastic energy usage in human walking. Journal of Applied Physiology 99:603–608

Ishikawa M, Niemela E, Komi PV 2005b The interaction between fascicle and tendinous tissues in short contact stretch–shortening cycle exercise with varying eccentric intensities. Journal of Applied Physiology 99:217–223

Ishikawa M, Pakaslahti J, Komi PV 2007 Medial gastrocnemius muscle behaviour during human running and walking. Gait and Posture 25(3):380–384

Jones C, Allen T, Talbot J, Morgan DL, Proske U 1997 Changes in the mechanical properties of human and amphibian muscle after eccentric exercise. European Journal of Applied Physiology 76(1):21–31

Jones DA, Rutherford OM 1987 Human muscle strength training: the effects of three different regimes and the nature of the resultant changes. Journal of Physiology 391:1–11

Kamen G, Knight CA 2004 Training–related adaptations in motor unit discharge rate in young and older adults. Journal of Gerontology A–59:1334–1338

Kaneko M 1970 The relationship between force, velocity and mechanical power in human muscle. Research Journal of Physical Education Japan 14:141–145

Kaneko M 1974 The dynamics of human muscle. Kyorinshoin Book Company, Tokyo (in Japanese)

Kaneko M, Fuchimoto T, Toji H, Suei, K 1983 Training effect of different loads o the force–velocity relationship and mechanical

power output in human muscles. Scandinavian Journal of Sport Sciences 5:50–55

Kawakami Y, Abe T, Fukunaga T 1993 Muscle–fiber pennation angles are greater in hypertrophied than in normal muscles. Journal of Applied Physiology 74:2740–2744

Kawakami Y, Muraoka T, Ito S, Kanehisa H, Fukunaga T 2002 In vivo muscle fibre behaviour during counter–movement exercise in humans reveals a significant role for tendon elasticity. Journal of Physiology 540:635–646

Kjaer M 2004 Role of extracellular matrix in adaptation of tendon and skeletal muscle to mechanical loading. Physiological Reviews 84:649–698

Koh TJ, Herzog W 1998 Eccentric training does not increase sarcomere number in rabbit dorsiflexor muscles. Journal of Biomechanics 31:499–501

Komi PV 1973 Measurement of the force–velocity relationship in human muscle under concentric and eccentric contraction. In: Jokl E (ed) Medicine and sport, biomechanics III. Karger, Basel, 8, 224–229

Komi PV 1975 Faktoren der Mueskelkraft und Prinzipien des Krafttrainings. Leistunsgsport 1:3–6

Komi PV 1983 Elastic potentiation of muscles and its influence on sport performance. In: Baumann W (ed) Biomechanik und Sportliche Leistung. Verlag Karl Hofmann, Schorndorf, 59–70

Komi PV 1984 Physiological and biomechanical correlates of muscle function: effects of muscle structure and stretch–shortening cycle on force and speed. Exercise and Sport Sciences Reviews 12:81–121

Komi PV 1986 Training of muscle strength and power: interaction of neuromotoric, hypertrophic and mechanical factors. International Journal of Sports Medicine 7(Suppl):10–15

Komi PV 1990 Relevance of in–vivo force measurements to human biomechanics. Journal of Biomechanics 23(Suppl 1):23–34

Komi PV 1992 Stretch–shortening cycle. In: Komi PV (ed) Strength and power in sport. Blackwell Scientific Publications, Oxford, 169–179

Komi PV 2000 Stretch–shortening cycle: a powerful model to study normal and fatigue muscle. Journal of Biomechanics 33:1197–1206

Komi PV, Belli A, Huttunen V, Bonnefoy R, Geyssant A, Lacour JR 1996 Optic fibre as a transducer of a tendomuscular forces. European Journal of Applied Physiology 72:278–280

Komi PV, Bosco C 1978 Utilization of stored elastic energy in leg extensor muscles by men and women. Medicine and Science in Sports 10:261–265

Komi PV, Buskirk ER 1972 Effect of eccentric and concentric muscle conditioning on tension and electrical activity of human muscle. Ergonomics 15(4):417–434

Komi PV, Gollhofer A 1997 Stretch reflex can have an important role in force enhancement during SSC–exercise. Journal of Applied Biomechanics 13:451–460

Komi PV, Gollhofer A, Schmidtbleicher D, Frick U 1987 Interaction between man and shoe in running: consideration for more comprehensive measurement approach. International Journal of Sports Medicine 8(3):196–202

Komi PV, Ishikawa M 2006 In–vivo interaction of fascicles and tendons as measured by the optic fiber and ultrasonographic technique. In: Rainoldi A, Minetto MA, Merletti R (eds) Biomedical engineering in exercise and sports. Edizioni Minerva Medica, Torino, 3–15

Komi PV, Rusko H 1974 Quantitative evaluation of mechanical and electrical changes during fatigue loading of eccentric and concentric work. Scandinavian Journal of Rehabilitation Medicine (Suppl 3):121–126

Konradsen L, Ravn JB, Sorensen AI 1993 Proprioception of the ankle: the effect of anaesthetic blockade of ligament receptors. Journal of Bone and Joint Surgery 75-B:433–436

Kraemer WJ, Keuning M, Ratamess NA, Volek JS, McCormick M, Bush JA, Nindl BC, Gordon SE, Mazzetti SA, Newton RU, Gómez AL,

Wickham RB, Rubin MR, Häkkinen K 2001 Resistance training combined with bench–step aerobics enhances women's health/fitness profile. Medicine and Science in Sports and Exercise 33:259–269

Kyröläinen H, Avela J, McBride JM, Koskinen S, Andersen JL, Sipilä S, Takala TE, Komi PV 2004 Effects of power training on mechanical efficiency in jumping. European Journal of Applied Physiology 91:155–159

Lacour M, Barthelemy J, Borel L, Magnan J, Xerri C, Chays A, Ouaknine M 1997 Sensory strategies in human postural control before and after unilateral vestibular neurotomy. Experimental Brain Research 115(2):300–310

Lam T, Anderschitz M, Dietz V 2006 Contribution of feedback and feedforward strategies to locomotor adaptations. Journal of Neurophysiology 95:766–773

Lephart SM, Rieman BL, Fu FH 2000 Introduction to sensorymotor system. In: Lephart SM Fu FH (eds) Proprioception and neuromuscular control in joint stability. Human Kinetics, Champaign, IL, 1–5

Lynn R, Morgan DL 1994 Decline running produces more sarcomeres in rat vastus intermedius muscle fibers than does incline running. Journal of Applied Physiology 77:1439–1444

McComas AJ 1996 Skeletal muscle form and function, Human Kinetics, Champaign, IL

MacDougall JD 2003 Hypertrophy and hyperplasia. In: Komi PV (ed) Strength and power in sport, 2nd edn. Blackwell, Oxford, 252–264

Maganaris CN, Baltzopoulos V, Sargeant AJ 1998 In vivo measurements of the triceps surae complex architecture in man: implications for muscle function. Journal of Physiology 512:603–614

Malisoux L, Francaux M, Nielens H, Theisen D 2006 Stretch–shortening cycle exercises: an effective training paradigm to enhance power output of human single muscle fibers. Journal of Applied Physiology 100:771–779

Mester J, Kleinöder H, Yue Z 2006 Vibration training: benefits and risks. Journal of Biomechanics 39:1056–1065

Mester J, Spitzenpfeil P, Yue Z 2003 Vibration loads: potential for strength and power development. In: Komi PV (ed) Strength and power in sport, 2nd edn. Blackwell Science, Oxford, 488–501

Mevill–Jones G, Watt DGD 1971 Observations on the control of stepping and hopping movements in man. Journal of Physiology 219:709–727

Mirkov DM, Nedeljkovic A, Milanovic S, Jaric S 2004 Muscle strength testing: evaluation of tests of explosive force production. European Journal of Applied Physiology 91:147–154

Morgan DL 1990 New insights into the behavior of muscle during active lengthening. Biophysical Journal 57(2):209–221

Moritani T 2003 Motor unit and motoneurone excitability during explosive movement. In: Komi PV (ed) Strength and power in sport, 2nd edn. Blackwell Science, Oxford, 27–49

Moritani T, deVries HA 1979 Neural factors versus hypertrophy in the time course of muscle strength gain. American Journal of Physical Medicine 58:115–130

Moritani T, Muro M 1987 Motor unit activity and surface electromyogram power spectrum during increasing force of contraction. European Journal of Applied Physiology and Occupational Physiology 56:260–265

Moritani T, Yoshitake Y 1998 The use of electromyography in applied physiology. Journal of Electromyography and Kinesiology 8:363–381

Narici MV, Binzoni T, Hiltbrand E, Fasel J, Terrier F, Cerretelli P 1996 In vivo human gastrocnemius architecture with changing joint angle at rest and during graded isometric contraction. Journal of Physiology 496:287–297

Nordlund MM, Thorstensson A 2007 Strength training effects of whole body vibration? Scandinavian Journal of Medicine and Science in Sports 17:12–17

Park HS, Martin BJ 1993 Contribution of the tonic vibration reflex to muscle stress and muscle fatigue. Scandinavian Journal of Work Environment and Health 19:35–42

Pearson RS 1958 An EMG investigation on coordination of the activity of antagonist muscles in man during the development of a motor habit. Pavlov Journal of Higher Nervous Activity 8:13–23

Phillips SM 2000 Short–term training: when do repeated bouts of resistance exercise become training? Canadian Journal of Applied Physiology 25(3):185–193

Phillips SM, Tipton KD, Aarsland A, Wolf SE, Wolfe RR 1997 Mixed muscle protein synthesis and break down after resistance exercise in humans. American Journal of Physiology 273:E99–E107

Reeves ND, Narici MV, Maganaris CN 2003 Behavior of human muscle fascicles during shortening and lengthening contractions in vivo. Journal of Applied Physiology 95(3):1090–1096

Rehn B, Lidström J, Skoglund J, Lindström B 2007 Effects of leg muscular performance from whole-body vibration exercise: a systematic review. Scandinavian Journal of Medicine and Science in Sports 17:2–11

Rennie MJ, Tipton KD 2000 Protein and amino acid metabolism during and after exercise and the effect of nutrition. Annual Review of Nutrition 20:457–483

Ribot–Ciscar E, Bergenheim M, Albert F, Roll JP 2003 Proprioceptive population coding of limb position in humans. Experimental Brain Research 149:512–519

Roberts TJ, Marsh RL, Weyand PG, Taylor CR 1997 Muscular force in running turkeys: the economy of minimizing work. Science 275:1113–1115

Roll JP, Bergenheim M, Ribot–Ciscar E 2000 Proprioceptive population coding of two–dimensional limb movements in humans. II. Muscle spindle feedback during 'drawing–like' movements. Experimental Brain Research 134:311–321

Romaiguère P, Vedel JP, Azulay JP, Pagni S 1991 Differential activation of motor units in the wrist extensor muscles during the tonic vibration reflex in man. Journal of Physiology 444:645–667

Roy RR, Monti RJ, Lai A, Edgerton VR 2003 Skeletal muscle and motor unit architecture: effect on performance. In: Komi PV (ed) Strength and power in sport, 2nd edn. Blackwell Science, Oxford, 27–49

Sale DJ 2003 Neural adaptation to strength training. In: Komi PV (ed) Strength and power in sport, 2nd edn. Blackwell Science, Oxford, 281–314

Schmalbruch H, Lewis DM 2000 Dynamics of nuclei of muscle fibers and connective tissue cells in normal and denervated rat muscles. Muscle and Nerve 23:617–626

Seger JY, Arvidsson B, Thorstensson A 1998 Specific effects of eccentric and concentric training on muscle strength and morphology in humans. European Journal of Applied Physiology 79:49–57

Semmler JG 2002 Motor unit synchronization and neuromuscular performance. Exercise and Sport Sciences Reviews 30:8–14

Shepstone TN, Tang JE, Dallaire S, Schuenke MD, Staron RS, Phillips SM 2005 Short–term high– vs. low–velocity isokinetic lengthening training results in greater hypertrophy of the elbow flexors in young men. Journal of Applied Physiology 98:1768–1776

Souza F, Ishikawa M, Vilas–Boas JP, Komi PV 2007 Intensity– and muscle–specific fascicle behavior during human drop jumps. Journal of Applied Physiology 102:382–389

Street SF 1983 Lateral transmission of tension in frog myofibres: a myofibrillar network and transverse cytoskeletal connections are possible transmitters. Journal of Cellular Physiology 14:346–364

Thorstensson A 1976 Muscle strength, fiber types and enzyme activities in man. Acta Physiologica Scandinavica 433(Suppl):1–44

Tihanyi J, Apor P, Fekete G 1982 Force–velocity–power characteristics and fiber composition in human leg extensor muscles. European Journal of Applied Physiology 48:331–343

Tropp H 1986 Pronator muscle weakness in functional instability of the ankle joint. International Journal of Sports Medicine 7:291–294

Trotter JA, Purslow PP 1992 Functional morphology of the endomysium in series fibered muscles. Journal of Morphology 212:109–122

Van Cutsem M, Duchateau J, Hainaut K 1998 Changes in single motor unit behaviour contribute to the increase in contraction speed after dynamic training in humans. Journal of Physiology 513:295–305

Walshe AD, Wilson GJ 1997 The influence of musculotendinous stiffness on drop jump performance. Canadian Journal of Applied Physiology 22:117–132

Westing SH, Cresswell AG, Thorstensson A 1991 Muscle activation during maximal voluntary eccentric and concentric knee extension. European Journal of Applied Physiology 62:104–108

Whitehead NP, Allen TJ, Morgan DL, Proske U 1998 Damage to human muscle from eccentric exercise after training with concentric exercise. Journal of Physiology 512:615–620

Whitehead NP, Weerakkody NS, Gregory JE, Morgan DL, Proske U 2001 Changes in passive tension of muscle in humans and animals after eccentric exercise. Journal of Physiology 533(2): 593–604

Wilkie DR 1950 The relation between force and velocity in human muscle. Journal of Physiology 110:249

Wilkie DR 1968 Muscle. St Martin's Press, New York, 28

Williams PE, Goldspink G 1971 Longitudinal growth of striated muscle fibres. Journal of Cell Science 9:751–767

Chapter 5

Central and neuromuscular fatigue

Janet L. Taylor   Paavo V. Komi   Caroline Nicol

Chapter 5 is presented in two halves, with the first addressing central fatigue and concentrating on isometric exercise of a single limb. The second half focuses on neuromuscular fatigue during exercise that involves the stretch–shortening cycle (Chapter 4), which occurs during natural activities (running and hopping), and includes eccentric and concentric components.

1 CENTRAL FATIGUE

1.1 Introduction

In voluntary tasks, muscle contraction results from a chain of processes starting in the brain. Most directly, descending output from the motor cortex activates spinal motoneurons, which in turn activate muscle fibres (Figure 5.1). Thus, the force generated depends not only on properties of the muscle, but also on activation by the nervous system. Muscle fatigue can be defined as any exercise-induced reduction in the ability of a muscle to generate force or power (Gandevia 2001). In humans, it can be measured as a fall in the force of a maximal voluntary contraction. During sustained or repetitive muscle action, processes that contribute to fatigue begin at each level of the motor pathway. The inability to continue a task (task failure or limit of endurance) is the culmination of these ongoing processes.

Muscle fatigue can be divided into two aspects (Figure 5.1): peripheral fatigue, which includes processes at or distal to the neuromuscular junction (Chapter 6); and central fatigue, which includes more proximal processes, and is defined as a progressive reduction in voluntary activation of muscle during exercise (Gandevia 2001). That is, despite maximal voluntary effort, the motor units are not driven fast enough to generate maximal force. Alterations in intrinsic motoneuron properties, sensory feedback or descending drive can contribute to central fatigue. The contribution of descending drive can be explored with stimulation of the motor cortex during maximal voluntary efforts. This technique identifies supraspinal fatigue (a component of central fatigue), which is defined as fatigue produced by failure to generate output from the motor cortex (Gandevia 2001).

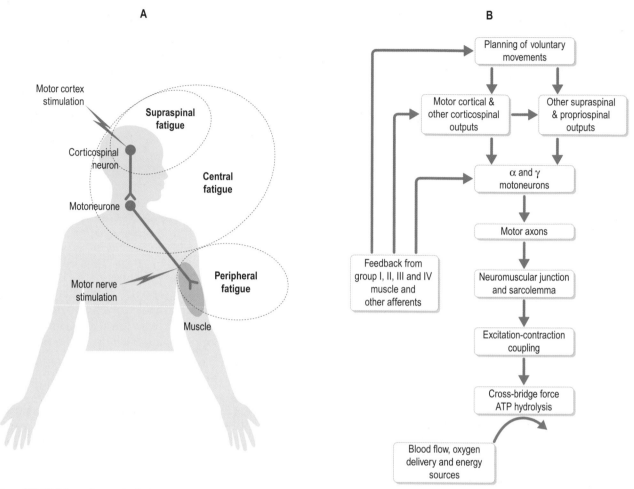

Figure 5.1 (A) Division of muscle fatigue into peripheral and central fatigue by motor nerve stimulation. Supraspinal fatigue is a subset of central fatigue. (B) The chain of processes leading to voluntary movement. Feedback from muscle afferents is shown going to the motoneurons, the motor cortex and premotor areas. Adapted from Gandevia (2001) with permission.

Central fatigue occurs during all kinds of exercise, including whole-body exercise and dynamic actions. However, its demonstration relies on sensitive measurements of muscle output, so it is most easily investigated during isometric contractions. The first half of this chapter will concentrate on such fatigue, describing both the techniques used to demonstrate its existence, and its contributing mechanisms. It is important to realise that only some changes in the nervous system, that occur during fatiguing exercise, impair muscle output, and can therefore be thought of as central fatigue.

1.2 Motor unit firing rates during fatiguing exercise

When a motor unit fires repetitively, its muscle fibre properties change. Initially, muscle fibres are potentiated and their ability to generate force is increased. With continued firing, the fibres become fatigued. They generate less force and their contractile properties are altered. The timing and degree of these changes depend on fibre type, with low-threshold fibres generally showing less potentiation and fatigue. For the successful performance of voluntary tasks, drive to the muscle must account for the ongoing changes in contractile properties.

In an isometric maximal voluntary contraction (MVC), the task is to generate as much instantaneous force as possible. Thus, all motor units in the agonist muscles should fire fast enough to maintain fused contractions. In a sustained MVC, force drops immediately, due to peripheral fatigue, and it is generally accepted that motor unit firing rates also fall (Figure 5.2; Gandevia 2001).

The 'muscle wisdom' hypothesis proposed that this fall in firing rate does not contribute to fatigue, but that it matches fatigue-related slowing of muscle contraction and relaxation (Marsden et al. 1983). Lower firing frequencies would still maintain fused contractions of the slowed muscle, and would minimise failure of neuromuscular transmission. However, there appears to be no direct link between changes in contractile properties and motor unit firing rates (Bigland-Ritchie et al. 1992, Garland et al. 1997). In sustained MVCs, motor unit firing rates fall below the

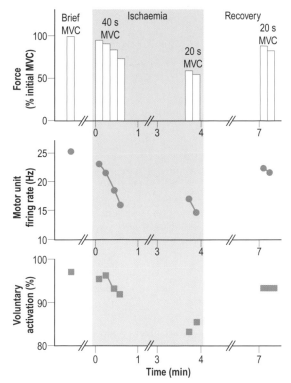

Figure 5.2 Force, motor unit firing rates and voluntary activation during voluntary isometric knee extensor activation. During a sustained maximal voluntary contraction (MVC; 40 s), maximal voluntary force, motor unit firing rates and voluntary activation fall. With the limb held ischaemic by an inflated cuff, a rest period does not allow recovery. It is proposed that sensory feedback from the muscle keeps motor unit firing and voluntary activation low. When blood flow resumes, rest results in peripheral and central recovery. Redrawn from Woods et al. (1987) with permission.

optimal rate to generate maximal force, and some motor units stop firing altogether (Gandevia 2001, Fuglevand & Keen 2003, Peters & Fuglevand 1999). Thus, this lack of neural drive to the muscle contributes to fatigue.

During submaximal, isometric voluntary actions, changes in motor unit firing are more complex because voluntary drive can vary to compensate for changes in muscle properties. For example, to compensate for fatigue in active muscle fibres, voluntary drive increases to recruit additional motor units, and this should increase firing rates of the active units. However, motor unit firing rates are reported to increase, stay the same or decrease (e.g. Carpentier et al. 2001, Garland et al. 1994). Presumably, the response of individual motor units depends on the intrinsic properties of the motoneurons, their specific history of activity and combined afferent and descending input. With longer contractions, there is progressive peripheral fatigue and increases in voluntary drive until the target force can no longer be maintained, despite maximal effort.

1.3 Fatigue and neuromuscular transmission

Reduced electrical activity of muscle (electromyogram) is sometimes suggested as evidence for central fatigue. During sustained MVCs, electromyogram amplitude falls and, although it increases during fatiguing submaximal contractions, it remains less than maximal at the limit of endurance (Gandevia 2001). One explanation is that voluntary activation of the muscle is impaired, with less than maximal motor unit recruitment or firing rates. However, changes in neuromuscular transmission must also be considered.

The electromyographic response to peripheral nerve stimulation (M-wave) is often used as an indicator of failure of neuromuscular transmission (Chapter 4). Conduction block in the terminal motor axons or neuromuscular junction is unlikely to be important in voluntary contractions, as stimulation of individual motor axons at high frequency does not decrease the M-wave (Chan et al. 1998). However, impairment clearly occurs during high-frequency stimulated activation of whole muscle (Bigland-Ritchie et al. 1979, Fuglevand & Keen 2003). This is probably due to altered propagation of the muscle fibre action potential along the sarcolemma. In fatigue, conduction velocity slows and the amplitude of the action potential can decrease, with depolarisation of the muscle fibre membrane through the accumulation of extracellular potassium (Sjøgaard 1996). The action potential may then be insufficient to depolarise the t-tubules and bring about excitation–contraction coupling (Chapter 6). However, some reduction in amplitude can occur before force is impaired (Fuglevand & Keen 2003). Thus, submaximal electromyogram amplitudes during maximal efforts are not unequivocal evidence of central fatigue, as the peripheral effects of activity can also reduce the electromyogram.

1.4 Evidence of central fatigue

1.4.1 Voluntary activation measured with peripheral nerve or muscle stimulation

Measurements of voluntary activation use the principle that motor units not engaged by voluntary drive during a voluntary contraction can be activated by electrical stimulation of the nerve or muscle. The increment in force so produced (superimposed or interpolated twitch) is inversely related to the strength of the muscle action (Merton 1954).

In the method known as twitch interpolation, voluntary activation is quantified by comparing the superimposed twitch to the twitch evoked in the resting muscle by the same stimulus. Although a model of twitch interpolation predicts a linear relationship between voluntary force and the superimposed twitch (Herbert & Gandevia 1999), the relationship is often non-linear in practice, with larger increases in force for smaller changes in activation at high forces (Figure 5.3; Allen et al. 1998, Behm et al. 2001). Mechanisms suggested for this non-linearity include differential

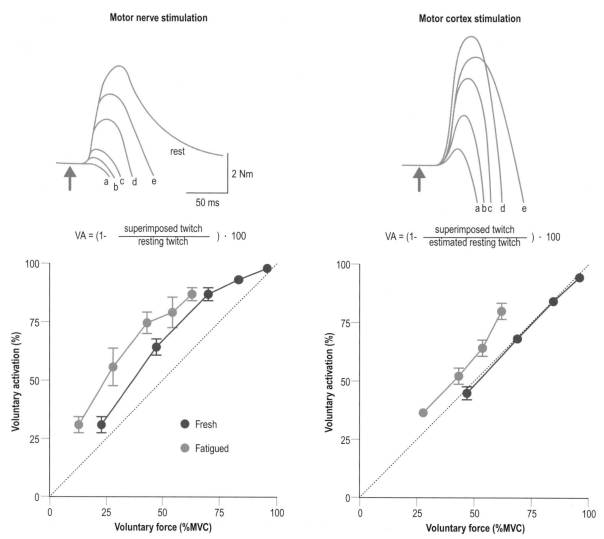

Figure 5.3 Voluntary activation of the elbow flexors with superimposed twitches evoked by motor nerve stimulation or motor cortex stimulation (arrows). The top panels show twitches evoked during brief isometric activation at 100% (a), 90% (b), 75% (c), 50% (d) and 25% (e) of maximal voluntary contraction (MVC) in one subject. The background forces are offset to allow comparison of the twitches. On the left are responses to motor nerve stimulation of biceps and brachialis, including a twitch evoked from the resting muscle (rest). To calculate voluntary activation (VA) the size of the superimposed twitch is compared to the size of the resting twitch. On the right are responses evoked from all elbow flexors using transcranial magnetic (motor cortex) stimulation. To calculate voluntary activation, the size of a resting twitch is estimated by extrapolation of a linear regression of superimposed twitch size against voluntary force for contractions >50% MVC. The superimposed twitch is then compared to the estimated resting twitch. The lower panels show voluntary activation for a group of subjects, when the muscle was fresh or fatigued, such that maximal voluntary force had fallen by 40%. Voluntary activation measured with motor nerve stimulation shows a curvilinear relationship to voluntary force (left), while that measured with motor cortex stimulation shows a linear relationship. From Todd et al. (2003) with permission.

activation of the tested muscles, non-isometric action and stimulation of antagonists.

Voluntary activation is also measured using the central activation ratio (Behm et al. 2001, Kent-Braun & Le Blanc 1996). In this technique, a train of stimuli is delivered during a contraction. The voluntary force prior to stimulation is compared to the total force (voluntary plus evoked) during stimulation. The major drawback is that the comparison is likely to overestimate voluntary activation, unless all synergists can be stimulated maximally. Trains of stimuli can also

evoke inhibitory reflexes between synergists, reducing the voluntary contribution to force (Naito et al. 1996).

1.4.2 Voluntary activation during maximal efforts

Superimposed twitches can commonly be evoked in normal subjects, even during maximal isometric efforts. A superimposed twitch indicates that, despite maximal voluntary effort, either not all motor units were recruited or not all units were firing fast enough to generate maximal force at the moment of stimulation (Merton 1954). That is, voluntary activation was <100%. Voluntary activation has been tested for knee extensors, elbow flexors and extensors, ankle plantar and dorsiflexors, the diaphragm, hand muscles, abdominal muscles and masseter (Gandevia 2001, Shield & Zhou 2004). In most muscles, some subjects can achieve 100% activation in some contractions, but blanket reports of 100% activation for any muscle group should be regarded with suspicion.

Voluntary activation is commonly reported as 85–95% for the knee extensors, and >95% for the elbow flexors and extensors. Recent studies also show high activation of the plantarflexors (>95%), with even higher activation of dorsiflexors. Voluntary activation has also been measured during dynamic (concentric and eccentric) actions. It is similar in maximal concentric and isometric actions but is lower during eccentric activity (Babault et al. 2001, Gandevia et al. 1998).

1.4.3 Voluntary activation during fatiguing exercise

During fatiguing exercise, the ability to maximally activate the fatigued muscle falls. This progressive decline is the marker of central fatigue, and has been demonstrated in knee extensors, ankle plantar and dorsiflexors, elbow flexors, diaphragm and hand muscles with various exercise protocols. During a sustained isometric MVC, voluntary force falls. Peripheral fatigue reduces the muscle's ability to generate force. At the same time, the force increment evoked by a superimposed stimulus grows. Thus, subjects have a reduced ability to drive the muscle maximally (Figure 5.2). At the end of a 90–180 s MVC, voluntary activation falls by 10–15% (Gandevia et al. 1996, Rattey et al. 2005).

The central activation ratio shows similar reductions (from 0.94 to 0.78) in ankle dorsiflexors during a 4 min MVC (Kent-Braun 1999). Central fatigue also develops when isometric MVCs are performed intermittently in a fatiguing protocol, with falls of voluntary activation of up to 20% reported for the ankle plantarflexors (Kawakami et al. 2000). No studies have directly compared central fatigue in sustained and intermittent tasks, although holding the muscle ischaemic greatly increases both peripheral and central fatigue (Russ & Kent-Braun 2003).

Central fatigue also occurs with submaximal efforts (Figure 5.4, motor nerve stimulation). For instance, voluntary activation measured from brief MVCs during a sustained submaximal effort shows that central fatigue develops progressively, even in efforts as weak as 15%

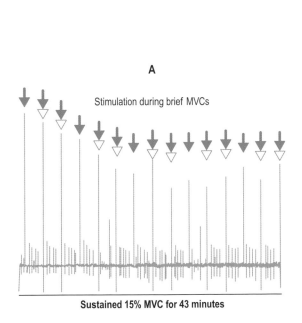

A

Stimulation during brief MVCs

Sustained 15% MVC for 43 minutes

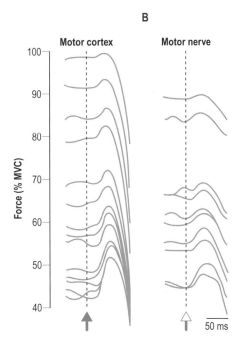

B

Figure 5.4 Central and supraspinal fatigue during a sustained isometric 15% MVC (elbow flexors, one subject). (A) Continuous record of elbow flexor force (target: 15% MVC) held throughout a 43-min trial. Brief maximal voluntary contractions (MVC) were performed at 3 min intervals, with force decline indicating fatigue. Stimuli were delivered to the motor cortex (filled arrows), or to the motor cortex and the motor nerve (open arrows) during each MVC. When motor nerve stimuli were given, a few seconds rest followed the MVC to allow a resting twitch to be evoked. Other stimuli delivered between the MVCs are seen as deviations from 15% MVC force. (B) Left traces show the increments in force (superimposed twitches) evoked by motor cortex stimulation. Their increase as maximal voluntary force falls indicates supraspinal fatigue. Right traces show superimposed twitches evoked by motor nerve stimulation. Their progressive increase indicates central fatigue. Data from Søgaard et al. (2006).

MVC, with substantial falls in voluntary activation (up to 25%; Søgaard et al. 2006). Intermittent submaximal fatiguing protocols sometimes produce falls in voluntary activation, and reports of central fatigue during concentric actions are also variable. It is not clear whether these differences are due to different muscles, different loads, speed of movement or duty cycle. With similar decreases in MVC in the knee extensors, central fatigue was less after concentric than isometric exercise, but was still evident (Babault et al. 2006). Eccentric actions often result in muscle damage as well as fatigue, so that maximal voluntary force can be reduced for days, with voluntary activation lower for up to 24 h, and increased central fatigue during sustained MVCs (Endoh et al. 2005, Prasartwuth et al. 2005).

1.5 Evidence of supraspinal fatigue

1.5.1 Voluntary activation measured with motor cortical stimulation

Transcranial magnetic stimulation over the motor cortex can evoke a short-latency, excitatory response in most muscles. The stimulus activates corticospinal neurons both directly and synaptically, by activation of other cortical neurons. These descending corticospinal volleys activate motoneurons and thus, produce a response in the muscle. The motor response is seen in the electromyogram (motor evoked potential) and is accompanied by a muscle twitch. Under some circumstances, cortical stimulation can elicit a superimposed twitch during voluntary contractions, providing a measure of voluntary activation (Gandevia et al. 1996, Todd et al. 2003). However, a problem with transcranial magnetic stimulation is that the stimulation is not sufficiently focal to activate just one muscle group, so that some antagonist stimulation is likely.

The technique has been best described for the elbow flexors, and is successful because the flexors are more easily activated by cortical stimulation than the extensors and are approximately twice as strong. This minimises the antagonist contribution to the superimposed twitch (Todd et al. 2003). For the elbow flexors, the relationship between increments in force evoked by cortical stimulation and voluntary force is linear for contractions of >50% MVC, but not for weaker contractions, because of lower cortical and motoneuronal excitability (Figure 5.3). Thus, it is not appropriate to calculate voluntary activation by comparing the superimposed twitch to the twitch evoked when the muscle is at rest. This difficulty can be circumvented by extrapolation of the linear regression between the superimposed twitch and voluntary force for contractions >50% MVC to estimate twitch amplitude when force is zero (Todd et al. 2003, 2004). This estimated resting twitch is then used to calculate voluntary activation.

1.5.2 Cortical stimulation during maximal efforts

Voluntary activation measured with motor cortex stimulation is not equivalent to that measured with peripheral stimulation. The occurrence of a superimposed twitch to transcranial magnetic stimulation during a maximal effort implies that some motor cortical output was not sufficient to drive the motoneurons or the muscle maximally, but some output remained untapped by the voluntary effort (Gandevia 2001, Gandevia et al. 1996, Taylor et al. 2006).

It is possible for voluntary activation to be lower when measured with peripheral stimulation than magnetic stimulation. For example, if corticospinal input to the motoneurons is limited by pathology, then peripheral stimulation would show low activation, whereas voluntary activation measured by transcranial stimulation could be high, if no extra corticospinal output was available.

On the contrary, it is theoretically impossible for voluntary activation measured with cortical stimulation to be worse than that measured with motor nerve stimulation, since impairments in voluntary activation shown by the former method are a subset of the latter. In practice, the relationship of voluntary activation to contraction strength is curvilinear for peripheral nerve stimulation, and linear for cortical stimulation, so values derived by these techniques are not easily compared (Taylor et al. 2006, Todd et al. 2003). Superimposed twitches evoked by transcranial magnetic stimulation have been demonstrated in the elbow flexors, elbow extensors and adductor pollicis during brief maxi-mal efforts (Gandevia 2001). This suggests that a supraspinal component to submaximal voluntary activation is common.

1.5.3 Motor cortical stimulation during fatiguing exercise

During fatiguing exercise, maximal voluntary activation measured with transcranial magnetic stimulation declines. Motor cortical output becomes less able to drive the motoneurons and muscles maximally, although there is additional output available that is not employed voluntarily, but can be elicited with transcranial stimulation. This component of central fatigue has been called supraspinal fatigue (Gandevia et al. 1996, Taylor et al. 2006). It has been demonstrated by an increase in the size of the superimposed twitch evoked by cortical stimulation during sustained and intermittent isometric MVCs (elbow flexors), as well as during bouts of maximal concentric and eccentric actions (Gandevia et al. 1996, Löscher & Nordlund 2002, Taylor et al. 2000). Sustained, submaximal isometric contraction also results in progressive supraspinal fatigue, tested during occasional brief MVCs (Figure 5.4; motor cortex; Søgaard et al. 2006). Superimposed twitches, evoked by transcranial and motor nerve stimulation, tend to increase in parallel in fatiguing exercise. However, they differ after eccentric exercise designed to cause muscle damage (Taylor et al. 2006). Because the relationship between voluntary activation measured by cortical stimulation and voluntary force remains linear with fatigue for medium to high contraction strengths, it is possible to estimate the proportion of force loss attributable to supraspinal fatigue (Taylor et al. 2006, Todd et al.

2003; Figure 5.3). This varies from ~25% during a 2 min MVC, to ~40% during a 40 min 15% MVC.

1.6 Effects of fatigue at the spinal level

As discussed above, motor unit firing rates decrease during fatiguing MVCs. This reduction is more than required to match changing contractile properties of the muscle, as is shown by the progressive failure of voluntary activation. Motor unit firing rates depend on motoneuron properties, and on the excitatory and inhibitory inputs to the motoneurons. These inputs include descending drive, recurrent inhibition and afferent feedback from the periphery. During fatiguing exercise, all of these can change and influence motor unit firing rates (Gandevia 2001).

1.6.1 Intrinsic properties of motoneurons

Motoneurons fire repetitively when their cell bodies are stimulated with a maintained current. However, over a period of constant stimulation, some motoneurons stop firing and others slow their firing rates (Spielmann et al. 1993). This process is known as late adaptation, and is more pronounced in larger, higher-threshold motoneurons. After current injection, the motoneurons recover quickly (~2 min rest). Evidence of adaptation to synaptic inputs is less clear. In humans, when the firing rates of targeted single motor units are maintained voluntarily for 10 min, additional motor units are recruited. This implies that subjects increase descending drive to maintain the firing rate of the target unit, which has become less responsive during repetitive activation; this is consistent with adaptation (Johnson et al. 2004).

1.6.2 Recurrent inhibition

Renshaw cells in the spinal cord are excited by the firing of motoneurons via collateral axon branches. They inhibit the motoneurons (recurrent inhibition) and could slow motor unit firing. However, the role of recurrent inhibition in the control of motoneuron firing rates in fatigue remains unclear. In humans, it may be decreased during sustained submaximal contractions but increased during MVCs. With experimental activation of muscle nociceptors, rather than physiological activation by fatigue, recurrent inhibition is increased in humans but decreased in animal studies.

1.6.3 Influence of sensory input

The afferents most likely to change during fatiguing exercise, and thus contribute to central fatigue, are those in the muscle. These include muscle spindle afferents (group Ia and II), Golgi tendon organ afferents (group Ib), group II and III afferents (mechanically sensitive) and group III and IV afferents (chemically sensitive or respond to noxious mechanical events).

During voluntary efforts, muscle spindle afferents provide excitatory input to homonymous motoneurons through oligosynaptic pathways. Thus, decreased spindle input could slow motor unit firing rates. With maintained actions, spindle afferent firing falls (Macefield et al. 1991). In addition, presynaptic inhibition of Ia afferents by group III and IV afferents, or by homosynaptic depression, may also decrease the excitatory support of spindle afferents to the motoneurons (Pettorossi et al. 1999). Golgi tendon organs, which signal muscle force, are unlikely to contribute to motoneuron slowing, as their inhibition to the contracting muscle is reduced during sustained voluntary contractions (Zytnicki et al. 1990).

Mechanically sensitive, non-spindle muscle afferents (groups II and III) fire with muscle action, stretch and non-noxious pressure, whereas other group III and group IV afferents fire with noxious pressure or with chemical stimulation (e.g. potassium, lactic acid, bradykinin, arachidonic acid and adenosine triphosphate (Kaufman et al. 2002). The firing of both types of afferents is enhanced by ischaemia, and both mediate cardiovascular reflex responses to exercise (Chapter 1). During contractions, mechanically sensitive afferents fire initially whereas the group IV afferents fire later as metabolites accumulate (Kaufman et al. 2002).

The hypothesis that small-diameter muscle afferents inhibit motoneurons during fatigue is supported by human studies, in which muscles were maintained ischaemic at the end of a fatiguing contraction (Figure 5.2, Woods et al. 1987). In this condition, motor unit firing rates during MVCs remain low. This strongly indicates that feedback from the muscle is responsible for low motor unit firing rates in fatigue, and the most likely candidates are the small-diameter afferents. However, animal studies show that group III and IV muscle afferents have mixed effects on motoneurons. They tend to inhibit extensor motoneurons but excite the flexors. Humans also show inhibition of the extensors, but excitation of the flexors for muscles about the elbow (Martin et al. 2006). Thus, small-diameter muscle afferents may contribute to the inhibition of motoneurons in some muscles but not in others.

1.6.4 Descending drive

The demonstration of supraspinal fatigue with motor cortical stimulation indicates that descending drive from the motor cortex becomes suboptimal during fatigue (Gandevia et al. 1996, Taylor et al. 2006). However, it does not provide a measure of whether the absolute level of descending drive has changed; this is discussed below.

In summary, during isometric fatiguing exercise, repetitive activation alters the intrinsic properties of motoneurons so that they are less responsive to input. Small-diameter muscle afferents may inhibit some motoneuron pools and excite others, and excitatory drive from muscle spindle afferents falls. Descending drive becomes suboptimal. Decreased excitation, increased inhibition or altered intrinsic properties could all slow motor unit firing. However, when motoneuron excitability is tested by stimulation of the corticospinal tract during sustained MVCs, the size of the evoked muscle response falls with fatigue (Butler et al. 2003). This is consistent with effective inhibition of motoneurons, rather than a decrease of excitatory drive alone. In the elbow flexors, the maintained firing of small-diameter muscle afferents by muscle ischaemia does not prevent recovery of the response (Butler et al. 2003). Thus, by exclusion, changes in intrinsic motoneuron properties with repetitive activation are likely to be an important contributor to decreased motoneuron excitability, and a slowing of firing rates during fatigue.

1.7 Effects of fatigue at the motor cortex

Firing of neurons in the primary motor cortex tends to increase with the force of muscle action, although this is not a simple relationship (Ashe 1997). Imaging shows that motor cortex activity increases during fatiguing tasks in which submaximal target forces are maintained (Liu et al. 2003), whereas activity first increases but then decreases during sustained maximal efforts. Although this finding suggests a late decrease in descending drive which could contribute to central fatigue, these signals represent not only motor activity, but also sensory input and its processing, as well as cardiorespiratory responses to exercise, and are difficult to interpret. With similar fatigue produced by intermittent MVCs motor cortical activity does not change significantly, although supraspinal fatigue is likely to be present (Liu et al. 2005, Taylor et al. 2000).

1.7.1 Responses to cortical stimulation

Changes in the electromyographic responses to transcranial magnetic stimulation have been observed with muscle fatigue (Taylor & Gandevia 2001). During submaximal fatiguing contractions, the motor evoked potential increases in size as more motor units are recruited to maintain a target force. This is consistent with increased cortical and motoneuronal excitability with increases in voluntary activity. During fatiguing MVCs, the motor evoked potential also increases in size but responses to subcortical stimulation are reduced (Butler et al. 2003, Taylor et al. 1996). Thus, the increase represents extra output evoked from the cortex and implies increased motor cortical excitability. However, transcranial magnetic stimulation activates inhibitory neurons in the cortex concurrently with excitatory neurons and the silent period, an inhibitory response that follows the motor evoked potential, increases in duration, and suggests increased intracortical inhibition during fatiguing MVCs. In contrast, a different measure of intracortical inhibition, tested with paired-pulse transcranial magnetic stimulation in short breaks between fatiguing contractions, decreases with fatigue (Benwell et al. 2006, Maruyama et al. 2006). These changes appear not to contribute directly to central fatigue, as the altered electromyographic responses can be dissociated from voluntary activation in a number of circumstances (Gandevia et al. 1996, Søgaard et al. 2006).

There are also changes in motor evoked potentials when the muscle is at rest after exercise. Potentials are initially facilitated and then depressed. Postcontraction depression can last for >60 min, and its duration is related to the intensity and duration of the preceding exercise. Again, there is no clear functional consequence of the depression. Motor evoked potentials are not depressed if measured during a weak contraction and dexterity is not impaired (Humphry et al. 2004, Lazarski et al. 2002).

1.7.2 Influence of sensory input

As discussed above, sensory feedback from contracting muscle changes during the development of fatigue, and these changes depend on the type of exercise. Muscle spindle afferents have an excitatory influence on the motor cortex (e.g. Stuart et al. 2002). Therefore, falls in muscle spindle firing during sustained isometric contractions are likely to reduce excitatory drive to the motor cortex. Effects of small-diameter muscle afferents have been investigated through intramuscular injection of hypertonic saline, which causes muscle pain. A reduction in motor evoked potentials in the resting muscle indicates decreased motor cortical excitability, although motoneuron excitability is also reduced (Le Pera et al. 2001, Svensson et al. 2003). Motor evoked potentials were not changed during voluntary contraction (Romaniello et al. 2000), but experimental muscle pain can reduce maximal voluntary force (Graven-Nielsen et al. 1997). Similarly, when the firing of small-diameter muscle afferents is maintained by muscle ischaemia at the end of a fatiguing contraction, voluntary activation measured by transcranial magnetic stimulation remains reduced, although motor evoked potentials and the silent period recover (Gandevia et al. 1996). Thus, it seems likely that small-diameter muscle afferents have a role in supraspinal fatigue.

In summary, although descending drive from the motor cortex becomes suboptimal during fatigue, the level of drive cannot be easily measured. That is, drive could increase during fatigue, but still be inadequate due to other changes at a spinal level. Changes in excitability and intracortical inhibition of the motor cortex are associated with fatiguing contractions, but do not directly contribute to supraspinal fatigue.

1.8 Other influences on central fatigue

1.8.1 Exercise of another muscle

Fatiguing voluntary efforts on one side can alter voluntary activation of homologous muscles on the other side of the body. This crossover of central fatigue is small for muscles of the upper limb (Zijdewind et al. 1998), but is more significant in the leg (Rattey et al. 2005). Transcranial magnetic stimulation has shown some evidence of changes in the ipsilateral cortex following fatiguing exercise, with effects confined to the muscle homologous to that fatigued (Humphry et al. 2004). Within a limb, exercise of biceps that produced altered responses to transcranial stimulation did not produce similar changes in hand muscles (Humphry et al. 2004, Taylor et al. 1996). However, voluntary activation of quadriceps is reduced by fatigue of back muscles (Hart et al. 2006).

1.8.2 Combined motor and cognitive tasks

When a cognitive task is performed at the same time as a motor task, the effect on the cognitive task depends on the type and level of exercise (Tomporowski 2003). With exercise to exhaustion, performance on most cognitive tasks becomes impaired. Moderate exercise improves some cognitive tasks (e.g. reaction time, visual recognition), but decreases performance in others. With isometric action of hand muscles, speed and accuracy in a choice reaction time task performed with the other hand are impaired (Lorist et al. 2002, Zijdewind et al. 2006). Impairment is greater with a stronger effort, but is even worse if the contracting hand is fatigued. Thus, muscle fatigue may influence cognitive performance (Lorist et al. 2002). In the same task, variability of force production in the sustained effort was increased compared to when it was performed alone, but endurance time was not altered. This implies that increased cognitive demands can impair motor performance but may not alter central fatigue.

1.8.3 Whole–body exercise

During whole-body exercise, performance is constrained by systemic factors which do not apply in single-limb exercise. These include cardiovascular and respiratory limits, as well as temperature, fluid and fuel regulation (Chapters 1, 2, 6, 7, 10.1 and 19). The exact nature of the exercise determines how each of these factors interacts with muscle fatigue and leads to cessation of exercise. Central fatigue has been demonstrated by stimulation of the knee extensors during isometric MVCs after running, cycling and skiing (Millet & Lepers 2004). It did not depend on the duration of the exercise, but was more pronounced when subjects exercised to exhaustion.

With exercise in temperate conditions, fatigue is not seen in muscles that did not exercise. For example, handgrip is unaffected after running (Seaward & Clarke 1992). Thus, even with whole-body exercise, central fatigue is not necessarily generalised. However, for exercise-induced or passive hyperthermia, unexercised muscles show impaired voluntary activation, if activated for more than a few seconds (Nybo & Secher 2004). Thus, a high core temperature can contribute to increased central fatigue (Chapter 27.2).

Comparison of arterial and venous concentrations shows that the brain extracts more oxygen, glucose and lactate from the blood during intense exercise (Dalsgaard 2005, Nybo & Secher 2004). That is, the metabolic activity of the brain is increased. If subjects become hypoglycaemic during prolonged submaximal whole-body exercise, a fall in glucose utilisation by the brain indicates that its metabolic activity decreases. In this condition, subjects show greater failure of voluntary activation during a sustained MVC. Thus, inadequate substrate for maintained firing of neurons may contribute to central fatigue in some circumstances.

A role in central fatigue has been proposed for the serotonergic system, which mediates functions such as arousal, temperature regulation, activation of the hypothalamic-pituitary axis, and has descending effects on motoneurons. Cerebral levels of serotonin are increased with exercise, and it is suggested this may play a part in fatigue. In animals, pharmacological interventions show that high levels of serotonin reduce endurance time. In humans, some studies have shown that serotonin reuptake inhibitors increase perceived effort and decrease endurance time, but others have not reproduced this effect (Newsholme & Blomstrand 2006). Furthermore, the links between exercise and increased serotonin synthesis are doubtful (Fernstrom & Fernstrom 2006).

Other potential factors that may contribute to altered brain function and fatigue during exercise include monoamines, cytokines, endogenous opioids, ammonia and glutamine (Nybo & Secher 2004). However, it is not clear what interaction there is between the changes associated with prolonged whole-body exercise and the progressive failure of voluntary activation that defines central fatigue in single-limb voluntary efforts, and which can occur with maximal actions sustained over short time periods, or with weak actions sustained for many minutes.

1.9 Summary and conclusions

Fatiguing maximal and submaximal isometric voluntary actions of a single muscle group result in a progressive failure of the ability of the nervous system to drive muscles maximally. Motoneuron adaptation to repetitive activation probably decreases their response to synaptic input. Decreased muscle spindle feedback and increased small-diameter muscle afferent input may also contribute to slowing of motoneuron firing rates. Stimulation of the motor cortex shows that descending drive becomes suboptimal. Changes in afferent feedback alter excitability of the motor cortex and may act on circuits that generate motor cortical output to impair voluntary activation. Systemic changes associated with whole-body exercise can increase central fatigue, but are not necessary for the occurrence of central or supraspinal fatigue. In sustained maximal and submaximal isometric actions involving a single limb, central fatigue can account for 25–40% of the loss of force.

2 NEUROMUSCULAR FATIGUE OF EXHAUSTIVE STRETCH–SHORTENING CYCLE EXERCISE

2.1 Introduction

In Chapter 4, the basic concepts of muscle function were introduced, including the stretch–shortening cycle, a natural form of muscle function. This information is also important for understanding the complexity of neuromuscular fatigue, when studied in natural conditions. The mechanisms of muscle fatigue examined in the preceding section and

Chapter 6 are pertinent to fatigue during exhaustive stretch–shortening cycle activities. However, the latter form of fatigue has many unique features, and these are the emphasis of this section.

2.2 Basic concepts

2.2.1 Stretch–shortening cycle versus pure eccentric and concentric actions

The stretch–shortening cycle is a series of consecutive muscle actions (Figure 5.5), commencing with preactivation (100–200 ms prior to ground contact). The preactivation amplitude is a function of both the expected impact load, with a positive relationship observed between running velocity and gastrocnemius preactivation (Komi et al. 1987a,b), and the rebound intensity (Chapter 4). The greatest electromyographic activity is, however, measured during the braking phase, with some muscles experiencing eccentric action. The final functional (push-off) phase is usually performed through concentric activation but with very low electromyographic activity. The nature of this phase resembles a recoil action, resulting in low metabolic activity but high mechanical efficiency (Chapter 4). In the legs, running, jumping and hopping are typical examples of stretch–shortening cycle actions.

With regard to fatigue, one can easily see that the loading characteristics are clearly different from isolated isometric, concentric or eccentric actions. Indeed, the stretch–shortening cycle is characterised by high impact forces that are often repeated over long durations (e.g. >20,000 ground contacts during marathon running). These impact loads (braking forces) are accompanied by loading of the reflexes that are involved in both length-feedback (muscle spindles) and force-feedback (Golgi tendon organs) control of muscular forces. In addition, and in common with isolated concentric and eccentric actions, the stretch–shortening cycle stresses skeletal muscle metabolically. The magnitude of metabolic stress is dependent on the velocity of stretch (eccentric), and the coupling time between stretch and shortening (concentric phase).

2.2.2 Can stretch reflexes play a role in stretch–shortening cycle exercise?

Stretch reflexes are sensitive to exhaustive stretch–shortening cycle fatigue. The functional significance of this sensitivity depends on whether stretch reflexes are operative, and functionally meaningful, in stretch–shortening cycle activities. In normal movements with high electromyographic activity, the magnitude and net contribution of reflex regulation of muscle force are difficult to assess.

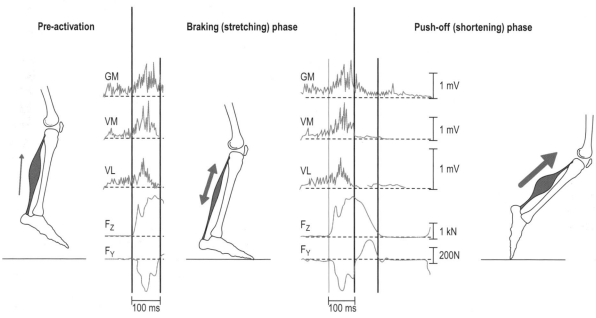

Figure 5.5 The stretch–shortening cycle during the functional contact phase of running, illustrating simultaneously recorded vertical (F_z) and horizontal (F_y) ground reaction forces, together with electromyographic activities of gastrocnemius medialis (GM), vastus medialis (VM) and lateralis (VL) muscles. The large arrow indicates ground contact, and vertical lines denote the end of braking and push-off phases, respectively. Note gastrocnemius medialis shows high preactivation, with all muscles showing low activity during push-off. Data from Mero & Komi (1986).

The task becomes much easier when studying relatively slow passive dorsiflexions, where stretch reflex-induced force enhancement is reportedly 200–500% greater than in the pure passive force (Nicol & Komi 1998, Nicol et al. 2003). These measurements also revealed electromechanical delays of 10–12 ms, providing a rational basis for calculating whether there is sufficient time for stretch reflexes to be activated. Since the duration of a simple stretch reflex loop is 40 ms, the maximum delay between the initial stretch and subsequent reflex-induced force potentiation would be ~50–55 ms. In running, the first ground contact indicates the initial stretch, with contact times ranging between 90–100 ms (sprinting) and ~250 ms (marathon running; Mero & Komi 1986). The duration of the braking and push-off phases decreases with increasing running speed. The stretch reflex contribution will then occur at the end of the braking phase for slow running, but may extend to the push-off phase during sprinting. These calculations confirm that there is ample time for stretch reflexes to be instrumental in force and power enhancement, and to play a significant role in human locomotion. Accordingly, reflex responses have been observed in numerous studies for several muscles (Komi & Gollhofer 1997).

Thus, it seems the muscle stretch is powerful enough to induce sufficient muscle spindle afferent activation. This is illustrated in Figure 4.7 of Chapter 4. If spindle activation occurs, then stretch reflexes contribute to the motor output by making the push-off phase more powerful. This can facilitate an immediate and smooth transition from the pre-activated and eccentrically stretched muscle–tendon unit to the concentric push-off. However, to confirm the role of the stretch reflex in force and power enhancement, it must be demonstrated that the fascicles are actually stretched during the braking phase of the cycle.

Ultrasonography has been successfully used to show the gastrocnemius fascicles are stretched for a short time, immediately upon ground contact (Ishikawa et al. 2006). This muscle was thought to demonstrate fascicle shortening during braking (Fukunaga et al. 2001), based on measurements of relatively low (40–50 Hz) image frequency. However, Ishikawa et al. (2006b) used higher frequency sampling (96 Hz) and observed the early appearance of fascicle lengthening (Figure 5.6).

2.3 Stretch–shortening cycle fatigue

What do these observations mean with regard to fatigue? They can be considered not only as basic phenomena but also as opportunities to examine parameters of stretch–shortening cycle fatigue. In such fatigue, the impact loads are repeated over time, stressing the metabolic, mechanical and neural components. However, it is the stretch–shortening cycle fatigue model in particular that causes disturbances in stretch-reflex activation and, consequently, provides an excellent basis for studying neuromuscular adaptation to exhaustive exercise. Due to the complex

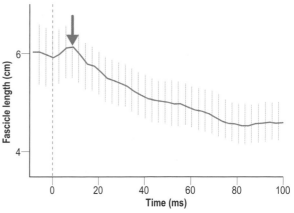

Figure 5.6 Average gastrocnemius fascicle length at a running velocity of 2.7 m.s^{-1} ($N = 7$), captured using B-mode ultrasonography (96 Hz). The dashed vertical line denotes the beginning of the ground contact. The arrow indicates the end of the fascicle stretch following the contact. This is believed to trigger a stretch-reflex. During the remaining ground contact, the fascicles shorten. Redrawn from Ishikawa et al. (2006) with permission.

nature of this type of fatigue, however, its definition is quite problematic.

Researchers are generally in agreement about the definition of fatigue during isometric or concentric exercises, although Gandevia (2001) has raised concerns about the accuracy of the various ways to define fatigue. We would suggest that, for the complex nature of stretch–shortening cycle fatigue, the definition of Asmussen (1979) may be applicable. This is based on a decreased muscle performance capacity, which is generally evident from a failure to maintain (or develop) a target force. We would add that, for stretch–shortening cycle fatigue, the performance decrement typically lasts for a few days and is bimodal in nature, with both large acute and delayed functional decrements. For such fatigue to develop, the individual must attain exhaustion, resulting in an inability to perform (or maintain) a stretch–shortening cycle task due to the associated muscle fatigue (Chapter 6).

2.3.1 Stretch–shortening cycle fatigue models and basic responses

There are several models for studying exhaustive stretch–shortening cycle exercise (Figure 5.7). For example, a sledge ergometer developed in our laboratory (Kaneko et al. 1984, Komi et al. 1987b) has been used to perform short-term, stretch–shortening exercises to induce fatigue in either the arms (Gollhofer et al. 1987ab) or legs (Nicol et al. 1996b). Another possibility is to use a longer-term exercise (marathon running) as the fatigue model. In these different models, exhaustion varies between 3 min and 3 h, with

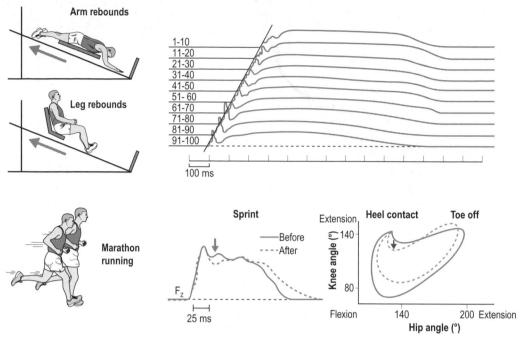

Figure 5.7 Schematic of the progression of stretch–shortening cycle fatigue induced by sledge rebound exercises (arms: Gollhofer et al. 1987b, legs: Nicol et al. 1996a) and marathon running (Nicol et al. 1991a,b). The force plate records in arm exercise (averaged over 10 successive contacts) show progressive increases in the impact peak and contact time. Marathon running shows a clear drop in peak force of the sprint force-time curve (Nicol et al. 1991a). The lower right graph shows the knee angle/hip angle diagram (Nicol et al. 1991b), demonstrating an increased knee flexion immediately after ground contact in the postmarathon situation.

fatigue development being progressive yet individual, with its timing being exercise mode dependent.

Disturbances in submaximal running kinematics and reduced running economy are not revealed with previous methods (Ftaiti et al. 2001, Kyröläinen et al. 2000, Nicol et al. 1991b). However, progressive development of contractile failure can be demonstrated using electromyographic analysis, even in submaximal running (Kyröläinen et al. 2001) and jumping (Regueme et al. 2005). For example, in marathon running (Nicol et al. 1991b), gait remains unchanged despite increased electromyographic activity of the leg extensors during the braking and push-off phases. Only in subjects with >40% reduction in knee extensor force production is there a clear gait modification. As fatigue progresses, electromyographic or joint kinematic changes occur during the preactivation phase, influencing the regulation of postlanding stiffness. This is usually associated with an increased ground impact force, possibly leading to a vicious circle through a reduced tolerance to stretch, resulting in a loss of elastic recoil and increased work during the push-off phase. Depending upon exercise intensity, this additional work may progressively reduce the capacity to maintain the task.

Figure 5.7 provides an example in which 100 stretch–shortening cycle repetitions (arm rebounding) were characterised by a gradual increase in the contact time of both the braking and push-off phases. There is also a progressive increase in the impact force and a decrease in the postimpact force. Similar observations have been reported in a maximal sprint test after a marathon run, with evidence indicating that changes in ground contact force are associated with problems in maintaining constant angular displacement during contact as fatigue progresses.

2.4 Bimodality of the stretch–shortening cycle fatigue response

Stretch–shortening cycle fatigue is usually associated with large acute and delayed changes in muscle mechanics and neuromuscular activation that may significantly influence the regulation of joint and muscle stiffness. Nicol et al. (2006) found that ~50% of studies of stretch–shortening cycle fatigue concentrated on the acute recovery phase (up to 2 h after exercise), whereas the others extended the investigation to the delayed recovery phase (up to 7 d). The longer recovery follow-up is important, as it reveals that fatigue-induced performance deterioration, and subsequent recovery, is a long process that usually occurs in a bimodal fashion. The delayed recovery phase is typically associated with delayed-onset muscle soreness.

However, delayed-onset muscle soreness related to stretch–shortening cycle fatigue disappears a few days prior to complete structural and functional recovery. It cannot therefore be used to reflect detailed recovery processes. Such muscle soreness has also been studied during eccentric fatigue (Clarkson & Newham 1995), which has helped development of several mechanistic explanations of stretch–shortening cycle fatigue and its recovery, with studies supporting the bimodal recovery concept (Faulkner et al. 1993, Komi 2000, MacIntyre et al. 1995).

This bimodality is characterised by an acute, primarily metabolically induced reduction in neuromuscular function, followed after a few hours by a short-term (fast) recovery, which is in turn followed by a secondary functional reduction with a slow recovery. However, this pattern is not always evident, especially if the fatigue protocol is not exhaustive. Consequently, fatigue protocols that use a fixed exercise duration may not reveal the true effects of stretch–shortening cycle fatigue, and differences in the type and intensity of the exercise may also affect data interpretation. In addition, since this bimodal pattern is widely variable among individuals, group-averaged changes may not always reveal meaningful fatigue patterns (Nicol et al. 2006).

2.4.1 Parallelism between mechanical and neural changes

Asmussen (1979) was among the first to suggest that fatigue-induced changes occur in parallel between mechanical and neural factors, and the results of stretch–shortening cycle fatigue studies confirm this interrelationship, revealing bimodal trends for both mechanical and neural indices. In fact, there is enough evidence to consider this interaction as neural mechanisms that compensate for contractile failure or protect fatigued muscles.

Neuromuscular fatigue induced by stretch–shortening cycle exercise has often been quantified using isometric MVC tests, with simultaneous recording of electromyographic activity (Nicol et al. 2006). Figure 5.8A illustrates the acute fatigue response, which is characterised by an immediate drop in both indices followed by a prolonged recovery period (Figure 5.8B).

Although maximal isometric tests often reveal the effects of stretch–shortening cycle fatigue, maximal dynamic tests seem more meaningful mechanistically. In dynamic tests involving slight or no ground impact, such as counter movements or squat jumps, no significant change is usually observed after fatigue. However, when those tests are maximal and involve high ground impact forces, significant acute (Nicol et al. 1991a) and delayed (Horita et al. 2003) reductions in performance have been reported. In these maximal situations, where stretch loads are high and muscle stiffness must be well regulated to meet the external loads, the decline in performance is typically characterised by a loss of resistance to impact (peak force reduction after impact; Avela et al. 1999). This is associated with clear electromyographic reductions during both the centrally programmed preactivation phase and the subsequent braking phase. Simultaneous reductions in the short-latency, stretch-reflex response imply that the electromyographic changes are both central and reflex in nature (Figure 5.9A).

These observations point to the existence of neural attempts to protect fatigued muscle in maximal stretch–shortening cycle testing conditions. They also support the findings of Gollhofer et al. (1987a) in arm muscles that protective neural mechanisms (reduced short-, medium- and long-latency components of the stretch reflex) only take place in the most extreme testing conditions. Supporting

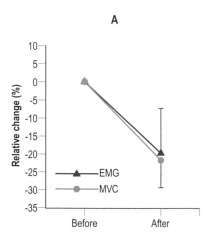

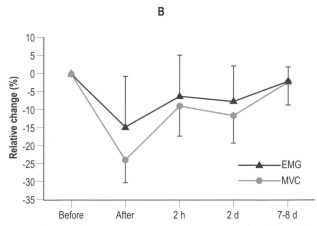

Figure 5.8 (A) Acute (relative) decrements in voluntary electromyographic (EMG) and maximal voluntary isometric force (MVC) following fatiguing stretch–shortening cycle exercise. Data compiled from 15 published articles using either knee extensor or plantarflexor muscles. (B) Acute and delayed changes in the same variables reported in seven studies. Note the bimodal recovery trends.

A

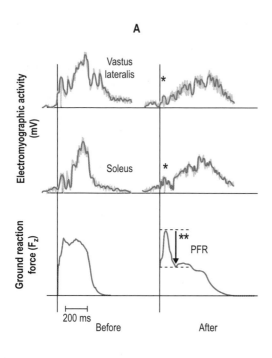

B

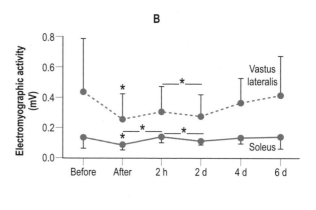

C

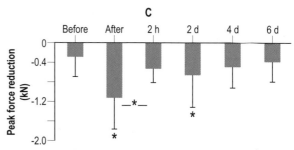

Figure 5.9 (A) Bimodal recovery of electromyographic activity and vertical ground reaction force over time, during 10 successive sledge rebounds performed before and after marathon running ($N = 7$). (B) Corresponding active short-latency reflex component of electromyographic activity. (C) Postlanding stiffness regulation as reflected by peak force reduction measured from ground reaction forces. Adapted from Avela et al. (1999) with permission.

the functional role of a prolonged reduction in the short-latency, stretch-reflex response, Avela et al. (1999) showed a parallel in bimodal changes between this reflex response and the ability to withstand high ground impact loads (Figure 5.9B). Nicol et al. (1996a), and more recently Dousset et al. (2007), were also able to show that the Hoffman reflex (H reflex), which is used to measure the level of spinal excitability, demonstrated a bimodal recovery pattern after similar exhaustive exercise. Avela et al. (1999) observed an acute reduction in the H/M-wave ratio, but with no secondary decline.

Bimodal recovery of the mechanical reflex response has also been reported when tested in passive stretch conditions after both short-term (sledge exercise) and long-term (10 km run) fatiguing exercise (Nicol et al. 2003). In the delayed recovery phase, the amplitude of reflex electromyographic activity induced by passive stretch showed a positive relationship with the corresponding mechanical response. This was reflected in the peak and mean torques, and the rate of relaxation. This implies that the electromyographic/force ratio could be maintained to a large degree during the 2–7 day recovery.

These observations are in agreement with the original suggestions of Asmussen (1979), and exemplify how changes in mechanical and neural indices occur in parallel

after exhaustive stretch–shortening cycle exercise. This parallelism during fatigue and recovery points to a coupling of the neural and mechanical factors. It must not be interpreted to mean that the fatigue response and subsequent recovery have a generalised, fixed pattern, since their time courses are very individual.

Nicol et al. (2003) and Kuitunen et al. (2004) have recently demonstrated great individual differences in the magnitude of changes in these variables, with some people only showing acute fatigue changes. Part of the reason for these individual differences lies in the difficulty in obtaining a sufficient number of measurement points to characterise the recovery profile for each person. Another reason is related to the problem of selecting the fatigue protocol such that each subject is loaded and exhausted similarly.

2.4.2 Fascicle–tendon interaction during stretch–shortening cycle fatigue

The stretch–shortening cycle refers to the entire muscle–tendon unit. However, recent studies using ultrasonography during different exercises have questioned the applicability of this definition to the fascicles and tendinous tissue (e.g. Ishikawa et al. 2007). It is usually monoarticular muscles (e.g. soleus, vastus lateralis) that demonstrate stretch–shortening cycle behaviour of the fascicles, similar to that of the muscle–tendon unit. Biarticular muscles (e.g. gastrocnemius) may exhibit more complex fascicle–tendon interactions, in some situations demonstrating fascicle lengthening in the early braking phase of ground contact.

Although the literature is not very comprehensive on this matter, the following observations have emerged (Asmussen 1979, Ishikawa et al. 2006). First, fascicle–tendon interaction is muscle specific for given stretch–shortening cycle tasks. Second, it is the impact load that determines fascicle behaviour (shortening or lengthening) in a muscle. Third, rebound intensity (submaximal versus maximal) after the braking phase has some influence on fascicle–tendon interaction by affecting tendon recoil in the final push-off phase. Future studies should continue to explore these problems so that fascicle–tendon interaction becomes better understood, as it plays an integral role in muscle stiffness regulation during locomotion.

These observations indicate that fascicle and tendon lengths (and related measures) are sensitive to stretch–shortening cycle fatigue, especially due to the repeated impact nature of such exercise. However, since only one study has examined this fascicle–tendon interaction (Ishikawa et al. 2007), it is too early to make generalisations. Nevertheless, this study was unable to confirm the existence of bimodality in fascicle variables after exhaustive exercise.

2.5 Potential mechanisms

The bimodal nature of fatigue recovery can be considered a characteristic of exhaustive stretch–shortening cycle exercise. However, the challenge lies in finding the underlying mechanisms of this process. Presumably, these involve both central and peripheral fatigue mechanisms, and should differ between the acute (<2 h) and delayed recovery phases.

In the acute phase, the easiest explanation for recovery could be that it follows metabolic recovery. That is, it is thought to be caused by the accumulation or depletion of metabolites or ions, either intra- or extracellularly (Chapter 6). It is noteworthy that none of the stretch–shortening studies have reported significant links between the exercise-induced metabolic and neuromuscular changes. We will thus concentrate on muscle damage, which is known to be involved in the other causes of force decline after repeated eccentric and stretch–shortening actions.

The second (delayed) and perhaps the more relevant recovery phase is usually related to the natural time course of inflammatory and remodelling processes related to muscle damage. This phase usually lasts for a few days and is associated with delayed-onset muscle soreness. However, it is noticeable that muscle soreness disappears before functional recovery is complete. This observation in particular raises interest regarding the potential effect of various parameters during the recovery period.

2.5.1 Potential influences of extra- and intrafusal muscle fibre damage, inflammation and remodelling

Long-lasting but reversible ultrastructural muscle damage is frequently reported after eccentric muscle actions (Lieber et al. 2002). Damage is evident from histological analysis, and indirectly from reductions in strength and range of motion, as increased plasma concentration of soluble muscle proteins (Nosaka & Clarkson 1996). However, these indirect indicators of muscle damage do not accurately reflect the magnitude of muscle damage. This is particularly true for serum creatine kinase activity (Fridén & Lieber 2001a).

The associated shift in the active length–tension relationship after eccentric fatigue (Jones et al. 1997, Komi & Rusko 1974) has been considered as one of the most reliable indicators of muscle damage (Whitehead et al. 2001). The shift of the peak of the length–tension relation has also been reported to contribute to the decline in force at the original optimum length (Brockett et al. 2001, Wood et al. 1993). There is no reason to doubt that this would also occur in the case of stretch–shortening cycle fatigue (Ishikawa et al. 2007).

It seems that the induced ultrastructural muscle damage is very small and localised, and differs in severity among muscles, depending upon their architecture and muscle fibre composition (Fridén & Lieber 2001b). In humans, fast-twitch fibres are considered to be more sensitive to damage than slow-twitch fibres (Fridén & Lieber 2001b, Fridén et al. 1983). Furthermore, fast-twitch fibres possess a reduced oxidative capacity, which is believed to result in failure of cross-bridge detachment during intensive exercise, thus leading to an inhomogeneous resistance to stretch among sarcomeres and muscle fibres (Fridén & Lieber 1992).

During intensive stretch–shortening cycle exercise, this would imply that local acidosis could favour the rapid development of sarcomere inhomogeneity, and enhance the damaging effect of the repeated impact loads. Although there is a lack of research in this area, it seems that the intersubject variability is quite large in the delayed functional decrements (Nicol et al. 2003, 2006). As illustrated by the protective effect of previous eccentric work (Nosaka et al. 2005), the training status of the subjects is also expected to play a major role in exercise-induced muscle damage.

With regard to the progressive ultrastructural changes, it is well documented that cytoskeletal and myofibrillar abnormalities are lower immediately after exercise, relative to those observed 2–3 days later (Newham et al. 1983a). After a marathon run, Hikida et al. (1983) demonstrated significant ultrastructural changes that peaked on days one and three, with some lasting until day seven. These observations are well supported by the rapid functional recovery, usually observed 1–2 h after exercise, followed by a secondary decline 1–2 days later. Interestingly, serum creatine kinase activity appears to be an indirect indicator of either fast- or slow-recovering subjects (Nicol et al. 2003). This is in line with our earlier findings relative to neuromuscular changes (Avela et al. 1999, Horita et al. 1999, Kyröläinen et al. 1998, Nicol et al. 2003). It is suggested that relative changes in serum creatine kinase may help to detect tissue inflammation and associated functional defects. Other indicators of exercise-induced inflammation include delayed changes in muscle stiffness and thickness, as well as delayed-onset muscle soreness.

The existence of the inflammatory model in purely eccentric fatigue has recently been challenged. Convincing evidence has been produced for a remodelling theory (Yu et al. 2003) that would explain the release of α-actinin, titin and nebulin, and most likely also some Z-disk and I-band associated proteins, in the early recovery phase. Provided that mechanical coupling does exist between extra- and intrafusal fibres, this finding may provide evidence to support the possibility of disturbances in the intrafusal fibres themselves. Leading to reduced muscle spindle sensitivity, this could contribute to the immediate reductions of both stretch-reflex sensitivity and the electromyographic response (Nicol et al. 1996b). According to Gregory et al. (2004), however, intrafusal fibres are not prone to damage of the kind seen in extrafusal fibres after eccentric work. Whether this notion applies to stretch–shortening cycle fatigue that involves much higher impact (stretch) loads than pure eccentric exercise remains to be seen.

Finally, muscle damage may be expected to have potential effects on neuromuscular transmission, action potential conduction along muscle fibres and excitation–contraction coupling (Warren et al. 2001). However, fatiguing stretch–shortening cycle exercises have not been studied extensively enough regarding this particular problem. For example, in the acute recovery phase, the reported effects are contradictory, both on the maximal M-wave and on low-frequency fatigue (Kuitunen et al. 2004, Martin et al. 2004, Millet et al. 2002, 2003, Place et al. 2004). Moreover, data concerning the delayed recovery phase are lacking, as only a few studies have examined these indices (i.e. Kuitunen et al. 2004, Martin et al. 2004). However, this should not be interpreted to mean that peripheral impairments are not important during stretch–shortening cycle fatigue.

2.5.2 Stiffness and thickness of the muscle–tendon unit

It is well known that, with pure eccentric fatigue, muscle volume increases after exercise (Howell et al. 1993, Murayama et al. 2000). This can be caused, among other things, by increased internal fluid pressure due to swelling (Crenshaw et al. 1994). However, swelling and stiffness do not change in parallel (Chleboun et al. 1998), and Ishikawa et al. (2006a) demonstrated this using ultrasound scanning following fatiguing exercise (Figure 5.10). Thus, if resis-

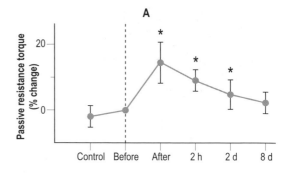

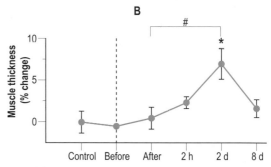

Figure 5.10 (A) Passive resistance of plantarflexors to dorsiflexion torque (relative to 'Before') measured during recovery from exhaustive stretch–shortening cycle exercise. (B) Changes in muscle thickness (triceps surae; relative to 'Before'). Note the peaks of the two curves occur at different times. Adapted from Ishikawa et al. (2006) with permission.

tance is measured in the resting situation, it may not necessarily reveal when the peak of muscle swelling occurs, with peaks for passive resistance to stretch and muscle thickness occurring immediately after, and 2 days after exercise (respectively). Note that the passive resistance to stretch remained elevated, even 2 days after exercise.

In the case of damaged elbow flexors due to eccentric fatigue, delayed changes in stiffness have frequently been reported in association with a reduced ability to fully flex or extend the joint (Clarkson et al. 1992). According to Whitehead et al. (2001), the rise in passive tension results from development of injury contractures in the damaged muscles. Ebbeling & Clarkson (1989) suggested there may be an abnormal accumulation of calcium inside the muscle cell, due to either a loss of sarcolemmal integrity or dysfunction of the sarcoplasmic reticulum.

The ultrasound method enables consideration of the potential influence of structural and mechanical parameters on the fascicle–tendon interaction (Fukunaga et al. 1996). Using such techniques, Ishikawa et al. (2006a) found fascicle lengths to be longer at day two in both passive (resting) and active (peak MVC) testing conditions. The active fascicle angle was smaller and there was no change in the net fascicle shortening. As there was a parallel drop in MVC, it was suggested that fascicles could not shorten sufficiently, due to the increased internal fluid pressure. This secondary decline in MVC torque was also attributed to the reduced compliance of tendinous tissues. Although this experiment demonstrated that changes in fascicle–tendon interactions may have considerable consequences on muscle function after stretch–shortening cycle fatigue, more studies are needed to understand their exact influence.

2.5.3 Delayed–onset muscle soreness

Sore muscles are often stiff and tender, and their ability to produce force is reduced for several days or weeks (Asmussen 1956, Komi & Rusko 1974, Komi & Viitasalo 1977, Murayama et al. 2000, Sherman et al. 1984). This soreness was suggested, as early as in 1902 (Hough), to be due to exercise-induced muscle damage.

Delayed-onset muscle soreness is characterised by a sensation of dull pain and discomfort, increasing in intensity during the first 2 days, remaining symptomatic for 1–2 days, then usually disappearing 5–7 days after exercise. However, muscle regeneration is still incomplete. At present it is known, however, that neither the degree nor timing of ultrastructural damage correlates well with respective changes in muscle soreness (Howell et al. 1993, Newham et al. 1983b). Part of this discrepancy may be explained by the fact that when peripheral tissues are damaged, the sensation of pain in response to a given stimulus is enhanced. This phenomenon (hyperalgesia) occurs first at the site of tissue damage, before spreading throughout other compartments (e.g. Bobbert et al. 1986). In addition, soreness is not constant, being mostly felt when the exercised limbs are extended or fully flexed, or when the muscles are palpated deeply (Howell et al. 1993). Even though stiffness has been reported to increase with a delayed time course that parallels that of muscle soreness (Jones et al. 1987), stiffness may peak earlier, and it often lasts much longer (Dousset et al. 2007, Howell et al. 1993).

2.6 Neural changes

With the progressive development of fatigue during stretch–shortening cycle exercise (Figure 5.7), a significant interaction has been demonstrated between prelanding activation and kinematics, and the resulting postlanding stiffness adjustment. These results emphasise the plasticity, as well as the efficacy, of neural adjustments during the early parts of fatiguing exercise. They may also explain why, in some studies that used very moderate-intensity exercise, the fatigue effects were minimal. The parallelism between activation and kinematic changes may persist during the recovery period. This would indicate the existence of neural failure or adjustments to contractile deterioration that could operate at different levels of the activation pathways. These variations may be explained as compensations for contractile failure (Gollhofer et al. 1987a, Komi &

Viitasalo 1977), as an optimisation of neural drive in proportion to contractile failure (muscle wisdom; Bigland-Ritchie et al. 1983) or as compounding contractile failure through inadequate neural drive (Gandevia et al. 1995).

2.7 Signs of central fatigue

In fatiguing stretch–shortening cycle exercise, in which muscle damage occurs, inadequate neural drive can be an attempt of the neuromuscular system to protect the muscle–tendon unit from additional damage (Regueme et al. 2005, 2007, Strojnik et al. 2001). If these adjustments reduce neural drive then, regardless of the mechanism, central fatigue will develop. Support for the central fatigue hypothesis during the recovery phase comes from results such as those shown in Figure 5.9, where bimodal (and parallel) decreases in electromyographic activity and force production are evident. Only a few studies have normalised electromyographic activity to the maximal M-wave amplitude, but results confirmed the occurrence of an acute (<30 min) reduction in central activation (Millet & Lepers 2004). Other methods, such as the ratio of the forces achieved with voluntary and electrically evoked (80 Hz) actions, and the activation deficit (Millet & Lepers 2004), confirmed this initial reduction. Additional support for the central fatigue hypothesis during the delayed recovery phase comes, however, from the few studies that observed 2–5 day reductions in the Hoffman reflex peak-to-peak amplitude and H/M-wave ratio (Dousset et al. 2007, Nicol et al. 1996a). This reduction in Hoffman reflex amplitude may include the possibility of supraspinal modulation of the α-motoneuron pool during fatigue.

As delayed-onset muscle soreness is characteristic of stretch–shortening cycle fatigue, one would expect that pain research would bring additional information on the possibilities of central activation failure. Although pain influence has not been measured directly in connection with such fatigue, its potential inhibitory effect has been demonstrated using experimental pain protocols. For example, the experimental muscle pain study of Graven-Nielsen et al. (1997) revealed no increase in the resting electromyographic activity, but a reduced activity in maximal voluntary contraction and changes in coordination during dynamic exercises. In accordance with the pain adaptation model (Lund et al. 1991), several studies reported increased antagonist and decreased agonist activity (Arendt-Nielsen et al. 1996, Sohn et al. 2000). More recently, transcranial magnetic stimulation techniques demonstrated that tonic muscle pain can induce an inhibition of the primary motor cortex (Le Pera et al. 2001). However, it is not currently possible to discuss the exact supraspinal influence of pain associated with stretch–shortening cycle fatigue. Since electromyographic activity recovers after the pain has dissipated, it is suggested that delayed-onset muscle soreness may contribute primarily to these electrical changes during the first 2–3 days after exercise.

2.8 Reflex adjustments of neural activation

Compared to only a few studies that have examined direct cortical influences, there are many reports concerning the fatigue effects of exhaustive stretch–shortening cycle exercise on peripheral neural inputs, especially on facilitation/inhibition of the spinal stretch reflexes (e.g. Figure 5.9). We would like to emphasise that the bimodality concept particularly applies to exercise-induced changes in the stretch-reflex response.

Central and peripheral influences are entwined in these changes in neuromuscular function. During the bimodal recovery period, acute structural and chemical changes in the periphery, and their subsequent inflammation and remodelling processes, will affect the afferent sensory pathways and these, in turn, will act within the nervous system on efferent activities. Evidence for the involvement of group III and IV muscle afferents comes from the finding that selective damage of these afferents (by application of capsaicin) abolishes the depression of the monosynaptic reflex induced by muscle fatigue (Brunetti et al. 2003). Thus, changes in feedback from the altered muscle will lead to altered central activation (either inhibition or facilitation), and should then lead to changes in the function of the neuromuscular system.

In the acute recovery phase, the immediate postexercise reduction in stretch-reflex amplitude measured either in passive or active conditions can be explained by simple metabolic fatigue, provided that the fatigue is exhaustive enough. It was originally suggested by Asmussen & Mazin (1978), and later supported by Bigland-Ritchie et al. (1986), that a reduction in neural activation could depend on some reflex response from the contracting muscle itself. This hypothesis was later challenged by Löscher et al. (1996) for sustained isometric contractions.

The nature of stretch–shortening cycle fatigue could, however, favour the intervention of such mechanisms. In the acute recovery phase, increased extracellular potassium, phosphate or lactic acid may stimulate muscle metaboceptors (Kaufman et al. 2002). This could explain the acute metabolic-induced reduction in stretch-reflex and H-reflex amplitudes, operating through presynaptic inhibition at the spinal level. As the muscle spindle and its intrafusal fibres also exhibit metabolic activity, and are reportedly susceptible to fatigue (Emonet-Denand & Laporte 1974), a parallel reduction in spindle sensitivity could lead to reduced Ia afferent input to the α-motoneurons (Fukami 1988). It is very likely that, since the eccentric part of the stretch–shortening cycle action induces a powerful loading of the muscle spindles, continuous and cyclic loading could also modify the γ-loop system. Due to methodological difficulties, it can only be hypothesised at present that direct and indirect fatigue effects on the fusimotor-muscle spindle system may exist. The rapid partial recovery within 1–2 h after exercise supports the metabolic nature of these acute neural changes. Within this area, one may question the role of the Golgi tendon organ during fatiguing stretch–shortening cycle exercise. Unfortunately, the literature lacks information about its potential role, e.g. as an inhibitory pathway, although presumably, the Golgi tendon organ should reliably signal changes in muscle tension after fatiguing exercise (Gregory et al. 2003).

In the delayed recovery phase, group III and IV muscle afferents can also play an important role (Mense & Meyer 1988). These polymodal afferents are sensitive to chemical, thermal and mechanical changes that are associated with exercise-induced muscle injury (Kniffki et al. 1978, Mense 1977). In these conditions, their activation may differ from those obtained using pure experimental pain protocols. Once activated, they release neuropeptides, which cause vasodilatation, oedema and the release of histamine. These processes then lead to a further, long-lasting activation of some of the sensory endings (Fields 1987). With regard to the slow conduction velocity of small muscle afferents (2.5–3.0 m.s^{-1}), their continuous activation by these polymodal stimuli supports their potential role in the delayed and prolonged recovery phase. In terms of their influence on neural activation, both facilitatory and inhibitory influences have been reported that may operate at different levels of the nervous system (Nicol et al. 2006).

2.9 Concluding comments

Stretch–shortening cycle exercise, when repeated to exhaustion, can load the neuromuscular system in a more complex and thorough way than any form of isolated muscle action. When sufficiently exhaustive, such fatigue is usually characterised by reversible muscle damage, with subsequent inflammation/remodelling processes associated with delayed-onset muscle soreness. These events have considerable influence on neuromuscular function including such indices as muscle structure, muscle mechanics, and joint and muscle stiffness.

In connection with these variables, the neural modifications are of considerable mechanistic interest, and the observation of a parallelism between mechanical and neural changes during and after stretch–shortening cycle fatigue is especially significant. Overall, this form of fatigue reduces performance in a bimodal fashion (acute and delayed). For example, stretch-reflex sensitivity is dramatically reduced immediately after exercise. The immediate reduction in performance is thought to follow metabolic fatigue, but the delayed recovery is more complex in nature.

It is suggested that this delay results from the influences of structural damage/remodelling of the muscle-tendon tissues, possibly including both the intra- and extrafusal fibres. Structural and functional recovery is long lasting and prevents an individual from performing normal exercise routines for several days. In some severe cases, the recovery period may exceed 10 days. The functional consequences and their coupling with muscle damage/remodelling induced by stretch–shortening cycle exercise are illustrated in Figure 5.11, with an emphasis upon the delayed recovery phase.

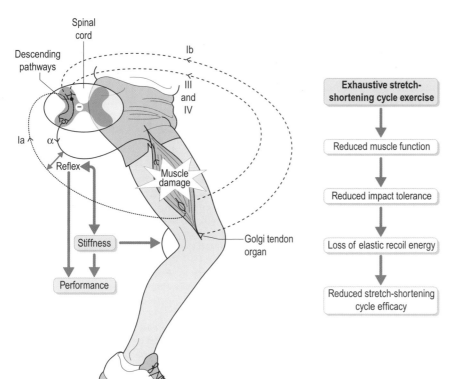

Exhaustive stretch-shortening cycle exercise

↓

Reduced muscle function

↓

Reduced impact tolerance

↓

Loss of elastic recoil energy

↓

Reduced stretch-shortening cycle efficacy

Figure 5.11 Schematic representation of the possible interaction between neural pathways and the events of mechanical failure during the delayed recovery phase from exhaustive stretch–shortening exercise. When the muscle deteriorates, it is characterised by reduced tolerance to repeated stretch loads, by a deterioration of elastic recoil and increased work during the push-off phase, so that the same functional outcome can be maintained. Modified from Horita (2000) with permission.

References

Allen GM, McKenzie DK, Gandevia SC 1998 Twitch interpolation of the elbow flexor muscles at high forces. Muscle and Nerve 21(3):318–328

Arendt-Nielsen L, Graven-Nielsen T, Svarrer H, Svensson P 1996 The influence of low back pain on muscle activity and coordination in gait: a clinical and experimental study. Pain 64:231–240

Ashe J 1997 Force and the motor cortex. Behavioural Brain Research 87(2):255–269

Asmussen E 1956 Observations on experimental muscle soreness. Acta Rheumatologica Scandinavica 2:109–116

Asmussen E 1979 Muscle fatigue. Medicine and Science in Sports and Exercise 11(4):313–321

Asmussen E, Mazin BA 1978 Central nervous component in local muscular fatigue. European Journal of Applied Physiology and Occupational Physiology 38:9–15

Avela J, Kyröläinen H, Komi PV, Rama D 1999 Reduced reflex sensitivity persists several days after long-lasting stretch–shortening cycle (SSC) exercise. Journal of Applied Physiology 86(4):1292–1300

Babault N, Pousson M, Ballay Y, Van Hoecke J 2001 Activation of human quadriceps femoris during isometric, concentric and eccentric contractions. Journal of Applied Physiology 91(6):2628–2634

Babault N, Desbrosses K, Fabre MS, Michaut A, Pousson M 2006 Neuromuscular fatigue development during maximal concentric and isometric knee extensions. Journal of Applied Physiology 100(3):780–785

Behm D, Power K, Drinkwater E 2001 Comparison of interpolation and central activation ratios as measures of muscle inactivation. Muscle and Nerve 24(7):925–934

Benwell NM, Sacco P, Hammond GR, Byrnes ML, Mastaglia FL, Thickbroom GW 2006 Short-interval cortical inhibition and corticomotor excitability with fatiguing hand exercise: a central adaptation to fatigue? Experimental Brain Research 170(2):191–198

Bigland-Ritchie B, Jones DA, Woods JJ 1979 Excitation frequency and muscle fatigue: electrical responses during human voluntary and stimulated contractions. Experimental Neurology 64(2):414–427

Bigland-Ritchie B, Johansson R, Lippold OC, Woods JJ 1983 Contractile speed and EMG changes during fatigue of sustained maximal voluntary contraction. Journal of Neurophysiology 50:313–324

Bigland-Ritchie BR, Dawson NJ, Johansson RS, Lippold OC 1986 Reflex origin for the slowing of motoneurone firing rates in fatiguing human voluntary contractions. Journal of Physiology 379:451–459

Bigland-Ritchie B, Thomas CK, Rice CL, Howarth JV, Woods JJ 1992 Muscle temperature, contractile speed and motoneuron firing rates during human voluntary contractions. Journal of Applied Physiology 73(6):2457–2461

Bobbert MF, Hollander AP, Huijing PA 1986 Factors in delayed onset muscular soreness of man. Medicine and Science in Sports and Exercise 18(1):75–81

Brockett CL, Morgan DL, Proske U 2001 Human hamstring muscles adapt to eccentric exercise by changing optimum length. Medicine and Science in Sports and Exercise 33:783–790

Brunetti O, Della Torre G, Lucchi ML, Chiocchetti R, Bortolami R, Pettorossi VE 2003 Inhibition of muscle spindle afferent activity during masseter muscle fatigue in the rat. Experimental Brain Research 52(2):251–262

Butler JE, Taylor JL, Gandevia SC 2003 Responses of human motoneurons to corticospinal stimulation during maximal voluntary contractions and ischemia. Journal of Neuroscience 23(32):10224–10230

Carpentier A, Duchateau J, Hainaut K 2001 Motor unit behaviour and contractile changes during fatigue in the human first dorsal interosseus. Journal of Physiology 534(Pt 3):903–912

Chan KM, Andres LP, Polykovskaya Y, Brown WF 1998 Dissociation of the electrical and contractile properties in single human motor units during fatigue. Muscle and Nerve 21(12):1786–1789

Chleboun GS, Howell JN, Conatser RR, Giesey JJ 1998 Relationship between muscle swelling and stiffness after eccentric exercise. Medicine and Science in Sports and Exercise 30(4): 529–535

Clarkson PM, Newham DJ 1995 Associations between muscle soreness, damage and fatigue. In: Gandevia SC, Enoka RM, McComas AJ, Stuart DG, Thomas CK (eds) Fatigue. Plenum Press, NewYork, 457–469

Clarkson PM, Nosaka K, Braun B 1992 Muscle function after exercise-induced muscle damage and rapid adaptation. Medicine and Science in Sports and Exercise 24(5):512–520

Crenshaw AG, Thornell LE, Fridén J 1994 Intramuscular pressure, torque and swelling for the exercise-induced sore vastus lateralis muscle. Acta Physiologica Scandinavica 152(3):265–277

Dalsgaard MK 2005 Fuelling cerebral activity in exercising man. Journal of Cerebral Blood Flow and Metabolism 26(6):731–750

Dousset E, Avela J, Ishikawa M, Kallio J, Kuitunen S, Kyröláinen H, Linnamo V, Komi PV 2007 Bimodal recovery pattern in human skeletal muscle induced by exhaustive stretch shortening cycle exercise. Medicine and Science in Sports and Exercise 39(3): 453–460

Ebbeling CB, Clarkson PM 1989 Exercise-induced muscle damage and adaptation. Sports Medicine 7(4):207–234

Emonet-Denand F, Laporte Y 1974 Selective neuromuscular block in extrafusal junctions of skeleton-fusimotor axons produced by high frequency repetitive stimulation. Comptes rendus hebdomadaires des séances de l'Académie des sciences. Série D: Sciences naturelles 279:2083–2085

Endoh T, Nakajima T, Sakamoto M, Komiyama T 2005 Effects of muscle damage induced by eccentric exercise on muscle fatigue. Medicine and Science in Sports and Exercise 37(7):1151–1156

Faulkner JA, Brooks SV, Opiteck JA 1993 Injury to skeletal muscle fibres during contractions: conditions of occurrence and prevention. Physical Therapy 73(12):911–921

Fernstrom JD, Fernstrom MH 2006 Exercise, serum free tryptophan and central fatigue. Journal of Nutrition 136(2):553S-559S

Fields HL 1987 Pain. McGraw-Hill, New York, 35

Fridén J, Lieber RL 1992 Structural and mechanical basis of exercise-induced muscle injury. Medicine and Science in Sports and Exercise 24(2):521–530

Fridén J, Lieber RL 2001a Serum creatine kinase level is a poor predictor of muscle function after injury. Scandinavian Journal of Medicine and Science in Sports 11(2):126–127

Fridén J, Lieber RL 2001b Eccentric exercise-induced injuries to contractile and cytoskeletal muscle fibre components. Acta Physiologica Scandinavica 171:321–326

Fridén J, Sjöström M, Ekblom B 1983 Myofibrillar damage following intense eccentric exercise in man. International Journal of Sports Medicine 4:170–176

Ftaiti F, Grélot L, Coudreuse JM, Nicol C 2001 Combined effects of heat stress, dehydration and exercise on neuromuscular function in humans. European Journal of Applied Physiology 84:87–94

Fuglevand AJ, Keen DA 2003 Re-evaluation of muscle wisdom in the human adductor pollicis using physiological rates of stimulation. Journal of Physiology 549(Pt 3):865–875

Fukami Y 1988 The effects of NH3 and CO2 on the sensory ending of mammalian muscle spindles: intracellular pH as a possible mechanism. Brain Research 463:140–143

Fukunaga T, Roy RR, Shellock FG, Hodgson JA, Edgerton VR 1996 Specific tension of human plantar flexors and dorsiflexors. Journal of Applied Physiology 80:158–165

Fukunaga T, Kubo K, Kawakami Y, Fukashiro S, Kanehisa H, Maganaris CN 2001 In vivo behaviour of human muscle tendon during walking. Proceedings of the Royal Society of London Series B 268:229–233

Gandevia SC 2001 Spinal and supraspinal factors in human muscle fatigue. Physiological Reviews 81(4):1725–1789

Gandevia SC, Allen GM, McKenzie DK 1995 Central fatigue. Critical issues, quantification and practical implications. Advances in Experimental Medicine and Biology 384:281–294

Gandevia SC, Allen GM, Butler JE, Taylor JL 1996 Supraspinal factors in human muscle fatigue: evidence for suboptimal output from the motor cortex. Journal of Physiology 490(Pt 2):529–536

Gandevia SC, Herbert RD, Leeper JB 1998 Voluntary activation of human elbow flexor muscles during maximal concentric contractions. Journal of Physiology 512(Pt 2):595–602

Garland SJ, Enoka RM, Serrano LP, Robinson GA 1994 Behavior of motor units in human biceps brachii during a submaximal fatiguing contraction. Journal of Applied Physiology 76(6):2411–2419

Garland SJ, Griffin L, Ivanova T 1997 Motor unit discharge rate is not associated with muscle relaxation time in sustained submaximal contractions in humans. Neuroscience Letters 239(1):25–28

Gollhofer A, Komi PV, Fujitsuka N, Miyashita M 1987a Fatigue during stretch–shortening cycle exercises. II. Changes in neuromuscular activation patterns of human skeletal muscle. International Journal of Sports Medicine 8(Suppl 1):38–47

Gollhofer A, Komi PV, Miyashita M, Aura O 1987b Fatigue during stretch–shortening cycle exercises: changes in mechanical performance of human skeletal muscle. International Journal of Sports Medicine 8:71–78

Graven-Nielsen T, Svensson P, Arendt-Nielsen L 1997 Effects of experimental muscle pain on muscle activaty and co-ordination during static and dynamic motor function. Electroencephalography and Clinical Neurophysiology 105:156–164

Gregory JE, Morgan DL, Proske U 2003 Tendon organs as monitors of muscle damage from eccentric contractions. Experimental Brain Research 151:346–355

Gregory JE, Morgan DL, Proske U 2004 Responses of muscle spindles following a series of eccentric contractions. Experimental Brain Research 157(2):234–240

Hart JM, Fritz JM, Kerrigan DC, Saliba EN, Gansneder BM, Ingersoll CD 2006 Reduced quadriceps activation after lumbar paraspinal fatiguing exercise. Journal of Athletic Training 41(1):79–86

Herbert RD, Gandevia SC 1999 Twitch interpolation in human muscles: mechanisms and implications for measurement of voluntary activation. Journal of Neurophysiology 82(5): 2271–2283

Hikida RS, Staron RS, Hagerman FC, Sherman WM, Costill DL 1983 Muscle fiber necrosis associated with human marathon runners. Journal of the Neurological Sciences 59:185–203

Horita T 2000 Stiffness regulation during stretch–shortening cycle exercise [dissertation]. University of Jyväskylä, Department of Biology of Physical Activity, Jyväskylä, Finland

Horita T, Komi PV, Nicol C, Kyröläinen H 1999 Effect of exhausting stretch–shortening cycle exercise on the time course of mechanical behaviour in the drop jump: possible role of muscle damage. European Journal of Applied Physiology and Occupational Physiology 79:160–167

Horita T, Komi PV, Hämäläinen I, Avela J 2003 Exhausting stretch–shortening cycle (SSC) exercise causes greater impairment in SSC performance than in pure concentric performance. European Journal of Applied Physiology 88:527–534

Hough T 1902 Ergographic studies in muscle soreness. American Journal of Applied Physiology 7:76–92

Howell JN, Chleboun G, Conatser R 1993 Muscle stiffness, strength loss, swelling and soreness following exercise-induced injury in humans. Journal of Physiology 464:183–196

Humphry AT, Lloyd-Davies EJ, Teare RJ, Williams KE, Strutton PH, Davey NJ 2004 Specificity and functional impact of post-exercise depression of cortically evoked motor potentials in man. European Journal of Applied Physiology 92(1–2):211–218

Ishikawa M, Dousset E, Avela J, Kyröläinen H, Kallio J, Linnamo V, Kuitunen S, Nicol C, Komi PV 2006 Changes in the soleus muscle architecture after exhausting stretch–shortening cycle exercise in humans. European Journal of Applied Physiology and Occupational Physiology 97(3):298–306

Ishikawa M, Pakaslahti J, Komi PV 2007 Medial gastrocnemius muscle behaviour during human running and walking. Gait and Posture 25(3):380–384

Johnson KV, Edwards SC, Van Tongeren C, Bawa P 2004 Properties of human motor units after prolonged activity at a constant firing rate. Experimental Brain Research 154(4):479–487

Jones DA, Newham DJ, Clarkson PM 1987 Skeletal muscle stiffness and pain following eccentric exercise of the elbow flexors. Pain 30:233–242

Jones C, Allen T, Talbot J, Morgan DL, Proske U 1997 Changes in the mechanical properties of human and amphibian muscle after eccentric exercise. European Journal of Applied Physiology and Occupational Physiology 76(1):21–31

Kaneko M, Komi PV, Aura O 1984 Mechanical efficiency of concentric and eccentric exercises performed with medium to fast contraction rates. Scandinavian Journal of Sports Sciences 6(1):15–20

Kaufman MP, Hayes SG, Adreani CM, Pickar JG 2002 Discharge properties of group III and IV muscle afferents. Advances in Experimental Medicine and Biology 508:25–32

Kawakami Y, Amemiya K, Kanehisa H, Ikegawa S, Fukunaga T 2000 Fatigue responses of human triceps surae muscles during repetitive maximal isometric contractions. Journal of Applied Physiology 88(6):1969–1975

Kent-Braun JA 1999 Central and peripheral contributions to muscle fatigue in humans during sustained maximal effort. European Journal of Applied Physiology and Occupational Physiology 80(1):57–63

Kent-Braun JA, Le Blanc R 1996 Quantitation of central activation failure during maximal voluntary contractions in humans. Muscle and Nerve 19(7):861–869

Kniffki KD, Mense S, Schmidt RF 1978 Responses of group IV afferent units from skeletal muscle to stretch, contraction and chemical stimulation. Experimental Brain Research 31:511–522

Komi PV 2000 Stretch–shortening cycle: a powerful model to study normal and fatigued muscle. Journal of Biomechanics 33: 1197–1206

Komi PV, Gollhofer A 1997 Stretch reflex can have an important role in force enhancement during SSC-exercise. Journal of Applied Biomechanics 33:1197–1206

Komi PV, Rusko H 1974 Quantitative evaluation of mechanical and electrical changes during fatigue loading of eccentric and concentric work. Scandinavian Journal of Rehabilitation Medicine 3(Suppl):121–126

Komi PV, Viitasalo JT 1977 Changes in motor unit activity and metabolism in human skeletal muscle during and after repeated eccentric and concentric contractions. Acta Physiologica Scandinavica 100:246–254

Komi PV, Gollhofer A, Schmidtbleicher D, Frick U 1987a Interaction between man and shoe in running: considerations for more comprehensive measurement approach. International Journal of Sports Medicine 8(3):196–202

Komi PV, Kaneko M, Aura O 1987b EMG activity of the leg extensor muscles with special reference to mechanical efficiency in concentric and eccentric exercise. International Journal of Sports Medicine 8(Suppl 1):22–29

Kuitunen S, Avela J, Kyröläinen H, Komi PV 2004 Voluntary activation and mechanical performance of human triceps surae muscle after exhaustive stretch–shortening cycle jumping exercise. European Journal of Applied Physiology 91:538–544

Kyröläinen H, Takala TES, Komi PV 1998 Muscle damage induced by stretch–shortening cycle exercise. Medicine and Science in Sports and Exercise 30(3):415–420

Kyröläinen H, Pullinen T, Candau R, Avela J, Huttunen P, Komi PV 2000 Effects of marathon running on running economy and kinematics. European Journal of Applied Physiology 82(4):297–304

Kyröläinen H, Belli A, Komi PV 2001 Biomechanical factors affecting running economy. Medicine and Science in Sports and Exercise 33(8):1330–1337

Lazarski JP, Ridding MC, Miles TS 2002 Dexterity is not affected by fatigue-induced depression of human motor cortex excitability. Neuroscience Letters 321(1–2):69–72

Le Pera D, Graven-Nielsen T, Valeriani M, Oliviero A, Di Lazzaro V, Tonali PA, Arendt-Nielsen L 2001 Inhibition of motor system excitability at cortical and spinal level by tonic muscle pain. Clinical Neurophysiology 112(9):1633–1641

Lieber R, Shah S, Fridén J 2002 Cytoskeletal disruption after eccentric contraction-induced muscle injury. Clinical Orthopaedics and Related Research 403(Suppl):S90–99

Liu JZ, Shan ZY, Zhang LD, Sahgal V, Brown RW, Yue GH 2003 Human brain activation during sustained and intermittent submaximal fatigue muscle contractions: an fMRI study. Journal of Neurophysiology 90(1):300–312

Liu JZ, Zhang L, Yao B, Sahgal V, Yue GH 2005 Fatigue induced by intermittent maximal voluntary contractions is associated with significant losses in muscle output but limited reductions in functional MRI-measured brain activation level. Brain Research 1040(1–2):44–54

Lorist MM, Kernell D, Meijman TF, Zijdewind I 2002 Motor fatigue and cognitive task performance in humans. Journal of Physiology 545(Pt 1):313–319

Löscher WN, Nordlund MM 2002 Central fatigue and motor cortical excitability during repeated shortening and lengthening actions. Muscle and Nerve 25(6):864–872

Löscher G, Cresswell AG, Thorstensson A 1996 Excitatory drive to the α-motoneuron pool during fatiguing submaximal contraction in man. Journal of Physiology 491:271–280

Lund JP, Donga R, Widmer CG, Stohler CS 1991 The pain-adaptation model: a discussion of the relationship between chronic musculoskeletal pain and motor activity. Canadian Journal of Physiology and Pharmacology 69(5):683–694

Macefield G, Hagbarth KE, Gorman R, Gandevia SC, Burke D 1991 Decline in spindle support to alpha-motoneurons during sustained voluntary contractions. Journal of Physiology 440: 497–512

MacIntyre DL, Reid WD, McKenzie DC 1995 Delayed muscle soreness: the inflammatory response to muscle injury and its clinical implications. Sports Medicine 20(1):24–40

Marsden CD, Meadows JC, Merton PA 1983 'Muscular wisdom' that minimizes fatigue during prolonged effort in man: peak rates of motoneuron discharge and slowing of discharge during fatigue. Advances in Neurology 39:169–211

Martin V, Millet GY, Martin A, Deley G, Lattier G 2004 Assessment of low-frequency fatigue with two methods of electrical stimulation. Journal of Applied Physiology 97:1923–1929

Martin PG, Smith JL, Butler JE, Gandevia SC, Taylor JL 2006 Fatigue-sensitive afferents inhibit extensor but not flexor motoneurons in humans. Journal of Neuroscience 26(18):4796–4802

Maruyama A, Matsunaga K, Tanaka N, Rothwell JC 2006 Muscle fatigue decreases short-interval intracortical inhibition after exhaustive intermittent tasks. Clinical Neurophysiology 117(4):864–870

Mense S 1977 Nervous outflow from skeletal muscle following chemical noxious stimulation. Journal of Physiology 267:75–88

Mense S, Meyer H 1988 Bradykinin-induced modulation of the response behaviour of different types of feline group III and IV muscle receptors. Journal of Physiology 398:49–63

Mero A, Komi PV 1986 Force-, EMG- and elasticity-velocity relationships at submaximal, maximal and supramaximal running speeds in sprinters. European Journal of Applied Physiology and Occupational Physiology 55(5):553–561

Merton PA 1954 Voluntary strength and fatigue. Journal of Physiology 123(3):553–564

Millet GY, Lepers R 2004 Alterations of neuromuscular function after prolonged running, cycling and skiing exercises. Sports Medicine 34(2):105–116

Millet GY, Lepers R, Maffiuletti NA, Babault N, Martin V, Lattier G 2002 Alterations of neuromuscular function after an ultramarathon. Journal of Applied Physiology 92:486–492

Millet GY, Martin V, Maffiuletti NA, Martin A 2003 Neuromuscular fatigue after a ski skating marathon. Canadian Journal of Applied Physiology 28(3):434–445

Murayama M, Nosaka K, Yoneda T, Minamitani K 2000 Changes in hardness of the human elbow flexor muscles after eccentric exercise. European Journal of Applied Physiology 82(5–6): 361–367

Naito A, Shindo M, Miyasaka T, Sun YJ, Morita H 1996 Inhibitory projection from brachioradialis to biceps brachii motoneurons in human. Experimental Brain Research 111(3):483–486

Newham DJ, McPhail G, Mills KR, Edwards RH 1983a Ultrastructural changes after concentric and eccentric contractions of human muscle. Journal of the Neurological Sciences 61:109–122

Newham DJ, Mills KR, Quigley BM, Edwards RH 1983b Pain and fatigue after concentric and eccentric muscle contractions. Clinical Science 64:55–62

Newsholme EA, Blomstrand E 2006 Branched-chain amino acids and central fatigue. Journal of Nutrition 136(1 Suppl):274S-276S

Nicol C, Komi PV 1998 Significance of passively induced stretch reflexes on Achilles tendon force enhancement. Muscle and Nerve 21:1546–1548

Nicol C, Komi PV, Marconnet P 1991a Fatigue effects of marathon-running on neuromuscular performance. I. Changes in muscle force and stiffness characteristics. Scandinavian Journal of Medicine and Science in Sports 1:10–17

Nicol C, Komi PV, Marconnet P 1991b Effects of marathon fatigue on running kinematics and economy. Scandinavian Journal of Medicine and Science in Sports 1:195–204

Nicol C, Komi PV, Avela J 1996a Stretch–shortening cycle fatigue reduces stretch-reflex response. In: Abstract book of the 1996 International Pre-Olympic Scientific Congress, July 10–14, Dallas, Texas, 108

Nicol C, Komi PV, Horita T, Kyröläinen H, Takala TE 1996b Reduced stretch-reflex sensitivity after exhaustive stretch–shortening cycle exercise. European Journal of Applied Physiology and Occupational Physiology 72(5–6):401–409

Nicol C, Kuitunen S, Kyröläinen H, Avela J, Komi PV 2003 Effects of long- and short-term fatiguing stretch–shortening cycle exercises on reflex EMG and force of the tendon-muscle complex. European Journal of Applied Physiology 90:470–479

Nicol C, Avela J, Komi PV 2006 Stretch–shortening cycle (SSC): a model to study naturally occurring neuromuscular fatigue. Sports Medicine 36(11):1–23

Nosaka K, Clarkson PM 1996 Changes in indicators of inflammation after eccentric exercise of the elbow flexors. Medicine and Science in Sports and Exercise 28(8):953–961

Nosaka K, Newton MJ, Sacco P 2005 Attenuation of protective effect against eccentric exercise-induced muscle damage. Canadian Journal of Applied Physiology 30(5):529–542

Nybo L, Secher NH 2004 Cerebral perturbations provoked by prolonged exercise. Progress in Neurobiology 72(4):223–261

Peters EJ, Fuglevand AJ 1999 Cessation of human motor unit discharge during sustained maximal voluntary contraction. Neuroscience Letters 274(1):66–70

Pettorossi VE, Della Torre G, Bortolami R, Brunetti O 1999 The role of capsaicin-sensitive muscle afferents in fatigue-induced modulation of the monosynaptic reflex in the rat. Journal of Physiology 515(Pt 2):599–607

Place N, Lepers R, Deley G, Millet GY 2004 Time course of neuromuscular alterations during a prolonged running exercise. Medicine and Science in Sports and Exercise 36(8):1347–1356

Prasartwuth O, Taylor JL, Gandevia SC 2005 Maximal force, voluntary activation and muscle soreness after eccentric damage to human elbow flexor muscles. Journal of Physiology 567(Pt 1): 337–348

Rattey J, Martin PG, Kay D, Cannon J, Marino FE 2005 Contralateral muscle fatigue in human quadriceps muscle: evidence for a centrally mediated fatigue response and cross-over effect. Pflügers Archiv 452(2):199–207

Regueme SC, Nicol C, Barthèlemy J, Grélot L 2005 Acute and delayed neuromuscular adjustments of the triceps surae muscle group to exhaustive stretch–shortening cycle fatigue. European Journal of Applied Physiology 93(4):398–410

Regueme SC, Barthèlemy J, Gauthier GM, Blin O, Nicol C 2007 Delayed influence of stretch–shortening cycle fatigue on the ankle static position sense. Scandinavian Journal of Medicine and Science in Sport Oct 17; [Epub ahead of print] PMID: 17944813

Romaniello A, Cruccu G, McMillan AS, Arendt-Nielsen L, Svensson P 2000 Effect of experimental pain from trigeminal muscle and skin on motor cortex excitability in humans. Brain Research 882(1–2):120–127

Russ DW, Kent-Braun JA 2003 Sex differences in human skeletal muscle fatigue are eliminated under ischemic conditions. Journal of Applied Physiology 94(6):2414–2422

Seaward BL, Clarke DH 1992 The effects of treadmill running on the isometric fatigue of the handgrip muscles. Journal of Sports Medicine and Physical Fitness 32(3):243–249

Sherman WM, Armstrong LE, Murray TM, Hagerman FC, Costill DL, Staron RC, Ivy JL 1984 Effect of a 42.2-km footrace and subsequent rest or exercise on muscular strength and work capacity. Journal of Applied Physiology 57:1668–1673

Shield A, Zhou S 2004 Assessing voluntary muscle activation with the twitch interpolation technique. Sports Medicine 34(4):253–267

Sjøgaard G 1996 Potassium and fatigue: the pros and cons. Acta Physiologica Scandinavica 156(3):257–264

Søgaard K, Gandevia SC, Todd G, Petersen NT, Taylor JL 2006 The effect of sustained low-intensity contractions on supraspinal fatigue in human elbow flexor muscle. Journal of Physiology 573(Pt 2):511–523

Sohn MK, Graven-Nielsen T, Arendt-Nielsen L, Svensson P 2000 Inhibition of motor unit firing during experimental muscle pain in humans. Muscle and Nerve 23:1219–1226

Spielmann JM, Laouris Y, Nordstrom MA, Robinson GA, Reinking RM, Stuart DG 1993 Adaptation of cat motoneurons to sustained and intermittent extracellular activation. Journal of Physiology 464:75–120

Strojnik V, Nicol C, Komi PV 2001 Fatigue during one-week tourist alpine skiing. In: Müller E, Schwameder H, Raschner C, Lindinger S, Kornexl E (eds) Science and skiing II. Kovac, Hamburg, 599–607

Stuart M, Butler JE, Collins DF, Taylor JL, Gandevia SC 2002 The history of contraction of the wrist flexors can change cortical excitability. Journal of Physiology 545(Pt 3):731–737

Svensson P, Miles TS, McKay D, Ridding MC 2003 Suppression of motor evoked potentials in a hand muscle following prolonged painful stimulation. European Journal of Pain 7(1):55–62

Taylor JL, Gandevia SC 2001 Transcranial magnetic stimulation and human muscle fatigue. Muscle and Nerve 24(1):18–29

Taylor JL, Butler JE, Allen GM, Gandevia SC 1996 Changes in motor cortical excitability during human muscle fatigue. Journal of Physiology 490(Pt 2):519–528

Taylor JL, Allen GM, Butler JE, Gandevia SC 2000 Supraspinal fatigue during intermittent maximal voluntary contractions of the human elbow flexors. Journal of Applied Physiology 89(1): 305–313

Taylor JL, Todd G, Gandevia SC 2006 Evidence for a supraspinal contribution to human muscle fatigue. Clinical and Experimental Pharmacology and Physiology 33(4):400–405

Todd G, Taylor JL, Gandevia SC 2003 Measurement of voluntary activation of fresh and fatigued human muscles using transcranial magnetic stimulation. Journal of Physiology 551(Pt 2):661–671

Todd G, Taylor JL, Gandevia SC 2004 Reproducible measurement of voluntary activation of human elbow flexors with motor cortical stimulation. Journal of Applied Physiology 97(1):236–242

Tomporowski PD 2003 Effects of acute bouts of exercise on cognition. Acta Psychologica 112(3):297–324

Warren GL, Ingalls CP, Lowe DA, Armstrong RB 2001 Excitation-contraction uncoupling: major role in contraction-induced muscle injury. Exercise and Sport Sciences Reviews 29(2):82–87

Whitehead NP, Weerakkody NS, Gregory JE, Morgan DL, Proske U 2001 Changes in passive tension of muscle in humans and animals after eccentric exercise. Journal of Physiology 533(2):593–604

Wood SA, Morgan DL, Proske U 1993 Effects of repeated eccentric contractions on structure and mechanical properties of toad sartorius muscle. American Journal of Physiology 265:C792–C800

Woods JJ, Furbush F, Bigland-Ritchie B 1987 Evidence for a fatigue-induced reflex inhibition of motoneuron firing rates. Journal of Neurophysiology 58(1):125–137

Yu JG, Furst DO, Thornell LE 2003 The mode of myofibril remodelling in human skeletal muscle affected by DOMS induced by eccentric contractions. Histochemistry and Cell Biology 119(5): 383–393

Zijdewind I, Zwarts MJ, Kernell D 1998 Influence of a voluntary fatigue test on the contralateral homologous muscle in humans. Neuroscience Letters 253(1):41–44

Zijdewind I, van Duinen H, Zielman R, Lorist MM 2006 Interaction between force production and cognitive performance in humans. Clinical Neurophysiology 117(3):660–667

Zytnicki D, Lafleur J, Horcholle-Bossavit G, Lamy F, Jami L 1990 Reduction of Ib autogenetic inhibition in motoneurons during contractions of an ankle extensor muscle in the cat. Journal of Neurophysiology 64(5):1380–1389

Chapter 6

Cellular mechanisms of skeletal muscle fatigue

David G. Allen Graham D. Lamb Håkan Westerblad

1 INTRODUCTION

High-intensity exercise leads to a rapid decline in muscle performance, known as fatigue. The most obvious consequence of fatigue is a decline in the tetanic force but, in addition, shortening velocity is reduced, and the time for relaxation is prolonged. In this chapter we will review possible causes of muscle fatigue, focusing mainly on the causes of a reduction in tetanic force; earlier reviews by ourselves and others can be consulted for other aspects of fatigue (Allen et al. 1995, Fitts 1994, Westerblad et al. 1991). Muscles are activated by a pathway that starts in the motor cortex, involves upper and lower motor neurons in the central nervous system, and traverses the neuromuscular junction before exciting the muscle. Clearly fatigue can potentially occur anywhere along this pathway, and the contributions of central fatigue are considered in Chapter 5 and have been extensively reviewed (Gandevia 2001). In the present chapter, we will only discuss fatigue within the muscle, which is usually the largest component.

Fatigue can be studied in a variety of preparations including intact animals, isolated muscles and isolated subcellular preparations. Each preparation has advantages and disadvantages; in the present chapter we concentrate particularly on isolated single fibres, and on skinned fibres whose surface membrane has been chemically or physically removed. Single fibres are uncomplicated by the mixture of fibre types that occurs in whole muscles, and in intact single fibres it is possible to measure intracellular ions simultaneously with mechanical performance. Skinned fibres have the advantage that the composition of solutions bathing the contractile proteins and the sarcoplasmic reticulum can be specified completely, so the effect of any particular metabolic change can be investigated in the absence of the multitude of changes that occur during fatigue. We believe this combination of methods is a particularly powerful way to address the cellular mechanisms of fatigue. Of course, when a fatigue mechanism is established in a simplified preparation, it is essential to determine what role, if any, it has in the fatigue observed in intact animals.

During fatigue induced by repeated short tetanic contractions, a characteristic pattern is observed in fast-twitch (type II) fibres: initially there is fast decline of tetanic force by 10–20% that is accompanied by an increase in tetanic free myoplasmic calcium concentration ($[Ca^{2+}]_i$; phase 1); then follows a period of relatively constant tetanic force (phase 2), accompanied by a slow decline in tetanic $[Ca^{2+}]_i$; finally there is rapid decline of both tetanic force and $[Ca^{2+}]_i$ (phase 3; Allen et al. 1995). Thus, the force decline in early fatigue (phase 1) is caused by impaired myofibrillar function, whereas the decline in late fatigue (phase 3) is caused by decreased sarcoplasmic reticulum calcium release. Note that slow (type I) fibres are relatively insensitive to fatigue (Bruton et al. 2003, Burke et al. 1973), and we therefore concentrate on fast-twitch fibres in the present account.

2 DECREASED MYOFIBRILLAR FORCE PRODUCTION

2.1 Lactate and hydrogen ion accumulation

Energy consumption in skeletal muscle fibres increases greatly during high-intensity exercise and, in fast-twitch fibres in particular, the energy consumption substantially exceeds the aerobic capacity of the cells, and a large fraction of the adenosine triphosphate (ATP) consumed is produced by anaerobic metabolism. Anaerobic breakdown of glycogen can lead to large increases in the intracellular concentrations of hydrogen ($[H^+]$) and lactate ions, and with vigorous exercise pH can decrease to ~6.5 and lactate concentration can reach 30 mM or higher (Fitts 1994). Although early studies indicated that low pH deleteriously affected the force production by the contractile apparatus and calcium (Ca^{2+}) release from the sarcoplasmic reticulum, more recent studies, conducted under more realistic physiological conditions, show that these effects are very small. In fact, the decrease in intracellular pH might help maintain muscle excitability (Nielsen et al. 2001). Also, the lactate is itself a valuable substrate for energy production (Brooks 1991).

Experiments with skinned fibres show that the presence of 30 mM lactate in the intracellular environment has virtually no effect on either Ca^{2+} sensitivity and maximum force production of the contractile apparatus, or on Ca^{2+} release by action potential stimulation (Posterino et al. 2001). Experiments with skinned fibres from rabbit muscle found that although maximum force production and maximum shortening velocity were substantially reduced when pH was lowered from 7.0 to 6.2 at a temperature of 10°C, they were affected comparatively little at 30°C, closer to normal body temperature (Pate et al. 1995). Comparable results have also been obtained in isolated muscle fibres (Westerblad et al. 1997) and whole muscles (Wiseman et al. 1996) from mouse. In regard to Ca^{2+} release, although isolated Ca^{2+} release channels are poorly activated by Ca^{2+} at ~pH 6.0 (Laver et al. 2000, Ma et al. 1988), the release channels in situ in skinned fibres are readily opened by activating the voltage sensors, the normal physiological trigger

(Lamb & Stephenson 1994, Lamb et al. 1992). Consistent with these findings, tetanic force production in mammalian muscle at close to physiological temperatures has been found to be little affected, or even increased, at low pH (Ranatunga 1987, Westerblad et al. 1997), and the rate of fatigue development is not increased at acid pH (Bruton et al. 1998, Kristensen et al. 2005, Zhang et al. 2006). Also, intracellular acidity can have a beneficial effect on muscle performance by reducing membrane chloride conductance, which enables continued action potential propagation even under the adverse ionic conditions that can occur with intense exercise (Nielsen et al. 2001, Pedersen et al. 2004, 2005); this issue will be discussed in more detail later.

The absence of any major deleterious effect of a low pH on muscle performance in isolated muscle preparations at close to physiological conditions offers a ready explanation for the lack of temporal correlation between force production and muscle pH when human subjects are recovering from fatiguing contractions (Sahlin & Ren 1989). It is also consistent with the conclusion of other studies in exercising humans, that elevated intracellular $[H^+]$ is not the major factor causing muscle fatigue (Bangsbo et al. 1996). Nevertheless, it should be noted that a rise in blood lactate is still a useful aid for assessing exercise performance. A marked increase in blood lactate is observed when muscles utilise anaerobic metabolism heavily, and this type of muscular activity usually leads to rapid fatigue development (Zhang et al. 2006). Thus, there is often a good correlation between fatigue and blood lactate, but this does not mean that the relationship is causative.

In conclusion, although lactate and hydrogen ions accumulate in muscle cells in some types of fatigue, neither appears to be the main cause of fatigue, at least in mammals at physiological temperatures.

2.2 Accumulation of inorganic phosphate ions

Creatine kinase catalyses the exchange of inorganic phosphate (P_i) between ATP and phosphocreatine (PCr) via the following reaction: $PCr + ADP + H^+ \rightleftharpoons Cr$ (creatine) $+ ATP$. During periods of high energy demand, phosphocreatine breaks down to creatine and P_i, while the ATP concentration remains almost constant until the phosphocreatine is close to exhaustion. Creatine has little effect on contractile function (Godt & Nosek 1989), whereas there are several mechanisms by which increased P_i may depress contractile function. The current view of cross-bridge function is that P_i is released in the transition from low-force, weakly attached cross-bridges to high-force, strongly attached cross-bridge states. This implies that the transition to the high-force states is hindered by increased P_i. Therefore, fewer cross-bridges would be in high-force states and the force production would decrease as P_i increases during fatigue development. In line with this, experiments on skinned fibres consistently show a reduced maximum Ca^{2+} activated force in the presence of elevated P_i (Millar &

Homsher 1990, Pate & Cooke 1989). Similar to the situation with decreased pH described above, the P_i-induced inhibition of cross-bridge force production becomes less marked as the temperature is increased (Coupland et al. 2001, Dantzig et al. 1992, Debold et al. 2004).

The effect of P_i on cross-bridge force production has been difficult to test in intact muscle cells, since it has proven difficult to alter myoplasmic P_i without imposing other metabolic changes as well. An experimental model that can be used in this regard is genetically modified mice that completely lack creatine kinase (CK) in their skeletal muscles ($CK^{-/-}$ mice; Steeghs et al. 1997). Fast-twitch skeletal muscle fibres of $CK^{-/-}$ mice display an increased myoplasmic P_i concentration at rest, and there is no significant further P_i accumulation during fatigue (Dahlstedt et al. 2000). The maximum Ca^{2+}-activated force of unfatigued $CK^{-/-}$ fast-twitch fibres is only about 70% of wild-type fibres and this can partly be explained by a P_i-induced depression of cross-bridge force production (Dahlstedt & Westerblad 2001). Furthermore, $CK^{-/-}$ fibres do not display the 10–20% reduction of maximum Ca^{2+}-activated force observed after about ten fatiguing tetani (phase 1; above), which has been ascribed to increased P_i (Dahlstedt et al. 2000). Even after 100 fatiguing tetani, force was not significantly affected in $CK^{-/-}$ fibres, whereas by this time force was reduced to <30% of the original in wild-type fibres. Additional support for a coupling between myoplasmic P_i concentration and force production in intact muscle cells comes from experiments where reduced myoplasmic P_i is associated with increased force production (Bruton et al. 1997, Phillips et al. 1993).

As discussed above, there is good experimental support for the notion that increased myoplasmic P_i decreases force production during fatigue by direct action on cross-bridge function. Altered cross-bridge function may also affect the force-$[Ca^{2+}]_i$ relationship via the complex interaction between cross-bridge attachment and thin (actin) filament activation (Gordon et al. 2000). A reduced myofibrillar Ca^{2+} sensitivity is frequently observed in skeletal muscle fatigue (Allen et al. 1995). Skinned fibre experiments have shown that increased P_i decreases the myofibrillar Ca^{2+} sensitivity (Martyn & Gordon 1992, Millar & Homsher 1990). Results from unfatigued $CK^{-/-}$ fibres, that display an increased myoplasmic P_i concentration at rest, also indicate an P_i-induced decrease in the myofibrillar Ca^{2+} sensitivity (Dahlstedt et al. 2001).

In conclusion, the fatigue-induced increase in P_i can reduce force production by decreasing both cross-bridge force production and myofibrillar Ca^{2+} sensitivity, though these effects are modest at mammalian physiological temperatures.

2.3 Reactive oxygen species

The most important reactive oxygen species (ROS) are super-oxide, hydrogen peroxide and hydroxyl radicals (Halliwell & Gutteridge 1998). Superoxide is produced in mitochondria as a by-product of oxidative phosphorylation and also by various enzymes including nicotinamide adenine dinucleotide-oxidase (NADPH oxidase), xanthine oxidase, lipo- and cyclooxygenases. Superoxide is moderately reactive and is rapidly broken down by superoxide dismutase to hydrogen peroxide. Superoxide has a negative charge and therefore does not easily cross membranes but may do so via anion channels (Lynch & Fridovich 1978, Turrens 2003). Hydrogen peroxide is less reactive than superoxide. It easily diffuses through cell membranes, and can act as a cellular messenger. Hydrogen peroxide can be broken down to the extremely reactive hydroxyl radical by free transition metals, such as Fe^{2+}, or by ultraviolet light. Hydroxyl radicals can damage proteins, DNA and cell membranes. Hydrogen peroxide is also broken down by catalase to water and oxygen, or by glutathione peroxidase, which produces water while converting reduced glutathione (GSH) to the oxidised form (GSSG). Given that the important ROS form a cascade, it is difficult to pinpoint whether a change in muscle function associated with ROS production is caused by the general redox status of the cell, represented by the ratio of GSH/GSSG or by a particular species of ROS. Furthermore, there is a complex interplay between ROS and reactive nitrogen species, and these (e.g. nitric oxide) can affect muscle function (Reid & Durham 2002).

Reactive oxygen species production is accelerated by muscle activity and increased temperature, both of which accompany intense exercise (Davies et al. 1982, Reid et al. 1992, Zuo et al. 2000). The clearest evidence that increased ROS production is contributing to muscle fatigue comes from studies in which ROS scavengers reduce the rate of fatigue. An early study utilised strips of diaphragm muscle perfused via their own circulation, and showed that intravenous injection of a general ROS scavenger (N-acetylcysteine) increased contractile force at the end of a period of intermittent 20 Hz stimulation (Shindoh et al. 1990). Subsequent studies have shown that both membrane-permeant ROS scavengers (Tiron, Tempol, DMSO) and membrane-impermeant scavengers (catalase, superoxide dismutase) can slow fatigue development (Moopanar & Allen 2005, Reid et al. 1992). This suggests that either both intracellular and extracellular ROS can influence fatigue, or that the ROS species involved are membrane permeant.

The magnitude of the improvement in fatiguing muscle performance by ROS scavengers is quite variable. One factor that contributes to this variability is the stimulation protocol employed. For instance, Reid et al. (1994) fatigued human muscles using intermittent tetani at either 40 Hz or 10 Hz. At 40 Hz, force decreased rapidly and N-acetylcysteine did not affect the rate of fatigue development, whereas at 10 Hz, fatigue occurred more slowly and N-acetylcysteine substantially decreased its rate of development. These results suggest that the mechanism of fatigue produced by low-frequency stimulation, possibly reduced Ca^{2+} release or reduced Ca^{2+} sensitivity, is sensitive to the effects of ROS.

Another factor that contributes to the variability in response to ROS scavengers is muscle temperature. For instance, mouse fibres fatigued at 22°C were unaffected by ROS scavengers, while the more rapid fatigue at 37°C was slowed by ROS scavengers (Moopanar & Allen 2005). This finding is probably a consequence of the temperature sensitivity of ROS production (Zuo et al. 2000).

As discussed above, there is strong evidence that ROS contribute to some models of fatigue, but our understanding of the mechanisms involved remains limited. In skinned fibres, a number of studies have characterised how myofibrillar function was affected by various exogenous ROS. Superoxide can reduce the maximum Ca^{2+}-activated force in skeletal muscle (Callahan et al. 2001, Darnley et al. 2001), while hydrogen peroxide can either increase maximum force (Darnley et al. 2001) or have little effect (Callahan et al. 2001, Lamb & Posterino 2003). Myofibrillar Ca^{2+} sensitivity was unaffected by application of various ROS in several studies (Callahan et al. 2001, Darnley et al. 2001). However, Lamb & Posterino (2003) showed that the effect of hydrogen peroxide on Ca^{2+} sensitivity depends on whether GSH is present or not. In the presence of GSH, application of hydrogen peroxide resulted in a marked increase in Ca^{2+} sensitivity followed by a slower fall. Given that GSH and GSSG are present in muscle and their ratio changes during exercise, this suggests that interactions between GSH and ROS are important for fatigue-induced ROS effects. Experiments on intact fibres showed similar results (Andrade et al. 1998); that is, application of hydrogen peroxide produced an initial increase in myofibrillar Ca^{2+} sensitivity followed by a decline. Interestingly, in a subsequent paper, Andrade et al. (2001) showed that these effects can be observed at very low concentrations of hydrogen peroxide (<nM), which raises the possibility that the effect might be mediated via activation of a signalling cascade, rather than a direct effect on the contractile filaments. Furthermore, Moopanar & Allen (2005, 2006) recently showed that the rapid force decrease during repeated tetanic contractions of single toe fibres at 37°C was caused by decreased myofibrillar Ca^{2+} sensitivity, and it could be prevented by preapplication of ROS scavengers and reversed by postapplication of dithiothreitol. These findings suggest that ROS cause conversion of free sulphydryl groups to disulphide bridges on a protein which regulates Ca^{2+} sensitivity (Moopanar & Allen 2006).

In conclusion, ROS production is accelerated during intense muscle activity and contributes to the development of fatigue, particularly at physiological temperatures. Currently it appears that myofibrillar Ca^{2+} sensitivity is the muscle parameter most sensitive to ROS, and that Ca^{2+} sensitivity is reduced by ROS during fatigue.

3 FATIGUE-INDUCED FAILURE OF SARCOPLASMIC RETICULUM CALCIUM RELEASE

Force production in a muscle fibre will decrease if there is inadequate release of intracellular Ca^{2+} from the sarcoplas-

mic reticulum, and this could occur for a number of reasons, including any or all of the following: (1) failure or deficiency in the spread of electrical excitation along the sarcolemma and into the transverse-tubular system; (2) reduced activation of the voltage-sensor molecules (dihydropyridine receptors) in the transverse-tubular system membrane; (3) disrupted or inadequate voltage-sensor stimulation of the Ca^{2+} release channel (ryanodine receptors) in the sarcoplasmic reticulum; (4) impaired function of ryanodine receptors; and (5) decreased sarcoplasmic reticulum Ca^{2+} concentration. In the following, we will review some mechanisms by which fatigue may decrease sarcoplasmic reticulum Ca^{2+} release.

3.1 Failure of action potential propagation into the transverse–tubular system

Normal tetanic contraction of a muscle fibre requires action potentials to propagate rapidly along the length of a muscle fibre, and then into and throughout the transverse-tubular (T-) system. Clear evidence of the existence and need for action potential propagation in the T-system has been obtained (Bezanilla et al. 1972, Nakajima & Gilai 1980), including the demonstration that action potential-induced twitch and tetanic force responses can be elicited by electrical stimulation, even in mechanically skinned fibres, where the sarcolemma has been peeled away and the T-system has sealed off to become an enclosed compartment (Posterino et al. 2000). These latter experiments also revealed that action potentials travel lengthwise inside a muscle fibre via the longitudinal tubular system which, though sparse in adult muscle (Franzini-Armstrong & Jorgensen 1994, Launikonis & Stephenson 2002), is sufficient to ensure electrical connection between adjacent sarcomeres. This arrangement is likely to help ensure that action potentials reach all parts of the tubular system throughout the fibre, even if conduction in some transverse tubules is blocked for some reason. This may be why the formation of local enlargements (vacuoles) in the T-system during exercise does not appear to have any major deleterious effect on force production in most circumstances (Lännergren et al. 1999, 2002).

If an isolated muscle fibre is continuously stimulated at a relatively high frequency, force declines quite rapidly (high-frequency fatigue), and there is reduced Ca^{2+} release in the centre of the fibre (Duty & Allen 1994, Westerblad et al. 1990), indicating that the voltage sensors there are not adequately activated. Cairns & Dulhunty (1995) have shown this is not due to dysfunction of the voltage sensors themselves, and is caused by inadequate activation of the voltage sensors by T-system action potentials. However, if the fibres are stimulated instead in a more physiological manner, by repeated short tetani, the peak force reached on successive tetani declines comparatively slowly (Westerblad & Lännergren 1986, Westerblad et al. 1990), and the reduction in intracellular $[Ca^{2+}]$ eventually occurring is homogenous across the fibre (Duty & Allen 1994, Westerblad et al. 1993), indicating that voltage-sensor activation is uniform throughout the T-system. As tetanic [Ca^{2+}] did not recover rapidly when these isolated fibres were given a break from the repeated stimulation, it is apparent that the reduction in Ca^{2+} release was not caused by alterations in the concentrations of ions in the tubular system and instead was likely to be due to metabolic or other changes inside the fibre.

However, in intact muscles in vivo there may be considerable changes in the ionic conditions, both extracellularly and intracellularly, and these may have much greater effect on excitability than in isolated fibres. The extracellular potassum concentration, close to fibres in well-perfused muscles working at high intensity, can rise from its normal level of ~4–5 mM to ~9 mM, and the rise in the T-system could be even greater (Sejersted & Sjøgaard 2000). This, together with the rise in intracellular sodium concentration occurring with prolonged exercise (Clausen 2003), will decrease the resting membrane potential of the muscle fibres and adversely affect action potential propagation, both of which could reduce the extent of voltage-sensor activation during tetanic stimulation (Cairns et al. 2003, Dulhunty 1992, Nielsen et al. 2004). If human muscle in vivo is subjected to continuous high-frequency stimulation, there is a marked decrease in force production, which is less marked if the frequency of stimulation is reduced. Studies of the electromyogram and the evoked action potential suggest that this type of fatigue is caused by failure of action potential propagation, probably mainly over the sarcolemma (Bigland-Ritchie et al. 1979, Jones 1996). During voluntary contractions, this failure in surface action potential conduction is avoided by a progressive reduction in the frequency of motor unit activation (Bigland-Ritchie et al. 1983). However, this decrease in action potential frequency has little effect on force production because it is approximately paralleled by a decrease in contraction fusion frequency (Balog et al. 1994). The decrease in the fusion frequency occurring with sustained activity comes about because of a slowing of relaxation. While this slowing of relaxation helps to counteract the reduced firing frequency, it can also impair muscle performance by reducing the ability to produce rapid alternating movements (Allen et al. 1995).

Propagation of action potentials along the surface membrane of a muscle appears not to limit performance in isolated fatigued muscle (Balog et al. 1994). Nonetheless, it is quite possible there is a chronic level of voltage-sensor inactivation and action potential propagation failure occurring within the T-system, and this may cause reduced Ca^{2+} release from the sarcoplasmic reticulum (Nielsen et al. 2004). One mechanism that can help prevent such action potential conduction failure and the consequent force loss, is the reduction in membrane chloride conductance that occurs when intracellular pH decreases in a muscle fibre, as this helps action potentials to continue to propagate, both

along the sarcolemma and within the T-system, despite even substantial increases in extracellular potassium concentration and the accompanying membrane depolarisation (Nielsen et al. 2001, Pedersen et al. 2004, 2005).

In conclusion, while external high-frequency stimulation can cause T-tubular action potential failure and fatigue, in vivo the risk of T-tubular failure is decreased by a gradual reduction of the motoneuron firing frequency. Moreover, acidosis may prevent the occurrence of T-tubular failure, by decreasing the chloride conductance.

3.2 Direct effects of metabolic changes on the sarcoplasmic reticulum calcium release channels

It has been claimed that adenosine triphosphate concentration ([ATP]) in muscle cells does not fall to very low levels during normal exercise (Fitts 1994). However, this claim was based largely on data of the average change in whole muscles or muscle homogenates, which are composed of fibre types with different metabolic profiles and recruitment patterns. Recently, Karatzaferi et al. (2001) measured phosphocreatine and ATP in individual fibres from the vastus lateralis muscle of human subjects immediately after a 25 s maximal cycling bout, and found that in most fibres containing the fastest myosin heavy chain isoform (type IIX), the [ATP] dropped from its resting level of 5–6 mM to between ~0.7 and 1.7 mM. Considering that the ATP is poorly buffered by the very low phosphocreatine levels in these conditions, the [ATP] in regions of high energy consumption may well have dropped to very low levels (<0.5 mM).

Adenosine triphosphate concentration in specialised local regions may differ substantially from the average cytoplasmic level (Korge & Campbell 1995). The triad junction, for example, where the T-system abuts the sarcoplasmic reticulum, is rich in glycolytic enzymes, and is evidently a region of highly localised production and consumption of ATP (Han et al. 1992). A substantial proportion of glucose evidently enters muscle cells via the T-system (Lauritzen et al. 2006), and many of the mitochondria deep in fibres are positioned adjacent to the triad junction. Many glycogen granules are also located in the same region. Thus, the triad junctional gap may act as an important local ATP-sensing region, stopping or reducing Ca^{2+} release and, as a result, ATP consumption when [ATP] drops very low. This would have the consequence that force production would decline; that is, the muscle would show fatigue. On the other hand, it could help prevent complete exhaustion of cellular ATP, which if it occurred could lead to cellular damage, owing to the development of localised rigor cross-bridges.

The sarcoplasmic reticulum Ca^{2+} release channels are inhibited by reduced ATP (Smith et al. 1985). A net breakdown of ATP will result in an increased concentration of free myoplasmic magnesium ([Mg^{2+}]$_i$), since ATP binds Mg^{2+} more strongly than does its breakdown products

(Blazev & Lamb 1999, Westerblad & Allen 1992a,b). Increased $[Mg^{2+}]_i$ has also been shown to inhibit sarcoplasmic reticulum Ca^{2+} release channels (Lamb & Stephenson 1991). Furthermore, the combination of reduced ATP and increased $[Mg^{2+}]_i$ has an additive effect (Blazev and Lamb 1999, Dutka and Lamb 2004, Owen et al. 1996). It is also possible that low [ATP] in the triad junction could inhibit the ATP-driven sodium-potassium (Na^+-K^+) pumps or open ATP-sensitive K^+ channels, and in this way prevent action potential propagation and the subsequent voltage-sensor activation of Ca^{2+} release.

During fatigue induced by intermittent tetani, $[Mg^{2+}]_i$ starts to increase at the time when tetanic $[Ca^{2+}]_i$ starts to fall, suggesting a causal relationship (Westerblad & Allen 1992a,b). However, the relationship between decreasing tetanic $[Ca^{2+}]_i$ and increasing $[Mg^{2+}]_i$ is lost after pharmacological inhibition of creatine kinase (Dahlstedt & Westerblad 2001), which shows that inhibition of the sarcoplasmic reticulum Ca^{2+} release by increased Mg^{2+}, and reduced ATP cannot be the sole mechanism involved.

In the absence of creatine kinase activity, changes in ATP and $[Mg^{2+}]_i$ during contraction should be larger and hence sarcoplasmic reticulum Ca^{2+} release more affected. Accordingly, with high-intensity intermittent tetanic stimulation (20 brief tetani at a duty cycle of 0.67), $[Ca^{2+}]_i$ decreased in muscle fibres from $CK^{-/-}$ mice while it increased in control fibres (Dahlstedt et al. 2000). In a subsequent study, the same authors showed that injection of creatine kinase into $CK^{-/-}$ fibres prevented the decrease in $[Ca^{2+}]_i$ during high-intensity stimulation, which strongly indicates the effect was due to the lack of creatine kinase and not some adaptive response to its deletion (Dahlstedt et al. 2003). However, with a less intense stimulation protocol (duty cycle 0.14), $CK^{-/-}$ muscle fibres were actually more fatigue resistant than muscles from their wild-type littermates (Dahlstedt et al. 2000), which to some extent can be explained by an increased aerobic power of $CK^{-/-}$ fibres.

In conclusion, direct inhibition of sarcoplasmic reticulum Ca^{2+} release channels by reduced ATP and increased $[Mg^{2+}]_i$ appears to be of greatest importance at the onset of high duty-cycle fatigue, whereas a role in later stages of fatigue remains uncertain.

3.3 Calcium–phosphate precipitation in the sarcoplasmic reticulum

A recently suggested mechanism of the decreased sarcoplasmic reticulum Ca^{2+} release in fatigue is that calcium-phosphate (Ca^{2+}-P_i) might precipitate within the sarcoplasmic reticulum, leading to a reduced amount of free Ca^{2+} available for release. The underlying theory is that during fatigue, inorganic phosphate (P_i) first accumulates in the myoplasm due to the breakdown of phosphocreatine via the creatine kinase reaction. Some P_i ions are then transported into the sarcoplasmic reticulum, where the Ca^{2+}-P_i solubility product is exceeded, precipitation occurs and the releasable pool of Ca^{2+} is reduced (Fryer et al. 1995, Inesi & de Meis 1989). Although Ca^{2+}-P_i precipitation has not been directly shown, strong indirect evidence for its existence has been presented, both in experiments on skinned fibres with intact sarcoplasmic reticulum exposed to high P_i solutions (Fryer et al. 1995), and with intact mouse fibres microinjected with P_i (Westerblad & Allen 1996).

Recent experiments have provided three lines of support for the Ca^{2+}-P_i precipitation mechanism in fatigue (Allen & Westerblad 2001, Allen et al. 2002a). First, the amount of Ca^{2+} in the sarcoplasmic reticulum that can be released by application of a high dose of caffeine or 4-choro-m-cresol is reduced in fatigued mouse (Westerblad & Allen 1991) and toad muscle fibres (Kabbara & Allen 1999). Both of these compounds act directly on the sarcoplasmic reticulum Ca^{2+} release channels, and a reduced response indicates that the Ca^{2+} available for release has been reduced. Second, measurement of the free $[Ca^{2+}]$ in the sarcoplasmic reticulum using a low-affinity Ca^{2+} indicator (fluo-5N) showed that it declined throughout a period of fatiguing stimulation, recovering afterwards (Kabbara & Allen 2001). Third, the decline of tetanic $[Ca^{2+}]_i$ during fatiguing stimulation was markedly delayed in fibres where the creatine kinase reaction was inhibited, either pharmacologically (Dahlstedt & Westerblad 2001) or genetically (Dahlstedt et al. 2000). In this case, fibre fatigue will occur without a significant accumulation of P_i in the myoplasm and hence Ca^{2+}-P_i precipitation will not occur. Intriguingly, $CK^{-/-}$ fibres injected with creatine kinase displayed the normal changes in tetanic $[Ca^{2+}]_i$ during fatigue; an early increase followed by a decrease (Dahlstedt et al. 2003). Thus, both the early fatigue-induced increase and the subsequent decrease in tetanic $[Ca^{2+}]_i$ appear directly related to phosphocreatine breakdown and P_i accumulation.

The sarcoplasmic reticulum membrane contains small conductance chloride channels that may conduct P_i (Ahern & Laver 1998, Laver et al. 2001). The probability that these channels are open increases at low [ATP], which is in accordance with the fact that P_i entry into the sarcoplasmic reticulum of skinned muscle fibres is inhibited by ATP (Posterino & Fryer 1998). There are several unresolved issues related to the Ca^{2+}-P_i precipitation hypothesis, which the above observations may help to explain. (1) Myoplasmic $[P_i]$ increases relatively early during fatiguing stimulation, while the decline of tetanic $[Ca^{2+}]_i$ generally occurs quite late. (2) In mouse fast-twitch fibres the decline of tetanic $[Ca^{2+}]_i$ temporally correlates with an increase in $[Mg^{2+}]_i$, which presumably stems from a net breakdown of ATP (Westerblad & Allen 1992a), and it is not obvious why Ca^{2+}-P_i precipitation in the sarcoplasmic reticulum should show a temporal correlation with ATP breakdown. The dependence of sarcoplasmic reticulum P_i channel permeability on [ATP] can provide an explanation for these issues, because the delayed decline in [ATP] will tend to make Ca^{2+}-P_i precipitation occur later than otherwise. Interestingly, in fibres where creatine kinase was pharmacologically inhibited,

$[Mg^{2+}]_i$ increased early during fatiguing stimulation and this was not associated with a decline of tetanic $[Ca^{2+}]_i$ (Dahlstedt & Westerblad 2001). Thus, the temporal correlation between declining tetanic $[Ca^{2+}]_i$ and increasing $[Mg^{2+}]_i$ is lost when myoplasmic P_i accumulation is prevented.

In conclusion, several lines of evidence show that Ca^{2+}-P_i precipitation in the sarcoplasmic reticulum can be a major cause of reduced tetanic $[Ca^{2+}]_i$ in the late stages of fatigue.

3.4 Failure of sarcoplasmic reticulum calcium release due to glycogen depletion

In prolonged endurance activities, muscle fatigue becomes more pronounced at about the time when muscle glycogen levels fall to low levels (Bergström et al. 1967). Studies on single mouse fibres have shown that glycogen content fell to ~25 % during fatigue caused by repeated tetani, and this coincided with reduced Ca^{2+} transients (Chin & Allen 1997). If the muscle fibre was allowed to recover in the absence of glucose, glycogen did not recover and there was limited recovery of tetanic force and $[Ca^{2+}]_i$. When restimulated with repeated tetani, the fibre fatigued much more rapidly. Similar results were obtained in a recent study on isolated mouse extensor digitorum longus (fast-twitch) muscles (Helander et al. 2002). These muscles were fatigued by repeated tetani, allowed to recover for 2 h in a bath with zero, normal or high extracellular glucose concentrations and then fatigued again. Muscles recovering in zero glucose had lower glycogen levels (~50% of the control) at the start of the second fatigue run, and fatigued more rapidly, regarding both tetanic force and $[Ca^{2+}]_i$. Thus, there is a correlation between the level of glycogen and the decrease of tetanic $[Ca^{2+}]_I$ during fatigue.

Electron microscopy of human muscle biopsies, obtained under control conditions and after exhaustive exercise, shows that, in fatigue, glycogen particles were preferentially depleted in the region of the transverse-tubular–sarcoplasmic reticulum junction. Furthermore, the more rapidly fatiguable fibres experienced greater depletion than fatigue-resistant fibres (Friden et al. 1989). These results suggest that glycogen depletion in the region of the transverse-tubular–sarcoplasmic reticulum junction may contribute to the failure of sarcoplasmic reticulum Ca^{2+} release during fatigue. Moreover, the ability of skinned toad muscle fibres to respond to depolarisation of the transverse-tubules correlated closely with the muscle glycogen content (non-soluble component; Stephenson et al. 1999). In these skinned fibre experiments, ATP and phosphocreatine were present in the bathing solutions, suggesting that the glycogen performed a structural rather than a metabolic role. In line with this, using intact mouse muscle fibres, we recently showed that the premature fatigue seen during a second fatigue run after recovery in the absence of glucose (described above) was not associated with a decline in [ATP] (Allen et al. 2002b).

In conclusion, depletion of glycogen during prolonged, exhausting exercise may contribute to fatigue by causing decreased sarcoplasmic reticulum Ca^{2+} release.

3.5 Disruption caused by elevated calcium ion concentration

After intense or prolonged exercise, muscle may show fatigue that lasts many hours or days, and because the reduction in force is relatively greater at low stimulus frequencies, it is commonly referred to as low-frequency fatigue (Edwards et al. 1977, Jones 1996, Westerblad et al. 1993). The reduced force response is due, in large part, to decreased Ca^{2+} release from the sarcoplasmic reticulum (Chin & Allen 1996, Chin et al. 1997, Westerblad et al. 1993). A number of studies have examined the properties of isolated sarcoplasmic reticulum obtained from muscles of animals and humans following various exercise regimes, and some report reductions in the sarcoplasmic reticulum Ca^{2+} release (Favero et al. 1993, Hill et al. 2001). However, in such studies, the Ca^{2+} release had to be triggered by non-physiological stimuli (typically by addition of silver ions), and the rate of Ca^{2+} release achieved this way was several orders of magnitude slower than when the voltage sensors activate the Ca^{2+} release channels. Given that voltage-sensor activation of Ca^{2+} release in intact fibres is frequently found to be quite unaffected by conditions that inhibit Ca^{2+} release in isolated sarcoplasmic reticulum channels (e.g. raised hydrogen and lactate concentrations, oxidation), the above studies do not provide convincing evidence that exercise-induced changes in the release channels themselves are the primary cause of either short-term or long-term reductions in Ca^{2+} release following exercise.

Experiments in isolated single fibres provide evidence that prolonged stimulation can cause long-term reductions in Ca^{2+} release, via a mechanism linked to elevated intracellular $[Ca^{2+}]$ (Bruton et al. 1996, Chin & Allen 1996, Chin et al. 1997). This mechanism is likely to be the same as the one described in skinned fibres, in which elevating intracellular $[Ca^{2+}]$ to very high levels (>10 μM) for a number of seconds (Lamb et al. 1995), or to more moderate levels (2–10 μM) for several minutes (Verburg et al. 2005, 2006) causes long-term disruption of voltage sensor-induced activation of the Ca^{2+} release channels. The involvement of Ca^{2+}-dependent proteases (e.g. calpains) in this process has been suggested, since the deleterious changes can be slowed or prevented in some circumstances by high concentrations (0.2–1.0 mM) of leupeptin, a calpain inhibitor (Duncan & Jackson 1987, Lamb et al. 1995, Verburg et al. 2005). However, in most circumstances, calpain inhibitors are ineffective in stopping the uncoupling between the voltage sensor and the Ca^{2+} release channel (Chin & Allen 1996, Lamb et al. 1995). The reason for this may be that calpains are not involved, or that the experimental conditions used did not allow calpain effects to be detected.

In conclusion, low-frequency fatigue appears to be largely due to Ca^{2+}-dependent damage to the Ca^{2+} release mechanism.

4 FUTURE PERSPECTIVES

Studies mainly from simplified muscle preparations have provided evidence for a range of different mechanisms contributing to fatigue. In humans it is easy to measure the changes in force production, and energy changes can be estimated by muscle biopsies or nuclear magnetic resonance studies, but this does not allow the identification of cellular mechanisms. A major challenge for the future is to establish which of the mechanisms identified in studies of isolated tissues contributes to fatigue in intact animals and humans, and whether there are other, as yet undiscovered, mechanisms. Clearly, the importance of different mechanisms will vary depending on whether the muscle activity is prolonged or brief, whether the required force is maximal or submaximal, and whether the contractions are isometric or involve shortening or lengthening. Diseases such as heart failure, anaemia and renal failure display excessive muscle fatiguability as prominent symptoms, and identification of the mechanisms involved represents an important step in the development of new therapeutic strategies.

Acknowledgements

We thank the Australian National Health and Medical Research Council, the Australian Research Council, the Swedish Medical Research Council, the Karolinska Institute and the Swedish National Center for Sports Research for research funding.

References

Ahern GP, Laver DR 1998 ATP inhibition and rectification of a Ca2+-activated anion channel in sarcoplasmic reticulum of skeletal muscle. Biophysical Journal 74:2335–2351

Allen DG, Westerblad H 2001 Role of phosphate and calcium stores in muscle fatigue. Journal of Physiology 536:657–665

Allen DG, Lännergren J, Westerblad H 1995 Muscle cell function during prolonged activity: cellular mechanisms of fatigue. Experimental Physiology 80:497–527

Allen DG, Kabbara AA, Westerblad H 2002a Muscle fatigue: the role of intracellular calcium stores. Canadian Journal of Applied Physiology 27:83–96

Allen DG, Lännergren J, Westerblad H 2002b Intracellular ATP measured with luciferin/luciferase in isolated single mouse skeletal muscle fibres. Pflügers Archiv European Journal of Physiology 443:836–842

Andrade FH, Reid MB, Allen DG, Westerblad H 1998 Effect of hydrogen peroxide and dithiothreitol on contractile function of single skeletal muscle fibres from the mouse. Journal of Physiology 509:565–575

Andrade FH, Reid MB, Westerblad H 2001 Contractile response of skeletal muscle to low peroxide concentrations: myofibrillar calcium sensitivity as a likely target for redox-modulation. FASEB Journal 15:309–311

Balog EM, Thompson LV, Fitts RH 1994 Role of sarcolemma action potentials and excitability in muscle fatigue. Journal of Applied Physiology 76:2157–2162

Bangsbo J, Madsen K, Kiens B, Richter EA 1996 Effect of muscle acidity on muscle metabolism and fatigue during intense exercise in man. Journal of Physiology 495:587–596

Bergström J, Hermansen L, Hultman E, Saltin B 1967 Diet, muscle glycogen and physical performance. Acta Physiologica Scandinavica 71:140–150

Bezanilla F, Caputo C, Gonzalez-Serratos H, Venosa RA 1972 Sodium dependence of the inward spread of activation in isolated twitch muscles of the frog. Journal of Physiology 223:507–523

Bigland-Ritchie B, Jones DA, Woods JJ 1979 Excitation frequency and muscle fatigue: electrical responses during human voluntary and stimulated contractions. Experimental Neurology 64:414–427

Bigland-Ritchie B, Johansson R, Lippold OC, Smith S, Woods JJ 1983 Changes in motoneurone firing rates during sustained maximal voluntary contractions. Journal of Physiology 340:335–346

Blazev R Lamb GD 1999 Low [ATP] and elevated [Mg^{2+}] reduce depolarization-induced Ca^{2+} release in mammalian skeletal muscle. Journal of Physiology 520:203–215

Brooks GA 1991 Current concepts in lactate exchange. Medicine and Science in Sports and Exercise 23:895–906

Bruton JD, Lännergren J, Westerblad H 1996 Effects of repetitive tetanic stimulation at long intervals on excitation-contraction coupling in frog skeletal muscle. Journal of Physiology 495:15–22

Bruton JD, Wretman C, Katz A, Westerblad H 1997 Increased tetanic force and reduced myoplasmic [P(i)] following a brief series of tetani in mouse soleus muscle. American Journal of Physiology. Cell Physiology 272:C870–C874

Bruton JD, Lännergren J, Westerblad H 1998 Effects of CO_2-induced acidification on the fatigue resistance of single mouse muscle fibers at 28 degrees C. Journal of Applied Physiology 85:478–483

Bruton JD, Tavi P, Aydin J, Westerblad H, Lännergren J 2003 Mitochondrial and myoplasmic [Ca^{2+}] in single fibres from mouse limb muscles during repeated tetanic contractions. Journal of Physiology 551:179–190

Burke RE, Levine DN, Trairis P, Zajac FE 1973 Physiological types and histochemical profiles in muscle motor units of the cat gastrocnemius. Journal of Physiology 234:723–748

Cairns SP, Dulhunty AF 1995 High-frequency fatigue in rat skeletal muscle: role of extracellular ion concentrations. Muscle and Nerve 18:890–898

Cairns SP, Buller SJ, Loiselle DS, Renaud JM 2003 Changes of action potentials and force at lowered [Na^+]o in mouse skeletal muscle: implications for fatigue. American Journal of Physiology. Cell Physiology 285:C1131-C1141

Callahan LA, She ZW, Nosek TM 2001 Superoxide, hydroxyl radical and hydrogen peroxide effects on single-diaphragm fiber contractile apparatus. Journal of Applied Physiology 90:45–54

Chin ER, Allen DG 1996 The role of elevations in intracellular Ca^{2+} concentration in the development of low frequency fatigue in mouse single muscle fibres. Journal of Physiology 491:813–824

Chin ER, Allen DG 1997 Effects of reduced muscle glycogen concentration on force, Ca^{2+} release and contractile protein function in intact mouse skeletal muscle. Journal of Physiology 498:17–29

Chin ER, Balnave CD, Allen DG 1997 Role of intracellular calcium and metabolites in low-frequency fatigue in mouse skeletal muscle. American Journal of Physiology. Cell Physiology 272:C550–C559

Clausen T 2003 Na$^+$-K$^+$ pump regulation and skeletal muscle contractility. Physiological Reviews 83:1269–1324

Coupland ME, Puchert E, Ranatunga KW 2001 Temperature dependence of active tension in mammalian (rabbit psoas) muscle fibres: effect of inorganic phosphate. Journal of Physiology 536:879–891

Dahlstedt AJ, Westerblad H 2001 Inhibition of creatine kinase reduces the fatigue-induced decrease of tetanic [Ca^{2+}]$_i$ in mouse skeletal muscle. Journal of Physiology 533:639–649

Dahlstedt AJ, Katz A, Wieringa B, Westerblad H 2000 Is creatine kinase responsible for fatigue? Studies of isolated skeletal muscle deficient in creatine kinase. FASEB Journal 14:982–990

Dahlstedt AJ, Katz A, Westerblad H 2001 Role of myoplasmic phosphate in contractile function of skeletal muscle studies on creatine kinase deficient mice. Journal of Physiology 533:379–388

Dahlstedt AJ, Katz A, Tavi P, Westerblad H 2003 Creatine kinase injection restores contractile function in creatine-kinase-deficient mouse skeletal muscle fibres. Journal of Physiology 547:395–403

Dantzig JA, Goldman YE, Millar NC, Lacktis J, Homsher E 1992 Reversal of the cross-bridge force-generating transition by photogeneration of phosphate in rabbit psoas muscle fibres. Journal of Physiology 451:247–278

Darnley GM, Duke AM, Steele DS, MacFarlane NG 2001 Effects of reactive oxygen species on aspects of excitation-contraction coupling in chemically skinned rabbit diaphragm muscle fibres. Experimental Physiology 86:161–168

Davies KJ, Quintanilha AT, Brooks GA, Packer L 1982 Free radicals and tissue damage produced by exercise. Biochemical and Biophysical Research Communications 107:1198–1205

Debold EP, Dave H, Fitts RH 2004 Fiber type and temperature dependence of inorganic phosphate: implications for fatigue. American Journal of Physiology. Cell Physiology 287:C673-C681

Dulhunty AF 1992 The voltage-activation of contraction in skeletal muscle. Progress in Biophysics and Molecular Biology 57:181–223

Duncan CJ, Jackson MJ 1987 Different mechanisms mediate structural changes and intracellular enzyme efflux following damage to skeletal muscle. Journal of Cell Science 87:183–188

Dutka TL, Lamb GD 2004 Effect of low cytoplasmic [ATP] on excitation-contraction coupling in fast-twitch muscle fibres of the rat. Journal of Physiology 560:451–468

Duty S, Allen DG 1994 The distribution of intracellular calcium concentration in isolated single fibres of mouse skeletal muscle during fatiguing stimulation. Pflügers Archiv European Journal of Physiology 427:102–109

Edwards RHT, Hill DK, Jones DA, Merton PA 1977 Fatigue of long duration in human skeletal muscle after exercise. Journal of Physiology 272:769–778

Favero TG, Pesssah IN, Klug GA 1993 Prolonged exercise reduces Ca^{2+} release in rat skeletal muscle sarcoplasmic reticulum. Pflügers Archiv European Journal of Physiology 422:472–475

Fitts RH 1994 Cellular mechanisms of muscle fatigue. Physiological Reviews 74:49–94

Franzini-Armstrong C, Jorgensen AO 1994 Structure and development of E-C coupling units in skeletal muscle. Annual Review of Physiology 56:509–534

Friden J, Seger J, Ekblom B 1989 Topographical localization of muscle glycogen: an ultrahistochemical study in the human vastus lateralis. Acta Physiologica Scandinavica 135:381–391

Fryer MW, Owen VJ, Lamb GD, Stephenson DG 1995 Effects of creatine phosphate and P$_i$ on Ca^{2+} movements and tension development in rat skinned skeletal muscle fibres. Journal of Physiology 482:123–140

Gandevia SC 2001 Spinal and supraspinal factors in human muscle fatigue. Physiological Reviews 81:1725–1789

Godt RE, Nosek TM 1989 Changes in the intracellular mileiu with fatigue or hypoxia depress contraction of skinned rabbit skeletal and cardiac muscle. Journal of Physiology 412:155–180

Gordon AM, Homsher E, Regnier M 2000 Regulation of contraction in striated muscle. Physiological Reviews 80:853–924

Halliwell B, Gutteridge JMC 1998 Free radicals in biology and medicine, 3rd edn. Oxford University Press, Oxford

Han J-W, Thieleczek R, Varsanyi M, Heilmeyer LMG 1992 Compartmentalized ATP synthesis in skeletal muscle triads. Biochemistry 31:377–384

Helander I, Westerblad H, Katz A 2002 Effects of glucose on contractile function, [Ca^{2+}]$_i$ and glycogen in isolated mouse skeletal muscle. American Journal of Physiology. Cell Physiology 282: C1306–C1312

Hill CA, Thompson MW, Ruell PA, Thom JM, White MJ 2001 Sarcoplasmic reticulum function and muscle contractile character following fatiguing exercise in humans. Journal of Physiology 531:871–878

Inesi G, de Meis L 1989 Regulation of steady state filling in sarcoplasmic reticulum: roles of back-inhibition, leakage and slippage of the calcium pump. Journal of Biological Chemistry 264:5929–5936

Jones DA 1996 High- and low-frequency fatigue revisited. Acta Physiologica Scandinavica 156:265–270

Kabbara AA, Allen DG 1999 The role of calcium stores in fatigue of isolated single muscle fibres from the cane toad. Journal of Physiology 519:169–176

Kabbara AA, Allen DG 2001 The use of fluo-5N to measure sarcoplasmic reticulum calcium in single muscle fibres of the cane toad. Journal of Physiology 534:87–97

Karatzaferi C, de Haan A, Ferguson RA, van Mechelen W, Sargeant AJ 2001 Phosphocreatine and ATP content in human single muscle fibres before and after maximum dynamic exercise. Pflügers Archiv European Journal of Physiology 442:467–474

Korge P, Campbell KB 1995 The importance of ATPase microenvironment in muscle fatigue: a hypothesis. International Journal of Sports Medicine 16:172–179

Kristensen M, Albertsen J, Rentsch M, Juel C 2005 Lactate and force production in skeletal muscle. Journal of Physiology 562:521–526

Lamb GD, Posterino GS 2003 Effects of oxidation and reduction on contractile function in skeletal muscle fibres of the rat. Journal of Physiology 546:149–163

Lamb GD Stephenson DG 1991 Effects of Mg^{2+} on the control of Ca^{2+} release in skeletal muscle fibres of the toad. Journal of Physiology 434:507–528

Lamb GD, Stephenson DG 1994 Effects of intracellular pH and [Mg^{2+}] on excitation-contraction coupling in skeletal muscle fibres of the rat. Journal of Physiology 478:331–339

Lamb GD, Recupero E, Stephenson DG 1992 Effect of myoplasmic pH on excitation-contraction coupling in skeletal muscle fibres of the toad. Journal of Physiology 448:211–224

Lamb GD, Junankar PR, Stephenson DG 1995 Raised intracellular [Ca^{2+}] abolishes excitation-contraction coupling in skeletal muscle fibres of rat and toad. Journal of Physiology 489:349–362

Lännergren J, Bruton JD, Westerblad H 1999 Vacuole formation in fatigued single muscle fibres from frog and mouse. Journal of Muscle Research and Cell Motility 20:19–32

Lännergren J, Westerblad H, Bruton JD 2002 Dynamic vacuolation in skeletal muscle fibres after fatigue. Cell Biology International 26:911–920

Launikonis BS, Stephenson DG 2002 Tubular system volume changes in twitch fibres from toad and rat skeletal muscle assessed by confocal microscopy. Journal of Physiology 538:607–618

Lauritzen HP, Ploug T, Prats C, Tavare JM, Galbo H 2006 Imaging of insulin signaling in skeletal muscle of living mice shows major role of T-tubules. Diabetes 55:1300–1306

Laver DR, Eager KR, Taoube L, Lamb GD 2000 Effects of cytoplasmic and luminal pH on Ca^{2+} release channels from rabbit skeletal muscle. Biophysical Journal 78:1835–1851

Laver DR, Lenz GKE, Dulhunty AF 2001 Phosphate ion channels in the sarcoplasmic reticulum of rabbit skeletal muscle. Journal of Physiology 537:763–778

Lynch RE, Fridovich I 1978 Permeation of the erythrocyte stroma by superoxide radical. Journal of Biological Chemistry 253:4697–4699

Ma J, Fill M, Knudson CM, Campbell KP, Coronado R 1988 Ryanodine receptor of skeletal muscle is a gap junction-type channel. Science 242:99–102

Martyn DA, Gordon AM 1992 Force and stiffness in glycerinated rabbit psoas fibers. Effects of calcium and elevated phosphate. Journal of General Physiology 99:795–816

Millar NC, Homsher E 1990 The effect of phosphate and calcium on force generation in glycerinated rabbit skeletal muscle fibers: a steady-state and transient kinetic study. Journal of Biological Chemistry 265:20234–20240

Moopanar TR, Allen DG 2005 Reactive oxygen species reduce myofibrillar Ca^{2+}-sensitivity in fatiguing mouse skeletal muscle at 37°C. Journal of Physiology 564:189–199

Moopanar TR, Allen DG 2006 The activity-induced reduction of myofibrillar Ca2+ sensitivity in mouse skeletal muscle is reversed by dithiothreitol. Journal of Physiology 571:191–200

Nakajima S, Gilai A 1980 Radial propagation of muscle action potential along the tubular system examined by potential-sensitive dyes. Journal of General Physiology 76:751–762

Nielsen OB, de Paoli F, Overgaard K 2001 Protective effects of lactic acid on force production in rat skeletal muscle. Journal of Physiology 536:161–166

Nielsen JJ, Mohr M, Klarskov C, Kristensen M, Krustrup P, Juel C, Bangsbo J 2004 Effects of high-intensity intermittent training on potassium kinetics and performance in human skeletal muscle. Journal of Physiology 554:857–870

Owen VJ, Lamb GD, Stephenson DG 1996 Effect of low [ATP] on deploarization-induced Ca^{2+} release in skeletal muscle fibres of the toad. Journal of Physiology 493:309–315

Pate E, Cooke R 1989 Addition of phosphate to active muscle fibers probes actomyosin states within the powerstroke. Pflügers Archiv European Journal of Physiology 414:73–81

Pate E, Bhimani M, Franks-Skiba K, Cooke R 1995 Reduced effect of pH on skinned rabbit psoas muscle mechanics at high temperatures: implications for fatigue. Journal of Physiology 486:689–694

Pedersen TH, Nielsen OB, Lamb GD, Stephenson DG 2004 Intracellular acidosis enhances the excitability of the working muscle. Science 305:1144–1147

Pedersen TH, de Paoli F, Nielsen OB 2005 Increased excitability of acidified skeletal muscle: role of chloride conductance. Journal of General Physiology 125:237–246

Phillips SK, Wiseman RW, Woledge RC, Kushmerick MJ 1993 The effect of metabolic fuel on force production and resting inorganic phosphate levels in mouse skeletal muscle. Journal of Physiology 462:135–146

Posterino GS, Fryer MW 1998 Mechanisms underlying phosphate-induced failure of Ca^{2+} release in single skinned skeletal muscle fibres of the rat. Journal of Physiology 512:97–108

Posterino GS, Lamb GD, Stephenson DG 2000 Twitch and tetanic force responses and longitudinal propagation of action potentials in skinned skeletal muscle fibres of the rat. Journal of Physiology 527 (Pt 1):131–137

Posterino GS, Dutka TL, Lamb GD 2001 L(+)-lactate does not affect twitch and tetanic responses in mechanically skinned mammalian muscle fibres. Pflügers Archiv European Journal of Physiology 442:197–203

Ranatunga KW 1987 Effects of acidosis on tension development in mammalian skeletal muscle. Muscle and Nerve 10:439–445

Reid MB, Durham WJ 2002 Generation of reactive oxygen and nitrogen species in contracting skeletal muscle: potential impact on aging. Annals of the New York Academy of Sciences 959:108–116

Reid MR, Haack KE, Franchek KM, Valberg PA, Kobzik L, West MS 1992 Reactive oxygen in skeletal muscle I. Intracellular oxidant kinetics and fatigue in vitro. Journal of Applied Physiology 73:1797–1804

Reid MB, Stokic DS, Koch SM, Khawli FA, Leis AA 1994 N-acetylcysteine inhibits muscle fatigue in humans. Journal of Clinical Investigation 94:2468–2474

Sahlin K, Ren JM 1989 Relationship of contraction capacity to metabolic changes during recovery from a fatiguing contraction. Journal of Applied Physiology 67:648–654

Sejersted OM, Sjøgaard G 2000 Dynamics and consequences of potassium shifts in skeletal muscle and heart during exercise. Physiological Reviews 80:1411–1481

Shindoh C, DiMarco A, Thomas A, Manubay P, Supinski G 1990 Effect of N-acetylcysteine on diaphragm fatigue. Journal of Applied Physiology 68:2107–2113

Smith JS, Coronado R, Meissner G 1985 Sarcoplasmic reticulum contains adenine nucleotide-activated calcium channels. Nature 316:446–449

Steeghs K, Benders A, Oerlemans F, de Haan A, Heerschap A, Ruitenbeek W, Jost C, van Deursen J, Perryman B, Pette D, Brückwilder M, Koudijs J, Jap P, Veerkamp J, Wieringa B 1997 Altered Ca^{2+} responses in muscles with combined mitochondrial and cytosolic creatine kinase deficiencies. Cell 89:93–103

Stephenson DG, Nguyen LT, Stephenson GMM 1999 Glycogen content and excitation-contraction coupling in mechanically skinned muscle fibres of the cane toad. Journal of Physiology 519:177–187

Turrens JF 2003 Mitochondrial formation of reactive oxygen species. Journal of Physiology 552:335–344

Verburg E, Murphy RM, Stephenson DG, Lamb GD 2005 Disruption of excitation-contraction coupling and titin by endogenous Ca^{2+}-activated proteases in toad muscle fibres. Journal of Physiology 564:775–790

Verburg E, Dutka TL, Lamb GD 2006 Long-lasting muscle fatigue: partial disruption of excitation-contraction coupling by elevated cytosolic Ca^{2+} concentration during contractions. American Journal of Physiology. Cell Physiology 290:C1199-C1208

Westerblad H, Allen DG 1991 Changes of myoplasmic calcium concentration during fatigue in single mouse muscle fibers. Journal of General Physiology 98:615–635

Westerblad H, Allen DG 1992a Myoplasmic free Mg^{2+} concentration during repetitive stimulation of single fibres from mouse skeletal muscle. Journal of Physiology 453:413–434

Westerblad H, Allen DG 1992b Myoplasmic Mg^{2+} concentration in Xenopus muscle fibres at rest, during fatigue and during metabolic blockade. Experimental Physiology 77:733–740

Westerblad H, Allen DG 1996 The effects of intracellular injections of phosphate on intracellular calcium and force in single fibres of mouse skeletal muscle. Pflügers Archiv European Journal of Physiology 431:964–970

Westerblad H, Lännergren L 1986 Force and membrane potential during and after fatiguing, intermittent tetanic stimulation of single Xenopus fibres. Acta Physiologica Scandinavica 128:369–378

Westerblad H, Lee JA, Lamb AG, Bolsover SR, Allen DG 1990 Spatial gradients of intracellular calcium in skeletal muscle during fatigue. Pflügers Archiv European Journal of Physiology 415:734–740

Westerblad H, Lee JA, Lännergren J, Allen DG 1991 Cellular mechanisms of fatigue in skeletal muscle. American Journal of Physiology 261:C195–209

Westerblad H, Duty S, Allen DG 1993 Intracellular calcium concentration during low-frequency fatigue in isolated single fibers of mouse skeletal muscle. Journal of Applied Physiology 75:382–388

Westerblad H, Bruton JD, Lännergren J 1997 The effect of intracellular pH on contractile function of intact, single fibres of mouse muscle declines with increasing temperature. Journal of Physiology 500:193–204

Wiseman RW, Beck TW, Chase PB 1996 Effect of intracellular pH on force development depends on temperature in intact skeletal muscle from mouse. American Journal of Physiology. Cell Physiology 40:C878–C886

Zhang SJ, Bruton JD, Katz A, Westerblad H 2006 Limited oxygen diffusion accelerates fatigue development in mouse skeletal muscle. Journal of Physiology 572:551–559

Zuo L, Christofi FL, Wright VP, Liu CY, Merola AJ, Berliner LJ, Clanton TL 2000 Intra- and extracellular measurement of reactive oxygen species produced during heat stress in diaphragm muscle. American Journal of Physiology. Cell Physiology 279: C1058–C1066

Chapter **7**

Performance limitations due to substrate availability

Mark Hargreaves

1 INTRODUCTION

The immediate energy source for skeletal muscle actin–myosin cross-bridge cycling during exercise is adenosine triphosphate (ATP). In addition, ATP is required for a number of energy-dependent cellular processes that have a fundamental role in excitation-contraction coupling, such as sodium and potassium exchange across the sarcolemma and transverse-tubule, and calcium release and re-uptake by the sarcoplasmic reticulum. Since the intramuscular stores of ATP are relatively small (~5 mmol·kg^{-1} wet muscle), other metabolic pathways responsible for the generation of ATP must be activated to maintain contractile activity and delay the onset of intramuscular fatigue (Chapters 5 and 6). These energy pathways are summarised in Table 7.1.

Phosphocreatine (PCr) is a high-energy compound, stored in greater amounts (~20 mmol·kg^{-1}) in skeletal muscle, which can be rapidly degraded during intense exercise to provide energy for ATP resynthesis. ATP can also be formed directly from adenosine diphosphate, in a reaction catalysed by adenylate kinase. The degradation of glucose units, derived primarily from intramuscular glycogen stores, to lactic acid generates more ATP than PCr degradation, albeit at a slower rate. These substrate-level phosphorylation reactions are not dependent upon oxygen availability, but are maximally active during high-intensity exercise of short duration, where power outputs are typically much greater than can be supported by oxidative phosphorylation. As exercise duration increases, with a concomitant reduction in exercise intensity, oxidative phosphorylation provides the majority of ATP for contracting skeletal muscle, with both carbohydrates (muscle glycogen, blood glucose) and lipids (intramuscular triglyceride, plasma free fatty acids) providing the major substrates for this process. The relative contribution of carbohydrates and lipids is influenced by the exercise intensity and duration, preceding diet and substrate availability, endurance-training status and environmental conditions.

The availability of ATP for energy-dependent cellular processes, or phosphocreatine, muscle glycogen, blood

Table 7.1 Metabolic pathways in skeletal muscle that contribute to ATP utilisation and resynthesis during exercise

ATP utilisation:

$ATP + H_2O \rightarrow ADP + P_i + H^+ + energy$

ATP resynthesis:

(i) Substrate level phosphorylation (anaerobic)

$PCr + ADP + H^+ \rightarrow ATP + creatine$

$2ADP \rightarrow ATP + AMP$

$Glycogen + 3ADP + 3P_i \rightarrow 3ATP + 2\ lactate + 2H^+$

(ii) Oxidative phosphorylation

$Glucose + 6O_2 + 36ADP \rightarrow 36ATP + 6CO_2 + 6H_2O$

$Palmitate + 23O_2 + 130ADP \rightarrow 130ATP + 16CO_2 + 16H_2O$

glucose and free fatty acids for ATP production, is critical for the maintenance of skeletal muscle force and power production during exercise. Depletion of these substrates is likely to contribute to the development of fatigue, and is one factor among many (Chapters 5 and 6) that limits exercise performance. It should be noted that substrate depletion during exercise occurs simultaneously with the accumulation of metabolic by-products (e.g. adenosine diphosphate, inorganic phosphate, hydrogen and lactate ions, and reactive oxygen species), and these may also be involved in the development of fatigue during exercise. The potential role of these metabolic by-products in limiting exercise performance was discussed in more detail in the previous chapter.

2 ADENOSINE TRIPHOSPHATE

Given the importance of ATP for cellular function, one might expect that its intramuscular concentration ([ATP]) would be reasonably well protected during even the most intense exercise, so as to avoid complete cellular ATP depletion. Indeed, when measured in whole-muscle samples, [ATP] is reduced by only ~30–40% following intense electrical stimulation (Spriet et al. 1987), maximal cycling exercise (Hargreaves et al. 1998, Spriet et al. 1989, Withers et al. 1991) and sprint running (Cheetham et al. 1986).

One interpretation of this apparent ATP protection is that it demonstrates the effectiveness of the various metabolic pathways in generating ATP, albeit at a rate slower than its utilisation, and also with reduced exercise performance. Alternatively, global muscle ATP measurements may not be a true reflection of the [ATP] in critical loci within the muscle, either in individual muscle fibres or near the sites of maximal ATP utilisation (i.e. cross-bridges, sarcolemma, transverse-tubules, sarcoplasmic reticulum and their respective ATPases). Indeed, it has been observed that [ATP] in fast-twitch (type II) muscle fibres following intense exercise is lower than in slow-twitch (type I) muscle fibres in some (Casey et al. 1996b, Karatzaferi et al. 2001) but not all studies (Greenhaff et al. 1994, Söderlund & Hultman 1991). This

may partly explain the greater fatiguability of the type II fibres, and the decline in power output when they can no longer contribute to force generation (Casey et al. 1996b). Studies in skinned, single muscle fibres demonstrate that low [ATP] impairs excitation-contraction coupling and force production (Blazev & Lamb 1999, Dutka & Lamb 2004, Owen et al. 1996), effects that are potentiated by the concomitant increases in sarcoplasmic magnesium, adenosine diphosphate and inorganic phosphate (Blazev & Lamb 1999, Dutka & Lamb 2004).

Thus, local ATP depletion in the vicinity of the sarcoplasmic reticulum calcium release channels and calcium ATPase, and the sarcolemmal and transverse-tubular sodium-potassium ATPases, could produce fatigue before all of the ATP within the muscle cell is consumed. While this reduces exercise performance, it also protects the cell from the negative effects of total ATP depletion (rigor and cellular damage). During prolonged, strenuous exercise when there is a major reliance on oxidative phosphorylation for energy production, muscle ATP levels are reduced only slightly (Sahlin et al. 1990, 1997), or not at all at the point of fatigue (Ball-Burnett et al. 1991, Febbraio & Dancey 1999, McConell et al. 1999).

3 PHOSPHOCREATINE

Whereas intramuscular [ATP] is reasonably well maintained during exercise, the major role of PCr degradation is to preserve ATP availability. It is not surprising, therefore, that intramuscular PCr concentration ([PCr]) can be reduced to very low levels following intense electrical stimulation (Spriet et al. 1987), maximal cycling exercise (Hargreaves et al. 1998, Spriet et al. 1989, Withers et al. 1991) and sprint running (Cheetham et al. 1986). This is seen in both type I and II muscle fibres (Casey et al. 1996b, Karatzaferi et al. 2001, Söderlund & Hultman 1991), although a greater reduction in [PCr] in type II fibres was observed following maximal treadmill running (Greenhaff et al. 1994).

The decline in power output during maximal exercise is associated with the reduction in intramuscular [PCr], and results in a greater reliance on glycolysis and oxidative phosphorylation (Figure 7.1; Parolin et al. 1999), processes that generate ATP more slowly than PCr degradation. In addition, the recovery of power output during maximal exercise is closely correlated with the resynthesis of PCr (Bogdanis et al. 1995). Furthermore, prevention of PCr resynthesis, an oxygen-dependent process, by circulatory occlusion will result in lower work output during maximal cycling (Trump et al. 1996).

Collectively, these studies demonstrate the importance of PCr for power output during maximal exercise. An increased PCr availability, especially in type II muscle fibres, may explain the ergogenic benefits of dietary creatine supplementation (Balsom et al. 1993, Casey et al. 1996a), although this is not a universal observation (McKenna et al. 1999, Snow et al. 1998). Significant reductions in muscle [PCr]

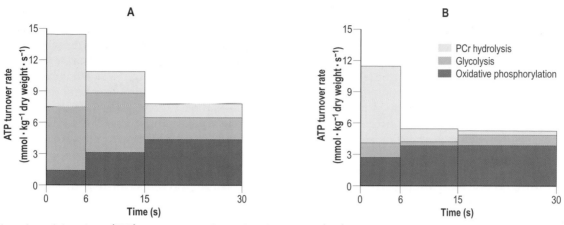

Figure 7.1 Adenosine triphosphate (ATP) turnover rate from phosphocreatine (PCr) hydrolysis, glycolysis and oxidative phosphorylation during the first (A) and third (B) bouts of maximal cycling exercise (from Parolin et al. 1999, with permission from the American Physiological Society).

have also been observed following prolonged, submaximal exercise (Febbraio & Dancey 1999, McConell et al. 1999, Sahlin et al. 1990, 1997, Tsintzas et al. 2001), which may partly reflect the lower glycogen availability at the point of fatigue, although the significance of a lower [PCr] in the aetiology of fatigue has been questioned (Febbraio & Dancey 1999).

4 MUSCLE GLYCOGEN

The importance of muscle glycogen for endurance exercise performance was confirmed in some of the first studies to obtain samples from human skeletal muscle, using percutaneous needle biopsy techniques before, during and after exercise. These early studies observed an association between muscle glycogen depletion and exhaustion during prolonged, strenuous exercise (Bergström & Hultman 1967, Hermansen et al. 1967), and demonstrated a direct relationship between pre-exercise muscle glycogen concentration and time to fatigue during prolonged, strenuous exercise (Bergström et al. 1967). These studies established the theoretical basis of glycogen (carbohydrate) loading, a nutritional strategy designed to increase muscle glycogen availability and enhance endurance exercise performance in athletic events lasting more than ~90 min (see Hawley et al. (1997) for review).

Subsequent studies demonstrated muscle fibre type selective glycogen depletion patterns, depending upon the exercise intensity and duration. Muscle glycogen was primarily depleted in type I muscle fibres during prolonged, submaximal exercise, with some glycogen utilisation in type II muscle fibres towards the latter stages of exercise (Gollnick et al. 1973a). In contrast, during high-intensity exercise, the type II muscle fibres were the first to become depleted of muscle glycogen (Gollnick et al. 1973b).

The underlying biochemical mechanism linking muscle glycogen depletion to fatigue has been postulated to be an inability to maintain a rate of ATP resynthesis that is sufficient to meet the energy demands of exercise, as reflected by an increase in intramuscular inosine monophosphate, an ATP breakdown product, and reduced PCr (Sahlin et al. 1990, 1997, Spencer et al. 1992). According to this hypothesis, a lower muscle pyruvate availability, secondary to muscle glycogen depletion, results in reduced substrate for both carbohydrate oxidation and the anaplerotic (restorative) reactions considered important to maintain tricarboxylic acid (Krebs) cycle intermediate levels, and the flux and delivery of carbohydrate-derived reducing equivalents to the electron transport chain (Sahlin et al. 1990, Spencer et al. 1992). The relationship between muscle glycogen and inosine monophosphate may be partly dependent on endurance training status (Baldwin et al. 1999).

In contrast, other studies have failed to observe consistent relationships between ATP, PCr, inosine monophosphate and muscle glycogen depletion (Baldwin et al. 2003, Ball-Burnett et al. 1991, Febbraio & Dancey, 1999), thereby raising the possibility that muscle glycogen depletion may induce fatigue via other mechanisms. Of note, the ability of single, mechanically skinned fibres to respond to depolarisation is correlated with the initial, intramuscular glycogen concentration (Stephenson et al. 1999), and glycogen depletion can impair sarcoplasmic reticulum calcium release (Chin & Allen 1997) and the ability to respond to depolarisation, even in the presence of optimal ATP availability (Stephenson et al. 1999). Since it is known that muscle glycogen is closely associated with the sarcoplasmic reticulum, it is possible that the glycogen concentration in this region may be crucial for excitation-contraction coupling, via both ATP-dependent and ATP-independent mechanisms.

While there is no question that glycogen availability is critical for endurance exercise performance, there is more debate on its importance for performance during high-intensity, sprint exercise. Perhaps not surprising, given the heavy reliance on glycolysis, very low, pre-exercise muscle glycogen concentration can impair high-intensity exercise performance (Casey et al. 1996c, Maughan et al. 1997).

Muscle glycogen loading has variable effects, with some studies showing no benefit for a single maximal exercise bout (Hargreaves et al. 1997), and others demonstrating improved performance (Maughan et al. 1997), especially if repeated bouts are undertaken (Balsom et al. 1999). While these effects may be mediated by muscle glycogen availability per se, it is possible that alterations in acid–base status, secondary to changes in dietary carbohydrate intake, may also play a role in extending exercise duration (Maughan et al. 1997).

5 BLOOD GLUCOSE

Although muscle glycogen is the major source of carbohydrates for oxidative phosphorylation during prolonged exercise, especially during intense, submaximal exercise, the uptake and oxidation of blood glucose can contribute significantly to oxidative energy metabolism (Romijn et al. 1993). Lowered blood glucose availability, or hypoglycaemia, is associated with the development of fatigue during prolonged strenuous exercise (Coggan & Coyle 1987, Coyle et al. 1983, 1986, McConell et al. 1999, Spencer et al. 1991, Tsintzas et al. 1996). Increasing blood glucose availability during exercise, via carbohydrate ingestion, is therefore an effective strategy for enhancing endurance performance, and is a common practice during such activities.

The mechanisms responsible for a more rapid fatigue development with hypoglycaemia are secondary to changes in blood glucose concentration, and include effects on carbohydrate oxidation and energy metabolism within contracting skeletal muscle, as well as changes in central nervous system function (e.g. perception of effort, motor drive; Chapter 5). These interactions dictate the ergogenic benefits of carbohydrate ingestion, which acts to maintain or increase blood glucose concentration and carbohydrate oxidation during prolonged, strenuous exercise (Figure 7.2; Coggan & Coyle 1987, Coyle et al. 1983, 1986).

The maintenance of carbohydrate oxidation is due to increased glucose uptake (McConell et al. 1994) at a time when muscle glycogen is low. This occurs with no effects on net muscle glycogen utilisation, at least during prolonged, strenuous cycling exercise (Coyle et al. 1986, Hargreaves & Briggs 1988). Some studies have observed reduced muscle glycogen utilisation during running exercise, notably in the type I fibres, following carbohydrate ingestion (Tsintzas et al. 1996), and this was associated with an attenuation of PCr hydrolysis in these fibres (Tsintzas et al. 2001). Irrespective of the mechanism that delays fatigue, an increased carbohydrate supply to contracting skeletal muscle results in improved energy metabolism, as reflected by lower muscle inosine monophosphate levels (McConell et al. 1999, Spencer et al. 1991).

An increased blood glucose availability also acts via the central nervous system, as reflected by the attenuation of exercise-induced increases in ratings of perceived exertion (Burgess et al. 1991, Nybo 2003, Nybo et al. 2003), and decreases in central nervous system activation during maximal isometric contractions following prolonged exercise (Nybo et al. 2003). These effects could be due to either maintenance of cerebral glucose supply (Nybo et al. 2003), an essential fuel for the central nervous system, or an attenuation of increases in plasma free tryptophan concentration, and tryptophan/branched chain amino acids concentration ratio (Davis et al. 1992). These latter parameters are considered important in determining the brain uptake of tryptophan and the subsequent production of serotonin, increases in the concentration of which are associated with fatigue (Davis et al. 1992).

6 FREE FATTY ACIDS

Even in the leanest of endurance athletes, the adipose tissue and intramuscular triglyceride stores are not limiting for endurance performance. That said, there may be situations where the supply of free fatty acids (non-esterified fatty acids) to skeletal muscle mitochondria limits fat oxidation. As exercise intensity increases, reduced adipose tissue blood flow can limit the delivery of plasma fatty acids to contracting skeletal muscle (Romijn et al. 1993, 1995). Increasing plasma fatty acid concentration during intense exercise, by infusing the triglyceride emulsion Intralipid® and heparin (to activate lipoprotein lipase), increases fat oxidation, but does not restore it to the maximal levels observed at more moderate exercise intensities (Romijn et al. 1995). This implies there are limitations to the uptake and oxidation of fatty acids by skeletal muscle. Potential limiting factors include, but are not restricted to: (1) reduced sarcolemmal fatty acid transport; (2) impaired mitochondrial uptake via the carnitine palmitoyl transferase reaction, secondary to reduced carnitine availability, or inhibition of carnitine palmitoyl transferase activity by enhanced glycolytic flux; and (3) inhibition of mitochondrial β-oxidation. Although increasing fatty acid availability and fat oxidation has the potential to reduce the reliance on carbohydrates during prolonged, strenuous exercise, the effects of such ergogenic interventions on exercise performance are equivocal (Burke & Hawley 2002, Hawley 2002; Chapter 32).

7 SUMMARY

The supply of ATP during muscle contraction is essential for excitation-contraction coupling, cross-bridge force generation and ionic homeostasis. Although muscle [ATP] is reasonably well protected during exercise, it may be suffi-

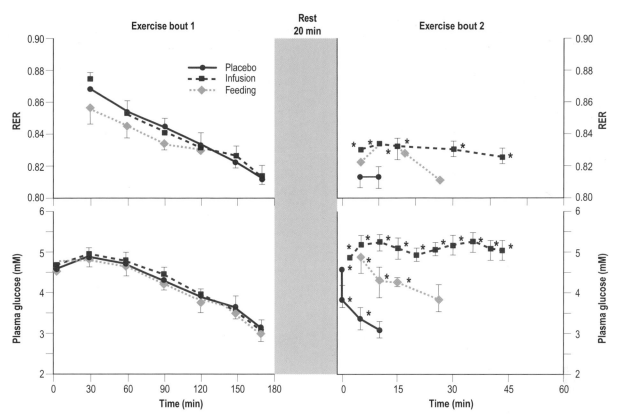

Figure 7.2 Respiratory exchange ratio (RER) and plasma glucose concentrations during consecutive cycling exercise bouts to fatigue, separated by a 20 min rest period. During the rest period and second bout of exercise, subjects were provided one of three treatments: glucose infusion; ingestion of a glucose solution; a placebo drink. **Symbols:** † denotes lower (P < 0.05) than 30 min value for all trials; * denotes different (P < 0.05) from the value at end of bout 1 for that trial (from Coggan & Coyle 1987, with permission from the American Physiological Society).

ciently reduced in specific loci within contracting skeletal muscle to impair these cellular processes. The regeneration of ATP via metabolic pathways within skeletal muscle is crucial for ongoing contractile activity. Critical substrates of these pathways that are depleted with exercise include PCr, muscle glycogen and blood glucose. Strategies to enhance their availability before, during and after exercise are often associated with reduced fatigue and enhanced exercise performance, and are discussed in more detail in

Chapters 32 and 33. The relative efficacy of such interventions will largely depend upon the duration and intensity of exercise (work), which determines the extent to which the availability of different substrates may limit performance. In general, PCr is primarily important during repeated exercise (work) bouts of high intensity but short duration, while the availability of muscle glycogen and blood glucose is crucial during prolonged, strenuous exercise lasting >60–90 min.

References

Baldwin J, Snow RJ, Carey MF, Febbraio MA 1999 Muscle IMP accumulation during fatiguing submaximal exercise in endurance trained and untrained men. American Journal of Physiology 277: R295–R300

Baldwin J, Snow RJ, Gibala MJ, Garnham A, Howarth K, Febbraio MA 2003 Glycogen availability does not affect the TCA cycle or TAN pools during prolonged, fatiguing exercise. Journal of Applied Physiology 94:2181–2187

Ball-Burnett M, Green HJ, Houston ME 1991 Energy metabolism in human slow and fast twitch fibres during prolonged cycle exercise. Journal of Physiology 437:257–267.

Balsom PD, Ekblom B, Söderlund K, Sjödin B, Hultman E 1993 Creatine supplementation and dynamic high-intensity intermittent exercise. Scandinavian Journal of Medicine and Science in Sports 3:143–149

Balsom PD, Gaitanos GC, Söderlund K, Ekblom B 1999 High-intensity exercise and muscle glycogen availability in humans. Acta Physiologica Scandinavica 165:337–345

Bergström J, Hultman E 1967 A study of the glycogen metabolism during exercise in man. Scandinavian Journal of Clinical and Laboratory Investigation 19:218–228

Bergström J, Hermansen L, Hultman E, Saltin B 1967 Diet, muscle glycogen and physical performance. Acta Physiologica Scandinavica 71:140–150

Blazev R, Lamb GD 1999 Low [ATP] and elevated [Mg^{2+}] reduce depolarization-induced Ca^{2+} release in rat skinned skeletal muscle fibres. Journal of Physiology 520:203–215

Bogdanis GC, Nevill ME, Boobis LH, Lakomy HKA, Nevill AM 1995 recovery of power output and muscle metabolites following 30 s of maximal sprint cycling in man. Journal of Physiology 482:467–480

Burgess ML, Robertson RJ, Davis JM, Norris JM 1991 RPE, blood glucose, and carbohydrate oxidation during exercise: effects of glucose feedings. Medicine and Science in Sports and Exercise 23:353–359

Burke LM, Hawley JA 2002 Effects of short-term fat adaptation on metabolism and performance of prolonged exercise. Medicine and Science in Sports and Exercise 34:1492–1498

Casey A, Constantin-Teodosiu D, Howell S, Hultman E, Greenhaff PL 1996a Creatine ingestion favourably affects performance and muscle metabolism during maximal exercise in humans. American Journal of Physiology 271:E31–E37

Casey A, Constantin-Teodosiu D, Howell S, Hultman E, Greenhaff PL 1996b Metabolic response of type I and II muscle fibres during repeated bouts of maximal exercise in humans. American Journal of Physiology 271:E38-E43

Casey A, Short AH, Curtis S, Greenhaff PL 1996c The effect of glycogen availability on power output and the metabolic response to repeated bouts of maximal, isokinetic exercise in man. European Journal of Applied Physiology 72:249–255

Cheetham ME, Boobis LH, Brooks S, Williams C 1986 Human muscle metabolism during sprint running. Journal of Applied Physiology 61:54–60

Chin E, Allen DG 1997 Effects of reduced muscle glycogen concentration on force, Ca^{2+} release and contractile protein function in intact mouse skeletal muscle. Journal of Physiology 498:17–29

Coggan AR, Coyle EF 1987 Reversal of fatigue during prolonged exercise by carbohydrate infusion or ingestion. Journal of Applied Physiology 63:2388–2395

Coyle EF, Hagberg JM, Hurley BF, Martin WH, Ehsani AA, Holloszy JO 1983 Carbohydrate feeding during prolonged strenuous exercise can delay fatigue. Journal of Applied Physiology 55:230–235

Coyle EF, Coggan AR, Hemmert MK, Ivy JL 1986 Muscle glycogen utilization during prolonged strenuous exercise when fed carbohydrate. Journal of applied Physiology 61:165–172

Davis JM, Bailey SP, Woods JA, Galiano FJ, Hamilton MT, Bartoli WP 1992 Effects of carbohydrate feedings on plasma free tryptophan and branched-chain amino acids during prolonged cycling. European Journal of Applied Physiology 65:513–519

Dutka TL, Lamb GD 2004 Effect of low cytoplasmic [ATP] on excitation-contraction coupling in fast-twitch muscle fibres of the rat. Journal of Physiology 560:451–468

Febbraio MA, Dancey J 1999 Skeletal muscle energy metabolism during prolonged, fatiguing exercise. Journal of Applied Physiology 87:2341–2347

Gollnick PD, Armstrong RB, Saubert CW, Sembrowich WL, Shepherd RE, Saltin B 1973a Glycogen depletion patterns in human skeletal muscle fibres during prolonged work. Pflügers Archives 344:1–12

Gollnick PD, Armstrong RB, Sembrowich WL, Shepherd RE, Saltin B 1973b Glycogen depletion pattern in human skeletal muscle fibres after heavy exercise. Journal of Applied Physiology 34:615–618

Greenhaff PL, Nevill ME, Soderlund K, Bodin K, Boobis LH, Williams C, Hultman E 1994 The metabolic responses of human type I and II muscle fibres during maximal treadmill sprinting. Journal of Physiology 478:149–155

Hargreaves M, Briggs CA 1988 Effect of carbohydrate ingestion on exercise metabolism. Journal of Applied Physiology 65:1553–1555

Hargreaves M, Finn JP, Withers RT, Halbert JA, Scroop GC, Mackay M, Snow RJ, Carey MF 1997 Effect of muscle glycogen availability on maximal exercise performance. European Journal of Applied Physiology 75:188–192

Hargreaves M, McKenna MJ, Jenkins DG, Warmington SA, Li JL, Snow RJ, Febbraio MA 1998 Muscle metabolites and performance during high intensity, intermittent exercise. Journal of Applied Physiology 84:1687–1691

Hawley JA 2002 Effect of increased fat availability on metabolism and exercise capacity. Medicine and Science in Sports and Exercise 34:1485–1491

Hawley JA, Schabort EJ, Noakes TD, Dennis SC 1997 Carbohydrate loading and exercise performance: an update. Sports Medicine 24–73–81

Hermansen L, Hultman E, Saltin B 1967 Muscle glycogen during prolonged severe exercise. Acta Physiologica Scandinavica 71:129–139

Karatzaferi C, de Haan A, Ferguson RA, van Mechelen W, Sargeant AJ 2001 Phosphocreatine and ATP content in human single muscle fibres before and after maximum dynamic exercise. Pflügers Archives 442:467–474

McConell GK, Fabris S, Proietto J, Hargreaves M 1994 Effect of carbohydrate ingestion on glucose kinetics during exercise. Journal of Applied Physiology 77:1537–1541

McConell GK, Snow RJ, Proietto J, Hargreaves M 1999 Muscle metabolism during prolonged exercise in humans: influence of carbohydrate availability. Journal of Applied Physiology 67:1083–1086

McKenna MJ, Morton J, Selig SE, Snow RJ 1999 Creatine supplementation increases muscle total creatine but not maximal intermittent exercise performance. Journal of Applied Physiology 87:2244–2252

Maughan RJ, Greenhaff PL, Leiper JB, Ball D, Lambert CP, Gleeson M 1997 Diet composition and the performance of high-intensity exercise. Journal of Sports Sciences 15:265–275

Nybo L 2003 CNS fatigue and prolonged exercise: effect of glucose supplementation. Medicine and Science in Sports and Exercise 35:589–594

Nybo L, Møller K, Pedersen BK, Nielsen B, Secher NH 2003 Association between fatigue and failure to preserve cerebral energy turnover during prolonged exercise. Acta Physiologica Scandinavica 179:67–74

Owen VJ, Lamb GD, Stephenson DG 1996 Effect of low [ATP] on depolarization-induced Ca^{2+} release in skeletal muscle fibres of the toad. Journal of Physiology 493:309–315

Parolin ML, Chesley A, Matsos MP, Spriet LL, Jones NL, Heigenhauser GJF 1999 regulation of skeletal muscle glycogen phosphorylase and PDH during maximal intermittent exercise. American Journal of Physiology 277:E890–E900

Romijn JA, Coyle EF, Sidossis LS, Gastaldelli A, Horowitz JF, Endert E, Wolfe RR 1993 Regulation of endogenous fat and carbohydrate metabolism in relation to exercise intensity and duration. American Journal of Physiology 265:E380–E391

Romijn JA, Coyle EF, Sidossis LS, Zhang X-J, Wolfe RR 1995 Relationship between fatty acid delivery and fatty acid oxidation during strenuous exercise. Journal of Applied Physiology 79:1939–1945

Sahlin K, Katz A, Broberg S 1990 Tricarboxylic acid cycle intermediates in human muscle during prolonged exercise. American Journal of Physiology 259:C834–C841

Sahlin K, Söderlund K, Tonkonogi M, Hirakoba K 1997 Phosphocreatine content in single fibres of human muscle after sustained submaximal exercise. American Journal of Physiology 273:C172–C178

Snow RJ, McKenna MJ, Selig SE, Kemp J, Stathis CG, Zhao S 1998 Effect of creatine supplementation on sprint exercise performance and muscle metabolism. Journal of Applied Physiology 84:1667–1673

Söderlund K, Hultman E 1991 ATP and phosphocreatine changes in single human muscle fibres after intense electrical stimulation. American Journal of Physiology 261:E737–E741

Spencer MK, Yan Z, Katz A 1991 Carbohydrate supplementation attenuates IMP accumulation in human muscle during prolonged exercise. American Journal of Physiology 261:C71–C76

Spencer MK, Yan Z, Katz A 1992 Effect of low glycogen on carbohydrate and energy metabolism in human muscle during exercise. American Journal of Physiology 261:C975–C979

Spriet LL, Söderlund K, Bergström M, Hultman E 1987 Anaerobic energy release in skeletal muscle during electrical stimulation in men. Journal of Applied Physiology 62:611–615

Spriet LL, Lindinger MI, McKelvie RS, Heigenhauser GJF, Jones NL 1989 Muscle glycogenolysis and H+ concentration during maximal intermittent cycling. Journal of Applied Physiology 66:8–13

Stephenson DG, Nguyen LT, Stephenson GMM 1999 Glycogen content and excitation-contraction coupling in mechanically skinned muscle fibres of the cane toad. Journal of Physiology 519:177–187

Trump ME, Heigenhauser GJF, Putman CT, Spriet LL 1996 Importance of muscle phosphocreatine during intermittent maximal cycling. Journal of Applied Physiology 80:1574–1580

Tsintzas O-K, Williams C, Boobis L, Greenhaff P 1996 Carbohydrate ingestion and single muscle fibre glycogen metabolism during prolonged running in men. Journal of Applied Physiology 81:801–809

Tsintzas K, Williams C, Constantin-Teodosiu D, Hultman E, Boobis L, Clarys P, Greenhaff P 2001 Phosphocreatine degradation in type I and type II muscle fibres during submaximal exercise in man: effect of carbohydrate ingestion. Journal of Physiology 537:305–311

Withers RT, Sherman WM, Clark DG, Esselbach PC, Nolan SR, Mackay MH, Brinkman M 1991 Muscle metabolism during 30, 60 and 90 s of maximal cycling on an air-braked ergometer. European Journal of Applied Physiology 63:354–362

Chapter 8

Genetics and human performance: natural selection and genetic modification

Geoffrey Goldspink   Cristiana P. Velloso

1 INTRODUCTION

For more than 99% of the existence of *Homo sapiens*, our species has been a hunter/gatherer. From a Darwinian point of view, the adaptability of muscle tissue was vitally important, as foraging for food required stamina for covering considerable distances, whereas establishing territory and warding off predators and rivals required strength. Therefore, there had to be a balance between strength, which is related to muscle mass, and the economic cost of carrying that mass over long distances. As conditions changed on a yearly or even a monthly basis, muscle mass could be increased when food, particularly meat, was more plentiful, and could also be metabolised to provide the protein required for survival, when food was scarce. In these conditions, the slow oxidative muscle fibres tend to be spared, and it is the fast-contracting fibres that atrophy in times of inanition. They recover rapidly, however, in response to resistance exercise and adequate nutrition. Therefore, there was natural selection pressure for adaptability dating back to our mammalian ancestors and predating *Homo sapiens*.

Muscle adaptability is critical to performance, as it is this that underlies the utility of different training protocols for both sports events (Chapter 4) and rehabilitation. From a physiological point of view, however, the functions of various systems, in addition to muscle, combine to determine athletic ability. For example, the East Africans, who have produced legendary long distance runners, tend to have not only a greater percentage of slow oxidative muscle fibres, but also a large lung volume, long legs and an efficient cardiovascular system (Saltin et al. 1995a,b). In that part of East Africa, cattle raiding on the wide semi-arid plains was a necessity, and natural selection apparently favoured those who could run well and for extended durations.

Nowadays, we study genetic constitution much more in terms of its impact on health, rather than from an evolutionary perspective. Many diseases are known to be due to mutations in specific genes (muscular dystrophy, cystic fibrosis, sickle cell anaemia), while for other diseases, for example breast cancer, it is the risk of developing the disease that is associated with particular genotypes. Unsurprisingly, many physical performance measures have also been correlated with genetic constitution, and altered expression of many genes has been shown to affect muscle mass and metabolism in animal models.

The human genome has now been sequenced and, somewhat surprisingly, there are only about 25,000 genes. We know, however, that there are more than 200,000 different proteins. This discrepancy is explained, in part, by the process of alternative splicing. In eukaryotes, genes are organised into introns and exons. These are simply nucleotide sequences that alternate along the length of a gene. When a gene is first transcribed from the genomic DNA into the primary messenger RNA (mRNA) transcript, both introns and exons are copied. The primary transcript undergoes several processing events in the nucleus to produce the mature mRNA that is exported to the cytoplasm to be translated into protein. Splicing results in the removal of sequences that are not present in the mature mRNA, and are therefore not translated into protein. These sequences are mostly introns but splicing can also result in the inclusion or exclusion of different exons from the mature mRNA. Alternative exon usage greatly increases the number of different proteins that can be coded by a single gene.

Proteins created by alternative splicing contain distinct amino acid sequences and, in many cases, different functional domains, and thus are likely to have different functions. In terms of function, there is also the possibility that slight differences in the sequence of nucleotide bases in the protein coding region of a gene make one variant of the gene, and its protein product, more effective than another when expressed. This can lead to differences in performance between individuals. Sequence variations that are maintained in a population at a frequency of 1% or higher are classified as polymorphisms. Around 90% of genetic variations in humans are due to single nucleotide polymorphisms. These can sometimes be silent and do not result in phenotypic differences. When a polymorphism is in a noncoding region of a gene (intron or untranslated region), it can affect gene regulatory sequences, thereby affecting gene expression levels, timing of expression and tissue specificity; it can also alter the splicing pattern, mRNA stability and the efficiency of protein translation. The effect of the polymorphism on performance may be direct, if the protein is important for physiological function, or indirect, if the protein or RNA regulates expression or function of other genes.

A long-standing question in exercise physiology is whether athletes are born or made. Genes play a role in determining the potential of an individual to excel at a particular physical activity, and that is at least as important as environmental factors, such as nutrition and training. It has been estimated from studies of closely related individuals subjected to a training programme that about 50% of maximal oxygen uptake (Bouchard et al. 1998, 1999), and that about 45% of cardiac output (An et al. 2000) and 67% of explosive muscle power (Calvo et al. 2002) are inherited.

There are several methods of identifying genes that play a role in athletic performance. An obvious course is to compare the genetic make-up of elite athletes to that of the general population. Selection for competitive athletics has unwittingly been indirect genetic selection, in that elite athletes participating in the same sports discipline are likely to be more physiologically and genetically homogenous than the general population, or even the population of elite athletes considered as a whole. A different approach involves comparing variations in a single candidate gene between athletes and non-athletes. Both approaches require careful selection of sizable populations to produce relevant results. Another consideration, given the genetic heterogeneity of the human population, is that variations in functional groups of genes, rather than in individual genes, are likely to be most revealing when trying to link genotype to performance.

At present, there is considerable effort based on the use of cDNA microarrays to study changes in gene expression in response to exercise. This technique enables the simultaneous analysis of hundreds of genes, including splice variants, and potentially offers the prospect of screening and selecting individuals with appropriate responses to training for specific events. In human exercise physiology, only a few studies have been published, with none comparing elite athletes and normal individuals. These types of study have been useful, however, in understanding muscle wasting in medical conditions in which there are obvious effects on muscle mass and muscle strength (Chapter 30). This approach has also been extended to measuring proteins as well as other small molecules by using mass spectrometry and, as these methods are automated, a great deal of data can be derived. When this is coupled with powerful computer analyses, different patterns of metabolites and signalling molecules can be recognised. This approach has been called 'metabolomics'.

We live in exciting and challenging times. The developments of biomedicine, in particular gene therapy, will result in the introduction and manipulation of genes for treatment of various inherited as well as acquired conditions. Although the potential benefits of the technology are immense, the prospect of genotyping and genetic manipulation of human embryos cannot be ignored. A more immediate threat is gene doping for enhancing athletic performance using gene therapy methods developed for a range of medical conditions. In this chapter, we review our knowledge of how genotype is linked to physical performance, and the function of key genes that are likely candidates for manipulation in the practice of gene doping (the ethics of this, and other practices are discussed in the introduction to section 6).

2 GENOTYPE AND PERFORMANCE

Physical performance ultimately involves the integration of several variables, but two physiological systems stand out as key determinants: the cardiorespiratory and musculoskeletal systems. Thus, genes that are known to affect these systems are likely to play a role in performance. It has been estimated that a single gene accounts for 40% of the variation in oxygen uptake (Feitosa et al. 2002), and two genes for 37% of the variation in heart rate in response to training (An et al. 2003). There is currently, however, no example of a gene in which the presence of a particular variant or mutation is proven incontestably to determine elite athletic status.

The accumulation of evidence from various sources, such as genetic linkage studies, functional studies and in vitro and animal studies identifying the biological role of different genes, has nevertheless provided some candidates that show significant associations with performance traits and have plausible biological mechanisms of action (MacArthur & North 2005). Due to the nature of these studies, which involve statistical association of genotype with function, there is always a chance that the findings, though statistically significant, may not actually be functionally relevant. Two genes for which there appear to be particularly strong genetic linkage data are angiotensin-converting enzyme and actinin 3. In these genes, particular polymorphisms (variations in gene sequence) have been associated with endurance and strength.

2.1 Angiotensin–converting enzyme gene and different alleles

The angiotensin-converting enzyme (ACE) is part of the renin-angiotensin system, and is involved in regulating vasoconstriction as well as salt and body fluid balance. Angiotensinogen is cleaved by renin to produce angiotensin I. ACE catalyses the conversion of angiotensin into the vasoconstrictor angiotensin II and degrades the vasodilator bradykinin. ACE inhibitors are commonly used in the treatment of heart disease.

The ACE gene has been intensively studied in the context of cardiac and circulatory diseases, and different alleles have been associated with strength and endurance performance. The variation in the ACE gene involves the absence or presence of a 287 base pair sequence in one of the introns of the gene. Since this sequence variation is present in an intron, and introns are normally excluded during splicing, it would not be expected to have effects on the phenotype of the protein. However, the allele containing the 287 base pair sequence (I-insertion allele) and the allele in which the 287 base pair sequence is absent (D-deletion allele), code for enzymes with different activities. In humans, individuals with the DD genotype have plasma ACE activities that are approximately 1.5–2 times higher than those of II individuals (Rigat et al. 1990). Several population association studies, where the genotype of one population is compared with that of another, have indicated an increased association of the I-insertion allele with successful endurance athletes (Gayagay et al. 1998), and individuals with a greater ability to ascend to high altitudes without supplemental oxygen (Montgomery et al. 1998). The D allele, on the other hand, occurs with greater frequency in individuals who respond well to strength training (Folland et al. 2000) and athletes who participate in short-distance events (Woods et al. 2001).

The D allele was originally associated with human cardiac hypertrophy following exercise, and might be linked with the regulation of skeletal muscle mass (Montgomery et al. 1997). Some studies, however, have also failed to show a link between ACE and performance but many of these have been criticised based on the criteria used for population selection. If the population studied is very heterogeneous in terms of gender, race and competitive discipline, it is likely that significant variations will be masked, particularly when the polymorphism is present with large frequency in the general population. At present, the jury is still out on ACE, but undoubtedly many more studies will be performed. It would be highly relevant to show a cause and effect relationship between strength and ACE activity in animal or human models, perhaps by demonstrating reversible effects on strength or endurance by modulating ACE expression or activity.

2.2 Actinin 3

The protein product of the actinin 3 gene is located at the Z line of type II muscle fibres and serves to anchor actin filaments. There is a null allele due to a nonsense mutation that results in an absence of expression of the protein. Approximately 18% of the world's population is homozygous for this allele (Mills et al. 2001). The null allele is less frequently expressed in athletes specialising in power disciplines than in either endurance athletes or a control population of healthy non-athletes (Yang et al. 2003). In contrast, the null allele was found to occur with significantly higher frequencies in endurance athletes than in controls. Little published data exists for actinin 3, and the effects of its absence on muscle function are not known. Likewise, there are no animal data showing a cause and effect relationship between either actinin 3 expression and improved power generation, or lack of actinin 3 expression and greater endurance. Therefore, the association of the genotype with athletes of a particular discipline, though strong, remains an interesting observation.

Many other gene polymorphisms have been associated with muscle strength, body composition and cardiovascular function, with more associations revealed on a weekly basis (MacArthur & North 2005), but a convincing cause and effect relationship has yet to be demonstrated. In order to affect performance, changes in gene sequence or expression patterns, whether naturally occurring or due to manipulation, should have key functional outcomes: increasing the generation of power or increasing endurance. Some events require a combination of these attributes. In the next sections, some of the genes that have proven functional effects (in humans or animal models) on the muscular and the cardiorespiratory systems will be highlighted.

3 REGULATION OF MUSCLE MASS

3.1 Autocrine and endocrine growth factors: growth hormone and IGF-I

3.1.1 The growth hormone and IGF-I axis

The somatomedin hypothesis originated in the 1950s in an effort to understand how somatic growth was regulated by a protein secreted by the pituitary gland (pituitary-derived growth hormone). This did not act directly on its target tissues to promote growth, but through intermediary substances, particularly insulin-like growth factor I (IGF-I; Daughaday & Reeder 1966). Much later, Green and collaborators (1985) proposed the dual effector hypothesis which suggested that growth hormone had direct effects on peripheral tissues, in addition to those mediated by circulating IGF-I.

The liver is the main source of circulating IGF-I and growth hormone upregulates not only the synthesis of IGF-I, but also that of IGF binding protein 3 and the acid-labile subunit. IGF binding protein 3, acid-labile subunit and IGF-I form a tripartite binding complex that stabilises IGF-I in the serum. As a result of tissue-specific gene deletion experiments in mice, the role of hepatic IGF-I on somatic growth has been questioned (Sjogren et al. 1999, Yakar et al.1999). An homologous recombination system was used to create a liver-specific deletion of the IGF-I gene, but allowed normal expression of this gene in other non-hepatic tissues, such as heart, muscle, fat, spleen and kidney. This liver-specific gene deletion of IGF-I reduced serum IGF-I levels relative to those found in control mice, but measurements of body size and individual organ weights showed no difference between the knockout animals and their wild-type littermates. Hence, postnatal growth and development was considered normal without the contribution of liver-derived IGF-I (Sjogren et al. 1999). This emphasises the importance of local IGF-I synthesis for organ growth.

Unquestionably, the growth hormone/IGF-I axis plays a role in postnatal growth and development. In pituitary dwarfs, the circulating levels of growth hormone are abnormally low and skeletal growth is suppressed. Abnormally increased stature occurs in gigantism, in which circulating growth hormone and IGF-I levels are abnormally high. In contrast to gigantism, acromegaly occurs primarily in middle-aged adults when excessive growth hormone is present, after fusion of the growth plates of the long bones. Consequently, it does not result in increased height. Rather, bones of the extremities and face are affected, and other organs including heart and liver may increase in size.

The circulating growth hormone and IGF-I concentrations peak during adolescence. With increasing age, however, there is a marked decline in the circulating growth hormone and a somewhat smaller decline in circulating IGF-I (Rudman et al. 1981). In young adults who are growth hormone deficient, the administration of recombinant human growth hormone (rhGH) has positive effects on muscle mass and function (Cuneo et al. 1991). Extended treatment of growth hormone-deficient adults not only increases muscle strength but also decreases body fat content (Beshyah et al. 1995). These findings have led to the belief that older individuals with decreased circulating growth hormone and IGF-I could benefit from growth hormone therapy, and have encouraged the illicit use of growth hormone among athletes, even those competing at secondary school level, in an attempt to enhance performance. There is, however, no evidence that growth hormone is anabolic in individuals with normal growth hormone endocrinology (Rennie 2003).

3.1.2 Genes regulating the growth hormone/IGF-I axis

Growth hormone is produced in a pulsatile manner. This, together with its short half-life, results in fluctuating serum growth hormone concentrations during the day. Growth hormone release is regulated by somatostatin, which is an inhibitory regulator, and growth hormone-releasing hormone, a positive regulator. Analogues of somatostatin are used to treat acromegalic patients, and the manipulation of growth hormone secretion has been studied in relation to treatment of pituitary dwarfs and other clinical conditions for which low growth hormone levels is a symptom.

Growth hormone also regulates itself via a negative feedback system, such that its administration often results in a shutdown of its endogenous production. The situation is more complex as analogues of growth hormone-releasing hormone occur naturally and are produced in tissues other than the pituitary. These are referred to as growth hormone secretagogues and include the orexigenic (appetite-inducing) hormone ghrelin, a newly discovered peptide with potent growth hormone releasing activity, originally isolated from the rat stomach. There is also a group of synthetic peptides (GHRPs) which are growth hormone secretagogues. The detection of these, as well as growth hormone, presents a major challenge for the anti-doping agencies.

The roles of circulating growth hormone and IGF-I, particularly with regard to muscle function in adult and later life, are still unclear. Some of the stimuli that affect growth hormone secretion are sleep, feeding and exercise. Since exercise induces growth hormone release, and athletes tend to have above-average baseline values, it is difficult to know which levels are considered to be optimal for performance in young healthy individuals. What is very apparent is that circulating growth hormone concentrations drop markedly during the ageing process and this is correlated with a significant drop in muscle mass. Despite this observation, systemic growth factors may be of relatively minor importance in muscle mass maintenance and hypertrophy. One study, for example, showed that the overloaded muscles in hypophysectomised rats were still able to hypertrophy despite significantly reduced circulating IGF-I levels (Adams & Haddad 1996). This finding, coupled with the simple observation that it is only challenged muscles which hypertrophy, highlights the importance of a local system of muscle adaptation.

3.1.3 Structure and regulation of the IGF–I gene

About 15 years ago, our group set about cloning the growth factor(s) involved in the local regulation of muscle mass using a technique known as differential display to compare mRNA expression. We initially used an animal model in which we could make a muscle grow rapidly. Previous work had shown that if tibialis anterior in the mature rabbit was electrically stimulated, whilst held in the stretched position by plaster cast immobilisation, it increased in mass by 30% within 7 days (Goldspink et al. 1992). The RNA in the stretched and stimulated muscles increased considerably, but most of this was ribosomal RNA. Using oligonucleotide primers and the RT-PCR technique, it was possible to detect an RNA transcript that was only expressed in the stretched and stimulated muscles, but not in resting control muscles. This was cloned and sequenced, and it became evident that it was derived from the insulin-like growth factor gene by alternative splicing. The terminology of the IGF-I is a problem when comparing humans and rodents and therefore we named this splice variant mechano growth factor, as it is expressed in response to mechanical stimulation (McKoy et al. 1999, Yang et al. 1996).

The human gene for IGF-I resides on the long arm of chromosome 12 (Brissenden et al. 1984, Tricoli et al. 1984). It spans a region of more than 95 kb of chromosomal DNA (de Pagter-Holthuizen et al. 1986, Gilmour 1994, Rotwein et al. 1986) and contains six exons which are spliced in different ways. The structure of the human IGF-I gene is shown in Figure 8.1. Exons one and two are alternative leader exons (Gilmour 1994, Tobin et al. 1990) with distinct transcription start sites, that are differentially spliced to the common exon three, and produce class one and two IGF-I mRNA transcripts respectively (Weller et al. 1993). Exons three and four code for the mature IGF-I peptide (A, B, C and D domains), the peptide that is found in blood and which binds to the IGF-I receptor, as well as the first 16 amino acids of the E-domain at the C-terminus of the protein. Exons five and six contain the sequences encoding the alternative parts of the E-domain and the 3′ untranslated regions, followed by alternative polyadenylation signals. Polyadenylation signals are sequences near which the mRNA is cleaved, and tracts of around 200 adenine nucleotides are added by the enzyme poly A polymerase. The function of the poly A tail of mRNA is to stabilise the mRNA and prevent its degradation. Thus, the alternative splicing of the primary IGF-I transcript may result in six or more different IGF-I mRNAs, that all encode the same mature IGF-I (exons three and four), but differ in sequences 5′ (exon one and two) and 3′ (exons five and six) to the IGF-I coding sequence (Daughaday & Rotwein 1989, Hepler & Lund 1990).

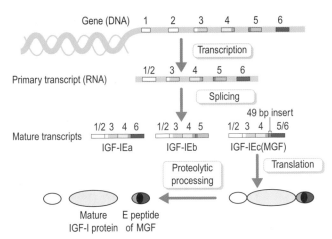

Figure 8.1 Splicing of the IGF-I gene. This gene contains six exons (top). The primary transcript contains exon 1 or 2 as well as the remaining exons. The spliced mRNAs for IGF-IEa, Eb and Ec are shown. During splicing of the mechano growth factor (IGF-IEc) mRNA, the insertion of a 49 base pair (bp) sequence from exon 5 leads to a reading frame shift, resulting in a different 3′ sequence that encodes a unique C-terminal peptide. The MGF propeptide is proteolytically cleaved to produce mature IGF-I and Ec peptide.

There is very little available data regarding the roles of the different 5′ IGF-I isoforms. Class II transcripts are more abundant than class I transcripts in the liver, and have been shown to be preferentially upregulated by growth hormone administration in sheep. Consequently, it has been suggested that class II transcripts encode the secreted form of the protein, since GH treatment increases circulating levels of IGF-I, whereas class I transcripts encode forms that remain localized to the tissue where it is produced. The experimental evidence to corroborate this hypothesis is lacking, and preliminary analyses of the class I and II sequences have not revealed any obvious signal sequences that would target class II transcripts for secretion. We have recently examined the effects of growth hormone administration on class I and II transcripts in muscles of young men but have not found upregulation of either class I or class II transcripts in this tissue. The young men did, however, have increased circulating IGF-I following growth hormone treatment. Based on these observations, we concluded that the expression of class I and class II transcripts is not regulated by growth hormone in human muscle. These observations do not exclude an effect of growth hormone on IGF-I isoform expression in the human liver, since tissue-specific responses may exist.

The translation of IGF-I transcripts that are alternatively spliced at the 3′ end would generate three proIGF-I proteins with different C-terminal domains: IGF-IEa, IGF-IEb and IGF-IEc (mechano growth factor). Of these proIGF-I proteins, IGF-IEb is the longest and contains 147 amino acid residues, IGF-IEa is the shortest with 105 amino acid residues, and IGF-Ec has 110 amino residues. As noted above, all three proteins contain the mature IGF-I peptide and share a common 16 amino acid sequence at the N-terminal portion of the E-domain. The E-domain of IGF-IEb shares homology with part of the E-domain of IGF-IEc. Both of these contain a potential heparin-binding site and a consensus nuclear localisation signal. Heparin is found in the blood, and the presence of a binding site for this molecule suggests that if the protein is secreted from the cell, it may be transported via the bloodstream to other sites in the body. Alternatively, the heparin binding may inhibit interaction of the molecule with its cell surface receptor and thus regulate its activity. The presence of the nuclear localisation signal, on the other hand, suggests that the protein may have a role in regulating nuclear events. Proteins that regulate the cell cycle possess nuclear localisation signals, and it is tempting to postulate that IGF-IEc may exert its effect of muscle cell proliferation, explained below, by interacting with cell cycle proteins. This remains to be demonstrated.

The sequence of mechano growth factor mRNA differs from that of IGF-IEa due to the presence of a 52 base pair insert in the rat and 49 base pair insert in the human. Amino acids are encoded by triplets of nucleotides called codons. As the length of the nucleotide insert that results in production of mechano growth factor is not a multiple of three, the coding sequence located 3' to the insert is shifted relative to that of IGF-IEa. This means that the amino acid sequence of the E-domains is entirely different. This has important functional consequences as the C-terminus is involved in the recognition of the binding proteins that stabilise and target these growth factors. Furthermore, in the case of mechano growth factor, this part of the peptide may act as a separate growth factor involved in inducing the proliferation of muscle progenitor cells involved in postnatal growth, maintenance and repair. The simplest model of muscle repair is that involving satellite cells and is illustrated in Figure 8.2. Mechano growth factor E peptide acts via a receptor distinct from the IGF-I receptor (Yang & Goldspink

2002) through which the anabolic effects of mature IGF-I are produced, including increased protein synthesis.

As well as having a different C-terminal peptide sequence, mechano growth factor expression kinetics are different from those of IGF-IEa. Haddad & Adams (2002) found that mechano growth factor expression peaks earlier than that of total IGF-I mRNA. Hill & Goldspink (2003) showed that following muscle damage, mechano growth factor is produced as a pulse lasting only 2 or 3 days, followed by longer lasting expression of IGF-IEa mRNA. This expression pattern is consistent with a role for mechano growth factor in activating satellite cell proliferation, and is in accord with in vitro observations. Skeletal muscle cells in culture, either transfected with the mechano growth factor cDNA or treated with the mechano growth factor E peptide, increased in number but remained as monocleated myoblasts (Yang & Goldspink 2002). If mechano growth factor prevents differentiation of myoblasts, then it would have to be down-regulated in order to allow the activated myoblasts to fuse with mature myofibres.

Intramuscular injection of full-length mechano growth factor cDNA inserted into a plasmid vector demonstrated that mechano growth factor is a potent inducer of muscle hypertrophy. A single injection resulted in a 25% increase in the fibre cross-sectional area of the injected muscle within 3 weeks (Goldspink 2001). Similar experiments using IGF-IEa have also been carried out using viral constructs which resulted in a 25% increase in muscle mass, but this took more than 4 months to develop (Musaro et al. 2001). Although these experiments are not strictly comparable, it would appear that mechano growth factor is more potent in activating muscle hypertrophy, possibly due to its effect on satellite cell proliferation.

3.1.4 Mechano growth factor in ageing and disease

The inability to maintain muscle mass is a consequence of both ageing, which may have a genetic component, and of hereditary muscle wasting diseases like muscular dystrophy. Age-related muscle loss (sarcopenia) is one of the most debilitating effects of ageing (Chapter 16). The work of Owino and collaborators (2001) indicated that muscles in old rats expressed much lower levels of mechano growth factor than those of younger animals, when surgically overloaded. Hameed and collaborators (2003a) showed elderly male volunteers were unable to upregulate mechano growth factor expression after exercise to the same extent as young subjects, when measurements were performed 150 minutes after an exercise bout. Mechano growth factor levels were upregulated, however, when measured 5 and 12 weeks after entry into a resistance training programme (Hameed et al. 2003b).

We found that administration of growth hormone, when combined with resistance exercise, considerably improved mechano growth factor mRNA levels in the thigh muscles of elderly subjects relative to either treatment alone. In contrast, IGF-IEa levels were not upregulated to a greater extent

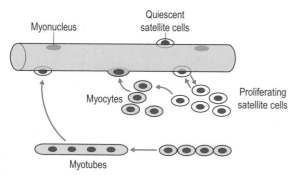

Figure 8.2 Muscle repair by satellite cells. The satellite cells lie between the basal lamina of the myofibre and the sarcolemma. Satellite cells can be activated by muscle damage or exercise and proliferate, whereas myofibre nuclei are postmitotic. Some satellite cells may return to a quiescent state, renewing the satellite cell pool, while others will differentiate and fuse with the damaged muscle fibre or form new myotubes by fusing with each other.

by combined resistance training and growth hormone administration than by growth hormone treatment alone. This led to the development of the hypothesis that growth hormone upregulates primary IGF-I transcripts that are normally spliced toward IGF-IEa. Mechanical signals (muscle activation and stretch) generated during resistance exercise then cause splicing towards mechano growth factor.

Interestingly, a statistical correlation was observed between baseline expression levels of mechano growth factor but not of IGF-IEa, with the cross-sectional area of the thigh musculature. There is evidence that mechano growth factor is a neuronal survival factor (Aperghis et al. 2004). One possibility is that expression levels of mechano growth factor influence the survival of muscle fibres damaged during the lifetime of the organism, and thus individuals with higher expression levels retain more fibres as they age. It may be also that higher baseline levels of mechano growth factor expression result in increase motoneuron survival, better muscle innervation, and thus size, with increasing age.

Muscle loss is a major problem in certain hereditary diseases. It has been suggested that in dystrophic muscles there is an inability to produce mechano growth factor in response to mechanical overload (Goldspink et al. 1996). The systemic type of IGF-IEa is produced by dystrophic muscle. If mechano growth factor upregulation is indeed required to ensure muscle fibre repair and survival, then understanding its role seems to be very relevant to understanding the aetiology and development of possible treatment in these muscle-wasting conditions.

3.2 Negative regulation of muscle mass: myostatin

In addition to positive regulators of muscle growth, there is also a factor that negatively affects muscle size. It is called myostatin and has attracted much attention in recent years. This gene was discovered in a breed of cattle, called the Belgian Blue, in which a myostatin-inactivating mutation is responsible for the double muscle phenotype of these animals which exhibit massive muscle hypertrophy (McPherron & Lee1997). Myostatin belongs to the transforming growth factor β (TGF-β) family of growth factors, but its expression is restricted to muscle tissue (McPherron et al. 1997). The striking phenotype of the myostatin knockout mouse is an increase in muscle mass (200% relative to wild-type littermates), but although some increase in muscle strength occurs, this is not commensurate with the increased muscle mass. The hypertrophy is associated primarily with a greater number of myocytes during embryological development, giving rise to a greater number of myofibres. In addition, these myofibres are also larger than those of wild-type controls.

Like circulating IGF-I, myostatin is synthesised as a propeptide that undergoes proteolytic cleavage to generate the biologically active molecule. Myostatin, however, is released from cells in a latent state that is still bound to the cleaved portion of the propeptide. In vitro, myostatin can also bind follistatin, follistatin-related gene and growth and differentiation factor-associated serum protein-1, all of which also inhibit its activity. It is hypothesised that myostatin is activated in a site-specific manner by the action of locally expressed proteases, which cleave the inhibitory molecules. Recent research using a knockout mouse indicates that myostatin suppresses muscle growth by maintaining the satellite cells in a quiescent state (McCroskery et al. 2003). Inactivation of myostatin by several methods, including antibody injections, results in muscle hypertrophy, whereas injection of myostatin into adult mice results in muscle loss.

It is not clear to what extent myostatin expression and activity are influenced by local and systemic growth factors. Although the relationship between growth factors and myostatin has yet to be determined, there is energising evidence that IGF-I, and particularly mechano growth factor levels, become elevated when myostatin levels are decreased. Indeed, it has been shown that resistance training in humans results in a decrease in myostatin and a commensurate increase in IGF-I and cyclin D1, which is upregulated in proliferating satellite cells (Kim et al. 2005). Although the satellite cell seems the likely target for myostatin activity, increased protein synthesis in cultured myotubes treated with myostatin has also been observed.

A key observation for human physiologists is that an inactivating mutation of myostatin has been found in humans. In a recent case, a male child with inactive myostatin showed remarkable muscular development and above-average strength (Schuelke et al. 2004). It will be interesting to see whether his strength and muscle development remain above average, and whether he becomes involved in competitive sports. Despite the ability of myostatin to affect muscle when modulated both pre- and post-natally, association studies of myostatin polymorphisms and human muscle traits have not yielded any significant associations (Huygens et al. 2005). Methods of inactivating myostatin are being explored as a treatment for muscular dystrophy and other muscle-wasting conditions such as cachexia and sarcopenia. Thus, myostatin inhibitors have the potential for misuse for enhancing athletic performance, as do IGF-I and growth hormone.

4 GENES REGULATING OXYGEN DELIVERY AND UTILISATION

4.1 Genes regulating muscle fibre type and metabolism

4.1.1 Myogenic regulatory factors

Myogenic regulatory factors are transcription factors that have received considerable attention as they are fundamental to muscle development. In the embryo, mesodermal cells receive signals that induce them to commit to the myogenic lineage; committed myogenic cells will only differentiate into muscle tissue. Once in the limb buds, myoblasts undergo extensive proliferation. During myogenesis, proliferation and differentiation are mutually exclusive, and the myoblasts withdraw from the cell cycle before fusing into primary myofibres. The primary myofibres act as a scaffold for other myoblasts that fuse to form secondary myofibres around the same time as the muscle becomes innervated. Maturation of the myofibres results in replacement of embryonic myosin heavy chain protein with adult fast and slow isoforms. Since the nuclei in adult myofibres are unable to enter the cell cycle and proliferate, the requirement for new nuclei in muscle repair, maintenance and hypertrophy is met by satellite cells. Satellite cells are essentially adult myoblasts but with a different embryonic history, and are present on adult myofibres in a quiescent state. However, the cells become activated following exercise, muscle damage or degeneration. Developmental muscle differentiation is recapitulated in satellite cells as they proliferate and fuse with existing fibres or with each other to form new myofibres (Figure 8.2). Over the last two decades, great progress has been made in unravelling the signals involved in regulating embryonic and adult myogenesis.

There are four myogenic regulatory factors: Myf5, MyoD, myogenin and MRF4/Myf6. Gene knockout experiments have revealed that the expression of either MyoD or Myf5 is required for establishment of the myogenic lineage in mice. The knockout animals for either MyoD or Myf5 have normal musculature, but the double knockout has no skeletal muscle at all (Rudnicki et al. 1993). Expression of myogenin is required for differentiation and maturation of the fibres, since the knockout animals have myoblasts in the limb but very few myofibres (Hasty et al. 1993, Nabeshima et al. 1993). Myogenin seems to be able to compensate for the lack of MRF4 expression and thus the MRF4 knockout does not have an obvious muscle phenotype. In quiescent satellite cells, MyoD and Myf5 expression is undetectable, but these factors are expressed following satellite cell activation.

The myogenic regulatory factors are helix-loop-helix proteins that bind to a regulatory element called the E-box or CANNTG motif. One or more E-boxes are present in muscle-specific genes, including those of myosin light chains 1 and 3 (Wentworth et al. 1991), troponin (Lin & Konieczny 1992), cardiac actin (Sartorelli et al. 1990) and creatine kinase (Lassar et al. 1989). Exercise results in upregulation of these transcription factors in humans, as they are involved in the regulation of muscle gene transcription during adaptation and remodelling, as well as satellite cell activation and differentiation. No effects of overexpression of these myogenic regulatory factors on muscle cell size have been reported, but they may be involved in the regulation of fibre type. In adult muscles, it is known that expression of the myogenic regulatory factor MyoD is highest in the fast fibres, and myogenin is highest in slow fibres. Overexpression of the latter in transgenic mice increased the levels of oxidative enzymes in fast muscles, although it did not induce a switch in myosin heavy chain types (Hughes et al. 1999). Therefore, myogenic regulatory factors like myogenin may play a role in fibre phenotype maintenance or conversion, though they do not seem to induce hypertrophy.

4.1.2 PGC1α and fatigue resistance changes

At Harvard University, Lin et al. (2002) overexpressed a factor in transgenic mice that is involved in mitochondrial biogenesis (PGC1α), and found the muscle fibres in these animals, in addition to containing more mitochondria, were much redder in colour than those of control mice, due to a higher myoglobin content. In addition, the transgenic mice had a higher ratio of slow- to fast-type fibres and were more fatigue resistant. Although there was a 10% increase in type I fibres in these mice, this cannot be regarded as a mechanism of muscle fibre type conversion, since the animals are overexpressing this factor throughout embryonic development. Therefore, the fibres may have developed as type I rather than transitioning from fast to slow at some stage during the embryonic development of the animal. The ability to transform the metabolic and contractile characteristics of type II fibres into those of type I fibres is desirable for athletes interested in increasing their endurance.

Some light now has been shed on the regulation of fibre type using cultured muscle cells. The fast to slow transition seems to be associated with calcium transients and involves the calcineurin pathway. Calcineurin is a calcium-sensitive serine/threonine phosphatase, which is activated in response to sustained low-amplitude levels of calcium, but not by transient spikes of high amplitude (Dolmetsch et al. 1997). This is correlated with motoneuron stimulation patterns of slow and fast fibres. In slow fibres, calcium concentrations are maintained between 100 and 300 nM via frequent motoneuron stimulation. Fast fibres, in contrast, have a lower resting calcium concentration, but higher intracellular peaks of short duration are reached during contraction. This model is in accord with the data for muscles fibre type conversion in vivo in which continuous, low-frequency electrical stimulation (Pette & Staron 1997) and stretch, with or without electrical stimulation (Goldspink et al. 1992), switch on the slow-type genes.

Other factors have also been associated with slow fibre types. Comparison of strains of mice that have postural problems with normal mice has permitted the identification of molecules that are predominantly expressed by type I muscle fibres (McKoy et al. 2005). This research showed that the gene Ankrd2 was responsive to muscle stretch and was associated with the expression of slow-type myosin. The cDNA of Ankrd2, or copy DNA which is reverse transcribed from a mature mRNA molecule, can now be inserted into a gene expression vector, a virus or plasmid and introduced into muscle tissue. Gene expression from cDNA is similar to that from genomic DNA, except that it is normally much more abundant since the promoter and regulatory sequences in vectors are designed for this purpose. Thus the effect of Ankrd2 expression or overexpression in fast muscle fibres, where it is not normally found, can now be studied.

4.1.3 PPARδ and endurance

Recent work on the genetic manipulation of the peroxisome proliferator-activated receptor δ (PPARδ) gene, particularly at the Salk Institute California (Wang et al. 2004), gives insight into how whole-body metabolism can markedly improve athletic performance. The team produced a transgenic mouse (Marathon Mouse) that can run twice as far and for twice as long as normal mice. Genetic manipulation of the peroxisome proliferator-activated receptor altered metabolism of the animal so that it had a leaner body and its muscle fibres had more mitochondria and myoglobin, thus being able to use and store more oxygen.

The significance of this work for manipulating performance in adult animals is open to question since the embryonic development of the transgenic mice occurred in the presence of excessive levels of the protein. The ability to induce fibre type conversion and increased fatigue resistance in adult animals rather than developing embryos thus needs to be demonstrated. Significantly, treatment of wild-type mice with the PPARδ-specific agonist GW501516 for 10 days resulted in upregulation of genes for slow fibre contractile proteins, mitochondrial biogenesis and oxidative metabolism. Whether the drug treatment also resulted in improved fatigue resistance was not determined. It will be interesting to see whether PPARδ agonists will be used by endurance athletes.

From the point of view of muscle mass and fibre type regulation, we need to determine how the above factors are regulated by mechanical signals as well as paracrine, autocrine and endocrine signals, and how they in turn regulate the expression of specific genes. It will also be very enlightening to determine the cross-talk of positive and negative regulatory signalling pathways (Figure 8.3). Potentially, any gene that affects muscle mass or metabolism may be used by those wishing to manipulate skeletal muscle physiology.

4.2 Genes regulating the oxygen–carrying capacity of blood: erythropoietin

Erythropoietin is widely used to treat anaemia. It is a glycoprotein that binds to the erythropoietin receptor on erythroid precursor cells, stimulating them to proliferate and differentiate into erythrocytes. Constitutively elevated erythropoietin causes erythrocytosis, increasing red blood cell counts. Provided no other underlying complications exist, this leads to an increase in the oxygen-carrying capacity of blood. This has obvious consequences for oxygen delivery to tissues and the performance of endurance tasks. Elevated endogenous erythropoietin secretion is one reason for training at altitude (Chapter 25), since synthesis of

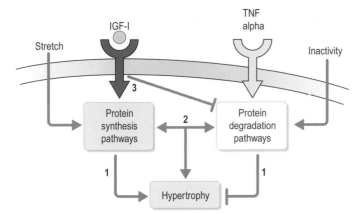

Figure 8.3 Cross-talk of signalling pathways in muscle hypertrophy and atrophy. Mechanical (stretch) and paracrine/autocrine (IGF-I) signals stimulate protein synthesis, whereas other signals (inactivity and cytokine tumour necrosis factor α, produced in disease states) stimulate protein breakdown. The cross-talk between signals may occur at different levels with signals being additive, such that (1) hypertrophy occurs if protein synthesis is stimulated to a greater extent than protein breakdown (2); the signalling proteins are shared or interact, such that a net hypertrophy or atrophy signal is produced (3); the same signal may stimulate one pathway and inhibit another. This has been shown to be the case for IGF-I which both stimulates protein synthesis and inhibits protein breakdown.

erythropoietin by kidney cells is stimulated by hypoxia. In addition, controlled trials have demonstrated that erythropoietin administration can affect maximal aerobic power and performance (Birkeland et al. 2000). Indeed, the illicit use of erythropoietin by athletes is notorious, particularly among cyclists, as came to light in the 1998 Tour de France and again prior to the Tour in 2006.

An athlete with natural but supraphysiological haemoglobin concentrations is the cross-country skier Eero Montirana, three times Olympic gold medallist. This confers on him an exceptional oxygen-carrying capacity and endurance capabilities. In his family, erythrocytosis exists in more than 30 individuals, all descendants from a couple born in the 1850s. The clinical condition is mild, and though haemoglobin concentrations are remarkably high (30% greater than average), erythropoietin in serum is low or low-normal. It turns out that the phenotype is due to a mutation in the erythropoietin receptor gene resulting in premature termination and truncation of the protein product, such that the 70 amino acids downstream of the mutation are missing (de la Chapelle et al. 1993). These amino acids code for the cytoplasmic domain of the receptor involved in the downregulation of erythropoietin receptor function. Thus, the mutant receptor is overactive.

The use of recombinant erythropoietin (or analogues) is risky because the increased number of red cells elevates blood viscosity and this can reduce blood flow to organs and blood clots can form more easily. Erythropoietin is also a candidate for gene therapy to treat chronic anaemia and this may be a future avenue of administration of the protein.

5 NATURE VERSUS GENE DOPING: CAN ATHLETES BE MADE IN THE LABORATORY?

Gene therapy has been intensively investigated for many years and there are currently thousands of clinical trials under way. On the whole, the results of these trials have been disappointing, largely due to the fact that gene delivery seems to be inefficient. This was an unexpected outcome, as gene therapy has proven effective in rodent and primate models. Currently, much of the research is focused on improving the delivery method, including making virus vectors both safer and able to carry larger genes, increasing efficiency of plasmid transfection and engineering both viral and plasmid vectors to target specific cells and tissues, by coating the vectors with proteins that bind to tissue-specific receptors or putting the gene under the regulation of a promoter that only functions in a specific tissue type.

The technique of gene therapy is not without its risks. Viral vectors, especially adenoviral vectors, are associated with large immune responses. It is also possible that an immune response is generated to the inserted protein. This is one of the limiting factors in expressing dystrophin in children with Duchenne muscular dystrophy, and in trials of erythropoietin, it has led to development of autoimmune anaemia. In addition, some viruses insert their genome into the host DNA. This can lead to insertional mutagenesis where an endogenous gene or a regulatory sequence of an endogenous gene is affected. When this happens near oncogenes, it can lead to the development of cancers. This has been observed in treatment for immunodeficiencies in both adults and children.

Nevertheless, the potential benefits of the technology are immense, and the reported complications, though serious, are relatively rare. At present gene doping remains a banned practice for athletes but the time may come when the possibility of treating injuries with gene therapy will become a reality. Will this be allowed or will gene therapy for tissue repair and regeneration be made available to the general population but not to athletes? What about designer babies? If we are eventually allowed to use gene therapy in embryos to treat inherited diseases like muscular dystrophy or to reduce the risk of cardiac myopathy and cancer, can transgenic children that have exceptional endurance or strength be far behind? These are questions that may have to be addressed eventually, and for which the answers may change as technology advances and as the values of society change. At present, gene therapy will only be used for the postnatal treatment of life-threatening and debilitating diseases, and the question does not apply. Nevertheless, the practice of gene doping is nascent and on the list of banned practices for enhancing athletic performance by the World Anti-Doping Agency. Thus, there is

now a requirement for developing tests for the detection of gene doping.

5.1 Detection of doping, including gene doping

The number of cases in which athletes have been shown to have taken substances that improve performance has escalated in recent years. This may in part be due to better and more extensive testing, but also because the prestige and monetary rewards are much greater, and the use of such substances to gain a small improvement in speed or stamina are even more tempting. Nevertheless, the involvement in doping devalues sports events and undermines the very essence of fair competition. It may be that the attraction of professional sport will diminish if it is perceived that one cannot excel without the use of these substances. The general public, who support these events financially, may become disillusioned if they believe what they are watching is the effectiveness of different enhancing substances, rather than genuine athletic ability. Unfortunately, there is much money to be made by supplying these substances via the counter-culture of small companies and individuals that supply licensed and non-licensed drugs. Excessive use of these substances is often associated with serious and sometimes fatal consequences, but this does not deter many athletes when striving to obtain that gold medal. The World Anti-Doping Agency has in recent years accredited several laboratories around the world for testing for banned substances. They are now justifiably concerned about the use of gene doping. Gene doping is merely gene therapy by another name, and as we develop the latter for treating bona fide medical purposes, the possibility for misuse will increase.

The detection of introduced genes will not be easy. A likely route for delivery is intramuscular injection of a vector, and the products of the genes introduced might never enter the circulation. Trying to find the site of injection would be like looking for a needle in a haystack, and even if the site of injection could be identified, it would require that a biopsy sample be taken from that region of the muscle. However, if a muscle biopsy sample is available, one of several strategies can be used to identify the presence of an engineered gene. Independent of whether a viral or plasmid vector is used to transfer the gene, there might be sequences that have to be included for production of the vector or improving efficiency of expression that are distinct from naturally occurring sequences. Or it might be that vectors developed for medical applications on a commercial scale will contain a sequence to identify the laboratory where it is produced (DNA tag). There is a risk that the vectors will reach other tissues besides muscle. It may be possible, therefore, to take oral swabs of mucosal cells or to use white blood cells to test for the gene vector. Mucosal cells are routinely used for gender determination and blood samples are now routinely taken after major events. The analyses of these samples for the presence of engineered genes or delivery vectors can be carried out using the polymerase reaction PCR, which is incredibly sensitive, as it can amplify one copy of a specific DNA sequence by over a million times within 20 minutes. Indeed, such a test could be carried out several years after the event in which the competitors are suspected of having cheated and the athletes retrospectively deprived of their medals. The possibility of retrospective punishment is perhaps the biggest deterrent to the use of currently undetectable substances by competitive athletes.

Recent advances in mass spectrometry and gene array technologies have allowed large-scale analyses of differential protein and gene expression in different tissues under different physiological conditions. Molecular signatures for these conditions are now being developed that encompass variations of hundreds of proteins or mRNAs that are specific to certain physiological states. Researchers in the UK are now developing a system of analysing serum samples by mass spectrometry and sophisticated computer analyses involving artificial neural networks. In our collaboration with Nottingham Trent University and HFL (formerly Horse Forensics Laboratories), it has been found that animals and human subjects that have been doped with growth hormone have a pattern of metabolites in their serum that is different from non-doped controls. The prospects of using this new approach for detecting doping therefore look encouraging. Initially, its use might be limited to screening large numbers of samples for those that have patterns of metabolites that are not normal. These suspicious samples could then be submitted to more specific tests that would be incontestable in a court of law. The application of this technique would be useful for detecting gene doping as well as alterations caused by novel drugs.

Finally, it has been suggested that athletes could be required to carry a proteomic passport that would chart the profile of each individual, during the course of his or her competitive career. Thus, the interindividual variability, due to factors such as gender, age, ethnicity, body composition, nutrition and exercise status, that limits the sensitivity of current tests could be circumvented. The battle against doping is not lost yet.

6 CONCLUSION

Advances in molecular genetics and proteomics enable us to monitor the way individuals train and how they may be selected for competition in different athletic events. They also enable us to detect those who are cheating in order to achieve their moment of glory. It is therefore important that every sports scientist has some basic knowledge of genes and how genes determine our innate ability to excel, as well as how training programmes can be designed to ensure that the key genes affecting performance are optimally expressed to achieve this aim and ensure a healthy lifestyle.

References

Adams GR, Haddad F 1996 The relationships among IGF-1, DNA content and protein accumulation during skeletal muscle hypertrophy. Journal of Applied Physiology 81(6):2509–2516

An P, Rice T, Gagnon J, Leon AS, Skinner JS, Bouchard C, Rao DC, Wilmore JH 2000 Familial aggregation of stroke volume and cardiac output during submaximal exercise: the HERITAGE Family Study. International Journal of Sports Medicine 21:566–572

An P, Borecki IB, Rankinen T, Pérusse L, Leon AS, Skinner JS, Wilmore JH, Bouchard C, Rao DC 2003 Evidence of major genes for exercise heart rate and blood pressure at baseline and in response to 20 weeks of endurance training: the HERITAGE Family Study. International Journal of Sports Medicine 24:492–498

Aperghis M, Johnson IP, Cannon J, Yang SY, Goldspink G 2004 Different levels of neuroprotection by two insulin-like growth factor-I splice variants. Brain Research 1009(1–2):213–218

Beshyah SA, Freemantle C, Shahi M, Anyaoku V, Merson S, Lynch S, Skinner E, Sharp P, Foale R, Johnston DG 1995 Replacement treatment with biosynthetic human growth hormone in growth hormone-deficient hypopituitary adults. Clinical Endocrinology 42(1):73–84

Birkeland KI, Stray-Gundersen J, Hemmersbach P, Hallen J, Haug E, Bahr R 2000 Effect of rhEPO administration on serum levels of sTfR and cycling performance. Medicine and Science in Sports and Exercise 32(7):1238–1243

Bouchard C, Daw EW, Rice T, Pérusse L, Gagnon J, Province MA, Leon AS, Rao DC, Skinner JS, Wilmore JH 1998 Familial resemblance for VO2max in the sedentary state: the HERITAGE Family Study. Medicine and Science in Sports and Exercise 30:252–258

Bouchard C, An P, Rice T, Skinner JS, Wilmore JH, Gagnon J, Pérusse L, Leon AS, Rao DC 1999 Familial aggregation of VO2max response to exercise training: results from the HERITAGE Family Study. Journal of Applied Physiology 87:1003–1008

Brissenden JE, Ullrich A, Francke U 1984 Human chromosomal mapping of genes for insulin-like growth factors I and II and epidermal growth factor. Nature 310(5980):781–784

Calvo M, Rodas G, Vallejo M, Estruch A, Arcas A, Javierre C, Viscor G, Ventura JL 2002 Heritability of explosive power and anaerobic capacity in humans. European Journal of Applied Physiology 86:218–225

Cuneo RC, Salomon F, Wiles CM, Hesp R, Sonksen PH 1991 Growth hormone treatment in growth hormone-deficient adults. I. Effects on muscle mass and strength. Journal of Applied Physiology 70(2):688–694

Daughaday WH, Reeder C 1966 Synchronous activation of DNA synthesis in hypophysectomized rat cartilage by growth hormone. Journal of Laboratory and Clinical Medicine 68(3):357–368

Daughaday WH, Rotwein P 1989 Insulin-like growth factors I and II. Peptide, messenger ribonucleic acid and gene structures, serum and tissue concentrations. Endocrine Reviews 10(1):68–91

de la Chapelle A, Traskelin AL, Juvonen E 1993 Truncated erythropoietin receptor causes dominantly inherited benign human erythrocytosis. Proceedings of the National Academy of Sciences of the United States of America 90(10):4495–4499

de Pagter-Holthuizen P, van Schaik FM, Verduijn GM, van Ommen GJ, Bouma BN, Jansen M, Sussenbach JS 1986 Organization of the human genes for insulin-like growth factors I and II. FEBS Letters 195(1–2):179–184

Dolmetsch RE, Lewis RS, Goodnow CC, Healy JI 1997 Differential activation of transcription factors induced by Ca2+ response amplitude and duration. Nature 386(6627):855–858

Feitosa MF, Gaskill SE, Rice T, Rankinen T, Bouchard C, Rao DC, Wilmore JH, Skinner JS, Leon AS 2002 Major gene effects on exercise ventilatory threshold: the HERITAGE Family Study. Journal of Applied Physiology 93(3):1000–1006

Folland J, Leach B, Little T, Hawker K, Myerson S, Montgomery H, Jones D 2000 Angiotensin-converting enzyme genotype affects the response of human skeletal muscle to functional overload. Experimental Physiology 85(5):575–579

Gayagay G, Yu B, Hambly B, Boston T, Hahn A, Celermajer DS, Trent RJ 1998 Elite endurance athletes and the ACE I allele – the role of genes in athletic performance. Human Genetics 103(1): 48–50

Gilmour RS 1994 The implications of insulin-like growth factor mRNA heterogeneity. Journal of Endocrinology 140(1):1–3

Goldspink G 2001 Method of treating muscular disorders. United States Patent No. US 6,221,842 B1

Goldspink G, Scutt A, Loughna P, Wells D, Jaenicke T, Gerlach GF 1992 Gene expression in skeletal muscle in response to mechanical signals. American Journal of Physiology 262:R326–R363

Goldspink G, Yang SY, Skarli M, Vrbova G 1996 Local growth regulation is associated with an isoform of IGF-I that is expressed in normal muscles but not in dystrophic muscles. Journal of Physiology 496P:162

Green H, Morikawa M, Nixon T 1985 A dual effector theory of growth-hormone action. Differentiation 29(3):195–198

Haddad F, Adams GR 2002 Selected contribution: acute cellular and molecular responses to resistance exercise. Journal of Applied Physiology 93(1):394–403

Hasty P, Bradley A, Morris JH, Edmondson DG, Venuti JM, Olson EN, Klein WH 1993 Muscle deficiency and neonatal death in mice with a targeted mutation in the myogenin gene. Nature 364(6437):501–506

Hameed M, Orrell RW, Cobbold M, Goldspink G, Harridge SDR 2003a Expression of IGF-I splice variants in young and old human skeletal muscle after high resistance exercise. Journal of Physiology 547:247–254

Hameed M, Lange KH, Andersen JL, Schjerling P, Kjaer M, Harridge SD, Goldspink G 2003b The effect of recombinant human growth hormone and resistance training on IGF-I mRNA expression in the muscles of elderly men. Journal of Physiology 555:231–240

Hepler JE, Lund PK 1990 Molecular biology of the insulin-like growth factors. Relevance to nervous system function. Molecular Neurobiology 4(1–2):93–127

Hill M, Goldspink G 2003 Expression and splicing of the insulin-like growth factor gene in rodent muscle is associated with muscle satellite (stem) cell activation following local tissue damage. Journal of Physiology 549:409–418

Hughes SM, Chi MM, Lowry OH, Gundersen K 1999 Myogenin induces a shift of enzyme activity from glycolytic to oxidative metabolism in muscles of transgenic mice. Journal of Cell Biology 145(3):633–642

Huygens W, Thomis MA, Peeters MW, Aerssens J, Vlietinck R, Beunen GP 2005 Quantitative trait loci for human muscle strength: linkage analysis of myostatin pathway genes. Physiological Genomics 22(3):390–397

Kim JS, Cross JM, Bamman MM 2005 Impact of resistance loading on myostatin expression and cell cycle regulation in young and older men and women. American Journal of Physiology. Endocrinology and Metabolism 288(6):E1110–E1119

Lassar AB, Buskin JN, Lockshon D, Davis RL, Apone S, Hauschka SD, Weintraub H 1989 MyoD is a sequence-specific DNA binding protein requiring a region of myc homology to bind to the muscle creatine kinase enhancer. Cell 58(5):823–831

Lin H, Konieczny SF 1992 Identification of MRF4, myogenin and E12 oligomer complexes by chemical cross-linking and two-dimensional gel electrophoresis. Journal of Biological Chemistry 267(7):4773–4780

Lin J, Wu H, Tarr PT, Zhang CY, Wu Z, Boss O, Michael LF, Puigserver P, Isotani E, Olson EN, Lowell BB, Bassel-Duby R, Spiegelman BM 2002 Transcriptional co-activator PGC-1 alpha drives the formation of slow-twitch muscle fibres. Nature 418(6899):797–801

Macarthur DG, North KN 2005 Genes and human elite athletic performance. Human Genetics 116(5):331–339

McCroskery S, Thomas M, Maxwell L, Sharma M, Kambadur R 2003 Myostatin negatively regulates satellite cell activation and self-renewal. Journal of Cell Biology 162(6):1135–1147

McKoy G, Ashley W, Mander J, Yang SY, Williams N, Russell B, Goldspink G 1999 Expression of insulin-like growth factor-I splice variant and structural genes in rabbit skeletal muscle induced by stretch and stimulation. Journal of Physiology 516:583–592

McKoy G, Hou Y, Yang SY, Vega Avelaira D, Degens H, Goldspink G, Coulton GR 2005 Expression of Ankrd2 in fast and slow muscles and its response to stretch are consistent with a role in slow muscle function. Journal of Applied Physiology 98(6):2337–2343

McPherron AC, Lawler AM, Lee SJ 1997 Regulation of skeletal muscle mass in mice by a new TGF-beta superfamily member. Nature 387(6628):83–90

McPherron AC, Lee SJ 1997 Double muscling in cattle due to mutations in the myostatin gene. Proceeding of the National Academy of Sciences of the United States of America 94(23):12457–12461

Mills M, Yang N, Weinberger R, Vander Woude DL, Beggs AH, Easteal S, North K 2001 Differential expression of the actin-binding proteins, alpha-actinin-2 and -3, in different species: implications for the evolution of functional redundancy. Human Molecular Genetics 10(13):1335–1346

Montgomery HE, Clarkson P, Dollery CM, Prasad K, Losi MA, Hemingway H, Statters D, Jubb M, Girvain M, Varnava A, World M, Deanfield J, Talmud P, McEwan JR, McKenna WJ, Humphries S 1997 Association of angiotensin-converting enzyme gene I/D polymorphism with change in left ventricular mass in response to physical training. Circulation 96(3):741–747

Montgomery HE, Marshall R, Hemingway H, Myerson S, Clarkson P, Dollery C, Hayward M, Holliman DE, Jubb M, World M, Thomas EL, Brynes AE, Saeed N, Barnard M, Bell JD, Prasad K, Rayson M, Talmud PJ, Humphries SE 1998 Human gene for physical performance. Nature 393(6682):221–222

Musarò A, McCullagh K, Paul A, Houghton L, Dobrowolny G, Molinaro M, Barton ER, Sweeney HL, Rosenthal N 2001 Localized IGF-I transgene expression sustains hypertrophy and regeneration in senescent skeletal muscle. Nature Genetics 27:195–200

Nabeshima Y, Hanaoka K, Hayasaka M, Esumi E, Li S, Nonaka I, Nabeshima Y 1993 Myogenin gene disruption results in perinatal lethality because of severe muscle defect. Nature 364(6437): 532–532

Owino V, Yang SY, Goldspink G 2001 Age-related loss of skeletal muscle function and the inability to express the autocrine form of insulin-like growth factor-1 (MGF) in response to mechanical overload. FEBS Letters 506:259–263

Pette D, Staron RS 1997 Mammalian skeletal muscle fiber type transitions. International Review of Cytology 170:143–223

Rennie MJ 2003 Claims for the anabolic effects of growth hormone: a case of the emperor's new clothes? British Journal of Sports Medicine 37(2):100–105

Rigat B, Hubert C, Alhenc-Gelas F, Cambien F, Corvol P, Soubrier F 1990 An insertion/deletion polymorphism in the angiotensin I-converting enzyme gene accounting for half the variance of serum enzyme levels. Journal of Clinical Investigation 86(4):1343–1346

Rotwein P, Pollock KM, Didier DK, Krivi GG 1986 Organization and sequence of the human insulin-like growth factor I gene. Alternative RNA processing produces two insulin-like growth factor I precursor peptides. Journal of Biological Chemistry 261(11):4828–4832

Rudman D, Kutner MH, Rogers CM, Lubin MF, Fleming GA, Bain RP 1981 Impaired growth hormone secretion in the adult population: relation to age and adiposity. Journal of Clinical Investigation 67: 1361–1369

Rudnicki MA, Schnegelsberg PN, Stead RH, Braun T, Arnold HH, Jaenisch R 1993 MyoD or Myf-5 is required for the formation of skeletal muscle. Cell 75(7):1351–1359

Saltin B, Larsen H, Terrados N, Bangsbo J, Bak T, Kim CK, Svedenhag J, Rolf CJ 1995a Aerobic exercise capacity at sea level and at altitude in Kenyan boys, junior and senior runners compared with Scandinavian runners. Scandinavian Journal of Medicine and Science in Sports 5:209–221

Saltin B, Kim CK, Terrados N, Larsen H, Svedenhag J, Rolf CJ 1995b Morphology, enzyme activities and buffer capacity in leg muscles of Kenyan and Scandinavian runners. Scandinavian Journal of Medicine and Science in Sports 5:222–230

Sartorelli V, Webster KA, Kedes L 1990 Muscle-specific expression of the cardiac alpha-actin gene requires MyoD1, CArG-box binding factor and Sp1. Genes and Development 4(10): 1811–1822

Schuelke M, Wagner KR, Stolz LE, Hübner C, Riebel T, Kömen W, Braun T, Tobin JF, Lee SJ 2004 Myostatin mutation associated with gross muscle hypertrophy in a child. New England Journal of Medicine 350(26):2682–2688

Sjögren K, Liu JL, Blad K, Skrtic S, Vidal O, Wallenius V, LeRoith D, Törnell J, Isaksson OG, Jansson JO, Ohlsson C 1999 Liver-derived insulin-like growth factor I (IGF-I) is the principal source of IGF-I in blood but is not required for postnatal body growth in mice. Proceedings of the National Academy of Sciences of the United States of America 96(12):7088–7092

Tobin G, Yee D, Brunner N, Rotwein P 1990 A novel human insulin-like growth factor I messenger RNA is expressed in normal and tumor cells. Molecular Endocrinology 4(12):1914–1920

Tricoli JV, Rall LB, Scott J, Bell GI, Shows TB 1984 Localization of insulin-like growth factor genes to human chromosomes 11 and 12. Nature 310(5980):784–786

Wang YX, Zhang CL, Yu RT, Cho HK, Nelson MC, Bayuga-Ocampo CR, Ham J, Kang H, Evans RM 2004 Regulation of muscle fiber type and running endurance by PPARdelta. PLoS Biology 2(10): e294. Erratum in: PLoS Biology 2005;3(1):e61

Weller PA, Dickson MC, Huskisson NS, Dauncey MJ, Buttery PJ, Gilmour RS 1993 The porcine insulin-like growth factor-I gene: characterization and expression of alternate transcription sites. Journal of Molecular Endocrinology 11(2):201–211

Wentworth BM, Donoghue M, Engert JC, Berglund EB, Rosenthal N 1991 Paired MyoD-binding sites regulate myosin light chain gene expression. Proceedings of the National Academy of Sciences of the United States of America 88(4):1242–1246

Woods D, Hickman M, Jamshidi Y, Brull D, Vassiliou V, Jones A, Humphries S, Montgomery H 2001 Elite swimmers and the D allele of the ACE I/D polymorphism. Human Genetics 108(3):230–232

Yakar S, Liu JL, Stannard B, Butler A, Accili D, Sauer B, LeRoith D 1999 Normal growth and development in the absence of hepatic insulin-like growth factor I. Proceedings of the National Academy of Sciences of the United States of America 96(13):7324–7329

Yang SY, Goldspink G 2002 Different roles of the IGF-IEc peptide (MGF) and mature IGF-I in myoblast proliferation and differentiation. FEBS Letters 522:156–160

Yang SY, Alnaqeeb M, Simpson H, Goldspink G 1996 Cloning and characterisation of an IGF-I isoform expressed in skeletal muscle subjected to stretch. Journal of Muscle Research and Cell Motility 17:487–495

Yang N, MacArthur DG, Gulbin JP, Hahn AG, Beggs AH, Easteal S, North K 2003 ACTN3 genotype is associated with human elite athletic performance. American Journal of Human Genetics 73(3):627–631

Chapter 9

Detraining, bed rest and adaptation to microgravity

Marco V. Narici   Claire E. Stewart   Pietro E. di Prampero

1 INTRODUCTION

Skeletal muscle is highly adaptable, rapidly responding to stresses associated with growth, the maintenance of posture, extreme athletic performance and the repair of injury. In addition, skeletal muscle also declines in mass and function with age (Chapter 16), disuse (Chapter 28) and disease.

2 REGULATORS OF SKELETAL MUSCLE MASS IN HEALTH

Human skeletal muscle is derived at approximately week six of gestation, when precursor skeletal muscle cells or myoblasts (muscle cells determined with respect to myogenic phenotype) develop. After a period of proliferation, these cells fuse with one another (weeks 7–9 of gestation) to form multinucleated myofibres. This transformation depends upon muscle-specific transcription factors belonging to the myogenic regulatory factor family of genes (Pownall et al. 2002). Myoblasts continue to be added to these myotubes throughout gestation, allowing them to expand in both length and girth. At approximately 10 weeks, innervation of the fibres occurs and muscle gradually converts to adult-type myosins. By 24 weeks, it is believed that fibre numbers are set, with any further cross-sectional growth occurring as a consequence of hypertrophy. This is dependent not only on nuclear acquisition from resident undifferentiated muscle stem cells, but also on de novo protein synthesis. The capacity for nuclei to be recruited and to enable protein synthesis is dependent upon the recognition of anabolic signals that are altered with loading, for example the insulin-like growth factors (I and II).

A number of factors also induce atrophy. These include: interleukin-1, tumour necrosis factor α and also myostatin, which is associated with atrophy of microgravity, AIDS and ageing. In contrast to hypertrophy, conditions leading to atrophy are associated with myoblast cell death and ubiquitin-mediated protein degradation.

2.1 Skeletal muscle stem cells

The primary function of skeletal muscle is force generation, achieved by the synchronous activation of bundles of highly specialised myofibres. The generation and functional specialisation of such fibres are achieved through terminal differentiation, which is dependent upon the establishment of a specific configuration of expressed genes that defines cellular identity and function. Zammit & Beauchamp (2001) proposed that the cost of such a high degree of specialisation is the loss of the ability of muscle to proliferate. Consequently, the capacity to generate new myonuclei for myofibre repair, growth or replacement is dependent upon the persistence of a reservoir of undifferentiated cells.

2.1.1 Satellite cells: proliferation and differentiation

Satellite cells (myosatellite cells) were first identified by Mauro (1961) and, defined on the basis of their geographical location in mature muscles (beneath basal lamina close to the plasmalemma), it is these cells that enable muscle growth and regeneration to occur (Mauro 1961). Following muscle trauma, overuse or increased tension, satellite cells become activated, proliferate and co-express myogenic factors (Qu-Petersen et al. 2002). Ultimately, these cells fuse to existing muscle fibres during regeneration of damaged muscle (Seale & Rudnicki 2000). Some daughter cells remain in this undifferentiated state, providing a life-long source of new nuclei.

Normally, mitosis ceases in adult muscle satellite cells, but becomes activated in response to cellular damage, trauma or various adaptation stimuli (e.g. physical training). Hepatocyte growth factor is an integral mediator of satellite cell activation (Anastasi et al. 1997), while other growth factors, endothelial and insulin-like growth factors (Johnson & Allen 1995) facilitate the subsequent increase in satellite cell numbers. Following multiple divisions, a proportion of daughter satellite cells (myoblasts or muscle precursor cells) undergo terminal differentiation and become incorporated into mature muscle fibres (Zammit & Beauchamp 2001). Those that do not differentiate re-enter a quiescent state and replenish the satellite cell pool. Therefore, satellite cells are a population of precursors that provide a reserve capacity to replace differentiated, postmitotic cells.

Animal experiments have shown that older muscles are injured more easily and regenerate more slowly than younger muscles (impaired functional recovery; Goldspink & Harridge 2004). There is increasing evidence that the growth factor(s) that activate muscle stem cells are produced at lower levels in aged muscle following exercise. For example, Owino et al. (2001) assessed the response of insulin-like growth factor I signalling, and the capacity of the skeletal muscle (plantaris and soleus) to adapt to mechanical overload, using synergistic muscle ablation in young, mature and aged rats. This produced hypertrophy and activation of satellite cells, particularly in young rats. In contrast, older muscles were less able to respond, showing a lower expression of the local splice variant mechano growth factor (a stimulant for muscle satellite cell division). This implies that replenishment of the muscle satellite stem cell pool is important for the maintenance of muscle mass and function. Evidence suggests that this stem cell pool does not run out of satellite cells during normal ageing, but the pool is not adequately replenished in aged muscles (Renault et al. 2002).

Thus, when considering satellite cell activation, proliferation and differentiation, it is essential to address the molecular events underlying these processes. Key myogenic regulatory factors (MRFs) Myf5 and MyoD control the conversion of satellite cells to muscle precursor cells and cell cycle entry of satellite cells. Secondary MRFs (myogenin and MRF4) modulate terminal differentiation: precursor cells to myofibre (Arnold & Winter 1998). The expression profile of the myogenic regulatory factors in the satellite cell lineage is analogous to the programme manifested during embryonic myogenesis (Seale et al. 2001).

Myogenic regulatory factors reveal differential regulation patterns during the cell cycle. Withdrawal from the cell cycle and the onset of differentiation are associated with high expression of MyoD and low expression of Myf5 (Kitzmann et al. 1998). Conversely, high expression of the latter may be incompatible with both cell cycle progression and differentiation (Cornelison et al. 2000). Therefore, the expression of these regulatory factors determines the proportion of satellite cells within each phase of muscle development: quiescence, activation, proliferation and differentiation (Zammit & Beauchamp 2001).

Satellite cells and their regulators therefore play an essential role in muscle maintenance, regeneration, hypertrophy and postnatal growth, and their ability to repair or regenerate skeletal muscle is unequivocal. While satellite cell number is efficiently maintained during early adult life, the chronic demand for new myonuclei culminates in a reduction in satellite cell numbers in aged muscle (Gibson & Schultz 1983). Such an inability to maintain the satellite cell pool at equilibrium suggests an eventual decrease in the efficiency of self-renewal over time. An understanding of and an ability to manipulate this decline with age may realise the potential for adult muscle stem cells in treating wasting disorders, including those associated with disuse, detraining and microgravity.

2.2 Skeletal muscle homeostasis

Skeletal muscle satellite cells are therefore important modulators contributing to muscle homeostasis. Under normal conditions, young individuals maintain a homeostatic muscle equilibrium characterised by constant mass and protein content, albeit with fluctuations due to altered metabolic demands. In this state, protein synthesis and degradation are in balance (Szewczyk & Jacobson 2005). In order for hypertrophy or atrophy to occur, perturbations in this stability are evoked. For example, the transition into hypertrophy requires not only stem cell recruitment but protein turnover, in which synthesis exceeds degradation, a state accomplished by adjustments in the rates of one or both processes. Biochemical signals (growth factors, cytokines) are predominantly responsible for altering protein metabolism. In the simplest sense, signals that decrease protein degradation or increase synthesis potentially induce hypertrophy and oppose atrophy. Importantly, protein turnover also allows the qualitative remodelling of muscle fibres (section 3.1.2), enabling myosin heavy chain isoform alterations (Baldwin & Haddad 2002). Protein turnover, therefore, provides the mechanisms essential for regulating the amount and type of proteins in muscle, and the adaptability required to accommodate environmental stresses.

2.2.1 Skeletal muscle homeostasis: transcription and translation

Protein synthesis is regulated at transcriptional and post-translational levels. Gene expression and protein levels can be controlled at several points along the synthetic pathway, with the rate of gene transcription, changes in the processing of mRNA and the rate of mRNA translation affecting protein abundance. Independent of mRNA abundance or protein synthesis, mechanisms involving protein degradation are considered central to post-translational modifications of protein availability (Baldwin & Haddad 2002).

As we age, changes in our genome integrity, gene expression, translation efficiency and post-translational modifications of proteins are all instrumental in the muscle-wasting process. In older (>60 y) compared with younger adults (<35 y), decreased synthesis of mixed muscle proteins in the quadriceps reflects a reduction in the synthesis rates of myofibrillar (Welle et al. 1993) but not sarcoplasmic proteins (Balagopal et al. 1997). The synthesis of myosin heavy chains is dramatically reduced in the absence of transcriptional rate changes (Balagopal et al. 1997, Welle et al. 1993). Importantly, major declines occur in the fractional rates of protein synthesis in middle-aged (54 y) compared with young adults (24 y), but thereafter tend to increase with advancing age (Rooyackers et al. 1996), suggesting that while declines in protein synthesis may be important in the initiation of muscle loss, they do not contribute to the gradual erosion of muscle protein into old age. These studies suggest that protein degradation is more important in older individuals (Chapter 16).

2.2.2 Skeletal muscle homeostasis: mechanical load, protein synthesis and degradation

All biological materials are constantly in a state of flux, with every protein having its own steady-state exchange rate that varies from seconds to weeks. For the expression of any protein to be altered, a highly specific adaptation stimulus (Chapter 21) must be applied at sufficient intensity, duration and frequency. Generally, stimuli are intermittent (e.g. resistance training), yet application of continuous overload

stresses may elicit a greater hypertrophic response (Baldwin & Haddad 2002). Under regimens of intermittent training, the adaptive response will not, however, follow predicted kinetics for protein turnover (as is the case in chronic unloading: microgravity). Therefore, our understanding of adaptation stimuli for optimising hypertrophic cellular adaptations is incomplete.

Despite these caveats, studies are being performed to assess the critical threshold stimulus (e.g. mechanical force) required to affect the flow of genetic information and to culminate in optimal hypertrophy. Indeed, recent animal models suggest that ~50 near-maximal, high-resistance contractions, performed in a single training session, will increase mRNA and contractile protein synthesis. This stimulus does, however, need to be sufficiently repeated (12–15 sessions) at short intervals (every other day) to induce a net gain in contractile protein mass and increase fibre cross-sectional area (Baldwin & Haddad 2001, 2002, Smerdu et al. 1994).

The balance between the rates of protein synthesis and degradation in muscle determines its ultimate protein content, and thus its size and functional capacity. While we strive to glean an understanding of the mechanisms governing protein synthesis, good models of protein degradation do exist, with three proteolytic pathways (lysosomal, calcium dependent and ubiquitin dependent) reportedly active in skeletal muscle.

Skeletal muscle contains few lysosomes and the major lysosomal enzymes (cathepsins) do not appear to contribute significantly to protein degradation (Attaix et al. 2005). Furthermore, very few reports suggest either increased activity or mRNA levels of these enzymes in muscle wasting. Finally, lysosomes are not thought to be major contributors to myofibrillar degradation. The second proteolytic pathway involves the calcium-dependant calpains, which are thought to be involved in the degradation of sarcomeric proteins (Huang & Forsberg 1998). However, like lysososmal enzymes, there is scant evidence documenting their systematic activation in muscle loss with ageing, and they are not responsible for myofibrillar protein breakdown.

Most protein degradation in mammalian cells requires adenosine triphosphate, and involves the polypeptide cofactor ubiquitin and the ATP-dependent proteasome (Beehler et al. 2006). This ubiquitin–proteasome system normally functions to ensure the quality of intracellular proteins, preventing potentially toxic accumulation of damaged proteins. Indeed, signalling pathways converging on ubiquitin ligases will ultimately determine whether muscle protein synthesis or degradation predominates.

In mammalian cells, the ubiquitin–proteasome-dependent pathway normally catalyses the breakdown of short-lived proteins. In skeletal muscle, it is also responsible for the breakdown of long-lived myofibrillar proteins (Attaix et al. 2005). The contractile proteins of skeletal muscle are among the most stable of all proteins, having half-lives of 10 (myosin heavy chain) to 20 (actin) days, when maintained within the sarcomere (Russell et al. 2000). However, if either of these molecules is removed from its protection within an intact filament, it is susceptible to rapid degradation via the ubiquitin pathway, within a new half-life of minutes. This system is one of the primary proteolytic pathways implicated in skeletal muscle atrophy under catabolic conditions. Indeed, in examples of chronic catabolic diseases, increased expression or transcription of the muscle specific ubiquitin ligases has been reported (Attaix et al. 2005). While these changes are associated with increased rates of substrate ubiquitination and increased proteasome activity, once again, information pertaining to this pathway and its role in detraining, disuse and microgravity is limited.

Other important, unanswered questions concerning protein synthesis and degradation in skeletal muscle prevail. For example, what fosters the unravelling of filaments, in order that degradation of actin and myosin may follow? Removal of load is believed to play a key role. Indeed, this is witnessed in spaceflight (Chapter 26), artificial dispersion of tissues into culture or the inhibition of contraction, all of which are sufficient to reduce myosin heavy chain and actin content of myocytes with an associated disappearance of sarcomeres (Byron et al. 1996). These are, however, reversible events, with an increase in load or activity, enhancing reassembly of the sarcomere (Simpson et al. 1996) and protein stability.

2.2.3 Skeletal muscle homeostasis: hormonal control

When assessing muscle homeostasis, it is not sufficient to consider only transcription, translation, synthesis and degradation; one must also contemplate the extracellular regulators of these processes. Indeed, there is a complex network of cross-talk activities between anabolic hormones (e.g. growth hormone, insulin-like growth factors, testosterone), inflammatory cytokines (e.g. interleukins, tumour necrosis factor α) and the intracellular pathways mediating the signals governing muscle homeostasis.

Resistance exercise elicits acute hormonal responses believed to be critical for tissue growth, remodelling and strength increases. It is these changes, rather than chronic modifications in resting hormonal concentrations, that are believed to elicit the hypertrophic responses (Kraemer & Ratamess 2005). If an adequate adaptation stimulus is present (Chapter 21), anabolic hormones (e.g. growth hormone and testosterone) peak 15–30 min after resistance training. Protocols high in volume, moderate to high in intensity, using short rest intervals and stressing a large muscle mass, tend to produce the greatest acute hormonal elevations (Kraemer & Ratamess 2005), and are similar to those necessary for adequate protein synthesis. Other anabolic hormones such as insulin (secretion is regulated by blood glucose and amino acid levels (Chapter 30)) and insulin-like growth factor I (IGF-I; hepatic secretion occurs in response to growth hormone elevations) are also critical to skeletal muscle growth.

2.2.3.1 Skeletal muscle homeostasis: hormonal control – testosterone

Testosterone replacement therapy stimulates muscle protein synthesis and improves the reutilisation of amino acids (Ferrando et al. 2002b). Testosterone-induced hypertrophy is associated with a parallel increase in satellite cell numbers (Sinha-Hikim et al. 2003), and is reported to impact directly on IGF-I production and responsiveness (Urban et al. 1995). Circulating testosterone and IGF-I concentrations correlate positively with muscle mass; declining as we age and with muscle wastage (Davidson et al. 1983, Pfeilschifter et al. 1996). Indeed, in men, elevated testosterone and IGF-I concentrations are inversely correlated with sarcopenia (Payette et al. 2003).

2.2.3.2 Skeletal muscle homeostasis: hormonal control – IGF-I

The insulin-like growth factors form part of a complex regulatory system consisting of two growth factors (IGF-I and IGF-II), the type I and type II cell surface receptors, specific high-affinity binding proteins and proteases, as well as other interacting molecules (Holly et al. 2000). IGF-I and IGF-II have a broad range of functions in the embryo, foetus and adult. The relevance of the insulin-like growth factor system has been demonstrated in vivo, where ligand or receptor knockout (in mice) results in neonatal death, primarily as a consequence of skeletal muscle hypoplasia (Stewart & Rotwein 1996). Indeed, insulin-like growth factors are implicated in several aspects of muscle development, mediating myoblast proliferation, survival and terminal differentiation (Florini et al. 1996).

Binding of the insulin-like growth factors to the IGF-I receptor stimulates intrinsic tyrosine kinase activity, and activates a signalling cascade that culminates in de novo protein synthesis (Rommel et al. 2001). Additionally, the insulin-like growth factors can increase the diameter of myotubes, suppress protein degradation and increase amino acid uptake (Rommel et al. 2001).

In humans, the circulating and intramuscular concentrations of IGF-I and the responsiveness of muscle to IGF-I are reduced in most medical conditions where circulating cytokines are elevated and muscle wasting is evident. Indeed, pro-inflammatory cytokines, at concentrations often found in the elderly, interfere with IGF-I gene and protein expression and the capacity of IGF-I to stimulate protein synthesis and maintain muscle mass.

In contrast to skeletal muscle loss in adults, hypertrophy is characterised by an increase in the size of individual myofibres occurring as an adaptive response to load-bearing exercise and enhanced protein synthesis (Glass 2003b). IGF-I is believed to induce hypertrophy by stimulating the phosphatidylinositol 3-kinase-protein kinase-B (also known as Akt; PI3K-Akt) pathway, resulting in the downstream transcription and translation of proteins (Bodine et al. 2001). This enables new contractile filaments to be added to existing muscle fibres, increasing force generation. In a feedforward control loop (Chapter 18), increased muscle work stimulates IGF-I expression and induces hypertrophy through the autocrine and paracrine mechanisms (Harridge 2003).

In rodent models, local overexpression of IGF-I in skeletal muscle stimulates myofibre hypertrophy, and maintains muscle mass and strength during ageing (Barton-Davis et al. 1998). IGF-I mRNA and protein are expressed in newly replicating rat skeletal myoblasts following ischaemic or toxic injury (Caroni & Schneider 1994, Jennische & Hansson 1987), and IGF-I and -II gene expression is induced as an early event in work-induced hypertrophy in hypophysectomised rats (DeVol et al. 1990). Importantly, these studies implicate insulin-like growth factors as local regulators of growth and regeneration, independent of the growth hormone axis.

Exercise increases muscle mass in rodents, with regular treadmill running resulting in a 25% increase in muscle cross-sectional area. This response is doubled in IGF-I transgenic mice (Paul & Rosenthal 2002) and blocked in mice expressing an inactive IGF-I receptor (Fernandez et al. 2002). Substantiating these findings, Brahm et al. (1997) demonstrated a net release of IGF-I during one-legged dynamic extension, where arteriovenous differences were measured across the working muscle. This local production of IGF-I suggests its importance in autocrine/paracrine function with regard to satellite cell activation, protein synthesis and ultimately for muscle maintenance.

2.2.4 Skeletal muscle homeostasis: cytokines

While testosterone and the insulin-like growth factors are positive regulators of muscle mass, elevated concentrations of interleukin-2, -6 and tumour necrosis factor α are associated with accelerated muscle loss and reduced strength and function (Payette et al. 2003). These cytokines cause muscle mass losses by inhibiting nuclear factor κβ (NF-κβ), activating the ubiquitin–proteasome system and promoting muscle cell apoptosis (Sharma & Anker 2002). The release of cytokines increases with age, and appears to play a role in the ageing process (Ershler & Keller 2000). Furthermore, both androgen and oestrogen deficiencies may upregulate proinflammatory cytokines (Joseph et al. 2005). Elevated levels of these cytokines, along with low concentrations of anabolic hormones, are believed to synergistically contribute to sarcopenia (Baumgartner et al. 1999), with elevated cytokines and reduced insulin-like growth factors being independent risk factors of mortality.

2.2.5 Skeletal muscle homeostasis: myostatin

Myostatin (also known as growth and differentiation factor 8) is a member of the transforming growth factor β superfamily, playing a key role in muscle homeostasis by controlling the proliferation of precursor cells. Furthermore, it promotes differentiation of multipotent mesenchymal stem cells into the adipogenic lineage and inhibits myogenesis (Artaza et al. 2005). The importance of myostatin was first demonstrated in knockout mice, which display marked increases in muscle mass (McPherron et al. 1997). These findings have been substantiated in humans, with increased muscle mass reported in a boy with a mutation in the myostatin gene (Schuelke et al. 2004). Furthermore, myostatin expression is increased in muscle atrophy associated with human immunodeficiency virus infection (Gonzalez-Cadavid et al. 1998), and following prolonged bed rest (Zachwieja et al. 1999b). Although the mechanisms governing the loss of skeletal muscle mass during spaceflight are not well understood, myostatin may be a potentially negative factor. Indeed, in rodent models, muscle atrophy during spaceflight is associated with increased myostatin mRNA and protein levels, and decreased IGF-II mRNA levels. These changes are normalised upon restoration of normal gravity, suggesting that reciprocal changes in the expression of myostatin and IGF-II may contribute to the multifactorial pathophysiology of muscle atrophy during spaceflight (Lalani et al. 2000).

2.3 Cell signalling

IGF-I and IGF-II are unique in their ability to stimulate both myoblast proliferation and terminal differentiation (Singleton & Feldman 2001), with IGF-I receptor (IGF-IR) signalling playing a critical role in these processes. Binding of IGF-I to its receptor induces its conformational change, resulting in its transphosphorylation, activation and phosphorylation of insulin receptor substrate 1, ultimately triggering the activation of signalling pathways crucial for cell proliferation and survival, and the mediation of three effects of IGF-I on skeletal muscle: fusion of myoblasts into myotubes; resistance to apoptosis; and anabolism (Singleton & Feldman 2001). Early studies suggested that IGF-I activates the lipid kinase, PI3K and Akt which results in mammalian target of rapamycin (mTOR) phosphorylation and its subsequent activation.

Substantiating these findings, Bodine et al. (2001) demonstrated that Akt and p70S6 kinase are involved not only in regulating cell growth, proliferation and the translational upregulation of mRNAs, but also in hypertrophy. As this pathway regulates several aspects of protein synthesis, these data implicate translational control of protein production as a key component underlying the hypertrophic response. Parallel studies examining the regulators of disuse atrophy induced by hindlimb suspension once again point to roles for Akt and p70S6 kinase. Levels of both enzymes decline during the development of atrophy, but are restored during recovery. Furthermore, forced expression of Akt culminates in increased muscle mass, even in the absence of weight-bearing activity (Bodine et al. 2001). Together these studies support a role for insulin-like growth factor-stimulated signalling pathways culminating in protein synthesis and growth. Figure 9.1 summarises some of the signalling pathways important in the regulation of muscle homeostasis.

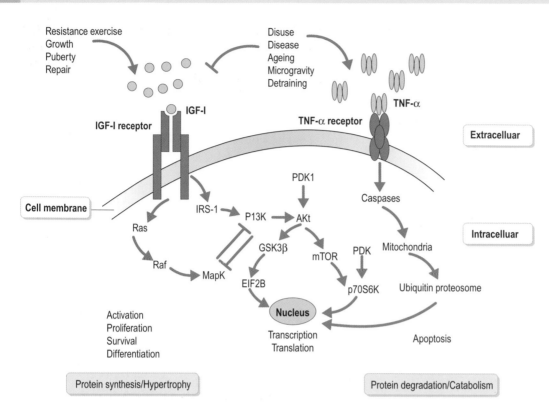

Figure 9.1 Regulators of skeletal muscle mass. In skeletal muscle, the MAP kinase and PI3K-Akt pathways control growth, survival and hypertrophy following IGF–I stimulation, whereas the caspase and ubiquitin proteasome pathways regulate cell death and catabolism following cytokine activation. Abbreviations: eIF-2B, eukaryotic translation initiation factor 2B; GSK3b, glycogen-synthase kinase 3b; IGF–I, insulin-like growth factor I; IRS, insulin receptor substrate; MapK, mitogen activate protein kinase; mTOR, mammalian target of rapamycin; p70S6K, p70 S6 kinase; PDK, phosphoinositide-dependent protein kinase; PI3K, phosphatidyl-inositol-3 kinase; TNF, tumour necrosis factor.

2.3.1 Cell signalling: PI3K and Akt

PI3K is a lipid kinase that phosphorylates phosphatidylinositol (4,5)-biphosphate, producing phosphatidylinositol-(3,4,5)-trisphosphate (Matsui et al. 2003), which mediates the activation of two kinases: Akt1 and phosphoinositide-dependent protein kinase (Kozma & Thomas 2002). Three isoforms of Akt exist, but in skeletal muscle it is Akt1 which is phosphorylated and thereby activated by PDK1. Once activated, Akt1 phosphorylates an ever increasing set of substrates, including proteins that block apoptosis and induce protein synthesis, gene transcription and cell proliferation (Matsui et al. 2003).

Activation of the mammalian target of rapamycin increases protein translation via two pathways: stimulating p70S6K and inhibiting phosphorylated heat- and acid-stable protein (PHAS1), which is a negative regulator of a translation initiation factor (Hara et al. 1997, 2002). Hence, stimulation of p70S6K and blockade of the phosphorylated heat- and acid-stable protein might represent potential routes to increasing protein synthesis and hypertrophy.

Glycogen synthase kinase 3β (GSK3β) is another downstream substrate of Akt1 implicated in hypertrophy (Glass 2003a). GSK3β can block protein translation (Hardt & Sadoshima 2002). However, phosphorylation of Akt inactivates GKS3β. Therefore, inhibition might induce hypertrophy by stimulating protein synthesis. Since a dominant, negative form of GSK3β can induce hypertrophy in skeletal myotubes (Rommel et al. 2001), it is potentially an attractive target hypertrophic agent.

Contractile activity (exercise) has been demonstrated to stimulate Akt signalling. Furthermore, mechanical tension may be a part of the mechanism by which contraction activates Akt in fast-twitch muscles. The PI3K/Akt/p70S6K pathway appears critical for maintaining protein in skeletal muscle and for inducting hypertrophy. Indeed, Li et al. (2003) suggested that, in ageing muscle, there is a general decrease in PI3K/Akt/p70S6K activity, associated with an increased resistance to p70S6K phosphorylation, due to lower IGF-I receptor numbers and reduced Akt1 phosphorylation. In context, this would suggest that older people might be less adaptable (responsive) to exercise than younger people. However, Hasten et al. (2000) reported similarly increased fractional rates of myosin heavy chain and mixed muscle protein synthesis in younger (23–34 y) and older (74–84 y) individuals, following 2 weeks of resistance training. Furthermore, many recent studies have examined strength adaptation and hypertrophy in old and very old people (Chapter 16). In general, these studies show that isometric strength and muscle cross-sectional area respond to training in a similar manner to young people (Harridge et al. 1999). Consequently, the effect of exercise on the insulin-like growth factor system in old versus young people requires clarifying. However, regardless of these caveats, signalling through Akt, directly following the binding of IGF-I to its receptor or indirectly via testosterone, is associated positively with muscle protein synthesis (Morley et al. 2005). Phosphorylation and activation of Akt may therefore be considered as a potential target for muscle-wasting conditions, including those associated with detraining, bed rest and microgravity.

2.4 Summary

When considering muscle homeostasis and potential therapeutic regulators of muscle loss, it is imperative that we have an understanding of the mechanisms governing skeletal muscle degeneration and regeneration. Whether interventions for skeletal muscle atrophy are exercise, hormonal or drug based, it is essential that we understand what impact altering one system (e.g. synthesis) has on the long-term response of another (e.g. degradation). Furthermore, many conditions cause protein degradation or at least reduce protein synthesis (Figure 9.1). Therefore, we need to devise parallel research models to determine whether microgravity, disuse, disease and ageing share similar mechanisms, albeit with different temporal patterns. While research is progressing in the fields of ageing and disease, our understanding of the mechanisms governing muscle atrophy at altitude, under microgravity or with disuse lags behind.

3 EFFECTS OF DETRAINING AND INACTIVITY: CELLULAR ADAPTATIONS

3.1 Single fibre atrophy

Disuse during microgravity (spaceflight, Chapter 26), limb suspension, immobilisation or bed rest leads to a rapid decrease in muscle mass (atrophy). In animals, the magnitude of atrophy is generally fibre-type specific. Postural muscles normally contain a higher proportion of type I (slow-twitch) fibres, and are more prone to atrophy (soleus, vastus intermedius, adductor longus) than non-postural muscles that contain a higher proportion of type II (fast-twitch) fibres (Ohira et al. 1992, Tischler et al. 1993). In rats, a decrease in muscle mass of up to 37% has been found after just one week of spaceflight (Russian Cosmos and US Shuttle missions).

In humans, based on short-term spaceflight, it has been suggested that type II fibres are at least as, if not more, susceptible to atrophy than type I fibres (Fitts et al. 2001). For instance, the type II fibres of vastus lateralis display greater atrophy after an 11-day spaceflight (Edgerton et al. 1995). Similarly, after a 17-day Space Shuttle flight, the cross-sectional area of type II fibres in soleus was reduced by 26%, with a 15% reduction for the type I fibres (Widrick et al. 1999).

However, quite a different picture emerges when recent data from prolonged bed rest are analysed. After a 12-week bed rest, the cross-sectional areas of type I and II fibres in vastus lateralis decreased by 35% and 20% (respectively), and by 42% and 25% in soleus (Rudnick et al. 2004). Similarly, vastus lateralis type I fibre diameter decreased by 15%, while type II decreased by 8% following an 84-day bed rest (Trappe et al. 2004). Therefore, it seems that in rodents and humans, type I fibres are more susceptible to disuse atrophy.

3.2 Myosin heavy chains

In response to spaceflight and hindlimb suspension (rats), a shift from slow to fast myosin heavy chain isoforms occurs (Baldwin & Haddad 2001). These adaptations involve a downregulation of the type I myosin heavy chain, together with a de novo expression of the type IIx myosin heavy chain. Data obtained during an 84-day bed rest study show that this phenotypic shift also occurs in humans, resulting in a 2.8-fold increase in the type I/IIa myosin heavy chain ratio (Trappe et al. 2004). Furthermore, the proportion of hybrid fibres co-expressing more than one isoform increases from 13–14% (before bed rest) to 49% (Trappe et al. 2004). These transformations are qualitatively similar to those observed in animals and humans following spinal cord injury (Andersen et al. 1996) or spinal transection (Talmadge 2000, Talmadge et al. 1999), indicating that the fast myosin heavy chain is the default phenotype towards which fibres progress, with denervation or prolonged inactivity. However, in humans, the time course of these transformations is about three times longer than in animals (Baldwin & Haddad 2002).

3.3 Single fibre contractile properties

Animal and human data show significant microgravity adaptations in single-fibre contractile properties. These changes concern the following variables: peak force, force per unit (cross-sectional) area, maximal unloaded contractile velocity and force-power characteristics.

3.4 Peak force and force per unit cross-sectional area

Peak force in single fibres of soleus (rat) decreased by 25% after 14 days, and 45% after 18.5 days of spaceflight (Fitts et al. 2000). Scanty data exist on the effects of spaceflight on single-fibre force per unit area. However, hindlimb suspension experiments show a significant decrease with unloading, with a 17% reduction after just 7 days of a 3-week hindlimb suspension in rats (McDonald & Fitts 1995). Similarly, in humans, force per unit area (soleus) decreased by 4% after a 17-day spaceflight that included in-flight preventative exercise (Widrick et al. 1999). These findings are also confirmed by prolonged unloading, showing a 40% and ~25% reduction in myosin heavy chain I fibre force per unit area after 42 and 84 days of bed rest, respectively (Larsson et al. 1996). The reasons for this decline in single fibre-specific tension have been attributed to a reduction in myofibrillar protein density, suggesting a reduction in the number of cross-bridges, rather than reduced force exerted by each cross-bridge (D'Antona et al. 2003). It seems unlikely that this reduced specific tension was due to a selective loss of actin (observed with spaceflight and suspected to cause an increase in lattice spacing), since force per unit area has been found to be maintained, even in the presence of selective actin loss (Widrick et al. 1999). However, other mechanisms, such as calcium kinetics or fibre damage, cannot be excluded.

3.5 Maximum unloaded velocity

The shifts in myosin heavy chain composition should affect maximal unloaded contractile velocity. Both rat and human experiments support this, showing increased maximal unloaded contractile velocity of the calf muscle following spaceflight (Caiozzo et al. 1996, Widrick et al. 1999). This effect is very marked, with increases evident in rat soleus after just 6 (14%) and 14 days (20%) of spaceflight. These effects were associated with an increased expression of type IIx myosin heavy chain isoforms and decreased expression of the type I isoform.

In humans, Widrick et al. (1999) reported an increase in soleus fibres maximal unloaded contractile velocity (30%) and shortening velocity (44%) after a 17-day spaceflight. These increases indicate that an elevated shortening velocity of the plantarflexors is not simply due to an increased expression of IIx fibres, but also to a change in shortening velocity of the individual fibres (Fitts et al. 2001). The cause of these changes is still unclear but it may be related to a disproportionate loss of actin, known to occur in rats with microgravity exposure (Riley et al. 2000). It has been suggested that the selective loss of actin would lead to an increase in myofilament spacing (otherwise known as 'lattice spacing'). As a result, the cycling cross-bridges would be expected to detach sooner, and because of a reduction in internal drag, maximal unloaded contractile velocity would be increased.

However, conflicting findings are apparent following prolonged bed rest. For instance, Trappe et al. (2004) reported decreased myosin heavy chain I (21%) and IIa fibres (6%) in human vastus lateralis after 84 days of bed rest. Despite this contrast, these results support the observations of Larsson et al. (1996) and Widrick et al. (2002) since, upon closer scrutiny, it appears that an increase in maximal unloaded contractile velocity is primarily evident when preventive (physical) countermeasures were performed, whereas a decrease in maximal unloaded contractile velocity seems to occur when countermeasures are not used. Thus, habitual muscle activity plays an important role in modulating shortening velocity.

3.6 Peak power

Single-fibre peak power decreases following actual and simulated microgravity. In rats, soleus peak power decreased by 16–20% after 6–14 day of spaceflight (Caiozzo et al. 1994, 1996). This occurred despite a 14–20% increase in shortening velocity, indicating the loss of power was consequential to the loss in force.

Little evidence is available on the effect of spaceflight on human single fibres. Nevertheless, Widrick et al. (1999) reported peak power declined by ~20% (soleus type I fibres) in two crew members of a 17-day Space Shuttle mission. In two other crew members, the increase in shortening velocity was high enough to compensate for the loss of force, and as a result, peak power remained unchanged.

A clearer picture emerges from the Toulouse bed rest study (Trappe et al. 2004). In six subjects undergoing bed rest only, the composite single-fibre power (soleus) decreased by 23%, whereas in six subjects performing regular resistive exercise, peak power was maintained. This suggests that resistive exercise plays an important role in maintaining muscle power by increasing maximal unloaded contractile velocity.

4 EFFECTS OF DETRAINING AND INACTIVITY: WHOLE-MUSCLE ADAPTATIONS

4.1 Muscle atrophy and composition

The results of human and animal studies performed in simulated or actual microgravity consistently show that skeletal muscle undergoes substantial atrophy, due to a decrease in fibre size, with no change in fibre number (Roy et al. 1987, Templeton et al. 1984, Thomason & Booth 1990). Furthermore, atrophy was considerably greater in postural muscles, but with substantial differences among these muscles. In general, the plantarflexors experience the largest volume decrease, followed in decreasing order by the dorsiflexors, knee extensors, knee flexors and the intrinsic lower back muscles (LeBlanc et al. 1997).

Whereas common agreement exists regarding this general picture, the time course of atrophy is less well documented. On the whole, the picture emerging from bed rest studies, combined with unloading models, suggests that the time course of atrophy follows an exponential function (Figure 9.2), such that after ~120 days of simulated microgravity, muscle attains a constant mass that is ~70% of its pre-exposure value. In fact, the 90-day Toulouse bed rest study elicited a 30% loss in calf muscle mass. Thus, this process may be even faster than predicted from the analysis of the above cross-sectional data.

This observation generates considerable concern since, from a clinical point of view, a loss of lean body mass greater than 40% is associated with an increased risk of death (Roubenoff 2001). However, since these observations were derived from changes in postural muscles during extended bed rest without preventive countermeasures, their application to spaceflight with countermeasures or with high-intensity physical activity is unwarranted.

For both simulated and actual microgravity, muscle atrophy is due to an imbalance in protein turnover (Thomason & Booth 1990). Indeed, during the first 2 weeks of hindlimb suspension in rats, protein synthesis decreased and degradation increased. In the following 2 weeks, an equilibrium was again achieved between synthesis and

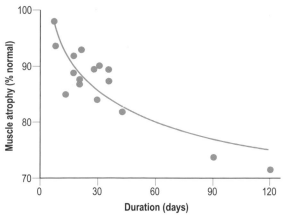

Figure 9.2 Calf muscle atrophy due to unloading in actual or simulated microgravity (unilateral lower limb suspension, bed rest or spaceflight).

4.2 Muscle architecture

Similar to senile sarcopenia (Narici & Maganaris 2006), disuse atrophy in humans also entails a decrease in fascicle length and pennation angle (Bleakney & Maffulli 2002, Kawakami et al. 2000, Narici & Cerretelli, 1998, Reeves et al. 2002). After 90 days of strict bed rest, pennation angle and fascicle length of the gastrocnemius were found to decrease by 10% and 13%, respectively, in those not performing exercise countermeasures (Reeves et al. 2002). Participants who performed high-intensity resistive exercise every 3 days showed a partial mitigation of muscle atrophy, and adverse changes in muscle architecture were only marginally smaller than the non-exercise group (fascicle length 7%; pennation angle 13%), indicating a greater volume of exercise would be required to prevent atrophy. These findings suggest that changes in muscle architecture associated with disuse involve a loss of sarcomeres, both in parallel (reduced cross-sectional area) and in series (reduced fascicle length) and, as such, would be expected to play significant roles in the loss of muscle force and power.

4.3 Force and power

Several human studies have reported substantial decreases in muscle strength with bed rest or other simulations (Berg & Tesch 1996, Berg et al. 1991, 1993, 1997, LeBlanc et al. 1988). For example, after 42 days of bed rest, the maximal strength of the lower limbs muscles decreased by ~30% (Berg & Tesch 1996). No changes in time to peak tension or relaxation half-time were found after 17 days of bed rest (Narici et al. 1997), whereas in the same conditions, the ratio of tetanic force to cross-sectional area decreased significantly (8% and 13 %, respectively). This has been previously observed (Berg & Tesch 1996, Dudley et al. 1989, LeBlanc et al. 1988) and may be due to a reduction in fibre-specific tension, due to decreased myofibrillar density, reduced neuromotor drive, reduced electromechanical coupling efficiency or an increase in the amount of non-contractile tissue.

After the Skylab missions, the maximal force of several muscle groups (quadriceps, trunk flexors and extensors) showed relative decreases from 6.5% to 25%, depending on muscle group and flight duration. In addition, since crews performed physical exercise to minimise deconditioning, these results are difficult to interpret in terms of underlying muscle fibre function. Nevertheless, this substantial muscle force decline was accompanied by an even greater fall in maximal muscle power. Indeed, data obtained from the Euromir 94 and 95 missions show that the maximal explosive power of the lower limbs was reduced to ~67% after 31 days and to ~45% after 180 days (Antonutto et al. 1991, 1998, 1999). At variance with these data, maximal power developed during all-out bouts on a cycle ergometer was reduced to a lesser extent, attaining ~75% of preflight power, regardless of the flight duration. Since, in the same subjects,

degradation, stabilising protein content, albeit at a lower level (Loughna et al. 1987, Thomason et al. 1989).

As discussed in section 2.2, the loss of muscle mass necessarily involves a disruption of muscle homeostasis.

In humans, data from spaceflight and bed rest studies indicate that the loss of muscle mass is due to a depression in protein synthesis, rather than increased degradation. Indeed, after 3 months on the Mir space station, whole-body protein synthesis decreased by 45% (Stein et al. 1999). At the same time, protein degradation decreased. Hence, it seems the loss of muscle mass during spaceflight is primarily due to decreased protein synthesis (Ferrando et al. 2002a).

While it is difficult to exclude the effects of decreased caloric intake, there is evidence of a direct effect of microgravity per se on protein synthesis. Indeed, experiments performed during spaceflight on cultured avian muscles cells showed that microgravity directly depressed protein synthesis (Vandenburgh et al. 1999). These observations on changes in protein turnover with spaceflight are similar to those made during short-term bed rest. After 14 days of strict bed rest in young healthy volunteers, whole-body protein synthesis decreased by 14% and skeletal muscle protein synthesis by ~50% (Ferrando et al. 1996). This depression in protein synthesis was also demonstrated by investigating its stimulation synthesis in response to a labelled amino acid infusion, during 14 days of strict bed rest (Biolo et al. 2004). During bed rest, the net amino acid deposition (synthesis minus degradation) into body protein was 8% lower than that observed in ambulatory subjects, highlighting the reduction in protein anabolism caused by bed rest.

lower limb muscle mass decreased only 9–13%, irrespective of the flight duration, these data suggest that a large fraction of the decline in maximal power, at least during the very short explosive efforts, may be due to the effects of weightlessness on motor unit recruitment pattern, electromechanical efficiency and predisposition to muscle damage (Antonutto et al. 1991, 1998, 1999, di Prampero & Narici 2003).

This view is similar to hypogravitational ataxia hypothesis (Grigoriev & Egorov 1991) and the large fall of maximal explosive power seems to be a specific characteristic of spaceflight, and may not be easily reproduced using bed rest. Indeed, after 42 days of strict bed rest, the maximal explosive power was reduced to 76% of preflight (Ferretti et al. 2001), compared with 67% after 31 days of spaceflight featuring 2 h of exercise per day (as above). These observations support the hypothesis that the absence of gravity, favouring smooth and delicately balanced muscle actions, brings about a substantial rearrangement of the motor control system that is responsible, to a large extent, for the observed decline in the maximal explosive power. This rearrangement does not seem to manifest itself during bed rest or, if it does, it appears to be markedly less effective since the pull of gravity is not abolished but simply shifted 90° (di Prampero & Narici 2003).

4.4 Muscle fatiguability

Whilst in rats, weightlessness and hindlimb suspension have been shown to increase fatigability (soleus muscle; McDonald et al. 1992), little is known concerning human muscle fatigability in either actual or simulated microgravity. However, Narici et al. (2003b) found plantarflexor fatigue, assessed using electrically evoked contractions, increased considerably (~16%) after a 17-day spaceflight, persisting during recovery. Several possible factors may contribute to this phenomenon: an increased expression of heavy chain (fast) myosin (Widrick et al. 1999), a reduced ability to oxidise fatty acids and increased carbohydrate and glycogen utilisation, and reduced muscle blood flow during exercise (Jasperse et al. 1999).

4.5 Tendon mechanical properties

Despite the critical importance of tendons for movement, their adaptation to prolonged disuse has received little attention. Recently, however, changes in tendon mechanical properties in response to simulated microgravity (long-term bed rest) and spinal cord injury have been described.

Tendon stiffness, length and cross-sectional area were measured in 18 young, healthy males before and after 90 days of bed rest; nine subjects performed resistive exercise (calf raise and leg press, every 3 days) and nine underwent bed rest only. Gastrocnemius tendon stiffness (58%) and Young's modulus (57%) both decreased in the latter group, but not muscle cross-sectional area. Despite the intensive resistive exercise of the former group, tendon stiffness (37%) and Young's modulus also decreased (38%; Reeves et al. 2005). These findings showed that unloading caused a decrease in tendon stiffness, due to altered tendon material properties but not tendon dimensions, and that a very large volume of resistive exercises is needed to protect the tendon from disuse adaptation.

In the second disuse paradigm, patellar tendon mechanical properties were compared between men affected by spinal cord injury, and able-bodied men. Tendon stiffness and Young's modulus were lower by 77% and 59% in the former group, and cross-sectional area was also 17% smaller but without differences in tendon length (Maganaris et al. 2006).

4.6 Muscle damage

Evidence exists that simulated and actual microgravity result in a greater susceptibility to damage upon reloading the muscles. Such damage is characterised by eccentric contraction-like lesions, showing smeared and less dense Z-bands, and a lesioned endomysium. In addition, the presence of helical polyribosomes, indicating active protein synthesis, suggests activation of repair processes. Accompanying microcirculatory changes and interstitial oedema lead to muscle swelling. However, evidence of a greater susceptibility to muscle damage following spaceflight is sparse, although it is plausible that muscle atrophy, and a selective loss of contractile or structural proteins (titin, desmin, dystrophin; Fitts et al. 2001), make muscles susceptible to damage, since a greater relative load would be experienced when weight bearing is resumed.

This hypothesis seems in line with the observations of a continuous fall in human plantarflexor tetanic torque, despite a progressive reversal of muscle atrophy, during the recovery phase following spaceflight (Narici et al. 2003a).

4.7 Neural drive, muscle activation capacity, unilateral versus bilateral motor tasks

Chronic electromyographic (EMG) recordings, obtained with intramuscular electrodes during prolonged hindlimb suspension (animals; 1–4 wk), show a rapid decrease in antigravity muscle activity (plantarflexors), commencing within the first week. There is also a slight increase in non-antigravity muscle activity (tibialis anterior), due to stretching of those muscles (Edgerton & Roy 1994).

In humans, there is little available evidence concerning chronic EMG activity following prolonged bed rest or spaceflight. However, there is a marked increase in the total EMG activity of tibialis anterior and soleus, with no change in gastrocnemius medialis activity during a 17-day spaceflight (Edgerton et al. 2001). As far as maximal EMG activity is concerned, a 44% decrease in knee extensor activity has been found after 42 days of bed rest, suggesting decreased neural drive.

These observations are in line with those of Duchateau & Hainaut (1987) who reported a significant decrease in

EMG activity of the thumb after a 6-week forearm immobilisation. It seems that prolonged disuse leads to a decrease in maximal neural drive to the muscle. In the initial phases of unloading, this effect seems to be related to a decrease in afferent activity (De-Doncker et al. 2005). However, other mechanisms, such as a decrease in activation capacity, may explain the long-term decrease in EMG activity during prolonged disuse, with a 33% deficit in central activation found following a 5-week bed rest (Duchateau 1995).

Most microgravity studies focus on unilateral muscle function. However, when comparing the deficit in muscle power generated during bilateral muscle activation (maximal leg extensions) to that produced during unilateral contractions (cycling), the deficit in power was far greater for the bilateral movement. This is attributed to the effects of weightlessness on motor unit recruitment pattern, electromechanical efficiency and predisposition to muscle damage (Antonutto et al. 1991, 1998, 1999, di Prampero & Narici 2003).

The observation of a greater fall in power in the bilateral suggests a larger reduction in motor unit recruitment for the bilateral motor task. It has been known for some time that the force exerted by a single limb during a maximal bilateral contraction is less than that generated during a maximal unilateral contraction (Howard & Enoka 1991). It therefore seems possible that this bilateral deficit phenomenon may be accentuated with disuse.

5 COUNTERMEASURES

Several approaches have been proposed to combat skeletal muscle atrophy and the functional deterioration associated with spaceflight, and an absence of weight-bearing (zero gravity), and seven such methods will now be discussed. However, the efficacy of these methods in preventing or ameliorating skeletal muscle changes has not been thoroughly evaluated. Nevertheless, and regardless of the mechanism(s) responsible for the negative impact of spaceflight and weightlessness on skeletal muscle, countermeasures are imperative for maintaining crew health and mobility during long-duration space missions. Many astronauts/cosmonauts have carried out these activities in-flight, yet they invariably suffered from strength losses on return to Earth. Unfortunately, since countermeasure activities were not logged, rather little has been learned from past spaceflights.

5.1 Aerobic exercise

In-flight cycle ergometer exercise is typically used to maintain cardiovascular function, yet this is ineffective for maintaining musculoskeletal function simply because the mechanical load provided by aerobic exercise programmes is too low to prevent muscle atrophy, let alone induce muscle hypertrophy. For instance, results from a 30-day bed rest study show that 30 min of cycle ergometer exercise,

performed 5 d·wk^{-1}, failed to prevent muscle wasting and weakness, compared to non-exercising controls (Greenleaf et al. 1989). Similarly, daily supine cycle ergometry exercise for 60 min at 40% of maximal aerobic power did not protect against either muscle or strength loss in individuals subjected to a 20-day bed rest (Suzuki et al. 1994). It would appear that aerobic exercise has little to offer as a countermeasure to weightlessness.

5.2 Resistance exercise

Part of the decrease in muscle mass observed with spaceflight and physical inactivity is due to reduced protein synthesis (Ferrando et al. 2002a). Healthy subjects confined to bed rest for 2 weeks, who also performed knee extensor and ankle extensor resistance exercise every other day (five sets of 6–10 repetitions at ~80% of maximum), were able to maintain protein synthesis, whilst those who did no training showed decreased strength, muscle mass and protein synthesis. However, isometric strength and neural activation were reduced (Bamman et al. 1997, 1998, Ferrando et al. 1997).

A protective effect of resistive (flywheel) training on soleus muscle mass and protein synthesis has also been shown in rats (Fluckey et al. 2002). This mode of training is based on concentric and eccentric contractions against a flywheel (Berg & Tesch 1998), and has been used for the prevention of muscle atrophy and weakness in simulated microgravity, unilateral lower limb suspension and bed rest. For instance, quadriceps muscle atrophy, induced by 5 weeks of lower limb suspension, was prevented by four sets of seven maximal concentric and eccentric knee extensions, performed 2–3 times per week (Tesch et al. 2004).

However, in humans, the soleus muscle shows limited predisposition to work-induced hypertrophy, especially when compared to the quadriceps. For instance, whereas high-intensity flywheel exercise performed twice per week during a 90-day bed rest study fully prevented quadriceps atrophy, it only partially mitigated atrophy of soleus (Alkner & Tesch 2004). This limited predisposition to hypertrophy of human soleus is also confirmed by findings of a poor increase in protein synthesis of this muscle in response to an acute resistive exercise bout (Trappe et al. 2004). Taken together, these results suggest that resistive exercise is presently the method of choice for mitigating or even preventing the negative effects of unloading on skeletal muscle. However, significant differences in the response to training exist among muscles, and the causes thereof warrant further investigation.

5.3 Penguin suit exercise

This method was introduced by Russian space scientists, and consists of a body suit in which elastic bands are sewn to maintain a constant stretching load on the antigravity muscles. It is difficult to judge whether this type of (passive) stimulus is effective for combating muscle atrophy and weakness during disuse. However, in a small group of subjects ($N = 4$), bedridden for ~120 days, the size of muscle fibres in soleus appeared to be maintained after performing a single, daily 10 h bout with modest loading (~10 kg) using the Penguin suit (Ohira et al. 1999). While such results may sound promising, no hard conclusions may be drawn from observations made on such a small sample, and it seems unlikely that such low loads will prove effective in preventing muscle wasting and weakness of the large antigravity muscles.

5.4 Pharmacological interventions

For some time, clenbuterol (a β2-adrenergic agonist) has been used on farm animals to boost muscle mass, with chronic administration inducing hypertrophy by increasing protein synthesis (Wineski et al. 2002). Although its precise mode of action is not clear, clenbuterol has also been found to reduce disuse muscle atrophy in hindlimb-suspended rats (Apseloff et al. 1993) and orthopaedic patients (Maltin et al. 1993). Thus, it has been proposed as a therapeutic tool to combat muscle wasting in patients with neuromuscular disorders (Lynch et al. 2001). Recently, clenbuterol has been used in heart failure patients in an attempt to promote myocardial recovery (George et al. 2006). Although it failed to improve cardiac muscle mass and function, it significantly increased skeletal muscle mass and strength. Clearly, insufficient information is available to conclude whether or not it may represent a viable pharmacological aid against disuse muscle atrophy in space and on Earth but these results warrant further investigations.

Similarly, testosterone administration has also been proposed as a countermeasure against muscle atrophy and weakness (section 2.2.3.1), since it increases protein synthesis in young and elderly adults (Ferrando et al. 1998, Urban et al. 1995). However, in a 28-day bed rest study, testosterone administration was found to preserve protein balance but not muscle strength, presumably due to the absence of muscle activity (Zachwieja et al. 1999a). Recent observations that resistive exercise during a 30-day bed rest depresses testosterone level (Wade et al. 2005) challenge this possibility, suggesting that a synergistic action of exercise plus testosterone may not exist during bed rest or that high volumes of low-intensity exercise may be needed to prevent muscle loss in these conditions. Hence, further research concerning these mechanisms is required.

Considerable attention has also been given to IGF-I, a possible prophylactic measure against muscle wasting during microgravity exposure. Although low IGF-I concentrations are associated with muscle wasting (Spate & Schulze 2004, Wang et al. 2005; section 2.2.3), no protective effects have been found in transgenic mice overexpressing human IGF-I, which exhibited similar atrophy to normal mice during 14-day hindlimb suspension (Criswell et al. 1998).

Also, intramuscular IGF-I mRNA concentrations do not to differ between space-exposed rats and ground-control rats, whereas IGF-II levels were depressed. In the same study, myostatin concentration was significantly increased during spaceflight. This indicates that levels of negative regulators of muscle mass are increased with spaceflight, while those of the positive regulators are depressed (Lalani et al. 2000). Hence, further research is needed to develop a clearer understanding of these interrelationships and the role of growth factors in muscle atrophy during spaceflight.

5.5 Lower–body negative pressure

The use of lower-body negative pressure, alone or combined with simultaneous exercise, has been proposed as an in-flight countermeasure. It has been suggested that forces applied to the limbs during negative pressure may simulate those involved in weight bearing on Earth (Hargens et al. 1991, Murthy et al. 1994). This is, however, quite dubious, since it is unlikely that the application of such a low-intensity load, for a short duration, would prevent muscle atrophy. Although it has been suggested that a regimen comprising such low-intensity negative pressure with isokinetic exercise may limit strength loss and muscle wasting during bed rest, it remains to be established whether negative pressure alone contributes to this effect (Germain et al. 1995).

5.6 Electrical stimulation

Transcutaneous electrical muscle stimulation has been tested as a countermeasure against muscle atrophy and weakness during a 30-day bed rest study (Duvoisin et al. 1989). In this investigation, subjects were treated twice daily, every third day, with unilateral electrical stimulation ($N = 3$, 60 Hz frequency, 0.30 ms pulse width, 4 s train). The results showed a smaller decrease in strength and muscle mass in the treated limb. Although these results showed a mitigation of muscle atrophy and weakness, electrical stimulation did not prevent these conditions. Furthermore, no comparison was made between the effects of electrical stimulation and voluntary activation. Also, in a recent hindlimb suspension study in rats, daily transcutaneous electrical stimulation plus hindlimb suspension, did not provide protection against muscle atrophy, when compared to rats exposed to hindlimb suspension only (Yoshida et al. 2003). Although electrical stimulation has the advantage of standardising muscle activation and duration, when compared to voluntary activation, it requires high stimulation currents, and these are quite uncomfortable.

5.7 Artificial gravity: centrifuges and cycling in space

Since chronic exposure to gravitational force on Earth is sufficient to prevent muscle atrophy, it has been hypothesised that the introduction of Earth-like gravity in a space station may prove useful for preventing muscle deconditioning. Currently, two methods have been proposed for exercising with Earth-like gravity: conditioning with centrifuges and cycling along the inner wall of the space module.

5.7.1 Countermeasures based on centrifuges

On Earth, experiments have been performed using short- and long-arm centrifuges aiming to evaluate the different levels and durations of gravitational acceleration (g) needed to prevent cardiovascular and muscular deconditioning. In hindlimb-suspended rats, the application of 1 G for 4 h·d^{-1} prevented atrophy in soleus, while increasing the accelerational forces to 2.6 g provided no additional benefit (Zhang et al. 2003).

In humans, the application of alternating days of artificial (centrifuge-induced) gravity and intensive aerobic training (90% maximal heart rate) maintains muscle size during 20 days of bed rest (Akima et al. 2005). Total thigh muscle volume was maintained, relative to a 9% decrease in non-exercising, bed rest controls. While the maximum voluntary contraction force of the knee extensors decreased by 7% in the countermeasure group, it was 23% lower in the control subjects. These results seem very promising. However, the minimum intensity and duration of the gravitational acceleration still need to be established.

5.7.2 Cycling in space

Training protocols under microgravity do not prevent a substantial deconditioning of the cardiovascular system (Antonutto & di Prampero 2003). To minimise deconditioning, Antonutto et al. (1991) proposed gravity simulation using a twin-bike exercise system. The system consists of two bicycles that move at the same speed, but in opposite directions, along the inner wall of a cylindrically shaped space module (di Prampero 2000; Figure 9.3). The circular trajectories induce positive centrifugal acceleration vectors oriented through each subject (head-to-feet; +Gz).

Assuming barometric pressure and temperature inside the space capsule are similar to those on Earth, and a radius of gyration of 2 m (conventional space module), the generation of 1 G at the feet would elicit a tangential velocity of 4.5 m·s^{-1}. The corresponding mechanical power and oxygen uptake would be 75 W and 1.2 L·min^{-1}.

The twin-bike system should also be effective in protecting against cardiovascular deconditioning, because the weight of the blood column induced by centrifugal acceleration acts throughout the circulatory system, as is the case on Earth. Indeed, at any level in the circulatory system, the prevailing pressure is given by the sum of the pressure generated by the heart plus (or minus) the hydrostatic component, with the latter being gravity dependent. The twin-bike system creates an ability to reestablish the hydrostatic component when in space, albeit intermittently.

When riding the twin-bike system, slight head movements may lead to simultaneous rotations of the semicircular canals about more than one axis. This state, and the resulting sensory conflict, is one of the major determinants of acute motion sickness. This possibility was tested on six healthy males pedalling a cycle ergometer (50 W, 20 min) fixed to one arm of a human centrifuge, set to rotate at 21 rev·min^{-1}, yielding an angular velocity close to that required in the twin-bike system to attain 1 G at the subject's feet (Antonutto et al. 1993). The subject kept his head still or moved it in varying degrees of rolling, pitching or yawing actions, whilst rating acute motion sickness symptoms. Only one subject suffered a mild level of motion sickness. Thus, the discomfort deriving from the rotating environment necessary to generate artificial gravity is reasonably low and well tolerated.

A

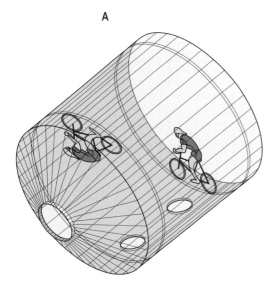

B

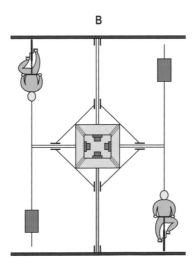

Figure 9.3 (A) Cyclists moving along the inner wall of a cylindrically shaped space module, generating an acceleration vector and mimicking gravity. (B) A schematic depiction of the twin-bike system in which the thick lines represent the walls of the space module. Reproduced with permission from Antonutto et al. (1991), di Prampero (2000).

5.8 Summary

Both animal and human muscles undergo significant wasting and strength loss during microgravity exposures. Muscle atrophy mainly affects the antigravity muscles, but strength and power losses tend to exceed that of muscle size, both at the whole-muscle and single-fibre levels. Cellular and neural mechanisms seem to contribute to this phenomenon, but also the presence of muscle damage caused by reloading of muscles in 1 G cannot be excluded.

Several countermeasures have been proposed, some based on pharmacological interventions, some on aerobic exercises and others on resistive exercises or artificial gravity. Most methods have yielded positive results in terms of combatting either muscular or cardiovascular deconditioning. However, one of the main challenges for the future will be that of identifying an intervention that may simultaneously ameliorate muscular, cardiovascular and vestibular deconditioning. In this respect, exercising in artificial gravity seems promising.

References

Akima H, Katayama K, Sato K, Ishida K, Masuda K, Takada H, Watanabe Y, Iwase S 2005 Intensive cycle training with artificial gravity maintains muscle size during bed rest. Aviation and Space Environmental Medicine 76:923–929

Alkner BA, Tesch PA 2004 Knee extensor and plantar flexor muscle size and function following 90 days of bed rest with or without resistance exercise. European Journal of Applied Physiology 93:294–305

Anastasi S, Giordano S, Sthandier O, Gambarotta G, Maione R, Comoglio P, Amati P 1997 A natural hepatocyte growth factor/scatter factor autocrine loop in myoblast cells and the effect of the constitutive Met kinase activation on myogenic differentiation. Journal of Cell Biology 137:1057–1068

Andersen JL, Mohr T, Biering-Sorensen F, Galbo H, Kjaer M 1996 Myosin heavy chain isoform transformation in single fibres from m. vastus lateralis in spinal cord injured individuals: effects of long-term functional electrical stimulation (FES). Pflügers Archiv 431:513–518

Antonutto G, di Prampero PE 2003 Cardiovascular deconditioning in microgravity: some possible countermeasures. European Journal of Applied Physiology 90:283–291

Antonutto G, Capelli C, di Prampero PE 1991 Pedalling in space as a countermeasure to microgravity deconditioning. Microgravity Quarterly 1:93–101

Antonutto G, Linnarsson D, di Prampero PE 1993 On-Earth evaluation of neurovestibular tolerance to centrifuge simulated artificial gravity in humans. Physiologist 36:S85–S87

Antonutto G, Bodem F, Zamparo P, di Prampero PE 1998 Maximal power and EMG of lower limbs after 21 days spaceflight in one astronaut. Journal of Gravitational Physiology 5:63–66

Antonutto G, Capelli C, Girardis M, Zamparo P, di Prampero PE 1999 Effects of microgravity on maximal power of lower limbs during very short efforts in humans. Journal of Applied Physiology 86:85–92

Apseloff G, Girten B, Walker M, Shepard DR, Krecic ME, Stern LS, Gerber N 1993 Aminohydroxybutane bisphosphonate and clenbuterol prevent bone changes and retard muscle atrophy respectively in tail-suspended rats. Journal of Pharmacology and Experimental Therapeutics 264:1071–1078

Arnold HH, Winter B 1998 Muscle differentiation: more complexity to the network of myogenic regulators. Current Opinion in Genetics and Development 8:539–544

Artaza JN, Bhasin S, Magee TR, Reisz-Porszasz S, Shen R, Groome NP, Meerasahib MF, Gonzalez-Cadavid NF 2005 Myostatin inhibits myogenesis and promotes adipogenesis in C3H 10T(1/2) mesenchymal multipotent cells. Endocrinology 146:3547–3557

Attaix D, Mosoni L, Dardevet D, Combaret L, Mirand PP, Grizard J 2005 Altered responses in skeletal muscle protein turnover during aging in anabolic and catabolic periods. International Journal of Biochemistry and Cell Biology 37:1962–1973

Balagopal P, Rooyackers OE, Adey DB, Ades PA, Nair KS 1997 Effects of aging on in vivo synthesis of skeletal muscle myosin heavy-chain and sarcoplasmic protein in humans. American Journal of Physiology 273:E790–E800

Baldwin KM, Haddad F 2001 Effects of different activity and inactivity paradigms on myosin heavy chain gene expression in striated muscle. Journal of Applied Physiology 90:345–357

Baldwin KM, Haddad F 2002 Skeletal muscle plasticity: cellular and molecular responses to altered physical activity paradigms. American Journal of Physical Medicine and Rehabilitation 81:S40–S51

Bamman MM, Hunter GR, Stevens BR, Guilliams ME, Greenisen MC 1997 Resistance exercise prevents plantar flexor deconditioning during bed rest. Medicine and Science in Sports and Exercise 29:1462–1468

Bamman MM, Clarke MS, Feeback DL, Talmadge RJ, Stevens BR, Lieberman SA, Greenisen MC 1998 Impact of resistance exercise during bed rest on skeletal muscle sarcopenia and myosin isoform distribution. Journal of Applied Physiology 84:157–163

Barton-Davis ER, Shoturma DI, Musaro A, Rosenthal N, Sweeney HL 1998 Viral mediated expression of insulin-like growth factor I blocks the aging-related loss of skeletal muscle function. Proceedings of the National Academy of Science of the USA 95:15603–15607

Baumgartner RN, Waters DL, Gallagher D, Morley JE, Garry PJ 1999 Predictors of skeletal muscle mass in elderly men and women. Mechanisms of Ageing and Development 107:123–136

Beehler BC, Sleph PG, Benmassaoud L, Grover GJ 2006 Reduction of skeletal muscle atrophy by a proteasome inhibitor in a rat model of denervation. Experimental Biology and Medicine (Maywood) 231:335–341

Berg HE, Tesch PA 1996 Changes in muscle function in response to 10 days of lower limb unloading in humans. Acta Physiologica Scandinavica 157:63–70

Berg HE, Tesch PA 1998 Force and power characteristics of a resistive exercise device for use in space. Acta Astronautica 42:219–230

Berg HE, Dudley GA, Haggmark T, Ohlsen H, Tesch PA 1991 Effects of lower limb unloading on skeletal muscle mass and function in humans. Journal of Applied Physiology 70:1882–1885

Berg HE, Dudley GA, Hather B, Tesch PA 1993 Work capacity and metabolic and morphologic characteristics of the human quadriceps muscle in response to unloading. Clinical Physiology 13:337–347

Berg HE, Larsson L, Tesch PA 1997 Lower limb skeletal muscle function after 6 wk of bed rest. Journal of Applied Physiology 82:182–188

Biolo G, Ciocchi B, Lebenstedt M, Barazzoni R, Zanetti M, Platen P, Heer M, Guarnieri G 2004 Short-term bed rest impairs amino acid-induced protein anabolism in humans. Journal of Physiology 558:381–388

Bleakney R, Maffulli N 2002 Ultrasound changes to intramuscular architecture of the quadriceps following intramedullary nailing. Journal of Sports Medicine and Physical Fitness 42:120–125

Bodine SC, Stitt TN, Gonzalez M, Kline WO, Stover GL, Bauerlein R, Zlotchenko E, Scrimgeour A, Lawrence JC, Glass DJ, Yancopoulos GD 2001 Akt/mTOR pathway is a crucial regulator of skeletal muscle hypertrophy and can prevent muscle atrophy in vivo. Nature Cell Biology 3:1014–1019

Brahm H, Piehl-Aulin K, Saltin B, Ljunghall S 1997 Net fluxes over working thigh of hormones, growth factors and biomarkers of bone metabolism during short lasting dynamic exercise. Calcified Tissue International 60:175–180

Byron KL, Puglisi JL, Holda JR, Eble D, Samarel AM 1996 Myosin heavy chain turnover in cultured neonatal rat heart cells: effects of [Ca2+]i and contractile activity. American Journal of Physiology 271:C01447–C01456

Caiozzo VJ, Baker MJ, Herrick RE, Tao M, Baldwin KM 1994 Effect of spaceflight on skeletal muscle: mechanical properties and myosin isoform content of a slow muscle. Journal of Applied Physiology 76:1764–1773

Caiozzo VJ, Haddad F, Baker MJ, Herrick RE, Prietto N, Baldwin KM 1996 Microgravity-induced transformations of myosin isoforms and contractile properties of skeletal muscle. Journal of Applied Physiology 81:123–132

Caroni P, Schneider C 1994 Signaling by insulin-like growth factors in paralyzed skeletal muscle: rapid induction of IGF1 expression in muscle fibers and prevention of interstitial cell proliferation by IGF-BP5 and IGF-BP4. Journal of Neuroscience 14:3378–3388

Cornelison DD, Olwin BB, Rudnicki MA, Wold BJ 2000 MyoD(−/−) satellite cells in single-fiber culture are differentiation defective and MRF4 deficient. Developmental Biology 224:122–137

Criswell DS, Booth FW, DeMayo F, Schwartz RJ, Gordon SE, Fiorotto ML 1998 Overexpression of IGF-I in skeletal muscle of transgenic mice does not prevent unloading-induced atrophy. American Journal of Physiology 275:E373–E379

D'Antona G, Pellegrino MA, Adami R, Rossi R, Carlizzi CN, Canepari M, Saltin B, Bottinelli R 2003 The effect of ageing and immobilization on structure and function of human skeletal muscle fibres. Journal of Physiology 552:499–511

Davidson JM, Chen JJ, Crapo L, Gray GD, Greenleaf WJ, Catania JA 1983 Hormonal changes and sexual function in aging men. Journal of Clinical Endocrinology and Metabolism 57:71–77

De-Doncker L, Kasri M, Picquet F, Falempin M 2005 Physiologically adaptive changes of the L5 afferent neurogram and of the rat soleus EMG activity during 14 days of hindlimb unloading and recovery. Journal of Experimental Biology 208:4585–4592

DeVol DL, Rotwein P, Sadow JL, Novakofski J, Bechtel PJ 1990 Activation of insulin-like growth factor gene expression during work-induced skeletal muscle growth. American Journal of Physiology 259:E89–E95

di Prampero PE 2000 Cycling on Earth, in space, on the Moon. European Journal of Applied Physiology 82:345–360

di Prampero PE, Narici MV 2003 Muscles in microgravity: from fibres to human motion. Journal of Biomechanics 36:403–412

Duchateau J 1995 Bed rest induces neural and contractile adaptations in triceps surae. Medicine and Science in Sports and Exercise 27:1581–1589

Duchateau J, Hainaut K 1987 Electrical and mechanical changes in immobilized human muscle. Journal of Applied Physiology 62:2168–2173

Dudley GA, Gollnick PD, Convertino VA, Buchanan P 1989 Changes of muscle function and size with bedrest. Physiologist 32:S65–S66

Duvoisin MR, Convertino VA, Buchanan P, Gollnick PD, Dudley GA 1989 Characteristics and preliminary observations of the influence of electromyostimulation on the size and function of human skeletal muscle during 30 days of simulated microgravity. Aviation and Space Environmental Medicine 60:671–678

Edgerton VR, Roy RR 1994 Neuromuscular adaptation to actual and simulated weightlessness. Advances in Space Biology and Medicine 4:33–67

Edgerton VR, Zhou MY, Ohira Y, Klitgaard H, Jiang B, Bell G, Harris B, Saltin B, Gollnick PD, Roy RR, Day MK, Greenisen M 1995 Human fiber size and enzymatic properties after 5 and 11 days of spaceflight. Journal of Applied Physiology 78:1733–1739

Edgerton VR, McCall GE, Hodgson JA, Gotto J, Goulet C, Fleischmann K, Roy RR 2001 Sensorimotor adaptations to microgravity in humans. Journal of Experimental Biology 204:3217–3224

Ershler WB, Keller ET 2000 Age-associated increased interleukin-6 gene expression, late-life diseases and frailty. Annual Review of Medicine 51:245–270

Fernandez AM, Dupont J, Farrar RP, Lee S, Stannard B, Le Roith D 2002 Muscle-specific inactivation of the IGF-I receptor induces compensatory hyperplasia in skeletal muscle. Journal of Clinical Investigation 109:347–355

Ferrando AA, Lane HW, Stuart CA, Davis-Street J, Wolfe RR 1996 Prolonged bed rest decreases skeletal muscle and whole body protein synthesis. American Journal of Physiology 270:E627–E633

Ferrando AA, Tipton KD, Bamman MM, Wolfe RR 1997 Resistance exercise maintains skeletal muscle protein synthesis during bed rest. Journal of Applied Physiology 82:807–810

Ferrando AA, Tipton KD, Doyle D, Phillips SM, Cortiella J, Wolfe RR 1998 Testosterone injection stimulates net protein synthesis but not tissue amino acid transport. American Journal of Physiology 275: E864–E871

Ferrando AA, Paddon-Jones D, Wolfe RR 2002a Alterations in protein metabolism during space flight and inactivity. Nutrition 18:837–841

Ferrando AA, Sheffield-Moore M, Yeckel CW, Gilkison C, Jiang J, Achacosa A, Lieberman SA, Tipton K, Wolfe RR, Urban RJ 2002b Testosterone administration to older men improves muscle function: molecular and physiological mechanisms. American Journal of Physiology. Endocrinology and Metabolism 282:E601–E607

Ferretti G, Berg HE, Minetti AE, Moia C, Rampichini S, Narici MV 2001 Maximal instantaneous muscular power after prolonged bed rest in humans. Journal of Applied Physiology 90:431–435

Fitts RH, Riley DR, Widrick JJ 2000 Physiology of a microgravity environment invited review:microgravity and skeletal muscle. Journal of Applied Physiology 89:823–839

Fitts RH, Riley DR, Widrick JJ 2001 Functional and structural adaptations of skeletal muscle to microgravity. Journal of Experimental Biology 204:3201–3208

Florini JR, Ewton DZ, Coolican SA 1996 Growth hormone and the insulin-like growth factor system in myogenesis. Endocrine Reviews 17:481–517

Fluckey JD, Dupont-Versteegden EE, Montague DC, Knox M, Tesch P, Peterson CA, Gaddy-Kurten D 2002 A rat resistance exercise regimen attenuates losses of musculoskeletal mass during hindlimb suspension. Acta Physiologica Scandinavica 176:293–300

George I, Xydas S, Mancini DM, Lamanca J, DiTullio M, Marboe CC, Shane E, Schulman AR, Colley PM, Petrilli CM, Naka Y, Oz MC, Maybaum S 2006 Effect of clenbuterol on cardiac and skeletal muscle function during left ventricular assist device support. Journal of Heart and Lung Transplantation 25:1084–1090

Germain P, Guell A, Marini JF 1995 Muscle strength during bedrest with and without muscle exercise as a countermeasure. European Journal of Applied Physiology. Occupational Physiology 71:342–348

Gibson MC, Schultz E 1983 Age-related differences in absolute numbers of skeletal muscle satellite cells. Muscle and Nerve 6:574–580

Glass DJ 2003a Molecular mechanisms modulating muscle mass. Trends in Molecular Medicine 9:344–350

Glass DJ 2003b Signalling pathways that mediate skeletal muscle hypertrophy and atrophy. Nature Cell Biology 5:87–90

Goldspink G, Harridge SD 2004 Growth factors and muscle ageing. Experimental Gerontology 39:1433–1438

Gonzalez-Cadavid NF, Taylor WE, Yarasheski K, Sinha-Hikim I, Ma K, Ezzat S, Shen R, Lalani R, Asa S, Mamita M, Nair G, Arver S, Bhasin S 1998 Organization of the human myostatin gene and expression in healthy men and HIV-infected men with muscle wasting. Proceedings of the National Academy of Science of the USA 95:14938–14943

Greenleaf JE, Bernauer EM, Ertl AC, Trowbridge TS, Wade CE 1989 Work capacity during 30 days of bed rest with isotonic and isokinetic exercise training. Journal of Applied Physiology 67:1820–1826

Grigoriev AI, Egorov AD 1991 The effects of prolonged spaceflights on the human body. Advances in Space Biology and Medicine 1:1–35

Hara K, Yonezawa K, Kozlowski MT, Sugimoto T, Andrabi K, Weng QP, Kasuga M, Nishimoto I, Avruch J 1997 Regulation of eIF-4E BP1 phosphorylation by mTOR. Journal of Biological Chemistry 272:26457–26463

Hara K, Maruki Y, Long X, Yoshino K, Oshiro N, Hidayat S, Tokunaga C, Avruch J, Yonezawa K 2002 Raptor, a binding partner of target of rapamycin (TOR), mediates TOR action. Cell 110:177–189

Hardt SE, Sadoshima J 2002 Glycogen synthase kinase-3beta: a novel regulator of cardiac hypertrophy and development. Circulation Research 90:1055–1063

Hargens AR, Whalen RT, Watenpaugh DE, Schwandt DF, Krock LP 1991 Lower body negative pressure to provide load bearing in space. Aviation and Space Environmental Medicine 62:934–937

Harridge SD 2003 Ageing and local growth factors in muscle. Scandinavian Journal of Medicine and Science in Sports 13:34–39

Harridge SD, Kryger A, Stensgaard A 1999 Knee extensor strength, activation and size in very elderly people following strength training. Muscle and Nerve 22:831–839

Hasten DL, Pak-Loduca J, Obert KA, Yarasheski KE 2000 Resistance exercise acutely increases MHC and mixed muscle protein synthesis rates in 78–84 and 23–32 yr olds. American Journal of Physiology. Endocrinology and Metabolism 278:E620–E626

Holly JM, Perks CM, Stewart CE 2000 Overview of insulin-like growth factor physiology. Growth Hormone and IGF Research 10(Suppl A): S8–S9

Howard JD, Enoka RM 1991 Maximum bilateral contractions are modified by neurally mediated interlimb effects. Journal of Applied Physiology 70:306–316

Huang J, Forsberg NE 1998 Role of calpain in skeletal-muscle protein degradation. Proceedings of the National Academy of Science of the USA 95:12100–12105

Jasperse JL, Woodman CR, Price EM, Hasser EM, Laughlin MH 1999 Hindlimb unweighting decreases ecNOS gene expression and endothelium-dependent dilation in rat soleus feed arteries. Journal of Applied Physiology 87:1476–1482

Jennische E, Hansson HA 1987 Regenerating skeletal muscle cells express insulin-like growth factor I. Acta Physiologica Scandinavica 130:327–332

Johnson SE, Allen RE 1995 Activation of skeletal muscle satellite cells and the role of fibroblast growth factor receptors. Experimental Cell Research 219:449–453

Joseph C, Kenny AM, Taxel P, Lorenzo JA, Duque G, Kuchel GA 2005 Role of endocrine-immune dysregulation in osteoporosis, sarcopenia, frailty and fracture risk. Molecular Aspects of Medicine 26:181–201

Kawakami Y, Muraoka Y, Kubo K, Suzuki Y, Fukunaga T 2000 Changes in muscle size and architecture following 20 days of bed rest. Journal of Gravitational Physiology 7:53–59

Kitzmann M, Carnac G, Vandromme M, Primig M, Lamb NJ, Fernandez A 1998 The muscle regulatory factors MyoD and myf-5 undergo distinct cell cycle-specific expression in muscle cells. Journal of Cell Biology 142:1447–1459

Kozma SC, Thomas G 2002 Regulation of cell size in growth, development and human disease:PI3K, PKB and S6K. Bioessays 24:65–71

Kraemer WJ, Ratamess NA 2005 Hormonal responses and adaptations to resistance exercise and training. Sports Medicine 35:339–361

Lalani R, Bhasin S, Byhower F, Tarnuzzer R, Grant M, Shen R, Asa S, Ezzat S, Gonzalez-Cadavid NF 2000 Myostatin and insulin-like growth factor-I and -II expression in the muscle of rats exposed to the microgravity environment of the NeuroLab space shuttle flight. Journal of Endocrinology 167:417–428

Larsson L, Li X, Berg HE, Frontera WR 1996 Effects of removal of weight-bearing function on contractility and myosin isoform composition in single human skeletal muscle cells. Pflügers Archiv 432:320–328

LeBlanc A, Gogia P, Schneider V, Krebs J, Schonfeld E, Evans H 1988 Calf muscle area and strength changes after five weeks of horizontal bed rest. American Journal of Sports Medicine 16:624–629

LeBlanc A, Rowe R, Evans H, West S, Shackelford L, Schneider V 1997 Muscle atrophy during long duration bed rest. International Journal of Sports Medicine 18(Suppl 4):S283–S285

Li M, Li C, Parkhouse WS 2003 Age-related differences in the des IGF-I-mediated activation of Akt-1 and p70 S6K in mouse skeletal muscle. Mechanisms of Ageing and Development 124:771–778

Loughna PT, Goldspink DF, Goldspink G 1987 Effects of hypokinesia and hypodynamia upon protein turnover in hindlimb muscles of the rat. Aviation and Space Environmental Medicine 58: A133–A138

Lynch GS, Hinkle RT, Faulkner JA 2001 Force and power output of diaphragm muscle strips from mdx and control mice after clenbuterol treatment. Neuromuscular Disorders 11:192–196

McDonald KS, Delp MD, Fitts RH 1992 Fatigability and blood flow in the rat gastrocnemius-plantaris-soleus after hindlimb suspension. Journal of Applied Physiology 73:1135–1140

McDonald KS, Fitts RH 1995 Effect of hindlimb unloading on rat soleus fiber force, stiffness and calcium sensitivity. Journal of Applied Physiology 79:1796–1802

McPherron AC, Lawler AM, Lee SJ 1997 Regulation of skeletal muscle mass in mice by a new TGF-beta superfamily member. Nature 387:83–90

Maganaris CN, Reeves ND, Rittweger J, Sargeant AJ, Jones DA, Gerrits K, De Haan A 2006 Adaptive response of human tendon to paralysis. Muscle and Nerve 33:85–92

Maltin CA, Delday MI, Watson JS, Heys SD, Nevison IM, Ritchie IK, Gibson PH 1993 Clenbuterol, a beta-adrenoceptor agonist, increases relative muscle strength in orthopaedic patients. Clinical Science (London) 84:651–654

Matsui T, Nagoshi T, Rosenzweig A 2003 Akt and PI 3-kinase signaling in cardiomyocyte hypertrophy and survival. Cell Cycle 2:220–223

Mauro A 1961 Satellite cell of skeletal muscle fibers. Journal of Biophysics, Biochemistry and Cytology 9:493–495

Morley JE, Kim MJ, Haren MT 2005 Frailty and hormones. Reviews in Endocrine and Metabolic Disorders 6:101–108

Murthy G, Watenpaugh DE, Ballard RE, Hargens AR 1994 Exercise against lower body negative pressure as a countermeasure for cardiovascular and musculoskeletal deconditioning. Acta Astronautica 33:89–96

Narici M, Cerretelli P 1998 Changes in human muscle architecture in disuse-atrophy evaluated by ultrasound imaging. Journal of Gravitational Physiology 5:73–74

Narici MV, Maganaris CN 2006 Adaptability of elderly human muscles and tendons to increased loading. Journal of Anatomy 208:433–443

Narici MV, Kayser B, Barattini P, Cerretelli P 1997 Changes in electrically evoked skeletal muscle contractions during 17-day spaceflight and bed rest. International Journal of Sports Medicine 18(Suppl 4):S290–S292

Narici M, Kayser B, Barattini P, Cerretelli P 2003a Effects of 17-day spaceflight on electrically evoked torque and cross-sectional area of the human triceps surae. European Journal of Applied Physiology 90:275–282

Narici MV, Maganaris CN, Reeves ND, Capodaglio P 2003b Effect of aging on human muscle architecture. Journal of Applied Physiology 95:2229–2234

Ohira Y, Jiang B, Roy RR, Oganov V, Ilyina-Kakueva E, Marini JF, Edgerton VR 1992 Rat soleus muscle fiber responses to 14 days of spaceflight and hindlimb suspension. Journal of Applied Physiology 73:51S–57S

Ohira Y, Yoshinaga T, Ohara M, Nonaka I, Yoshioka T, Yamashita-Goto K, Shenkman BS, Kozlovskaya IB, Roy RR, Edgerton VR 1999 Myonuclear domain and myosin phenotype in human soleus after bed rest with or without loading. Journal of Applied Physiology 87:1776–1785

Owino V, Yang SY, Goldspink G 2001 Age-related loss of skeletal muscle function and the inability to express the autocrine form of insulin-like growth factor-1 (MGF) in response to mechanical overload. FEBS Letters 505:259–263

Paul AC, Rosenthal N 2002 Different modes of hypertrophy in skeletal muscle fibers. Journal of Cell Biology 156:751–760

Payette H, Roubenoff R, Jacques PF, Dinarello CA, Wilson PW, Abad LW, Harris T 2003 Insulin-like growth factor-1 and interleukin 6 predict sarcopenia in very old community-living men and women: the Framingham Heart Study. Journal of the American Geriatric Society 51:1237–1243

Pfeilschifter J, Scheidt-Nave C, Leidig-Bruckner G, Woitge HW, Blum WF, Wüster C, Haack D, Ziegler R 1996 Relationship between circulating insulin-like growth factor components and sex hormones in a population-based sample of 50- to 80-year-old men and women. Journal of Clinical Endocrinology and Metabolism 81:2534–2540

Pownall ME, Gustafsson MK, Emerson CP Jr 2002 Myogenic regulatory factors and the specification of muscle progenitors in vertebrate embryos. Annual Review of Cell and Developmental Biology 18:747–783

Qu-Petersen Z, Deasy B, Jankowski R, Ikezawa M, Cummins J, Pruchnic R, Mytinger J, Cao B, Gates C, Wernig A, Huard J 2002 Identification of a novel population of muscle stem cells in mice: potential for muscle regeneration. Journal of Cell Biology 157:851–864

Reeves NJ, Maganaris CN, Ferretti G, Narici MV 2002 Influence of simulated microgravity on human skeletal muscle architecture and function. Journal of Gravitational Physiology 9:153–154

Reeves ND, Maganaris CN, Ferretti G, Narici MV 2005 Influence of 90-day simulated microgravity on human tendon mechanical properties and the effect of resistive countermeasures. Journal of Applied Physiology 98:2278–2286

Renault V, Thornell LE, Eriksson PO, Butler-Browne G, Mouly V 2002 Regenerative potential of human skeletal muscle during aging. Aging Cell 1:132–139

Riley DA, Bain JL, Thompson JL, Fitts RH, Widrick JJ, Trappe SW, Trappe TA, Costill DL 2000 Decreased thin filament density and length in human atrophic soleus muscle fibers after spaceflight. Journal of Applied Physiology 88:567–572

Rommel C, Bodine SC, Clarke BA, Rossman R, Nunez L, Stitt TN, Yancopoulos GD, Glass DJ 2001 Mediation of IGF-1-induced skeletal myotube hypertrophy by PI(3)K/Akt/mTOR and PI(3)K/Akt/GSK3 pathways. Nature Cell Biology 3:1009–1013

Rooyackers OE, Adey DB, Ades PA, Nair KS 1996 Effect of age on in vivo rates of mitochondrial protein synthesis in human skeletal muscle. Proceedings of the National Academy of Science of the USA 93:15364–15369

Roubenoff R 2001 Origins and clinical relevance of sarcopenia. Canadian Journal of Applied Physiology 26:78–89

Roy RR, Bello MA, Bouissou P, Edgerton VR 1987 Size and metabolic properties of fibers in rat fast-twitch muscles after hindlimb suspension. Journal of Applied Physiology 62:2348–2357

Rudnick J, Püttmann B, Tesch PA, Alkner B, Schoser BG, Salanova M, Kirsch K, Gunga HC, Schiffl G, Lück G, Blottner D 2004 Differential expression of nitric oxide synthases (NOS 1–3) in human skeletal muscle following exercise countermeasure during 12 weeks of bed rest. FASEB Journal 18:1228–1230

Russell B, Motlagh D, Ashley WW 2000 Form follows function:how muscle shape is regulated by work. Journal of Applied Physiology 88:1127–1132

Schuelke M, Wagner KR, Stolz LE, Hübner C, Riebel T, Kömen W, Braun T, Tobin JF, Lee SJ 2004 Myostatin mutation associated with gross muscle hypertrophy in a child. New England Journal of Medicine 350:2682–2688

Seale P, Rudnicki MA 2000 A new look at the origin, function and 'stem-cell' status of muscle satellite cells. Developmental Biology 218:115–124

Seale P, Asakura A, Rudnicki MA 2001 The potential of muscle stem cells. Developmental Cell 1:333–342

Sharma R, Anker SD 2002 Cytokines, apoptosis and cachexia:the potential for TNF antagonism. International Journal of Cardiology 85:161–171

Simpson DG, Sharp WW, Borg TK, Price RL, Terracio L, Samarel AM 1996 Mechanical regulation of cardiac myocyte protein turnover and myofibrillar structure. American Journal of Physiology 270:C1075–C1087

Singleton JR, Feldman EL 2001 Insulin-like growth factor-I in muscle metabolism and myotherapies. Neurobiology of Disease 8:541–554

Sinha-Hikim I, Roth SM, Lee MI, Bhasin S 2003 Testosterone-induced muscle hypertrophy is associated with an increase in satellite cell number in healthy, young men. American Journal of Physiology. Endocrinology and Metabolism 285:E197–E205

Smerdu V, Karsch-Mizrachi I, Campione M, Leinwand L, Schiaffino S 1994 Type IIx myosin heavy chain transcripts are expressed in type IIb fibers of human skeletal muscle. American Journal of Physiology 267:C1723–C1728

Spate U, Schulze PC 2004 Proinflammatory cytokines and skeletal muscle. Current Opinion in Clinical Nutrition and Metabolic Care 7:265–269

Stein TP, Leskiw MJ, Schluter MD, Donaldson MR, Larina I 1999 Protein kinetics during and after long-duration spaceflight on MIR. American Journal of Physiology 276:E1014–E1021

Stewart CE, Rotwein P 1996 Growth, differentiation and survival: multiple physiological functions for insulin-like growth factors. Physiological Reviews 76:1005–1026

Suzuki Y, Kashihara H, Takenaka K, Kawakubo K, Makita Y, Goto S, Ikawa S, Gunji A 1994 Effects of daily mild supine exercise on physical performance after 20 days bed rest in young persons. Acta Astronautica 33:101–111

Szewczyk NJ, Jacobson LA 2005 Signal-transduction networks and the regulation of muscle protein degradation. International Journal of Biochemistry and Cell Biology 37:1997–2011

Talmadge RJ 2000 Myosin heavy chain isoform expression following reduced neuromuscular activity:potential regulatory mechanisms. Muscle and Nerve 23:661–679

Talmadge RJ, Roy RR, Edgerton VR 1999 Persistence of hybrid fibers in rat soleus after spinal cord transection. Anatomic Record 255:188–201

Templeton GH, Padalino M, Manton J, Glasberg M, Silver CJ, Silver P, DeMartino G, Leconey T, Klug G, Hagler H, Sutko JL 1984 Influence of suspension hypokinesia on rat soleus muscle. Journal of Applied Physiology 56:278–286

Tesch PA, Trieschmann JT, Ekberg A 2004 Hypertrophy of chronically unloaded muscle subjected to resistance exercise. Journal of Applied Physiology 96:1451–1458

Thomason DB, Booth FW 1990 Atrophy of the soleus muscle by hindlimb unweighting. Journal of Applied Physiology 68:1–12

Thomason DB, Biggs RB, Booth FW 1989 Protein metabolism and beta-myosin heavy-chain mRNA in unweighted soleus muscle. American Journal of Physiology 257:R300–R305

Tischler ME, Henriksen EJ, Munoz KA, Stump CS, Woodman CR, Kirby CR 1993 Spaceflight on STS-48 and earth-based unweighting produce similar effects on skeletal muscle of young rats. Journal of Applied Physiology 74:2161–2165

Trappe S, Trappe T, Gallagher P, Harber M, Alkner B, Tesch P 2004 Human single muscle fibre function with 84 day bed-rest and resistance exercise. Journal of Physiology 557:501–513

Urban RJ, Bodenburg YH, Gilkison C, Foxworth J, Coggan AR, Wolfe RR, Ferrando A 1995 Testosterone administration to elderly men increases skeletal muscle strength and protein synthesis. American Journal of Physiology 269:E820–E826

Vandenburgh H, Chromiak J, Shansky J, Del Tatto M, Lemaire J 1999 Space travel directly induces skeletal muscle atrophy. FASEB Journal 13:1031–1038

Wade CE, Stanford KI, Stein TP, Greenleaf JE 2005 Intensive exercise training suppresses testosterone during bed rest. Journal of Applied Physiology 99:59–63

Wang H, Casaburi R, Taylor WE, Aboellail H, Storer TW, Kopple JD 2005 Skeletal muscle mRNA for IGF-IEa, IGF-II and IGF-I receptor is decreased in sedentary chronic hemodialysis patients. Kidney International 68:352–361

Welle S, Thornton C, Jozefowicz R, Statt M 1993 Myofibrillar protein synthesis in young and old men. American Journal of Physiology 264:E693–E698

Widrick JJ, Knuth ST, Norenberg KM, Romatowski JG, Bain JL, Riley DA, Karhanek M, Trappe SW, Trappe TA, Costill DL, Fitts RH 1999 Effect of a 17 day spaceflight on contractile properties of human soleus muscle fibres. Journal of Physiology 516(Pt 3):915–930

Widrick JJ, Trappe SW, Romatowski JG, Riley DA, Costill DL, Fitts RH 2002 Unilateral lower limb suspension does not mimic bed rest or spaceflight effects on human muscle fiber function. Journal of Applied Physiology 93:354–360

Wineski LE, von Deutsch DA, Abukhalaf IK, Pitts SA, Potter DE, Paulsen DF 2002 Muscle-specific effects of hindlimb suspension and clenbuterol in mature male rats. Cells Tissues Organs 171:188–198

Yoshida N, Sairyo K, Sasa T, Fukunaga M, Koga K, Ikata T, Yasui N 2003 Electrical stimulation prevents deterioration of the oxidative capacity of disuse-atrophied muscles in rats. Aviation and Space Environmental Medicine 74:207–211

Zachwieja JJ, Smith SR, Lovejoy JC, Rood JC, Windhauser MM, Bray GA 1999a Testosterone administration preserves protein balance but not muscle strength during 28 days of bed rest. Journal of Clinical Endocrinology and Metabolism 84:207–212

Zachwieja JJ, Smith SR, Sinha-Hikim I, Gonzalez-Cadavid N, Bhasin S 1999b Plasma myostatin-immunoreactive protein is increased after prolonged bed rest with low-dose T3 administration. Journal of Gravitational Physiology 6:11–15

Zammit P, Beauchamp J 2001 The skeletal muscle satellite cell:stem cell or son of stem cell? Differentiation 68:193–204

Zhang LF, Sun B, Cao XS, Liu C, Yu ZB, Zhang LN, Cheng JH, Wu YH, Wu XY 2003 Effectiveness of intermittent -Gx gravitation in preventing deconditioning due to simulated microgravity. Journal of Applied Physiology 95:207–218

Chapter **10**

Topical debates

Chapter 10.1

Maximal exercise: is it limited centrally or peripherally?

Peter D. Wagner   Niels H. Secher

The question of what sets the limits to human performance has intrigued both the lay and scientific communities for a long time. What is it that makes an individual a winner as opposed to a runner-up? In most sports, the quantitative difference between first and second place has become very small. Winning an Olympic 1500 m race by 1 m is a clear victory when you see it on television, but it represents a margin of only 0.07%. No physiological measurement system can resolve differences down to this level, enabling an explanation of the difference between the winner and runner-up. Moreover, psychological (motivational) factors must play at least as important a role as physiological characteristics in gaining that 1 m advantage.

Rather than try to discuss performance, which embodies both physiological and psychological elements, in this chapter, the physiological underpinnings of central and peripheral limits to the performance of maximal exercise will be discussed. The focus is upon high-intensity exercise, such that work rate either increases incrementally (ramp forcing function), or starts and remains at such an intensity as to elicit volitional fatigue, enabling the quantification of peak power generation and peak aerobic power (maximal oxygen uptake). This discussion will further be limited to endurance exercise, whilst very brief, intense exercise (weightlifting, sprinting) have an entirely different set of limiting factors that are beyond the scope of this chapter.

Essential background material is contained within each of the preceding chapters, along with the accompanying debates and also the introduction to Section 3. Readers may also find Chapter 14.2 to be instructive. Part A of this chapter contains an overview of the central limits to maximal exercise, whilst Part B presents the case that peripheral factors are at least as important as the central limits. However, it must be noted that, across individuals, modes of exercise and exercise intensities, the limits to maximal exercise will vary.

Part A: Central limitations to maximal exercise
Niels Secher

1 INTRODUCTION

There are many limiting factors to human performance and their mutual contribution varies not only with the muscle mass involved in exercise, but also with the circumstances under which a given task is performed. For example, work with one hand elicits pain in the forearm and is considered to be limited by local metabolic factors, since no strain is imposed on ventilation or central circulation. Yet, intense exercise (weightlifting) can be supported by a Valsalva-like manoeuvre that, besides stabilising the spine, briefly increases mean arterial pressure and perfusion pressure to working muscles. Equally, it is a common experience that work performed over the head (painting) elicits fatigue and local pain, while lowering the arm relieves the discomfort. Since circulation is not supported by the gravitational force of a siphon that would drag blood along the vasculature, veins collapse when raised above the level of the heart (Dawson et al. 2004), and perfusion pressure depends on the mean arterial pressure at the level of the active tissue. Thus, arm blood flow during overhead work is limited by the hydrostatic restraint on arterial flow. In the giraffe, for example, the mean arterial pressure necessary to adequately perfuse the brain is about twice that observed in humans. However, it is open to discussion whether the limited ability of the muscle pressor reflex (Mitchell et al. 1983) or a Valsalva-like manoeuvre (Clifford et al. 1994) to raise mean arterial pressure sufficiently to provide for adequate perfusion pressure to muscles can be interpreted as a central limitation to performance.

Most often, considerations on the importance of central and peripheral limitations to performance address dynamic exercise and, specifically, factors limiting whole-body exercise. For each such circumstance, experiments can be designed to evaluate the relative importance of one or several variables. Furthermore, the integrated response can be evaluated by the formalism developed by Wagner (Part B of this chapter).

2 PROLONGED EXHAUSTIVE EXERCISE

Many studies describe exercise to exhaustion, but the definition of such a state remains elusive. Following exhaustive exercise, blood lactate concentration is typically lower in a laboratory-based experiment (15 mM) than after a championship race (30 mM), where arterial pH also reaches its lowest value (6.74; Nielsen 1999). Such lactate levels indicate an extreme effort but do they represent exhaustion? When Pheidippides reported to Athens (490 bc) of the victory over the Persians at the battle of Marathon, he died after running 35 km, but after first having asked Sparta for help (running 400 km), according to the legend, in full uniform. With that degree of exhaustion, death is by cardiac insufficiency, because the blood volume of the heart increases from ~30% to ~50%. This has been demonstrated is an animal model (rat; Figure 10.1.1), with recovery over 2–3 days.

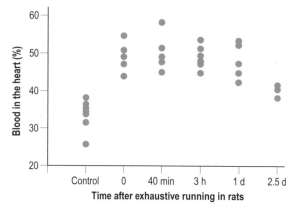

Figure 10.1.1 Blood in the heart (rat) following exhaustive running. From Secher (1921).

Athletes are not forced into a similar degree of exhaustion but so-called cardiac fatigue may be detected following prolonged exercise (e.g. 4 h rowing), with an attenuated heart rate response to administration of sympathomimetic drugs. Most likely, exercise is terminated because of fading motivation, heat stress (when brain temperature reaches 41°C; Nybo & Secher 2004; Chapters 27.1 and 27.2) or intramuscular glycogen depletion (Karlsson & Saltin 1971; Chapter 7) and, ultimately, in astrocytes providing energy to the neurones (Dalsgaard 2006). So-called central fatigue (Chapter 5) affects recruitment of slow-twitch rather than fast-twitch muscle fibres (Secher 1992), and is characterised by an inability to maintain a smooth movement pattern, as is well known for myasthenic patients.

3 PULMONARY LIMITATIONS TO EXERCISE

With exhaustive exercise of shorter duration, oxygen delivery to the working muscles becomes a critical limitation. The lungs' membrane diffusion capacity of about $600 \text{ mL·min}^{-1}\text{·kPa}^{-1}$ may not be sufficient to secure oxygen delivery during maximal, whole-body exercise in athletes. Accordingly, in spite of the alveolar oxygen tension (P_AO_2) being raised by hyperventilation, arterial oxygen tension (P_aO_2) decreases. Because of the Bohr effect on the oxyhaemoglobin dissociation curve, reduction of pH by lactate further reduces arterial oxygen saturation (Chapter 2), as observed during maximal exercise where a value of 90% is typical (Nielsen et al. 1999). On the other hand, the Bohr effect is curtailed when P_aO_2 is maintained, while breathing oxygen-enriched air. Saturation is then restored to near resting levels and maximal oxygen uptake ($\dot{V}_{O_{2max}}$) increases accordingly, indicating a 5–10% pulmonary limitation to performance. Athletes who possess an extraordinarily large pulmonary vital capacity (~7 L), with a record of 9.1 L (Secher 1983) are more suitable for events with a large anaerobic contribution to work.

4 CARDIAC OUTPUT AND MUSCLE BLOOD FLOW

Cardiac output ($\dot{Q}$) follows lung diffusion in the cascade of oxygen delivery to working muscles (Chapter 1). During exercise, cardiac output increases in proportion to work rate and oxygen uptake, with the slope for the latter being close to 5 (Mitchell et al. 1958). Ultimately, however, this slope decreases because of an insufficient preloading of the heart (Mortensen et al. 2005). Also, the increase in cardiac output during exercise demonstrates a remarkably interindividual variation, with difference of up to 100% being evident between the smallest and the largest outputs, with that variation having a genetic background (Snyder et al. 2006).

Haematocrit has a further influence on cardiac output or regional blood flow (González-Alonso et al. 2004). At low haematocrits (e.g. anaemia), blood flow is high, suggesting that oxygen delivery or venous oxygen saturation is the regulated variable (Krantz et al. 2005; Chapter 1). Conversely, a given oxygen uptake creates little reduction in haemoglobin saturation when haemotocrit is high and a low flow is maintained. Nitric oxide and adenosine triphosphate (ATP) are liberated from haemoglobin when it is deoxygenated, inducing vasodilatation and indicating that haemoglobin contributes to the control of blood flow (González-Alonso et al. 2002).

Yet, it may be that the ability of the heart to increase its output is limited, since following β1-adrenergic blockade, and during intense exercise, there is an insufficient preload. Under such circumstances, leg blood flow is reduced by sympathetic vasoconstriction, as indicated by an enhanced noradrenaline spill over from the working legs (Pawelczyk et al. 1992). Equally, when the ability to increase cardiac output is affected by heart disease, leg blood flow is attenuated during exercise (Schmidt et al. 1995). The key role of cardiac output in regulating leg blood flow in cardiac patients is underscored when the former is elevated by digitalis administration and leg blood flow is similarly enhanced.

Across varying abilities to increase cardiac output, mean arterial pressure is regulated at a remarkably stable state, suggesting that it is the primarily regulated circulatory variable (Chapters 1 and 18). Mean arterial pressure is attenuated very little by the vascular adjustments accompanying endurance training, including an enormous increase in vascular conductance during exercise (Clausen 1976). Mean arterial pressure is regulated via feedback from the arterial baroreceptors, with their main influence being the modulation of total peripheral resistance (Ogoh et al. 2003a). The pressure that is regulated is determined by the central nervous system (feedforward or central command; Gallagher et al. 2001a), the muscle pressor reflex (Gallagher et al. 2001b) and the central blood volume (Ogoh et al. 2003b). Each of these influences on the arterial baroreflex is modified by endurance training, thus explaining why the mean arterial pressure response to exercise is attenuated. Following training, work becomes easier, the increased muscle blood flow attenuates the muscle pressor reflex, and an elevated blood volume enhances the central blood volume and filling of the heart (Chapter 27.3).

The regulated pressure is achieved mainly by increasing cardiac output, compensating for the large reduction in total peripheral resistance associated with exercise. Blood used to

enhance muscle blood flow (Pawelczyk et al. 1992), and central blood volume, is recruited from the splanchnic region by vasoconstriction (Perko et al. 1998). This is a prerequisite for pressure regulation (Dela et al. 2003). However, if the increase in cardiac output is not large enough to maintain the blood pressure, vasoconstriction is induced not only within the splanchnic region but also to working muscles and the brain (Ide & Secher 2000). Indeed, this dominance of pressure regulation over other regulatory mechanisms becomes most evident when exercising in the heat (Chapter 19).

5 MUSCLE BLOOD FLOW DURING WHOLE-BODY EXERCISE

Maintenance of an adequate mean arterial pressure during exercise can be problematic, especially when several muscle groups are involved. To evaluate the influence of muscle mass on the control of muscle blood flow, it is convenient to compare limb blood flow during arm and leg exercise. In such a comparison, light handgrip or other forms of arm exercise has no influence on blood flow to the working leg. However, at higher upper limb exercise intensities, a marked increase in sympathetic activity occurs, and leg blood flow is reduced (Saito et al. 1992, Secher et al. 1977). In the reverse situation, where leg exercise is added to ongoing arm-cranking exercise, the result is similar with a reduction in arm oxygenation and flow when the load on the legs is large (Volianitis et al. 2004).

Because blood flow to working skeletal muscle is under the control of the arterial baroreflex, that aims to regulate mean arterial pressure, skeletal muscles are seldom allowed to manifest their potential for flow. When intense exercise is performed with several muscle groups, attenuation in muscle blood flow is reflected in an attenuated muscle diffusion for oxygen (Figure 10.1.2; Volianitis et al. 2004), illus-

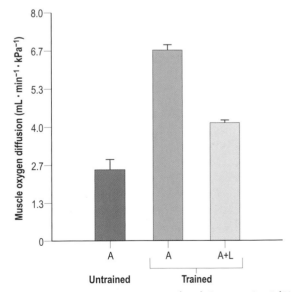

Figure 10.1.2 Muscle oxygen diffusion (arm) for untrained ($N = 8$) and trained rowers ($N = 7$) during arm cranking, and with combined leg exercise and arm cranking. Data (mean $\pm$ SE) from Volianitis et al. (2004).

trating a reduced capillary recruitment. The metabolic potential of the muscle is not challenged during whole-body exercise; instead it is limited by the convective flow and oxygen that the muscles receive. This is in striking contrast to the regulation of cerebral blood flow. While cerebral capillary oxygenation increases during activation (Ide & Secher 2000), muscle oxygenation decreases during exercise.

Part B: An equivalent role for peripheral limitations to maximal exercise
Peter Wagner

1 INTRODUCTION

Given the focus of this chapter, the essential question for debate becomes, under the circumstances described within the general introduction, what limits maximal oxygen uptake? In Part A, it was proposed that maximal oxygen uptake is limited centrally, while I will reason that it is limited not only by central factors, but that peripheral factors are just as important. Indeed, I will show that every step of the oxygen delivery pathway (Weibel 1984) contributes to defining peak aerobic power for a given individual.

First, we need to settle on what we mean by central and peripheral. This is not as trivial as it sounds. The term central may refer to the central nervous system and the role it may possibly play as an overall governor of the maximal intensity of exercise (Chapter 10.2), or it may refer to central cardiopulmonary components of the oxygen transport system or to both. Peripheral is also not a crystal clear concept. Where does central end and peripheral begin? Lung function is clearly wholly central, until one realises that the amount of oxygen that can diffuse from alveolar gas into pulmonary capillary blood is affected by the level of oxygen in the mixed venous blood returning from the tissues (Wagner 1982). This, in turn, reflects the ability of muscles to extract oxygen from the blood and transport it to the mitochondria. Thus, a peripheral structure (muscle) has a well-described effect on lung function. So too, cardiovascular function is an integrated outcome of heart (central) and vascular (peripheral) structure and function. In addition, increasing cardiac output positively affects convective delivery of oxygen around the body, but at the same time may impair diffusive loading of oxygen in the lungs (central) as well as diffusive unloading of oxygen in the muscles (peripheral) by reducing capillary transit time for red blood cells (Chapter 2).

Rather than dwell on the definitions of central and peripheral factors (because they are hopelessly intertwined, as must now be clear), it makes more sense to reframe the question in terms of the principal delivery and utilisation functions required to get oxygen from the air to the mitochondria, and to produce ATP. These are, in sequence:

1. alveolar ventilation
2. alveolar-capillary oxygen diffusion
3. loading oxygen onto haemoglobin
4. delivery of oxygenated blood to the muscles (blood flow)
5. diffusion of oxygen from muscle microvessels to the mitochondria
6. production of ATP through oxidative phosphorylation.

Although not listed as a biological function, the inspired oxygen concentration also affects maximal oxygen uptake, as demonstrated on many occasions (Knight et al. 1993, Wagner et al. 1996c, Welch 1982, 1987). On the other hand, heterogeneity in (a) ventilation and blood flow in the lungs (Chapter 2), and (b) metabolic rate and blood flow in the muscles will (reasonably) be considered insufficient to affect oxygen delivery in health, and will thus be ignored (because the analysis to follow would be impossibly complicated).

Accordingly, the question now becomes: do any of these steps influence the maximal oxygen uptake that an individual can attain? The answer is that each and every step can be limiting, and this is the core concept in this chapter. The reason why each step plays a role is that the transition from extracting oxygen from the air to producing ATP is a serially linked process (six steps above), much like a bucket brigade. No step can be bypassed. Suppose we have a real bucket brigade made up of six people. Suppose all six are of equal size, but one is recovering from a broken arm and can handle only very light buckets. Because the system is strictly an in-series system, the number of buckets passed down the line per minute cannot exceed the capacity of the weakest step. Now replace this weak link with a giant who is twice as strong as the other five. His extra strength is of little help because the other five cannot keep up. Thus, a singularly weak link significantly impairs delivery, while an especially strong link on its own does little to augment delivery.

This analogy is not really adequate when one delves more deeply into oxygen delivery. A bucket brigade is a unidirectional process, where the overall function is not affected by downstream actions beyond the last step. Oxygen delivery, however, forms a closed loop, in which blood sent to the muscles then returns to the lungs for more oxygen. This difference is significant, because it makes the performance of the lungs, in part, dependent on the oxygenation state of venous blood. This one example implies a complex interaction that exists among all six steps of this process.

So now the question becomes, given the multiple steps and their complex interactions, what is the relative (quantitative) importance of each step in determining maximal oxygen uptake? Central to this debate is evaluating the importance of factors that are traditionally regarded as central (steps 1–4), versus those thought of as peripheral factors (steps 5 and 6). Because of the complex interactions among the six factors, no simple or unique quantitative answer can be given without further analysis. Experiments to address this question are difficult to design because of these interactions, and so theoretical modelling has a role to play, because of the ability to understand both the primary and the secondary effects of changes at each delivery step. Thus, building a mathematical model that integrates these functions offers an analytical approach that will predict the influence of each factor; such a model exists (Wagner 1993, 1996a).

Before applying this model to this debate, it should be pointed out that an abundance of experimental evidence exists to show that changing the performance of any one of the above steps of the oxygen pathway will affect maximal oxygen uptake. This evidence is systematically reviewed in several places, most recently in this book (Chapter 1), and also in Wagner et al. (1997) and will therefore not be repeated here. Suffice it to say that changes in the inspired oxygen partial pressure, alveolar ventilation, alveolar-capillary diffusion, cardiac output/muscle blood flow, haemoglobin concentration and oxygen binding, diffusion of oxygen from muscle capillaries to mitochondria and the mitochondrial capacity to use oxygen have individually been shown to affect maximal oxygen uptake, and hence exercise capacity.

2 INTEGRATION BETWEEN CENTRAL AND PERIPHERAL FACTORS

Perhaps the easiest way to understand how the delivery components affect maximal oxygen uptake is visually, using the Fick diagram (Wagner 1996b; Chapter 1, Figure 1.10). Oxygen uptake (ordinate) is plotted against muscle venous oxygen partial pressure (abscissa), based on two separate mass conservation laws, which both happen to bear the name of Adolph Fick (Fick 1855), a 19th-century German scientist.

The first law is better known as the Fick Principle, which expresses muscle oxygen uptake ($\dot{V}_{O_2}$) as the product of blood flow ($\dot{Q}$) and the arteriovenous oxygen concentration difference. Thus:

Equation 1a: $\dot{V}_{O_2} = \dot{Q} \cdot [C_aO_2 - C_vO_2]$

where:

C_aO_2 and C_vO_2 = arterial and muscle venous oxygen concentrations (respectively).

Ignoring physically dissolved oxygen, which contributes less than 2% to total circulating oxygen, equation 1a can be reexpressed by describing blood concentrations in terms of their components – haemoglobin concentration ([Hb]) and oxygen saturation:

Equation 1b: $\dot{V}_{O_2} = 1.39 \cdot \dot{Q} \cdot [Hb] \cdot [S_aO_2 - S_vO_2]$

where:

S_aO_2 and S_vO_2 = arterial and muscle oxygen saturation (respectively).

The second law is Fick's Law of Diffusion and reduced to its simplest form and applied to diffusion of oxygen between the muscle capillaries and the mitochondria, it becomes:

Equation 2: $\dot{V}_{O_2} = DMO_2 \cdot [P_cO_2 - P_{mit}O_2]$

where:

DMO_2 = whole-muscle diffusing capacity for oxygen
P_cO_2 and $P_{mit}O_2$ = mean muscle capillary (determined by integrating along the capillary from arterial to venous end) and mitochondrial oxygen tension (respectively).

Equations 1 and 2 describe quite different physical processes (convective oxygen delivery by the blood and diffusive oxygen delivery within muscle), but they both quantify the net flux of oxygen ($\dot{V}_{O_2}$). The critical concept is that in a steady state, both equations must result in the same oxygen uptake. Per unit time, the amount of oxygen removed from blood (Equation 1) equals the amount moved subsequently by diffusion (Equation 2). Figure 10.1.3 shows these two equations graphically (Fick diagram), based on typical data for a normal subject exercising maximally.

For Equation 1, we first have to determine the oxygen tension corresponding to oxygen concentration, using the oxyhaemoglobin dissociation curve. This explains the sigmoid shape of curve representing Equation 1 in the figure. Equation 1 states that, for any given set of values for cardiac output, haemoglobin concentration and oxygen saturation, the amount of oxygen unloaded per unit time is a unique function of muscle venous oxygen tension (P_vO_2), because of the requirement that mass (oxygen) be conserved. This curve has a negative slope, with its highest point (arterial oxygen delivery; top left) at a P_vO_2 of zero (100% oxygen extraction). At this point, oxygen uptake would equal all of the oxygen delivered in the arterial blood. Its lowest point (bottom right) occurs when no oxygen is extracted from the blood ($P_vO_2 = P_aO_2$). In life, neither extreme is observed.

For Equation 2, it turns out that the mean muscle capillary oxygen tension (P_cO_2) is closely and proportionally related to muscle P_vO_2. So if we set mean muscle P_cO_2 to

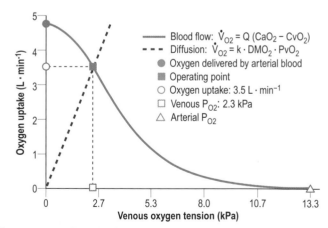

Figure 10.1.3 Relationships between oxygen uptake and muscle venous oxygen tension for a normal, maximally exercising subject, as given by the Fick Principle and Fick's Law of diffusion (Chapter 1): the Fick diagram. Cardiac output in this example is taken to be 23 L·min⁻¹, haemoglobin concentration as 15 g·100 mL⁻¹ and arterial oxygen tension to be 13.3 kPa. Mass conservation requires that oxygen uptake is the value at their intersection.

equal P_vO_2 (times a proportionality constant), we also can plot oxygen uptake from Equation 2 on this diagram as a function of muscle P_vO_2. An important approximation is that mitochondrial oxygen tension is close enough to zero to be ignored. This simplification is reasonable because P_aO_2 is ~13.3 kPa, muscle P_vO_2 ~2.7 kPa and P_cO_2 is therefore in the range of 5.3–6.7 kPa. Mitochondrial oxygen tension, on the other hand, must be less than that in the muscle cytoplasm, which has been determined from measurements of myoglobin oxygen saturation to be about 0.4–0.5 kPa during heavy exercise (Richardson et al. 1995). Thus, Equation 2 becomes a straight line with positive slope, passing through the origin, with its slope reflecting muscle oxygen-diffusing capacity.

Because both equations quantify oxygen uptake, there is only one point in the diagram at which oxygen uptake and muscle P_vO_2 (given by both equations) are simultaneously the same, thus allowing mass conservation for oxygen: the operating point (solid square) at the intersection of the two relationships. When the determining variables (cardiac output, haemoglobin concentration, oxygen saturation, muscle oxygen-diffusing capacity) are those measured at maximal exercise, the operating point defines maximal oxygen uptake. In Figure 10.1.3, for the data used, maximal oxygen uptake must be 3.5 L·min^{-1} and muscle P_vO_2 must be 2.3 kPa.

Since the shape and position of the solid Fick Principle line depend on haemoglobin concentration, the oxyhaemoglobin dissociation curve, cardiac output and arterial oxygen saturation, it should be evident that the operating point will shift, depending on the values of these variables. Importantly, they reflect heart, blood and pulmonary function. In the same way, the slope of the Fick's Law line depends on muscle diffusing capacity, such that changes will independently affect the operating point, and thus maximal oxygen uptake. The critical conclusion from Figure 10.1.3 is that changes in any of the oxygen delivery variables must affect maximal oxygen uptake.

3 RELATIVE IMPORTANCE OF EACH DELIVERY STEP IN LIMITING MAXIMAL AEROBIC POWER

Figure 10.1.4 shows the consequence for maximal oxygen uptake of reducing just one variable (cardiac output) by 25%. The Fick Principle line shifts downwards in accord with Equation 1, lowering the operating point, and the maximal oxygen uptake must fall (from 3.5 to 2.9 L·min^{-1}). Figure 10.1.5 shows the corresponding effect of reducing muscle diffusing capacity by 25%. The operating point again shifts downwards because the slope of the Fick's Law line is decreased by 25% and maximal oxygen uptake is reduced essentially as much as when cardiac output falls by the same percentage (3.0 versus 2.9 L·min^{-1}).

Thus, when oxygen delivery components are individually decreased from normal, it is apparent from these examples that the effect on maximal oxygen uptake of reducing

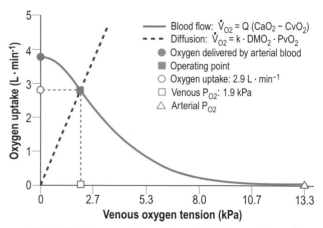

Figure 10.1.4 Fick diagram from Figure 10.1.3 but with cardiac output reduced by 25%, with oxygen uptake reduced (intersection point).

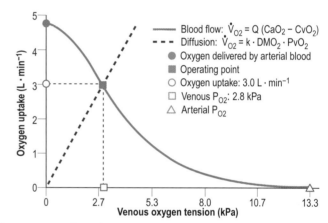

Figure 10.1.5 Fick diagram from Figure 10.1.3, but with muscle oxygen-diffusing capacity reduced by 25%.

these so-called central factors is almost the same as equivalent reductions in peripheral factors. Thus, the diffusion of oxygen within muscle is almost as important (quantitatively) as blood flow.

To this point, the analysis shown in these figures has accounted for the first five oxygen delivery steps, but it has ignored the sixth delivery step – producing ATP through oxidative phosphorylation. In the absence of an oxygen delivery limitation, a muscle must exhibit some maximal metabolic capacity to use oxygen to produce ATP. Two possibilities therefore exist. The first, as implied by the analysis in the above figures, is that mitochondrial metabolic capacity exceeds oxygen delivery capacity, which therefore limits the maximal (actual) oxygen uptake as described. However, the second possibility is that mitochondrial metabolic capacity is insufficient to use all of the oxygen that could be transported by the processes of convection and diffusion.

Figure 10.1.6 shows both of these scenarios. If the maximal mitochondrial capacity to use oxygen were 4 L·min^{-1}, actual maximal oxygen uptake would be indeed 3.5 L·min^{-1}, as

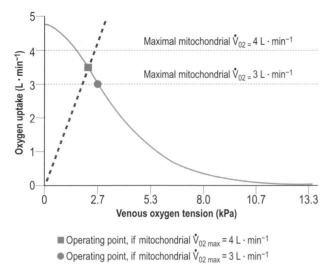

Operating point, if mitochondrial $\dot{V}_{O_2 \, max} = 4 \, L \cdot min^{-1}$
Operating point, if mitochondrial $\dot{V}_{O_2 \, max} = 3 \, L \cdot min^{-1}$

Figure 10.1.6 Fick diagram for the subject in Figure 10.1.3, but now indicating the effects of two different maximal mitochondrial metabolic (oxygen uptake) limits: 3 and 4 L·min⁻¹. In the former case, maximal oxygen uptake (solid circle) is limited by, and to, mitochondrial capacity. In the latter, maximal oxygen delivery is less than metabolic capacity, such that transport limits maximal oxygen uptake (solid square).

presented previously (Figure 10.1.3), because delivery capacity is less than metabolic capacity. However, for the same delivery capacity, if metabolic capacity were only 3 L·min⁻¹, this, and not oxygen delivery, would define the limit on actual maximal oxygen uptake. To conserve mass, the operating point would have to remain on the Fick Principle line, but would move to a lower point (solid circle). Neither convective nor diffusive oxygen delivery is any longer contributing to limit oxygen uptake. Thus, cardiac output could be doubled, and maximal oxygen uptake would not improve. All that would happen is that muscle P_vO_2 would increase, because the extra oxygen delivered would not be used.

These four figures provide conceptual examples of the integration of all delivery steps in determining maximal oxygen uptake. To obtain a more quantitative sense of the relative importance of each of the delivery steps over a wide range of increases and decreases, Figure 10.1.7 is presented. The upper panel assumes a metabolic capacity of 4 L·min⁻¹, in the absence of an oxygen limitation, while the lower panel is for a metabolic capacity of 3 L·min⁻¹. The results are based on prior analytical formulations of the integrated transport system (Wagner 1993), and use the same normal data as Figure 10.1.3. Maximal (actual) oxygen uptake is plotted as a function of each oxygen delivery variable indicated, altered one at a time, relative changes in each variable given to allow a direct comparison of variables having widely different absolute values.

This figure allows two major conclusions. First, the effects on maximal oxygen uptake of changes in any of the oxygen delivery variables are quite similar, across a wide range of values, generalising the conclusion from the above exam-

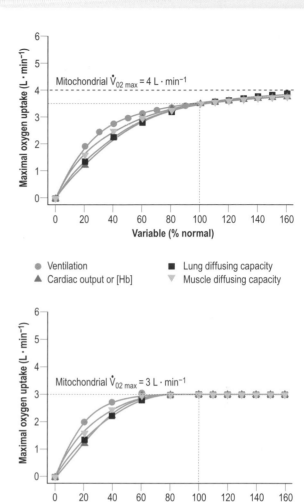

● Ventilation
▲ Cardiac output or [Hb]
■ Lung diffusing capacity
▼ Muscle diffusing capacity

Figure 10.1.7 Effects of changes in all oxygen delivery variables (one at a time) on maximal oxygen uptake when maximal mitochondrial metabolic (oxygen uptake) capacity is 4 L·min⁻¹ (upper panel) and 3 L·min⁻¹ (lower panel). All variables affect maximal oxygen uptake similarly. Increases in oxygen delivery capacity increase maximal oxygen uptake only slightly (upper panel) or not at all (lower panel), while reductions impair oxygen uptake considerably.

ples. Second, increases in the value of any one delivery variable have little beneficial effect on maximal oxygen uptake, while the same percentage reduction in the variable has a more substantial negative impact.

4 CONCLUSION

An analysis of oxygen delivery and utilisation, using these simple, robust quantitative approaches, clearly reveals that every step of the oxygen delivery pathway will affect maximal oxygen uptake. Moreover, the quantitative influence of each step is quite similar over a wide range of changes. While there is no doubt that central cardiopulmonary factors are important determinants of maximal oxygen uptake, it should be evident that peripheral factors are just as important, and there is a wealth of experimental evidence to support this conclusion.

References

Clausen JP 1976 Circulatory adjustments to dynamic exercise and effect of physical training in normal subjects and in patients with coronary artery disease. Progress in Cardiovascular Diseases 18:459–495

Clifford PS, Hanel B, Secher NH 1994 Arterial blood pressure response to rowing. Medicine and Science in Sports and Exercise 26:715–719

Dalsgaard MK 2006 Fuelling cerebral activity in exercising man. Journal of Cerebral Blood Flow and Metabolism 26:731–750

Dawson EA, Secher NH, Dalsgaard MK, Ogoh S, Yoshiga CC, González-Alonso J, Steensberg A, Raven PB 2004 Standing up to the challenge of standing: a siphon does not support cerebral blood flow in humans. American Journal of Physiology 287:R911–R914

Dela F, Mohr T, Jensen CM, Haahr HL, Secher NH, Biering-Sørensen F, Kjaer M 2003 Cardiovascular control during exercise: Insight from spinal cord-injured humans. Circulation 107:2127–2133

Fick A 1855 Über diffusion. Poggendorff's Annalen der Physik und Chemie 94:59–86

Gallagher KM, Fadel PJ, Strømstad M, Ide K, Smith SA, Querry RG, Raven PB, Secher NH 2001a Effect of partial neuromuscular blockade on carotid baroreflex function during exercise in humans. Journal of Physiology 533:861–870

Gallagher KM, Fadel PJ, Strømstad M, Ide K, Smith SA, Querry RG, Raven PB, Secher NH 2001b Effect of exercise pressor reflex activation on carotid baroreflex function during exercise in humans. Journal of Physiology 533:871–880

González-Alonso J, Olsen DB, Saltin B 2002 Erythrocyte and the regulation of human skeletal muscle blood flow and oxygen delivery. Circulation Research 91:1046–1055

González-Alonso J, Dalsgaard MK, Osada T, Volianitis S, Dawson EA, Yoshiga CC, Secher NH 2004 Brain and central haemodynamic and oxygenation during maximal exercise in humans. Journal of Physiology 557:331–342

Ide K, Secher NH 2000 Cerebral blood flow and metabolism during exercise. Progress in Neurobiology 61:397–414

Karlsson J, Saltin B 1971 Diet, muscle glycogen and endurance performance. Journal of Applied Physiology 31:203–206

Knight DR, Schaffartzik W, Poole DC, Hogan MC, Bebout DE, Wagner PD 1993 Effects of hyperoxia on maximal leg O_2 supply and utilization in men. Journal of Applied Physiology 75(6):2586–2594

Krantz T, Warberg J, Secher NH 2005 Venous oxygen saturation during norvolaemic haemodilution in the pig. Acta Anaesthesiologica Scandinavica 49:1149–1156

Mitchell JH, Sproule BJ, Chapman CB 1958 The physiological meaning of the maximal oxygen intake test. Journal of Clinical Investigation 37:538–547

Mitchell JH, Kaufman MP, Iwamoto G 1983 The exercise pressor reflex: its cardiovascular mechanisms and central pathways. Annual Review of Physiology 45:229–242

Mortensen SP, Dawson EA, Yoshiga CC, Dalsgaard MK, Damsgaard R, Secher NH, González-Alonso J 2005 Limitations to systemic and locomotor limb muscle oxygen delivery and uptake during maximal exercise in humans. Journal of Physiology 566:273–285

Nielsen HB 1999 pH after competitive rowing: the lower physiological range? Acta Physiologica Scandinavica 165:113–114

Nielsen HB, Boushel R, Madsen P, Secher NH 1999 Cerebral desaturation during exercise reversed by O_2 supplementation. American Journal of Physiology 277:H1045–H1052

Nybo L, Secher NH 2004 Cerebral perturbations provoked by prolonged exercise. Progress in Neurobiology 72:223–261

Ogoh S, Fadel PJ, Nissen P, Jans Ø, Selmer C, Secher NH, Raven PB 2003a Carotid baroreflex-mediated changes in cardiac output and total vascular conductance during exercise in humans. Journal of Physiology 550:317–324

Ogoh S, Volianitis S, Nissen P, Wray DW, Secher NH, Raven PB 2003b Carotid baroreflex responsiveness to head-up tilt induced central hypovolaemia: effect of aerobic fitness. Journal of Physiology 551:601–608

Pawelczyk JA, Hanel B, Pawelczyk RA, Warberg J, Secher NH 1992 Leg vasoconstriction during dynamic exercise with reduced cardiac output. Journal of Applied Physiology 73:1838–1846

Perko MJ, Nielsen HB, Skak C, Clemmesen JO, Schroeder TV, Secher NH 1998 Mesenteric, coeliac and splanchnic blood flow in humans during exercise. Journal of Physiology 513:907–913

Richardson RS, Noyszewski EA, Kendrick KF, Leigh JS, Wagner PD 1995 Myoglobin O_2 desaturation during exercise: evidence of limited O_2 transport. Journal of Clinical Investigation 96:1916–1926

Saito M, Kagaya A, Ogita F, Shinohara M 1992 Changes in muscle sympathetic nerve activity and calf blood flow during combined leg and forearm exercise. Acta Physiologica Scandinavica 146:449–456

Schmidt TA, Bundgaard H, Olesen HL, Secher NH, Kjeldsen K 1995 Digoxin affects potassium homeostasis during exercise in patients with heart failure. Cardiovascular Research 29:506–511

Secher K 1921 Eperimentelle Untersuechungenüber den Einfluß der Anstrennungen auf die Größe des Herzens. Zeitschrift für die gesamte eperimentelle Medizin 14:113–129

Secher NH 1983 The physiology of rowing. Journal of Sports Sciences 1:23–53

Secher NH 1992 Central nervous influence on fatigue. In: Shepherd RJ, Åstrand P-O (eds) The Olympic book of endurance sports. Blackwell, London, 96–107

Secher NH, Clausen JP, Klausen K, Noer I, Trap-Jensen J 1977 Central and regional circulatory effects of adding arm exercise to leg exercise. Acta Physiolologica Scandinavica 100:288–297

Snyder EM, Beck KC, Dietz NM, Eisenach JH, Joyner MJ, Turner ST, Johnson BD 2006 ARG16GLY polymorism of the beta-2 adrenergic receptor is associated with differences in cardiovascular function at rest and during exercise in humans. Journal of Physiology 571:121–130

Volianitis S, Yoshiga CC, Nissen P, Secher NH 2004 Effect of fitness on arm vascular and metabolic responses to upper body exercise. American Journal of Physiology 286:H1736–H1741

Wagner PD 1982 Influence of mixed venous PO_2 on diffusion of O_2 across the pulmonary blood-gas barrier. Clinical Physiology 2:105–115

Wagner PD 1993 Algebraic analysis of the determinants of VO_2max. Respiration Physiology 93:221–237

Wagner PD 1996a A theoretical analysis of factors determining VO_2max at sea level and altitude. Respiration Physiology 106(3):329–343

Wagner PD 1996b Determinants of maximal oxygen transport and utilization. Annual Review of Physiology 58:21–50

Wagner PD, Erickson BK, Seaman J, Kubo K, Hiraga A, Kai M, Yamaya Y 1996c Effects of altered FIO_2 on maximum VO_2 in the horse. Respiration Physiology 105:123–134

Wagner PD, Hoppeler H, Saltin B 1997 Determinants of maximal oxygen uptake. In: Crystal RG, West JB, Barnes PJ, Cherniack NS, Weibel ER (eds) The lung: scientific foundations, 3rd edn. Raven Press, New York, 1585–1593

Weibel ER 1984 The pathway for oxygen. Structure and function in the mammalian respiratory system. Harvard University Press, Cambridge, MA

Welch HG 1982 Hyperoxia and human performance: a brief review. Medicine and Science in Sports and Exercise 14(4):253–262

Welch HG 1987 Effects of hypoxia and hyperoxia on human performance. Exercise and Sports Sciences Reviews 15:191–221

Chapter 10.2

Human performance and maximal aerobic power

Timothy D. Noakes Björn Ekblom

INTRODUCTION

In preceding chapters, there has been extensive discussion of the central and peripheral causes of fatigue. It is clear that fatigue has many causes, with the importance of specific causal agents varying from one physiological state to another, and across modes and intensities of exercise. In this chapter, space has been allocated to debating a theory that challenges historical and contemporary theories of fatigue: the central governor model. It will be argued that, during exercise of increasing intensity, fatigue may also be associated with a centrally mediated regulation of exercise intensity (pacing). This theory does not exclude other causes of fatigue (e.g. catastrophe theory), but aims to highlight the possibility that other theories may not have included appropriate consideration for such central mechanisms. The central governor model is then refuted.

Several chapters form essential background reading for this discussion (e.g. Chapter 5). Indeed, the current chapter, in many respects, is a parallel discussion of the debate in Chapter 10.1, and there is also overlap with the introduction of Section 3, both of which deal with factors that may limit maximal aerobic power. However, herein readers will also find a discussion related to predicting human endurance performance on the basis of aerobic power measures.

Part A: The central governor model
Timothy D. Noakes

1 INTRODUCTION

Attempts to predict athletic performance from aerobic power began at the start of the previous century, based on a model developed by A.V. Hill (1920s), which predicts this form of exercise is limited by a peripherally based, metabolite-induced failure of skeletal muscle contractile function, independent of reduced muscle activation by the central nervous system; peripheral fatigue (Chapters 5, 6, 10.1 and 10.3). This model was critically dependent on the observations of Fletcher and Hopkins, who studied lactate concentrations in frog muscle, stimulated to induce fatigue, reporting a strong association between lactic acid production, fatigue and anaerobiosis (Needham & Baldwin 1949). They discovered that plunging samples into ice-cold alcohol immediately inactivated glycogenolysis, preventing lactic acid accumulation.

Hill and colleagues proposed that performance during high-intensity exercise was terminated by skeletal muscle anaerobiosis, resulting from reduced skeletal muscle blood flow accompanying myocardial ischaemia (Noakes 1998). Such anaerobiosis ultimately prevented the neutralisation of lactic acid, impairing skeletal muscle relaxation, and causing the involuntary termination of exercise. This logic led to the catastrophe theory (Noakes & St Clair Gibson 2004), which posits that exercise terminates when intracellular homeostasis is lost (Chapter 6), and the universal adoption of this peripheral fatigue model has encouraged the belief that all forms of exercise-induced fatigue result from the failure of cellular homeostasis, occurring when the biological capacity of the organ(s) has been exceeded.

Thus, one interpretation is that the limits of human aerobic exercise occur when cardiac output peaks, setting the upper limit for oxygen delivery (González-Alonso & Calbet 2003, Mitchell & Saltin 2003, Mortensen et al. 2005, Noakes et al. 2004), and driving anaerobic metabolism and lactate accumulation (see Chapter 10.3). The ability to perform maximal aerobic exercise can therefore be predicted by measuring the maximal cardiac output or its surrogate, peak or maximal oxygen uptake (maximal aerobic power; $V_{O_{2max}}$).

It is my argument that the Hill model cannot explain how physiological function is regulated during exercise, and that maximal aerobic power is influenced by movement economy (efficiency) and peak work rate. Thus, the fastest endurance athletes are often those who are the most economical and achieve the highest peak work rates during maximal exercise, regardless of the actual maximal aerobic power achieved. A more likely explanation for the factors predicting human performance is provided by a model in which fatigue forms part of a regulated, anticipatory response, coordinated centrally, with the ultimate goal being to preserve homeostasis (Noakes et al. 2005, St Clair Gibson & Noakes 2004). Thus, there are two reasons why it is not possible to predict human performance on the basis of maximal aerobic power.

First, the model on which this prediction is based is too simplistic, and based on a process of reductionism in which the limiting factors are usually reduced to one or two, typically cardiovascular variables such as the maximum cardiac output (González-Alonso & Calbet 2003, Mortensen et al. 2005, Noakes et al. 2004) and the capacity to extract oxygen (Mitchell & Saltin 2003). But there is little evidence to support the theory that maximal exercise terminates because of an oxygen delivery failure (Noakes et al. 2004). Rather, we have argued that human exercise performance is regulated in anticipation, by an intelligent complex system (St Clair Gibson & Noakes 2004, Tucker et al. 2006a).

Indeed, the crucial weakness of this reductionist model is that it allows no role for the brain and factors such as motivation, mental toughness, experience, pharmacological manipulations (Sgherza et al. 2002, Watson et al. 2005) or even hypnosis or music on human performance. Most importantly, this model fails completely to include a feedforward loop from brain to muscle, which initially establishes the work output, and hence the metabolic rate from the beginning of the exercise bout. Rather, it seems to consider only the direct effect of chemical changes in muscle which cause muscular fatigue and the termination of exercise. But how did the muscle contract in the first place? Did this occur in the absence of feedforward drive from the motor cortex? As a result, this model includes no explanation for the role of anticipation of what is to come. Yet how are we to explain the different paces at which we choose to exercise?

Since pacing is determined from the very first step in a race (e.g. 100 m versus 1000 km), it has to be an anticipatory response. Similarly, the decision of exactly when to terminate any exercise bout must be made by the central nervous system (Kayser 2003). There is now clear evidence that this decision is planned shortly after the onset of the exercise bout, regardless of its duration (Noakes 2004, Tucker et al. 2006a). Yet, we persist in our belief that anticipation can play no part in determining our biological response to exercise, and that only the poisonous products of skeletal muscle metabolism, acting directly in those muscles and influenced by oxygen delivery, determine that response. It is a devotion to a foundation myth that defies logical explanation (Noakes 2005a).

Second, even if Hill's model is correct, predictions based on it presume that the predictive power of aerobic power measurements are independent of all other factors. Yet, we showed that a better predictor of running performance was the peak power achieved during a maximal exercise test and not the peak oxygen uptake (Noakes et al. 1990). In part, this can be explained by individual differences in exercise economy and probably by differences in skeletal muscle contractility and recruitment (Noakes 2003). Thus, even if oxygen delivery was the sole determinant of athletic performance, it would remain a less than optimal predictor if individual differences in economy and peak power production are not considered.

2 WHY THE REDUCTIONIST MODEL OF HUMAN PERFORMANCE LIMITS CANNOT BE CORRECT

The popular view is that fatigue during most forms of exercise is due to a peripherally based, metabolite-induced failure of skeletal muscle contractile function (peripheral fatigue), independent of skeletal muscle activation from the motor cortex (central fatigue). This view is referred to as the cardiovascular, anaerobic or catastrophic model. In this model, lactic acid acts as a peripheral regulator that impairs skeletal muscle function (e.g. relaxation) leading to fatigue and involuntary exercise termination. In fact, Hill believed that lactic acid initiated muscle contraction (Noakes 1998) and his model predicts that the failure to remove the excess lactic acid would cause exercise to terminate as a result of skeletal muscle rigor. Yet, to my knowledge, no athletic competition has yet been lost by an athlete who developed skeletal muscle rigor. But, more to the point is that Hill's writings were so influential that, for the past 80 years, exercise physiologists have indeed taught that athletics is purely energetics and biochemistry (Bassett & Howley 2000). Forgotten has been the process of muscle stimulation, the feed-forward component of motor control (Kayser 2003, St Clair Gibson & Noakes 2004). So to begin this debate, I present the evidence showing the weaknesses of the Hill model.

2.1 Contention 1: The Hill model, as currently taught, is not the model Hill believed

The catastrophic model is depicted in Figure 10.2.1. Hill believed that during high-intensity, short-duration exercise, the maximal cardiac output was achieved, resulting in myocardial ischaemia and decline in cardiac output. This falling cardiac output resulted in inadequate oxygen delivery to the exercising muscles, leading to anaerobiosis (Noakes 1988, 1997, 1998, 2000). The initiating cause of skeletal muscle anaerobiosis is myocardial failure, secondary to a limiting of myocardial oxygen delivery that threatens a potentially catastrophic myocardial ischaemia.

Since Hill presumed that uncontrolled myocardial ischaemia would cause irreversible heart damage, he proposed the existence of a governor, which acted by reducing the pumping capacity of the heart during ischaemia. This component of the Hill model disappeared from subsequent generations of textbooks, following the demise of *Bainbridge's Textbook of Physiology* (Bainbridge 1931), which records how Hill's ideas were embraced by David Dill and colleagues at the Harvard Fatigue Laboratory (Dill 1938).

The pivotal event in the universal acceptance of Hill's model occurred when Taylor et al. (1955) proposed that a plateau in oxygen uptake can be identified in most (94%) humans during laboratory testing. But the crucial impor-

tance of that study is that it was based on the acceptance (Noakes 1988, 1997, 1998, 2000, 2003) by these authors of Hill's core belief that an oxygen deficiency alone (whether in the heart or skeletal muscles) limits maximal exercise. As a result, the plateau phenomenon became entrenched as the virtual marker of a hypothetical intracellular event (anaerobiosis), secondary to a plateau in cardiac output and myocardial ischaemia. This is the central pillar of the Hill model and the basis for the belief that performance can be predicted solely from tests of aerobic power.

2.2 Contention 2: The Hill model makes six absolute predictions, none of which has been shown to be true

2.2.1 Prediction 1

If the development of oxygen deficiency in the active muscles is the exclusive factor limiting maximum exercise performance, and if the plateau phenomenon is the external marker of anaerobiosis, then a plateau must occur in 100% of subjects at exhaustion during each progressive exercise test. However, this fails to occur in >50% of progressive exercise tests (Noakes & St Clair Gibson 2004). The point is that if exercise at the subject's limit of tolerance terminates without evidence for an abrupt plateau (in each exercise test), then there is no reason to continue the belief in Hill's original theory. Without a plateau, the theory loses its foundation (no plateau equals no anaerobiosis) and oxygen delivery does not limit maximal exercise. That there may be an absolute and reproducible maximal rate of oxygen consumption in each individual is not relevant to this argument. According to the complex system model (St Clair Gibson & Noakes 2004), the activation of any number of regulatory controls other than skeletal muscle anaerobiosis could explain this finding.

2.2.2 Prediction 2

Skeletal muscle anaerobiosis must develop at exhaustion during maximum exercise. Presently, no study has conclusively established that skeletal muscle hypoxia or anaero-

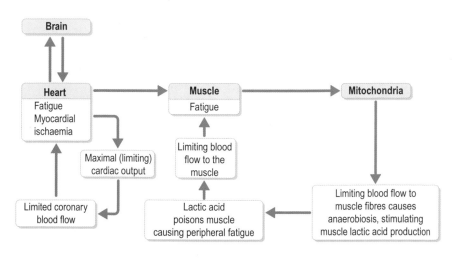

Figure 10.2.1 The catastrophic model in which the development of myocardial ischaemia leads to skeletal muscle anaerobiosis, lactic acidosis and muscle fatigue. From Grubbström et al. (1991), used with permission.

biosis develops during voluntary exercise in humans (Noakes & St Clair Gibson 2004). Rather, the published evidence indicates that the intracellular oxygen tension does not reach critically low values, despite large changes in the external work rate (Noakes & St Clair Gibson 2004). Such findings are incompatible with Hill's interpretation that the maximal exercise is limited by skeletal muscle anaerobiosis. Hence the conclusion must be that maximal exercise terminates for reasons other than anaerobiosis.

2.2.3 Prediction 3

To maximise skeletal muscle blood flow and oxygen delivery, cardiac output must always be maximum at fatigue since the heart is the slave to the oxygen demands of exercising muscles. This prediction stems from the conclusion that most circulatory adaptations are designed to increase muscle blood supply during exercise (McDowall 1938), and studies showing that, at rest, muscle blood flow is regulated to insure a constant oxygen delivery (González-Alonso et al. 2006). The assumption is that the same regulation must exist during exercise. If this is correct, then oxygen delivery to satisfy exercising muscle demands must be the principal focus of the heart. But there are a number of findings that show that this peripheral regulation, present during mild–moderate exercise, cannot also be the most important controller during maximum exercise.

If maximum oxygen uptake is limited by a maximum cardiac output, then the latter must also plateau during maximum exercise. However, with two notable exceptions (González-Alonso & Calbet 2003, Mortensen et al. 2005), the literature shows that cardiac output increases linearly with work rate up to the maximal oxygen uptake, with no evidence of a plateau (Noakes & St Clair Gibson 2004). If anything, cardiac function appears to be enhanced at maximal work rates, especially in trained athletes (Noakes & St Clair Gibson 2004). The studies showing a plateau in cardiac output used an exercise protocol in which work rate increased from low to maximal within 5 min: non-steady state conditions. Stroke volume fell in these experiments, whereas central venous pressure rose, indicating the onset of myocardial failure, which is unusual for maximal exercise (Noakes & St Clair Gibson 2004).

An especially important prediction of the Hill model is that cardiac output must always be high under conditions of hypoxia or anaemia, when cardiac output becomes the only factor that can maintain a maximum oxygen delivery. Thus, if the heart is indeed the slave to the peripheral muscles, then the maximum cardiac output cannot ever be lower, for example, in hypoxia or anaemia than in normoxia or normocythaemia, unless the function of the heart is itself altered either directly or indirectly, by those states. But maximum cardiac output is reduced under those conditions (Noakes & St Clair Gibson 2004). Furthermore, this same effect is present during single-legged exercise in hypoxia (Noakes & St Clair Gibson 2004), when the peak cardiac output is decidedly submaximal.

Finally, Calbet et al. (2002, 2003, 2004) have shown that, despite a 36% increase in haemoglobin concentration (Calbet et al. 2002) and a 37–54% increase in oxygen delivery (Calbet et al. 2003), induced by altitude acclimatisation, neither maximal oxygen uptake nor peak work rate increased during subsequent maximal exercise testing at altitude (5260 m). Nor did plasma volume expansion influence these variables (Calbet et al. 2004). These observations indicate that factors other than cardiac output and oxygen delivery determine maximum exercise performance and aerobic power during hypoxia (Noakes et al. 2004). In contrast, Amann et al. (2006) have shown that the extent of skeletal muscle recruitment is progressively reduced with increasingly severe hypoxia, as predicted by the central governor model (Kayser 2003, Noakes et al. 2004). Hence, the low maximal cardiac output at altitude and in other conditions is due to low levels of skeletal muscle recruitment by the motor cortex, causing a low demand for blood flow.

2.2.4 Prediction 4

Models of peripheral fatigue predict there must always be recruitment of all motor units in the active limbs at fatigue. A graphic used to illustrate factors that may limit the maximum oxygen uptake is shown in Figure 10.2.2. However, lacking from this figure is the central nervous system necessary to recruit skeletal muscle motor units, that is, the feedforward component that must be present in any model of human movement.

Whilst Figures 10.2.1 and 10.2.2 provide a valid depiction of the predictions of the catastrophic model, either is correct only if there is always complete motor unit recruitment, since if <100% of the motor units are active at fatigue, then it is difficult to understand how a peripheral fatigue mechanism can regulate the function of fibres that are not actively contracting, as they have yet to be recruited by the central nervous system, or how it can prevent recruitment of additional quiescent fibres by the central nervous system in order to overcome 'fatigue' or exhaustion. Recruitment of those fibres would allow exercise to continue longer, resulting in a higher oxygen uptake. Thus, if motor unit recruitment is <100%, then a peripheral fatigue mechanism cannot be assumed, unless a limitation within the central nervous system has first been excluded. But if motor unit recruitment is unknown, one cannot exclude the possibility that an inability to recruit additional motor units limits maximal oxygen uptake. Thus, it may not be an oxygen delivery limitation, but an oxygen demand limitation.

Several studies have shown that fatigue during maximum exercise to exhaustion occurs when <100% of the motor units in the tested limbs have been recruited. First, studies show that electromyographic activity, and the number of motor units recruited, is lower at exhaustion during maximum exercise at altitude than at sea level (Noakes & St Clair Gibson 2004); fatigue precedes 100% recruitment. Furthermore, increasing the oxygen content of the inspired air during exercise at altitude improves performance by

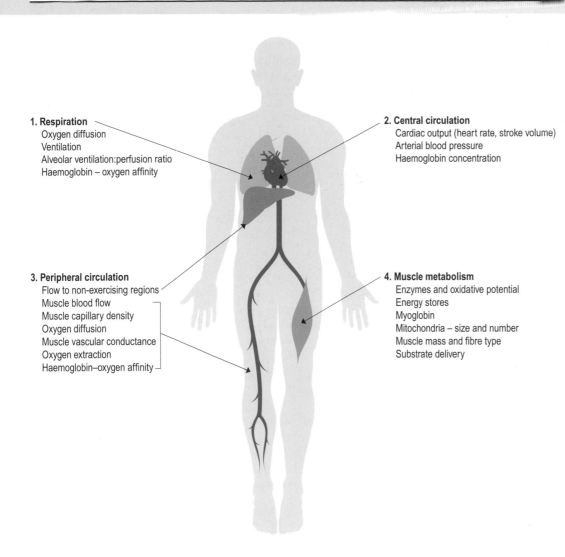

Figure 10.2.2 A popular depiction of the factors believed to limit the maximum oxygen consumption. Missing are the central (brain) and peripheral nervous systems without which exercise is impossible. From Hammond et al. (1992), used with permission.

1. Respiration
  Oxygen diffusion
  Ventilation
  Alveolar ventilation:perfusion ratio
  Haemoglobin – oxygen affinity

2. Central circulation
  Cardiac output (heart rate, stroke volume)
  Arterial blood pressure
  Haemoglobin concentration

3. Peripheral circulation
  Flow to non-exercising regions
  Muscle blood flow
  Muscle capillary density
  Oxygen diffusion
  Muscle vascular conductance
  Oxygen extraction
  Haemoglobin–oxygen affinity

4. Muscle metabolism
  Enzymes and oxidative potential
  Energy stores
  Myoglobin
  Mitochondria – size and number
  Muscle mass and fibre type
  Substrate delivery

increasing electromyographic activity in the exercising limbs (Kayser et al. 1994). Second, exercise-induced contrast shifts in magnetic resonance images indicate that only 40–90% of the motor units in lower limb muscles are recruited during progressive running to exhaustion (Noakes & St Clair Gibson 2004).

Therefore, there is no conclusive evidence that all of the available motor units are recruited at the point of maximal oxygen uptake during whole-body exercise in normoxia. Without such evidence, it is not possible to exclude the central nervous system from determining maximal exercise performance, either partially or wholly.

2.2.5 Prediction 5

Fatigue must always develop when a similar concentration of peripheral (inhibiting) metabolites has been reached. This prediction would seem to be disproved by the lactate paradox of high altitude (Noakes & St Clair Gibson 2004), in which fatigue occurs at different blood lactate concentrations during exercise at different altitudes, by the finding that patients with chronic diseases terminate exercise at low blood lactate concentrations (Noakes & St Clair Gibson

2004), and by the observation that interventions (endurance training, oxygen therapy) allow higher blood lactate concentrations and higher work rates, and hence a greater motor unit recruitment, after the intervention. Conversely, anaemia causes exercise termination at lower blood lactate concentrations (Noakes & St Clair Gibson 2004). Hence, these studies dissociate a specific blood or muscle lactate concentration and fatigue development (see Chapters 6 and 10.3).

More significantly, Nielsen et al. (2001) showed that lactic acid restores normal function to isolated rat soleus muscle, whose function has been impaired by perfusion with an elevated potassium concentration. The authors conclude that lactate accumulation protects against muscular fatigue (Chapter 6). Similarly, Pedersen et al. (2004) found that intracellular acidosis increased the excitability of intramuscular tubules, thereby maintaining normal excitation-contraction coupling despite intracellular potassium accumulation.

This multifaceted role would be most probable if lactate is one of the preferred fuels for skeletal muscle metabolism (Gladden 2004), as it is for cardiac muscle when blood lactate concentrations are elevated (Noakes & St Clair Gibson 2004). It seems paradoxical that the preferred fuel for the maximally working heart is supposedly toxic to the maximally working skeletal muscle (Figure 10.2.1). One also wonders why respiratory muscles are not affected by lactic acid during maximal exercise. Hence, if lactic acid is not the peripheral regulator predicted by Hill, then another mechanism must insure that muscles terminate exercise before they develop rigor.

2.2.6 Prediction 6

Fatigue must always be absolute. If it is the accumulation of metabolites that causes fatigue, then their accumulation must lead to the onset of an absolute fatigue, which requires recovery and metabolite removal before exercise can again begin (St Clair Gibson & Noakes 2004). This forms the basis for studies evaluating the effects of different recovery periods on metabolism and exercise performance, since it is presumed the two are casually linked (Noakes & St Clair Gibson 2004). Yet, these studies clearly show that fatigue is not absolute since, regardless of the level of exhaustion, exercise can always be continued in a subsequent bout, albeit at a lower intensity. Indeed, Hargreaves et al. (1998) found performance was the same in the first and final bouts of exercise, regardless of the amount of exercise undertaken in between, suggesting a pacing strategy (Ansley et al. 2004, Kay et al. 2001) that regulated the exercise intensity throughout exercise.

Thus, it is a common observation that even the most exhausted marathon runner can, at any time, choose to walk rather than to continue running. Hence those metabolites believed to cause peripheral fatigue must have only a partial effect. To my knowledge, no one has yet chosen to explain how such constrainers act only partially. Furthermore, the absolute fatigue requirement is at variance with what happens during competition in which athletes usually speed up in the last 10% of races lasting more than about 2 minutes (Noakes & St Clair Gibson 2004, Tucker et al. 2006b).

2.3 Contention 3: If oxygen uptake limits maximum aerobic exercise, individual differences in the economy of movement reduce the accuracy of predicting performance

2.3.1 Peak work rate and fatigue resistance

Peak work rate and the ability to sustain a high percentage of that mode-specific work rate (fatigue resistance) are the best predictors of performance during that activity. However, based on the assumption that oxygen delivery limits aerobic exercise, the maximal aerobic power test is the most frequently used predictor of athletic ability. It is assumed that a greater oxygen transport capacity would delay the onset of anaerobic conditions and fatigue. There is now sufficient experience to prove that these predictions have not been fulfilled.

First, amongst elite athletes with quite similar performances, maximal oxygen uptake can vary quite dramatically (Table 10.2.1). For example, Steve Prefontaine and Frank Shorter differed substantially in maximal aerobic power (by 16%), yet they had 1 (1.6 km) and 3 mile (4.8 km) times that differed by <8 s (3.4%) and <0.2 s. If maximal oxygen uptake is the sole explanation for differences in performance, then Prefontaine should have been much better at all distances. Similarly, despite a substantially higher maximal aerobic power, Joan Benoit's marathon times were not faster than Derek Clayton's, who held the world marathon record despite a relatively poor maximal aerobic power. These examples indicate this index becomes a less effective predictor of performance as distance increases. The alternative paradox is that some athletes with quite similar maximal oxygen uptake have quite different running performances. Compare the performances of Craig Virgin, Alberto Salazar, Grete Waitz and Cavin Woodward (ultramarathoner; Table 10.2.1).

Thus, the maximal aerobic power test, whilst being an excellent predictor of performance in athletes of very widely varying abilities, is a less effective predictor for longer duration events, due to its relatively short duration

Table 10.2.1 Maximum oxygen uptake and performance (data from Noakes 2003)

Athlete	Country	Major performance	$\dot{V}O_{2max}$
Steve Prefontaine	USA	03:54.6 1 mile	84 mL·kg^{-1}·min^{-1}
Craig Virgin	USA	2:10:26 marathon	81 mL·kg^{-1}·min^{-1}
Joan Benoit	USA	2:24:52 marathon	78 mL·kg^{-1}·min^{-1}
Alberto Salazar	USA	2:08:13 marathon	76 mL·kg^{-1}·min^{-1}
Cavin Woodward	U.K.	2:19:50 marathon	74 mL·kg^{-1}·min^{-1}
Grete Waitz	Norway	2:25:29 marathon	73 mL·kg^{-1}·min^{-1}
Frank Shorter	USA	2:10:30 marathon	71 mL·kg^{-1}·min^{-1}
Derek Clayton	Australia	2:08:34 marathon	69 mL·kg^{-1}·min^{-1}

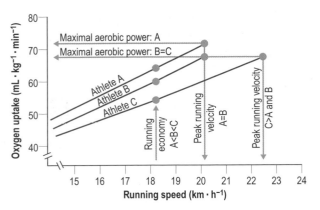

Figure 10.2.3 Running economy, peak treadmill running speed and maximal oxygen uptake in three runners (A, B, C). According to the Hill model, runner A will be the best; according to the central governor model, runner C will perform the best.

and high intensity (it lacks specificity). However, its poor predictive qualities for more elite athletic performance may stem from differences in both the economy of movement and peak work rate during maximal exercise (Noakes 2003).

To explain this phenomenon, Figure 10.2.3 compares oxygen uptake at submaximal speeds (economy) and maximal running velocity of three runners. Runner C is the most economical and also achieves the highest peak treadmill velocity, but with a maximal oxygen uptake equal to that of runner B but lower than runner A (least economical). When runners A and B reach peak running speeds, runner A has a higher oxygen uptake. It has been shown that the best athletes are usually also the most economical (Noakes 1988). Conley & Krahenbuhl (1980) studied 12 runners whose best 10 km times were closely bunched (30:31 to 33:33 min). Maximal oxygen uptake ranged from 67 to 78 mL·kg^{-1}·min^{-1} and could not predict 10 km times. However, there was an excellent correlation between submaximal running economy and 10 km times; the most economical runners had the fastest times. The authors concluded that a high maximal oxygen uptake helped each athlete gain membership of this elite group, but within this group, running economy determined success.

I would interpret those data somewhat differently. Athletes with different running economies and a similar maximal aerobic power must differ in peak speeds (Figure 10.2.3; B versus C). Thus, the crucial physiological data are peak treadmill running velocities subjects achieved during a maximal, progressive exercise test. There are now many studies showing that peak treadmill running velocity is at least as good a predictor of running performance as any other variable, and substantially superior to maximal aerobic power (Lacour et al. 1991, Morgan et al. 1989, Noakes et al. 1990, Scott & Houmard 1994). Thus, according to these predictions, runner C would be the fastest at any distance. The low maximal oxygen uptake is a reflec-

tion of a superior running economy, with superior performance being related to an ability to achieve the highest peak running speed. The athlete in Table 10.2.1 who most closely fits this description would be Derek Clayton, one of the most economical runners studied, with a relatively low maximal oxygen uptake, but who held the marathon world record. Similar differences in economy also account for variations in the performance of adolescents (Chapter 15).

2.3.2 Differences in fatigue resistance

One of the most interesting recent phenomena in athletics has been the rise of East African runners, especially Kenyans and Ethiopians, to dominance in the 3000 m steeplechase and 12 km cross-country events (Pitsiladis et al. 2007). Currently, Kenyans win 40–50% of medals in international competitions for distances from 800 m to the marathon. No international sport has ever been dominated to such an extent by athletes from one country.

Studies of Kenyan runners have so far failed to provide a definitive physiological answer for their manifest superiority as distance runners (Pitsiladis et al. 2007). The only other study of elite (South) African runners (Coetzer et al. 1993) reported physiological data from one of the best groups of distance and middle-distance runners yet evaluated. Running performances of both groups were similar at race distances up to 3 km, but the distance runners became significantly better at the longer distances. The distance runners were lighter and smaller, with a slightly lower proportion of type I muscle fibres, but they were able to run substantially faster at all distances >5 km, despite having a maximal aerobic power equivalent to the middle-distance runners. Thus, they were able to sustain a substantially higher proportion of their maximal oxygen uptake when racing. Thus, superior performance was explained by superior fatigue resistance. Other studies have also found that (South) African distance runners have superior fatigue resistance when compared to sub-elite Caucasian runners of similar abilities (Bosch et al. 1990, Harley & Noakes 2006, Weston et al. 1999).

Maximal aerobic power may be unable to discriminate between good and superior performance in events lasting more than a few minutes; the majority of sporting events. This failure stems from the inability to measure or predict fatigue resistance during prolonged submaximal exercise on the basis of measures taken during a test of progressive, maximal exercise lasting only a few minutes.

The concept that endurance athletes differ in their fatigue resistance is not new. What has perhaps not always been appreciated is that physiological factors determining maximal oxygen uptake and the sustained (relative) exercise intensity ($\dot{V}_{O_{2max}}$%) during prolonged exercise might be quite different. Thus, a high maximal oxygen uptake value does not guarantee the capacity to sustain a high exercise intensity and vice versa. A possible explanation for differences in running performance may be differences in the sustainable exercise intensity. The possible reasons for this ability have recently been reviewed according to a complex, but not a reductionist model of human performance (Harley & Noakes 2006).

3 CONCLUSION

An unfortunate consequence of the Hill catastrophic model is that it encouraged scientists to believe that a single physiological function, in particular oxygen delivery and consumption, limits exercise and determines performance. This reductionist approach (Noakes 2005b) has fostered the concept that a single laboratory test can be used to predict competitive ability.

I have advanced three reasons why such a test cannot predict performance. First, there is no evidence that oxygen delivery limits exercise performance (Noakes & St Clair Gibson 2004). Rather, a more probable model is that exercise performance is regulated centrally and in anticipation by a complex, intelligent system (Noakes et al. 2005, St Clair Gibson & Noakes 2004, Tucker et al. 2006a): the central governor model. Second, humans differ in running economy, fatigue resistance, and peak work rates. Third, the best athletes are those with a superior physiology and better able to maintain homeostasis despite very high metabolic rates, heat production and eccentric muscle loading. This allows sustained higher rates of muscle recruitment from muscles with superior contractility (Harley & Noakes 2006, Nummela et al. 2006). Hence they exhibit superior fatigue resistance, but that resistance is set by the brain on the basis of an anticipatory response, learned in training and previous competitions and modified in response to what is happening during exercise.

This central governor model is the converse of the Hill model. Perhaps, were Hill alive today, he would be the first to agree. For in 1933, he wrote:

> In the case of bodily movement the nervous system is the steersman, who has to compound all the messages – the nerve waves – he receives to form one general impression on which to act . . . The continual reaction between muscles, nerves, end-organs and central nervous system is the physiological basis of muscular skill and on its smooth and efficient working depend many of the things that mankind finds worthy of accomplishment. (Hill 1965, p.117)

Part B: A response to the central governor model
Björn Ekblom

1 INTRODUCTION

The central governor model is presented as a theory in which overall physical performance is regulated by the subconscious brain. This model states that, during strenuous exercise and increasing fatigue, the neuronal output from the brain is controlled so that if the brain estimates, by some mechanism, that the physical strain will be too hard for important organs and physiological systems, then neuronal output is reduced to avoid serious failure of general homeostasis (e.g. cardiac ischaemia). This model is built more on criticism of the commonly accepted catastrophic model than scientific proof for a central governor. Even if some aspects of the central governor model and critiques of catastrophic model are valid, the former cannot explain, in my view, all of the physiological consequences that lead to fatigue and termination of severe exercise.

Fatigue and performance decrement can be explained by factors anywhere from the brain to the muscle (Chapters 1, 2, 5, 6, 7 and 10.1). Central fatigue involves activities of the central nervous system, the base for the central governor and central cardiorespiratory functions (e.g. pumping and oxygen delivery), while peripheral fatigue mainly refers to peripheral nervous system, signal transduction, gas exchange, energy turnover and force production. However, there is no clear boundary separating central and peripheral factors (Chapter 10.1). Energy availability through oxygen transport is of vital importance for the whole fatigue spectrum, but is mostly related to the periphery. Since the central governor model is supposed to influence maximal aerobic power, which has long been regarded as the most important factor for both cardiorespiratory and overall endurance performance, I will focus on the central governor model as an explanation of the limitation of maximal aerobic power and also present my view of what limits aerobic power.

Every type of physical activity has its unique performance capacity profile. Different types of performances depend on, and are explained by different physiological, psychological and environmental factors, but the dependence and importance of each factor for performance in athletic pursuits are widely variable. For instance, in endurance sports, the physiological profile for elite performances may, from a naive perspective, look very similar. But athletes, trainers and exercise physiologists know that the physiological demands differ widely across endurance events. Thus, the best cross-country runners and skiers are seldom the best track runners or road cyclists, despite some common physiological capacities.

This event-related specificity of critical (limiting) physiological factors is illustrated in track running, where there is no close cross-over of elite performance between neighbouring distances (200 and 800 m or 400 and 1500 m). This performance specificity among individuals was exemplified by Noakes. If we also add the complexity of the interaction among factors determining overall physical performance, we simply cannot expect to find a good correlation between a single physiological factor (e.g. maximal oxygen uptake) and endurance performance. Noakes also stresses this, and most exercise physiologists, although not all sports scientists, accept this fact. But the same must also be true for the central governor model. The task and factor specificity in different physiological performances makes it difficult to believe that fatigue, across all types of physical performances, is regulated and determined by a single factor: the subconscious brain. There are, of course, different substances, liberated from active muscles (metabolites), and also some reflex systems that can report to the brain and, thus, act as messengers (feedback; Chapter 18) between the working muscles and the central command. But these mechanisms must vary considerably across different types of work and so their role, as factors responsible for fatigue, must also vary.

One line of argument for the central governor model is the pacing strategy (Gibson et al. 2006). For me, this is a fairly simplistic argument. Any experienced runner knows (the conscious brain) that one cannot start a 1 km race with 100 m speed. The fact that fatigue can be sensed by the brain does not mean that a central governor controls fatigue. Observe children when they compete in endurance races. Their inexperience makes them run very fast to start with, but after a while they must reduce their speed or stop. If the subconscious brain regulates the pace strategy and fatigue development, then this would not happen. Or are there differences between children and adults in this respect? If so, at which age does the subconscious brain take over?

An important part of the central governor model is that neuronal output is reduced during maximal exercise to avoid serious disturbances in cardiac function and, thus, maximal aerobic power is regulated and limited by the subconscious brain (Gibson & Noakes 2004, Noakes 1997). According to this model, maximal oxygen uptake is only a consequence of the amount of work that the heart is allowed to perform by the governor, and not a consequence of oxygen delivery to the periphery reaching its maximum during maximal exercise involving large muscle groups. On the other hand, if maximal oxygen uptake depends on the central circulation during maximal exercise, then what is the bottleneck? Furthermore, how do we know that the muscles can accept all of the oxygen delivered during maximal exercise and that there is not a peripheral limitation? These questions will be addressed below.

2 ARE THERE SIGNS OF CARDIAC ISCHAEMIA DURING SEVERE EXERCISE?

I am not aware of any study that has observed heart muscle ischaemia or signs thereof, during severe exercise in healthy subjects during normal conditions, not even at extreme (simulated) altitudes corresponding to Mt Everest (Malconian et al. 1990, Reeves el al 1987). This can, of course, be a proof of the protecting effect of a central governor against cardiac ischaemia. But the basic prerequisite for ischaemia during severe exercise is that the heart's metabolic capacity is utilised to its maximum and myocardial blood flow is also maximal. But this is not the case for two reasons.

First, three studies have shown there is a reserve in myocardial blood flow and myocardial oxygen uptake during

maximal exercise (Grubbström et al. 1991, 1993, Kaijser et al. 1993). These experiments reduced the oxygen content of coronary blood during maximal exercise by breathing either 12% or 15% oxygen, and compared data with that obtained during normoxia. The resulting hypoxaemia was almost totally met by a compensatory increase (35%) in coronary sinus blood flow and a slightly more complete oxygen extraction, so that myocardial oxygen uptake was almost maintained at the same level during both hypoxaemia and normoxaemia (Figure 10.2.4). At this point, there was also a lactate release from the heart muscle in the hypoxaemic state. Thus, during maximal exercise in normoxia, myocardial blood flow was not maximal and there were no signs of anaerobic energy turnover, as with hypoxaemia. It was concluded that the heart has a coronary flow reserve that can be used during severe stress.

Second, this finding is supported by a recent experiment from our laboratory (Brink-Elfegoun et al. 2006). We measured cardiac output and blood pressure during two different maximal, combined arm–leg exercise bouts (average 387 and 426 W, respectively). Maximal oxygen uptake, as well as peak heart rate and cardiac output, were the same in each exercise bout, but mean arterial and systolic (but not diastolic) pressures were higher during the heavier exercise bout. Myocardial oxygen uptake is indicated by the product of cardiac output or heart rate times blood pressure (Kitamura et al. 1972, Nelson et al. 1974). This index was higher during the higher work rate, indicating greater cardiac strain and, consequently, myocardial oxygen uptake must also have been higher. Thus, at the lower maximal work rate, creating the same maximal oxygen uptake as the higher one, myocardial oxygen uptake and blood flow were not maximal.

Both of these studies indicate that there is a cardiac reserve capacity for oxygen uptake and blood flow during

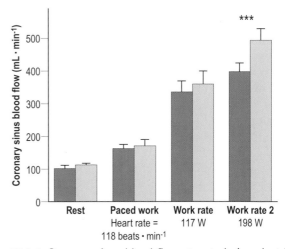

Figure 10.2.4 Coronary sinus blood flow at rest, during electrical stimulation of heart rate at rest (paced work) and during submaximal (work rate 1) and maximal exercise (work rate 2) breathing air (filled bars) and 15% oxygen in nitrogen: *** denotes P < 0.001. Adapted from Grubbström et al. (1990) with permission.

normal conditions, even during maximal exercise. Thus, the prerequisite for myocardial ischaemia, during maximal exercise in normal conditions in healthy subjects, and for the central governor model does not exist.

3 MAXIMAL AEROBIC POWER

The limitations of maximal aerobic power have been an issue of debate since Hill & Lupton (1923) first discussed the topic, with many theories subsequently being hypothesised. Hoppeler et al. (1987) proposed a peripheral limitation, in which the skeletal muscle oxidative capacity, mainly total mitochondrial volume, limits maximal oxygen uptake. Further support for a limitation due to mitochondrial oxygen extraction was forwarded by Wagner and colleagues (Richardson et al. 1995, Wagner 1992). These theories have been rejected by some researchers (see below), as well as the peripheral limitation theory from Clausen (1976), who suggested that the vasodilatation in relation to cardiac output sets the upper limits for maximal oxygen transport. A 'symmorphosis' theory was presented by Weibel's group (Taylor & Weibel 1981, Taylor et al. 1987), suggesting there was no single limiting factor, since all links in the oxygen delivery system chain are in harmony and designed so that each step just meets the functional demand. Their view was supported by di Prampero (1985, 2003), who analysed these links, as resistances in Ohm's Law, during severe dynamic exercise. The greatest resistance to oxygen delivery was attributed to central circulation but other links also played a role.

The theory of a harmonised oxygen transport chain during maximal exercise is in line with the view I advocate, in which the oxygen transported from the left ventricle to the periphery (cardiac output ($\dot{Q}$) times oxygen content of arterial blood (CaO_2)) is the basic determinant for maximal aerobic power ($\dot{V}_{O_2max}$). Thus, changes in different factors within the oxygen delivery chain, such as variations in haemoglobin concentration ([Hb]), oxygen content of inspired air (F_IO_2), arterial oxygen saturation (S_aO_2), or the type of exercise may only modify the aerobic power obtained under optimal conditions. As Bassett & Howley (1997) point out, a plateau in oxygen uptake (relative to increasing rate of work) is not necessary for establishing a cardiovascular limitation but, in most cases, it helps. Therefore, in my view, maximal aerobic power is the highest oxygen uptake obtained under optimal conditions (e.g. combined arm and leg incremental exercise) with minimal arterial desaturation, and during which oxygen uptake levels off. Uphill running and combined arm and leg exercise will result in an oxygen uptake plateau for most healthy subjects: maximal oxygen uptake. However, when oxygen uptake fails to plateau (e.g. cycling), oxygen uptake is often 5–10% lower than its true maximal level (Bergh et al. 1976, Stenberg et al. 1967). This is best described as a peak oxygen uptake ($\dot{V}_{O_2peak}$)

This difference between maximal and peak oxygen uptake is essential, not only for the value obtained but for the question regarding limitations of maximal oxygen uptake. For instance, using findings and interpretations from studies of peak data is, in most cases, irrelevant to the discussion of maximal limitations. It has been argued that the peripheral, intramuscular 'black box', which includes factors such as the inhomogeneity of blood flow, oxygen unloading, tissue oxygenation and phosphocreatine recovery rate, could be a candidate for limiting aerobic power. It might be of interest when peak oxygen uptake is the base for discussion but not, in my view, when maximal oxygen uptake is being considered. For detailed discussion of different limiting factors see: di Prampero (1985, 2003), Bassett & Howley (1997), Roberts (2001), Chapter 10.1. In the following subsections, short comments are provided regarding these limitations, along with primary source materials.

3.1 Is there a peripheral limitation?

The answer is both 'yes' and 'no'. The former is quite evident when small muscle groups (e.g. one leg exercise, arms only) are activated, but also in some cases where only an oxygen uptake peak is achieved. But which arguments and facts are available concerning the latter?

3.1.1 Muscle blood flow capacity

Muscle blood flow capacity and oxygen uptake during exercise were studied by Andersen & Saltin (1985), using a single-leg kick model during incremental (graded) exercise. They found that peak muscle blood flow and oxygen uptake were ~2.5 and 0.35 $L·kg^{-1}·min^{-1}$ (respectively). Extrapolated to whole-body exercise (running uphill or combined arm and leg exercise), this means that when ~25–30 kg of skeletal muscle are active, the potential for muscle blood flow and oxygen uptake would be up to 75 and 10 $L·min^{-1}$ (respectively), and far above the highest values obtained for these measures.

3.1.2 Total mitochondrial volume

Hoppeler et al. (1987) proposed that skeletal muscle oxidative capacity, mainly total mitochondrial volume, limits maximal oxygen uptake. When only the arms are working maximally, normal subjects can reach ~70% of their true, whole-body maximal oxygen uptake (Bergh et al. 1976). However, adding maximal arm to maximal leg work only marginally enhances maximal oxygen uptake, although the total mitochondrial volume is increased substantially (Bergh et al. 1976, Stenberg et al. 1967). Nor are there any differences in maximal cardiac output between maximal leg and maximal combined arm and leg exercise, despite a higher total muscle mass being engaged in exercise (Stenberg et al. 1967).

3.1.3 Total muscle aerobic enzyme capacity

The theory that enzyme capacity could limit maximal aerobic power was challenged when arterial oxygen content was increased during maximal exercise. This was achieved by increasing haemoglobin concentration through autologous blood reinfusion (Buick et al. 1980, Ekblom et al. 1972a), or more slowly through injections of erythropoietin (Ekblom & Berglund 1991) or increasing the oxygen content of breathing gases (Ekblom et al. 1975). These experiments increased maximal oxygen uptake but without increasing maximal cardiac output (Ekblom et al. 1976, Kanstrup & Ekblom 1982). Thus, mitochondrial enzymes did not limit aerobic power, since they used the additional oxygen delivered to increase oxygen uptake.

There are clear indications that whole-body oxygen uptake and total skeletal muscle blood flow can exceed levels typically observed during incremental (maximal) exercise. In addition, there are overwhelming facts that suggest that neither total mitochondrial volume nor muscle aerobic enzyme capacities limit maximal aerobic power.

3.2 A central cardiovascular limitation

3.2.1 Changing arterial oxygen content and maximal cardiac output
Reductions in oxygen delivery during maximal exercise, either through carbon monoxide blockade of haemoglobin (Ekblom & Huot 1972, Ekblom et al. 1975) or anaemia (Celsing et al. 1987, Ekblom et al. 1976), do not elicit central cardiovascular compensations for reduced oxygen delivery, and maximal oxygen uptake is reduced in concordance with arterial oxygen content.

3.2.2 Blockade of the autonomic nervous system
A pharmacological blockade of sympathetic receptors reduces heart rate, but oxygen uptake is unchanged during submaximal exercise. During maximal exercise, this blockade decreases peak heart rate and peak cardiac output. Since stroke volume is marginally changed, maximal aerobic power is decreased. Peripheral blood flow is affected (Pawelczyk et al. 1992); however, parasympathetic blockade with atropine has no effect on central circulation during maximal, but increases heart rate during submaximal exercise (Ekblom et al. 1972b).

3.2.3 Blood volume
Endurance-trained athletes with high aerobic power generally have large blood volumes, in parallel with higher stroke volume and maximal cardiac output (Ekblom & Hermansen 1968). Acute reductions of blood volume decrease maximal oxygen uptake through reductions in diastolic function (Krip et al. 1997). When blood volume is increased with haematocrit held constant (autologous reinfusion), maximal oxygen uptake increases. However, the effects of plasma volume expansion (lower haematocrit) are less clear (Chapter 27.3). In untrained subjects, plasma volume expansion increases stroke volume and maximal cardiac output and, despite haemodilution, aerobic power is increased (Coyle et al. 1990). On the other hand, a corresponding plasma expansion in trained subjects may increase stroke volume and maximal cardiac output to some extent, but cannot compensate for the haemodilution affect, with only marginal changes in maximal oxygen uptake being observed (Kanstrup & Ekblom 1984, Warburton et al. 1999). The conclusion is that blood volume changes in untrained subjects can increase maximal oxygen uptake due to their suboptimal blood volume in relation to diastolic function of the heart (preload). The trained subjects have already an increased and optimal blood volume, resulting from endurance training (Kanstrup & Ekblom 1982, Krip et al. 1997).

3.2.4 Training and detraining
The main difference between endurance-trained athletes and sedentary individuals is maximal stroke volume, which explains the marked difference in maximal cardiac output (Ekblom & Hermansen 1968), while there are no major differences in arterial oxygen content or arteriovenous oxygen differences between the groups. Improvements of aerobic power with endurance training are mediated through increased stroke volume, which increases cardiac output, since maximal heart rate and the arteriovenous oxygen difference are not greatly affected (Ekblom et al. 1968, Saltin et al. 1968). However, endurance training of small (local) muscle groups (one arm or leg) improves exercise-specific peak oxygen uptake, but does not improve whole-body aerobic power (Saltin et al. 1976). Accordingly, decreases in aerobic power with prolonged bed rest (Chapter 9), and its subsequent restoration with training, are mainly explained by stroke volume changes (Saltin et al. 1968).

3.2.5 Then what is the bottleneck?
Since maximal oxygen uptake seems to be tightly linked to stroke volume during maximal exercise, apart from variations in arterial oxygen content and the factors discussed above, then what limits maximal cardiac output? This question was studied by two groups, using animal models (Hammond et al. 1992, Stray-Gundersen et al. 1986). The hypothesis was tested that the pericardium limits stroke volume and cardiac output during maximal exercise. Prior to, and some weeks after removing the pericardium, submaximal and maximal exercise, was carried out on a treadmill. In both studies, stroke volume during submaximal and maximal exercise increased (Figure 10.2.5). Since peak heart rate was unchanged by the operation, then both maximal cardiac output and oxygen uptake increased. Of interest was that in one experiment, the arterial oxygen content was unchanged and, therefore, the arteriovenous oxygen difference during maximal exercise after the pericardiectomy was increased (Hammond et al. 1992). These observations favour the view that a total peripheral muscle blood flow reserve exists during maximal exercise. Another important finding was that arterial blood pressure during maximal exercise was not changed after the surgery. Evidently, the strict regulation of blood pressure during maximal exercise was maintained despite a 30% increase in maximal cardiac output.

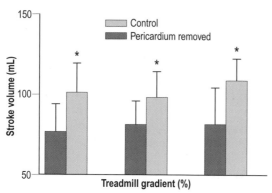

Figure 10.2.5 Stroke volume as a function of treadmill grade (fixed running speed) with (control) and without the pericardium: * denotes P < 0.05. Adapted from Hammond et al. (1992) with permission.

4 CONCLUSION

The focus of this discussion has been on maximal aerobic power. The first part of this discussion is a critique of the central governor model and its inability to explain the limitations of maximal aerobic power. There is no prerequisite for a model built on the assumption that the subconscious brain limits cardiac function during maximal exercise, and thereby prevents cardiac ischaemia. During normal conditions, even during maximal exercise, the reserve capacity of the heart is such that it eliminates any risk of cardiac ischaemia.

The question is then: 'what limits maximal oxygen uptake?'. Three views have been discussed across this and the preceding chapter: central cardiovascular, peripheral gas exchange and central governor theories. It is this author's contention that, under normal conditions, whilst performing whole-body exercise, maximal aerobic power in physically active subjects is primarily limited by oxygen delivery to peripheral muscles, although arterial desaturation and the type of work may modify this maximal value. However, in the sedentary subject, and in conditions during which only peak oxygen uptake is obtained, blood volume, as well as some peripheral factors, may modify maximal oxygen uptake. In both cases, during normal conditions, the pericardium seems to be a primary factor that affects maximal oxygen uptake.

References

Amann M, Eldridge MW, Lovering AT, Stickland MK, Pegelow DF, Dempsey JA 2006 Arterial oxygenation influences central motor output and exercise performance via effects on peripheral locomotor muscle fatigue in humans. Journal of Physiology 575(Pt 3):937–952

Andersen P, Saltin B 1985 Maximal perfusion of skeletal muscle in man. Journal of Physiology 366:233–249

Ansley L, Robson PJ, St Clair GA, Noakes TD 2004 Anticipatory pacing strategies during supramaximal exercise lasting longer than 30 s. Medicine and Science in Sports and Exercise 36(2):309–314

Bainbridge FA 1931 The physiology of muscular exercise. Longmans, Green, London

Bassett DR Jr, Howley ET 1997 Maximal oxygen uptake; 'classical' versus 'contemporary' viewpoints. Medicine and Science in Sports and Exercise 29:591–603

Bassett DR Jr, Howley ET 2000 Limiting factors for maximum oxygen uptake and determinants of endurance performance. Medicine and Science in Sports and Exercise 32(1):70–84

Bergh U, Kanstrup I-L, Ekblom B 1976 Maximal oxygen uptake during exercise with various combinations of arm and leg work. Journal of Applied Physiology 41:191–196

Bosch AN, Goslin BR, Noakes TD, Dennis SC 1990 Physiological differences between black and white runners during a treadmill marathon. European Journal of Applied Physiology. Occupational Physiology 61(1–2):68–72

Brink-Elfegoun T, Kaijser L, Gustafsson T, Ekblom B 2006 Maximal oxygen uptake is not limited by a Central Nervous System Governor. Journal of Applied Physiology 102:781–786

Buick FJ, Gledhill N, Froese AB, Spriet L, Meyers FC 1980 Effect of induced erythrocythemia on aerobic work capacity. Journal of Applied Physiology 48:636–642

Calbet JA, Radegran G, Boushel R, Sondergaard H, Saltin B, Wagner PD 2002 Effect of blood haemoglobin concentration on VO2 max and cardiovascular function in lowlanders acclimatised to 5260 m. Journal of Physiology 545(Pt 2):715–728

Calbet JA, Boushel R, Radegran G, Sondergaard H, Wagner PD, Saltin B 2003 Why is VO2 max after altitude acclimatization still reduced despite normalization of arterial O2 content? American Journal of Physiology. Regulatory, Integrative and Comparative Physiology 284(2):R304-R316

Calbet JA, Radegran G, Boushel R, Sondergaard H, Saltin B, Wagner PD 2004 Plasma volume expansion does not increase maximal cardiac output or VO2 max in lowlanders acclimatized to altitude. American Journal of Physiology. Heart and Circulation Physiology 287(3):H1214-H1224

Celsing F, Svedenhag J, Pihlstedt P, Ekblom B 1987 Effects of anaemia and stepwise-induced polycythemia on maximal aerobic power in individuals with high and low hemoglobin concentrations. Acta Physiologica Scandinavica 129:47–54

Clausen JP 1976 Circulatory adjustment to dynamic exercise and effects of physical training in normal subjects and in patients with coronary artery disease. Progress in Cardiovascular Diseases 18:459–495

Coetzer P, Noakes TD, Sanders B, Lambert MI, Bosch AN, Wiggins T, Dennis SC 1993 Superior fatigue resistance of elite black South African distance runners. Journal of Applied Physiology 75(4):1822–1827

Conley DL, Krahenbuhl GS 1980 Running economy and distance running performance of highly trained athletes. Medicine and Science in Sports and Exercise 12(5):357–360

Coyle EF, Hopper MK, Coggan AR 1990 Maximal oxygen uptake relative to plasma volume. International Journal of Sports Medicine 11:116–119

di Prampero PE 1985 Metabolic and circulatory limitations to VO2 max at the whole animal level. Journal of Experimental Biology 115:319–331

di Prampero PE 2003 Factors limiting maximal performance in humans. European Journal of Applied Physiology 90:420–429

Dill DB 1938 Life, heat and altitude. Harvard University Press, Cambridge, MA

Ekblom B, Berglund B 1991 Effect of erythropoietin administration on maximal aerobic power in man. Scandinavian Journal of Medicine and Science in Sports 1:88–93

Ekblom B, Hermansen L 1968 Cardiac output in athletes. Journal of Applied Physiology 25:619–625

Ekblom B, Huot R 1972 Response to submaximal and maximal exercise at different levels of carboxyhemoglobin. Acta Physiologica Scandinavica 86:474–482

Ekblom B, Åstrand P-O, Saltin B, Stenberg J, Wallström BM 1968 Effect of training of circulatory response to exercise. Journal of Applied Physiology 24:518–528

Ekblom B, Goldbarg A, Gullbring B 1972a Response to exercise after blood loss and reinfusion. Journal of Applied Physiology 33:175–180

Ekblom B, Goldbarg A, Kilbom Å, Åstrand P-O 1972b Effect of atropine and propanolol on the oxygen transport system during exercise in man. Scandinavian Journal of Clinical and Laboratory Investigations 30:35–43

Ekblom B, Huot R, Stein EM, Thorstensson A 1975 Effect of changes in arterial oxygen content on circulation and physical performance. Journal of Applied Physiology 39:71–75

Ekblom B, Wilson G, Åstrand P-O 1976 Central circulation during exercise after venesection and reinfusion of red blood cells. Journal of Applied Physiology 40:379–383

Gibson AC, Noakes TD 2004 Evidence for complex system intregration and dynamic neural regulation of skeletal muscle recruitment during exercise in humans. British Journal of Sports Medicine 38:797–806

Gibson AC, Lambert EV, Rauch LH, Tucker R, Baden DA, Foster C, Noakes TD 2006 The role of information processing between the brain and peripheral physiological systems in pacing and perception of effort. Sports Medicine 36:705–722

Gladden LB 2004 Lactate metabolism: a new paradigm for the third millennium. Journal of Physiology 558(Pt 1):5–30

González-Alonso J, Calbet JA 2003 Reductions in systemic and skeletal muscle blood flow and oxygen delivery limit maximal aerobic capacity in humans. Circulation 107(6):824–830

González-Alonso J, Mortensen SP, Dawson EA, Secher NH, Damsgaard R 2006 Erythrocytes and the regulation of human skeletal muscle blood flow and oxygen delivery: role of erythrocyte count and oxygenation state of haemoglobin. Journal of Physiology 572(Pt 1):295–305

Grubbström J, Berglund B, Kaijser L 1991 Myocardial lactate release and lactate metoblism at rest and during exercise with reduced arterial oxygen content. Acta Physiologica Scandinavica 142:467–474

Grubbström J, Berglund B, Kaijser L 1993 Myocardial oxygen supply and lactate metabolism during marked arterial hypoxaemia. Acta Physiologica Scandinavica 149:303–310

Hammond HK, Frances CW, Bhargava V, Shabetai R 1992 Heart size and maximal cardiac output are limited by the pericardium. American Journal of Physiology 263:1675–1681

Hargreaves M, McKenna MJ, Jenkins DG 1998 Muscle metabolites and performance during high-intensity, intermittent exercise. Journal of Applied Physiology 84(5):1687–1691

Harley Y, Noakes TD 2006 Studies of physiological and neuromuscular function of black South African distance runners, in East African running: toward a cross-disciplinary perspective Routledge, London, 159–198

Hill AV 1965 Trails and trials in physiology. Edward Arnold. London

Hill AV, Lupton H 1923 Muscular exercise, lactic acid, and the supply and utilization of oxygen. Quarterly Journal of Medicine 16:135–171

Hoppeler, H, Kayar SR, Claassen H, Uhlmann E, Karas RH 1987 Adaptive variation in the mammalian respiratory system in relation to energetic demand. III. Skeletal muscles; setting the demand for oxygen. Respiratory Physiology 21:1463–1470

Kaijser L, Grubbström J, Berglund B 1993 Myocardial lactate release during prolonged exercise under hypoxaemia. Acta Physiologica Scandinavica 149:427–433

Kanstrup I-L, Ekblom B 1982 Acute hypervolemia, cardiac performance and aerobic power during exercise. Journal of Applied Physiology 52:1186–1191

Kanstrup I-L, Ekblom B 1984 Blood volume and hemoglobin concentration as determinants of maximal aerobic power. Medicine and Science in Sports and Exercise 16:256–262

Kay D, Marino FE, Cannon J, St Clair GA, Lambert MI, Noakes TD 2001 Evidence for neuromuscular fatigue during high-intensity cycling in warm, humid conditions. European Journal of Applied Physiology 84(1–2):115–121

Kayser B 2003 Exercise starts and ends in the brain. European Journal of Applied Physiology 90(3–4):411–419

Kayser B, Narici M, Binzoni T, Grassi B, Cerretelli P 1994 Fatigue and exhaustion in chronic hypobaric hypoxia: influence of exercising muscle mass. Journal of Applied Physiology 76(2):634–640

Kitamura K, Jorgensen CR, Gobel FL, Taylor HL, Wang Y 1972 Hemodynamic correlates of myocardial oxygen consumption during upright exercise. Journal of Applied Physiology 32:516–522

Krip B, Gledhill N, Jamnik V, Warburton D 1997 Effect of alteration in blood volume on cardiac function during maximal exercise. Medicine and Science in Sports and Exercise 29:1469–1476

Lacour JR, Padilla-Magunacelaya S, Chatard JC, Arsac L, Barthelemy JC 1991 Assessment of running velocity at maximal oxygen uptake. European Journal of Applied Physiology. Occupational Physiology 62(2):77–82

McDowall RJS 1938 The control of the circulation of the blood. Longmans, Green, London

Malconian M, Rock P, Hultgren H, Donner H, Cymerman A, Groves B, Reeves J, Alexander J, Sutton J, Nitta M 1990 Operation Everest II: the electrocardiogram at rest and exercise during a simulated ascent of Mt Everest. American Journal of Cardiology 65:1475–1480

Mitchell JH, Saltin B 2003 The oxygen transport system and maximal oxygen uptake. In: Exercise physiology. Oxford University Press, Oxford, 255–291

Morgan DW, Baldini FD, Martin PE, Kohrt WM 1989 Ten kilometer performance and predicted velocity at VO2max among well-trained male runners. Medicine and Science in Sports and Exercise 21(1):78–83

Mortensen SP, Dawson EA, Yoshiga CC, Dalsgaard MK, Damsgaard R, Secher NH, González-Alonso J 2005 Limitations to systemic and locomotor limb muscle oxygen delivery and uptake during maximal exercise in humans. Journal of Physiology 566(Pt 1):273–285

Needham J, Baldwin E 1949 Hopkins and biochemistry 1861–1947. Wheffer and Sons, London

Nelson RR, Gobel FL, Jorgensen CR, Wang K, Wang Y, Taylor HL 1974 Hemodynamic predictors of myocardial oxygen consumption during static and dynamic exercise. Circulation 50:1179–1189

Nielsen OB, de Paoli F, Overgaard K 2001 Protective effects of lactic acid on force production in rat skeletal muscle. Journal of Physiology 536(Pt 1):161–166

Noakes TD 1988 Implications of exercise testing for prediction of athletic performance: a contemporary perspective. Medicine and Science in Sports and Exercise 20(4):319–330

Noakes TD 1997 Challenging beliefs: ex Africa semper aliquid novi: 1996 J.B. Wolffe Memorial Lecture. Medicine and Science in Sports and Exercise 29(5):571–590

Noakes TD 1998 Maximal oxygen uptake: 'classical' versus 'contemporary' viewpoints: a rebuttal. Medicine and Science in Sports and Exercise 30(9):1381–1398

Noakes TD 2000 Physiological models to understand exercise fatigue and the adaptations that predict or enhance athletic performance. Scandinavian Journal of Medicine and Science in Sports 10(3):123–145

Noakes TD 2003 Lore of running. Human Kinetics, Champaign, IL

Noakes TD 2004 Linear relationship between the perception of effort and the duration of constant load exercise that remains. Journal of Applied Physiology 96(4):1571–1572

Noakes TD 2005a How does a foundational myth become sacred scientific dogma? The case of A.V. Hill and the anaerobiosis controversy. In: Philosophy and the sciences of exercise, health and sport. Routledge, London, 56–84

Noakes TD 2005b Counterpoint: positive effects of intermittent hypoxia (live high: train low) on exercise performance are/are not mediated primarily by augmented red cell volume. Journal of Applied Physiology 99:2453–2462

Noakes TD, St Clair Gibson A 2004 Logical limitations to the 'catastrophe' models of fatigue during exercise in humans. British Journal of Sports Medicine 38(5):648–649

Noakes TD, Myburgh KH, Schall R 1990 Peak treadmill running velocity during the VO2 max test predicts running performance. Journal of Sports Science 8(1):35–45

Noakes TD, Calbet JA, Boushel R, Søndergaard H, Rådegran G, Wagner PD, Saltin B 2004 Central regulation of skeletal muscle recruitment explains the reduced maximal cardiac output during exercise in hypoxia. American Journal of Physiology. Regulatory, Integrative and Comparative Physiology 287(4):R996-R999

Noakes TD, St Clair Gibson A, Lambert EV 2005 From catastrophe to complexity: a novel model of integrative central neural regulation of effort and fatigue during exercise in humans: summary and conclusions. British Journal of Sports Medicine 39(2):120–124

Nummela AT, Paavolainen LM, Sharwood KA, Lambert MI, Noakes TD, Rusko HK 2006 Neuromuscular factors determining 5 km running performance and running economy in well-trained athletes. European Journal of Applied Physiology 97(1):1–8

Pawelczyk JA, Hanel B, Pawelczyk PA, Warberg J, Secher NH 1992 Leg vasoconstriction during dynamic exercise with reduced cardiac output. Journal of Applied Physiology 73:1838–1846

Pedersen TH, Nielsen OB, Lamb GD, Stephenson DG 2004 Intracellular acidosis enhances the excitability of working muscle. Science 305(5687):1144–1147

Pitsiladis Y, Bale J, Sharp C, Noakes TD 2007 East African running. Routledge, London, 2007

Reeves JT, Groves BM, Sutton JR, Wagner PD, Cymerman A, Malconian MK, Rock PB, Young PM, Houston CS 1987 Operation Everest II: preservation of cardiac function at extreme altitude. Journal of Applied Physiology 63:531–539

Richardson RS, Noyszewski EA, Kendrick KF, Leigh JS, Wagner PD 1995 Myoglobin O_2 desaturation during exercise. Evidence for limited O_2 transport. Journal of Clinical Investigations 96:1916–1926

Robergs RA 2001 An exercise physiologist's 'contemporary' interpretations of the 'ugly and creaking edifices' of the VO_2max concept. Journal of Exercise Physiology 4:1–44

Saltin B, Blomqvist G, Mitchell JH, Johnson RL, Wildenthal K Jr, Chapman CB 1968 Response to exercise after bed rest and after training. A longitudinal study of adaptive changes in oxygen transport and body composition. Circulation 37/38 (Suppl VII):1–78

Saltin B, Nazar K, Costill DL, Stein E, Jansson E, Essen B, Gollnick D 1976 The nature of the training responce: peripheral and central adaptations of one legged exercise. Acta Physiologica Scandinavica 96:289–305

Scott BK, Houmard JA 1994 Peak running velocity is highly related to distance running performance. International Journal of Sports Medicine 15(8):504–507

Sgherza AL, Axen K, Fain R, Hoffman RS, Dunbar CC, Haas F 2002 Effect of naloxone on perceived exertion and exercise capacity during maximal cycle ergometry. Journal of Applied Physiology 93(6):2023–2028

St Clair Gibson A, Noakes TD 2004 Evidence for complex system integration and dynamic neural regulation of skeletal muscle recruitment during exercise in humans. British Journal of Sports Medicine 38(6):797–806

Stenberg J, Åstrand P-O, Ekblom B, Royce J, Saltin B 1967 Hemodynamic response to work with different muscle groups, sitting and supine. Journal of Applied Physiology 22:61–70

Stray-Gundersen J, Musch TI, Haidet GC, Swain DP, Ordway GA, Mitchell JH 1986 The effects of pericardiectomy on maximal oxygen comsumption and maximal cardiac output in untrained dogs. Circulation Research 58:523–530

Taylor C, Weibel E 1981 Design of the mammalian respiratory system I. Problem and strategy. Respiratory Physiology 44:1–10

Taylor HL, Buskirk E, Henschel A 1955 Maximal oxygen uptake as an objective measure of cardio-respiratory performance. Journal of Applied Physiology 8:73–80

Taylor C, Karas R, Weibel E, Hoppeler H 1987 Adaptive variation in the mammalian respiratory system in relation to energetic demand. Respiratory Physiology 69:1–127

Tucker R, Marle T, Lambert EV, Noakes TD 2006a The rate of heat storage mediates an anticipatory reduction in exercise intensity during cycling at a fixed rating of perceived exertion. Journal of Physiology 574(Pt 3):905–915

Tucker R, Lambert MI, Noakes TD 2006b An analysis of pacing strategies during men's world record performances in track athletics. International Journal of Sports Physiology and Performance 1:233–245

Wagner PD 1992 Gas exchange and peripheral diffusion limitation. Medicine and Science in Sports and Exercise 24:54–58

Warburton DER, Gledhill N, Jamnik VK, Kirp B, Card N 1999 Induced hypervolemia, vardiac function, VO_{2max} and performance in elite cyclists. Medicine and Science in Sports and Exercise 31:800–808

Watson P, Hasegawa H, Roelands B, Piacentini MF, Looverie R, Meeusen R 2005 Acute dopamine/noradrenaline reuptake inhibition enhances human exercise performance in warm, but not temperate conditions. Journal of Physiology 565(Pt 3):873–883

Weston AR, Karamizrak O, Smith A, Noakes TD, Myburgh KH 1999 African runners exhibit greater fatigue resistance, lower lactate accumulation, and higher oxidative enzyme activity. Journal of Applied Physiology 86(3):915–923

Chapter 10.3

The anaerobic threshold: fact or misinterpretation?

Michael I. Lindinger   Brian J. Whipp

'The term anaerobic threshold (Wasserman & McIlroy 1964) seems to polarise investigators into those who believe it to be a milestone in advancing the understanding of exercise bioenergetics and those who believe it to be a millstone. Much of the confusion, however, can be traced to two conceptual cruces: what exactly is meant by "anaerobic" and by "threshold"?' (BJW). In this chapter, a point–counterpoint approach will be undertaken, in which the scientific evidence from both sides of this debate will be reviewed. First will be the case that the term is a misrepresentation of the available scientific evidence, and that an anaerobic threshold does not exist. Next, the case will be presented that the regional intramuscular oxygen partial pressures within exercising tissues may indeed fall below the critical oxygen delivery threshold at the cellular level. Each author will then provide rebuttal statements.

Part A: A physiological misinterpretation
Michael Lindinger

1 INTRODUCTION

The anaerobic threshold is a conceptual approach developed to determine the exercise intensity at which arterial blood lactate concentration began to increase sharply, during an incremental running or cycling test (Wasserman & McIlroy 1964). During such tests, blood lactate accumulation was attributed to inadequate oxygen delivery to contracting muscle which, in turn, resulted in increased rates of glycolysis and lactate production. Thus, one might be able to determine the work rate at which metabolic acidosis commenced (Wasserman et al. 1973). Subsequently, this threshold has been defined as the highest oxygen uptake ($\dot{V}_{O_2}$) beyond which lactate begins accumulating in the blood, causing a metabolic acidosis (Wasserman & Whipp 1975). Whilst easily measured, albeit not without some variability, the anaerobic threshold actually represents the exercise intensity at which the net release of lactate from contracting skeletal muscle exceeds its clearance (turnover; see Chapter 1: the metabolic hypothesis). Thus, the anaerobic threshold is a lactate threshold.

The initial purpose for using the anaerobic threshold was to determine the upper limit of aerobic exercise in cardiac patients (Wasserman & McIlroy 1964). Soon after the initial description of the concept (Jones & Ehrsam 1982, Myers & Ashley 1997), many researchers examined ways of applying it to normal populations, with the aim of quantifying aerobic power and as a yardstick for assessing endurance training programmes (Jones & Ehrsam 1982, Svedahl & MacIntosh 2003).

Based on our current understanding of muscle physiology, the conceptual basis for the anaerobic threshold was, at best, incomplete. Full consideration must be given to mechanisms of both lactate appearance in arterial blood and its clearance from venous and arterial blood. Within contracting muscles, lactate production, and the apparent threshold are functions of glyolytic pyruvate production, pyruvate dehydrogenase activity, lactate dehydrogenase activity, monocarboxylate transporter activity and intercellular lactate shuttling. With respect to non-contracting tissues (lactate clearance), the apparent threshold is also a function of these enzyme and transporter activities in cells taking up lactate and oxidising pyruvate.

It is now recognised that all cell types, including the brain (Aubert et al. 2005), take up and use lactate as an energy substrate. It is also recognised that lactate is a preferred substrate by skeletal muscle (Miller et al. 2002). Thus, many cellular and molecular mechanisms determine the anaerobic threshold, and the regulation of these mechanisms is complex. Within an individual, each mechanism may be independently or co-dependently regulated in both the short and long term (gene regulation and expression). Indeed, Jones & Ehrsam (1982) noted that blood lactate concentration and oxygen uptake are dependent variables, affected by different factors among people. Within individuals, some of these factors, unrelated to either lactate release or disposal, include prior exercise, diet, muscle glycogen stores, hydration, motivational and thermal state, and mode of exercise, as it determines the active muscle mass. As an example, provision of a lactate infusion during exercise markedly alters variables related to the anaerobic threshold (Miller et al. 2005). Accordingly, many factors can independently affect the anaerobic threshold, with this influence varying over time. Thus, the threshold within an individual is variable, unless many of these factors can be controlled.

Svedahl & MacIntosh (2003) highlighted two key limitations of the anaerobic threshold concept. First, is the difficulty in providing a reliable, accurate and standardised operational threshold measurement. Thus, because the threshold cannot be measured, it has been necessary to use variables such as arterial blood lactate concentration or oxygen uptake, and several different operational measures have been developed: maximal lactate steady state, lactate threshold, lactate minimum speed, onset of blood lactate accumulation and ventilatory threshold (Svedahl & MacIntosh 2003). Second, intramus-

cular lactate production can be substantial even when oxygen availability is sustained, and this has been repeatedly demonstrated over the past 50 years (Connett et al. 1990, Hogan 2001, Richardson et al. 1998, Stainsby et al. 1991).

Perhaps the greatest limitation of the anaerobic threshold concept, and the reason why it is a misrepresentation, is that within contracting muscle, there is no anaerobic threshold. That is, there does not exist a rate of energy demand that causes a switch from aerobic to anaerobic metabolism – an explicit prerequisite of any threshold.

Based on the experimental research approaches of Connett et al. (1990) and Hogan et al. (1992, Hogan 2001), it is highly likely that, in normal individuals, all muscle activity occurs in the presence of an adequate tissue oxygen delivery. Rest to work transitions, and transitions from lower to higher work rates are accompanied by abrupt increases in adenosine triphosphate (ATP) demand, which are transiently met through the hydrolysis of phosphocreatine and increased rates of glycogenolysis and glycolysis. When work rates are ramped up in a continuous fashion, as opposed to discrete steps, there is no abrupt stepwise increase in ATP demand, and ATP demand should increase more as a continuous function. Under these conditions, it is very important to understand that ATP production occurs in the presence of adequate tissue oxygenation (Connett et al. 1990); cells are neither anaerobic nor hypoxic.

Glycolytic ATP production is the mechanism by which energy, provided in the form of muscle glycogen or blood-borne glucose, is made available to the cell. On the pyruvate removal side, pyruvate dehydrogenase activity is a major determinant of intramuscular pyruvate accumulation. At the onset of exercise, there is a latency to the allosteric upregulation of pyruvate dehydrogenase (Spriet et al. 2000), and abrupt increases in ATP demand imposed by stepwise work transitions result in glycolytic pyruvate production exceeding its removal through pyruvate dehydrogenase. This results in the conversion of pyruvate to lactate by lactate dehydrogenase. The lactate dehydrogenase isozyme in glycolytic muscle favours this conversion, facilitating an increase in mitochondrial redox potential (Connett et al. 1990), removing lactate from the cell by export through monocarboxylate transporters (Bonen 2000). In oxidative muscle, the reverse occurs, with lactate dehydrogenase converting lactate, which enters these cells via monocarboxylate transporters, to pyruvate, thus aiding the clearance of lactate from the circulation (Brooks 2000). It may be concluded that even in glycolytic muscle there is no insufficiency of oxygen delivery, yet lactate can be produced at elevated rates, and therefore an anaerobic threshold does not exist in these fibres.

Attempts have been made to correlate the metabolic acidosis associated with blood lactate accumulation with hyperventilation (reduced arterial carbon dioxide partial pressure). Specifically, in the region of the anaerobic threshold, there occurs an abrupt increase in the minute ventilation with respect to the oxygen uptake. This point was first described by Owles (1930; Owles point) and subsequently termed the ventilation threshold (Jones & Erhsam 1982) or the ventilatory threshold (Svedahl & MacIntosh 2003), and was attributed to increased carbon dioxide output relative to oxygen uptake. The former was thought to reflect acidification of arterial blood and associated proton-mediated stimulation of chemoreceptor drive (Lahiri & Forster 2003). This, too, appears to have been an oversimplification of physiological processes and was initially based on a few easily measured variables.

During exercise, there is a modest temporal dissociation between the lactate and ventilatory thresholds (Jones & Ehrsam 1982, Svedahl & MacIntosh 2003), as one might expect on the basis of the varied and complex mechanisms outlined above. The drive to ventilate is similarly more complex than represented by an acidification of arterial blood resulting from the accumulation of lactate. Increased metabolic carbon dioxide production, as well as that generated from proton bicarbonate buffering within extracellular fluids, also has acidifying effects, and contributes to the increased carbon dioxide production. The exercise-induced increase in plasma protein concentration also contributes to acidification of plasma.

During exercise, ventilation is driven by many variables, including increased arterial hydrogen ion concentration ([H⁺]), with the former buffering the latter by reducing arterial carbon dioxide partial pressure. Ventilation is not only reliant on [H⁺]. Importantly, increases in arterial osmolality have been shown to be crucial to the control of ventilation during exercise (Jennings 1994). This increase is primarily due to a net flux of ion-poor fluid from the vascular compartment into contracting skeletal muscle (Harrison 1985, Lindinger et al. 1994). Increased carbon dioxide release occurs from contracting muscles, increasing venous carbon dioxide partial pressure and [H⁺], and this carbon dioxide is ultimately eliminated at the lungs. Thus, the stimulus for hyperventilation at the anaerobic threshold is not increased arterial [H⁺]. Indeed, the acidifying effect of increased plasma lactate concentration at the anaerobic threshold can be more than offset by a reduction in arterial carbon dioxide, although this often does not change appreciably at this exercise intensity (Miller et al. 2005).

2 CONCLUSION

Despite these limitations of the anaerobic threshold concept, it has been extensively used and continues to be an important aerobic power assessment technique for both clinical and athletic subjects. The problem, and this is what has spawned considerable debate over the decades, is determining what the anaerobic threshold represents mechanistically. Contrary to the initial suggestion (Wasserman & McIlroy 1964), the anaerobic threshold does not represent inadequate delivery of oxygen to contracting skeletal muscle cells. Many studies have demonstrated increased blood lactate accumulation in the presence of adequate muscle perfusion and oxygen delivery. The concept of anaerobic threshold has served out its useful purpose, and should be replaced with meaningful, operational definitions of aerobic performance.

Part B: The anaerobic threshold: Yes, no, maybe!
Brian Whipp

1 INTRODUCTION

The major concerns with the anaerobic threshold seem to be the implicit synonymy between lactate-yielding and anaerobic on the one hand, and the evidence for, and the criterion used for discriminating, a variable that supportably partitions the response of a relevant variable-of-interest into one that does not change at all (or changes minimally), and one that does change systematically (or begins to change at an appreciably greater rate).

While the cause(s) of the anaerobic threshold (with lactate, lactic acidosis, gas exchange and ventilatory as competing adjectival descriptors) remains the subject of continuing dispute, its consequences are less so. The anaerobic threshold is one of the indices that partition a subject's oxygen uptake capability into intensity domains (e.g. light, moderate, heavy). As these domain partitions occur at such widely differing percentages of the maximum oxygen uptake ($\dot{V}_{O_{2max}}$) among subjects, this effectively nullifies the use of relative intensities (e.g. % ($\dot{V}_{O_{2max}}$) as valid descriptors of exercise intensity (see Chapter 27.2); common intensities should be characterised by common metabolic strain profiles. The threshold, therefore, is one of the determinants of exercise tolerance; in patients with heart disease, it is also a component index of life expectancy (Gitt et al. 2002).

2 DETERMINANT(S)

Two of the concerns related to terminology can be dispensed with readily. First, is the increased blood and muscle lactate concentration of anaerobic origin? Yes! It is the consequence of a process that does not directly involve the utilisation of oxygen and so, in this sense, it is anaerobic, regardless of whether it is also results from a simultaneous lack of oxygen. Second, is there any work rate at which an anaerobic process does not contribute to the energy transfer? No! Phosphocreatine concentration decreases in muscles, even at the lightest work rates; reflecting anaerobic energy transfer. Thus, there can be no anaerobic threshold in this sense. But this is not the sense in which the term is conventionally used. Rather, it is considered to represent a metabolic rate above which anaerobic (lactate-related) energy transfer mechanisms systematically begin to supplement the predominantly aerobic processes (Wasserman et al. 2005).

The issue then resolves to: (1) whether the increase in lactate concentration is due to an inadequate oxygen supply at the cytochrome oxidase terminus of the electron transport chain, hence justifying the anaerobic qualification; or (2) whether increased lactate concentration begins abruptly, hence justifying threshold terminology.

3 METABOLIC OR LACTIC ACIDOSIS?

Because of its dissociation constant, there is virtually no lactic acid per se formed in the contracting muscles at any work rate. What is formed are the dissociated products: lactate and hydrogen (H^+) ions. Robergs et al. (2004), consequently, rail against the use of the term lactic acidosis, asserting that not only is lactic acid not the source of the increased proton production, but ATP hydrolysis is a major contributor to additional sources of proton production. While the former is justifiable, its force erodes when the term lactic acidosis is recognised in many, if not most, usages to be shorthand for the lactate-associated metabolic acidosis (Whipp 1994). The latter is not so justifiable. While ATP hydrolysis yields a proton (Chapter 7, Table 7.1), the ATP concentration in contracting muscles changes little, if at all, even at high work rates. Even more decisive is the fact that phosphocreatine breaks down to creatine and inorganic phosphate, thus contributing to ATP stability whilst consuming protons. The result is a transient alkalosis (not acidosis).

Proton dissociation from acids also occurs higher in the glycolytic chain. Pyruvic acid is an order of magnitude more highly dissociated than lactic acid, although its concentration is an order of magnitude or so less (Keul et al. 1967, Wasserman et al. 1985). However, the degree of proton dissociation at these steps may be considered merely transitional. Thus, while acids other than lactic (including ionic changes) can contribute to the net proton load, Kemp (2005) and Lindinger et al. (2005) remind us that most of the glycolytic protons appear at a rate of one proton per lactate molecule, and that lactate accumulation directly contributes to intracellular acidosis. This being the case, increased lactate ion concentration justifiably serves as a proxy for metabolic acidosis, but not necessarily acidaemia. This notion is bolstered by the demonstration that if there is not an increase in lactate concentration during exercise, neither is there a metabolic acidosis in individuals deficient in the myophosphorylase b (McArdle's syndrome; Hagberg et al. 1982, O'Dochartaigh et al. 2004).

4 A THRESHOLD?

The lactate-associated protons are exposed to a pool of buffers, including protein-linked histidine residues, inorganic phosphate and bicarbonate that constrain the consequent fall of pH. The amount trapped is a function of both available buffer concentration and its dissociation constant. In fact, the initial 0.3–0.5 mM of the lactate increase is domi-nated by buffers other than bicarbonate (Visser et al. 1964, Wasserman et al. 2005), but it does provide more than 90% of the buffering, yielding one molecule of carbon dioxide for each molecule of bicarbonate and hydrogen lost:

Equation 1: $H^+ + HCO_3^- \rightarrow H_2CO_3 \rightarrow H_2O + CO_2$

As [H^+] increases, bicarbonate concentration falls and carbon dioxide production increases, resulting in an obligatory increase in carbon dioxide output at the lung ($\dot{V}_{CO_2}$). As the temporal dissociation between carbon dioxide production and its alveolar appearance is also manifest within a delay between muscle oxygen uptake ($\dot{Q}_{O_2}$) and its alveolar equivalent ($\dot{V}_{O_2}$), a gas exchange index of the onset of the metabolic acidosis is properly characterised as a metabolic rate rather than a work rate (watts). This is because the work rate during an incremental test increases during this delay by an amount that is incrementation rate dependent.

But it is not just that extra-aerobic carbon dioxide is formed in these reactions; the increase is quantitatively large (see Whipp 1994), making carbon dioxide output analysis, as a function of oxygen uptake, such a good functional index of the onset of the metabolic acidosis. However, it is important to recognise that the extra volume of CO_2 produced (V_{CO_2} versus $\dot{V}_{CO_2}$) under these conditions is a direct function of the bicarbonate decrease in the vascular and muscle compartments. Any contribution from non-bicarbonate buffering mechanisms, while important for [H^+] regulation, does not produce extra carbon dioxide. The rate at which extra carbon dioxide is produced ($\dot{V}_{CO_2}$) will be a function of the rate at which bicarbonate falls; the more rapid the lactate elevation, the greater the increase in carbon dioxide production. This accounts for carbon dioxide production and the respiratory exchange rate being appreciably higher at a given oxygen uptake, in the period of increasing blood lactate, during rapid incremental exercise, compared to tests in which increments are relatively slow (Whipp & Mahler 1980).

It is necessary, however, that to appropriately subserve the relevant threshold function, carbon dioxide production must also increase with a clearly discriminatory profile. This it does! But there is a proviso. It must be verified that the discernibly additional carbon dioxide is of bicarbonate origin. That is, true hyperventilation must be ruled out. Fortunately, this can be convincingly achieved using gas exchange criteria (Whipp et al. 1986). Mass balance considerations dictate that the arterial carbon dioxide partial pressure ($PaCO_2$) can only be regulated if there is a precise proportional relationship between the ventilatory equivalent for carbon dioxide ($\dot{V}_E/\dot{V}_{CO_2}$) and the physiological dead space fraction of the breath (V_D/V_T):

Equation 2: $P_aCO_2 = 863/(\dot{V}E/\dot{V}CO_2) \cdot (1-V_D/V_T)$

The decreasing ventilatory equivalent for carbon dioxide, evident early during an incremental test, appropriately matches the reducing dead space fraction. But, as the latter is usually minimal at the lactate threshold, hyperventilation requires the former to increase. This rarely occurs until a much higher work rate. Instead, the relative constancy or small continued decrease of the ventilatory equivalent for carbon dioxide over this range rules out hyperventilation as causing an increased slope of the carbon dioxide output to oxygen uptake relationship. The lack of a decrease in arterial and end-tidal carbon dioxide partial pressures supports this contention. Furthermore, an absence of hyperventilation during this phase provides a region of isocapnic buffering (Wasserman et al. 2005, Whipp et al.1989), crucial to establishing that the extra-aerobic carbon dioxide output is of bicarbonate origin. Accordingly, the profile of the carbon dioxide output to oxygen uptake relationship, during an appropriately designed incremental exercise test, provides a justifiable index of a threshold of bicarbonate decrease; one that is closely linked to increased lactate concentration.

Having established that this gas exchange profile is consistent with a lactate concentration threshold, one must now consider whether this threshold is reflective of an anaerobic source.

5 AN ANAEROBIC THRESHOLD?

Brooks (1985) and his colleagues (e.g. Gladden 2004) have been the contemporary champions of the importance of the lactate clearance-to-production relationship in determining lactate concentration (see also Barr & Himwich 1923). Lactate serves an important thermodynamic function, supplementing the mitochondrially produced ATP fuelling muscle activation. But lactate is also a viable oxidative energy substrate for glyconeogenesis, locally and in regions to which it is transferred (lactate shuttle; e.g. nearby fibres in the same muscle, other muscles, the liver). It is important therefore to distinguish between the production rate of lactate and its consequent concentration in blood. This reflects, in addition, its transport out of the cell (Brooks 2000, Juel 2001), its volume and kinetics of distribution, and the dynamics of its subsequent metabolism. This, and the small pyruvate-linked component, presumably accounts for the instances in which the profile of arterial lactate concentration does not show an acceptably sharp rate of change; although the lactate-to-pyruvate ratio, considered to be an index of the cellular redox state, does change more abruptly under these conditions (Wasserman et al. 1985).

Thus, the issue is not that intramuscular lactate production at low work rates does not increase, but whether there is an anaerobic basis for the rapid increase in the venous lactate concentration, that is subsequently discernible in arterial blood. The resolution of this hinges on the mitochondrial oxygen partial pressure within lactate-producing tissues, in the context of a critical partial pressure for mitochondrial oxidative phosphorylation. But accessing this information in exercising humans presents a formidable technical challenge. The critical partial pressure is commonly given, from isolated mitochondrial studies, to be ≤ 0.13 kPa (≤ 1 mmHg). Recent evidence, however, has suggested that, in some cells, mitochondrial respiratory rates may begin to decline at a partial pressure that is 2–3 times higher (Richardson et al. 1999, Wilson et al. 1977). In vivo mitochondrial metabolism in human muscles may be significantly compromised at a partial pressure four times greater (Richardson et al. 1999). Thus, providing conclusive evidence that critical levels are attained within exercising muscle is by no means straightforward. Other evidence, usually heavily assumption laden, has therefore been marshalled to cast light on the likelihood.

For example, the lactic acidosis of muscular exercise can be defensibly justified as being oxygen related, based on the demonstration that the four causes of tissue hypoxia (hypoxic, stagnant, anaemic, histotoxic) lead to increased blood lactate concentration (Wasserman 1994). Furthermore, when oxygen is added to the inspirate, the onset of the lactic acidosis is delayed and lactate concentration at a given high work rate is reduced. However, the terms oxygen related and anaerobic are not synonymous.

Unfortunately, measures of oxygen uptake are not very helpful when seeking evidence of insufficient intramuscular oxygen, because it lacks the necessary sensitivity (Whipp et al. 1995), and the presence of excess oxygen uptake at work rates is associated with a lactic acidosis (Whipp & Rossiter 2004). The partial pressure of oxygen in blood was thought useful for this purpose. However, it has been argued (Brooks 1986) that this is unlikely to be limiting, because femoral venous partial pressure during high-intensity leg exercise only falls to ≥ 2.7 kPa (20 mmHg; Keul et al. 1972). More recently, it has been demonstrated that the femoral venous partial pressure actually falls to about this value at the lactate threshold (Stringer et al. 1994, Wasserman et al. 2005), being maintained at this level up to the limit of tolerance due to the rightward shift of the oxyhaemoglobin dissociation curve. This, it has been argued, is consistent with the attainment of critical partial pressures in the capillaries and mitochondria. Thus, we have equivalent venous oxygen partial pressures being used as evidence for and against an anaerobic cause of lactic acidosis.

However, unless we are asked to accept that a single value exists for the oxygen partial pressures of all the vascular beds that drain into the femoral-venous sampling site (and not all exercising muscle blood does drain into this site), then regional variations in end- and mean-capillary partial pressures are likely to exist, with some regions being lower, and potentially appreciably so, as conceded by Keul et al. (1972, p.66). In fact, as there is convincing evidence demonstrating a wide range of metabolic rate to blood flow ratios and phosphocreatine and H^+ concentrations, both between and within exercising muscles (Richardson et al. 2002, Rossiter et al. 2004), inferences regarding the presence of critical intramuscular partial pressures from femoral venous sampling seem unjustified.

Others have attempted to establish a representative mean intramuscular oxygen partial pressure from its relationship with the desaturation of myoglobin (Richardson et al. 1999). These authors concluded that maximal mitochondrial metabolism appeared compromised when the intracellular partial pressure fell below ~0.5 kPa (4 mmHg). Conley et al. (2000) noted relatively constant intracellular partial pressures over work rates from ~50–100% of peak aerobic power (~0.4 kPa, 3 mmHg), concluding that skeletal muscle cells do not become anaerobic as lactate concentrations suddenly rise, because the intracellular oxygen partial pressure is preserved at a constant level. However, these data did not demonstrate a constant level, but an average partial pressure having a standard deviation of ~0.1 kPa (1 mmHg). Furthermore, this was not just an average but the average of averages, including plausible variations only within the type I and IIa fibres.

This criticism, however, cannot be levelled at the pivotal studies of Connett et al. (1986) and Honig et al. (1984) who studied oxymyoglobin saturation muscle slices to establish whether regional oxygen partial pressure variations included the critical value for mitochondrial oxygen use. They failed to demonstrate such regions. Honig et al. (1984), however, did demonstrate regions with partial pressures <0.26 kPa (2 mmHg) during intense exercise. One wonders how much earlier such values might be established, in the context of the relatively stable average tissue partial pressures reported over the range of work rates during which blood lactate was increasing (Conley et al. 2000, Richardson et al. 1999). A concern also attends the value used for the P_{50} of oxymyoglobin, since recent work considers a value almost 50% lower to be a better estimate at 37°C (Schenkman et al. 1997). This being the case, the myoglobin-to-oxygen partial pressure transform would be consistent with an even lower oxygen partial pressure. Nevertheless, the certainty of the conclusion totters if the critical mitochondrial partial pressure under physiological conditions during high-intensity exercise was to be 0.26 kPa or more. And what happens with type IIb muscle fibres? Therefore, on the basis of current evidence, it cannot conclusively be disproved that some proportion of mitochondrial cells may have a local oxygen concentration that limits the cellular respiration rate (Brown 1992).

Finally, Duhaylongsod et al. (1993) demonstrated that the concentration of oxidised mitochondrial cytochrome a,a3 fell progressively with increasing work rate. They concluded that maximal exercise would lead to a nearly complete cytochrome reduction, secondary to an inadequate oxygen supply. Chillingly, the value at maximum exercise was found not to significantly differ from that observed at death!

6 CONCLUSION

The author is aware of no study that has convincingly demonstrated that the mean intramuscular tissue oxygen partial pressure, during exercise at intensities associated with a metabolic (lactic) acidosis, is decreased to levels below that commonly cited to be necessary to impair aerobic energy transfer. Thus, on these grounds, an anaerobic cause for the lactic acidosis seems to be unsustainable. But so much important physiology lurks behind such a categorical statement. The mean tissue oxygen partial pressure does not properly represent the distribution extremes of regions of widely varying metabolic functioning, and these may include regions with considerably lower values. Also the frame of reference for the critical partial pressure needs to be convincingly established for mitochondria in their exercising *milieu*, rather than in in vitro suspensions under highly unphysiological conditions.

And so, in the context of these uncertainties regarding the anaerobic threshold, one wonders where the certain find the certainty.

Part C: Rebuttal
Michael Lindinger

At best, the anaerobic threshold is only one of many rudimentary descriptors of human exercise performance, whether it is for clinically compromised individuals or high-performance athletes. The anaerobic threshold does not provide a mechanistic basis upon which to explain exercise performance. There are good reasons for its use as a descriptive indicator of performance, several of which have been outlined in Professor Whipp's description.

Despite attempts to describe the consequences of the anaerobic threshold, none have been provided. Rather, a series of exercise intensity domains have been constructed for which the anaerobic threshold has been termed a relevant descriptive index. The use of these domains to support the anaerobic threshold fails, because they were not constructed independently of the anaerobic threshold; rather, they are part of the same descriptive construct, and do not provide a mechanistic basis for exercise performance.

The well-known linear relationship between oxygen uptake and exercise intensity has been neglected and it clearly shows the high dependence of oxygen uptake on the increasing mass of exercising muscle and frequency of its activation. The linear nature of this relationship provides no indication of an oxygen limitation to muscle contractile activity at exercise intensities well above the anaerobic threshold. The assertion that the threshold is one of the determinants of exercise tolerance is unsupported amongst normal subjects, who are capable of tolerating exercise at very high intensities for variable and extended durations, and this is a function of many factors, of which the anaerobic threshold remains a poor descriptive determinant.

By admission, Professor Whipp acknowledges there is no anaerobic threshold because anaerobic processes (glycolysis, phosphocreatine degradation) contribute to ATP production at all work rates. Glycolytic lactate production always supplements the ongoing, predominantly aerobic processes even in resting muscle, and to imply that this is not systematic is erroneous. As such, the term anaerobic threshold is a descriptive misnomer that provides little mechanistic insight into cellular energy provision.

Phosphocreatine degradation is not associated with the anaerobic threshold and reference to its degradation as a net proton consumer, in the context of glycolytic proton production, is misleading. Phosphocreatine degradation occurs well in advance of marked increases in glycolytic activity, specifically during the rest to work transitions and with appreciable step transitions in work rate. Furthermore, Kemp's assertion that most glycolytic protons come from glycolysis and the production of lactate is erroneous, as discussed by Hochachka & Mommsen (1983), Gevers & Dowdle (1963) and Lindinger et al. (2005). While it is true that, in the minds of many individuals, lactate serves as a proxy for the metabolic acidosis, it is recognised that lactate is only one of many contributors. Indeed, according to anaerobic threshold theory, one would infer, based on recent results from exercise conditioning of McArdles' patients (Haller et al. 2006), that these patients should exhibit increases in the anaerobic (lactate) threshold. However, these changes do not occur in such patients.

One of the fundamental problems with the initial and ongoing descriptions of the anaerobic threshold is that of comparing increases in whole-blood lactate concentration with that of plasma bicarbonate concentration. The apparent 1:1 stoichiometry for this has proven convenient for descriptions of the anaerobic threshold (Beaver et al. 1986), but it fails to recognise a mechanism. Indeed, when one compares the rise in plasma lactate concentration with the decrease in plasma bicarbonate concentration, the increase in the former significantly exceeds that of the latter, by a factor of ~1.3. This discrepancy is because the anaerobic threshold concept cannot account for key roles of the erythrocytes in carbon dioxide, lactate, chloride and proton transfer and transport (Greco & Solomon 1997, Lindinger & Grudzien 2003). With respect to the carbon dioxide system and plasma bicarbonate concentration, a clear distinction must be made between carbon dioxide and water produced at elevated rates within mitochondria of contracting muscle cells, and the carbon dioxide generated by bicarbonate buffering of protons. This distinction is hidden in Whipp's description, and the reader is left with the misleading impression that all of the increase in carbon dioxide production occurs as a result of bicarbonate buffering. However, this increase is a function of both respiratory chain carbon dioxide production and proton buffering by extracellular bicarbonate. The increase in the former is directly proportional to the increase in muscle oxygen uptake, such that only that component of carbon dioxide production due to bicarbonate buffering of protons can be associated with an anaerobic threshold.

A third of Professor Whipp's article deals with the probability of skeletal muscle experiencing periods of mitochondrial hypoxia at exercise intensities approaching, at and above the anaerobic threshold. The evidence provided by several cited groups in both sections of this chapter at best supports a probability (suggestion) that mitochondrial hypoxia may occur at exercise intensities well above the anaerobic threshold. For example, it has been speculated that oxygen delivery may be inadequate, with consequent mitochondrial hypoxia, during maximal contractile activity in highly oxidative canine gracilis muscle (Duhaylongsgod et al. 1993). However, there is as yet no such evidence at lower exercise intensities.

So what is the anaerobic threshold? It does represent a mismatch between glycolytic lactate production and pyruvate conversion to acetyl Co-A. The evidence to date supports the idea that no oxygen limitation exists at the onset of this mismatch. Mechanistically, one must turn one's attention to the regulation of enzyme activities at and downstream of pyruvate dehydrogenase.

Part D: Rebuttal
Brian Whipp

My article itself is a rebuttal of Dr Lindinger's well-written and concise representation of the contra-anaerobic threshold argument(s). The percipient reader, however, cannot have failed to notice the absence of any consideration of the criterion value necessary to determine whether or not there is an anaerobic contribution to the lactate production at high work rate (not, of course, that all need be), and also to what extent the extant literature actually provides the evidence to resolve the issue. I will refrain from warranted challenge to his comments on the ventilatory control aspects as, while important, they are tangential to the core issue. He sees the currently available evidence as sufficient to justify a decisive 'no' in answer to the question of whether there is an anaerobic threshold during muscular exercise. To which I contend, not so; not justifiably decisive. Not a decisive 'yes', I concede, but not a 'no' either. But the evidence that has convinced him I find not to be convincing. To be decisively dispositive of the controversy, two crucial issues must be resolved. (1) What is the critical oxygen partial pressure necessary to sustain mitochondrial oxygen utilisation under the real in situ conditions of heavy-intensity exercise? (2) Are there regions (possibly small) of the muscle fibres (regardless of type) that infringe upon this level? I contend that the answers to these questions are not currently known. It is important in science that the link between implication and inference not be stretched beyond the breaking point.

References

Aubert A, Costalat R, Magistretti PJ, Pellerin L 2005 Brain lactate kinetics: modelling evidence for neuronal lactate uptake upon activation. Proceedings of the National Academy of Sciences 102(45):16448–16453

Barr DP, Himwich HE 1923 Studies in the physiology of muscular exercise. II. Comparison of arterial and venous blood following vigorous exercise. Journal of Biological Chemistry 55:525–538

Beaver WL, Wasserman K, Whipp BJ 1986 Bicarbonate buffering of lactic acid generated during exercise. Journal of Applied Physiology 60(2):472–478

Bonen A 2000 Lactate transporters (MCT proteins) in heart and skeletal muscles. Medicine and Science in Sports and Exercise 32(4):778–789

Brooks GA 1985 Lactate: glycolytic product and oxidative substrate during sustained exercise in mammals – the 'lactate shuttle'. In: Gilles R (ed) Comparative physiology and biochemistry: current topics and trends, vol A, respiration-metabolism-circulation. Springer, Berlin, 208–218

Brooks GA 1986 Lactate production under fully aerobic conditions: the lactate shuttle during rest and exercise. Federation Proceedings 45:2924–2929

Brooks GA 2000 Intra- and extra-cellular lactate shuttles. Medicine and Science in Sports and Exercise 32:790–799

Brown GC 1992 Control of respiration and ATP synthesis in mammalian mitochondria and cells. Biochemical Journal 284:1–13

Conley KE, Ordway GA, Richardson RS 2000 Deciphering the mysteries of myoglobin in striated muscle. Acta Physiologica Scandinavica 168:623–634

Connett RJ, Gayeski TEJ, Honig CR 1986 Lactate efflux is unrelated to intracellular PO_2 in working red skeletal muscle in situ. Journal of Applied Physiology 61:402–408

Connett RJ, Honig CR, Gayeski TE, Brooks GA 1990 Defining hypoxia: a systems view of VO2, glycolysis, energetics and intracellular PO2. Journal of Applied Physiology 68(3):833–842

Duhaylongsod FG, Griebel JA, Bacon DS, Wolfe WG, Piantadosi CA 1993 Effects of muscle contraction on cytochrome a,a_3 redox state. Journal of Applied Physiology 75:790–797

Gevers W, Dowdle E 1963 The effect of pH on glycolysis in vitro. Cinical Science 25:343–349

Gitt AK, Wasserman K, Kilkowski C, Kleemann T, Kilkowski A, Bangert M, Schneider S, Schwarz A, Senges J 2002 Exercise anaerobic threshold and ventilatory efficiency identify heart failure patients for high risk of early death. Circulation 106:3079–3084

Gladden LB 2004 Lactate metabolism: a new paradigm for the third millennium. Journal of Physiology 558:5–30

Greco FA, Solomon AK 1997 Kinetics of chloride-bicarbonate exchange across the human red blood cell membrane. Journal of Membrane Biology 159(3):197–208

Hagberg JM, Coyle EF, Carroll JE, Miller JM, Martin WH, Brooke MH 1982 Exercise hyperventilation in patients with McArdle's Disease. Journal of Applied Physiology 52:991–994

Haller RG, Wyrick P, Taivassalo T, Vissing J 2006 Aerobic conditioning: an effective therapy in McArdle's disease. Annals of Neurology 59(6):922–928

Harrison MH 1985 Effects on thermal stress and exercise on blood volume in humans. Physiological Reviews 65(1):149–209

Hochachka PW, Mommsen TP 1983 Protons and anaerobiosis. Science 219(4591):1391–1397

Hogan MC 2001 Fall in intracellular PO(2) at the onset of contractions in Xenopus single skeletal muscle fibers. Journal of Applied Physiology 90(5):1871–1876

Hogan MC, Arthur PG, Bebout DE, Hochachka PW, Wagner PD 1992 Role of O2 in regulating tissue respiration in dog muscle working in situ. Journal of Applied Physiology 73(2):728–736

Honig CR, Gayeski TEJ, Federspiel W, Clark A Jr, Clark P 1984 Muscle O_2 gradients from hemoglobin to cytochrome: new concepts, new complexities. Advances in Experimental Medicine and Biology 169:23–38

Jennings DB 1994 Respiratory control during exercise: hormones, osmolality, strong ions and PaCO2. Canadian Journal of Applied Physiology 19(3):334–349

Jones NL, Ehrsam RE 1982 The anaerobic threshold. In: Terjung RL (ed) Exercise and sport sciences reviews, volume 10. American College of Sports Medicine, The Franklin Institute Press, Philadelphia, 49–83

Juel C 2001 Current aspects of lactate exchange: lactate/H+ transport in human skeletal muscle. European Journal of Applied Physiology 86:12–16

Kemp G 2005 Lactate accumulation, proton buffering and ph change in ischemically exercising muscle. American Journal of Physiology. Regulatory, Integrative and Comparative Physiology 289: R895–R901

Keul J, Keppler D, Doll E 1967 Lactate/pyruvate ratio and its relation to oxygen pressure in arterial, coronarvenous and femorolovenous blood. Archives of Internal Physiology and Biochemistry 75:573–578

Keul J, Doll E, Keppler D 1972 Oxidative energy supply. In: Energy metabolism of human muscle. University Park Press, Baltimore, MD

Lahiri S, Forster RE 2nd 2003 CO_2/H^+ sensing: peripheral and central chemoreception. International Journal of Biochemistry and Cell Biology 35(10):1413–1435

Lindinger MI, Grudzien SP 2003 Exercise-induced changes in plasma composition increase erythrocyte Na+,K+-ATPase but not Na+-K+-2Cl- cotransporter, activity to stimulate net and unidirectional K+ transport in humans. Journal of Physiology 553(Pt 3):987–997

Lindinger MI, Spriet LL, Hultman E, Putman T, McKelvie RS, Lands LC, Jones NL, Heigenhauser GJ 1994 Plasma volume and ion regulation during exercise after low- and high-carbohydrate diets. American Journal of Physiology 266(6 Pt 2):R1896–R1906

Lindinger MI, Kowalchuk JM, Heigenhauser GJ 2005 Applying physicochemical principles to skeletal muscle acid-base status. American Journal of Physiology, Regulatory, Integrative and Comparative Physiology 289(3):R891–R894

Miller BF, Fattor JA, Jacobs KA, Horning MA, Navazio F, Lindinger MI, Brooks GA 2002 Lactate and glucose interactions during rest and exercise in men: effect of exogenous lactate infusion. Journal of Physiology 544(Pt 3):963–975

Miller BF, Lindinger MI, Fattor JA, Jacobs KA, Leblanc PJ, Duong M, Heigenhauser GJ, Brooks GA 2005 Hematological and acid-base changes in men during prolonged exercise with and without sodium-lactate infusion. Journal of Applied Physiology 98:856–865

Myers J, Ashley E 1997 Dangerous curves. A perspective on exercise, lactate and the anaerobic threshold. Chest 111(3):787–795

O'Dochartaigh CS, Ong HY, Lovell SM, Riley MS, Patterson VH, Young IS, Nicholls DP 2004 Oxygen consumption is increased relative to work rate in patients with McArdle's disease. European Journal of Clinical Investigation 34:731–737

Owles WH 1930 Alterations in the lactic acid content of the blood as a result of light exercise and associated changes in the CO_2-combining power of the blood and in alveolar CO_2 pressure. Journal of Physiology 69:214–237

Richardson RS, Noyszewski EA, Leigh JS, Wagner PD 1998 Lactate efflux from exercising human skeletal muscle: role of intracellular PO2. Journal of Applied Physiology 85(2):627–634

Richardson RS, Leigh JS, Wagner PD, Noyszewski EA 1999 Cellular PO_2 as a determinant of maximal mitochondrial O_2 consumption in trained human skeletal muscle. Journal of Applied Physiology 87:325–331

Richardson RS, Noyszewski EA, Haseler LJ, Bluml S, Frank LR 2002 Evolving techniques for the investigation of muscle bioenergetics and oxygenation. Biochemical Society Transactions 30:232–237

Robergs RA, Ghiasvand F, Parker D 2004 Biochemistry of exercise-induced metabolic acidosis. American Journal of Physiology. Regulatory, Integrative and Comparative Physiology 287: R502–R516

Rossiter HB, Whipp BJ, Ward SA, McIntyre DJ, Griffiths JR, Howe FA 2004 The heterogeneity of intramuscular metabolism using simultaneous ^{31}P 2D-CSI and pulmonary oxygen uptake (VO$_2$) during incremental knee-extensor exercise in humans. Proceedings of the International Society of Magnetic Resonance in Medicine 12:773

Schenkman KA, Marbel DR, Burns DH, Feigl EO 1997 Myoglobin oxygen dissociation by multiwavelength spectroscopy. Journal of Applied Physiology 68:2369–2372

Spriet LL, Howlett RA, Heigenhauser GJ 2000 An enzymatic approach to lactate production in human skeletal muscle during exercise. Medicine and Science in Sports and Exercise 32(4):756–763

Stainsby WN, Brechue WF, O'Drobinak DM 1991 Regulation of muscle lactate production. Medicine and Science in Sports and Exercise 23(8):907–911

Stringer WW, Wasserman K, Casaburi R, Porszasz J, Maehara, French W 1994 Lactic acidosis as a facilitator of oxyhemoglobin dissociation during exercise. Journal of Applied Physiology 76:1462–1467

Svedahl K, MacIntosh BR 2003 Anaerobic threshold: the concept and methods of measurement. Canadian Journal of Applied Physiology 28(2):299–323

Visser BF, Kreuknet J, Maas H 1964 Increase of whole blood lactic acid concentration during exercise as predicted from pH and PCO$_2$ determinations. Pflügers Archiv 281:300–304

Wasserman K 1994 Coupling of external to cellular respiration during exercise: the wisdom of the body revisited. American Journal of Physiology 266:E519–E539

Wasserman K, McIlroy MB 1964 Detecting the threshold of anaerobic metabolism in cardiac patients during exercise. American Journal of Cardiology 14:844–852

Wasserman K, Whipp BJ, Koyal SN, Beaver WL 1973 Anaerobic threshold and respiratory gas exchange during exercise. Journal of Applied Physiology 35:236–243

Wasserman K, Whipp BJ 1975 Exercise physiology in health and disease. American Review of Respiratory Disease 112:219–249

Wasserman K, Beaver WL, Davis JA, Pu JZ, Heber D, Whipp BJ 1985 Lactate, pyruvate and lactate-to-pyruvate ratio during exercise and recovery. Journal of Applied Physiology 59:935–940

Wasserman K, Hansen JE, Sue DY, Stringer WW, Whipp BJ 2005 Principles of exercise testing and interpretation. Lea and Febiger, Philadelphia

Whipp BJ 1994 The bioenergetic and gas-exchange basis of exercise testing. Clinics in Chest Medicine 15:173–192

Whipp BJ, Mahler M 1980 Dynamics of gas exchange during exercise In: West JB (ed) Pulmonary gas exchange, vol. II. Academic Press, New York, 33–96

Whipp BJ, Rossiter HB 2004 The kinetics of oxygen uptake: physiological inferences from the parameters. In: Jones AM, Poole DC (eds) Oxygen uptake kinetics in health and disease. Routledge, London, 64–94

Whipp BJ, Ward SA, Wasserman K 1986 Respiratory markers of the anaerobic threshold. Advances in Cardiology 35:47–64

Whipp BJ, Davis JA, Wasserman K 1989 Ventilatory control of the 'isocapnic buffering' region in rapidly-incremental exercise. Respiration Physiology 76:357–368

Whipp BJ, Lamarra N, Ward SA 1995 Obligatory anaerobiosis resulting from oxygen uptake-to-blood flow ratio dispersion in skeletal muscle: a model. European Journal of Applied Physiology 71:147–152

Wilson DF, Erecinska M, Drown C, Silver IA 1977 Effect of oxygen tension on cellular energetics. American Journal of Physiology 233: C135–C140

SECTION 2

Gender differences

Section introduction: Current limits of physiological knowledge: the legacy of male–based physiology

Sarah A. Nunneley

Although women now play key roles as both scientists and subjects in exercise physiology, the legacy of its all-male origins remains embedded in most physiology courses and textbooks. The prevailing, if unstated, assumption is that the standard human is male; compared to that standard, women are found to be not only smaller but also subtly different with respect to metabolism, and more difficult to study due to variations in their hormonal *milieu* (Shephard 2000a). In fact, some still call women (slightly more than half of the human race) a 'special population' (Marolf et al. 2001). In the next few pages, we will take a look at this conundrum, based in part on the author's experience with human experimentation over the past 35 years, a period of great change in attitudes toward women and their physical capabilities in work, sport and adventure.

How we got here

Modern physiology emerged as a distinct discipline during the 19th century. In those days, science was generally an amateur's subject pursued by gentlemen with a classical education and personal wealth, or a well-to-do patron to support their work. Although women sometimes assisted or were unacknowledged partners in scientific endeavours, science wore a male face. Furthermore, educated men viewed women as 'the weaker sex', creatures with limited physical capacity who might suffer harm if allowed to undertake rigorous studies (Newcomer 1959). Work outside the home was for men, while women supervised the household, bore children and were confined to bed for a prolonged period after each birth. The male arbiters of science and empire ignored the fact that in other parts of the world (or, for that matter, among their own peasantry), women not only bore the children, but were full partners in the never-ending physical work required for subsistence; such women did not have time to rest after normal childbirth, but instead strapped the babies onto their backs and resumed work.

Blinkered by the attitudes of their class and time, the proto-physiologists who sought to understand the effects of physical work (Section 1) and environmental stress (Section 4) saw no reason to study women. Thus, in physiology, as in language, the standard was male: human, mankind, man-like, subsuming women under the pronoun 'he' in statements that referred to both genders. Despite the rise of higher education for women beginning in the mid-19th century, male monopolisation of physiology continued through the Industrial Revolution and two World Wars. However, those very upheavals drew women out of their domestic settings and into the world of work, including tasks in heavy industry that had been previously regarded as being beyond their capabilities. The result was a gradual change in social attitudes that, among other things, encouraged physiologists to begin systematic studies of women in work and sport. These matters are further discussed at the beginning of Chapter 11.

Early studies of female subjects often concerned measurement of passive characteristics such as body composition and basal metabolism, but experimenters gradually began to address physical activity (Åstrand 1952). During the early 1970s, the topics of interest expanded to include issues related to fitness, training effects and thermal tolerances (Drinkwater 1973, Nunneley 1978). Data from healthy young women (college students) were compared to earlier findings from healthy young men, leading to the conclusion that women had a low capacity for physical exertion and responded poorly to heat stress, thus confirming the expectations of the time. The largely unrecognised caveat was that the male subjects had been military recruits and college students, who normally participated in strenuous work and sports, while female college students at that time rarely engaged in vigorous exercise (Nunneley 1978). Thus, while the findings represented norms for their respective populations, they did not address women's physiological capacities per se. The blinkers were still on.

In the US, growing interest in women's inherent physiological characteristics coincided with the rise of feminism in the 1960s, followed by the 1972 passage of Title IX (USA), legislation that opened the door to collegiate sports for women; other nations made comparable changes. A contemporaneous liberating factor was the ready availability of exogenous hormones that allowed women to control their reproductive lives, and even reschedule their menstrual cycles. Physiologists began to adjust their calculations to allow for gender-related variables, such as lean body mass, and in some cases studied exercise effects simultaneously in groups of men and women matched for variables such as body size or heat acclimatisation, and found that some of the presumed gender differences in response to stress were actually by-products of body build and lifestyle. Humans are not a dimorphic species: with respect to many physical and physiological characteristics, men and women can be represented by two bell-shaped curves that have different amplitudes and mean values, but nevertheless overlap. Thus, for occupations that involve physical exertion, it makes more sense to set rational requirements for individual capacity (Chapter 14.1), rather than to arbitrarily exclude women while admitting small or unfit men.

The male-controlled world of big-time sport was very slow to change: the US Amateur Athletics Union did not allow women to participate in long-distance running until 1971 and the Olympic Committee waited until 1984 to establish a women's marathon. Since then, many social and financial barriers have fallen, and enough women have been exposed to sport in schools and colleges to allow the emergence of elite female athletes with access to high-quality coaching; as a result, records for female athletes have improved rapidly and come ever closer to those for men, as discussed in Chapters 11 and 14.2.

As we now know, young women's physiology varies subtly over time with their natural menstrual cycles and the use of contraceptive hormone regimens, and more radically when they become pregnant (Chapters 11 and 12). Furthermore, strenuous physical training, combined with efforts to control body mass, can flatten the normal hormone curve and produce the female athlete triad (Chapter 11). These variations can make the study of women and exercise more complex than similar studies of men although, in many cases, the physiological effects of the hormone cycle are so subtle that they can only be demonstrated under rigorously controlled laboratory conditions. In many studies, the division between luteal and follicular phases has been estimated simply by asking the subject how many days it has been since she last started menstruating, and assuming this cycle in this woman is 28 days (Chapter 11). Of course, the cycle ends as women age (menopause), producing a sudden loss of reproductive hormones, and related physiological changes that have no parallel in the gradual decline of testosterone that occurs in ageing men. Only recently have physiologists begun to study the effects of exercise and training in postmenopausal women (Chapter 13).

Where we are

Even today, most basic physiology textbooks treat women as an afterthought. In lectures, as in texts, the presentation is based on that shibboleth, the 70 kg man. From him, students learn the standard values for cardiac output, oxygen uptake, heat production and water requirements, and he is the basis for the calculation of therapeutic dosages and the resultant packaging of pharmaceuticals. Of course, calculations can be adjusted for body size, but women are not just small men. For instance, lean women have more body fat than lean men (Chapter 11), and resistance training in women increases strength without the accompanying muscle mass seen in men (Shephard 2000a). Nevertheless, these are all variations on a theme, in the sense that women are members of the same species as men, with essentially similar physiological responses to stress. Efforts to adapt protective equipment for use by women have unplanned pay-offs in accommodating small men, including large segments of Asian male populations, whose body size is typically smaller than men in the West.

Judging from current journal articles, physiologists fall into three camps in their approaches to women and exercise. Some feel that every experiment involving women should be controlled for the menstrual cycle, preferably by studying each female subject twice under each experimental condition to collect data for both the follicular and luteal phases. One must then also decide how to deal with subjects who are taking exogenous hormones or who have no regular cycles. The sheer laboriousness of such studies often sends investigators into the second camp: those who avoid the problem by studying only male subjects. Justifications for this dodge include: (a) lack of time or funding for double (follicular and luteal) studies, (b) alleged inability to obtain female subjects, (c) the absence (or scarcity) of women in the population of interest, (d) lack of privacy or other feminine amenities in the study setting, or (e) fear that the women might be pregnant (see below). A more pragmatic viewpoint leads to the third experimental design, in which both male and female subjects are included, perhaps in the same proportion as in the population of interest, and the women's hormonal status is ignored on the grounds that the effects are too subtle to alter the results or that the activity under investigation goes on without reference to that cycle.

Studies of pregnant women raise ethical issues because the experiment necessarily involves a foetus that is incapable of assenting to participation, and this concern radiates to all women of reproductive age, because they might be pregnant without knowing it (Shephard 2000b). This can lead to either extreme caution in using female subjects or their avoidance altogether. The former approach can be seen in protocols where female volunteers for stressful experiments had to attend briefings and sign documents informing them of potential risks to a foetus (including unknown risks), affirm that they were not trying to become pregnant and were using reliable contraception or abstaining from sex, and submit a urine sample for pregnancy testing on the morning of each day they participated in the experiment. Avoidance of the problem was standard prac-

tice for decades in pharmaceutical testing in the US; exclusive use of male volunteers assured that no foetus would be exposed to the test substance. This prevented scientists from learning the specific therapeutic needs of women for heart disease and other important medical conditions.

The editors of this textbook have chosen to use the term gender with regard to the distinction between men and women. That is a legitimate decision, but it is worth mentioning some points related to terminology. As set forth in any good dictionary, 'sex' refers to the division of a species into males and females, according to their reproductive functions, and in humans relates to the presumed presence of either one or two X chromosomes in the individual's genome. On the other hand, 'gender' refers to the state of being male or female in a social or cultural context and has, of course, become a complex issue in a world where sex-change operations are possible and cross-dressing may be acceptable. Use of gender in physiology is logical because it allows for the fact that volunteer subjects self-designate themselves as men or women, and at the same time avoids confusion (or innuendo) regarding sex as a behaviour (Laner 2000). In a related issue, 'male' and 'female' may be used as nouns with respect to animals, but should only be used as adjectives when referring to humans, for whom the appropriate nouns are boys/men and girls/women.

The chapters in this section summarise the current state of our knowledge regarding exercise physiology in women. We know much more than we did even a decade ago, but many questions remain, and we need to establish a balance between the study of hormone effects for their own sake and the practical aspects that affect real-world activities. As noted in Chapter 13, complete understanding of inherent gender differences in response to exercise must await studies of men and women who have led equally active lives from childhood through to maturity and old age.

References

Åstrand P-O 1952 Experimental studies of working capacity in relation to sex and age. Munksgaard, Copenhagen, 1–171

Drinkwater BL 1973 Physiological responses of women to exercise. In: Wilmore JH (ed) Exercise and sport sciences reviews. Academic Press, New York, 125–153

Laner MR 2000 'Sex' versus 'gender': a renewed plea. Sociological Inquiry 70(4):462–474

Marolf GA, Kuhn A, White RD 2001 Exercise testing in special populations: athletes, women, and the elderly. Primary Care 2001 28(1):55–72, vi

Newcomer M 1959 A century of higher education for women. Harper and Brothers, New York, 26–28

Nunneley SA 1978 Physiological responses of women to thermal stress: a review. Medicine and Science in Sports 10(4):250–255

Shephard RJ 2000a Exercise and training in women, Part I: influence of gender on exercise and training responses. Canadian Journal of Applied Physiology Feb 25(1):19–34

Shephard RJ 2000b Exercise and training in women, Part II: influence of menstrual cycle and pregnancy. Canadian Journal of Applied Physiology Feb 25(1):35–54

Chapter 11

Exercise, work and stress in adolescent and adult women

Denise L. Smith   Patricia C. Fehling   Jeffrey O. Segrave

Humans have been obsessed with measuring and portraying the human body throughout history. Perhaps the most famous recording of the human body is Leonardo da Vinci's *Vitruvian Man*. But how does the female body compare to this representation of the male body? In addition to curiosity and intrigue about the human body, there has been considerable attention paid across the millennium to differences between males and females in terms of physical capabilities. This chapter will briefly review the history of women in work and sport, compare the structure and function of males and females, report on literature comparing the physical performance and physiological function of males and females, and discuss differences in physical performance and physiological function as they relate to the menstrual cycle.

1 HISTORY OF WOMEN IN WORK AND EXERCISE

1.1 Women and work

Work is a common element of every society, a requisite for survival and one often predicated on a gender-based division of labour. Throughout history, women have performed strenuous work, whether in the cotton fields of the American south, the paddy fields of Asia, the agricultural allotments of ancient Egypt or around the hearths and homes of the domestic domain in virtually every culture. In preindustrial Western societies, the family typically served as the fundamental economic and social unit, and women cooked and cleaned, made and mended clothes, manufactured and maintained articles in common daily use, performed household duties and cared for the children. Women of low social class and minority status invariably performed even more arduous work, sometimes working outside the house in traditional masculine fields, and often serving as indentured domestic servants.

The transformation from a predominantly agrarian, rural economy to an industrial urban society ushered in a new era in women's work, and the rise of the factory economy separated the world of work from the world of the home. While men typically assumed responsibility as wage earners and worked outside the home, women became primarily supporters and nurturers, and worked inside the home. In the US, the cult of true womanhood defined women in aesthetic and domestic terms, and biological and social arguments rationalised and justified women as being ill suited to the rigours of the workplace.

The gradual emergence of women in the paid workforce was furthered by the advent of World Wars I and II. The needs of the war machine and the shortage of male workers necessitated the employment of women in traditionally male-dominated occupations, and although the post-World War II work environment was generally hostile to women, the decades of the 1950s and 1960s, in particular, witnessed a dramatic increase in the number of older, married women in the labour market. In concert with a variety of powerful ideological, political, social and economic forces, the post-industrial, globalised economy has more recently wrought profound new changes in the nature of women's work. No longer restricted to the home, women have emerged in significant numbers as a viable and productive component of national workforces in both white- and blue-collar occupations, including many physically demanding trades. This latter topic is further developed within Chapter 14.1.

1.2 Women and sport performance

As in the world of work, women's sporting experiences have ultimately reflected larger sociocultural issues of gender roles, power relations, cultural expectations, women's quest for gender equality, meanings of cultural performances and conceptions about the body. Historically, programmes for women in sport have significantly differed from those of men, and have typically been more limited in number and style.

Despite such limitations, women have often remained physically active. In Egypt, ancient hieroglyphics depict women participating in aerobic exercise, dancing, swimming and a variety of ball games. Although not allowed to compete in, or even attend, the Olympic Games of ancient Greece, women established their own programme of competition called the Herean Games. In the Middle Ages and during the Renaissance, women engaged in archery, dancing, horse riding, skating and various ball activities.

Given traditional patriarchal beliefs about gender relations and societal divisions of labour in the 19th-century US, women's involvement in sport was largely sporadic, informal, invariably co-educational and limited to non-strenuous, lady-like and recreational activities. The most popular activities were archery, bowling, croquet, bicycling, tennis and golf. The mid-19th century Victorian formulation of women as being passive, gentle, delicate, submissive and nurturing largely consigned women to the domestic realm. In addition, many physicians counselled women against participation in competitive sport and strenuous physical exertion on the grounds that it might hinder their home-making responsibilities, compromise their child-bearing capabilities (Chapter 12), damage their bodies and tarnish their social image.

Throughout the course of the early 20th century, burgeoning industrialisation, urbanisation, the advent of world war and evolving conceptions of women's physical capacities enhanced women's entrée into the world of sport. As a result, the single most dramatic change in organised competitive sport and fitness during the past century has been the increased participation of girls and women. This development was precipitated by new opportunities in private and public programmes, government equal rights legislation, the global women's rights movement, the health and fitness movement, increased media coverage of women in sport and women athletes as role models (Coakley 2004). Today, women compete in greater numbers and in a wider variety of sports than ever before in recreational, school, college and professional settings. Women now constitute approximately 40% of the competitors in the Olympic Games.

1.2.1 Sport records

Despite the expanded opportunities for women in competitive sport, most researchers would generally agree that in most sports, if men and women competed against one another, men would typically emerge victorious (Chapters 14.2 and 15). The superiority of men is predicated on the fact that men are generally stronger than women, have greater cardiovascular power and have a larger proportion of lean body (muscle) mass. However, in some sports, such as running and swimming, the gap between men and women is closing, as women increasingly receive the benefits of improved training methods and coaching, greater societal acceptance and enhanced participation rates.

Chapter 14.2 contains a more detailed discussion of this gender gap, but consider briefly the following examples. In the 100 m, the 1932 women's World Record (11.9 s) was 17% slower than the men's record (10.2 s). By 2006, the gap had dropped to 7.4%, as the women's record fell to 10.49 s, compared to men, whose record was now 9.77 s. In the 400 m, the gap has narrowed even more dramatically, from a 38.3% differential in 1932 to a 10.2% differential in 2005. The World Records in the 100 m freestyle swim reflect similar trends. In 1905, women swam 100 m in 95.0 s, compared to 65.8 s for men, a 44.4% difference. In 2006, the gender difference was reduced to 11.7%: 53.42 s versus 47.84 s. In 1984, the first year that women officially competed in the Olympic marathon, Joan Benoit won the race in 2:24:52, while Portugal's Carlos Lopez ran it in 2:09:21, an 11.8% difference. Today, the world record for the women's marathon is 2:15:25 and for the men's marathon 2:04:55, an 8.6% differential. The current gap between men's and women's records in certain sports has stabilised at about a 10–15% differential. The question then becomes: Are we simply awaiting a further surge in women's participation in sport and exercise, or are the current differences a function of biology? While recognising the impact of cultural forces on women's levels of physical activity, we will, in this chapter, focus on physiological differences.

2 STRUCTURAL AND PHYSIOLOGICAL DIFFERENCES BETWEEN MALES AND FEMALES

Detailed discussion of the physiological limits to exercise and adaptations to training stimuli is presented within Section 1, while environmental influences are described in Section 4. In this chapter, we restrict discussion to gender-based differences alone, focusing upon postpubertal variations. Readers are directed to Chapter 15 for a discussion on anatomical and physiological differences in the prepubertal years.

2.1 Morphology

2.1.1 Body mass and stature

Adult males are heavier, taller and have less body fat and a greater skin surface area than females. Data from the National Health and Nutrition Examination Survey indicate that males are, on average, 15.5–19.3% heavier than females (MacDowell et al. 2005). Body mass patterns throughout the adult years are similar between males and females, but then increase during the fourth decade, briefly plateauing in the fifth, and finally declining through to the eighth decade. Between the seventh and eighth decades, females lose approximately 10% of body mass, while males lose approximately 8% (McDowell et al. 2005).

Males are approximately 8–9% taller than females across each decade. The height pattern for each gender is similar from the second to the eighth decade: height is relatively constant through to the fourth decade; thereafter, both genders experience a 0.7–2.0% loss every decade from the fifth through to the eighth (McDowell et al. 2005). This reduction in stature is primarily attributable to structural changes within the vertebral column.

2.2 Body composition

Males are heavier primarily because they have more lean body mass (muscle) than females, who generally have a higher percentage of fat. The average body fat for young males and females, 18–30 years, is approximately 13% and 26% respectively, increasing to 18% and 29% in those 31–50 years of age (Plowman & Smith 2003).

As part of the Health ABC longitudinal study, Katsiaras et al. (2005) measured 1512 black and white males ($N = 713$) and females ($N = 799$), aged 70–79 years. Overall, the males were heavier (81.0 ± 12.6 kg versus 68.7 ± 13.5 kg), taller (1.73 ± 0.06 m versus 1.59 ± 0.06 m), had less body fat ($28.6 \pm 5.2\%$ versus $39.2 \pm 5.7\%$) and had a greater lean body mass (57.2 ± 7.1 kg versus 40.9 ± 5.9 kg). Additionally, males had greater quadriceps and hamstring cross-sectional areas (CT scan). Males also had significantly less subcutaneous adipose tissue than females (47.1 ± 19.8 cm^2 versus $104.2 \pm$ 42.0 cm^2; CT scan data) in the mid-thigh region, but there was no difference in intramuscular adipose content: 9.6 ± 6.3 cm^2 (males) versus 9.8 ± 5.7 cm^2 (females).

2.2.1 Skeletal health and function

Bone mineral content is accrued throughout childhood, remaining constant in the early adult years for both men and women. After this plateau, there is an age-related decrease during middle age, that accelerates for women around the menopausal years (Chapter 13). On an absolute basis, men have a greater bone mineral content (3100–3500 g versus 2300–2700 g), larger bones and thicker cortices (Bailey et al. 1999), but there is no gender difference in the density of cortical bone (Khan et al. 2001). The greater bone mineral content is due, in large part, to greater calcium content, which results in a generally greater bone (mineral) density for males (Khan et al. 2001).

Both genders experience an age-related loss in bone mineral content and bone density, but there is a gender difference in the rate of cortical bone loss. After menopause, women experience an annual bone density loss of ~2.5–2.7% (predominantly from cortical sites), while men lose 0.8–1.0% during the same period (Khan et al. 2001). However, no gender difference is apparent in the rate of trabecular bone loss. In females, cortical bone becomes thinner due to an increased endosteal bone resorption, with little gain in the periosteal surface of the cortex. In males, there is a higher rate of periosteal acquisition and decrease in endosteal resorption, enhancing bone strength and decreasing susceptibility to fractures. This may explain the higher incidence of bone fractures among elderly women (Khan et al. 2001).

Beck et al. (2000) studied musculoskeletal strength in female ($N = 693$) and male ($N = 626$) US Marine Corps recruits. Overall, the females had significantly lower size-adjusted bone strength in the lower extremities, with both the section modulus and bone strength being 4.4% lower.

2.2.2 Lean body mass

Males have a greater lean body mass than females. The average 79 kg male has approximately 31 kg of muscle mass, whereas the average 57 kg female has approximately 20 kg of muscle mass (McArdle et al. 2001). While these absolute differences are well documented, the potential gender difference in muscle architecture, a difference that is linked to the quality of muscle strength and power, is less understood.

Abe et al. (1998) studied female ($N = 29$) and male athletes ($N = 22$) to describe gender differences in muscle architecture and the role that architecture played in muscle mass. The male athletes had a greater muscle layer thickness at all sites except the anterior thigh. Katsiaras et al. (2005), on the other hand, reported that males had greater amounts of muscle mass (cross-sectional area) at the mid-thigh than females. Abe et al. (1998) found that male athletes had a greater fascicle pennation angle than female athletes (triceps, vastus lateralis, gastrocnemius), but no significant differences were evident for fascicle length. It appears that the greater lean body mass of males is not the result of muscle architectural differences, but rather greater amounts of tissue.

Marras et al. (2001) studied the gender difference in the spine-loading trunk muscles in 20 females (25.0 ± 7.2 years) and 10 males (26.4 ± 5.5 years). Males had a significantly greater mass in the latissimus dorsi, erector spinae and external oblique muscles, but there were no significance differences in the masses of the rectus abdominis, internal oblique, psoas major or quadratus lumborum.

2.2.3 Fat mass

The pattern of fat distribution with greater deposits in the central (visceral) region is referred to as the android fat distribution. This is more common in men (Campaigne 1990), while the gynoid fat distribution (more peripheral) is more common in women. It is the android (visceral) adiposity pattern that is linked to several chronic disease risk factors, including, hyperinsulinaemia, insulin resistance, hypercholesterolaemia and hypertension (American College of Sports Medicine 2006, Chapters 28 and 30).

Clasey et al. (1997) used single-slice, abdominal CT scans to compare visceral (intraabdominal) fat in older and younger men and women. The authors reported that each age group of men had greater amounts of visceral fat than women (men 127.0 cm^2 and 44.1 cm^2; women 107.6 cm^2 and 33.6 cm^2 for older and younger subjects respectively).

2.2.4 Indirect measures of adiposity

Indirect measures of body composition should be treated with caution. While these indices can provide useful population data, extensive individual variability can invalidate the assumptions that underpin these measures, rendering compositional analysis from surface observations highly questionable. Nevertheless, we can use population statistics to draw some useful gender comparisons.

Waist circumference measures correlate well with adiposity in both genders; a circumference >115 cm is strongly associated with obesity (American College of Sports Medicine 2006). From 20 to 80 years, males have an approximately 6–8% larger waist circumference (MacDowell et al. 2005). This increased abdominal adiposity is known as the android fat distribution. For both genders, waist circumference increases from 20 through to 60 years, with an average change ranging from 2% to 4%. Both genders lose ~1.5% in the seventh decade and 3–4% in the eighth decade (McDowell et al. 2005). This pattern of increase and subsequent loss is similar to that observed for body mass.

The National Health and Nutrition Examination Survey found that males have less subcutaneous fat than females at the triceps (30–42% less across 2nd–8th decades), reflecting peripheral adiposity, and subscapula sites (12.2% less in the second decade to 2.1% less in the seventh decade; McDowell et al. 2005), reflecting central adiposity. The pattern for skinfold thickness is also similar with both genders gaining thickness (approximately 3–9% per decade) from the second through to the seventh decade (McDowell et al. 2005).

2.3 Muscle strength, power and adaptation

When comparing the genders for strength and power, it is important to consider whether absolute or relative comparisons are being made. Due to larger overall stature, men are stronger and more powerful than women on an absolute basis. On average, females are approximately two-thirds as strong as men, with a larger gap in upper-body strength measures, as compared to the lower body (Lauback 1976). When reported on a relative basis, strength differences are reduced, particularly for lower-body strength. When comparisons are made using either fat-free mass or muscle cross-sectional area, the gender differences largely disappear (Hurley & Hagberg 1998). This tells us that inherent, gender-related differences in motor unit function do not exist. Instead, since strength is a function of cross-sectional area, strength differences may be attributed to absolute variations in muscle size.

Similarly, women are less powerful than men on an absolute basis, but when these measurements are adjusted for lean body mass differences, the difference is again decreased (Baechle & Earle 2000). Lindle et al. (1997) found evidence that males appear to rely more upon the ability of muscle to store and utilise elastic energy, while females rely more upon neural factors during powerful activities.

These gender differences, however, tell us nothing about the ability of muscle tissue to respond to the repeated application of adaptation stimuli (resistance training). However, in general, it is thought that changes in neural, muscular and viscoelastic properties of muscle contribute to increased muscle strength in both genders as a result of resistance training.

Staron et al. (1994) trained 20 males and 14 females for 8 weeks, using a lower-body, progressive resistance programme. Strength was assessed at baseline and after every 2 weeks of training. Both genders increased absolute strength, but this was always greater for the males. However, relative strength changes (corrected for fat-free mass) were similar. The main gender difference was an apparent and rapid decrease in the percentage of type IIb fibres in the females within the first 2 weeks (12–21%). A similar response was observed in the males after 4 weeks of training. Experimental evidence shows that muscle fibre types are determined by the innervating motor unit, and can only change type following reinnervation. However, the histochemical properties are plastic and responsive to training stimuli, giving the impression that some fibres have taken on the characteristics of another phenotype.

Although strength adaptations were similar between genders, the mechanism by which these changes occurred may be different. Males appear to have a more favourable hormonal response, with changes in circulating testosterone (increased) and cortisol (decreased) promoting muscular hypertrophy. This response is less evident in females. Thus, it is possible that females have a more pronounced neural adaptation to resistance training, while males experience greater structural (cross-sectional area) changes.

Krivickas et al. (2006) analysed single-fibre and whole-muscle power production in older males and females (65–78 years). The females were 82% as strong in knee extension, 83% as strong in double leg press, 68% as powerful in knee extension and 75% as powerful in the double leg press when compared with males. Using biopsies obtained from vastus lateralis, they measured fibre size, cross-sectional area, shortening velocity (isometric and isotonic) and myosin heavy chain composition. No gender differences were detected for any of the single-fibre analyses.

With ageing, within- and between-gender differences in muscle function are evident (Chapter 16). For example, Lindle et al. (1997) found evidence that older females ($N = 7$; mean age 70 years) had greater stretch-shortening cycle enhancement than younger females and older and younger males. Additionally, the females in this study had superior muscle quality (peak force per unit muscle mass) for eccentric peak torque than males. Lynch et al. (1999) studied 225 males and 278 females (19–93 years; Baltimore Longitudinal Study of Aging). As expected, males had greater absolute peak torque and muscle mass across age groups. Although muscle quality differed at the arm between genders, with ageing, males lost muscle quality at greater rates than females; leg muscle quality changed at the same rate as both genders aged.

2.4 Pulmonary function

2.4.1 Lung volumes and minute ventilation

Before puberty, the vital capacity of boys is approximately 8% greater than in girls, as are its contributory volumes (Cotes 1979). However, all lung volumes and capacities are directly related to body stature and mass. Thus, when normalised, there is little difference across genders for most pulmonary function variables, either before or after puberty (Cotes 1979).

Adult males have approximately 30% greater maximal respiratory flows than females (Åstrand 1952, Schwartz et al. 1988). At a given absolute workload or oxygen uptake, women demonstrate a greater minute ventilation (Figure 11.1), which is achieved through both a greater tidal volume and breathing frequency (Cotes 1979). However, since lung volumes are typically smaller in women, it is mechanically more efficient to achieve this ventilation via increases in breathing frequency.

Minute ventilation responses to maximal exercise for males and females aged 4–20+ years are presented in Figure 11.1. As children mature, maximal minute ventila-

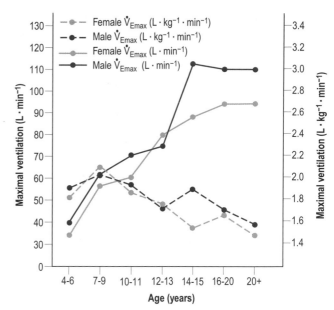

Figure 11.1 Pulmonary minute ventilation responses (absolute and relative) for males and females during maximal treadmill exercise as children age to adulthood. Based on data from Åstrand (1952).

tion increases, when recorded in absolute units ($L\cdot min^{-1}$), with males achieving greater values than females, particularly after puberty. When expressed on a relative basis ($L\cdot min^{-1}\cdot kg^{-1}$), it gradually declines from about 7 years until adulthood, with equivalent changes observed in both genders (Åstrand 1952).

2.4.2 Respiratory gas exchange

Respiratory gas exchange is affected by several variables: alveolar surface area, alveolar-arterial oxygen partial pressure gradient, blood haemoglobin concentration, thickness of the alveolar membrane and pulmonary capillary blood volume and flow. It appears, based on animal data, that when normalised to mass, adult females of the same age have a 20% greater alveolar surface area than men (Massaro et al. 1985).

There is no difference in arterial partial pressure of oxygen between the genders, although women have a higher 2,3-diphosphoglycerate concentration relative to their haemoglobin concentration, which shifts the oxygen dissociation curve rightward, possibly compensating for a lower haemoglobin concentration (Pate et al. 1985, Tate & Holtz 1998). However, women also maintain a marginally lower carbon dioxide partial pressure than men, which may act to counter this effect, eliciting a slight leftward displacement. This latter difference is most pronounced during pregnancy, when the sensitivity of the chemoreceptors is affected by progesterone.

2.5 Cardiovascular function

2.5.1 Heart size and volume

Women have smaller hearts, based on total mass and smaller left ventricular mass, wall thickness and end-diastolic cavity dimensions. These differences, however, are largely stature dependent.

A large study involving echocardiographic analysis of more than 600 normotensive, non-obese subjects, aged 4 months to 70 years, showed progressive age-related increases in absolute, or height and body surface area-adjusted, heart masses (de Simone et al. 1995). Gender differences in absolute or normalised heart masses emerged at the same time of life that height and body mass differences emerged, and are sustained across all adult ages. This study strongly suggests that left ventricular mass, like height and body mass, increases with age, irrespective of gender.

Aerobic (endurance) training is associated with positive adaptations in cardiac muscle and the heart (George et al. 1999). These adaptations occur primarily as an adaptation to increased ventricular load or volume overload and are similar in magnitude for both males and females. Resistance training is associated with increased left ventricular wall and septal thicknesses. These changes are thought to result from elevated myocardial work to overcome increased afterload (mean arterial pressure), but are diminished, or even become non-existent, when normalised to body size.

Pelliccia et al. (1996) studied male (N > 700) and female (N > 600) athletes of similar age, training intensity and sport participation (including 27 different sports). The authors reported that left ventricular dimensions and mass were significantly less in female athletes compared to male athletes (left ventricular end-diastolic dimension 54.2 mm versus 48.9 mm; left ventricular wall thickness 10.1 mm and 8.1 mm; left ventricular mass 206 g versus 133 g). This large-scale study demonstrated that female athletes display mild but statistically significant cardiac hypertrophy, as has been previously demonstrated for men. The greater wall thickness and left ventricular mass in males remained even after normalisation for height or body surface area. However, the dimension of the left ventricular cavity at end-diastole, and hence apparent end-diastolic volume, was larger in female athletes when normalised for body surface area.

A number of cross-sectional studies that utilised normally active (non-athletes) participants (de Simone et al. 1991, N = 110; Hense et al. 1998, N = 1371, Deague et al. 2000, N = 3000) have reported that the left ventricular mass index (left ventricular mass normalised for body surface area) is significantly greater in males than females, as are the posterior wall and intraventricular septum thicknesses. These morphological differences were not associated with significant gender differences in the rates, or extent, of diastolic filling of the heart. Therefore, in relation to ventricular mass, the left ventricular end-diastolic volume appears to be higher in both trained and untrained women than in their male counterparts. A study of young males and females using magnetic resonance imaging also found lower heart mass, cardiac output and stroke volume in females at rest, with marginally lower heart rates in the males (Marcus et al. 1999).

2.5.2 Blood volume

Women have a lower blood volume than men, even when normalised for body mass or fat-free body mass. Blood volume differences of over $5\ mL \cdot kg^{-1}$ are largely attributable to a lower red cell mass in females (Fortney et al. 1994, Wiebe et al. 1998). In healthy subjects, whole-blood viscosity is greater in males than in females; however, there is no gender difference in plasma viscosity, suggesting that the difference in whole-blood viscosity in men is due to their higher haematocrit (de Simone et al. 1991), and may contribute to the greater left ventricular mass index by increasing cardiac work.

A lower haematocrit in women results in a lower haemoglobin concentration and oxygen-carrying capacity. However, the driving force for oxygen delivery, arterial oxygen partial pressure, is not different between genders.

Given menstrual blood loss, women are likely to have a higher proportion of juvenile red blood cells. This could contribute to the lower fragility of red blood cells in females. Lower viscosity is also evident even when normalised for the difference in haematocrit (Kameneva et al. 1999), and this may help to improve oxygen delivery.

Endurance training causes an increase in red blood cell volume, due to the stimulation of erythropoiesis and increased plasma and total blood volumes (Green et al. 1999). During protracted exercise, progressive plasma loss occurs. However, the decrease in plasma volume occurs rapidly, causing rapid increases in haematocrit and haemoglobin concentration (Myhre et al. 1985). Indeed, plasma volume reduction occurs within the first 15 min of exercise, across a wide variety of air temperatures (Maw et al. 1998). The markedly lower haematocrit and haemoglobin concentrations found in females at rest are sustained throughout protracted exercise, and no significant differences in percentage mass loss are observed between males and females. The early reduction in plasma volume during exercise is due not to fluid loss but to its redistribution within the body, and is comparable in males and females.

2.5.3 Cardiac function

In untrained subjects, females display a higher heart rate ($\sim$20 $b \cdot min^{-1}$) when exercising at a low but equal workload (50 watts) compared to men (Wilmore et al. 2001). After 20 weeks of endurance training, exercising heart rate is reduced in both genders, with a greater reduction evident in females. It seems that males generally have a greater functional heart rate reserve, but this reserve is enhanced by training in both genders. At low workloads, small and comparable increases in stroke volume accompany training in both males and females, but at higher workloads, both training and gender differences are enhanced (Wilmore et al. 2001).

In a study of left ventricular function, Adams et al. (1987) reported that males and females had similar left ventricular ejection fractions at rest (gated blood-pool angiography). However, females had a smaller increase in ejection fraction and a lower maximal ejection fraction during supine exercise than did their male counterparts. While there were no differences in peak heart rate, the males exhibited a significantly higher peak systolic blood pressure during exercise. This was the major contributor to a small but significant increase in the rate pressure product, indicating that males have a higher myocardial oxygen uptake (consumption) at peak exercise than females. These differences in supine cardiac function were related to the work intensity that was absolutely greater in the males.

2.6 Metabolism

Metabolism collectively refers to the energy transformations that occur in the body, that are fuelled through chemical energy consumed as food. The caloric balance equation is the summation of energy (caloric) intake and expenditure, such that if the energy supply exceeds expenditure, then the body is in a positive balance and its mass will increase. Total energy expenditure (Chapter 32) is determined by the basal (resting) metabolic rate, diet-induced thermogenesis (heat production) and exercise-induced metabolic heat production (Chapter 19). Over a 24 h period, these components typically, and respectively, account for 60–75%, 7–13% and 15–30% of the total energy expenditure (Chapter 32), which tends to be higher in males (Adams 1967, Phillips et al. 1993, Tarnopolsky et al. 2001). However, when normalised for fat-free mass, this difference is no longer significant.

2.6.1 Basal and resting metabolic rate
Basal metabolic rate is defined as the energy expenditure required to sustain bodily functions in the waking (after 8 h sleep) rested state (30 min supine), when the individual is fasted (12 h), at normal body temperature and not stressed (physically or pharmacologically). Resting metabolic rate is a less stringent measure that quantifies energy expenditure while an individual is resting quietly in the supine position (30 min).

Although both basal and resting metabolic rates are higher (23–42%) in men than women, this difference is largely attributable to the greater body mass of males, and the normalised basal (resting) metabolic rate (Figure 11.2) rarely differs by more than 5% (Arciero et al. 1993, Berg 1991, Dionne et al. 1999, Horton et al. 1998, Lemmer et al. 2001). It should be noted, however, that the apparent age-related reduction in basal metabolic rate is, to some extent, an artefact (Chapter 16). That is, such data primarily reflect changes in the masses of our metabolically least active

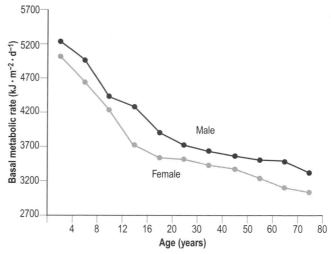

Figure 11.2 Maximal oxygen uptake and body mass for males and females aged 6–75 years. Modified from Shvartz & Reibold (1990) with permission.

tissues when at rest (adipose and muscle). When data are normalised to the masses of our most active tissues (brain, heart, kidneys, liver), this artefact is removed.

2.6.2 Fat and carbohydrate oxidation
The respiratory exchange ratio is the whole-body ratio of carbon dioxide produced, divided by oxygen consumed. Under steady-state conditions, this represents the relative use of carbohydrates and fats as energy sources, and varies from 0.7 to 1.0, representing a continuum from 100% fat to 100% carbohydrate utilisation. During resting states, on a mixed diet, the respiratory exchange ratio is about 0.83–0.85. During steady-state exercise, the ratio is typically 0.90–0.95.

In endurance-trained exercising individuals, females display significantly lower respiratory exchange ratios than males of similar training backgrounds during either a fixed-distance (Tarnopolsky et al. 1990) or a fixed-time run (Lamont et al. 2001, Phillips et al. 1993). This indicates a relatively greater use of fats as an energy source, which has a glycogen-sparing effect (Tarnopolsky et al. 1990). Several studies have documented women's greater reliance on fat as an energy source during submaximal endurance exercise, in both trained and untrained subjects, and using a variety of exercise modes (Froberg & Pederson 1984, Horton et al. 1998, Lamont et al. 2001, Phillips et al. 1993, Tarnopolsky et al. 1995). These metabolic differences are not attributable to either menstrual phase (follicular versus luteal) or menstrual status (eumenorrhoeic versus amenorrhoeic; De Souza et al. 1990).

2.6.3 Oxygen uptake during maximal exercise
Maximal oxygen uptake (aerobic power) is the ability to take in, transport and use oxygen during maximal exercise

(Chapters 1, 2, 10.1 and 10.2). Given the difficulties in ensuring that a maximal value has been achieved during testing, peak values are often reported. Since peak aerobic power is also body mass dependent, then gender differences typically favour males (Figure 11.3).

When maximal oxygen uptake is expressed in absolute terms (L·min^{-1}) males have approximately 30–60% higher values (Åstrand 1952, Shephard et al. 1988, Sparling 1980). Prior to puberty, these values are very similar (Chapter 15), and, in adults, when normalised for body size (relative terms: mL·kg^{-1}·min^{-1}), the differences decrease to 20–30%. Normalising to fat-free mass further reduces the differences (0–15%; Sparling 1980). However, if the fat-free body mass is indirectly measured, then interpreting the physiological significance of such normalisation may be very difficult.

It is also worth noting that considerable within- and between-gender variability in maximal oxygen uptake means that significant overlap exists between the genders. Thus, highly trained females often have higher maximal oxygen uptake values than normally active males (Wells & Plowman 1983). Finally, given the historical bias influencing participation in strenuous physical training, it is not clear to what extent differences in maximal oxygen uptake reflect biological or cultural differences between the genders.

2.7 Endocrine function

The endocrine system plays an integral role in the regulation of normal physiology, responding to the changing demands of the external and internal environments (Section 4). Hormones participate in the regulation of metabolism, body fluids and electrolyte balance (Chapters 18 and 19), and also provide the stimulus for maturation, growth, reproduction and development. This section outlines gender differences in the primary hormones responsible for these functions (Table 11.1).

2.7.1 Pituitary–adrenal axis (cortisol)

The hypothalamo-pituitary axis links the nervous and endocrine systems and is responsive to either perceived or real stress (Earle et al. 1999, Petrides et al. 1997, Wigger & Neumann 1999). The pituitary gland is divided into two distinct components: the anterior (adenohypophysis) and posterior pituitary (neurohypophysis). Adrenocorticotropin is released from the anterior pituitary in response to

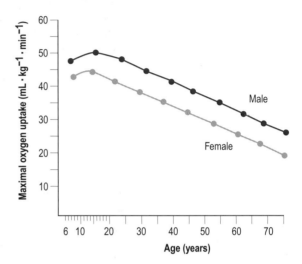

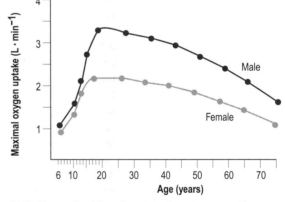

Figure 11.3 Normalised basal metabolic rate across the age span. Calculated from Brownell et al. (1987) and Elwyn et al. (1989).

Table 11.1 Plasma concentrations of several key hormones in resting men and women

Hormone	Men	Women	References
Cortisol (fasting)	50–250 µg·mL^{-1}	50–250 µg·mL^{-1}	Norman & Litwack 1997
Insulin	6–12 µU·mL^{-1}	6–12 µU·mL^{-1}	Galbo et al. 1975, Gustafson & Kalkhoff 1982, Hellstrom et al. 1996
Glucagon	42–90 pg·mL^{-1}	43–85 pg·mL^{-1}	Davis et al. 2000, Gustafson & Kalkhoff 1982
Adrenaline	70–100 pg·mL^{-1}	45–80 pg·mL^{-1}	Mills et al. 1996, Sanchez et al. 1980
Noradrenaline	300–400 pg·mL^{-1}	300–358 pg·mL^{-1}	Galbo et al. 1975, Mills et al. 1996, Sanchez et al. 1980
Growth hormone	1.0–6.0 mg·mL^{-1}	2.0–6.0 mg·mL^{-1}	Lang et al. 1987, Kraemer et al. 1993, Norman & Litwack 1997
Aldosterone	85 pg·mL^{-1}	Luteal: 85 pg·mL^{-1} Follicular: 156 pg·mL^{-1}	Stachenfeld et al. 1999
Vasopressin	1.4–1.7 pg·mL^{-1}	1.2–1.6 pg·mL^{-1}	Stachenfeld et al. 1999, Takamata et al. 2000

corticotropin-releasing hormone from the hypothalamus, and elicits secretion of cortisol into the circulation.

Cortisol, a steroid hormone, is secreted in response to stress, and exhibits diurnal variability that is generally similar between the genders (Born et al. 1995, Gelfin et al. 1995). Exercise stimulates cortisol secretion, which is related to the relative intensity (>60%) and duration of exercise (Inder et al. 1998, Kanaley et al. 2001), with a greater release associated with longer and more intense exercise (Galbo 1983, Kuoppasalmi et al. 1980). Secretion is also influenced by the type of exercise and the fitness level of the individual exercising. Endurance training lowers the basal level of cortisol in men and increases testosterone concentration, thus increasing the testosterone:cortisol ratio.

2.7.2 Adrenal function: catecholamine response

Catecholamines (adrenaline (epinephrine) and noradrenaline (norepinephrine)), a class of hormones responsible for adrenergic stimulation, are secreted by the adrenal medulla in response to fight or flight situations. Adrenergic stimulation has powerful systemic vasoconstrictor effects, and exerts both positive inotropic and chronotropic effects. Thus, cardiac output is elevated and redistributed away from visceral structures to the exercising muscles. Furthermore, catecholamines stimulate lipolysis and glycogenolysis, both of which support exercise.

At rest, there appear to be no gender differences in plasma catecholamine concentrations (Hellstrom et al. 1996, Laitinen et al. 1998, Pullinen et al. 1999, Rauste-von Wright et al. 1981). However, for both genders, plasma catecholamine concentrations increase dramatically with exercise (Gustafson & Kalkhoff 1982, Pullinen et al. 1999), with the change being directly related to exercise intensity (Galbo et al. 1975). Circulating concentrations rapidly decline after the cessation of exercise.

The adrenaline response appears to be higher in males, regardless of exercise mode (Davis et al. 2000, Gustafson & Kalkhoff 1982, Marliss et al. 2000, Sanchez et al. 1980). Noradrenaline has also been reported to be higher in males in response to endurance and isometric exercise (Davis et al. 2000, Gustafson & Kalkhoff 1982, Sanchez et al. 1980). However, these results should be viewed cautiously since several authors have failed to replicate these observations under similar conditions (Favier et al. 1983, Hellstrom et al. 1996, Pullinen et al. 1999). In trained subjects, the difference in catecholamine responses to exercise between the genders is reduced, although men still tend to have a higher concentration of circulating adrenaline at the end of prolonged exercise (Tarnopolsky et al. 1990).

2.7.3 Effect of insulin and glucagon on metabolism

Insulin and glucagon are the primary hormones involved in regulating carbohydrate metabolism and blood glucose concentration (Chapter 30), although cortisol and growth hormone also play an integral role. Insulin and glucagon

have reciprocal actions, with the former increasing glucose storage, while glucagon mobilises glucose for metabolism.

Plasma insulin concentrations decrease during work intensities >50% of peak aerobic power. The inhibiting action of exercise on glucose-mediated insulin secretion is also directly related to the duration of exercise. However, the increased need for glucose in active muscle, and increased adrenergic activity during exercise lead to a suppression of insulin secretion (Järhult & Holst 1979, Tarnopolsky et al. 1990). Adaptation to endurance training has been shown to attenuate the insulin response (Gyntelberg et al. 1977) and improve fatty acid utilisation and gluconeogenesis during submaximal exercise. Generally, there is little evidence of gender-related differences in the insulin response to exercise (Marliss et al. 2000), for either trained or untrained individuals (Friedmann & Kindermann 1989).

Glucagon is secreted in response to low blood glucose concentrations and increased plasma protein and fatty acid concentrations. Glucagon is catabolic, mobilising glucose and promoting glycogenolysis and lipolysis, resulting in increased metabolic rate (Frayn 1996, Norman & Litwack 1997). The rate of glucagon secretion is related to the rate of decline in blood glucose concentration. Accordingly, prolonged exercise promotes glucagon secretion, which declines during recovery as blood glucose is restored (Galbo et al. 1975, Marliss et al. 2000, Tarnopolsky et al. 1990). However, the relative exercise intensity, as well as blood glucose and catecholamine concentrations, also affect its secretion (Galbo et al. 1975). When comparing the genders, no differences have been found in glucagon secretion at rest or in response to exercise (Amiel et al. 1993, Galassetti et al. 2001).

2.7.4 Fluid balance (aldosterone and vasopressin)

Fluid and electrolyte balance is controlled hormonally, primarily through the actions of aldosterone and antidiuretic hormone (arginine vasopressin). Exercise increases plasma renin secretion, instigating aldosterone secretion. This process may be enhanced by increases in adrenocorticotropin and plasma potassium (Galbo 1983).

There are relatively few investigations that focus on gender differences in aldosterone secretion during exercise. There appears to be no gender difference in circulating aldosterone during maximal exercise (Stachenfeld et al. 1996), in either trained or untrained subjects (Crofton et al. 1986, Freund et al. 1987). While an increase in aldosterone has been shown in women during prolonged, dehydrating exercise, there was considerable variability in the response during the menstrual cycle, despite thorough control of hydration state, posture and timing of experiments (Stachenfeld et al. 1999).

Antidiuretic hormone secretion increases during exercise (Altemus et al. 2001, Inder et al. 1998), especially at intensities >60% of peak aerobic power, or exercise resulting in reduced plasma volume and increased plasma osmolality (Convertino & Greenleaf 1980). However, the stimuli for this release are not well understood. What is known is that increases in body core temperature, when accompanied by dehydration and increased plasma osmolality, will enhance secretion (Stachenfeld et al. 1996, 1999).

Stachenfeld et al. (1996) found no gender-related differences in circulating antidiuretic hormone concentration at rest, or during endurance cycling that elicited a 3% decrease in body mass (dehydration). However, the females displayed a delayed recovery in plasma antidiuretic hormone after exercise, although this was offset by a faster recovery in circulating aldosterone.

2.7.5 Reproductive function

One of the most obvious physiological differences between the genders is the circulating concentrations of the sex hormones (testosterone, oestrogen and progesterone). While men and women produce all three hormones, gender-based differences in secretion rates affect a variety of tissues, in particular skeletal muscle and adipose tissues, thus explaining many of the structural and morphological differences that account for variations in physical performance between the genders. Accordingly, males develop greater muscle mass, largely because of the anabolic effects of testosterone, whereas females have proportionally more fat, due to the relative lack of testosterone and greater concentrations of oestrogen and progesterone. Table 11.2 summarises gender differences in these hormones, with female concentrations given for the midfollicular and midluteal phases (Bonen et al. 1991, 1992, Nicklas et al. 1989, Tarnopolsky 1999).

Testosterone is produced primarily by the Leydig cells in the testes, with small amounts produced by the adrenal cortex in both genders. Circulating testosterone in women is only ~10% of that observed in men, with this being metabolised within adipose tissue (Ginsburg et al. 2001, Häkkinen & Pakarinen 1995, Weiss et al. 1983). Blood concentrations of testosterone are regulated by negative feedback inhibition of both luteinising hormone and gonadotropin-releasing hormone. Testosterone secretion is elevated in the prenatal male foetus and shortly after birth. Thereafter, the onset of puberty is influenced by the pituitary-gonadal system, and the resultant large increase in testosterone secretion triggers sexual maturation and stimulates growth. Testosterone secretion declines in later life, although it does not fall to levels seen in prepubescent males (Norman & Litwack 1997, Tarnopolsky 1999).

Testosterone has an anabolic effect on protein synthesis, promoting general body growth and the development of the male secondary sexual characteristics. It increases growth by increasing the synthesis and breakdown of proteins, resulting in muscular development beyond that observed in the female, as well as increasing skin thickness, body hair growth and vocal cord changes. Testosterone also leads to closure of the epiphyseal plates of the long bones. The later onset of puberty in males (~2 years) primarily accounts for gender differences in height. Hence, testosterone is responsible for the primary difference in body morphology between males and females.

Most studies examining the effect of exercise on testosterone secretion use resistance training as the experimental model (Häkkinen & Pakarinen 1995, Häkkinen et al. 1990, Kraemer et al. 1993, Weiss et al. 1983). However, some researchers have investigated the impact of endurance exercise in both genders (Ginsburg et al. 2001, Keizer et al. 1987c, Keizer et al. 1989).

An acute bout of resistance exercise increases circulating testosterone in men, with minimal impact in women (Häkkinen & Pakarinen 1995, Staron et al. 1994, Weiss et al. 1983). Weiss et al. (1983) demonstrated a 21.6% greater increase in testosterone in males compared to females, during sustained isometric handgrip to fatigue. Similarly, Häkkinen & Pakarinen (1995) found a tenfold greater testosterone concentration in males following heavy resistance exercise.

In response to resistance training (adaptation) programmes, males demonstrate elevated resting testosterone concentrations (Staron et al. 1994). However, Häkkinen et al. (1990) found no significant change in plasma testosterone concentration in seven physically active women. There were large interindividual differences among the women that correlated well with differences in power development. These correlations have not been demonstrated in men and may represent an important indicator of muscular power and strength trainability in women (Häkkinen et al. 1990).

Males have a significant gender-related response to endurance training that is not seen in females. Nevertheless, endurance-trained females do show greater increases in circulating testosterone during exhausting aerobic exercise, and this exceeds that found in untrained women (Keizer et al. 1987b). Furthermore, differences in testosterone secretion patterns have been reported in trained and

Table 11.2 Basal sex hormone concentrations

Hormone	Male	Female follicular phase	Female luteal phase
Testosterone (nmol·L^{-1})	~18.2	~0.87	~1.21
Oestrogen (pmol·L^{-1})	22.0–88.1	36.7–183.5	440.4–1376.2
Progesterone (nmol·L^{-1})	<1.90	0.32–4.74	7.9–88.5

untrained women during the follicular and luteal phases (Keizer et al. 1987a, b). However, the increase in the basal testosterone in trained females does not equate with that observed in endurance-trained males (Keizer et al. 1987a). After endurance events, testosterone levels decline, with one study demonstrating a greater decrease in males compared to females (Ginsburg et al. 2001).

Oestrogen is produced primarily by the ovaries, with small amounts produced by the adrenal cortex in both genders. During pregnancy, large quantities of oestrogen are secreted by the placenta. Three types of oestrogen are present in significant concentrations in the plasma of females: 17β-oestrodiol, oestrone and oestriol. The primary oestrogen secreted by the ovaries is 17β-oestrodiol and is the usual research focus. It has an oestrogenic potency 12 times that of oestrone and 80 times that of oestriol (Guyton & Hall 2000).

Oestrogen influences many bodily systems, often in intricate and complex ways that involve interactions with other hormones. Like testosterone, oestrogen plays important reproductive roles and is instrumental in developing primary and secondary sex characteristics. Oestrogen causes proliferation and growth of the tissues of the uterus, fallopian tubes and external genitalia. It also increases osteoblast activity, thereby causing increased bone mineral density, and it causes the epiphyses of long bones to fuse and stop growing. Oestrogens influence protein deposition, causing a slight increase in total body protein, and resulting in large gender differences in fat deposition. These differences constitute a primary characteristic of the female body composition. Oestrogen also increases metabolic rate, but this effect is only about one-third as potent as the effect of testosterone. Substrate metabolism is also modified by oestrogen, which enhances glycogen storage and increases lipolysis and the utilisation of fatty acids (Frankovich & Lebrun 2000). Fluid and electrolyte balance is modified by oestrogen, causing sodium and water retention by the tubules of the kidney. This effect is small and of questionable physiological significance. However, it may be quite pronounced during pregnancy, resulting in considerable body fluid retention. Oestrogen also affects the cardiovascular system, including: enhancing platelet aggregation and thrombosis, decreasing fibrinolytic activity, decreasing total cholesterol and low-density lipoprotein concentrations, and possibly mediating vasodilatation (Frankovich & Lebrun 2000).

Progesterone is secreted by the corpus luteum, and in the normal, non-pregnant female is only secreted in significant amounts during the latter half of the menstrual cycle. Humans secrete two types of progestins: progesterone and 17α-hydroxyprogesterone. However, progesterone is by far the more potent and is typically measured and reported in the literature. It plays an important role in the ovarian and uterine cycles, particularly secretory changes in the endometrium, and it increases fallopian tube secretion, promotes

breast development and modulates uterine contractions. Progesterone appears to be responsible for the increase in core temperature during the luteal phase of the menstrual cycle (0.3–0.4°C), increased minute ventilation and augmented ventilatory responses to hypoxia and hypercapnia (Kleitman & Ramsaroop 1948). It is also possible that progesterone plays a role in fluid retention during the luteal phase via complex feedback mechanisms involving aldosterone and the renin–angiotensin system (Fortney 1996, Frankovich & Lebrun 2000). These changes may affect the manner in which women respond to environmental stresses (Section 4).

3 MENSTRUAL FUNCTION AND PERFORMANCE

The menstrual cycle involves the cyclic, monthly and rhythmical fluctuations in the secretion of oestrogen and progesterone, and the corresponding physical changes in the ovaries and other sexual organs. It has historically been cited as one of the reasons why women could not perform certain occupations or athletic events. In this section, we briefly review the physiology of the menstrual cycle and research literature related to its influence upon physical performance and physiological function.

3.1 The menstrual cycle

The menstrual cycle lasts ~28 days and, based on ovarian events, is typically divided into two phases: the follicular (preovulation) and luteal (postovulation) phases. Ovulation occurs at the midpoint of the cycle, at approximately day 14. The follicular phase begins with menses and ends with ovulation, whereas the luteal phase begins with ovulation and ends with the beginning of the menstrual flow (menstruation; Figure 11.4). These events are hormonally controlled, with considerable interindividual variability in the hormonal fluctuations during the menstrual cycle (Figure 11.5).

During menstruation, the uterus sheds the outermost portion of the endometrium, in response to declining concentrations of oestrogen and progesterone, signalling commencement of the follicular phase. The endometrial tissue and some blood pass through the vagina as the menstrual flow. Normal menses lasts ~3–5 days, resulting in the loss of ~40 mL of blood and ~35 mL of serous fluid (Guyton & Hall 2000). Following menses, the ovarian follicle grows, producing increasing amounts of oestrogen and stimulating the endometrial regeneration (proliferative phase). Ovulation occurs at the end of the follicular phase, in response to a sudden increase in luteinising hormone, with the ruptured follicle converted into the corpus luteum, which then produces progesterone to initiate the luteal phase. The endometrium increases in size and complexity in preparation for implantation of an embryo. Towards the end of the luteal phase, the corpus luteum begins to

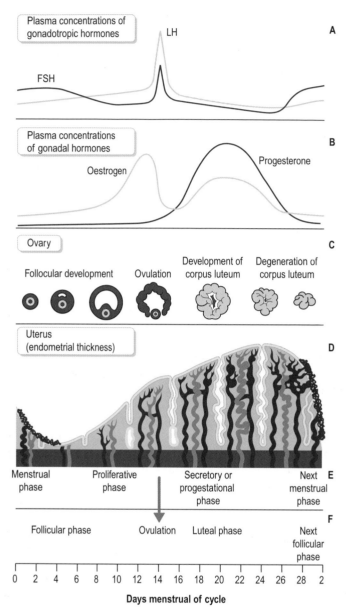

Figure 11.4 Correlation between hormonal levels and cyclical ovarian and uterine changes. Modified from Sherwood (1997) with permission.

degenerate, causing a decrease in progesterone secretion and endometrial degeneration, leading to menstruation.

3.2 The effects of the menstrual cycle on physiological function

3.2.1 The menstrual cycle and cardiovascular function

During exercise, oxygen delivery to the working muscles is elevated by increasing heart rate and stroke volume (cardiac output), and by redistributing blood away from less critical visceral organs (Chapter 1). The menstrual cycle appears not to have a significant impact on these mechanisms (De Souza et al. 1990, Dombovy et al. 1987, Eston & Burke 1984,

Garlick & Bernauer 1968, Higgs & Robertson 1981, Jurkowski et al. 1981, Lebrun et al. 1995, Nicklas et al. 1989).

3.2.2 Effect of menstrual cycle on respiratory function

During exercise, ventilation is increased to satisfy the metabolic oxygen demands of the working muscles. Several authors have reported that maximal minute ventilation is not significantly different between the follicular and luteal phase of the menstrual cycle (Bemben et al. 1995, De Souza et al. 1990, 1991, Dombovy et al. 1987, Hackney et al. 1994, Lebrun et al. 1995). In contrast, Jurkowski et al. (1981) reported that minute ventilation, in response to a maximal cycle ergometer test, was greater (approximately 8 L·min^{-1}) in the luteal phase than in the follicular phase. Schoene et al. (1981) have also reported that the hypoxic and hypercapnic ventilatory responses at rest, and the ventilatory equivalent during maximal exercise were higher in the luteal than in the follicular phase.

3.2.3 Effect of menstrual cycle on metabolic responses

The majority of researchers who have investigated exercise substrate utilisation have failed to detect differences associated with phases of the menstrual cycle (Bonen et al. 1983, De Souza et al. 1990, Galliven et al. 1997, Kanaley et al. 1992b, Nicklas et al. 1989). Similarly, Nicklas et al. (1989) took muscle biopsies from the vastus lateralis of six eumenorrhoeic women during the midfollicular and midluteal phases before and after cycling to exhaustion, and found no difference in glycogen utilisation between the phases.

There is, however, some evidence that substrate utilisation may be affected by the phase of the menstrual cycle. Dombovy et al. (1987) studied eight eumenorrhoeic athletes during a maximal cycle ergometer test and reported that the subjects had a lower respiratory exchange ratio during the luteal phase compared to the follicular phase, suggesting that they were relying more heavily upon fat utilisation during exercise in the luteal phase. However, these changes must be interpreted cautiously. Due to the sensitivity of carbon dioxide production to changes in breathing pattern, the exchange ratio can only be used to reflect cellular metabolism under steady-state conditions. Nevertheless, Hackney et al. (1994) also found the respiratory exchange ratio to be lower during the luteal phase, this time during 10 min of exercise at 35% and 60% of maximal aerobic power. These authors also reported that muscle glycogen utilisation was greater in the follicular phase, when subjects cycled for 60 min at 70% of maximal aerobic power (Hackney 1999). Lamont et al. (1987) reported significantly larger protein utilisation (based on urea nitrogen excretion) during the luteal phase, when 60 min of moderate-intensity exercise was performed.

In general, there appears to be no difference between the menstrual phases in the blood glucose response to exercise (Bonen et al. 1983, Kanaley et al. 1992b, Nicklas et al. 1989). For example, Galliven et al. (1997) investigated eight eumen-

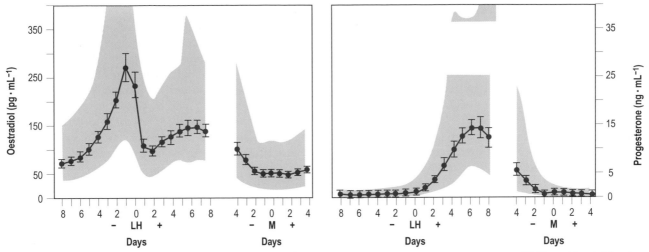

Figure 11.5 Concentration fluctuations in oestrogen (oestradiol), progesterone, follicle-stimulating hormone (FSH) and luteinising hormone (LH). Modified from Landgren et al. (1980) with permission.

orrhoeic non-athletes cycling at 70% of maximal aerobic power for 20 min. Plasma glucose was sampled every 10 min throughout the exercise period and during recovery. Plasma glucose concentrations were greater in the luteal phase after 20 min of exercise and for the first 20 min of recovery. However, the net integrated glucose response was not significantly different across phases of the menstrual cycle. Furthermore, there was no phase affect on the respiratory exchange ratio, implying that substrate utilisation was not significantly affected.

Many researchers have used blood lactate concentrations to evaluate metabolic responses. While it is correct that one of the end-products of glycolysis is lactic acid, its appearance in the blood reflects substrate turnover (production versus removal), which is affected by many factors other than metabolism (see Chapters 6, 7 and 10.3 for detailed discussions on this topic). Accordingly, such observations need to be interpreted cautiously, particularly if neither production nor removal was quantified.

Several groups have reported no effect of menstrual cycle phase on lactate responses to either submaximal or maximal exercise (Bonen et al. 1983, De Souza et al. 1990, Dombovy et al. 1987, Eston & Burke 1984, Kanaley et al. 1992b). Others, however, have reported a lower lactate response to exercise during the luteal phase (Jurkowski et al. 1981, Lavoie et al. 1987). For instance, Jurkowski et al. (1981) studied nine eumenorrhoeic women cycling at three different intensities (33%, 66% and to exhaustion at 90% of maximal aerobic power). These authors reported that the lactate response to the lightest exercise was not phase dependent, whereas exercise at 66% and 90% resulted in lower blood lactate concentrations in the luteal phase. Another group reported that recovery lactate concentrations were significantly lower in the luteal phase following a run to exhaustion (McCracken et al. 1994).

Hormonal differences that may influence metabolic responses to exercise have also been investigated. In general, researchers have reported no effect of menstrual phase on cortisol (Bonen et al. 1983, De Souza et al. 1991, Galliven et al. 1997, Kanaley et al. 1992a), adrenocorticotropic hormone (De Souza et al. 1991), prolactin (De Souza et al. 1991) or growth hormone response to exercise (Kanaley et al. 1992b). However, one group reported higher cortisol concentrations during the luteal phase, following 90 min of exercise, performed after a 24-h low-carbohydrate diet (Lavoie et al. 1987). Another group reported a greater growth hormone response during midcycle (near ovulation) than during menstruation (Hansen & Weeke 1974).

3.2.4 The menstrual cycle and muscular function

The influence of menstrual function on the contractile characteristics of muscle and measures of muscle function appear to be minimal, although some authors have reported phase-related differences. There are reports of greater strength in the premenstrual phase, improved handgrip endurance during the ovulatory phase (Petrofsky et al. 1976), greater handgrip strength during the follicular phase and greater handgrip strength during menses (Davies et al. 1991).

More recent studies have also reported conflicting results. Sawar et al. (1996) studied a group of women (weekly) throughout two menstrual cycles, and reported handgrip and quadriceps strength to be greater at midcycle (days 12–18) than during either the follicular or luteal phases. They also reported a significant, midcycle slowing of muscle relaxation and an increase in fatigability. Phillips et al. (1996) studied trained and untrained females, finding a significant increase (10%) in maximal voluntary force (adductor pollicis) during the follicular phase and a decrease at ovulation. In contrast, Greeves et al. (1999) found quadriceps strength was greater in the luteal phase.

In contrast, many studies have failed to detect differences in either strength or contractile properties of muscle between the menstrual phases (DiBrezzo et al. 1991, Gür 1997, Higgs & Robertson 1981, Janse de Jonge et al. 2001, Lebrun et al. 1995, White & Weekes 1998). For example, Janse de Jonge et al. (2001) investigated 15 subjects throughout the menstrual cycle, ensuring maximal force generation by superimposing electrical stimulation upon maximal voluntary activation. This group found no significant effect of the menstrual cycle on isometric handgrip and quadriceps strength, isokinetic (knee) extension and flexion torque or fatigue, or on various contractile characteristics of the quadriceps.

3.3 The menstrual cycle and physical performance

Concomitant with the increasing number of women participating in sport, fitness activities and strenuous physical work, there has been an increase in research aimed at delineating how the menstrual cycle affects physical performance. However, there is still a paucity of valid and reliable evidence concerning this relationship.

Since oestrogen and progesterone fluctuations may affect metabolism, respiration and muscle function and thermoregulation, some researchers have speculated that physical performance may vary across the menstrual cycle. While most authors have reported that neither maximal aerobic power nor time to exhaustion is affected by the phase of the menstrual cycle (Bemben et al. 1995, De Souza et al. 1990, 1991, Dombovy et al. 1987, Stephenson et al. 1982a, b), a few have noted a slightly higher maximal aerobic power during the follicular phase. For example, Schoene et al. (1981) reported that maximal aerobic power was higher in the follicular phase for untrained compared to trained women, while Lebrun et al. (1995) found a slightly higher maximal aerobic power during the follicular phase of highly trained endurance athletes.

While researchers have reported that submaximal oxygen uptake at a given workload is not affected by the menstrual cycle (De Souza et al. 1990, Dombovy et al. 1987, Galliven et al. 1997, Gamberale et al. 1975, Hackney et al. 1994, Kanaley et al. 1992b), time to exhaustion, at a submaximal intensity, has been variously reported. For instance, while some have found no effect of menstrual cycle phase (Dombovy et al. 1987, McCracken et al. 1994), others have reported greater endurance during the luteal phase (Jurkowski et al. 1981, Nicklas et al. 1989). Effort sense during submaximal exercise appears to be unaffected by phase of the menstrual cycle (Higgs & Robertson 1981, Nicklas et al. 1989, Stephenson et al. 1982b).

4 EXERCISE AND MENSTRUAL FUNCTION

The average age of puberty for females in the US is 12.8 years (Harlan et al. 1980), and it is not uncommon for female athletes to exhibit a later onset of menarche or to experience a loss of menses (amenorrhoea) during intensive training (Hager 2002). Amenorrhoea refers to the absence or cessation of the menstrual cycle, with primary amenorrhoea diagnosed when menarche has not occurred by 16 years or the secondary sexual characteristics are not present by the age of 14, and secondary amenorrhoea being the absence of menses for greater than 3 consecutive months after the onset of menarche. Oligomenorrhoea describes intermittent menses (Hager 2002). There are four general forms of amenorrhoea: psychogenic amenorrhoea (due to psychological and emotional disturbances, e.g. anorexia nervosa); stress amenorrhoea (due to prolonged physical stress, e.g. concentration camp exposure); lactogenic amenorrhoea (due to hormonal changes accompanying breast feeding); and exercise-induced (athletic) amenorrhoea. In this section, the focus is upon the last form, with an emphasis upon the female athletic triad, a combination of nutritional, hormonal and skeletal health aspects of amenorrhoea.

4.1 Athletic amenorrhoea

It has been well established that physical activity is necessary to maintain a healthy skeleton, but it is also known that excessive levels of physical activity are associated with amenorrhoea and the loss of bone density. Originally, it was hypothesised that exercise-induced amenorrhoea was due to oestrogen deficiencies and elevated circulating cortisol. This hypothesis was accepted until the early 1990s, when it was discovered that anorexic, amenorrhoeic women had similar endocrine disturbances (hypercortisolaemia, growth hormone resistance and low triiodothyronine) to amenorrhoeic athletes. The energy availability hypothesis suggests that the trigger for disruptions in the hormonal profile in the hypothalamic-pituitary pathway in amenorrhoea is not exercise stress, but reduced energy availability (Chapter 32). This hypothesis suggests that the decrease in energy availability disrupts the secretion of gonadotropin-releasing hormone (American College of Sports Medicine 2007).

Loucks et al. (1998) studied the frequency and amplitude of luteinising hormone secretion in two groups of women (physically active versus sedentary), in response to two energy-controlled diets (40 and 190 kJ·kg LBM^{-1}·day^{-1}). There was a decrease of 10% in luteinising hormone frequency and a 36% decrease in luteinising hormone secretion amplitude in the low-energy condition for the physically active subjects. When compared to the sedentary group, this represented a 60% blunting of the hormonal response. Two case studies also support the energy availability theory (Fredericson & Kent 2005, Zanker et al. 2004). Both reported that a substantial gain in body mass (20–34%) resulted in significant gains in bone density (17–25%). Support for this theory is now widespread, and it appears that an energy deficit, not exercise stress per se, is the primary cause of hypothalamic dysfunction in physically active women who experience amenorrhoea (Loucks 2003).

Leptin is known to regulate basal metabolic rate and is an indicator of nutritional status and fatness (Nattiv et al. 2002). Leptin receptors have been located in the hypothalamus and these are thought to be linked to the control of gonadotropin-releasing hormone secretion. Also, leptin receptors have been identified in bone, and it is plausible that leptin may be the common link in a yet unidentified mechanism linking amenorrhoea, low energy availability and bone loss. This tripartite relationship is known as the female athletic triad.

4.2 Female athletic triad

The female athletic triad constitutes one of the primary health concerns for women in sport. The interrelationship and confluence of disordered eating, amenorrhoea and osteoporosis in physically active women may cause potentially serious medical conditions. It is also important to note that each component of the triad occurs on a continuum, and that each can range from very mild to very severe (American College of Sports Medicine 2007).

Cobb and colleagues (2003) examined 91 competitive female long-distance runners (18–25 years). Sixty-four percent of the subjects were classified as eumenorrhoeic, 26% were oligomenorrehoeic and 10% were classified as amenorrhoeic. Diet and nutritional status were assessed using the Eating Disorder Inventory, menstrual history was assessed and bone density was measured using dual energy X-ray absorptiometry. Of the subjects classified as having elevated disordered eating scores ($N = 23$), 65% were either oligomenorrhoeic or amenorrhoeic, while only 27% of the subjects with normal eating scores had menstrual dysfunction. Additionally, the oligomenorrhoeic and amenorrhoeic subjects had 3–5% lower bone density scores for the lumbar spine, total hip and total body, when compared with the eumenorrhoeic group. A comparison of the disordered eating and bone density scores revealed that subjects with elevated eating disorder scores, but with regular menses, had lower bone densities than subjects with normal eating scores. This study provides solid evidence for a significant interrelationship among the three components of the triad. The authors suggest that not only does the female athletic triad exist, but it may not be as apparent as previously thought. The women in this study were not extremely lean (amenorrhoeic subjects were ~22% body fat). Thus, it may not be easy to diagnose this condition on the basis of excessive leanness. Rigorous screening for eating disorders, menstrual irregularities and low bone mass is therefore recommended.

Disordered eating may result from external pressures to achieve an unrealistically lean physique, either through social or sporting contexts. The spectrum of disordered eating can range from caloric restriction to the use of diet pills, laxatives, diuretics, vomiting and fasting, and affects ~3% of the US female population (Nattiv et al. 2002). A metaanalysis of 34 studies ($N = 2459$ athletes, $N = 8858$ controls) revealed that athletes are at greater risk for disordered eating, particularly those engaged in gymnastics, swimming, running and dancing (Smolak et al. 2000).

Osteoporosis is a disease in which there is a significant decrease in the bone density, leading to an increased risk of non-traumatic bone fracture. Osteoporosis is normally associated with ageing (Chapters 13 and 16), but it is also evident in some female athletes, manifesting itself in stress fractures (Nattiv et al. 2002). Athletes who have a known history of amenorrhoea or disordered eating should have a bone density scan. Early detection of osteopenia (loss of bone mass), or osteoporosis, can lead to early recognition and treatment. Perhaps more commonly, individuals who enter the stage of normal, age-related bone loss with already low bone density are particularly prone to serious health consequences, including compression fractures of the spine and fractures of the hip.

Treatment for osteopenia in young female athletes is not well established, but several goals should drive the treatment plan. Steps should be taken to initiate or re-establish normal menstruation and, in some cases, to ensure a proper diet. The latter involves both caloric and macronutrient considerations. Treatment to normalise menstrual function may include oral contraceptives or oestrogen replacement therapy, although it has been shown that this treatment alone does not cause, or ensure, a regain of bone density (Zanker et al. 2004). If high volumes of intense exercise are part of the daily regimen, then both the volume and intensity of exercise should be reduced until other treatments have become effective, with reductions in training and body mass gains facilitating significant increases in bone density (Fredericson & Kent 2005, Zanker et al. 2004).

References

Abe T, Brechue WF, Fujita S, Brown JB 1998 Gender difference in FFM accumulation and architectural characteristics of muscle. Medicine and Science in Sport and Exercise 30(7):1066–1070

Adams WC 1967 Influence of age, sex and body weight on the energy expenditure of bicycle riding. Journal of Applied Physiology 22:539–545

Adams KF, Vincent LM, McAllister SM, el-Ashmawy H, Sheps DS 1987 The influence of age and gender on left ventricular response to supine exercise in asymptomatic normal subjects. American Heart Journal 113:732–742

Altemus M, Roca C, Galliven E, Romanos C, Deuster P 2001 Increased vasopressin and adrenocorticotropin responses to stress in the midluteal phase of the menstrual cycle. Journal of Clinical Endocrinology and Metabolism 86:2525–2530

American College of Sports Medicine 2006 ACSM's guidelines for exercise testing and prescription, 7th edn. Lippincott Williams and Wilkins, Philadelphia

American College of Sports Medicine 2007 Position stand on the female athletic triad. Medicine and Science in Sport and Exercise 39:1867–1882

Amiel SA, Maran A, Powrie JK, Umpleby AM, Macdonald IA 1993 Gender differences in counterregulation to hypoglycaemia. Diabetologia 36:460–464

Arciero P, Goran M, Poehlman E 1993 Resting metabolic rate is lower in women than in men. Journal of Applied Physiology 75:2514–2520

Åstrand P-O 1952 Experimental studies of physical working capacity in relation to sex and age. Munksgaard, Copenhagen

Baechle TR, Earle RW 2000 Essentials of strength training and conditioning, 2nd edn. Human Kinetics, Champaign, IL

Bailey DA, McKay HA, Mirwald RA, Crocker PR, Faulkner RA 1999 A six-year longitudinal study of the relationship of physical activity to bone mineral accrual in growing children: the university of Saskatchewan bone mineral accrual study. Journal of Bone and Mineral Research 14:1672–1679

Beck TJ, Ruff CB, Shaffer RA, Betsinger K, Trone DW, Brodine SK 2000 Stress fracture in military recruits: gender differences in muscle and bone susceptibility factors. Bone 27:437–444

Bemben DA, Salm PC, Salm AJ 1995 Ventilatory and blood lactate responses to maximal treadmill exercise during the menstrual cycle. Journal of Sports Medicine and Physical Fitness 35:257–562

Berg KE 1991 Comparison of energy expenditure in men and women at rest and during exercise recovery. Journal of Sports Medicine and Physical Fitness 31:351–356

Bonen A, Haynes FJ, Watson-Wright W, Sopper MM, Pierce GN, Low MP, Graham TE 1983 Effect of menstrual cycle on metabolic responses to exercise. Journal of Applied Physiology 55:1506–1513

Bonen A, Haynes FJ, Graham TE 1991 Substrate and hormonal responses to exercise in women using oral contraceptives. Journal of Applied Physiology 70:1917–1927

Bonen A, Campagna P, Gilchrist L, Young DC, Beresford P 1992 Substrate and endocrine responses during exercise at selected stages of pregnancy. Journal of Applied Physiology 73:134–142

Born J, Ditschuneit I, Schreiber M, Dodt C, Fehm HL 1995 Effects of age and gender on pituitary-adrenocortical responsiveness in humans. European Journal of Endocrinology 132:705–711

Brownell KD, Steen SN, Wilmore JH 1987 Weight regulation practices in athletes: analysis of metabolic and health effects. Medicine and Science in Sports and Exercise 19(6):546–556

Campaigne BN 1990 Body fat distribution in females: metabolic consequences and implications for weight loss. Medicine and Science in Sport and Exercise 22(3):291–297

Clasey J, Bouchard C, Wideman CL, Kanaley J, Teates CD, Thorner MO, Hartman ML, Weltman A 1997 The influence of anatomical boundaries, age and sex on the assessment of abdominal visceral fat. Obesity Research 5:395–401

Coakley J 2004 Sports in society: issues and controversies, 8th edn. McGraw-Hill, Boston

Cobb KL, Bachrach LK, Greendale G, Marcus R, Neer RM, Nieves J, Sowers MF, Brown BW Jr, Gopalakrishnan G, Luetters C, Tanner HK, Ward B, Kelsey JL 2003 Disordered eating, menstrual irregularity and bone mineral density in females runners. Medicine and Science in Sport and Exercise 35(5):711–719

Convertino VA, Greenleaf JE 1980 Role of thermal and exercise factors in the mechanisms of hypovolemia. Journal of Applied Physiology 48:657–664

Cotes JE 1979 Lung function assessment and application in medicine. Blackwell Scientific, Oxford

Crofton JT, Dustan H, Share L, Brooks DP 1986 Vasopressin secretion in normotensive black and white men and women on normal and low sodium diets. Journal of Endocrinology 108:191–199

Davies BN, Elford JC, Jamieson KF 1991 Variations in performance in simple muscle tests at different phases of the menstrual cycle. Journal of Sports Medicine and Physical Fitness 31:532–537

Davis SN, Galassetti P, Wasserman DH, Tate D 2000 Effects of gender on neuroendocrine and metabolic counterregulatory responses to exercise in normal man. Journal of Clinical Endocrinology and Metabolism 85:224–230

de Simone G, Devereux RB, Roman MJ, Ganau A, Chien S, Alderman MH, Atlas S, Laragh JH 1991 Gender differences in left ventricular anatomy, blood viscosity and volume regulatory hormones in normal adults. American Journal of Cardiology 68:1704–1708

de Simone G, Devereux RB, Daniels SR, Meyer RA 1995 Gender differences in left ventricular growth. Hypertension 26:979–983

De Souza MJ, Maguire MS, Rubin KR, Maresh CM 1990 Effects of menstrual phase and amenorrhea on exercise performance in runners. Medicine and Science in Sports and Exercise 22:575–580

De Souza MJ, Maguire MS, Maresh CM, Kraemer WJ, Rubin KR, Loucks AB 1991 Adrenal activation and prolactin response to exercise in eumenorrheic and amenorrheic runners. Journal of Applied Physiology 70:2378–2387

Deague JA, Wilson CM, Grigg LE, Harrap SB 2000 Increased left ventricular mass is not associated with impaired left ventricular diastolic filling in normal individuals. Journal of Hypertension 18:757–762

DiBrezzo R, Fort IL, Brown B 1991 Relationships among strength, endurance, weight and body fat during three phases of the menstrual cycle. Journal of Sports Medicine and Physical Fitness 31:89–94

Dionne I, Despres JP, Bouchard C, Tremblay A 1999 Gender difference in the effect of body composition on energy metabolism. International Journal of Obesity and Related Metabolic Disorders 23:312–319

Dombovy ML, Bonekat HW, Williams TJ, Staats BA 1987 Exercise performance and ventilatory response in the menstrual cycle. Medicine and Science in Sports and Exercise 19:111–117

Earle TL, Linden W, Weinberg J 1999 Differential effects of harassment on cardiovascular and salivary cortisol stress reactivity and recovery in women and men. Journal of Psychosomatic Research 46:125–141

Elwyn DH, Askanazi J, Kinney JM, Bursztein SE 1989 Energy metabolism, indirect calorimetry and nutrition. Williams and Wilkins, Baltimore, MD

Eston RG, Burke EJ 1984 Effects of the menstrual cycle on selected-responses to short-constant load exercise. Journal of Sports Sciences 2:145–153

Favier R, Pequignot JM, Desplanches D, Mayet MH, Lacour JR, Peyrin L, Flandrois R 1983 Catecholamines and metabolic responses to submaximal exercise in untrained men and women. European Journal of Applied Physiology. Occupational Physiology 50:393–403

Fortney SM 1996 Hormonal control of fluid balance in women during exercise. In: Buskirk ER, Puhl SM (eds) Body fluid balance: exercise and sport. CRC Press, Boca Raton, FL, 231–258

Fortney SM, Turner C, Steinmann L, Driscoll T, Alfrey C 1994 Blood volume responses of men and women to bed rest. Journal of Clinical Pharmacology 34:434–439

Frankovich RJ, Lebrun CM 2000 Menstrual cycle, contraception and performance. Clinics in Sports Medicine 19:251–271

Frayn KN 1996 Metabolic regulation: a human perspective. Portland Press, London

Fredericson M, Kent K 2005 Normalization of bone density in a previously amenorrheic runner with osteoporosis. Medicine and Science in Sport and Exercise 387(9):1481–1486

Freund BJ, Claybaugh JR, Dice MS, Hashiro GM 1987 Hormonal and vascular fluid responses to maximal exercise in trained and untrained males. Journal of Applied Physiology 63:669–675

Friedmann B, Kindermann W 1989 Energy metabolism and regulatory hormones in women and men during endurance exercise. European Journal of Applied Physiology. Occupational Physiology 59:1–9

Froberg K, Pederson P 1984 Sex differences in endurance capacity and metabolic response to prolonged, heavy exercise. European Journal of Applied Physiology 52:446–450

Galassetti P, Mann S, Tate D, Neill RA, Wasserman DH, Davis SN 2001 Effect of morning exercise on counterregulatory responses to subsequent, afternoon exercise. Journal of Applied Physiology 91:91–99

Galbo H 1983 Hormonal and metabolic adaptation to exercise. Thieme-Stratton, Stuttgart

Galbo H, Holst JJ, Christensen NJ 1975 Glucagon and plasma catecholamine responses to graded and prolonged exercise in man. Journal of Applied Physiology 38:70–76

Galliven EA, Singh A, Michelson D, Bina S, Gold, PW, Deuster PA 1997 Hormonal and metabolic responses to exercise across time of day and menstrual cycle phase. Journal of Applied Physiology 83:1822–1831

Gamberale F, Strindberg L, Wahlberg I 1975 Female work capacity during the menstrual cycle: physiological and psychological reactions. Scandinavian Journal of Work, Environment and Health 1:120–127

Garlick MA, Bernauer EM 1968 Exercise during the menstrual cycle: variations in physiological baselines. Research Quarterly 39:533–542

Gelfin Y, Lerer B, Lesch KP, Gorfine M, Allolio B 1995 Complex effects of age and gender on hypothermic, adrenocorticotrophic hormone and cortisol responses to ipsapirone challenge in normal subjects. Psychopharmacology 120:356–364

George KP, Gates PE, Whyte G, Fenoglio RA, Lea R 1999 Echocardiographic examination of cardiac structure and function in elite cross trained male and female alpine skiers. British Journal of Sports Medicine 33:93–98

Ginsburg GS, O'Toole M, Rimm E, Douglas PS, Rifai N 2001 Gender differences in exercise-induced changes in sex hormone levels and lipid peroxidation in athletes participating in the Hawaii ironman triathlon. Ginsburg-gender and exercise-induced lipid peroxidation. Clinica Chimica Acta 305:131–139

Green HJ, Carter S, Grant S, Tupling R, Coates G, Ali M 1999 Vascular volumes and hematology in male and female runners and cyclists. European Journal of Applied Physiology and Occupational Physiology 79:244–250

Greeves JP, Cable NT, Reilly T 1999 The relationship between maximal muscle strength and reproductive hormones during the menstrual cycle. 4th Annual Congress of the European College of Sport Science, Rome, Italy

Gür H 1997 Concentric and eccentric isokinetic measurements in knee muscles during the menstrual cycle: a special reference to reciprocal moment ratios. Archives of Physical Medicine and Rehabilitation 78:501–505

Gustafson AB, Kalkhoff RK 1982 Influence of sex and obesity on plasma catecholamine response to isometric exercise. Journal of Clinical Endocrinology and Metabolism 55:703–708

Guyton AC, Hall JE 2000 Textbook of medical physiology. WB Saunders, Philadelphia

Gyntelberg F, Rennie MJ, Hickson RC, Holloszy JO 1977 Effect of training on the response of plasma glucagon to exercise. Journal of Applied Physiology. Respiratory, Environmental and Exercise Physiology 43:302–305

Hackney AC 1999 Influence of oestrogen on muscle glycogen utilization during exercise. Acta Physiologica Scandinavica 167:273–274

Hackney AC, McCracken-Compton MA, Ainsworth B 1994 Substrate responses to submaximal exercise in the midfollicular and midluteal phases of the menstrual cycle. International Journal of Sport Nutrition 4:299–308

Hager WD 2002 Common gynecologic problems. In: Ireland ML, Nattiv A (eds) The female athlete. Saunders, Philadelphia, 113–117

Häkkinen K, Pakarinen A 1995 Acute hormonal responses to heavy resistance exercise in men and women at different ages. International Journal of Sports Medicine 16:507–513

Häkkinen K, Pakarinen A, Kyrolainen H, Cheng S, Kim DH, Komi P 1990 Neuromuscular adaptations and serum hormones in females during prolonged power training. International Journal of Sports Medicine 11:91–98

Hansen AP, Weeke J 1974 Fasting serum growth hormone levels and growth hormone responses to exercise during normal menstrual cycles and cycles of oral contraceptives. Scandinavian Journal of Clinical and Laboratory Investigation 34:199–205

Harlan WR, Harlan EA, Grillo GP 1980 Secondary sex characteristics of girls 12 to 17 years of age: the US health examination survey. Journal of Pediatrics 96:1074–1078

Hellstrom L, Blaak E, Hagstrom-Toft E 1996 Gender differences in adrenergic regulation of lipid mobilization during exercise. International Journal of Sports Medicine 17:439–447

Hense HW, Gneiting B, Muscholl M, Broeckel U, Kuch B, Doering A, Riegger GA, Schunkert H 1998 The associations of body size and body composition with left ventricular mass: impacts for indexation in adults. Journal of the American College of Cardiology 32:451–457

Higgs SL, Robertson LA 1981 Cyclic variations in perceived exertion and physical work capacity in females. Canadian Journal of Applied Sport Sciences - Journal Canadien des Sciences Appliquees au Sport 6:191–196

Horton TJ, Pagliassotti MJ, Hobbs K, Hill JO 1998 Fuel metabolism in men and women during and after long-duration exercise. Journal of Applied Physiology 85:1823–1832

Hurley BF, Hagberg JM 1998 Optimizing health in older person: aerobic or strength training? Exercise and Sport Sciences Reviews 26:61–89

Inder WJ, Hellemans J, Swanney MP, Prickett TC, Donald RA 1998 Prolonged exercise increases peripheral plasma acth, crh and avp in male athletes. Journal of Applied Physiology 85:835–841

Janse de Jonge XAK, Boot CRL, Thom JM, Ruell PA, Thompson MW 2001 The influence of menstrual cycle phase on skeletal muscle contractile characteristics in humans. Journal of Physiology 530:161–166

Järhult J, Holst J 1979 The role of the adrenergic innervation to the pancreatic islets in the control of insulin release during exercise in man. Pflügers Archiv - European Journal of Physiology 383:41–45

Jurkowski JE, Jones NL, Toews CJ, Sutton JR 1981 Effects of menstrual cycle on blood lactate, O2 delivery and performance during exercise. Journal of Applied Physiology. Respiratory, Environmental and Exercise Physiology 51:1493–1499

Kameneva MV, Watach MJ, Borovetz HS 1999 Gender difference in rheologic properties of blood and risk of cardiovascular diseases. Clinical Hemorheology and Microcirculation 21:357–363

Kanaley JA, Boileau RA, Bahr JA, Misner JE, Nelson RA 1992a Cortisol levels during prolonged exercise: the influence of menstrual phase and status. International Journal of Sports Medicine 13:332–336

Kanaley JA, Boileau RA, Bahr JA, Misner JE, Nelson RA 1992b Substrate oxidation and gh responses to exercise are independent of menstrual phase and status. Medicine and Science in Sports and Exercise 24:873–880

Kanaley JA, Weltman JY, Pieper KS, Weltman A, Hartman ML 2001 Cortisol and growth hormone responses to exercise at different times of day. Journal of Clinical Endocrinology and Metabolism 86:2881–2889

Katsiaras A, Newman AB, Kriska A, Brach J, Krishnaswami S, Feingold E, Kritchevsky SB, Li R, Harris TB, Schwartz A, Goodpaster BH 2005 Skeletal muscle fatigue, strength and quality in the elderly: the health ABC study. Journal of Applied Physiology 99:210–216

Keizer HA, Beckers E, de Haan J, Janssen GM, Kuipers H, van Kranenburg G, Geurten P 1987a Exercise-induced changes in the percentage of free testosterone and estradiol in trained and untrained women. International Journal of Sports Medicine 8:151–153

Keizer HA, Kuipers H, de Haan J, Beckers E, Habets L 1987b Multiple hormonal responses to physical exercise in eumenorrheic trained and untrained women. International Journal of Sports Medicine 8:139–150

Keizer HA, Kuipers H, de Haan J, Janssen GM, Beckers E, Habets L, van Kranenburg G, Geurten P 1987c Effect of a 3-month endurance training program on metabolic and multiple hormonal responses to exercise. International Journal of Sports Medicine 8:154–160

Keizer H, Janssen GM, Menheere P, Kranenburg G 1989 Changes in basal plasma testosterone, cortisol and dehydroepiandrosterone sulfate in previously untrained males and females preparing for a marathon. International Journal of Sports Medicine 10:S139–145

Khan K, McKay H, Kannus P, Bailey D, Wark J, Bennell K 2001 Physical activity and bone health. Human Kinetics, Champaign, IL

Kleitman N, Ramsaroop A 1948 Periodicity in body temperature and heart rate. Endocrinology 43:1–20

Kraemer WJ, Fleck SJ, Dziados JE, Harman EA, Marchitelli LJ, Gordon SE, Mello R, Frykman PN, Koziris LP, Triplett NT 1993 Changes in hormonal concentrations after different heavy-resistance exercise protocols in women. Journal of Applied Physiology 75:594–604

Krivickas LS, Fielding RA, Murray A, Callahan D, Johansson A, Dorer DJ, Frontera WR 2006 Sex differences in single muscle fiber power in older adults. Medicine and Science in Sport and Exercise 38(1):57–63

Kuoppasalmi K, Naveri H, Harkonen M, Adlercreutz H 1980 Plasma cortisol, androstenedione, testosterone and luteinizing hormone in running exercise of different intensities. Scandinavian Journal of Clinical and Laboratory Investigation 40:403–409

Laitinen T, Hartikainen J, Vanninen E, Niskanen L, Geelen G, Lansimies E 1998 Age and gender dependency of baroreflex sensitivity in healthy subjects. Journal of Applied Physiology 84:576–583

Lamont LS, Lemon PWR, Bruot BC 1987 Menstrual cycle and exercise effects on protein catabolism. Medicine and Science in Sports and Exercise 19:106–110

Lamont LS, McCullough MJ, Kalhan SC 2001 Gender differences in leucine, but not lysine, kinetics. Journal of Applied Physiology 91:357–362

Landgren BM, Unden AL, Diczfalusy E 1980 Hormonal profile of the cycle in 68 normally menstruating women. Acta Endocrinologica 94:89–98

Lang I, Schernthaner G, Pietschmann P, Kurz R, Stephenson JM, Templ H 1987 Effects of sex and age on growth hormone response to growth hormone-releasing hormone in healthy individuals. Journal of Clinical Endocrinology and Metabolism 65:535–540

Lauback L 1976 Comparative muscles strength of men and women: a review of the literature. Aviation, Space and Environmental Medicine 4:534–542

Lavoie JM, Dionne N, Helie R, Brisson GR 1987 Menstrual phase cycle dissociation of blood glucose homeostasis during exercise. Journal of Applied Physiology 62:1084–1089

Lebrun CM, McKenzie DC, Prior JC, Taunton JE 1995 Effects of menstrual cycle phase on athletic performance. Medicine and Science in Sports and Exercise 27:437–444

Lemmer JT, Ivey FM, Ryan AS, Martel GF, Hurlbut DE, Metter JE, Fozard JL, Fleg JL, Hurley BF 2001 Effect of strength training on resting metabolic rate and physical activity: age and gender comparisons. Medicine and Science in Sports and Exercise 33:532–541

Lindle RS, Metter EJ, Lynch NA 1997 Age and gender comparisons of muscle strength in 654 women and men aged 20–93 yr. Journal of Applied Physiology 83(5):1581–1587

Loucks AB 2003 Energy availability, not body fatness, regulates reproductive function in women. Exercise and Sport Sciences Reviews 31:144–148

Loucks AB, Verdun M, Heath EM 1998. Lower energy availability, not stress of exercise, alters LH pulsatility in exercising women. Journal of Applied Physiology 84:37–46

Lynch NA, Metter EJ, Lindle RS, Fozard JL, Tobin J, Roy TA, Fleg JL, Hurley BF 1999 Muscle quality. I. Age-associated differences between arm and leg muscle group. Journal of Applied Physiology 86(1):188–194

McArdle WD, Katch FI, Katch VL 2001 Exercise physiology, energy, nutrition and human performance. Lippincott Williams and Wilkins, Philadelphia

McCracken M, Ainsworth B, Hackney AC 1994 Effects of the menstrual cycle phase on the blood lactate responses to exercise. European Journal of Applied Physiology. Occupational Physiology 69:174–175

McDowell MA, Fryar CD, Hirsch R, Ogden CL 2005 Anthropometric reference data for children and adults: U.S. population, 1999–2002. Advance data from vital and health statistics: no 361. National Center for Health Statistics, Hyattsville, MD

Marcus JT, DeWaal LK, Gotte MJ, van der Geest RJ, Heethaar RM, Van Rossum AC 1999 Mri-derived left ventricular function parameters and mass in healthy young adults: relation with gender and body size. International Journal of Cardiac Imaging 15:411–419

Marliss EB, Kreisman SH, Manzon A, Halter JB, Vranic M, Nessim SJ 2000 Gender differences in glucoregulatory responses to intense exercise. Journal of Applied Physiology 88:457–466

Marras WS, Jorgensen MJ, Granata KP, Wiand B 2001 Female and male trunk geometry: size and prediction of the spine loading trunk muscles derived from MRI. Clinical Biomechanics 16:38–46

Massaro D, Teich N, Maxwell S 1985 Postnatal development of alveoli: regulation and evidence for a critical period in rats. Journal of Clinical Investigation 76:1297–1305

Maw GJ, Mackenzie IL, Taylor NAS 1998 Body-fluid distribution during exercise in hot and cool environments. Acta Physiologica Scandinavica 163:297–304

Mills PJ, Ziegler MG, Nelesen RA, Kennedy BP 1996 The effects of the menstrual cycle, race and gender on adrenergic receptors and agonists. Clinical Pharmacology and Therapeutics 60:99–104

Myhre LG, Hartung GH, Nunneley SA, Tucker DM 1985 Plasma volume changes in middle-aged male and female subjects during marathon running. Journal of Applied Physiology 59:559–563

Nattiv A, Callahan LR, Kehman-Sherstinsky A 2002 The female athletic triad. In: Ireland ML, Nattiv A (eds) The female athlete. WB Saunders, Philadelphia, 223–235

Nicklas BJ, Hackney AC, Sharp RL 1989 The menstrual cycle and exercise: performance, muscle glycogen and substrate responses. International Journal of Sports Medicine 10:264–269

Norman AW, Litwack G 1997 Hormones, 2nd edn. Academic Press, San Diego, CA

Pate RR, Barnes C, Miller W 1985 A physiological comparison of performance-matched female and male distance runners. Research Quarterly for Exercise and Sport 56:245–250

Pelliccia A, Maron B, Culasso F, Spataro A, Caselli G 1996 Athlete's heart in women. Echocardiographic characterization of highly trained elite female athletes. Journal of the American Medical Association 276:211–215

Petrides JS, Gold PW, Mueller GP, Singh A, Stratakis C, Chrousos GP, Deuster PA 1997 Marked differences in functioning of the hypothalamic-pituitary-adrenal axis between groups of men. Journal of Applied Physiology 82:1979–1988

Petrofsky JS, LeDonne DM, Rinehart JS, Lind AR 1976 Isometric strength and endurance during the menstrual cycle. European Journal of Applied Physiology. Occupational Physiology 35:1–10

Phillips SM, Atkinson SA, Tarnopolsky MA, MacDougall JD 1993 Gender differences in leucine kinetics and nitrogen balance in endurance athletes. Journal of Applied Physiology 75:2134–2141

Phillips SK, Sanderson AG, Birch KM, Bruce S, Woledge R 1996 Changes in maximal vountary force of human adductor pollicis muscle during the menstrual cycle. Journal of Physiology 496:551–557

Plowman S, Smith DS 2003 Exercise physiology for health, fitness and performance. Benjamin Cummings, San Francisco, CA

Pullinen T, Nicol C, MacDonald E, Komi PV 1999 Plasma catecholamine responses to four resistance exercise tests in men and women. European Journal of Applied Physiology. Occupational Physiology 80:125–131

Rauste-von Wright M, von Wright J, Frankenhaeuser M 1981 Relationships between sex-related psychological characteristics during adolescence and catecholamine excretion during achievement stress. Psychophysiology 18:362–370

Sanchez J, Pequignet JM, Peyrin L, Monod H 1980 Sex differences in the sympatho-adrenal response to isometric exercise. European Journal of Applied Physiology 45:147–154

Sawar R, Niclos BB, Rutherford OM 1996 Changes in muscle strength, relaxation rate and fatiguability during the human menstrual cycle. Journal of Physiology 493:267–272

Schoene RB, Robertson HT, Pierson DJ, Peterson AP 1981 Respiratory drives and exercise in menstrual cycles of athletic and nonathletic women. Journal of Applied Physiology. Respiratory, Environmental and Exercise Physiology 50:1300–1305

Schwartz JD, Katz SA, Fegley RW, Tockman MS 1988 Analysis of spirometric data from a national sample of healthy 6- to 24-year-olds (NHANES II). American Review of Respiratory Disease 138:1405–1414

Shephard RJ, Bouhel E, Vandewalle H, Monod H 1988 Muscle mass as a factor limiting physical work. Journal of Applied Physiology 64:1472–1479

Sherwood L 1997 Human physiology from cells to systems. Wadsworth Publishing, Belmont, CA

Shvartz E, Reibold RC 1990 Aerobic fitness norms for males and females aged 6 to 75 years: a review. Aviation and Environmental Physiology 61:3–11

Smolak L, Murnen SK, Ruble AE 2000 Female athletes with eating disorders: a meta-analysis. International Journal of Eating Disorders 27:371–380

Sparling PB 1980 A meta-analysis of studies comparing maximal oxygen uptake in men and women. Research Quarterly for Exercise and Sport 51(3):542–552

Stachenfeld NS, Gleim GW, Zabetakis PM, Nicholas JA 1996 Fluid balance and renal response following dehydrating exercise in well-trained men and women. European Journal of Applied Physiology. Occupational Physiology 72:468–477

Stachenfeld NS, DiPietro L, Kokoszka CA, Silva C, Keefe DL, Nadel ER 1999 Physiological variability of fluid-regulation hormones in young women. Journal of Applied Physiology 86:1092–1096

Staron RS, Karapondo DL, Kraemer WJ, Malicky ES, Falkel JE, Hagerman FC, Hikida RS 1994 Skeletal muscle adaptations during early phase of heavy-resistance training in men and women. Journal of Applied Physiology 76(3):1247–1255

Stephenson LA, Kolka MA, Wilkerson JE 1982a Metabolic and thermoregulatory responses to exercise during the human menstrual cycle. Medicine and Science in Sports and Exercise 14:270–275

Stephenson LA, Kolka MA, Wilkerson JE 1982b Perceived exertion and anaerobic threshold during the menstrual cycle. Medicine and Science in Sports and Exercise 14:218–222

Takamata A, Nose H, Kinoshita T 2000 Effect of acute hypoxia on vasopressin release and intravascular fluid during dynamic exercise in humans. American Journal of Physiology. Regulatory, Integrative and Comparative Physiology 279:R161–R168

Tarnopolsky M 1999 Gender differences in lipid metabolism during exercise and at rest. In: Tarnopolsky M (ed) Gender differences in metabolism: practical and nutritional implications. CRC Press, Boca Raton, FL, 179–199

Tarnopolsky LJ, MacDougall JD, Atkinson SA 1990 Gender differences in substrate for endurance exercise. Journal of Applied Physiology 68:302–308

Tarnopolsky MA, Atkinson SA, Phillips SM, MacDougall JD 1995 Carbohydrate loading and metabolism during exercise in men and women. Journal of Applied Physiology 78:1360–1368

Tarnopolsky MA, Zawada C, Richmond LB, Carter S, Shearer J, Graham T, Phillips SM 2001 Gender differences in carbohydrate loading are related to energy intake. Journal of Applied Physiology 91:225–230

Tate CA, Holtz RW 1998 Gender and fat metabolism during exercise: a review. Canadian Journal of Applied Physiology 23:570–582

Weiss LW, Cureton KJ, Thompson FN 1983 Comparison of serum testosterone and androstenedione responses to weight lifting in men and women. European Journal of Applied Physiology 50:413–419

Wells CL, Plowman SA 1983 Sexual differences in athletic performance: biological or behavioural? Physician and Sports Medicine 11(8):52–63

White MJ, Weekes C 1998 No evidence for change in the voluntary or electrically evoked contractile characteristics of the triceps surae during the human menstrual cycle. Journal of Physiology 506:199

Wiebe CG, Gledhill N, Warburton DE, Jamnik VK, Ferguson S 1998 Exercise cardiac function in endurance-trained males versus females. Clinical Journal of Sport Medicine 8:272–279

Wigger A, Neumann ID 1999 Periodic maternal deprivation induces gender-dependent alterations in behavioral and neuroendocrine responses to emotional stress in adult rats. Physiology and Behavior 66:293–302

Wilmore JH, Stanforth PR, Gagnon J, Rice T, Mandel S, Leon AS, Rao DC, Skinner JS, Bouchard C 2001 Cardiac output and stroke volume changes with endurance training: the Heritage Family Study. Medicine and Science in Sports and Exercise 33:99–106

Zanker CL, Cooke CB, Truscott JG, Oldroyd B, Jacobs HS 2004 Annual changes in bone density over 12 years in an amenorrheic athlete. Medicine and Science in Sport and Exercise 36(1):137–142

Chapter 12

Performance in the pregnant woman: maternal and foetal considerations

Michelle F. Mottola

1 INTRODUCTION

Pregnancy and aerobic conditioning are biological processes that involve striking physiological adaptations, and these may occur in the same or in opposite directions, depending on the specific variable being studied (Table 12.1). To illustrate this, consider cardiac function.

1.1 Cardiovascular adaptations

The resting cardiac output of a pregnant woman increases significantly in the first trimester (typically 4–5 L·min^{-1}; Pivarnik 1996) reflecting a 50% increase from non-pregnant values (Pivarnik et al. 1990), with smaller gradual increases until midway through the second trimester, after which cardiac output will plateau (Weissgerber & Wolfe 2006, Wolfe et al. 1989a). This early pregnancy-induced change is mediated by ovarian and placental hormones, and is observed in association with increases in aortic capacitance (Hart et al. 1986), a reduction in peripheral vascular resistance (Duvekot et al. 1993) and ventricular cavity dilation without an increase in wall thickness (Rubler et al. 1977). Evidence suggests that the maternal cardiovascular system is remodelled in early gestation by an oestrogen-mediated reduction in vascular tone leading to a primary reduction in afterload and increased venous capacitance (Duvekot et al. 1993), with the increase in ventricular cavity dimensions occurring at about the same time (Wolfe et al. 1999).

Aerobic conditioning, on the other hand, is thought to cause no change, or a slight increase in resting cardiac output in non-pregnant individuals (Wilmore et al. 2001). The early, pregnancy-induced changes in cardiac output are thought to occur in response to increases in resting heart rate (chronotropism), mediated by cardiovascular baroreflexes (Wolfe et al. 1999) caused by a decrease in vagal tone or an augmented sympathetic drive to the sinoatrial node (Pivarnik 1996), as most of the 15–20 beat increase in heart rate from non-pregnant values occurs during the first trimester (Wolfe et al. 1989a). Conversely, the resting heart rate is known to decrease in aerobically conditioned, non-pregnant individuals (Clausen 1977).

Table 12.1 Physiological responses to pregnancy (by trimester) and aerobic conditioning in the non-pregnant state as measured at rest (changes are relative to non-pregnant, sedentary state)

Variable	First trimester	Second trimester	Late pregnancy	Aerobic conditioning
Cardiac output (L·min^{-1})	↑↑	↑	–	– or ↑
Heart rate (beats·min^{-1})	↑↑	– or ↑	–	↓↓
Stroke volume (mL)	↑↑	– or ↑	–	↑↑
Blood volume (L)	↑↑	↑	–	↑
Oxygen uptake (mL·kg^{-1}·min^{-1})	–	↓	↓	↑

Data from Weissgerber & Wolfe 2006, Wolfe et al. 1989.

Increases in stroke volume facilitate the small rise in cardiac output in the second trimester (Spaanderman et al. 2000). However, the time course for serial changes in stroke volume during pregnancy remains controversial (Weissgerber & Wolfe 2006), possibly due to technical errors associated with stroke volume measurement, since, during pregnancy, this measurement is sensitive to body position (Wolfe et al. 1989a). Regardless, stroke volume has been shown to increase by approximately 10% at the end of the first trimester (Pivarnik et al. 1990). The mechanism for stroke volume increase is unknown and occurs before significant enhancement of maternal blood volume (Duvekot et al. 1993), which may increase up to 50% above non-pregnant values by late pregnancy (Pivarnik et al. 1994). It is suggested that the gradual increase in maternal plasma volume is caused by pregnancy-induced hormones that reduce peripheral vascular resistance, which in turn activates the renin-angiotensin-aldosterone system (Duvekot et al. 1993), leading to increased secretion of arginine vasopressin (antidiuretic hormone) and fluid retention to maintain blood pressure (Duvekot et al. 1993). Aerobic conditioning in non-pregnant individuals similarly increases stroke volume (Wilmore et al. 2001), but the mechanisms involved may not be the same.

1.2 Respiratory adaptations

Respiratory responses to pregnancy at rest are similar to those occurring in response to aerobic conditioning, but the mechanisms for these changes are quite different. Pregnancy-induced hormones cause a remodelling of the thoracic cage to a higher diaphragmatic midposition (Wolfe & Weissgerber 2003). As a result, the residual volume and expiratory reserve volume are both reduced, with an increase in inspiratory capacity, resulting in minimal effect on vital capacity (Ratigan 1983). One of the most substantial physiological changes due to pregnancy is an increase in respiratory sensitivity to carbon dioxide (Wolfe & Weissgerber 2003). This effect is observed early in the first trimester, causing an increase in tidal volume and minute ventilation, leading to a reduction in arterial carbon dioxide tension (P_aCO_2) and an augmentation in arterial oxygen tension (Heenan & Wolfe 2000, Wolfe et al. 1998). The stimulus for these effects is thought to be the pregnancy-induced increase in progesterone, a known breathing stimulant, and the oestrogen-mediated increase in hypothalamic progesterone receptors (Wolfe et al. 1998). Interestingly, these changes are accomplished with little or no change in respiratory frequency (Ohtake & Wolfe 1998). Although these early changes are not metabolically necessary, the first-trimester reductions in arterial carbon dioxide tension widen the maternal-foetal carbon dioxide gradient, creating a buffer zone to protect the foetus from acute elevations in maternal P_aCO_2 (Wolfe et al. 1998), and the early increase in maternal minute ventilation may prevent foetal hypercapnia and acidosis throughout pregnancy (Weissgerber et al. 2006a).

Many healthy pregnant women (with no history of cardiorespiratory disease) complain of respiratory discomfort (dyspnoea), especially in late pregnancy, both at rest and upon exertion (Milne et al. 1978). No definitive causes for this normal response have been reported in the literature because of considerable differences in study comparisons, and differences in specific instructions to subjects as to assessment of qualitative dimensions and the type of exertion employed (Jensen et al. 2007). Theories suggested for this phenomenon are maternal awareness of hyperventilation (Cugell et al. 1953), increased respiratory effort as a result of mechanical alterations of the respiratory system (Bader et al. 1959) or an increase in inspiratory effort that accompanies increased minute ventilation (Field et al. 1991). Perceptions of respiratory effort and dyspnoea appear to be reduced during submaximal steady-state exercise throughout gestation (Field et al. 1991). Again, no explanation exists for this effect, but it may be that temporal desensitisation to the sensory consequences of an augmented ventilatory drive, and relative hyperventilation may negate the expected increase in respiratory discomfort during cycle exercise (Jensen et al. 2007). It may also be possible that the maternal anatomical and mechanical adaptations of the respiratory system reduce airway resistance, preserve breathing mechanics and minimise the effort of ventilation and therefore reduce dyspnoea with the simultaneous increase in minute ventilation during exercise (Jensen et al. 2007).

Resting (relative) oxygen uptake (mL·kg^{-1}·min^{-1}) reflects the increase in body mass during pregnancy, and thus declines slightly during each trimester, whereas aerobic conditioning slightly increases resting oxygen uptake in non-pregnant individuals (Wolfe et al. 1989a).

1.3 Metabolic adaptations

Maternal blood glucose is the primary energy source for foetal-placental growth, and thus maternal metabolic adaptations ensure an adequate supply (Bauer et al. 1998). A cascade of hormonal events results in an increase in maternal blood glucose, with elevated release from the liver (drop in liver glycogen storage; Mottola & Christopher 1991), an increase in insulin production by the β cells (overworked pancreas; Catalano et al. 1991), an increase in insulin resistance at the skeletal muscle level (Buchanan et al. 1990) and a decrease in maternal peripheral utilisation of blood glucose (Lesser & Carpenter 1994). This normal insulin resistance at the muscle level ensures more maternal blood glucose for foetal usage, which can be as high as 30–50% in late gestation (Clapp 2002). Changes in β-cell responsiveness leading to insulin resistance occur in parallel with growth of the foetal-placental unit, and the release of hormones such as human placental lactogen, progesterone, cortisol and prolactin (Butte 2000). Maternal body fat is stored early in pregnancy (perhaps due to the lypogenic action of the increased insulin concentrations; Boden 1996), so that these adipose stores can be used for lypolysis in late pregnancy as an alternative fuel source, permitting the mother to conserve maternal glucose for foetal needs (Bessinger & McMurray 2003).

If the insulin resistance is excessive during pregnancy, gestational diabetes mellitus (carbohydrate intolerance of varying severity first described during pregnancy) is diagnosed, and management for this disease is initiated (Cowett et al. 1983). Many problems result from this condition, the most prominent of which is a large baby (≥4000 g), causing a difficult labour and delivery (Hiramatsu et al. 2000). The increase in newborn size is usually made up of body fat and the baby is born lethargic and unhealthy. In addition, baby growth is disproportional in that the shoulders grow larger than the head, leading to difficult delivery through the birth canal, frequently resulting in a caesarean section. Babies born to women with gestational diabetes may also be delivered with very low blood sugar concentrations. This is due to the high concentrations of circulating foetal insulin in response to the high glucose concentrations passing through the placenta into the foetal blood. Once the umbilical cord is cut, the high maternal blood glucose supply is cut off, while the foetal pancreas continues to deliver high concentrations of insulin into the foetal circulation. This results in low blood glucose concentrations at birth, and consequently these infants require an intravenous supply of glucose to increase blood concentrations. This insult to the foetal metabolic system at birth may place these infants at risk for developing type 2 diabetes later in life (Chapter 30), as well as an increased risk of developing type 2 diabetes in the mother (Ben-Haroush et al. 2003).

1.4 Thermoregulatory adaptations

Thermoregulation steadily improves during pregnancy, which is reflected by a gradual decline in rectal temperature (Clapp 1991, Linqvist et al. 2003), and the downward shift in the threshold body temperature for the initiation of sweating (Chapters 18 and 19), which results in evaporative heat loss commencing at a lower body temperature as pregnancy advances (Clapp 1991). The improved heat dissipation at rest may be due to decreased vascular tone with increased skin circulation (Jones et al. 1985), the increase in minute ventilation and plasma volume expansion (Clapp 1991). Maternal heat dissipation is important because foetal metabolism generates heat, and foetal temperature is dependent upon maternal temperature, foetal metabolism and uterine blood flow (Lindqvist et al. 2003).

These adaptations at rest, during pregnancy, represent complicated examples of the many changes occurring in a woman's body to support the growth and development of the foetus. Further readings summarise these pregnancy-induced alterations (Clapp 2006, Pivarnik 1996, Weissgerber & Wolfe 2006, Wolfe & Weissgerber 2003, Wolfe et al. 1994, 1989a). Based on these reviews, it is clear that the myriad of cardiovascular, respiratory, metabolic and thermoregulatory changes that occur when a woman becomes pregnant may affect her response to exercise (Pivarnik 1996), and these exercise responses may pose a potential conflict with foetal growth and development.

2 PERFORMANCE CAPACITY IN PREGNANT WOMEN

The maternal performance capacity for exercise depends on whether the activity is weight bearing or weight supported, whether the exercise is submaximal or maximal, and the initial fitness level of the participant.

2.1 Cardiorespiratory responses to exercise

Absolute maximal oxygen uptake (L·min^{-1}) is well preserved in pregnant women who maintain their customary levels of physical activity with advancing gestational age (Heenan et al. 2001, Lotgering et al. 1995, Sady et al. 1990), whereas maximal oxygen uptake as a function of body mass (mL·kg^{-1}·min^{-1}) usually declines as a result of pregnancy-related mass increases (Lotgering et al. 1991). This latter change has a significant impact on the interpretation of relative aerobic power changes following experimental treatments, with readers needing to carefully consider changes to both components (oxygen uptake and power) before interpreting such observations.

Maximal exercise stress testing is not recommended during pregnancy because of safety concerns, so few studies exist in which true maximal aerobic power has been accurately assessed in pregnant women. Most, if not all, of the studies examining maximal stress testing are actually using peak volitional fatigue by the participant as a proxy for maximal responses. Despite this, it is suggested that maximal exercise heart rate is moderately attenuated in mid-to-late pregnancy (Lotgering et al. 1991, 1992a). Since resting heart rate is already elevated, heart rate increases at a slower rate in response to increases in exercise intensity (Lotgering et al. 1992b, Sady et al. 1989, Pivarnik et al. 1990).

Pregnant women do not develop the typical training response in which there is a reduction in resting heart rate like healthy non-pregnant adults (Wolfe et al. 1999). This may be due to the dominance of the pregnancy withdrawal of cardiac (vagal) parasympathetic modulation during rest and during light exercise (Avery et al. 2001). However, training-induced bradycardia has been shown during heavy exercise in trained pregnant women (Ohtake & Wolfe 1998, Wolfe et al. 1999). This may be due to trained pregnant women having an attenuated catecholamine response to submaximal heavy exercise (Wolfe et al. 1999), in addition to a higher stroke volume (Pivarnik et al. 1990).

Functional cardiac (heart rate) reserve (calculated by subtracting resting heart rate from maximal heart rate) is reduced during pregnancy (Wolfe & Mottola 1993), due to pregnancy increasing the resting heart rate. As a result, the magnitude of heart rate reserve is also reduced during standard submaximal steady-state exercise (Wolfe et al. 1999), possibly due to a blunted sympathoadrenal response to strenuous exercise during pregnancy (Bonen et al. 1992). The practical implication of this reduced maximal heart rate reserve is that pulse rate measurement becomes less precise for monitoring and prescribing exercise intensity when one becomes pregnant, which may lead to overestimating the intensity at lower work rates and underestimating the intensity at the higher work rates (Wolfe & Weissgerber 2003).

Oxygen uptake at the ventilatory threshold (Owles point; an indicator of the onset of blood lactate accumulation) is not affected by pregnancy or advancing gestation (Heenan et al. 2000, Lotgering et al. 1995, Wolfe et al. 1994). The physiological significance of this is debated (see Chapters 6 and 10.3), so considerable caution must be exercised in its interpretation. For example, a change in the ventilatory threshold can occur independently of changes in metabolism, and pregnant women do display a mild hyperventilatory response at most levels of submaximal exercise (Jensen et al. 2007). However, this unaltered ventilatory threshold may indicate that pregnant women are able to perform submaximal work without blood lactic acid accumulation and fatigue (Wolfe & Weissgerber 2003). Maternal blood lactate accumulation following strenuous exercise is reported to be lower during pregnancy than in the non-pregnant condition, possibly due to the dilution of lactate in the expanded maternal blood volume (McMurray et al. 1988), or due to the utilisation of lactate as a metabolic fuel by the foetus and placenta (Battaglia & Meschia 1978). These observations reinforce the principle that blood lactate measures, in the absence of either production or removal indices, can be very difficult to interpret. One must also recall that blood lactate is not necessarily a metabolic index of fatigue, but may instead reflect the redistribution of energy which, through gluconeogenesis, is part of the energy shuttle among tissues (see Chapters 6, 7 and 10.3).

The efficiency of standard submaximal steady-state exercise for weight-supported activity is not changed by pregnancy or by advancing gestational age (Ohtake & Wolfe 1998), nor is peak oxygen uptake during upright cycle ergometry (McMurray et al. 1991). Semi-supine cycling has been shown to elicit similar stroke volumes and cardiac outputs to upright cycling in late pregnancy (O'Neill et al. 2006). In contrast, peak oxygen uptake during swimming (although body weight is supported) is reduced compared to land cycling (McMurray et al. 1991). These physiological differences may be associated with a decrease in peak ventilation due to immersion (McMurray et al. 1991; Chapters 22 and 23). For weight-bearing activities, such as walking or jogging, the energy requirement increases in proportion to maternal mass gain (Artal et al. 1989).

2.2 Metabolic responses to exercise

Maternal metabolic responses to exercise may differ depending upon the duration and intensity of exercise and the dietary profile (Bessinger & McMurray 2003). Maternal blood glucose concentrations during exercise have been shown to remain the same (Artal et al. 1981) or decline (Bonen et al. 1992, Giroux et al. 2006), and this response depends on the intensity of the exercise and the fitness of the individual. Although maternal blood glucose may decline during and after exercise, this effect appears transitional, eventually returning to preexercise values; however, maternal macronutrient intake (especially carbohydrates) is extremely important (Giroux et al. 2006).

3 FOETAL RESPONSES TO MATERNAL EXERCISE

The normal foetal response in a healthy pregnancy is an increase in foetal baseline heart rate (tachycardia), which is proportional to both the intensity and duration of maternal exercise (Clapp et al. 1993). The cause for this response is hypothesised to be a mild transient foetal hypoxia secondary to a relatively reduced uterine blood flow (Katz et al. 1990), increased foetal temperature and augmented foetal wakefulness (Clapp et al. 1993). Maximal (volitional fatigue) testing (acute response) in late gestation in low-risk (with no obstetric risk to mother or foetus) women leads to minimal changes in foetal heart rate (Macphail et al. 2000). Sustained bouts of maternal exercise have both acute and long-term effects on placental bed blood flow via the reduced uterine blood flow, as visceral blood flow is rerouted to the maternal exercising muscles (Lotgering et al. 1983b; see below). However, cycle ergometer exercise caused a decrease in placental resistance in recovery (Rafla 1999) and a drop in uterine artery resistance (Rafla & Etokowo 1998), suggesting that maternal exercise may increase umbilical (Rafla 1999) and uterine blood flow (Rafla & Etokowo 1998).

Regular maternal weight-bearing exercise (running, aerobics, stair-climbing) has been shown to stimulate midtrimester placental growth and size measured at birth (Clapp & Risk 1992, Clapp et al. 2002, Jackson et al. 1995). Placental size is important as it may reflect an increase in surface area that maintains the transfer of oxygen and substrates necessary for foetal well-being (Bergmann et al. 2004).

Pregnancy outcome, reflected in the size (usually mass) of the baby at birth, reflects the health and *milieu* of the uterine environment during gestation (Catalano & Ehrenberg 2006). Clinically, birth mass at a specific gestational age reflects the health of the baby, and whether various problems occurred during pregnancy that restricted or enhanced foetal growth and development. For example, a baby that is born small for gestational age (≤2500 g) represents severe growth restriction, and clinical intervention is necessary at delivery to ensure survival. A baby that is too large (macrosomia: ≥4000 g) for gestational age may be born to a woman with gestational diabetes and reflects problems with metabolic control in the maternal environment. Babies born at either end of the birthweight continuum (either too small or too large for gestational age) may be at increased risk for chronic diseases, such as obesity later in life (Oken & Gillman 2003). Birth mass is directly associated with the body mass index (BMI) seen later in adult life (Oken & Gillman 2003). This relationship can be represented by a J-shaped curve, with a slightly higher BMI in individuals born with a small mass, but a larger prevalence of overweight and obesity tends to occur in those born with greater mass (Catalano & Ehrenberg 2006).

Sustained weight-bearing modes of exercise conducted at moderate to high intensity have been shown to influence foetal-placental growth; these effects are time specific, and are dependent upon the frequency (Campbell & Mottola 2001), duration (Bell et al. 1995) and intensity (Clapp & Capeless 1990) of the exercise sessions (Clapp 2003). However, others have found no effect on birth mass as a result of maternal exercise (Duncombe et al. 2006, Lokey et al. 1991, Macphail et al. 2000, O'Neill et al. 2006)

4 POTENTIAL RISKS OF EXERCISE DURING PREGNANCY

During acute exercise in the non-pregnant condition, blood is redistributed from the splanchnic, renal and other visceral beds to the working muscles (Chapters 1 and 19), blood glucose is more heavily used as an energy source by the exercising muscles and body temperature may be elevated. These three factors may present potential risks to foetal growth and development (Figure 12.1). First, the sympathetically mediated blood redistribution from the viscera may include reduced blood flow to the uterus,

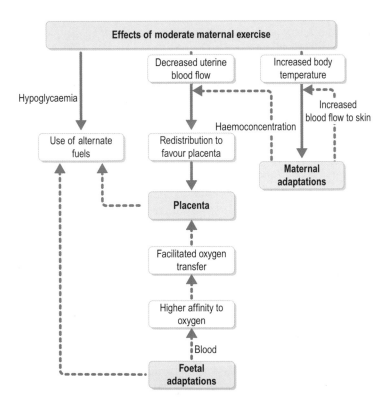

Figure 12.1 Maternal, placental and foetal adaptations occur in a low-risk medically prescreened pregnancy to protect the foetus from potential risks of maternal exercise. From Mottola & Wolfe (2000) with permission.

potentially leading to foetal hypoxia (decrease in oxygenation; Lotgering et al. 1983b). Second, maternal blood glucose is the major source of energy for foetal growth and development, and thus, maternal exercise may reduce the carbohydrate availability to the foetus (Mottola & Wolfe 2000). Third, elevated maternal body core temperature, accompanying endurance exercise, may change the normal thermal gradient for heat exchange between mother and foetus (Lotgering et al. 1983a). Heat is dissipated from high to low temperatures (Chapter 19) and thus, to maintain a thermal gradient from foetus to mother, the foetus is always about 0.6°C higher than the maternal body core temperature (Lotgering et al. 1983a). However, potential problems may occur during exercise because the gradient may shift due to elevated maternal core temperature, with the foetus becoming a partial recipient of the thermal energy generated during exercise. Teratogenic effects (abnormal foetal development) may occur in response to this increase in maternal heat, especially in the first trimester, when the foetus is most susceptible to developmental problems, with defects occurring in the central nervous system (Edwards et al. 2003).

Although these potential problems may raise concerns for the health of the foetus during maternal exercise, many pregnancy-induced adaptive mechanisms occur during a normal low-risk pregnancy from physiological changes to many maternal systems, and many protective mechanisms are also found in the foetus and placenta. These combine to reduce the risks of maternal exercise for the developing foetus.

There may be other potential effects of maternal exercise affecting the mother such as chronic fatigue, musculoskeletal injury and impact injury (repetitive and acute). Ligaments may become more prone to injury during pregnancy because of a circulating hormone called relaxin (Weiss et al. 1979). Relaxin loosens ligamentous connective tissue (at the symphysis pubis) as the body prepares for delivery of the foetus through the birth canal (Owens et al. 2002). Unfortunately, this hormone, because of its generalised distribution in maternal circulation, may affect other load-bearing joints that are prone to injury as a result of physical activity. In addition, some pregnant women may feel that they are more flexible with a wider range of motion in some joints, which would indicate that caution is advisable when using exercises to promote flexibility.

Very little scientific literature reports on muscle conditioning for pregnant women, as most of the studies investigate the physiological effects of aerobic exercise. Conventional wisdom and traditional medical advice have suggested that pregnant women avoid heavy lifting or straining, especially those activities which have a static or isometric exercise component (Avery et al. 1999). Theoretical risks of resistance exercise during pregnancy have included changes in maternal blood pressure, especially if the Valsalva manoeuvre is initiated (Lotgering et al. 1992b), initiation of premature labour (Durak et al. 1990) and tran-

sient foetal hypoxia (Green et al. 1988). High resistance exercise may reduce blood flow and oxygen supply to the uterus, which may cause a mild transient decrease in foetal oxygen concentrations (Avery et al. 1999), reflected by foetal bradycardia (Webb et al. 1991). Even with these potential risks in mind, few studies have examined the safety of strength conditioning exercises for the mother and the foetus.

Studies examining the maternal response to muscle conditioning activity have found that healthy pregnant women have not exhibited a hypertensive response to resistance exercise (Avery et al. 1999, Lotgering et al. 1992b, Webb et al. 1991). In addition, a stable foetal heart rate pattern during isotonic and isometric exercise has been reported in the literature (Avery et al. 1999, Lotgering et al. 1992b, Webb et al. 1991), while others revealed transient changes in foetal heart rate, especially during maternal exercise performed while lying on the back (supine position; Green et al. 1988, Nesler et al. 1988). The transient changes in foetal heart rate may be a reaction to a drop in uterine blood flow during supine exercise (Jeffreys et al. 2006). Thus, the literature would suggest that maternal strength conditioning exercises do not compromise maternal or foetal well-being in healthy pregnancies; however, exercises performed in the supine position should perhaps be avoided. Because of these potential risks, the guidelines below are based on common-sense principles, along with scientific, evidence-based research.

5 MATERNAL ADAPTATIONS

To counter the possible decrease in uteroplacental blood flow that may occur during maternal exercise, the mother has an increased plasma volume and erythrocyte count (haemoconcentration; McMurray et al. 1991; see also Chapter 27.3). These combine to increase oxygen transport to the placenta (Gilbert et al. 1985). In addition, pregnant women have been shown to maintain and even increase the oxygen saturation during short-term submaximal exercise (Pirhonen et al. 2003). The increase in blood volume facilitates an increase in blood flow to the skin for heat dissipation, thereby improving thermoregulation (Lindqvist et al. 2003). In addition, during mid to late pregnancy, the insulin resistance that develops in maternal skeletal muscle spares maternal blood glucose for foetal growth and development (Hay et al. 1983).

6 FOETAL ADAPTATIONS

Haemoglobin content, arterial oxygen placental bed blood flow, partial pressure and nutrient concentration of the maternal blood are important physiological determinants of the availability, or the rate of oxygen and substrate delivery to the maternal-placental-foetal interface (Clapp 2006). When uterine blood flow is decreased, blood entering the uterus is rerouted to favour the placenta and foetus, at the expense of the myometrium, ensuring adequate foetal oxygenation (Curet et al. 1976). Foetal haemoglobin has a higher affinity for oxygen, which also facilitates transplacental oxygen transfer (Gilbert et al. 1985). In addition, the foetal form of haemoglobin is insensitive to 2,3-diphosphoglycerate, which increases during anaerobic metabolism, and serves to reduce haemoglobin oxygen affinity. As a result, the foetal oxygen-haemoglobin dissociation curve lies to the left of the maternal curve, promoting better extraction of oxygen from haemoglobin at a given partial pressure (Gilbert et al. 1985). Furthermore, when maternal blood glucose concentrations are decreased, the placenta utilises maternal lactate for gluconeogenesis, and the foetus uses lactate as an alternative energy source for growth and development (Hay et al. 1983). Thus, in a normal low-risk pregnancy, the foetus is well protected against the potential risks of hypoxia and hypoglycaemia during maternal exercise. It has also been suggested that the foetal-placental interface is quite sensitive and responsive to an intermittent stimulus (maternal dietary intake and exercise) of either an increase or decrease in oxygen and substrate availability, rather than a persistent stimulus, and this intermittent stimulus produces beneficial growth effects (Clapp 2006).

7 MATERNAL EXERCISE GUIDELINES AND PRESCRIPTION

7.1 The need for medical prescreening

While the potential risks to the foetus may be offset by many protective mechanisms during pregnancy (Figure 12.1), no threshold has been identified for the intensity and duration of maternal exercise above which problems may occur (Figure 12.2). Because of this, it is important that medical prescreening occurs prior to exercise, to ensure a healthy, low-risk pregnancy. There appears to be a dose–response curve, in that as the quantity and quality of maternal exercise increase, the potential for these hypothetical risks also increases (Mottola & Wolfe 2000).

Current guidelines for exercise during pregnancy are considered appropriate for medically screened pregnant women who have no contraindications to exercise. Contraindications to exercise are listed in the medical prescreening document, and include both absolute and relative contraindications to exercise (Wolfe & Mottola 2002). The decision to exercise or not is made by medical personnel (Davies et al. 2003a, b).

The benefits of being active during pregnancy include an increase in metabolic and cardiopulmonary reserve, promotion of normal glucose tolerance and many psychological benefits to the mother (Figure 12.2; Mottola & Wolfe 2000), while increasing foetal and placental adaptations to ensure a healthy foetus (Clapp 2006). However, as Figure 12.2 suggests, there now is a potential problem at the other end of the spectrum, in the impact of chronic disease risk to both mother and offspring from a sedentary lifestyle. That is, the absence of an adequate habitual physical activity level, in which beneficial adaptive mechanisms occur, will ultimately lead to obesity, diabetes mellitus and cardiovascular disease in the future (Pivarnik et al. 2006; also see Chapters 28 and 30).

7.2 History of exercise guidelines

Prior to 1985, pregnant women were told by their healthcare providers to rest and not to engage in physical activ-

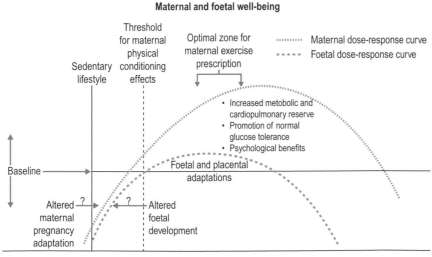

Figure 12.2 Maternal and foetal dose–response curves exist as the quantity and quality of maternal exercise increase from baseline. In a low-risk, medically prescreened pregnancy, an optimal zone for maternal exercise prescription is important because a threshold beyond which potential problems may occur has not yet been identified. However, there does appear to be a threshold of inactivity below which normal adaptive mechanisms do not occur, placing the mother and foetus at an increased disease risk for obesity, diabetes and cardiovascular disease because of a more sedentary lifestyle (Chapter 28). Modified from Wolfe et al. (1989a) with permission.

ity. These recommendations were based on concern for the developing foetus (Wolfe & Davies 2003). In the US, guidelines were published in 1985 in which conservative limits were placed on the maximal heart rate a pregnant woman should achieve while exercising (140 beats·min^{-1}), for 15 minutes duration (American College of Obstetricians and Gynecologists 1985), and it was suggested that previously sedentary women should not begin an exercise programme. These guidelines were controversial because there was no scientific basis for such conservative limits (Wolfe & Mottola 2000). Subsequent guidelines from the American College of Obstetricians and Gynecologists (1994 and 2002) ignored heart rate targets during exercise, and suggested that a pregnant woman with a low-risk pregnancy can participate in moderate exercise on most, if not all, days of the week for at least 30 minutes, with no heart rate limit.

In Canada, the PARmed-X for Pregnancy document was developed in 1996 (revised in 2002: www.csep.ca), and is based on scientific evidence that suggests that pregnant women who are medically prescreened and have no contraindications to exercise can safely exercise at 60–80% of their aerobic power (Wolfe & Davies 2003, Wolfe & Mottola 2000). This document contains a history questionnaire for the pregnant woman to complete, a list of contraindications to exercise (both relative and absolute) and guidelines for aerobic and muscular conditioning exercise, and a list of safety considerations, reasons to stop exercise and seek medical advice (Wolfe & Mottola 2002). The PARmed-X for Pregnancy has been endorsed by various professional bodies (American College of Sports Medicine 2005, Davies et al. 2003a,b, Stevenson 1997).

7.3 Aerobic exercise prescription

Once medical approval has been given, aerobic exercise prescription should be individualised for each pregnant participant. Women with low-risk pregnancies can begin an exercise programme in the second trimester, once fatigue and other pregnancy-induced discomforts have diminished.

Once regular physical activity has begun, frequency can be increased to 4–5 times per week. However, caution is indicated at five times per week, as Campbell & Mottola (2001) have shown that women who engaged in structured exercise five or more times per week in the last trimester were 4.6 times more likely to give birth to a low birthweight baby. In addition, at the other end of the spectrum, those women who engaged in structured activity two or less times per week were also more likely to deliver a baby with a low birth mass (Campbell & Mottola 2001). Thus, it is recommended that maintaining an exercise programme of 3–4 times per week is most beneficial.

The intensity of physical activity should be such that the heart rate remains within the target prescriptive zones (relative to the functional cardiac reserve) presented in Table

Table 12.2 Target heart rate (beats·min^{-1}) zones for aerobic exercise prescription during pregnancy based on age (years; PARmed-X for Pregnancy – Wolfe & Mottola 2002 with permission)

Age	Heart rate
<20	140–155
20–29	135–150
30–39	130–145
≥40	125–140

12.2 (Wolfe & Mottola 2002). These heart rate zones were modified from the heart rates of non-pregnant individuals for two reasons. First, heart rate during pregnancy is attenuated during maximal exercise, resulting in a significant decrease in the heart rate reserve (Wolfe & Mottola 1993). Second, the resting heart rate increases during pregnancy by about 15–20 beats·min^{-1} above non-pregnant values (Wolfe & Davies 2003). The safety and efficacy of this modified target pulse rate procedure have been verified in controlled studies (Ohtake & Wolfe 1998, Wolfe & Mottola 2000), and is deemed to be appropriate for normal-mass, active pregnant women (Mottola et al. 2006). An individual starting an exercise programme should begin at the lower end of the target heart rate range, while those women continuing an exercise programme can exercise at the upper end of the target heart rate range (Wolfe & Mottola 2002). Additional checks on appropriate intensity include using the rating of perceived exertion scale (Borg 1982), in which a range of 'somewhat hard' is appropriate for most pregnant women (Wolfe & Mottola 2002). In order to confirm the best intensity, these exercise heart rate prescriptions should be checked with the 'talk test', enabling a pregnant woman to carry on a conversation during exercise without being out of breath (Wolfe & Mottola 2002).

For healthy pregnant women just beginning an exercise session, 15 minutes at the target heart rate with a 10–15 min warm-up and a 10–15 min cool-down at a lower intensity is safe (Wolfe & Mottola 2002). The best time to progress to longer duration exercise is during the second trimester, by adding 2 min per week to the target exercise time until 30 min is reached (Davies et al. 2003a,b).

Women should choose activities that will minimise the loss of balance, risk of falling and foetal trauma (Davies et al. 2003a). The types of activities recommended are brisk walking, stationary cycling, swimming or aerobic activities that cause less impact to joints and ligaments (Davies et al. 2003b).

7.4 Prescription for muscular conditioning

The PARmed-X for Pregnancy includes precautions for muscle conditioning activity as well as examples of appropriate exercises (Wolfe & Mottola 2002). It would seem that the paucity of scientific studies examining the effects of muscle strength and conditioning during pregnancy, and the inconclusive results from some research indicate a need for further scientific investigation. Nevertheless, prescription for muscular conditioning includes full range of motion for all major muscle groups. The moving muscle group will increase in strength and endurance. One to two types of exercises should be used for each major muscle group for each side of the body. These areas should include: back and shoulders; chest and arms; legs and buttocks; abdominal and lower back muscles (body core support); and pelvic floor muscles. The supine position is to be avoided. Resistance exercise should include high repetitions (e.g. 12–15 repetitions without fatigue) with a comfortable mass, emphasising continuous breathing – exhaling on exertion and inhaling on relaxation (Brankston et al. 2004, Wolfe & Mottola 2002). During pregnancy, technique and proper breathing are extremely important to prevent injury. The Valsalva manoeuvre should be avoided during pregnancy as this may cause a change in blood pressure (Wolfe & Mottola 2002).

Four precautions are recommended for muscle conditioning exercise.

1. Avoid exercise in the supine position past 16 weeks of gestation, due to potential impingement of the pregnant uterus on the inferior vena cava (diminishing blood flow back to the heart) or the abdominal aorta (main blood supply to the uterine arteries; Ueland et al. 1969). The mechanisms that normally facilitate venous return, such as the muscle pump, are negated due to the heavy uterus impinging upon these vessels, and thus exercises while lying on the back are to be avoided.

2. Avoid exercise with rapid changes of direction and jarring of joints, due to a potential relaxation of ligaments and joint instability. This also includes caution for stretching activities, which should also be performed with caution to avoid ligament and joint injury.

3. Avoid abdominal exercise if diastasis recti (tearing of the connective tissue line or linea alba) occurs, as pregnancy progresses. This condition presents as a rippling or bulging along the abdominal midline, but its cause is not known. The rationale behind this guideline is logical. From a mechanical viewpoint, the pregnant abdomen will continue to increase in size. If the abdominal muscles, such as the rectus abdominis, the obliques and the transversus muscles, are continuously strengthened, the tear will occur at the weakest point as the abdomen increases in size, which will be the connective tissue. This will potentially cause more tearing of the linea alba and this condition may get worse, thus further strengthening of these abdominal muscles is not recommended once diagnosed (Bursch 1987).

4. Emphasise correct posture, which includes a neutral pelvic alignment. The enlarging uterus and breasts during pregnancy cause a forward shift in the centre of gravity, which may cause the shoulders to slump forward and increase the arch in the lower back (lordosis) (Heckman & Sassard 1994). Incorrect posture may lead to back and pelvic pain, and thus correct posture and a neutral pelvic alignment are recommended. To find a neutral pelvic alignment, the pregnant woman should stand with feet shoulder-width apart, knees slightly bent, with pelvic placement halfway between an accentuated lordosis and posterior pelvic tilt position (pushing the pelvis as far forward as possible). These extreme positions are to be avoided during pregnancy, while the neutral pelvic alignment is a comfortable position halfway between these two extremes.

7.5 Safety precautions and reasons to seek medical advice

Most health-care professionals agree that pregnant women should stop exercising and seek immediate medical advice if any adverse symptoms occur, as outlined in Table 12.3 (American College of Obstetricians and Gynecologists 2002, Davies et al. 2003a, Wolfe & Mottola 2002). While regular physical activity should be part of one's daily routine and the adverse consequences of the sedentary lifestyle are well established (Chapters 17.1, 28, 30 and 31.1), one must proceed with some caution when the health and well-being of the unborn child are challenged.

The pregnant woman should avoid exercise in hot, humid environments, since these offer more rigorous challenges to thermal homeostasis (Chapter 19), thereby placing the foetus under greater strain. Throughout the pregnancy, but particularly when regularly exercising, it is important to maintain proper nutrition and hydration (Giroux et al. 2006; Chapters 32 and 33). In addition, it is important to monitor the temperature of heated pools, as a warmer environment will augment the exercise-induced increase in maternal body core temperature and potentially compromise mater-

---

Table 12.3 Reasons to stop exercise and seek medical advice (Wolfe & Mottola 2002) with permission

- Persistent uterine contractions (>6–8 per hour)
- Bloody vaginal discharge
- Gush of fluid from vagina (suggesting ruptured membranes)
- Unexplained abdominal pain
- Sudden swelling of extremities (ankles, hands or face)
- Swelling, pain and redness in the calf of one leg (suggesting phlebitis)
- Persistent headaches or blurring of vision
- Unexplained dizziness or faintness
- Marked fatigue, chest pain or heart palpitations
- Failure to gain weight (<1 kg per month over last 2 trimesters)
- Absence of usual foetal movement (once detected)

nal and foetal thermoregulation (Mottola & Wolfe 2000). It is also recommended that athletic competition be avoided while pregnant (Wolfe & Mottola 2002).

Pregnant women are also cautioned against scuba diving, as the foetus is not protected against decompression sickness and gas embolism (Davies et al. 2003a; see also Chapter 23). Women should also be wary of exercise at high altitudes (above 2500 m; see Chapter 24), as appropriate acclimatisation is required to offset the effects of hypoxia on both the mother and the foetus (Artal et al. 1995, Huch 1996). In addition, resting uterine artery blood flow is lower in pregnant women who live at an altitude of 3100 m than in women who reside at 1600 m (Entin & Coffin 2004). This effect is likely to decrease further with maternal exercise at altitude.

8 SEDENTARY PREGNANT WOMEN

Aerobic power and exercise performance may be limited in sedentary pregnant women, particularly in those who were overweight prior to becoming pregnant (e.g. BMI > 25 $kg \cdot m^{-2}$; Mottola et al. 2006). Unfit women with peak aerobic power within the bottom 25th percentile had $\leqslant 21.0$ $mL \cdot kg^{-1} \cdot min^{-1}$ at age 20–29 years and $\leqslant 19.6$ $mL \cdot kg^{-1} \cdot min^{-1}$ at age 30–39 years (Mottola et al. 2006). The average body mass index of this cohort was 29.8 ± 1.2 $kg \cdot m^{-2}$ and 31.6 ± 1.0 $kg \cdot m^{-2}$, respectively. It has been suggested that the target heart rate zones found in the PARmed-X for Pregnancy document may be too difficult for sedentary pregnant women who are overweight, who have a lower peak aerobic power and who are beginning an exercise programme. New exercise target heart rate zones, based on age and fitness levels, were developed, being slightly lower for unfit pregnant women (129–144 $beats \cdot min^{-1}$ for 20–29 years and 128–144 $beats \cdot min^{-1}$ for 30–39 years). These targets would represent 60–80% of aerobic power (Mottola et al. 2006) and would replace the previous targets for this group of unfit women, but would still be used in conjunction with the other PARmed-X for Pregnancy guidelines. Improvements in submaximal exercise capacity can be made in overweight sedentary pregnant women who train at 50–60% of maximum predicted heart rate, starting in the second trimester (Santos et al. 2005).

9 FIT PREGNANT WOMEN

Fit women with peak aerobic power $\geqslant 27.2$ $mL \cdot kg^{-1} \cdot min^{-1}$ at ages 20–29 years and $\geqslant 26.1$ $mL \cdot kg^{-1} \cdot min^{-1}$ at ages 30–39 years have a higher aerobic power and greater exercise adaptations. These women have different target heart rate ranges representing 60–80% of peak aerobic power, with new heart rate zones of 145–160 $beats \cdot min^{-1}$ for women aged 20–29 years and 140–156 $beats \cdot min^{-1}$ for women 30–39 years. Again, these new target heart rate zones should be used in conjunction with the 'talk test' and the rating of perceived exertion scale, to confirm the appropriate and individualised exercise intensity (Mottola et al. 2006). Fit pregnant women should not train at intensities above 80% of their aerobic power because the threshold at which potential problems may occur has not been determined, and the risks to the developing foetus and risk of injury to the mother may outweigh the benefits gained at the higher exercise intensities. Because of this, pregnancy is not the time for engaging in athletic competition (Mottola 1998). High-intensity athletes are used to exercising through pain and discomfort, especially during competition. This is not necessarily appropriate for women who are pregnant as they may be ignoring pregnancy-induced changes (as mentioned above), and risks to the foetus, or to themselves, may be overlooked. In addition, competition usually produces augmented concentrations of circulating catecholamines, most of which may be metabolised by the mother; however, high circulating catecholamine concentrations may enhance uterine contractions (Bessinger & McMurray 2003), and about 15% may cross the placental barrier into foetal circulation (Artal et al. 1981). The consequences of this are unknown.

10 THE IMPORTANCE OF ACTIVE LIVING DURING PREGNANCY

With guidelines in place for medical prescreening and exercise prescription appropriate for low, average or high aerobic power (based on age), it is imperative that all pregnant women with low-risk pregnancies remain, or start being active during pregnancy. Promoting active living during pregnancy will have many benefits to both mother and foetus, such as healthy living habits, that will last a lifetime (Chapter 28). Pregnant women and women with young children have a strong influence on family life, and engagement of healthy eating habits and active lifestyle may be transferred to their children, hopefully diminishing potential health risks to the next generation. Prevention of excessive weight gain during pregnancy, through active living and prevention of weight retention after the baby is born, may be important strategies in helping to stem the obesity and diabetes epidemics facing our world today (Chapter 30).

11 FUTURE CONSIDERATIONS

It is clear that sedentary living and physical inactivity during pregnancy may cause increased risk for obesity, diabetes and cardiovascular disease later in life, for both the mother and her unborn child (Pivarnik et al. 2006, Weissgerber et al. 2006b). Armed with a medical prescreening tool with safe guidelines for aerobic and muscle conditioning exercises, exercise physiologists with an interest in special populations, such as pregnant women, can work closely with health-care and fitness professionals to provide healthy, low-risk pregnant women with active living programmes that will benefit them and their families.

References

American College of Obstetricians and Gynecologists 1985 Pregnancy and the postnatal period. ACOG Home Exercise Programs. American College of Obstetricians and Gynecologists, Washington, DC

American College of Obstetricians and Gynecologists 1994 Exercise during pregnancy and the postpartum period. ACOG Technical Bulletin 189:2–7

American College of Obstetricians and Gynecologists 2002 Opinion no. 267: exercise during pregnancy and the postpartum period. Obstetrics and Gynecology 99:171–173

American College of Sports Medicine 2004 Endorsements. Sports Medicine Bulletin 39(5)

Artal R, Platt L, Sperling M 1981 Exercise in pregnancy: maternal cardiovascular and metabolic responses in normal pregnancy. American Journal of Obstetrics and Gynecology 140:123–129

Artal R, Masak D, Khodiguian, N, Romem Y, Rutherford S, Wiswell R 1989 Exercise prescription in pregnancy:weight bearing vs non-weight bearing exercise. American Journal of Obstetrics and Gynecology 161:1464–1469

Artal R, Fortunato V, Welton A, Constantino N, Khodiguian N, Villabos L 1995 A comparison of cardiopulmonary adaptations to exercise in pregnancy at sea level and altitude. American Journal of Obstetrics and Gynecology 175:505–506

Avery N, Stocking K, Tranmer E, Davies G, Wolfe LA 1999 Fetal responses to maternal strength conditioning exercises in late gestation. Canadian Journal of Applied Physiology 24:362–376

Avery N, Wolfe LA, Amara C, Davies G, McGrath M 2001 Effects of human pregnancy on autonomic function above and below the ventilatory threshold. Journal of Applied Physiology 90:321–328

Bader R, Bader M, Rosse D 1959 The oxygen cost of breathing in dyspnoeic subjects as studied in normal pregnant women. Clinical Science (London) 18:223–235

Battaglia FC, Meschia G 1978 Principal substrates of the human fetus. Physiological Reviews 58:499–527

Bauer MK, Harding J, Bassett N, Breier B, Oliver M, Gallaher B 1998 Foetal growth and placental function. Molecular and Cellular Endocrinology 140:115–120

Bell R, Palma S, Lumley J 1995 The effect of vigorous exercise during pregnancy on birth-weight. Australian and New Zealand Journal of Obstetrics Gynaecology 35:46–51

Ben-Haroush A, Yogev Y, Hod M 2003 Epidemiology of gestational diabetes and its association with type 2 diabetes. Diabetic Medicine 21:103–113

Bergmann A, Zygmunt M, Clapp JF 2004 Running throughout pregnancy: effect on placental villous vascular volume and cell proliferation. Placenta 25:694–698

Bessinger R, McMurray R 2003 Substrate utilization and hormonal responses to exercise in pregnancy. Clinical Obstetrics and Gynecology 46: 467–478

Boden G 1996 Fuel metabolism in pregnancy and in gestational diabetes mellitus. Obstetrics and Gynecology Clinics of North America 23:1–10

Bonen A, Campagna P, Gilchrist L, Young D, Beresford P 1992 Substrate and endocrine responses to during exercise at selected stages of pregnancy. Journal of Applied Physiology 73:134–142

Borg GAV 1982 Psychophysical bases of perceived exertion. Medicine and Science in Sports and Exercise 14:377–381

Brankston GB, Mitchell E, Ryan E, Okun N 2004 Resistance exercise decreases the need for insulin in overweight women with gestational diabetes mellitus. American Journal of Obstetrics and Gynecology 190:188–193

Buchanan TA, Metzer B, Freinkel N 1990 Insulin sensitivity and B-cell responsiveness to glucose during late pregnancy in lean and moderately obese women with normal glucose tolerance or gestational diabetes. American Journal of Obstetrics and Gynecology 162:1008–1014

Bursch SG 1987 Interrater reliability of diastasis recti abdominis measurement. Physical Therapy 67:1077–1079

Butte N 2000 Carbohydrate and lipid metabolism in pregnancy: normal compared with gestational diabetes mellitus. American Journal of Clinical Nutrition 71(Suppl):1256S-1261S

Campbell MK, Mottola MF 2001 Recreational exercise and occupational activity during pregnancy and birth weight: a case-control study. American Journal of Obstetrics and Gynecology 184:403–408

Catalano PM, Ehrenberg HM 2006 The short- and long-term implications of maternal obesity on the mother and her offspring. British Journal of Obstetrics and Gynaecology 113:1126–1133

Catalano PM, Tyzbir E, Roman N 1991 Longitudinal changes in insulin release and insulin resistance in non-obese pregnant women. American Journal of Obstetrics and Gynecology 165:1667–1672

Clapp JF 1991 The changing thermal response to endurance exercise during pregnancy. American Journal of Obstetrics and Gynecology 165:1684–1689

Clapp JF 2002 Maternal carbohydrate intake and pregnancy outcome. Proceedings of the Nutrition Society 61:45–50

Clapp JF 2003 The effects of maternal exercise on fetal oxygenation and feto-placental growth. European Journal of Obstetrics, Gynaecology and Reproductive Biology 110:S80–85

Clapp JF 2006 Influence of endurance exercise and diet on human placental development and fetal growth. Placenta 27:527–534

Clapp JF, Capeless E 1990 Neonatal morphometrics after endurance exercise during pregnancy. American Journal of Obstetrics and Gynecology 163:1805–1811

Clapp JF, Risk K 1992 Effect of recreational exercise on midtrimester placental growth. American Journal of Obstetrics and Gynecology 183:1484–1488

Clapp JF, Little K, Capeless E 1993 Fetal heart rate response to sustained recreational exercise. American Journal of Obstetrics and Gynecology 168:198–206

Clapp JF, Kim H, Burciu B, Schmidt S, Petry K, Lopez B 2002 Continuing regular exercise during pregnancy: effect of exercise volume on fetoplacental growth. American Journal of Obstetrics and Gynecology 186:142–147

Clausen JP 1977 Effect of physical training on cardiovascular adjustments to exercise in man. Physiological Reviews 57:779–816

Cowett R, Susa J, Kahn C, Giletti B, Oh W, Schwartz R 1983 Glucose kinetics in nondiabetic and diabetic women during the third trimester of pregnancy. American Journal of Obstetrics and Gynecology 146:773–780

Cugell D, Frank N, Gaensler E, Badger T 1953 Pulmonary function in pregnancy. Serial observations in normal women. American Review of Tuberculosis and Pulmonary Diseases 67:568–597

Curet L, Orr J, Rankin J 1976 Effect of exercise on cardiac output and distribution of uterine blood flow in pregnant ewes. Journal of Applied Physiology 40:725–728

Davies G, Wolfe LA, Mottola MF, MacKinnon C 2003a Joint SOGC/CSEP Clinical Practice Guideline: Exercise in Pregnancy and the Postpartum Period. Journal of Obstetrics and Gynecology of Canada 25(6):516–22

Davies G, Wolfe LA, Mottola MF, MacKinnon C 2003b Joint SOGC/CSEP Clinical Practice Guideline: Exercise in Pregnancy and the Postpartum Period. Canadian Journal of Applied Physiology 28(3):329–341

Duncombe D, Skouteris H, Wertheim E, Kelly L, Fraser V, Paxton S 2006 Vigorous exercise and birth outcomes in a sample of recreational exercisers: a prospective study across pregnancy. Australian and New Zealand Journal of Obstetrics and Gynaecology 46:288–292

Durak E, Jovanovic-Peterson L, Peterson C 1990 Comparative evaluation of uterine response to exercise on five aerobic machines. American Journal of Obstetrics and Gynecology 162:754–756

Duvekot J, Cheriex E, Pieters F, Menheere P, Peeters L 1993 Early pregnancy changes in hemodynamics and volume homeostasis are consecutive adjustments triggered by a primary fall in systemic vascular tone. American Journal of Obstetrics and Gynecology 169:1382–1392

Edwards M, Saunders RD, Shiota K 2003 Effects of heat on embryos and foetuses. International Journal of Hyperthermia 19:295–324

Entin PL, Coffin L 2004 Physiological basis for recommendations regarding exercise during pregnancy at high altitude. High Altitude Medicine and Biology 5(3):321–324

Field S, Bell S, Cenaiko S, Whitelaw W 1991 Relationship between inspiratory effort and breathlessness in pregnancy. Journal of Applied Physiology 71:1987–1902

Gilbert RD, Lis L, Longo LD 1985 Temperature effects on oxygen affinity of human foetal blood. Journal of Developmental Physiology 7:299–304

Giroux I, Inglis S, Lander S, Gerrie S, Mottola MF 2006 Dietary intake, weight gain and birth outcomes of physically active pregnant women: a pilot study. Applied Physiology, Nutrition and Metabolism 31:483–489

Green RC, Schneider K, MacLennan A 1988 The foetal heart rate response to static antenatal exercises in the supine position. Australian Journal of Physiotherapy. 34:3–7

Hart MV, Morton MJ, Hosenpud J, Metcalfe J 1986 Aortic function during normal human pregnancy. American Journal of Obstetrics and Gynecology 154:887–891

Hay WW, Myers SA, Sparks JW, Wilkening RB, Meschia G, Battaglia FC 1983 Glucose and lactate oxidation rates in the fetal lamb. Proceedings of the Society for Experimental Biology and Medicine 173:553–563

Heckman JD, Sassard R 1994 Current concepts review: musculoskeletal considerations in pregnancy. Journal of Bone and Joint Surgery (Am) 76:1720–1730

Heenan AP, Wolfe LA 2000 Plasma acid-base regulation above and below the ventilatory threshold in late gestation. Journal of Applied Physiology 88:149–157

Heenan AP, Wolfe LA, Davies G 2001 Maximal exercise testing in late gestation: maternal responses. Obstetrics and Gynecology 97:127–134

Hiramatsu Y, Masuyama H, Mizutani Y, Kudo T, Oguni N, Oguni Y 2000 Heavy-for-date infants: their backgrounds and relationship with gestational diabetes. Journal of Obstetrics and Gynaecology Research 26:193–198

Huch R 1996 Physical activity at altitude in pregnancy. Seminars in Perinatology 20:303–314

Jackson MR, Gott P, Lye L, Ritche J, Clapp JF 1995 The effects of maternal aerobic exercise on human placental development: placental volumetric composition and surface areas. Placenta 16:179–191

Jeffreys R, Stepanchak W, Lopez B, Hardis J, Clapp JF 2006 Uterine blood flow during supine rest and exercise after 28 weeks of gestation. British Journal of Obstetrics and Gynaecology 113:1239–1247

Jensen D, Webb K, Wolfe LA, O'Donnell D 2007 Effects of human pregnancy and advancing gestation on respiratory discomfort during exercise. Respiratory Physiology and Neurobiology 156(1):85–93

Jones RL, Botti JJ, Anderson W, Bennett N 1985 Thermoregulation during aerobic exercise during pregnancy. Obstetrics and Gynecology 65:340–345

Katz V, McMurray R, Goodwin W, Cefalo R 1990 Nonweightbearing exercise during pregnancy on land and during immersion: a comparative study. American Journal of Perinatology 7:281–284

Lesser KB, Carpenter M 1994 Metabolic changes associated with normal pregnancy and pregnancy complicated by diabetes mellitus. Seminars in Perinatology 18:399–406

Lindqvist PG, Marsal K, Merlo M, Pirhonen J 2003 Thermal response to submaximal exercise before, during and after pregnancy: a longitudinal study. Journal of Maternal, Fetal and Neonatal Medicine 13:152–156

Lokey E, Tran Z, Wells C, Myers B, Tran A 1991 Effects of physical exercise on pregnancy outcomes: a meta-analytic review. Medicine and Science in Sports and Exercise 23:1234–1249

Lotgering F, Gilbert R, Longo L 1983a Exercise responses in pregnant sheep: blood gases, temperatures and fetal cardiovascular system. American Journal of Physiology 55:842–850

Lotgering F, Gilbert R, Longo L 1983b Exercise responses in pregnant sheep: oxygen consumption, uterine blood flow and blood volume. Journal of Applied Physiology 55:834–841

Lotgering F, Van Doorne M, Struijk P, Pool J, Wallenburg H 1991 Maximal aerobic exercise in pregnant women: heart rate, O_2 consumption, CO_2 production and ventilation. Journal of Applied Physiology 70:1016–1023

Lotgering F, Struijk P, Van Doorne M, Wallenberg H 1992a Errors in predicting maximal oxygen consumption in pregnant women. Journal of Applied Physiology 72:562–567

Lotgering F, van der Berg A, Struijk P, Wallenberg H 1992b Arterial pressure response to maximal isometric exercise in pregnant women. Obstetrics and Gynecology 166:538–542

Lotgering F, Struijk P, Van Doorne M, Spinnewijn W, Wallenburg H 1995 Anaerobic threshold and respiratory compensation in pregnant women. Journal of Applied Physiology 78:1772–1777

McMurray RG, Katz VL, Berry M, Cefalo RC 1988 The effect of pregnancy on metabolic responses during rest, immersion and aerobic exercise in the water. American Journal of Obstetrics and Gynecology 158:481–486

McMurray RG, Hackney AC, Katz V, Gall M, Watson WJ 1991 Pregnancy-induced changes in the maximal physiological responses during swimming. Journal of Applied Physiology 71(4):1454–1459

Macphail A, Davies G, Victory R, Wolfe LA 2000 Maximal exercise testing in late gestation: foetal responses. Obstetrics and Gynecology 96:565–570

Milne J, Howie A, Pack A 1978 Dyspnea during normal pregnancy. British Journal of Obstetrics and Gynaecology 85:260–263

Mottola MF 1998 Exercise and pregnancy – what do I tell my pregnant patient? In: Standish W (ed) Oxford textbook of sports medicine. Oxford University Press, New York, 779–786

Mottola MF, Christopher PD 1991 Effects of maternal exercise on liver and skeletal muscle glycogen storage in pregnant rats. Journal of Applied Physiology 71:1015–1019.

Mottola MF, Wolfe LA 2000 The pregnant athlete. In: Drinkwater BL (ed) Women in sport. Blackwell Science, Oxford, 194–207

Mottola MF, Davenport MH, Brun CR, Inglis SD, Charlesworth S, Sopper MM 2006 VO_{2peak} prediction and exercise prescription for pregnant women. Medicine and Science in Sports and Exercise 38(8):1389–1395

Nesler CL, Hassett S, Cary S, Brooke L 1988 Effects of supine exercise on fetal heart rate in the second and third trimesters. American Journal of Perinatology 5:159–163

Ohtake PJ, Wolfe LA 1998 Physical conditioning attenuates respiratory responses to steady-state exercise in late gestation. Medicine and Science in Sports and Exercise 30:17–27

Oken E, Gillman MW 2003 Foetal origins of obesity. Obesity Research 11:496–506

O'Neill M, Cooper K, Boyce E, Hunyor S 2006 Postural effects when cycling in late pregnancy. Women and Birth 19:107–111

Owens K, Pearson A, Mason G 2002 Symphysis pubis dysfunction: a cause of significant obstetric morbidity. European Journal of Obstetrics, Gynaecology and Reproductive Biology 105:143–146

Pirhonen J, Lindqvist P, Marsal K 2003 A longitudinal study of maternal oxygen saturation during short-term maternal exercise. Clinical Physiology and Functional Imaging 23:37–41

Pivarnik JM 1996 Cardiovascular responses to aerobic exercise during pregnancy and postpartum. Seminars in Perinatology 20(4):242–249

Pivarnik JM, Lee W, Clark S, Cotton D, Spillman M, Miller JF 1990 Cardiac output responses of primigravid women during exercise determined by the direct Fick technique. Obstetrics and Gynecology 75:954–959

Pivarnik JM, Mauer MB, Ayers N, Kirshon B, Dildy G, Cotton DB 1994 Effect of chronic exercise on blood volume expansion and hematologic indices during pregnancy. Obstetrics and Gynecology 83:265–269

Pivarnik JM, Chambliss HO, Clapp JF, Dugan SA, Hatch MC, Lovelady CA, Mottola MF, Williams MA 2006 Impact of physical activity during pregnancy and postpartum on chronic disease risk. Special Communications Roundtable Consensus Statement. Medicine and Science in Sports and Exercise 38(5):989–1006

Rafla N 1999 Umbilical artery flow velocity waveforms following maternal exercise. Journal of Obstetrics and Gynaecology 19:385–389

Rafla N, Etokowo G 1998 The effect of maternal exercise on uterine artery velocimetry waveforms. Journal of Obstetrics and Gynaecology 18:14–17

Ratigan TR 1983 Anatomic and physiologic changes of pregnancy: anesthetic considerations. American Association of Nurse Anesthetists Journal 51:38–42

Rubler S, Damani P, Pinto E 1977 Cardiac size and performance during pregnancy estimated with echocardiography. American Journal of Cardiology 40:534–540

Sady M, Carpenter M, Thomson P, Sady M, Haydon B, Coustan D 1989 Cardiovascular responses to cycle exercise during and after pregnancy. Journal of Applied Physiology 66:336–341

Sady M, Haydon B, Sady S, Carpenter M, Thompson P, Coustan D 1990 Cardiovascular response to maximal cycle exercise during pregnancy and at two and seven months postpartum. American Journal of Obstetrics and Gynecology 162:1181–1185

Santos IA, Stein R, Fuchs SC, Duncan BB, Ribeiro JP, Kroeff LR, Carballo MT, Schmidt MI 2005 Aerobic exercise and submaximal functional capacity in overweight pregnant women. Obstetrics and Gynecology 106:243–249

Spaanderman M, Meerten M, van Bussel M, Ekhart T, Peeters L 2000 Cardiac output increases independently of basal metabolic rate in early pregnancy. American Journal of Physiology. Heart Circulation and Physiology 278:H1585-H1588

Stevenson L 1997 Exercise in pregnancy: part 2 recommendations for individuals. Canadian Family Physician 43:107–111

Ueland K, Novy M, Peterson E, Metcalfe J 1969 Maternal cardiovascular dynamics. The influence of gestational age on the maternal cardiovascular response to posture and exercise. American Journal of Obstetrics and Gynecology 104:856–864

Webb KA, Wolfe LA, Lowe-Wylde S, Monga M 1991 A comparison of fetal heart rate (FHR) responses to maternal static and dynamic exercise. Medicine and Science in Sports and Exercise 23:S169

Weiss M, Nagelschmidt M, Struck H 1979 Relaxin and collagen metabolism. Hormones and Metabolism Research 11:408–410

Weissgerber TL, Wolfe LA 2006 Physiological adaptation in early pregnancy: adaptation to balance maternal-fetal demands. Applied Physiology, Nutrition and Metabolism 31:1–11

Weissgerber TL, Wolfe LA, Hopkins W, Davies G 2006a Serial respiratory adaptations and an alternate hypothesis of respiratory control in human pregnancy. Respiratory Physiology and Neurobiology 153:39–53

Weissgerber TL, Wolfe LA, Davies G, Mottola MF 2006b Exercise in the prevention and treatment of maternal-fetal disease: a review of the literature. Applied Physiology, Nutrition and Metabolism 31(6):661–674

Wilmore JH, Stanforth PR, Gagnon J, Rice T, Mandel S, Leon AS, Rao DC, Skinner JS, Bouchard C 2001 Cardiac output and stroke volume changes with endurance training: the Heritage Family Study. Medicine and Science in Sports and Exercise 33:99–106

Wolfe LA, Davies G 2003 Canadian guidelines for exercise in pregnancy. Clinical Obstetrics and Gynecology 46(2):488–495

Wolfe LA, Mottola MF 1993 Aerobic exercise in pregnancy: an update. Canadian Journal of Applied Physiology 18:119–147

Wolfe LA, Mottola MF 2000 Validation of guidelines for aerobic exercise in pregnancy. In: Kumbhare D, Basmajian JV (eds) Decision making in sports medicine. Churchill Livingstone, New York, 205–222

Wolfe LA, Mottola MF 2002 PARmed-X for Pregnancy. Canadian Society for Exercise Physiology, Ottawa, 1–4. Available online at: www.csep.ca

Wolfe LA, Weissgerber TL 2003 Clinical physiology of exercise in pregnancy: a literature review. Journal of Obstetrics and Gynecology of Canada 25(6):451–453

Wolfe LA, Ohtake PJ, Mottola MF, McGrath MJ 1989a Physiological interactions between pregnancy and aerobic exercise. Exercise and Sport Sciences Reviews 17:295–351

Wolfe LA, Hall P, Webb K, Goodman L, Monga M, McGrath M 1989b Prescription of aerobic exercise in pregnancy. Sports Medicine 8:273–301

Wolfe LA, Brenner IK, Mottola MF 1994 Maternal exercise, fetal well-being and pregnancy outcome. Exercise and Sports Sciences Reviews 22:145–194

Wolfe LA, Kemp J, Heenan A, Preston RJ, Ohtake PJ 1998 Acid-base regulation and control of ventilation in human pregnancy. Canadian Journal of Physiology and Pharmacology 76:815–827

Wolfe LA, Preston R, Burggraf G, McGrath M 1999 Effects of pregnancy and chronic exercise on maternal cardiac structure and function. Canadian Journal of Physiology and Pharmacology 77:909–917

Chapter **13**

Physiological bases of health-enhancing physical activity for postmenopausal women

Katriina Kukkonen-Harjula Tuula-Maria Asikainen

1 INTRODUCTION

It was only 35 years ago that the first evidence was published to show that postmenopausal women were responsive to physical training stimuli (Adams & de Vries 1973, Drinkwater 1973, Drinkwater et al. 1975, Kilbom & Astrand 1971). Today, it is universally agreed that older women are not only trainable, but actually need regular (habitual) physical exercise for health and well-being. Nevertheless, postmenopausal women have seldom been studied in randomised controlled trials, using physical activity as an intervention. Research in exercise physiology has concentrated on men, especially healthy, young and athletic men. When considering physical activity for postmenopausal women, one must take into consideration gender differences, effects of ageing and the physiological changes accompanying menopause.

Menopause refers to a natural, age-related decrease and, finally, loss of ovarian oestrogen production, leading to the cessation of menstruation. It is defined as the absence of menses for 12 consecutive months. At present, menopause occurs in Caucasian women around the age of 51–52 years. Menopause is preceded by a perimenopausal period, characterised by menstrual irregularity and hormonal variability, starting 2–8 years before and ending 1 year following the menopause, but typically lasting about 4 years.

This chapter will focus mainly on females in the early postmenopausal period (age 50–65 years), which occurs before old age (>65 years). This is an important phase in which increased physical activity in the sedentary woman's life may help to partially reverse adverse changes accompanying menopause, and preserve functional physiological capacity. After menopause, the effects of ageing start to appear more clearly, especially in inactive women. In this chapter training-induced effects on health-enhancing fitness (Bouchard & Shephard 1994), including the major cardiovascular risk factors in early postmenopause, are presented. This evidence is mostly based on randomised controlled trials, and on systematic reviews and meta-analyses. Finally, menopausal hormone therapy (with oestrogen only or combined with progestin) is discussed, as it may influence training responses, especially within the musculoskeletal system.

2 GENDER DIFFERENCES RELATED TO PHYSICAL ACTIVITY AND FITNESS

Until the age of ~12–14 years, boys and girls do not substantially differ in physiological responses to exercise (Chapter 15). This implies that basic bodily functions at rest and during exercise are similar between the genders. During puberty, hormonal alterations cause differences in body size, structures and functions. These are reviewed in detail in Chapter 11, with some key points referring to adulthood highlighted below.

There is great individual variation in morphology. On average, compared to adult males, women are approximately 13 cm shorter, weigh approximately 18 kg less and have approximately 8% %-units more fat, which is distributed more on the hips and thighs than abdominally (Wilmore & Costill 2004). Women have fewer and smaller muscle fibres than men, and the absolute muscle strength is approximately 30% less in the lower body and 50% less in the upper body. Women have a lower bone density, and there are also differences in bone and joint structure, posture and a more peripheral distribution of mass in women. For women of average stature, these result in a shorter stride length, a greater stride frequency and a higher mass-specific metabolic cost for walking at a set speed (Charkoudian & Joyner 2004). These differences may be disadvantageous when competing against men, but when exercising for health benefits, such inefficiencies affect the selection of suitable exercise mode and dose.

A wider pelvis, increased femoral anteversion and greater genu valgum and possible hormonal-based laxity of ligaments and joints, together with low muscle strength, are believed to predispose women to exercise-related leg injuries. For example, anterior cruciate ligament injury of the knee is more common in women (Belza & Warms 2004). On the other hand, when matched for muscle strength, women appear to tire more slowly and recover faster than men (Charkoudian & Joyner 2004).

Cardiorespiratory differences include, for example, a smaller heart size, stroke volume, blood volume and cardiac output, fewer red blood cells and less haemoglobin in women than in men. This leads to an approximately 10–30% smaller oxygen-carrying capacity and maximal aerobic power among women (Wilmore & Costill 2004), with circulatory differences also contributing to gender differences in endurance performance (Chapter 14.2). In addition, while lung capacity does not generally limit performance, ventilatory differences, such as smaller lung volumes and a lower capacity to oxygenate blood during intense exercise, combine to elicit exercise-induced arterial hypoxaemia more often in women than in men (Charkoudian & Joyner 2004, Hopkins & Harms 2004; Chapter 2).

Some metabolic differences also exist. For example, women use more fat and less carbohydrate to fuel exercise, at the same relative intensity during prolonged exercise, due to hormonal differences (Belza & Warms 2004). On the other hand, perhaps as a safeguard for potential pregnancy, reserves of body fat seem to be more resistant to the lipolytic demands of exercise in women than in men. This makes it more difficult to decrease body mass in overweight women. Hormonal differences might, in turn, influence cardiorespiratory responses to exercise, influence muscle damage caused by resistance training and affect thermoregulation during exercise (American College of Sports Medicine 1998a, Charkoudian & Joyner 2004, Belza and Warms 2004, Wilmore & Costill 2004). For a more detailed description of these interactions, see Chapter 11.

At the end of the 1990s, only 27% of US women aged 45–64 years regularly engaged in physical activity of light-moderate intensity (Bassuk & Manson 2003). Only 16% engaged in resistance exercise. The epidemiological information on habitual physical activity is based on self-reporting questionnaires, which have frequently been developed for men. However, there might be gender-related differences in physical activity patterns, with men being more active in structured exercise, while women are more involved in household and family care activities (Ainsworth 2000, Lawlor et al. 2002). Furthermore, some of the gender differences in physical activity, especially among older women, extend back to social and cultural restrictions on physical activity, previously imposed on girls and women. In the past, physical activity was not considered beneficial, or was even considered harmful for women. Thus, true gender differences cannot be fully appreciated until we have a generation of men and women who have had equal opportunities to be physically active across their entire lifespan.

3 AGEING, PHYSICAL ACTIVITY AND FITNESS

After menopause, the effects of ageing start to appear more clearly, especially in sedentary women. Chapter 16 focuses on the physiological consequences of ageing. However, to set the scene for the postmenopausal woman, some fundamental changes are highlighted. For example, height gradually decreases 1–3% after 35–40 years of age, due to intervertebral disc compression and postural changes. Body mass gradually increases from 20 years up to ~60 years, after which there is a tendency for mass reduction. Possible explanations for these changes during the menopausal transition are the loss of bone mass (osteopenia), increased body fatness and the loss of fat-free tissue mass (sarcopenia). Insulin resistance has typically increased at the time of menopause, but this is due more to ageing and mass gains than to the menopause per se. A healthy diet, with respect to total energy intake and saturated fat content, in combination with a sufficient physical activity habit may reduce these adverse changes, even up to very old age.

Bone mass develops during childhood and adolescence. Peak bone mass is finalised in the third decade of life, with physical training enhancing bone density and mass. Due to the decreasing production of oestrogen, bone mineral mass starts to decrease rapidly 2–3 years before the menopause, and continues until 5 years after menopause. Oestrogen has a central role in bone resorption and formation (Liu & Lebrun 2006), acting directly on bone cells through a specific receptor, but it also mediates the effects of other hormones. Oestrogen inhibits osteoclast formation and prolongs the action of osteoblasts and osteocytes, the net result being a reduction in bone turnover.

Both maximal aerobic power and capacity (total work performed) decline after the age of 20, decreasing ~1% per annum. Maximal heart rate decreases yearly by slightly less than 1 beat·min^{-1}. This is due to morphological and electrophysiological alterations in the cardiovascular system (Wilmore & Costill 2004). Maximal stroke volume, cardiac output and peripheral blood flow also decrease, and there is a loss of arterial wall elasticity. Respiratory function also decreases with ageing, as lung tissue loses its elasticity. However, for physically active people, this is not usually the primary limitation of aerobic power. Instead, this results partly from decreased habitual physical activity (see Chapters 9 and 28). Thus, this decline can possibly be slowed or at least postponed until very old age, by increasing habitual physical activity.

After 25–35 years of age, maximal muscle strength decreases and the responses of the nervous system steadily slow (Wilmore & Costill 2004). As women in general have a lower initial muscle strength than men, strength and also balance become the most important aspects of health-related fitness in the postmenopausal period. These characteristics ensure that routine and daily activities (e.g. rising from a chair and walking) can be performed without the risk of falling. Locomotion is essential for endurance training and also ensures that cardiovascular function is sustained (Guralnik et al. 2000). At the population level, the maintenance of an ability to walk comfortably is perhaps one of the key factors in the prevention of mobility-related disability. For instance, earlier cohort studies among middle-aged (Suni et al. 1998) and older populations (Guralnik et al. 2000, Malmberg et al. 2002) have shown a strong association between performance tests using walking and mobility-related function. Walking performance, measured by a 2 km walking test, is strongly associated with both maximal oxygen uptake (Oja et al. 1991) and musculoskeletal function (Suni et al. 1998), while a slow walking speed has been associated with an increased risk of falls (Guralnik et al. 2000, Luukinen et al. 1995).

Good musculoskeletal fitness has also been shown to be well correlated with decreased all-cause mortality (Rantanen 2003). When approaching old age, muscular strength, balance and the ability to walk assist in the preservation of adequate functional capacity for the requirements of everyday living and preventing falls (Ostir 1998).

Mobility limitations tend to appear earlier in ageing women than in men (Koskinen et al. 2004).

4 MENOPAUSE AND PHYSICAL ACTIVITY

Menopause results in a decreased cyclic secretion of oestrogen which, in addition to body mass gains, may also be associated with a rapid decline in aerobic power and endurance, muscle strength, balance and bone mineral density, especially in sedentary women. All these changes increase the risk of chronic, non-contagious diseases (Chapters 28 and 30), especially coronary heart disease, type 2 diabetes and osteoporotic fractures (Luoto 2006, Sowers & La Pietra 1995, Wilson 2003). In addition to decreased habitual physical activity, smoking is another central coronary risk factor. Thus, a decreased functional capacity, in combination with chronic diseases, may lead to an inability to stay mobile and to live an independent life when approaching old age (Chapter 31.1). Early postmenopausal women should therefore be made more aware of the need to preserve functional abilities, with the ultimate aim of physical activity promotion being to improve the quality of life and to prolong independent living (at home) in the elderly.

Interactions between physical activity, health, hormonal functional and ageing are complex (Copeland et al. 2004). For instance, when evaluating the effects of physical exercise, one has to differentiate between the acute responses and chronic (adaptive) training effects, and also take into account the exercise type (endurance versus resistance training). Indeed, the exact dose–response relationship of exercise and health-related fitness in postmenopausal women remains unknown. Decreasing circulating concentrations of anabolic hormones may be associated, for example, with musculoskeletal atrophy, loss of function and diminished health. On the other hand, physical activity itself might have a positive effect on circulating hormone concentrations, and also on the hormone actions themselves, due to changes in circulatory protein carriers and the hormone receptors at the target tissues. However, evaluating training responses on the basis of circulating hormone concentrations might be misleading, as local production of hormones and growth factors by muscles or adipose tissue may also take place.

4.1 Hormonal alterations accompanying menopause

The main hormone systems that show marked changes with age are the gonadal hormones (oestrogen and progesterone), adrenal steroids (dehydroepiandrostendione, DHEA, and its sulphate, DHEAS) and hormones of the growth hormone axis (insulin-like growth factor I) (Copeland et al. 2004). Compared with men, women experience more dramatic changes in endocrine function with ageing, especially during menopause. Menopause is characterised by a marked reduction of oestradiol production, resulting in oestrone becoming the primary circulating oestrogen. Menopause causes changes in the reproductive hormone axis (hypothalamus, pituitary, ovaries and uterus). It enhances the secretion of pituitary gonadotropins (follicle-stimulating hormone and luteinising hormone), which stimulate ovarian secretion of oestradiol and inhibin. On the other hand, progesterone secretion is not greatly affected by menopause.

In addition to oestrogen, the ovaries secrete testosterone, which is also produced in peripheral tissues through aromatisation of androstendione, DHEA and DHEAS. The circulating concentrations of testosterone decline with age, but menopause does not affect them dramatically. Testosterone is transported in the circulation by sex hormone-binding globulins, which means that only the unbound hormone is biologically active. DHEA is secreted by the adrenal glands and its secretion is not affected by menopause. Androstendione is secreted from the ovaries and the adrenals, and is converted to oestrone in the peripheral tissues, especially in adipose tissue.

In some postmenopausal women who have an active endurance exercise habit, serum oestrone concentration has been reported to be low, probably due to decreased adiposity. On the other hand, resistance training appears not to increase the serum concentrations of the sex steroid hormones (especially testosterone), even though muscle strength and mass are increased (Häkkinen et al. 2001). Thus, a low circulating testosterone concentration may be a limiting factor in training-induced muscle hypertrophy.

4.2 Hormone therapy and training adaptation

Based on longitudinal cohort studies during the latter half of the 20th century, hormone therapy, using oestrogen alone or combined with progestin, has been used in the prevention and treatment of coronary heart disease around the menopausal transition. This was based on the findings of its favourable effects on cardiovascular risk factors: lowering resting blood pressure and improving serum lipoprotein concentrations. However, randomised controlled trials on postmenopausal women did not confirm such results. On the contrary, there was an increased occurrence of cardiovascular events. In addition, the risk of breast cancer was increased. Thus, the disadvantageous effects of hormone therapy clearly exceeded its benefits in the prevention of osteoporosis (US Preventive Services Task Force 2005). At present, the only acceptable indication for this therapy is for the management of severe vasomotor symptoms (Burger et al. 2004).

Middle-aged women often gain weight, but this is more an age- and exercise-related phenomenon than a result of menopause. On the other hand, reduced circulating oestrogen (regardless of cause) is associated with a more central redistribution of adipose tissue, increasing both visceral and subcutaneous abdominal fat while reducing that in the gluteofemoral region. As the mass of metabolically active tissue declines, the resting metabolic rate also decreases in the perimenopause. These changes are further exacerbated by decreased physical activity, leading to a reduced muscle (lean body) mass. It seems that the peak weight gain occurs in the early postmenopause. On its own, hormone therapy (either oestrogen alone or combined with progestin) does not induce weight gain (Norman et al. 1999), but the effect on adipose redistribution has not been studied.

In younger women, training-induced elevations in cardiac stroke volume and maximal aerobic power are similar to those observed in men. However, in postmenopausal women, stroke volume does not increase with endurance physical training, although increases in maximal aerobic power have been found to be similar for both elderly men and women. This implies a difference in the exercise adaptation mechanism between the genders in older adults, which is believed to be due to an oestrogen deficiency, and is possibly related to the vasodilatory effect of oestrogen on arterial walls, especially at high exercise intensities (Charkoudian & Joyner 2004, Green et al. 2002).

Skeletal muscle performance, especially strength, starts to decrease in the perimenopausal phase. This is due to sarcopenia, which is partly oestrogen dependent. However, the exact mechanisms of how oestrogen acts on the muscle tissue and performance are not known (Sirola & Rikkonen 2005). Hormone therapy with oestrogen may partly reverse the adverse effects of sarcopenia (e.g. reduced strength). The evidence for this is based on a few randomised, placebo-controlled training studies, the results of which are not unequivocal (Sipilä & Poutamo 2003). Oestrogen is also believed to protect muscle from exercise-induced muscle damage (Belza & Warms 2004).

4.3 Hormone therapy and cardiovascular risk factors

The effects of hormone therapy (oestrogen alone or combined with progestin) are partly contradictory with reference to cardiovascular risk factors. Hormone therapy with oestrogen alone may decrease the circulating concentrations of total cholesterol, but increase those of high-density lipoprotein (HDL) cholesterol and triglycerides. However, the available evidence for these effects is scarce (Green et al. 2004, Haddock et al. 2000). In addition, the type of pharmacological hormones used, the phase of menopausal transition and the health status of the women can all affect these results. For example, the effects of hormone therapy on lipoprotein metabolism are varying and less consistent than those reported for bone density. In addition, polymorphic variations of key genes regulating lipid metabolism (e.g. apoE genotype) may interact with these hormones, making data interpretation difficult (Hagberg et al. 2003).

When hormone therapy is combined with physical training, interpretation is further complicated, due primarily to the limited number of studies conducted with postmenopausal women. However, epidemiological studies have reported that hormone therapy with oestrogen may be associated with an elevated maximal aerobic power. This association is most likely not causal, but instead is due to sociocultural aspects that may possibly have caused both increased physical activity and more frequent hormone therapy use. Nevertheless, hormone therapy does seem to improve muscle strength, balance and bone strength. The effects of hormone therapy and exercise training on other components of health-related fitness remain unclear, especially for body composition, resting blood pressure and serum lipoproteins. Indeed, research is required for women in different phases of the menopausal transition, and should involve both healthy women and those with cardiovascular disease risk factors. However, there are many favourable endurance training adaptations evident in postmenopausal women that occur independently of hormone therapy.

4.4 Effects of exercise training on menopausal symptoms

Menopausal symptoms include hot flushes, night sweating, sleep disturbance, urogenital problems and changes in mood. Hot flushes originate from altered hypothalamic temperature regulation (background information: Chapter 18). Physical activity may decrease vasomotor symptoms by modifying hypothalamic β-endorphin activity, the low level of which is associated with the pathogenesis. However, the available evidence is scarce and equivocal (Aiello et al. 2004, Wilbur et al. 2005). Most often, symptoms have been studied as secondary outcomes in trials with separate primary objectives, and the occurrence of menopausal symptoms has not been great. Physical activity may act indirectly by increasing the quality of life and thus improve general well-being, even though direct effects on the symptoms are not detected.

5 WORK-RELATED DEMANDS ON POSTMENOPAUSAL WOMEN

In developed countries, the working population >50 years of age will grow considerably in the near future. After 2010, the number of retired people >65 years will almost double from that of 1995, probably having a strong impact on working conditions and on the labour market. Many postmenopausal women are and will be working, with some working in physically demanding occupations (Chapter 14.1). The ability to do such work is a dynamic process, changing throughout life, and results from the interaction of various individual resources (e.g. health, physiological functional capacity, education, skills), working conditions and society (Ilmarinen & Rantanen 1999). Thus, the promotion of work ability must target several factors, such as physiological work demands and the environment, work organisation and the community, promotion of workers' health and functional capacity, and promotion of profes-

sional competence, which is strongly associated with the ability to work (Tuomi et al. 2001).

Each of the components of health-related physical fitness is relevant and important to a discussion of workers' functional capacity: morphology (stature, body mass, obesity), cardiorespiratory fitness and aerobic capacity (especially submaximal endurance), muscular strength and motor abilities. Gender and age differences might make postmenopausal women less suitable for physically demanding jobs in general, but individual variations might counteract some of the gender differences. Physical activity can also affect the health-related fitness of a female worker to such an extent that she might be more capable for the task than a sedentary male worker (Chapter 14.1). However, there are certain physiological limits that must be considered, and overloading of an elderly female worker must be avoided. Nevertheless, occupational physical activity could form an integral part of the habitual physical activity, resulting in improved health, providing the intensity, duration, frequency and total volume of the physical demand and rest are suitable for the worker.

6 PHYSICAL ACTIVITY AND CARDIOVASCULAR DISEASE

Coronary heart disease is often considered to occur predominantly in men, but this is only correct when comparing premenopausal women and men. In fact, coronary heart disease is the leading cause of death among pre- and post-menopausal women in the western world (Mosca et al. 2004). Physical inactivity is among the main risk factors for cardiovascular disease (Chapter 28).

Compared to men, premenopausal women have lower circulating concentrations of the atherogenic low-density lipoprotein cholesterol (LDL), especially the small dense LDL particles, and also total cholesterol. Such women also have higher serum concentrations of the antiatherogenic high-density lipoprotein (HDL) cholesterol. Both states are partly hormonally mediated. Postmenopausally, these lipoprotein concentrations change towards the male direction. From the age of 55 years, LDL cholesterol is higher in women than men (Mosca 2005), with serum lipoprotein(a) also increasing following menopause. The coronary risk associated with elevated triglycerides is more marked in women, and it has been suggested that HDL cholesterol is the most powerful predictor of the risk for cardiovascular disease in women (Mosca 2005). In particular, it is the antiatherogenic HDL_2 subfraction that decreases with age, while HDL_3 may increase (Carr 2003).

Elevated resting blood pressure is a coronary risk factor, also more prevalent in men than women in early adulthood. In developed countries blood pressure tends to increase with ageing, with systolic pressure rising until the eighth decade and diastolic until the sixth. From ~60 years onwards, women generally have higher blood pressure, but the causal mechanism is not clear.

Oguma & Shinoda-Tagawa (2004) conducted the first metaanalysis on the dose–response relationship of physical activity (PA) and cardiovascular disease in women, who were initially healthy, and most often were middle-aged. Cohort and case–control studies were included, physical activity was categorised into at least three levels and cardiovascular disease outcomes were related to either morbidity or mortality. Habitual physical activity was associated with a reduced risk of overall cardiovascular disease and also coronary heart disease and stroke in a dose–response fashion. In addition, higher levels of physical activity appeared not to be harmful. Walking 1 hour per week was chosen as a minimum dose (and possibly less) for reducing the overall risk of cardiovascular disease. However, these data did not permit a separate analysis regarding the postmenopausal phase. On average, the magnitude of the risk reduction was roughly 30%.

For men, the association between maximal aerobic power and cardiovascular disease is similar to that of physical activity, but few studies are available for women. Farrell et al. (2002) showed in 9925 women (20–79 years, mean age 43) that, after an 11-year follow-up, poor maximal aerobic power was a stronger predictor of all-cause mortality than body mass index. In this cohort, for the 40–49-year-old women to be classified as fit (above the 20th percentile), they had to have a maximal aerobic power >28.0 mL·min^{-1}·kg^{-1} (~8 METs). Such a goal is feasible with habitual endurance exercise (Chapter 17.2).

The first evidence-based guidelines for cardiovascular disease prevention for women were issued in 2004 (Mosca et al. 2004). Lifestyle approaches (diet, weight management, physical activity, smoking cessation) were recommended for all risk levels. The recommended physical activity level was 30 min of moderate-intensity exercise on most days. Of course, there are some adverse effects of exercise, such as sudden cardiac death, which is associated with strenuous exercise. However, the risk of such adverse events in women is lower than in men, with regular exercise further diminishing this risk (Whang et al. 2006). More common adverse training effects are orthopaedic injuries, also associated with strenuous exercise.

7 EXERCISE GUIDELINES TO IMPROVE FITNESS AND ENHANCE HEALTH

7.1 Cardiorespiratory fitness, body composition and musculoskeletal fitness

According to the exercise recommendations of the American College of Sports Medicine (1998a), to improve cardiorespiratory fitness and body composition, adults should exercise 3–5 d·wk^{-1} at 50–80% of the maximal oxygen uptake or functional heart rate reserves for 20–60 min continuously, or accumulate the same total amount of exercise in several daily bouts (minimum duration 10 min), which means expending approximately 2.9–8.4 MJ weekly (see

Chapter 17.1). Light-intensity training (i.e. <40% of reserve) is not considered effective for improving cardiorespiratory fitness (American College of Sports Medicine 1998a), although in the elderly and habitually sedentary people, it is assumed to have positive health effects. Interest in moderate-intensity exercise (40–60% of reserve), such as walking, has recently been growing because of its simplicity and safety. A frequency of 3 d·wk^{-1} is considered optimal for initially sedentary persons, since increasing the frequency to 5 d·wk^{-1} seems to have minimal additional impact upon maximal aerobic power.

According to the American College of Sports Medicine (1998a), resistance training should occur 2–3 d·wk^{-1} and include one set of 8–10 different exercises, focusing on the major muscle groups, with 8–12 repetitions for each exercise. For persons over 50–60 years, 10–15 repetitions with a lighter mass may be more appropriate, at least at the beginning, to avoid overexertion. Stretching should include appropriate static and dynamic techniques. For older adults (>65 years), the American College of Sports Medicine (1998b) emphasises training aimed at preserving or improving muscle mass and strength of lower extremities. This will help maintain balance and the ability to walk.

7.2 Health-enhancing physical activity and health-related fitness

Physical inactivity is almost as dangerous to one's health as smoking (Chapter 28). Therefore one must consider exercise from two perspectives: increasing cardiorespiratory fitness and health maintenance or improvement. In the recommendation for health-enhancing physical activity, it is assumed that even if the exercise dose does not improve cardiorespiratory fitness, it might have beneficial health effects (Pate et al. 1995). All adults should accumulate 30 min or more of moderate-intensity physical activity for most days (Chapter 17.1). Some of the health effects of endurance exercise training are assumed to be partly due to the acute effects of exercise, making it beneficial to exercise frequently. Daily exercise is also important in the formation of habitual behaviours.

The benefits of health-enhancing physical activity can be analysed using the concept of health-related fitness, introduced in the 1990s (Bouchard & Shephard 1994). The components of health-related fitness include: cardiorespiratory, musculoskeletal, neuromotor, morphological and metabolic components (Table 13.1). An adequate cardiorespiratory fitness is essential in the prevention of coronary heart disease and lowering of all-cause mortality. Musculoskeletal and neuromotor fitness, which include muscle strength and endurance, flexibility and postural control, are needed to preserve adequate physiological functional capacity, to ensure independent living in old age, and for fall prevention. Morphological fitness (body composition) includes adipose tissue and bone strength, which are important risk factors for coronary heart disease, type 2 diabetes, osteopo-

Table 13.1 Components of health-related fitness (modified after Bouchard & Shephard 1994) and methods of assessment

Component	Methods and outcomes of assessment
Cardiorespiratory fitness	
Maximal aerobic power	Maximal oxygen uptake, heart rate, work load, blood lactate, respiratory gases,
Submaximal cardiorespiratory (endurance) capacity	blood pressure
Musculoskeletal fitness	
Muscle strength and endurance	Muscle tests
Flexibility	Flexibility tests
Neuromotor fitness	
Postural control	Balance and coordination tests
Morphological fitness	
Adipose tissue	Body mass, body fat
Distribution of adipose tissue	Waist (and hip) circumference
Bone strength	Bone mineral density
Metabolic fitness	
Carbohydrate metabolism	Blood glucose and insulin
Lipid metabolism	Serum lipoproteins (HDL and LDL cholesterol, triglycerides)

HDL cholesterol, high-density lipoprotein cholesterol; LDL cholesterol, low-density lipoprotein cholesterol.

rosis and osteoporotic fractures. A sound metabolic fitness (i.e. normal carbohydrate and lipid metabolism) reduces the risk of coronary heart disease and type 2 diabetes.

8 HEALTH-RELATED FITNESS AND POSTMENOPAUSAL WOMEN

Exercise recommendations are based on both epidemiological evidence and clinical trials of exercise training which have, for the most part, been conducted on young or middle-aged men, and thus may not be fully applicable to postmenopausal women. To evaluate the relevance of these recommendations for postmenopausal women, additional data are needed, especially from randomised controlled trials in this age group. The following subsections summarise a systematic review of the existing evidence obtained from 30 randomised controlled trials (each lasting at least 8 weeks and having good methodological quality), conducted on early postmenopausal women and covering the years 1974–2004 (Asikainen 2006, Asikainen et al. 2004).

8.1 Cardiorespiratory fitness (aerobic power and capacity)

Maximal oxygen uptake (aerobic power) or other estimates of cardiorespiratory (aerobic or endurance) fitness were assessed in 20 studies with 1988 participants. The most frequently used exercise modes were walking, walking with other endurance training and endurance exercise combined with resistance training. In all but one of the studies, maximal oxygen uptake improved, with increases ranging from 2.2 to 7 mL·min^{-1}·kg^{-1} (4–32%); indirect estimations

revealed larger improvements. Such changes often reflect the pretreatment fitness of subjects, with less fit subjects being high responders.

The effects of endurance training on maximal oxygen uptake seem to be well documented for moderate-heavy intensity exercise among early postmenopausal women. However, there are no studies on light-intensity exercise, so the minimum exercise dose for improving aerobic power in this group is not known. In one study (Asikainen et al. 2002b) the smallest dose to improve aerobic power was walking at an intensity of 45% for an average of 45 min, 5 d·wk^{-1} for 24 weeks, corresponding to 6.3 MJ weekly, the intensity at the lower end, and the volume at the upper end of the ACSM recommendations.

Submaximal aerobic capacity (total work performed) was studied by only two groups. Improving this attribute is very relevant for sedentary women, since most daily tasks do not demand maximal effort and are more easily performed with good submaximal endurance. One study used exercise that was fractionated into two daily exercise bouts (Asikainen et al. 2002a). This proved to be as effective on submaximal aerobic capacity as one bout of continuous exercise. Only two studies subdivided subjects according to hormone therapy, and both found that each group had equal improve-ments in aerobic power.

8.2 Musculoskeletal fitness

8.2.1 Muscular strength
In a systematic review, 13 studies involving muscular strength or aerobic endurance training in 1317 participants were assessed (Asikainen 2006, Asikainen et al. 2004). In all

but two studies, muscular strength improved. It seems well documented that muscular strength in early postmenopausal women is trainable, with large improvements to be gained. See Chapter 11 for gender-related differences in strength adaptation.

8.2.2 Flexibility

The literature contains six studies (550 participants) in which flexibility training was assessed in postmenopausal women (Asikainen 2006, Asikainen et al. 2004). In three studies flexibility was improved. These studies used a supervised training programme of aerobic dancing or aerobic exercises combined with resistance training and stretching. In three studies no training effect was found. It seems that training can improve flexibility, though training may need supervision, at least initially. However, there were too few studies to draw conclusions concerning the best form of flexibility training.

8.3 Neuromotor fitness

Balance or coordination has been assessed in seven studies, using 719 postmenopausal women (Asikainen 2006, Asikainen et al. 2004). Four of these studies improved balance and coordination. These programmes consisted of resistance training or combined aerobic and resistance training or aerobic dance. High-impact jumping in combination with low-impact exercises was also effective. Improvements in balance and coordination in early postmenopausal women have been reported with programmes of low-impact aerobic dancing and walking combined with resistance training, with strength training alone, with aerobic dance and with high-impact jumping. Data indicate that balance and coordination may be improved by up to 14%. However, these attributes were reported in only a few studies, all using different exercise modes, so firm conclusions are therefore difficult to draw.

8.4 Morphological fitness

8.4.1 Adipose tissue

Astrup (1999) conducted a systematic review on postmenopausal women, to assess the relationship between body fat distribution and habitual physical activity. Cross-sectional studies revealed that women with high levels of physical activity had smaller amounts of both total and abdominal fat. In longitudinal studies, habitually active women were less likely to gain weight after menopause than sedentary women. There were few randomised controlled trials on exercise training, so the exercise dose necessary to prevent (or limit) weight gain with menopause remains unclear.

On average, exercise training alone can decrease body mass in overweight subjects by ~5 kg. Strong evidence from randomised controlled trials, on mostly overweight or obese men, showed a linear dose–response relationship between physical activity volume and weight loss after 16 weeks of training (Ross & Janssen 2001). However, training for more than 24 weeks failed to show a similar effect, due to low compliance. Nevertheless, there is strong evidence for other health benefits as a result of modest weight loss following training (Williams 2001), leading to decreased all-cause mortality.

Franz (2004) conducted a systematic review on weight reduction and maintenance in overweight women. She identified 17 randomised controlled trials (1291 women, predominantly premenopausal) lasting at least 1 year. For interventions using low-energy and low-fat diets, the mean weight loss of compliant subjects was 5.2 kg at 6 months and 6 kg at 12 months. The corresponding reductions in diet plus exercise interventions were 8.9 and 8.8 kg. However, the true changes in fat mass were not given. This difference is important since, when sedentary subjects commence exercise, they might gain weight through muscle mass gains, since muscle is more dense than adipose tissue. For all interventions, a weight loss plateau was observed about 6 months after the start of the trial.

Intraabdominal (visceral) obesity, postmenopausal oestrogen deficiency and physical inactivity are associated with reduced insulin sensitivity, impaired glucose homeostasis, lipoprotein impairments and hypertension. These conditions constitute the so-called (menopausal) metabolic syndrome (Carr 2003; Chapter 30). The metabolic syndrome enhances the risk for coronary heart disease and type 2 diabetes. Increased physical activity, and especially the loss of excessive visceral adipose tissue can reverse this syndrome.

We have performed a systematic review of the effects of exercise training on body composition across 21 studies and 2150 participants (Asikainen 2006, Asikainen et al. 2004). In the studies with overweight participants, walking, other aerobic training, resistance training or combinations of these exercise modes were used. Three studies with overweight participants used only exercise training, and weight losses were minimal: the means ranged from 0.1 to 2.0 kg in 12–52 weeks. However, the largest losses were obtained by the three studies that used dietary regimens, producing mean weight losses of 2–10 kg over the same duration.

8.4.2 Bone strength

Aerobic dance, weight-bearing training and resistance training for on average 12 months increased bone density in the spinal region, and walking had favourable effects in the hip in postmenopausal women aged 40–75 years (Bonaiuti et al. 2002). Contrary to this, a recent metaanalysis involving postmenopausal women (mean age 65 years), using individual patient data, found that physical training did not increase femoral neck bone density (Kelley & Kelley 2006).

In addition to healthy diet, physical activity can help in preventing the decline in bone mineral density in healthy postmenopausal women. To favourably affect bone strength, exercise should involve various modes, including weight bearing and resistance exercises (Borer 2005). It is important to include both lower- and upper-body segments, and activities should also include rapid movements with directional changes and a range of impact levels (e.g. aerobic dance and racket games).

However, in healthy, early postmenopausal women (not having osteopenia or osteoporosis), it has not been shown that an increase in bone density, achieved by either physical activity or with pharmacological treatment, is associated with a decreased risk for osteoporotic fractures (Delaney 2006).

When bone mineral density is increased or its rate of loss is slowed with physical training, there are also simultaneous favourable health-related fitness outcomes. These include muscle strength and balance. These attributes are important for improving walking ability and preventing accidental falls and fractures, which might compromise independent living in older age. In addition, nutritional aspects have to be taken into account to prevent osteoporosis. This means adequate intake of protein, calcium and vitamin D, and moderation of alcohol consumption. The cessation of smoking is also recommended.

Our systematic review, of exercise-induced changes in bone density and bone mineral content identified 16 studies involving 1373 postmenopausal women (Asikainen et al. 2004). Ten studies did not include women using hormone therapy, six did, and two studies stratified subjects by hormone therapy. The 12 methodologically high-quality studies, with most participants showing positive outcomes, used aerobic training combined with resistance training, high-impact circuit training and aerobic dance, high-impact training combined with alendronate medication or brisk walking. The changes in bone density were site specific and in the magnitude 0–2% in the exercise groups, while bone density in the controls decreased approximately 1% yearly. Hormone therapy and alendronate also had favourable effects on bone density.

8.5 Metabolic fitness

8.5.1 Glucose and insulin
We have also reviewed studies of changes in blood glucose and insulin concentrations in response to physical activity, in healthy postmenopausal women (Asikainen 2006, Asikainen et al. 2004). Only one study reported a small training effect for glucose but none for insulin. All training programmes improved maximal aerobic power and most also reduced adiposity. The only study that showed a minor effect on blood glucose concentration used an exercise dose of walking five times a week for 15 weeks, 30–60 min daily in either one or two bouts, at an intensity of 65% of maximal aerobic power (Asikainen et al. 2003).

8.5.2 Serum lipoprotein concentrations
Because of increased energy consumption during exercise, lipoprotein metabolism is also enhanced, as fatty acids are used as energy by the working muscles. Fats and cholesterol ingested are absorbed in the gut and transported to the liver, from where they are distributed to tissues through circulation as lipoproteins (combinations of cholesterol, cholesterol esters, triglycerides, phospholipids and various apoprotein particles as carriers). Serum lipoprotein subfractions can be analysed based on their biochemical characteristics, and are classified as very low-density lipoprotein (VLDL), low-density lipoprotein (LDL) and high-density lipoprotein (HDL) particles. Very low-density lipoprotein particles are produced in the liver and contain mainly triglycerides. They are metabolised in the circulation, resulting in the formation of atherogenic LDL particles (with apoprotein B). High-density lipoprotein particles (with apoprotein A) act as reverse cholesterol transporters to the liver. During physical exercise, more VLDL particles are needed for energy, and during their metabolism, serum HDL cholesterol concentrations are increased and those of VLDL triglycerides are decreased. Both of these lipoprotein changes are observed acutely, with the change in HDL cholesterol also reflecting a training response.

Serum concentrations of LDL cholesterol do not decrease due to training, unless the intake of saturated fats is simultaneously reduced. Concomitant reductions in adiposity may enhance the above changes (Williams 2001). However, dietary reductions in saturated fats may also cause a decrease in the antiatherogenic HDL cholesterol, though physical exercise combined with such a diet change may diminish this effect, especially if associated with weight reduction.

According to a metaanalysis of both randomised and non-randomised controlled trials, involving around 2300 subjects (mostly men), moderate-intensity endurance training increases the serum concentration of HDL cholesterol ~5% from baseline, and decreases the concentration of LDL cholesterol (~5%) and triglycerides (~4%) in healthy, sedentary individuals with no dietary changes (Leon & Sanchez 2001). Most of the studies prescribed 30 min or more of exercise per session at moderate to strenuous intensity on 3–5 d·wk^{-1}.

The threshold to improve serum lipoprotein concentrations seems to be a total weekly exercise energy expenditure of 5–6.3 MJ (the lower level for women) for a minimum of 12 weeks (Leon & Sanchez 2001). Endurance training may increase the serum HDL cholesterol levels (especially the HDL$_2$ fraction), if the training intensity is at least moderate (50–70% of maximal aerobic power), which can be achieved with brisk walking. However, individual training responses may vary greatly for the same training stimulus (Leon et al. 2002), partly due to genetic factors, and baseline lipoprotein concentrations also influence the response, with a lower HDL cholesterol baseline enabling a higher training response.

Total exercise energy expenditure (volume or dose) seems to be more crucial than exercise intensity alone. This was found in an 8-month jogging training study of overweight dyslipidaemic persons aged 40–65 (Kraus et al. 2002), of whom ~40% were postmenopausal women. The most marked beneficial effects on lipoprotein subfractions were observed with a weekly energy expenditure of 8.4 MJ at strenuous intensity. However, the length of the training period is also important. In one study, after 1 year of moderate-intensity training, lipoprotein changes were not observed among postmenopausal women, but improvements were evident after the second year (King et al. 1995). Furthermore, exercise alone may not be sufficient to improve serum lipoprotein concentrations if postmenopausal women are obese or clearly dyslipidaemic. In such cases, it is then prudent to introduce a low-fat and low-energy diet (Mohanka et al. 2006, Stefanick et al. 1991).

Kelley et al. (2004) performed a metaanalysis of 41 randomised controlled trials on aerobic exercise training and serum lipoproteins in 1715 adult women (mean age 42 years, range 20–76 years). There were postmenopausal women in 14 studies, of which only seven studies included women using hormone therapy. On average, training typically involved walking, with a frequency of four times weekly at a mean intensity of ~70% maximal aerobic power, lasting for 22 weeks. Mean attendance was 86% of the prescribed sessions, but compliance was only reported for 55% of the studies. After training, reductions were evident for fasting total cholesterol (2%), LDL cholesterol (3%) and triglycerides (5%), with a 3% increase in HDL cholesterol. Being pre- or postmenopausal, or using hormone therapy did not affect the magnitude of these changes. Kelley et al. (2005) also performed a metaanalysis of randomised controlled trials on aerobic training in persons >50 years. Twenty-two studies were found, with 1427 subjects, whose mean age was 63 years (range 55–78) and of whom 737 were female. On average, training resulted in an increase of 6% in HDL cholesterol and a reduction of 7% in the ratio of total to HDL cholesterol.

Most research has concentrated on aerobic exercise, and evidence for the effects of resistance training on serum lipoprotein profiles, especially for postmenopausal women, is scarce and partly contradictory, when compared to aerobic training (Durstine et al. 2001). This may partly be due to lower total energy consumption when compared to aerobic exercise of the same perceived intensity.

In conclusion, aerobic training generally increases the fasting serum concentration of HDL cholesterol while decreasing that of triglycerides. This profile change denotes a decreased risk for atherosclerosis. However, most of the favourable effects of training on cardiovascular disease risk factors have been found in men, with the minority of studies focusing on postmenopausal women. Furthermore, few studies have investigated lipoprotein and apoprotein subclasses and their metabolism in postmenopausal women (Kraus et al. 2002, Stefanick et al. 1991), in addition to assessments of body composition and dietary intake. For overweight, obese or dyslipidaemic women, aerobic exercise training seems to improve the lipoprotein profile. The use of diets that are low in saturated fats and total energy will further improve these results. However, the interaction of hormone therapy with exercise and diet, and its effect on lipoprotein concentrations are variable, with independent (main) effects being difficult to interpret.

8.5.3 Resting blood pressure

The recommendations for exercise and hypertension are that hypertensive adults engage in endurance exercise on most and preferably all days of the week (American College of Sports Medicine 2004). The intensity of exercise should be moderate (40–60% of reserve), with the lower intensity exercise being especially appropriate for elderly sedentary persons. Indeed, the recommendations are based on several metaanalyses on the positive effects of physical training on resting and ambulatory (24 h) blood pressure, in both normotensive and hypertensive adults.

Kelley (1999) performed a metaanalysis of ten randomised controlled trials on the effects of both aerobic training and blood pressure, in 732 women (average age 55 years, range 20–70 years). Five studies included 524 early postmenopausal subjects (50–65 years). Most subjects were not hypertensive. On average, endurance exercise involved walking (four times weekly for 31 weeks) at an intensity of 63% of maximal aerobic power for 39 min. Compliance averaged 78% in seven studies. After training, the net reduction for the resting systolic blood pressure was about 2%, and 1% for diastolic pressure. However, a subgroup analysis for subjects over 50 years revealed that the decrease in diastolic pressure was smaller. Kelley (1999) also suggested that the effects of exercise training may be less pronounced in women. Nevertheless, daily exercise of moderate intensity is important for early postmenopausal women, as it might help to prevent the menopause-related increase in blood pressure, partly resulting from increased adipose tissue.

The most recent and comprehensive metaanalyses involved endurance training (Cornelissen & Fagard 2005a) and resistance training (Cornelissen & Fagard 2005b). There were 72 randomised controlled trials on endurance training (Cornelissen & Fagard 2005a), with almost 4000 normotensive or hypertensive subjects (mean age 47 years), of whom less than half were women. After an average of 16 weeks training, the net decrease in the systolic pressure was −3.0 mmHg and −2.4 mmHg for diastolic pressure. In the normotensive subjects, the decrease was −2.4/−1.6 mmHg, and in the hypertensive subjects it tended to be larger (−6.9/−4.9 mmHg).

The mechanisms responsible for the training-induced decrease in the resting blood pressure include reductions in total peripheral resistance, reduced regional sympathetic outflow, decreased fat mass, decreased hyperinsulinaemia and reduced sodium reabsorption in the kidney. There is also the influence of acute, postexercise hypotension, in which the magnitude of the decrease ranges between 18–20 mmHg for the systolic and 7–9 mmHg for diastolic blood pressure (MacDonald 2002).

By far the most frequent exercise modes investigated have involved walking, running and cycling. However, there are few training studies on sedentary middle-aged people that have used swimming. Cox et al. (2006) studied walking and swimming in 116 normotensive, non-obese women. The mean age of subjects was 56 years (range 50–70) with ~65% being postmenopausal. Surprisingly, when compared to walking, supervised swimming training for 6 months increased both supine and standing systolic pressure by 4.4 mmHg and 6.0 mmHg, respectively. A similar increasing trend was observed for the diastolic pressures (1.4 and 1.8 mmHg). Swimming takes place in the supine position, in a non-gravity environment and employs more arm work. Thus, the effects of various exercise modes are not always directly interchangeable. The effects of water aerobics or water running on resting blood pressure have not been studied.

There are very few training studies that have explored the relationship between resistance training and blood pressure. Cornelissen & Fagard (2005b) found nine randomised controlled trials with ~350 subjects (mean age >69 years), of whom 39% were women. The net blood pressure decrease was 6.0 mmHg for the systolic and 4.7 mmHg for the diastolic pressure.

9 FRACTIONATED VERSUS CONTINUOUS EXERCISE

Exercise that involves several daily bouts (fractionated or discontinuous) rather than one continuous exercise session has been proposed in health-enhancing physical activity recommendations (American College of Sports Medicine 1998a, Pate et al. 1995; Chapter 17.1). However, so far there have been very few randomised controlled trials on this topic that have involved early postmenopausal women. Woolf-May et al. (1999) conducted a study on women aged 40–66 years (mean 54 years) walking 20–40 min in either one, two or three daily bouts. Across all age groups, equivalent fitness results were observed. However, LDL cholesterol decreased in both the long- and intermediate-bout groups, but not in the short-bout group. There were no HDL cholesterol changes in any of the exercise groups. For the subgroup of postmenopausal women, no serum lipoprotein changes took place.

Staffileno et al. (2001) studied the effects of intermittent, moderate-intensity training for 8 weeks in 18 hypertensive, postmenopausal women. They found that the systolic pressure was reduced by 8 mmHg and diastolic by 5 mmHg in the exercise group versus the controls. Unfortunately, the study design did not include a continuous exercise group with which to make comparisons.

Walking 5 d·wk^{-1} at an intensity of 65% of maximal aerobic power, expending 6.3 MJ in weekly exercise of either one or two daily bouts (combined with 10–15 min of moderate resistance training twice a week), increased maximal aerobic power and improved walking performance and lower-extremity strength (Asikainen et al. 2002b, 2006). However, training was not enough to improve muscular strength of the trunk or upper limbs, nor did it enhance postural control in healthy, sedentary early postmenopausal women. Fractionated exercise led to fewer exercise-related lower-extremity complaints, possibly due to enhanced postexercise recovery. This observation is of great practical significance.

10 CONCLUSION

A dose–response relationship has been found for elderly people, with low- to moderate-intensity exercise being safer than high-intensity exercise (American College of Sports Medicine 1998b). This relationship emphasises the need to use the lowest effective dose of exercise for improvement in components of health-related fitness for early postmenopausal women. The minimum intensity seems to be around 40–50% of the maximal oxygen uptake reserve (American College of Sports Medicine 1998a). In practice, this means approximately 30–60 min of moderate walking in either once- or twice-daily exercise bouts, 5 days per week, combined with a 15–20 min of resistance training, performed twice per week (Asikainen et al. 2006). To attain larger improvements and also to affect other health-fitness components, i.e. metabolic, musculoskeletal and neuromotor fitness, the exercise dose should be increased (Kohl 2001).

Whilst it is clear that increasing or maintaining physical activity, especially resistance training, is very important for early postmenopausal women to preserve physiological functional capacity when approaching old age (>65 years), there are many unanswered issues concerning the effects of increased physical activity on the health of early postmenopausal women. For instance, very few training studies have used light-intensity aerobic training, fractionated aerobic exercise or resistance training. Furthermore, few studies have quantified the effective exercise dose necessary to improve submaximal aerobic endurance (capacity), body composition (especially adiposity), flexibility and postural control, as well as carbohydrate and lipid metabolism in healthy early postmenopausal women. These important knowledge gaps need to be filled so that we can discover how best to optimise the health of ageing women.

References

Adams GM, de Vries HA 1973 Physiological effects of an exercise training regimen upon women aged 52 to 79. Journal of Gerontology 28(1):50–55

Aiello EJ, Yasui Y, Tworoger SS, Ulrich CM, Irwin ML, Bowen D, Schwartz RS, Kumai C, Potter JD, McTiernan A 2004 Effect of a yearlong, moderate-intensity exercise intervention on the occurrence and severity of menopause symptoms in postmenopausal women. Menopause 11(4):382–388

Ainsworth BE 2000 Challenges in measuring physical activity in women. Exercise and Sport Sciences Reviews 28(2):93–96

American College of Sports Medicine 1998a Position stand: the recommended quantity and quality of exercise for developing and maintaining cardiorespiratory and muscular fitness and flexibility in healthy adults. Medicine and Science in Sports and Exercise 30(6):975–991

American College of Sports Medicine 1998b Position stand: exercise and physical activity for older adults. Medicine and Science in Sports and Exercise 30(6):992–1008

American College of Sports Medicine 2004 Exercise and hypertension. Medicine and Science in Sports and Exercise 36(3):533–553

Asikainen T-M 2006 Exercise for health for early postmenopausal women. In search of the minimum effective dose among continuous and fractionated walking programs. Academic dissertation. University of Tampere, Finland. Available online at http://acta.uta.fi/pdf/951-44-6580-6.pdf (accessed 28 September 2007)

Asikainen TM, Miilunpalo S, Oja P, Rinne M, Pasanen M, Vuori I 2002a Walking trials in postmenopausal women: effect of one vs two daily bouts on aerobic fitness. Scandinavian Journal of Medicine and Science in Sports 12(2):99–105

Asikainen TM, Miilunpalo S, Oja P, Rinne M, Pasanen M, Uusi-Rasi K, Vuori I 2002b Randomized, controlled walking trials in postmenopausal women: the minimum dose to improve aerobic fitness? British Journal of Sports Medicine 36(3):189–194

Asikainen TM, Miilunpalo S, Kukkonen-Harjula K, Nenonen A, Pasanen M, Rinne M, Uusi-Rasi K, Oja P, Vuori I 2003 Walking trials in postmenopausal women: effect of low doses and exercise fractionization on coronary risk factors. Scandinavian Journal of Medicine and Science in Sports 13(5):284–292

Asikainen T-M, Kukkonen-Harjula K, Miilunpalo S 2004 Exercise for health for early postmenopausal women, a systematic review of randomized controlled trials. Sports Medicine 34(11):753–778

Asikainen TM, Suni JH, Pasanen ME, Oja P, Rinne MB, Miilunpalo SI, Nygård CH, Vuori IM 2006 Effect of brisk walking in 1 or 2 daily bouts and moderate resistance training on lower-extremity muscle strength, balance and walking performance in women who recently went through menopause: a randomized, controlled trial. Physical Therapy 86(7):912–923

Astrup A 1999 Physical activity and weight gain and fat distribution changes with menopause: current evidence and research issues. Medicine and Science in Sports and Exercise 31(11 Suppl):S564–S567

Bassuk SS, Manson JE 2003 Physical activity and cardiovascular disease prevention in women: how much is good enough? Exercise and Sport Sciences Reviews 31(4):176–181

Belza B, Warms C 2004 Physical activity and exercise in women's health. Nursing Clinics of North America 39(1):181–193, viii

Bonaiuti D, Shea B, Iovine R, Negrini S, Robinson V, Kemper HC, Wells G, Tugwell P, Cranney A 2002 Exercise for preventing and treating osteoporosis in postmenopausal women (Cochrane Review). Cochrane Database of Systematic Reviews, issue 2. CD000333

Borer KT 2005 Physical activity in the prevention and amelioration of osteoporosis in women: interaction of mechanical, hormonal and dietary factors. Sports Medicine 35(9):779–830

Bouchard C, Shephard RJ 1994 Physical activity, fitness and health: the model and key concepts. In: Bouchard C, Shephard RJ, Stephens T (eds) Physical activity, fitness and health. Human Kinetics, Champaign, IL, 77–88

Burger H, Archer D, Barlow D, Birkhäuser M, Calaf-Alsina J, Gambacciani M, Genazzani A, Hadji P, Iversen OE, Kuhl H, Lobo RA, Maudelonde T, e Castro MN, Notelovitz M, Palacios S, Paszkowski T, Peer E, Pines A, Samsioe G, Stevenson J, Skouby S, Sturdee D, de Villiers T, Whitehead M, Ylikorkala O 2004 Practical recommendations for hormone replacement therapy in the peri- and postmenopause. Climacteric 7(2):210–216

Carr MC 2003 The emergence of the metabolic syndrome with menopause. Journal of Clinical Endocrinology and Metabolism 88(6):2404–2411

Charkoudian N, Joyner MJ 2004 Physiologic considerations for exercise performance in women. Clinics in Chest Medicine 25(2):247–255

Copeland JL, Chu SY, Tremblay MS 2004 Ageing, physical activity and hormones in women – a review. Journal of Ageing and Physical Activity 12(1):101–116

Cornelissen VA, Fagard RH 2005a Effects of endurance training on blood pressure, blood pressure-regulating mechanisms and cardiovascular risk factors. Hypertension 46(4):667–675

Cornelissen VA, Fagard RH 2005b Effect of resistance training on resting blood pressure: a meta-analysis of randomized controlled trials. Journal of Hypertension 23(2):251–259

Cox KL, Burke V, Beilin LJ, Grove JR, Blanksby BA, Puddey IB 2006 Blood pressure rise with swimming versus walking in older women: the Sedentary Women Exercise Adherence Trial 2 (SWEAT 2). Journal of Hypertension 24(2):307–314

Delaney MF 2006 Strategies for the prevention and treatment of osteoporosis during early postmenopause. American Journal of Obstetrics and Gynecology 194(2 Suppl):S12–S23

Drinkwater BL 1973 Physiological responses of women to exercise. Exercise and Sports Sciences Reviews 1:125–153

Drinkwater BL, Horvath SM, Wells CL 1975 Aerobic power of females ages 10 to 68. Journal of Gerontology 30(4):385–394

Durstine JL, Grandjean PW, Davis PG, Ferguson MA, Alderson NL, DuBose KD 2001 Blood lipid and lipoprotein adaptations to exercise: a quantitative analysis. Sports Medicine 31(15):1033–1062

Farrell SW, Braun L, Barlow CE, Cheng YJ, Blair SN 2002 The relation of body mass index, cardiorespiratory fitness and all-cause mortality in women. Obesity Research 10(6):417–423

Franz MJ 2004 Effectiveness of weight loss and maintenance interventions in women. Current Diabetes Reports 4(5):387–393

Green JS, Stanforth PR, Gagnon J, Leon AS, Rao DC, Skinner JS, Bouchard C, Rankinen T, Wilmore JH 2002 Menopause, estrogen and training effects on exercise hemodynamics: the HERITAGE study. Medicine and Science in Sports and Exercise 34(1):74–82

Green JS, Stanforth PR, Rankinen T, Leon AS, Rao Dc D, Skinner JS, Bouchard C, Wilmore JH 2004 The effects of exercise training on abdominal visceral fat, body composition and indicators of the metabolic syndrome in postmenopausal women with and without estrogen replacement therapy: the HERITAGE family study. Metabolism 53(9):1192–1196

Guralnik JM, Ferrucci L, Pieper CF, Leveille SG, Markides KS, Ostir GV, Studenski S, Berkman LF, Wallace RB 2000 Lower extremity function and subsequent disability: consistency across studies, predictive models and value of gait speed alone compared with the short physical performance battery. Journals of Gerontology Series A: Biological Sciences and Medical Sciences 55A(4):M221–M231

Haddock BL, Marshak HP, Mason JJ, Blix G 2000 The effect of hormone replacement therapy and exercise on cardiovascular disease risk factors in postmenopausal women. Sports Medicine 29(1):39–49

Hagberg JM, McCole SD, Ferrell RE, Zmuda JM, Rodgers KS, Wilund KR, Moore GE 2003 Physical activity, hormone replacement therapy and plasma lipoprotein-lipid levels in postmenopausal women. International Journal of Sports Medicine 24(1):22–29

Häkkinen K, Pakarinen A, Kraemer WJ, Häkkinen A, Valkeinen H, Alen M 2001 Selective muscle hypertrophy, changes in EMG and force and serum hormones during strength training in older women. Journal of Applied Physiology 91(2):569–580

Hopkins SR, Harms CA 2004 Gender and pulmonary gas exchange during exercise. Exercise and Sport Sciences Reviews 32(2):50–56

Ilmarinen J, Rantanen J 1999 Promotion of work ability during ageing. American Journal of Industrial Medicine 36(S1):21–23

Kelley GA 1999 Aerobic exercise and resting blood pressure among women: a meta-analysis. Preventive Medicine 28(3):264–275

Kelley GA, Kelley KS 2006 Exercise and bone mineral density at the femoral neck in postmenopausal women: a meta-analysis of controlled clinical trials with individual patient data. American Journal of Obstetrics and Gynecology 194(3):760–767

Kelley GA, Kelley KS, Tran ZV 2004 Aerobic exercise and lipids and lipoproteins in women: a meta-analysis of randomized controlled trials. Journal of Women's Health (Larchmont) 13:1148–1164. Erratum in Journal of Womens Health (Larchmont) 2005;14:198

Kelley GA, Kelley KS, Tran ZV 2005 Exercise, lipids and lipoproteins in older adults: a meta-analysis. Preventive Cardiology 8(4):206–214

Kilbom A, Astrand I 1971 Physical training with submaximal intensities in women. II Effect on cardiac output. Scandinavian Journal of Clinical and Laboratory Investigation 28(2):163–175

King AC, Haskell WL, Young DR, Oka RK, Stefanick ML 1995 Long-term effects of varying intensities and formats of physical activity on participation rates, fitness and lipoproteins in men and women aged 50 to 65 years. Circulation 91(9):2596–2604

Kohl HW 2001 Physical activity and cardiovascular disease: evidence for a dose-response. Medicine and Science in Sports and Exercise 33(6 Suppl):S472–S483

Koskinen S, Sainio P, Gould R, Sutama T, Aromaa A and the Working Group for Functional Capacity 2004 Functional capacity and working capacity. In: Aromaa A, Koskinen S (eds) Health and functional capacity in Finland. Baseline results of the Health 2000 Examination Survey. National Public Health Institute B12/2004, Helsinki, Finland, 79–94. Available online at: www.ktl.fi/terveys2000/index.uk.html (accessed 25th September 2007)

Kraus WE, Houmard JA, Duscha BD, Knetzger KJ, Wharton MB, McCartney JS, Bales CW, Henes S, Samsa GP, Otvos JD, Kulkarni KR, Slentz CA 2002 Effects of the amount and intensity of exercise on plasma lipoproteins. New England Journal of Medicine 347(19):1483–1492

Lawlor DA, Taylor M, Bedford C, Ebrahim S 2002 Is housework good for health? Levels of physical activity and factors associated with activity in elderly women. Results from the British Women's Heart and Health Study. Journal of Epidemiology and Community Health 56(6):473–478

Leon AS, Sanchez OA 2001 Response of blood lipids to exercise training alone or combined with dietary intervention. Medicine and Science in Sports and Exercise 33(6 Suppl):S502–S515

Leon AS, Gaskill SE, Rice T, Bergeron J, Gagnon J, Rao DC, Skinner JS, Wilmore JH, Bouchard C 2002 Variability in the response of HDL cholesterol to exercise training in the HERITAGE Family Study. International Journal of Sports Medicine 23(1):1–9

Liu SL, Lebrun CM 2006 Effect of oral contraceptives and hormone replacement therapy on bone mineral density in premenopausal and perimenopausal women: a systematic review. British Journal of Sports Medicine 40(1):11–24

Luoto R 2006 Menopausal transition and chronic diseases. Current Women's Health Reviews 2(2):125–132

Luukinen H, Koski K, Laippala P, Kivela SL 1995 Risk factors for recurrent falls in the elderly in long-term institutional care. Public Health 109(1):57–65

MacDonald JR 2002 Potential causes, mechanisms and implications of post exercise hypotension. Journal of Human Hypertension 16(4):225–236

Malmberg JJ, Miilunpalo SI, Vuori IM, Pasanen ME, Oja P, Haapanen-Niemi NA 2002 A health-related fitness and functional performance test battery for middle-aged and older adults: feasibility and health-related content validity. Archives of Physical Medicine and Rehabilitation 83(5):666–677

Mohanka M, Irwin M, Heckbert SR, Yasui Y, Sorensen B, Chubak J, Tworoger SS, Ulrich CM, McTiernan A 2006 Serum lipoproteins in overweight/obese postmenopausal women: a one-year exercise trial. Medicine and Science in Sports and Exercise 38(2):231–239

Mosca L 2005 Management of dyslipidemia in women in the post-hormone therapy era. Journal of General Internal Medicine 20(3):297–305

Mosca L, Appel LJ, Benjamin EJ, Berra K, Chandra-Strobos N, Fabunmi RP, Grady D, Haan CK, Hayes SN, Judelson DR, Keenan NL, McBride P, Oparil S, Ouyang P, Oz MC, Mendelsohn ME, Pasternak RC, Pinn VW, Robertson RM, Schenck-Gustafsson K, Sila CA, Smith SC Jr, Sopko G, Taylor AL, Walsh BW, Wenger NK, Williams CL; American Heart Association; American College of Cardiology; American College of Nurse Practitioners; Amercian College of Obstetricians and Gynecologists; American College of Physicians; American Medical Women's Association; Association of Black Cardiologists; Centers for Disease Control and Prevention; National Heart, Lung and Blood Institute, National Institutes of Health; Office of Research on Women's Health; Sociey of Thoracic Surgeons; World Heart Federation 2004 Evidence-based guidelines for cardiovascular disease prevention in women. Journal of American College of Cardiology 43(5):900–921

Norman RJ, Flight IHK, Rees MCP 1999 Oestrogen and progestogen hormone replacement therapy for peri-menopausal and post-menopausal women: weight and body fat distribution. Cochrane Database of Systematic Reviews, Issue 3. CD001018

Oguma Y, Shinoda-Tagawa T 2004 Physical activity decreases cardiovascular disease risk in women: review and meta-analysis. American Journal of Preventive Medicine 26(5):407–418

Oja P, Laukkanen R, Pasanen M, Tyry T, Vuori I 1991 A 2-km walking test for assessing the cardiorespiratory fitness of healthy adults. International Journal of Sports Medicine 12:356–362

Ostir GV, Markides KS, Black SA, Goodwin JS 1998. Lower body functioning as a predictor of subsequent disability among older Mexican Americans. Journals of Gerontology Series A: Biological Sciences and Medical Sciences 53A(6):M491–M495

Pate R, Pratt M, Blair SN, Haskell WL, Macera CA, Bouchard C, Buchner D, Ettinger W, Heath GW, King AC, Kriska A, Leon AS, Marcus BH, Morris J, Paffenbarger RS, Patrick K, Pollock ML, Rippe JM, Sallis J, Wilmore JH 1995 Physical activity and public health. A recommendation from the Centers for Disease Control and Prevention and the American College of Sports Medicine. Journal of the American Medical Association 273(5):402–407

Rantanen T 2003 Muscle strength, disability and mortality. Scandinavian Journal of Medicine and Science in Sports 13(1):3–8

Ross R, Janssen I 2001 Physical activity, total and regional obesity: dose-response considerations. Medicine and Science in Sports and Exercise 33(6,Suppl):S521–S527

Sipilä S, Poutamo J 2003 Muscle performance, sex hormones and training in peri-menopausal and post-menopausal women. Scandinavian Journal of Medicine and Science in Sports 13(1):19–25

Sirola J, Rikkonen T 2005 Muscle performance after the menopause. Journal of the British Menopause Society 11(2):45–50

Sowers MR, La Pietra M 1995 Menopause: its epidemiology and potential association with chronic diseases. Epidemiologic Reviews 17(2):287–302

Staffileno BA, Braun LT, Rosenson RS 2001 The accumulative effects of physical activity in hypertensive postmenopausal women. Journal of Cardiovascular Risk 8(5):283–290

Suni JH, Oja P, Miilunpalo SI, Pasanen ME, Vuori IM, Bös K 1998 Health-related fitness test battery for adults: associations with perceived health, mobility and back function and symptoms. Archives of Physical Medicine and Rehabilitation 79(5):559–569

Tuomi K, Huuhtanen P, Nykyri E, Ilmarinen J 2001 Promotion of work ability, the quality of work and retirement. Occupational Medicine (London) 51(5):318–324

US Preventive Services Task Force 2005 Hormone therapy for the prevention of chronic conditions in postmenopausal women: recommendations from the US Preventive Services Task Force. Annals of Internal Medicine 142(10):855–860

Whang W, Manson JE, Hu FB, Chae CU, Rexrode KM, Willett WC, Stampfer MJ, Albert CM 2006 Physical exertion, exercise and sudden cardiac death in women. Journal of the American Medical Association 295(12):1399–1403

Wilbur J, Miller AM, McDevitt J, Wang E, Miller J 2005 Menopausal status, moderate-intensity walking and symptoms in midlife women. Research and Theory for Nursing Practice 19(2):163–180

Williams PT 2001 Health effects resulting from exercise versus those from body fat loss. Medicine and Science in Sports and Exercise 33 (6 Suppl.):S611–S621

Wilmore JH, Costill DL 2004 Physiology of sport and exercise, 3rd edn. Human Kinetics, Champaign, IL

Wilson MM 2003 Menopause. Clinics in Geriatric Medicine 19(3):483–506

Woolf-May K, Kearney EM, Owen A, Jones DW, Davison RC, Bird SR 1999 The efficacy of accumulated short bouts versus single daily bouts of brisk walking in improving aerobic fitness and blood lipid profiles. Health Education Research 14(6): 803–814

Wood PD, Stefanick ML, Williams PT, Haskell WL 1991 The effects on plasma lipoproteins of a prudent weight-reducing diet, with or without exercise, in overweight men and women. New England Journal of Medicine 325(7):461–466

Chapter 14

Topical discussions

Chapter 14.1

Physically demanding trades: can women tolerate heavy workloads?

Peter L. McLennan   Herbert Groeller   Denise L. Smith
Nigel A.S. Taylor

Anatomical and physiological differences between the genders and their functional significance during exercise stress, have been explored throughout this section. In this chapter, the evidence that some of these differences may affect women's ability (relative to men) to undertake physically demanding trades is briefly reviewed and the validity of the statement that 'women are not capable of performing heavy physical work' is scrutinised using the available scientific evidence. This chapter summarises an extended review (McLennan et al. 2001) in which meaningful gender differences that would assist in determining the capacity for women to undertake physically demanding work, from both military and industrial perspectives, were identified and described using more than 1200 literature sources.

1 FUNCTIONAL AND ANATOMICAL DIFFERENCES

On a population basis, women are generally of smaller stature and lighter mass than men of the same age (Chapter 11). These structural differences affect many morphological and functional characteristics, but at the same time, there is sufficient overlap between the genders to show that differences could often be identified more on grounds of physical stature rather than on the basis of gender.

In an occupational setting, absolute strength (the ability to move a fixed mass) appears to be a key requirement for successful task performance without incurring injury. Indeed, a long-term, load-bearing capability of up to 40 kg is often required in military and occupational settings (Sharp 1994). Men are stronger than women, but this performance discrepancy becomes negligible when strength is expressed relative to muscle cross-sectional area (Miller et al. 1993). Therefore, the primary basis for this difference is that, on average, women have lower absolute body and muscle masses (Gallagher & Heymsfield 1998) and a higher relative body fat mass. The average woman therefore will have greater difficulty in moving the same absolute load, compared to the average man (Gallagher & Heymsfield 1998). These variations in muscle mass and strength are predominantly mediated via between-gender differences in the secretion of the androgenic hormones (Wilmore 1982).

There are gender-based differences in the basal concentrations of circulating growth hormone and testosterone. The female sex hormones interact with these and other hormones, such as cortisol, and this may have some bearing on the results of many experiments. Therefore, to accurately determine the effects of variations in hormone concentrations between men and women, testing should occur in both the follicular and luteal phases of the menstrual cycle (see the introductory text to this section of chapters). Nevertheless, cardiovascular, hormonal and metabolic responses to exercise do not appear to be influenced by menstrual phase. The best designed and controlled studies indicate that menstrual cycle phase has no measurable effect on muscle strength, fatigability or other contractile properties (Janse de Jonge et al. 2001), and there appears to be little, if any, effect of the menstrual cycle on measures of aerobic performance (Galliven et al. 1997).

Men require a greater absolute energy intake and are capable of a greater maximum work output than women (Costill et al. 1979), again, largely due to a greater muscle mass. When carrying a heavy load, women must therefore work at a higher relative maximal aerobic power, with a greater energy cost, and will tend to fatigue earlier than men carrying the same absolute load (Chapter 27.2). However, strength performance is not solely determined by the quantity of the activated muscle mass, but is also a function of the manner in which, and the extent to which, that mass is used (Sale 1988). Thus, superior technique, which is unrelated to gender, can often compensate for lower strength in either gender.

During endurance exercise, women make greater use of stored fat as an energy source and tend to spare muscle glycogen (Tarnopolsky et al. 1990). This difference can potentially improve endurance across most work intensities. Therefore, if allowed to work at an equal relative intensity, women may display better endurance and superior fatigue resistance than men. Men and women will benefit from proper nutritional preparation for anticipated long-term activity and, to reduce fatigue at higher workloads, both need to establish greater stores of muscle glycogen. While this is readily achieved in men through carbohydrate loading, women must also increase their total energy intake (Walker et al. 2000), as they typically have a greater difficulty achieving a positive energy balance within an exercise environment, and this increases their relative fatigue risk. Increasing energy intake might best be achieved through liquid carbohydrate supplements, as solid carbohydrates can perversely suppress appetite.

With a high demand on upper-body strength in many occupational tasks and the relatively smaller upper-body muscle mass of women, training prescriptions that focus on upper-body strength and power may be of greater benefit for women than an emphasis on aerobic conditioning.

Indeed, women appear to be just as responsive as males to resistance training for increasing relative muscle mass and strength (Castro et al. 1995). A similar training prescription could also benefit men. However, the expression and enhancement of absolute strength are very specific to the movement patterns performed so, as movement patterns change or become more complex, differences in strength change from being muscle mass related to being more dependent on the efficiency and skill of the person performing the task (Kumar et al. 1995).

Absolute gender differences in walking gait make women more prone to overstriding during marching or formation movements, and more susceptible to injury when stride length is increased to match that of taller individuals. However, gait pattern does not appear to be inherently gender determined, as these gait variations disappear when expressed relative to height (Yamasaki et al. 1991). Thus, differences in gait appear to be stature based and stride length dependent, making shorter males also more vulnerable to injury. With additional differences in foot shape and size, women are poorly served by general-purpose footwear designed for men and may be more prone to injury, due especially to insufficient support around the heel and ankle (Wunderlich & Cavanagh 2001). These differences are entirely compensatable. For example, it is possible to compensate for a shorter stride length by modifying task performance parameters, and to overcome deficits induced by inadequate footwear by designing shoes to better fit women's feet.

Women have smaller absolute lung volumes than men (Hoffstein 1986), making it mechanically more efficient for them to increase breathing frequency than to increase breathing depth during exercise. However, this pattern is seen in all people with a smaller vital capacity. Women also have a lower ventilatory sensitivity to circulating carbon dioxide (Irsigler 1976), perhaps making them better able to conserve breathing-gas supplies when working under situations in which carbon dioxide accumulation might occur (Chapter 23).

Women have a lower blood volume and haematocrit, and thus will also have a lower total oxygen delivery potential (Chapters 11 and 14.2). The upper capacity of the blood for oxygen delivery to the exercising muscles may limit endurance exercise (Chapter 10.1). However, a more rapid oxygen dissociation in women (Tate & Holtz 1998) and the lower blood viscosity help compensate for the lower oxygen delivery potential by facilitating blood passage through the capillaries, and enhancing oxygen delivery to the tissues. Further gender differences include observations that men display higher blood pressure at rest, greater increases in blood pressure in response to physical and mental stress, and a greater likelihood to develop hypertension, vascular and heart disease than women (Lloyd-Jones et al. 1999). One contributor to these differences, a less reactive sympathetic nervous system, makes women less prone to muscle tremor and racing heart rate under stress, but more prone to fainting when changing posture or standing still for long periods.

During heat exposure (Chapter 19), gender differences appear to influence physiological responses, at least superficially. However, the majority of experimental evidence demonstrates that heat tolerance is more closely related to cardiovascular function and hydration state than it is to gender. Nevertheless, women have a much lower sweat rate than men (Nunneley 1978), and a higher body temperature threshold for the initiation of sweating (Cunningham et al. 1978). These differences make women more reliant upon convective and conductive cooling than upon evaporation, and therefore better suited to use peripheral blood redistribution for heat dissipation. The resultant typically higher skin temperature in women reduces dry heat transfer between the environment and skin (Frye & Kamon 1983), whilst simultaneously increasing cutaneous water vapour pressure and enhancing evaporative cooling. Women also appear better able to adjust sweat secretion in relation to skin wettedness, and so display greater sweating efficiency. The combination of these factors results in the tendency for women to better tolerate hot-humid conditions than men. Both genders adapt equally well to the heat (Chapter 21), with those women who have equivalent endurance and heat acclimation histories appearing to tolerate the combined effects of exercise and heat at least as well as men.

There appear to be three primary gender differences of physiological and functional significance during cold stress (Chapter 20). First, regional variations in the deposition of fat, in relation to other insulating tissues, result in men being better able to retain body heat during resting exposures, while women seem better equipped during exercise. This is due to the relatively greater lower-body muscular development (heat generation) and cutaneous adiposity (insulation) of women. However, increased muscle blood flow during exercise can negate the benefit of increased insulation. Second, during cold exposures, women have cooler skin temperatures due to the combined influences of cutaneous vasoconstriction and a more even deposition of subcutaneous adipose tissue. Women appear to be more sensitive to and less comfortable with these skin temperatures. Third, women show a reduced shivering response relative to men for an equivalent reduction in core temperature (Grucza et al. 1999). The mechanism behind this response is uncertain.

2 WORK–RELATED RISK CONSEQUENCES OF FUNCTIONAL DIFFERENCES

Many physiological and anatomical differences exist between the genders during the performance of physically demanding tasks. Some act to favour one gender over the other, but the majority of these differences do not appear to preferentially predispose one group to greater occupational risk. However, there are several variables that may affect occupational health. Of these factors, some are gender based (determined by gender) while others are gender related. The latter are associated with typically observed morphological and physiological differences between the genders (e.g. stature), but may apply equally to either gender.

A lower absolute strength for any person performing a fixed load-carriage task will place that person under greater physiological strain, for which there are several potentially adverse consequences. That individual will be working closer to the upper tolerance limit and will be more susceptible to premature fatigue. This is exacerbated by a greater relative reduction in muscle blood flow, which is due to vascular compression and is a function of relative force production (Rowell 1993). Both of these factors place the person closer to the task-related threshold of failure and predispose to a greater risk of injury. Furthermore, in the fatigued state, more subtle anatomical, physiological and biomechanical limitations may now become factors that jeopardise health and safety. While many work tasks can be modified or reengineered so that this risk may be reduced, there exists a parallel benefit to be derived from carefully prescribed exercise programmes to further reduce this risk.

Differences in lifting techniques between the genders appear not to influence the development of low back pain. Instead, specific actions, such as twisting and handling unexpected heavy loads, may play a greater role. Thus, whilst back pain may have a minimal relationship with gender under controlled conditions, less strong individuals, including most women, are potentially exposed to a greater risk of acute low back injury, especially under conditions where the terrain and load distribution may vary suddenly. Such individuals may be required to carry the same absolute load, but the relative load, and therefore its physical and physiological impact, is higher.

In the military, women sustain disproportionately more overuse injuries, and in particular stress fractures (Nelson et al. 1999). These injuries can account for about 75% of all injuries among women during basic combat training. Approximately 80% of military training injuries among women involve the lower body and are gender dependent. Data from the US Army (Jones et al. 1993) show that the most commonly diagnosed injuries for the men were low back pain (7.3%), tendonitis (6.5%) and sprains (4.8%), whilst in the women they were muscle strains (15.6%), stress fractures (12.3%) and sprains (5.9%). It should be noted, however, that the type of injury incurred is also dependent upon the sports played by women and their time of service. Furthermore, injury rates for male and female cadets are not significantly different later in their careers.

Despite similarities between men and women in general anatomy and physiology of the joint, women have a significantly higher incidence, and severity, of acute and chronic knee injuries, perhaps due to structural and biochemical variations (Mandelbaum et al. 2001). For instance, there are subtle gender differences in cartilage anatomy, biochemistry, metabolism and susceptibility to inflammation. Indeed, the knee joints of women respond differently over time to load-bearing activities, and females are found to be more likely to rupture the anterior cruciate ligament, even in gender-comparable sports. Whilst such injuries represent a sizeable health problem, there are numerous preventive measures that may help reduce the difference in gender risk.

The vertical alignment of the femur (Q-angle) may also be clinically relevant for physically active people with Q-angles greater than 20°. Such angles potentially predispose individuals to knee injury (Mandelbaum et al. 2001). Whilst fewer men have this trait, people from either gender who have a greater pelvic width are at increased risk. Therefore, the combination of a large Q-angle with subtle differences in knee structure and function may increase the risk of knee injuries in women.

The shape of women's feet differs significantly from that of men (Wunderlich & Cavanagh 2001). Accordingly, women's boots should not be designed as versions of men's footwear, scaled for optimal fit. Since appropriate footwear and fit are important for foot and lower-limb health, it is suggested that women supplied with incorrectly designed footwear will be exposed to significantly greater risk.

Finally, males have been shown to be slightly more stable than females to centre of gravity shifts (Davis 1983), with differences being independent of stature. Stability is also affected by load. Women have been shown to be less stable than males, and are at greater risk of trip and fall injuries associated with materials handling tasks. However, stability is, at least in part, a function of ankle sway, and it can be compensated through the use of adequate and supportive footwear.

3 PRACTICAL IMPLICATIONS

Table 14.1.1 illustrates the theoretical capabilities of women and men to undertake generic, physically demanding tasks. This table presents gender-specific variables for average females and males (aged 18–39 years), and a hypothetical woman (Female B), standardised to match the stature of the average man. That is, the attributes of this woman are scaled upwards in proportion to changes in stature. Below we explore three physically demanding tasks to illustrate how one may approach such comparisons across these individuals.

First, during heavy materials handling tasks, particularly those that require load carriage over extended distances, the average woman (Female A), and some men of smaller stature, will be at a distinct physical and physiological disadvantage relative to the average man. From a military perspective, such people will have a mechanical disadvantage during heavy pack marching (>30 kg), when scaling walls and when performing tasks that require rapid directional changes when carrying a fixed load. These individuals will be working closer towards their maximal limits, and this elevates fatigue and injury risks.

Second, when males and females (Female B) of similar physical dimensions are asked to perform an identical task, equal performance may result, but only if both participants are of equal muscle strength, efficiency, aerobic power and endurance. Since Female B will more frequently have less strong and powerful musculature, then the hypothetical woman will be working closer to the upper tolerance limit, and will be more susceptible to premature fatigue, placing her closer to the threshold of failure. This situation predisposes both average and standardised women to a significantly greater risk of injury, relative to the average man, particularly if the task is performed on a repetitive basis.

The average woman (Female A), and some men of smaller stature, may have a distinct physical and physiological advantage, relative to the average man, during the completion of some endurance-dependent tasks. A good military example of this is an underwater, endurance fin-swimming task. For instance, a smaller physical stature and a smaller muscle mass, particularly in the upper body, may result in reduced cross-sectional area and therefore less drag in the water. Consequently, the average female may require less energy to propel herself through the water than the average male. However, the fixed shape of the diving equipment will result in the female having to overcome relatively greater drag when fin swimming with breathing apparatus. Women will be better able to use fat stores during exercise. In addition, a potentially superior glycogen-sparing capability and increased efficiency during fin swimming may indicate that, at least during prolonged water activities, Female B will have a performance advantage over the average male.

The comparisons above are only superficial assessments of gender differences in performance capabilities in physically demanding tasks. An essential prerequisite for such comparisons is a detailed assessment of the physical demands of a task. This is beyond the scope of this chapter, but methodological details are available within the literature (e.g. Taylor & Groeller 2003). In the next chapter, this gender-comparison theme is continued, but from a slightly different perspective: the gender gap in elite sports performance.

Table 14.1.1 Physical characteristics of average women and men, and those of a standardised woman (Female B)

Variable	Female A	Male	Female B
Height (m)	1.64	1.77	1.77
Mass (kg)	61.9	77.0	77.0
Sum of six skinfolds (mm)	102	72	90
Flexibility: sit and reach (cm)	46.4	43.6	43.0
Strength: grip strength (kg)	30.7	50.6	40.0
Estimated maximal aerobic power $(mL \cdot kg^{-1} \cdot min^{-1})$	33.9	42.6	38.0

References

Castro MJ, McCann DJ, Shaffrath JD, Adams WC 1995 Peak torque per unit cross-sectional area differs between strength-trained and untrained young adults. Medicine and Science in Sports and Exercise 27:397–403

Costill DL, Fink W, Getchell L, Ivy J, Wizmann F 1979 Lipid metabolism in skeletal muscle of endurance-trained males and females. Journal of Applied Physiology 47:787–791

Cunningham DJ, Stolwijk JA, Wenger CB 1978 Comparative thermoregulatory responses of resting men and women. Journal of Applied Physiology 45:908–915

Davis PR 1983 Human factors contributing to slips, trips and falls. Ergonomics 26:51–59

Frye AJ, Kamon E 1983 Sweating efficiency in acclimated men and women exercising in humid and dry heat. Journal of Applied Physiology 54:972–977

Gallagher D, Heymsfield SB 1998 Muscle distribution: variations with body weight, gender and age. Applied Radiation and Isotopes 49:733–734

Galliven EA, Singh A, Michelson D, Bina S, Gold PW, Deuster PA 1997 Hormonal and metabolic responses to exercise across time of day and menstrual cycle phase. Journal of Applied Physiology 83:1822–1831

Grucza R, Pekkarinen H, Hanninen O 1999 Different thermal sensitivity to exercise and cold in men and women. Journal of Thermal Biology 24:397–401

Hoffstein V 1986 Relationship between lung volume, maximal expiratory flow, forced expiratory volume in one second and tracheal area in normal men and women. American Review of Respiratory Diseases 136:956–961

Irsigler GB 1976 Carbon dioxide response lines in young adults: the limits of the normal response. American Review of Respiratory Diseases 114:429–436

Janse de Jonge XAK, Boot CRL, Thom JM, Ruell PA, Thompson MW 2001 The influence of menstrual cycle phase on skeletal muscle contractile characteristics in humans. Journal of Physiology 530:161–166

Jones BH, Bovee MW, Harris JM, Cowan DN 1993 Intrinsic risk factors for exercise-related injuries among male and female army trainees. American Journal of Sports Medicine 21:705–710

Kumar S, Narayan Y, Bacchus C 1995 Symmetric and asymmetric two-handed pull-push strength of young adults. Human Factors 37:854–865

Lloyd-Jones PM, Larson MG, Beiser A, Levy D 1999 Lifetime risk of developing coronary heart disease. Lancet 353:89–92

McLennan PL, Gordon CJ, Thoicharoen P, Armstrong KA, Smith DL, Steele JR, Fogarty AL, Groeller H, Taylor NAS 2001 Anatomical, physiological and functional significance of gender differences. UOW-HPL-Report-005. Human Performance Laboratories, University of Wollongong. Department of Defence, Canberra, Australia, 1–151

Mandelbaum BR, Roos H, Lohmander S 2001 The female athlete's knee: meniscus, articular cartilage and osteoarthritis. In: Garrett WE, Lester GE, McGowan J, Kirkendall DT (eds) Women's health in sports and exercise. American Academy of Orthopaedic Surgeons, Rosemont, IL, 107–124

Miller AE, MacDougall JD, Tarnopolsky MA, Sale DG 1993 Gender differences in strength and muscle fiber characteristics. European Journal of Applied Physiology 66:254–562

Nelson BJ, Uhorchak JM, LeBoeuf, MK, Taylor DC 1999 Physical training and injury in female cadets at the United States Military Academy. Connecticut Medicine 63:653–655

Nunneley SA 1978 Physiological responses of women to thermal stress: a review. Medicine and Science in Sports 10:250–255

Rowell LB 1993 Human cardiovascular control. Oxford University Press, New York

Sale DG 1988 Neural adaptation to resistance training. Medicine and Science in Sports and Exercise 20:S135-S145

Sharp MA 1994 Physical fitness and occupational performance of women in the U.S. Army. Work 2:80–92

Tarnopolsky LJ, MacDougall JD, Atkinson SA, Tarnopolsky MA, Sutton JR 1990 Gender differences in substrate for endurance exercise. Journal of Applied Physiology 68:302–308

Tate CA, Holtz RW 1998 Gender and fat metabolism during exercise: a review. Canadian Journal of Applied Physiology 23:570–582

Taylor NAS, Groeller H 2003 Work-based assessments of physically demanding jobs: a methodological overview. Journal of Physiological Anthropology 22(2):73–81

Walker JL, Heigenhauser GJ, Hultman E, Spriet LL 2000 Dietary carbohydrate, muscle glycogen content and endurance performance in well-trained women. Journal of Applied Physiology 88:2151–2158

Wilmore JH 1982 Training for sport and activity. The physiological basis of the conditioning process. Allyn and Bacon, Boston

Wunderlich RE, Cavanagh PR 2001 Gender differences in adult foot shape: implications for shoe design. Medicine and Science in Sports and Exercise 33:605–611

Yamasaki M, Sasaki T, Torii M 1991 Sex difference in the pattern of lower limb movement during treadmill walking. European Journal of Applied Physiology 62:99–103

Chapter 14.2

Are women narrowing the gender gap in elite sport performance?

Alan M. Nevill Greg Whyte

1 INTRODUCTION

In Chapter 11, we saw briefly how women have more dramatically lowered their world records than men. It therefore must come as no surprise that the question 'are women narrowing the gap in elite sport performance?' has been the focus of a lively debate in the scientific literature. Indeed, Whipp & Ward (1992), in their provocative article entitled 'Will women soon outrun men?', fitted linear regression models to world record running speeds for both men and women recorded during the 20th century (distances 200 m, 400 m, 800 m, 1500 m and marathon) and highlighted when the men's and women's predicted world record speeds would converge. Not only did they report a narrowing of the gap between men's and women's running world record speeds but, assuming world records continue to rise at the same rate, suggested that women will overtake men early in the 21st century (or, in the case of the marathon, by 1998), based on a linear extrapolation of men's and women's fitted regression models. In a more recent study, Tatem et al. (2004) also employed linear regression to analyse male and female 100 m running times, and predicted that women would run as fast as men by the year 2156 in a time of 8.079 s.

However, these predictions have recently come under strong criticism (Nevill & Whyte 2005). Apart from the obvious error that women would run marathons faster than men by 1998, a number of confounding variables may have led to these predictions being erroneous. These include the move from hand-held to electronic timing, technological advancements, including track surfaces in the mid 1960s, and the significant performance gains observed during the period associated with the alleged systematic doping of athletes in the Eastern Bloc regimes. However, it is the use of linear regression modelling that results in potentially the greatest source of error in the evidence presented by Whipp & Ward (1992) and Tatem et al. (2004). Both used linear regression analyses, but the former modelled world record running speeds whilst the latter used world record running times. Clearly both models cannot be correct (if we assume one model is linear, say time, then the other has to be a hyperbolic curve: speed = distance/time). Furthermore, if we extrapolate the linear model of Tatem et al. (2004), the model predicts that, at some time in the future, humans will run negative world record times.

2 MODELLING WORLD RECORD SPEEDS

Careful inspection of men's and women's running and walking world record speeds over the 20th century indicates that more recent record speeds have begun to plateau (Cheuvront et al. 2006, Sparling et al. 1998). Indeed, Nevill & Whyte (2005) identified that many of the middle- and long-distance world record running speeds followed a flattened S-shaped curve, similar to the logistic curve, indicating that a slow rise in world record speeds earlier in the 20th century was followed by a period of acceleration, that was subsequently followed by a plateau in running speeds in recent years. A logistic curve used to model world record running speeds, as a function of date (the predictor variable), is given by:

Equation 1:   Speed $(m \cdot s^{-1})$ = min + (max − min) · exp(b · (date − y))/(1 + exp(b · (date − y)))

where: min and max = minimum (maximum) predicted, asymptotic world record speeds

b = rate at which the world record speeds accelerated during 20th century

y = centred year in which this acceleration was greatest.

The fitted logistic curve parameters (estimated using non-linear regression analysis; see Nevill & Whyte 2005) for men's and women's world records for 800 m, 1500 m, 5000 m, 10,000 m, marathon and 20 km walk are given in Table 14.2.1. Note that, by comparing the estimates with twice their standard errors, all parameters are significant. The men's and women's 10,000 m and 20 km running and walking world record speeds recorded during 20th century, plus the fitted logistic curves, are given in Figures 14.2.1 and 14.2.2, respectively.

For comparative purposes, we assessed the significance of the two additional logistic curve parameters, for both men and women over distances reported in Table 14.2.1, obtained by partitioning the explained variance from the logistic and linear models (ANOVA). The logistic curves fitted the data significantly better than the linear models, with the exceptions being the

Table 14.2.1 Predicted world record running speed $(m \cdot s^{-1})$ parameters (using the logistic curve) and standard errors (SE) for men and women

Race	Parameters	Men		Women	
		Estimate	SE	Estimate	SE
800 m	Lower asymptote (min)	6.93	0.15	5.72	0.11
	Upper asymptote (max)	8.00	0.11	7.17	0.12
	Beta (b)	0.05	0.02	0.10	0.02
	Centred year (y)	1946.99	5.68	1959.95	1.99
1500 m	Lower asymptote (min)	6.19	0.12	5.67	0.18
	Upper asymptote (max)	7.38	0.10	6.50	0.05
	Beta (b)	0.04	0.01	0.29	0.10
	Centred year (y)	1952.52	3.12	1971.43	1.57
5000 m	Lower asymptote (min)	5.55	0.12	5.47	0.03
	Upper asymptote (max)	6.83	0.17	5.75	0.01
	Beta (b)	0.04	0.01	1.05	0.43
	Centred year (y)	1965.69	4.33	1984.67	0.39
10,000 m	Lower asymptote (min)	5.33	0.05	5.11	0.15
	Upper asymptote (max)	6.37	0.05	5.66	0.05
	Beta (b)	0.06	0.01	0.49	0.26
	Centred year (y)	1959.54	1.90	1984.47	1.19
Marathon	Lower asymptote (min)	4.30	0.13	3.16	0.06
	Upper asymptote (max)	5.69	0.06	5.07	0.03
	Beta (b)	0.05	0.01	0.21	0.02
	Centred year (y)	1947.90	3.33	1972.26	0.44
20 km walk	Lower asymptote (min)	3.33	0.08	2.51	0.07
	Upper asymptote (max)	4.67	0.25	4.12	0.26
	Beta (b)	0.04	0.01	0.09	0.02
	Centred year (y)	1973.98	7.30	1979.27	4.02

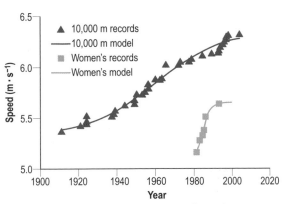

Figure 14.2.1 The 10,000 m running speed (m·s-1) world records recorded during the 20th century, plus the fitted logistic curves for men and women.

Table 14.2.2 Gender performance ratios (R) together with the ratios calculated from the predicted asymptotic (Asy) running speeds

Event/year	Women's/men's performance ratios (R)				
	1951	1967	1981	2006	Asy ratio
800 m	0.81	0.86	0.90	0.89	0.90
1500 m	*	0.83	0.91	0.89	0.88
5000 m	*	**	0.86	0.88	0.84
10,000 m	*	**	0.85	0.89	0.89
Marathon	0.66	0.69	0.88	0.92	0.89
20 km walk	0.77	0.75	0.80	0.89	0.88
mean	0.75	0.78	0.87	0.89	0.88

*Not run before 1967.
**Not run before 1981.

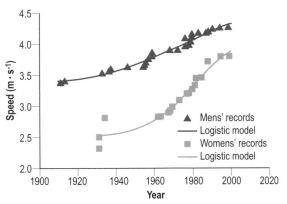

Figure 14.2.2 The 20 km walk speed (m·s-1) world records recorded during the 20th century, plus the fitted logistic curves for men and women.

men's 800 m and women's 10,000 m, where a lack of women's records prevented the latter F ratio reaching statistical significance.

3 COMPARING GENDER DIFFERENCES IN ATHLETIC PERFORMANCES

A number of authors have explored the gender differences in athletic performances during the second half of the 20th century. Furlong & Szreter (1975) were probably the first to observe a narrowing of the gap between men's and women's athletic performances from 1951 to 1967. The authors compared the world's best 20 male and 20 female athletic performances over 17 consecutive seasons, in eight athletic events (100 m, 200 m, 800 m, high jump and long jump, shot put, discus and javelin). To facilitate a gender comparison, Furlong & Szreter (1975) calculated a gender performance ratio for each event and season, where the mean speeds (distances) achieved by women were divided by the corresponding male performance (a ratio of 1.00 indicates no

difference). Their results identified a consistent narrowing of the gender gap, with the mean ratio increasing from 0.806 in 1951 to 0.830 in 1967, a gap narrowing of 2.4%.

Sparling et al. (1998) also compared gender differences in distance running performance over a 17-year period (1980–1996). The authors adopted the world best times and the 100th best times for both the 1500 m and marathon events for their data set. The magnitude and stability of gender differences were calculated (percentage difference), revealing women to be 11.1% and 11.2% slower for the 1500 m and marathon respectively. When expressed as gender performance ratios (Furlong & Szreter 1975), these become 0.89 and 0.89. We have calculated similar gender performance ratios, using world record speeds for the events listed in Table 14.2.1, for the years 1951, 1967, 1981 and 2006. These are presented in Table 14.2.2, together with ratios calculated from the predicted asymptotic running speeds reported in Table 14.2.1.

It is now clear that linear regression models used to describe world record progressions, recorded as either speeds or times, are questionable and, as such, should be treated with caution. A number of authors have observed that distance-running performances are beginning to reach a plateau (Cheuvront et al. 2006, Sparling et al. 1998) and consequently, non-linear models are more appropriate to describe such records. Indeed, here we demonstrate that a more biologically sound logistic, flattened S-shaped curve can be used to describe the middle- and long-distance world record performances. In general, all of the four-parameter logistic models fitted the data significantly better than the linear models and the upper asymptotic parameters indicate there are indeed limits to human running performance.

Previous authors (Tatem et al. 2004, Whipp & Ward 1992) might be forgiven for speculating that women will run faster than men, due to women's records reaching the steeper phase of the S-shaped curve more recently than men's. However, the stability of the running speeds for both genders over recent years has been a major contributor to the gender gap also reaching a plateau over the past 10 years (Table 14.2.2). The gender performance ratios derived from the asymptotic running speeds (0.88) also confirm the stability of the gender gap, being approximately 11% or 12% for middle- and long-distance running (and walking) events.

4 EXPLAINING THE GENDER DIFFERENCES

Gender differences for a wide range of physiological variables have been described within Chapter 11, and in Chapter 15 these are discussed with respect to youths. However, to establish the mechanisms underlying gender differences in running performance, an understanding of the determinants of endurance performance is crucial. Whilst much debate surrounds the prediction of endurance running performance, key determinants appear to be peak aerobic power, peak running velocity (maximal work rate), velocity at the lactate threshold (a concept debated within the literature: Chapter 10.3) and running economy (Chapter 10.2).

Maximal oxygen uptake (peak aerobic power) is determined by the product of maximal cardiac output and the maximal arteriovenous oxygen difference (Fick equation). Female athletes have smaller left ventricular cavities and left ventricular masses than males, in absolute and relative terms (Whyte et al. 2004). Smaller end-diastolic and blood volumes in female athletes result in a lower stroke volume at rest and during exercise, leading to a lower cardiac output in female athletes. Furthermore, female athletes have a 5–10% lower haemoglobin content, resulting in a reduced oxygen–carrying capacity, leading to a larger cardiac output at any level of submaximal oxygen uptake compared with males. Females also possess smaller absolute lung volumes and maximal expiratory flow rates. Even when scaled for stature, males possess larger airway diameters, lung volumes and diffusion surfaces (Sheel et al. 2004). The reduced oxygen-carrying capacity, smaller hearts and lungs, and higher body fat content result in a lower peak aerobic power in female athletes, even when scaled for body mass and adiposity (Cheuvront et al. 2006). Indeed, exercise-induced arterial hypoxaemia is believed to occur more often in women than in men (Hopkins & Harms 2004). Despite significant gender differences in peak aerobic power, running economy and lactate threshold appear unaffected by gender (Joyner 1993). Furthermore, fractional utilisation remains unchanged across time in trained individuals.

No gender differences exist for muscular strength, when expressed relative to muscle cross-sectional area. In absolute terms, however, men produce greater force, and this is associated with a greater muscle mass per unit of cross-sectional area. Noteworthy is the absence of gender differences in fibre type, fibre length, pennation angle and fascicle length. Peak running velocity is related to strength and, as such, male athletes are able to achieve higher peak running speeds than females, as evident within world record times.

Other gender-related factors that may result in performance differences include substrate utilisation and temperature regulation. Females use proportionately more lipids and less carbohydrate during low- and moderate-intensity exercise (Braun & Horton 2001), and such differences are associated with the function of the sex hormones, oestrogen and progesterone. The impact of these variations in substrate utilisation upon endurance running performance remains unclear; however, they are likely to be of greater importance as race duration increases.

Temperature regulation during exercise is crucial to maintain normal physiological function and running velocity. A number of factors impact upon heat production and heat dissipation during exercise (Chapter 19). For instance, female athletes generally possess a higher percentage of body fat that may act to reduce heat dissipation. Furthermore, females have a greater body surface area to mass ratio. Whilst this allows for greater heat dissipation when ambient temperature is below skin temperature, it may result in a greater rise in core temperature when ambient temperature is high. In addition, the menstrual cycle affects both core and skin temperatures at rest and during exercise, with increased circulating progesterone (luteal phase) leading to a core temperature increase of ~0.5°C, possibly also affecting the sweating threshold (Marsh & Jenkins 2002; see Chapter 18). These thermoregulatory differences may affect performance, particularly in hot-humid environments.

5 CONCLUSION

The data presented above indicate that an approximate 11–12% difference in endurance running performance exists between males and females. It is attractive to suggest that a single physiological determinant may account for this (e.g. 10% difference in haemoglobin content). However, this would be a gross oversimplification, as the determinants of running performance are multifactorial (Chapter 10.2). Furthermore, psychological, biomechanical and sociological factors may also have profound effects upon performance. Nevertheless, gender differences in the physiological factors that contribute to endurance performance are likely to represent a significant component in the present and future gender divide in world record times. Physiological manipulation, including pharmacology, surgery and gene therapy (Chapter 8), appears the only method by which women will further narrow the gap in elite sport performance.

References

Braun B, Horton T 2001 Endocrine regulation of exercise substrate utilization in women compared to men. Exercise and Sport Science Reviews 29:149–154

Cheuvront SN, Carter R, DeRuisseau, KC, Moffatt RJ 2006 Running performance differences between men and women. Sports Medicine 35(12):1017–1024

Furlong J, Szreter R 1975 The trend of the performance difference between leading men and women athletes, 1951–67. Statistician 24:115–128

Hopkins SR, Harms CA 2004 Gender and pulmonary gas exchange during exercise. Exercise and Sport Science Reviews 32(2):50–56

Joyner M 1993 Physiological limiting factors and distance running: influence of gender and age on record performances. Exercise and Sport Science Reviews 21:103–133

Marsh S, Jenkins D 2002 Physiological responses to the menstrual cycle. Sports Medicine 32:601–614

Nevill AM, Whyte G 2005 Are there limits to running world records? Medicine and Science in Sports and Exercise 37:1785–1788

Sheel A, Richards J, Foster G, Guenette J 2004 Sex differences in respiratory exercise physiology. Sports Medicine 34:567–579

Sparling PB, O'Donnell EM, Snow TK 1998 The gender difference in distance running performance has plateaued: an analysis of world rankings from 1980 to 1996. Medicine and Science in Sports and Exercise 30(12):1725–1729

Tatem AJ, Guerra CA, Atkinson PM, Hay SI 2004 Athletics: momentous sprint at the 2156 Olympics? Nature 431(7008):525

Whipp BJ, Ward SA 1992 Will women soon outrun men? Nature 355(6355):25

Whyte GP, George K, Sharma S, Firoozi S, Stephens N, Senior R, McKenna WJ 2004 The upper limit of physiologic cardiac hypertrophy in elite male and female athletes: the British experience. European Journal of Applied Physiology 31:592–597

SECTION **3**

Age

SECTION CONTENTS

Section introduction: Physical activity in the 21st century: challenges for young and old

Pietro E. di Prampero

In young adults, the span between the lower and upper limits of physical activity extends over more than two orders of magnitude in terms of intensity. Indeed, the energy requirement per unit of time of resting skeletal muscle is about 3 mL·kg^{-1}·min^{-1}, and it can increase to about 150–200 mL·kg^{-1}·min^{-1} at maximal aerobic power and to about eight times as much (1200–1600 mL·kg^{-1}·min^{-1}) during maximal explosive exercise lasting ~0.3 s. This large range decreases substantially with age, such that at 70 years, both maximal aerobic power and maximal explosive power per kg of active muscle are reduced to about 50% in both women and men, whereas the resting metabolism is essentially unchanged (Chapter 16).

The three chapters of this section deal with factors that affect the uppermost limits of physical activity during growth, maturation and ageing. The effects of regular exercise throughout life on health, life span and rate of ageing are also highlighted, and this topic is again a focus within Section 5.

When dealing with physical activity, we are very often interested in maximal performances. Therefore, the paragraphs that follow will be devoted to a brief summary of the factors setting maximal performances in track running, considered as a paradigmatic form of human locomotion, with the aim of identifying the key physiological processes that can be modified by growth, maturation or ageing. Readers should also consult Chapters 10.1 and 10.2 for further discussion on this topic.

Maximal running performances will be addressed considering the energy requirement for covering a given distance, on the one hand, and the maximal rate of metabolic energy output, on the other. Indeed, it is immediately apparent that the best performance time over a given distance is equal to the minimum time allowing the subject to obtain (from the energy-yielding mechanisms) the amount of energy necessary and sufficient for covering the distance at stake. This can be expressed formally (Equation 1), using the energy cost of locomotion per unit distance (C) and the overall amount of energy (E) necessary to cover the distance (d).

Equation 1: $E = C \cdot d$

After dividing both terms by the performance time (t_p) and rearranging (Equation 2a), it becomes immediately apparent that the speed over that distance ($V = d/t_p$) is set by the ratio of metabolic power ($\dot{E}$) to energy cost (at that speed). Thus, the maximal speed (V_{max}) attained by any given individual can be described by Equation 2b, where $\dot{E}_{max}$ is that person's maximal metabolic power.

Equation 2a: $d/t_p = V = \dot{E}/C$
Equation 2b: $V_{max} = \dot{E}_{max}/C$

ENDURANCE RUNNING

In wholly aerobic conditions, maximal metabolic power is proportional to the maximal oxygen uptake ($\dot{V}_{O_{2max}}$) and Equation 2b can be written to allow the derivation of the maximal endurance speed (V_{end}) for a given maximal fraction (F) of the maximal oxygen uptake that can be maintained throughout the exercise.

Equation 3: $V_{end} = F \cdot (\dot{V}_{O_{2max}}/C)$

Using Equation 3, di Prampero et al. (1986) calculated the maximal endurance speed for a group of runners taking part in a half or full marathon and in whom the maximal oxygen uptake and the energy cost of locomotion per unit distance (at the same average speed as observed during the competition) were also assessed. Data for the maximal sustainable fraction of the maximal oxygen uptake during racing were obtained from the literature. The results showed that the calculated average running speed (Equation 3) was not statistically different from the actual speed of performance. In addition, the three variables combined in Equation 3 explained 72% of the variability of the actual speed of performance, whereas either the first two (F and $\dot{V}_{O_{2max}}$) or the last two variables ($\dot{V}_{O_{2max}}$ and C) accounted for smaller fractions of the overall variability (58% and 62%, respectively).

Equation 3 shows that the well-known changes of maximal aerobic speed throughout life are due to the effects of growth, maturation and ageing on the three variables at stake. Numerous studies are devoted to the evolution of maximal aerobic power with age, and the reader is referred to the relevant chapters of this section. However, our knowledge of the evolution of the energy cost of locomotion per unit distance is much less detailed, with the general consensus being that it decreases with age, albeit at a decreasing rate, from about 5 years, to reach a constant value at puberty that is maintained throughout life (see MacDougal et al 1983), even if the data on elderly subjects are scanty. The data reported in Chapter 15 of this section are consistent with this general trend (Table S3.1).

The Cinderella of the three variables setting the maximal aerobic performance is the maximal sustainable exercise intensity (F), the evolution of which, with age, has not been systematically investigated, at least to my knowledge.

MIDDLE–DISTANCE RUNNING

When the energy requirement of the exercise is greater than an individual's maximal aerobic performance, the exercising muscles must rely on the anaerobic energy yield. This is provided by the net splitting of phosphocreatine, with a concomitant fall of its concentration in the working muscles and the net production of lactate, leading to an increase in

Table S3.1 The energy cost of locomotion was obtained from the ratio of net oxygen uptake (($\dot{V}_{O_2}$) above resting, and assumed to be 4 mL·kg^{-1}·min^{-1}) to speed (m·min^{-1}). It was also assumed that the anaerobic contribution was negligible and that, for the data at 5 and 15 years, maximal aerobic power was maintained at 100% throughout 1 mile (F = 1.0), a fact that may lead to a slight overestimation of the energy cost of locomotion in the 5-year-old group

Age (y)	V (m·min^{-1})	Net $\dot{V}_{O_2}$ (mL·kg^{-1}·min^{-1})	C (mL·kg^{-1}·m^{-1})
5°	116.9	46	0.390
7–9°°			0.240
9–11*	160	36.6	0.230
15°	222.4	46	0.206
≈20*	160	30.9	0.193

°Data calculated from best performances over 1609 m (1 mile).
°°From MacDougal et al. (1983).
*Data calculated from oxygen uptake during treadmill running at a constant speed (Maliszewski & Freedson 1996).

its concentration in the body fluids (see Chapter 10.3). The adenosine triphosphate concentration in the working muscle is essentially unchanged. Therefore, the maximal amount of anaerobic energy that the muscles can utilise (anaerobic stores capacity) is proportional to the sum of the maximal amount of phosphocreatine that can be hydrolysed, and the maximal amount of lactate that can be accumulated in the body fluids from rest to exhaustion. For exercises leading to exhaustion from about 50 s to about 10 min, the sum of these two energy sources is essentially constant. As a consequence, over this time range, the increase in metabolic power over and above the maximal aerobic power is larger with shorter times to exhaustion.

From a physiological as well as a factual perspective, the most satisfactory description of the relationship between the maximal metabolic power ($\dot{E}_{max}$), the maximal amount of energy that can be obtained from complete utilisation of the anaerobic stores (AnS) and the time to exhaustion (t_e), is Wilkie's (1980) modification of the hyperbolic model proposed by Scherrer & Monod (1960). In this model (Equation 4), all terms referring to energy or power are expressed in the same units, and the third term describes the fact that maximal oxygen uptake is not reached instantaneously at the onset of exercise but exponentially, with a time constant (τ). Thus, this third term describes the loss in metabolic power due to the oxygen deficit incurred at the onset of exercise.

Equation 4: $\dot{E}_{max} = AnS/te + (\dot{V}_{O_{2max}} - (\dot{V}_{O_{2max}} \cdot \tau(1 - e^{-te/\tau}))/t_e$

Using this equation, di Prampero et al (1993) calculated the individual relationships between the maximal metabolic power and the time to exhaustion or fatigue (Figure S3.1) for groups of athletes competing in track running, using the

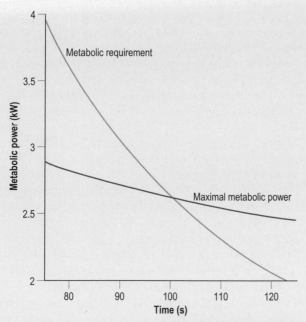

Figure S3.1 The metabolic power requirement of running 800 m (track) from a stationary start, as a function of the time, calculated from Equation 2c, assuming an average value of the energy cost of running of 0.182 mL·kg^{-1}·m^{-1} (3.8 J·kg^{-1}·m^{-1}). Maximal metabolic power for a top athlete of 70 kg body mass and 1.75 m stature is also reported on the same time axis and calculated from Equation 4, assuming a maximal oxygen uptake (above resting) of 74 mL·kg^{-1}·min^{-1} (25.8 W·kg^{-1}), a total capacity of the anaerobic energy store of 68 mL·kg^{-1} (1.4 kJ·kg^{-1}) and an oxygen uptake time constant of 10 s. The time at which the two functions are equivalent (intersect) is the theoretical best performance time for the subject considered over the distance in question. Reproduced from di Prampero (2003) with permission.

individually measured maximal oxygen uptakes, and the anaerobic store capacities from the literature for subjects of the same age and of similar athletic capacity. The assumption was also made that the time constant for oxygen uptake from a step forcing function (τ) was 10 s. In addition, using Equation 2, the metabolic power ($\dot{E}$) required to cover a given distance (d) in a given performance time (t_p) is given by the product of the energy cost of running (C) and the speed (V or d/t_p: Equation 2c). The former was determined in the same athletes for whom the individual maximal metabolic power and the time to exhaustion curves were obtained. The individual relationships between metabolic power and performance time could then be calculated (Figure S3.1).

Equation 2c: $\dot{E} = C \cdot V = C \cdot d / t_p$

Equations 4 and 2c made it possible to calculate, by graphical analysis (as in Figure S3.1) or by iterative procedures, the performance time, or time to exhaustion yielding a metabolic power that equals the maximal metabolic power.

This time was assumed to be the shortest possible time necessary for the athlete in question to cover the distance at stake. These calculations were repeated for several distances, corresponding to performance times from about 80 s to about 14 minutes, for all subjects. The best theoretical performance times so obtained were then compared to the actual best performance times obtained in the same season by the same athletes over the same distances (di Prampero 2003, di Prampero et al 1993). The agreement between theoretical and actual performance times turned out to be rather good, with the average ratio between actual and theoretical best performance times (over the distances of 800, 1000, 1500, 3000, 5000 m) ranging from 1.16 (SD 0.093) to 1.015 (SD 0.027).

A detailed discussion of the assumptions upon which the above analysis is based is beyond the scope of the current text, but interested readers should refer to the above references for such material. However, this line of reasoning shows that knowledge of the individual energy cost, together with that person's maximal metabolic power, is a necessary prerequisite to predict the energetic bottleneck setting the limit to the best performances in running. By analogy, the same approach can be applied to any form of locomotion in which the energy cost of locomotion is known as a function of the speed.

The physiological variables setting performance in the time window considered above (50 s to 10 min) also include the capacity of the anaerobic stores, and the time course of the oxygen uptake on-response at the onset of exercise. The effects of growth, maturation and ageing on maximal aerobic power are fairly well known, but our knowledge is less satisfactory concerning the energy cost of running, which must also include the metabolic power dissipated against air resistance, and to overcome inertia and accelerate the body from a stationary start to top speed. Whereas the former cannot be expected to change, once speed and body size are taken into account, the latter may well be affected by the mechanics of running. This, as discussed in Chapter 15, may well change with growth and maturation and, indeed, within the elderly. However, this remains largely unknown.

Of the last two factors that determine performance in the time range considered here, the time course of the oxygen uptake on-response, for a time to exhaustion of about 10 min, is responsible for only 1–2% of the maximal metabolic power. For exhaustion times of the order of 50 s, however, its role is larger and it depends on the time constant (τ) itself, accounting for about 24% of maximal metabolic power for a time constant of 24 s, 10% for time constant of 10 s. The data on this topic are rather scanty and difficult to interpret unequivocally, and will not be discussed further. However, its evolution throughout life is worth additional investigation, essentially because of its physiological relevance (see Lai et al. 2007).

Our knowledge of the evolution of maximal anaerobic capacity and of the corresponding maximal utilisation rate, with growth, maturation and ageing, as discussed Chapter 15, is still rather unsatisfactory, because of the conceptual difficulties in assessing anaerobic stores, and because of the methodological and ethical limits of such research, particularly when dealing with children.

THE FACTORS LIMITING MAXIMAL AEROBIC POWER

The maximal oxygen uptake plays a central role among the energy-yielding mechanisms. Therefore, the paragraphs that follow are devoted to an analysis of the factors limiting maximal aerobic power, particularly pertaining to the effects of growth, maturation and ageing. Readers should also consult Chapters 10.1 and 10.2 for additional discussion on this topic.

The problem will be addressed quantitatively by viewing the various steps of the oxygen cascade from the environment to the mitochondria as a number of resistances arranged in series, with each resistance (R_i) being overcome by a specific pressure gradient (ΔP_i; Shephard 1969). Under steady-state conditions, the oxygen flow through each resistance is equal to the overall flow (Equation 5) and the overall or total resistance (R_{tot}) to oxygen flow is given by the sum of all the individual resistances ($R_{tot} = \Sigma_1^n R_i$). Similarly, the overall pressure gradient from the environment to the mitochondria is equal to the sum of the individual pressure gradients. Then, at maximal oxygen flow, the total resistance to oxygen flow can be derived from a knowledge of the partial pressures of oxygen in the inspired air (P_IO_2) and in the mitochondria (P_mO_2; Equation 6a). If one takes as a first approximation that the mitochondria oxygen partial pressure is approximately zero, one can derive maximal oxygen uptake from the relationship between inspired oxygen partial pressure (P_IO_2) and total resistance to oxygen flow (R_{tot}; Equation 6b).

Equation 5: $\dot{V}_{O_2} = \Delta P_1/R_1 = \Delta P_2/R_2 = ... = \Delta P_n/R_n$
Equation 6a: $\dot{V}_{O_2max} = (P_IO_2 - P_mO_2)/R_{tot}$
Equation 6b: $\dot{V}_{O_2max} = P_IO_2/R_{tot}$

It seems useful to stress that we are dealing with resistances to oxygen flow and that the corresponding pressure gradients refer to the fall of oxygen partial pressure across the resistance in question. These equations show that if we know the inspired oxygen partial pressure, as well as the oxygen partial pressure difference across each resistance, together with the maximal oxygen uptake, the total resistance and each individual resistance to oxygen flow can be calculated. Furthermore, endurance training adaptations (Chapter 3) and several artificial manipulations (e.g. autologous reinfusion (blood doping), hypoxia (Chapter 24)), as well as growth, maturation and ageing, can each lead to changes in maximal oxygen uptake without any effects on the overall pressure difference from the environment to the mitochondria. Therefore, the changes of the total resistance to oxygen flow and of the individual resistances that are responsible for the changes of maximal aerobic power can also be pinpointed, provided that the oxygen partial pressure cascade across the various resistances is known. To this end, a set of five physiologically meaningful resistances will be identified, and the oxygen transport equations across each resistance will be made explicit (Equations 7–11 below). These concepts are also developed within Chapters 1 and 10.1.

The first step of the oxygen cascade is the convective transport of oxygen from the environment to the alveoli. From this relationship, one can derive oxygen uptake from alveolar ventilation ($\dot{V}_A$), the oxygen fractional concentrations (F_IO_2, F_AO_2) and partial pressures in the inspired and alveolar gas (P_IO_2, P_AO_2), and the transport coefficient of oxygen in gas (βg: 1.16 mL mm Hg^{-1} at 37°C; Equation 7). The convective transport from inspired to alveolar gas is followed by a diffusive flow of oxygen from the alveoli to the arterial blood (Equation 8), and this depends on a coefficient, which itself is a function of the diffusion capacity of the lungs (D^*_L), and on the alveolar to arterial partial pressure gradient (P_AO_2–P_aO_2). The lung and muscle tissue diffusion coefficients (D^*_T: Equation 10) are a function of, and are dimensionally, but not numerically, equal to the lung or tissue oxygen diffusion capacities (D_L and D_T). Indeed, these capacities are calculated as the differences between the alveolar and the integrated (average) partial pressure of oxygen for the lung capillaries (D_L), and the integrated (average) partial pressure of oxygen for the muscle capillaries and that of the tissue (D_T). The lung and muscle tissue diffusion coefficients (D^*_L and D^*_T) are obtained by replacing the respective capillary oxygen partial pressures with those for arterial blood (P_aO_2) and mixed-venous blood (P_vO_2). Accordingly, they are therefore dimensionally equal but substantially smaller than the corresponding lung or tissue oxygen diffusion capacities. This difference stems from the simplifying assumption on which this whole analysis is based. That is, the resistances to oxygen transport are arranged in series. Hence, the oxygen partial pressure at the end of one resistance must be equal to that at the beginning of the next resistance. For a detailed discussion on this topic, the reader is referred to di Prampero & Ferretti (1990).

Next, there is a convective transport process, which involves the cardiac output ($\dot{Q}$) and the average transport coefficient for oxygen in the blood (or the slope of the blood oxygen dissociation curve: $\beta b = (C_aO_2 - C_vO_2)/(P_aO_2 - P_vO_2)$. It should also be noted that, at variance with the transport coefficient of oxygen in gas, which is constant for any given temperature, the transport coefficient for oxygen in blood varies substantially under different experimental conditions because of the shape of the oxygen dissociation curve, a fact that will be briefly mentioned below and in Chapter 24. The last two steps of the oxygen cascade are the diffusive transport of oxygen from venous blood (P_vO_2) through the intracellular space (P_tO_2) to the mitochondria (P_mO_2), which are a function of tissue diffusion (D^*_T, see above) and the overall capacity of the mitochondria to consume oxygen (M).

Equation 7: $\dot{V}_{O_2} = \dot{V}_A \cdot (F_IO_2 - F_AO_2)$
$= \dot{V}_A \cdot \beta g \cdot (P_IO_2 - P_AO_2)$

Equation 8: $\dot{V}_{O_2} = D^*_L \cdot (P_AO_2 - P_aO_2)$

Equation 9: $\dot{V}_{O_2} = \dot{Q} \cdot (C_aO_2 - C_vO_2)$
$= \dot{Q} \cdot \beta b \cdot (P_aO_2 - P_vO_2)$

Equation 10: $\dot{V}_{O_2} = D^*_T \cdot (P_vO_2 - P_tO_2)$

Equation 11: $\dot{V}_{O_2} = M \cdot (P_tO_2 - P_mO_2)$

Equations 7–11 can be rearranged to make explicit the five major resistances to the oxygen flow from the environment to the mitochondria (Equation 5), thus allowing one to identify the physiological variables that modulate them. These five resistances are defined as follows, and are illustrated in Equations 12–16: ventilatory (R_V), lung diffusive (R_L), cardiovascular (R_Q), tissue diffusive (R_T), mitochondrial (R_M).

Equation 12: $R_V = (P_IO_2 - P_AO_2)/\dot{V}_{O_2} = 1/(\dot{V}_A \cdot \beta g)$

Equation 13: $R_L = (P_AO_2 - P_aO_2)/\dot{V}_{O_2} = 1/D^*_L$

Equation 14: $R_Q = (P_aO_2 - P_vO_2)/\dot{V}_{O_2} = 1/(\dot{Q} \cdot \beta b)$

Equation 15: $R_T = (P_vO_2 - P_tO_2)/\dot{V}_{O_2} = 1/D^*_T$
$= k_t/CSA$

Equation 16: $R_M = (P_tO_2 - P_mO_2)/\dot{V}_{O_2} = 1/M$
$= k_m/[SDA]$

where:

$\dot{V}_A$ and $\dot{Q}$ are at maximal exercise

CSA = cross-sectional area of skeletal muscle capillaries, assumed to be a measure of peripheral diffusion and perfusion

[SDA] = succinate dehydrogenase activity (or fractional mitochondrial volume), assumed to be proportional to mitochondrial oxydative capacity

k_t and k_m are constants necessary for dimensional coherence, and are given a value of 1.

This mathematical approach allowed di Prampero and co-workers (di Prampero 1985, 2003, di Prampero & Ferretti 1990, Ferretti & di Prampero 1995) to estimate changes within any of the above resistances, due to any given manipulation or external stress, from the measured changes of maximal oxygen uptake. Thus, the fractional limitation of maximal aerobic power, due to any given resistance (R_i/R_{tot}), could then be estimated. A detailed analysis and the corresponding calculations will not be reported here, and the interested reader is referred to the original papers where these are reported and discussed in detail. Suffice it to say that the results reported below were derived from data obtained when maximal oxygen uptake, maximal cardiac output, muscle capillary cross-section and mitochondrial succinate dehydrogenase activity were measured before and after the following interventions: endurance training performed with one or two legs; detraining (Chapter 9); blood withdrawal or reinfusion; or computer simulations mimicking maximal exercise at several different inspired oxygen partial pressures.

Table S3.2 Fractional limits to maximal oxygen uptake during exercise at sea level with large (L: cycling, running) or small muscle groups (S: one leg, arms), and at high altitude (5500 m), with large muscle groups only. Fractional limits downstream from the lung are reported in parentheses. At variance with the sea-level conditions, maximal oxygen uptake at high altitude is modulated by cardiovascular as well as by the ventilatory and peripheral resistances (see text for details)

Variable	Sea level		High altitude
	L	S	
$R_V + R_L$	0.36	0.36	0.36
R_Q	0.50 (0.75)	0.32 (0.50)	0.30
$R_T + R_M$	0.14 (0.25)	0.32 (0.50)	0.34

The results of these calculations are summarised below and in Table S3.2. During exercise with large muscle groups (two legs), the major factor limiting maximal oxygen uptake is the oxygen transport capacity, or the product of maximal cardiac output and the oxygen transport coefficient for blood. This is responsible for 70–75% of the factors limiting maximal oxygen uptake downstream of the lungs. Thus, an increase of 10% in this factor, as may be obtained through autologous reinfusion or the administration of erythropoietin, can be expected to lead to an acute (possibly transient) increase of about 7% in maximal aerobic power. The remaining 25–30% of the limits to maximal oxygen uptake are about equally partitioned between the two peripheral resistances: muscle perfusion and diffusion and mitochondrial capacity. Hence, an increase of 10% in either of these two factors can be expected to lead to an increase in maximal oxygen uptake of about 3%.

The data reported above were calculated neglecting the lung as a limiting factor (Chapters 1 and 2) and assuming that, downstream from the lung, the system is linear. However, about 30% of the overall resistance to oxygen flow during maximal exercise is situated at the lung level, since about one-third of the overall oxygen pressure drop from the environment to the mitochondria occurs between inspired air and arterial blood. However, under normoxia, the two resistances to oxygen flow due to the lung (R_V and R_L) cannot be considered as limiting factors, essentially because of the non-linearity of the system at the gas/blood interface. Indeed, in normoxia, the arterial point is located on the flat part of the oxygen dissociation curve. Hence, a decrease of the overall lung resistance, because of an increased alveolar ventilation or lung diffusing capacity, will be offset by an essentially equal increase of the cardiovascular resistance. This is so because the shift to the right of the arterial point will lead to a fall in the average slope of the oxygen dissociation curve, bringing about an increase in the cardiovascular resistance (Equation 14).

During exercise with small muscle groups, the weight of the cardiovascular resistance in setting maximal aerobic power decreases substantially (to about 50% of the total in the case of one-legged cycling), whereas the role of the periphery increases by the same amount. Again, perfusion and diffusion, and the mitochondrial capacity are about equally responsible for the overall peripheral resistance.

During exercise with large muscle groups in hypoxia, the lung becomes progressively more akin to a limiting factor, and the greater the hypoxic stimulus, the greater is this effect. This is so because the arterial point moves progressively towards the steeper part of the oxygen dissociation curve (Chapter 24). As a consequence, any changes in the ventilatory resistance are counteracted to a progressively lesser extent by the opposite changes of the cardiovascular resistance. Thus, the role of the cardiovascular resistance in hypoxia is reduced in direct proportion to the increased role of the lung.

In athletes characterised by a very large maximal oxygen uptake and cardiac output in normoxia, the situation is somewhat similar to that observed with mild hypoxia in less athletic subjects. Indeed, because of the very large maximal cardiac output in these athletes, the pulmonary capillary transit time is reduced to such an extent as to lead to a small, albeit significant desaturation of the arterial blood (arterial hypoxaemia) and this also brings the arterial point towards the steep part of the oxygen dissociation curve.

In conclusion, the main picture emerging from the above analysis is that of a set of factors that share the responsibility for setting a limit for the maximal oxygen uptake. Furthermore, the role of each individual factor can change dramatically with the characteristics of the exercise, the subject and the environment. For example, the overall resistance to oxygen flow during maximal exercise increases with age by the same amount by which maximal oxygen uptake falls. Since mitochondrial oxygen partial pressure can be assumed to be ≈ 0 in all cases, when breathing air at sea level, then the total resistance to oxygen flow can be estimated to be about 5.7 $kPa \cdot L^{-1} \cdot min^{-1}$ (43 $mmHg \cdot L^{-1} \cdot min^{-1}$) in a young (20 year old) moderately active male. In a similar hypothetical subject at 70 years, the total resistance to oxygen flow can be estimated to increase to about 10.5 $kPa \cdot L^{-1} \cdot min^{-1}$ (79 $mmHg \cdot L^{-1} \cdot min^{-1}$). These values were calculated assuming that the maximal oxygen uptake is 3.50 $L \cdot min^{-1}$ at age 20, and that it falls by 9% per decade (Chapter 17.2).

The effects of ageing on the distribution of the total resistance to oxygen flow among the five resistances identified above are rather difficult to disentangle. However, the relative weight of the overall pulmonary resistance can be expected to increase because of the widening of the alveolar to arterial oxygen partial pressure difference (Chapter 16). The resulting fall in the arterial oxygen tension may bring the arterial point closer to the steep part of the oxygen dissociation curve. So, in the elderly, the

Table S3.3 Average values for maximal oxygen uptake ($\dot{V}_{O_{2max}}$), and the ventilatory, cardiovascular, peripheral and total resistances to oxygen flow at age 20 and 70. The ratio of each individual resistance (R_i) to the total resistance (R_{tot}) is also reported at both ages, together with the ratio of each variable at age 70 to age 20. Data were calculated on the basis of the following simplifying assumptions: $P_iO_2 = 20$ kPa (150 mmHg), $P_aO_2 = 12.7$ kPa (95 mmHg: at age 20), 10.0 kPa (75 mmHg: at age 70); mixed venous oxygen partial pressure = 2.7 kPa (20 mmHg). See text for details and references

Age	20	R_i/R_{tot} 20	70	R_i/R_{tot} 70	R_i 70/R_i 20
$\dot{V}_{O_{2max}}$	3.50		1.90		0.53
$R_V + R_L$	15.9	0.37	39.5	0.50	2.48
R_Q	21.4	0.50	29	0.37	1.36
$R_T + R_M$	5.7	0.13	10.5	0.13	1.84
R_{tot}	43		79		1.84

overall pulmonary resistance may be more akin to a limiting factor in the usual sense of this term, as happens in elite athletes and in less athletic subjects in moderate hypoxia.

A rough estimate of the role of the other resistances can be made assuming that the haemoglobin concentration in the blood, and the shape of the oxygen dissociation curve do not change with age. The results of this line of reasoning are reported in Table S3.3, which shows that all resistances increase with age. Because of the widening of the alveolar to arterial oxygen partial pressure difference with age, the increase of the ventilatory resistance is substantially larger than the cardiovascular resistance. The increase of this last can be attributed to the fall of maximal cardiac output which, in turn, is directly proportional to the fall of maximal heart rate, since the stroke volume of the heart remains essentially unchanged with ageing (Chapter 16).

The relative distribution of the cardiovascular and the peripheral resistances downstream from the lung does not seem to change with age, since both at 20 years and at 70, the ratio of these resistances is of the order of 0.74–0.79. However, upon closer scrutiny, this may not be so straightforward. Indeed, in the age range 20–70 years, the muscle mass of the lower body in men decreases on average from 18.5 (SD 3.3) to 13.8 kg (SD 2.9; Janssen et al. 2000). As a first approximation, it seems reasonable to assume that, at the point of maximal oxygen uptake, the whole muscle mass of the lower body is maximally active. If this is so, it seems also reasonable to normalise the peripheral resistance, which is set by muscle perfusion and diffusion, and by mitochondrial capacity, to the lower-body muscle mass. These data show that the normalised peripheral resistances increase with age to a greater extent than do their absolute values. For example, the peripheral resistance per kg of the lower-body muscles increases by a ratio of 2.47, as compared to a ratio of 1.84 for their absolute values. This may indicate that the two peripheral resistances increase with age to a greater extent than reported in Table S3.3, which admittedly was calculated from assumed, rather than measured, oxygen partial pressures.

In children, all resistances can also be expected to be larger, and to decrease with age and maturation. The evolution thereof could be estimated along the same general lines described above.

CONCLUSION

This introduction was directed to a general discussion of the effects of ageing, growth and maturation on maximal performances, with running as a paradigmatic example thereof. However, any other form of locomotion could be treated along analogous lines. Furthermore, the same type of analysis could be applied, with the necessary adjustments, to submaximal exercise. For a more detailed discussion of the factors that limit maximal performances in humans, the reader is referred to Section 1 of this volume, wherein several chapters are devoted to these and related topics.

The general picture emerging from a perusal of the chapters of this section is that, whereas our knowledge of some of the problems at stake is satisfactory, in other cases, it is less so. A tentative summary of this state of affairs is reported in Table S3.4 which reflects the author's opinion and as such, should be taken with a grain of salt. Even so, it is hoped that this Table, together with the preceding paragraphs, will stimulate the reader to experimentally tackle the topics which, on the one hand, need deeper understanding and on the other, seem more directly applicable in practice.

I would like to conclude by highlighting the considerations reported in Chapters 17.1 and 17.2 of this section that, whereas the appropriate dose of exercise does not slow the rate of ageing, it does indeed help us live longer, healthier and (hopefully) happier lives.

Table S3.4 Synopsis of our knowledge of the evolution, with growth, maturation and ageing, of the physiological characteristics that affect human performance

Variable	Growth	Maturation	Ageing
$\dot{V}_{O_2max}$	Good	Good	Good
F	Scarce	Scarce	Scarce
C	Sufficient	Good	Sufficient
Anaerobic capacity	Scarce	Sufficient	Good
Anaerobic power	Scarce	Sufficient	Good
HR_{max}, $\dot{Q}_{max}$	Good	Good	Good
Muscle mass	Good	Good	Good
Muscle structure	Sufficient	Sufficient	Sufficient
Limits to $\dot{V}_{O_2max}$	Scarce	Scarce	Scarce
Gas exchange	Sufficient	Good	Good

$\dot{V}_{O_2max}$, maximal oxygen uptake; F, maximal fraction of maximal oxygen uptake that can be maintained as a function of the exercise duration; C, energy cost of running per kg body mass; HR_{max}, maximal heart rate; $\dot{Q}_{max}$, maximal stroke volume.

References

di Prampero PE 1985 Metabolic and circulatory limitations to V'O2max at the whole animal level. Journal of Experimental Biology 115:319–331

di Prampero PE 2003 Factors limiting maximal performance in humans. European Journal of Applied Physiology 90:420–429

di Prampero PE, Ferretti G 1990 Factors limiting maximal oxygen consumption in humans. Respiratory Physiology 80:113–128

di Prampero PE, Atchou G, Brückner J-C, Moia C 1986 The energetics of endurance running. European Journal of Applied Physiology 55:259–266

di Prampero PE, Capelli C, Pagliaro P, Antonutto G, Girardis M, Zamparo P, Soule RG 1993 Energetics of best performances in middle distance running. Journal of Applied Physiology 74:2318–2324

Ferretti G, di Prampero PE, 1995 Factors limiting maximal oxygen consumption: effects of acute changes in ventilation. Respiratory Physiology 99:259–271

Janssen I, Heymsfield SB, Wanf ZM, Ross R 2000 Skeletal muscle mass and distribution in 468 men and women aged 18–88 yr. Journal of Physiology 89:81–88

Lai N, Saidel GM, Grassi B, Gladden BL, Cabrera ME 2007 Model of oxygen transport and metabolism predicts effect of hyperoxia on canine muscle oxygen uptake dynamics. Journal of Applied Physiology 103:1366–1378

MacDougal JD, Roche PD, Bar-Or O, Moroz JR 1983 Maximal aerobic capacity of Canadian schoolchildren: prediction based on age related oxygen cost of running. International Journal of Sports Medicine 4:194–198

Maliszewski AF, Freedson PS 1996 Is running economy different between children and adults? Pediatric Exercise Science 8:351–360

Scherrer J, Monod H 1960 Le travail musculaire local et la fatigue chez l'homme. Journal de Physiologie (Paris) 52:419–501

Shephard RJ 1969 A non linear solution of the oxygen conductance equation: applications to performances at sea level and at altitude. Internationale Zeitschrift für angewandte Physiologie, einschlisslich Arbeitsphysiologie 27:212–225

Wilkie DR 1980 Equations describing power input by humans as a function of duration of exercise. In: Cerretelli P, Whipp BJ (eds) Exercise bioenergetics and gas exchange. Elsevier, Amsterdam, 75–80

Chapter 15

Physical performance in prepubescent and adolescent males and females: limits, benefits and problems

Thomas W. Rowland

Interest in youth-related exercise physiology has emerged in response to a variety of issues unique to the paediatric age group (Armstrong & Van Mechelen 2000, Bar-Or & Rowland 2004, Rowland 2005). Young athletes are engaging in increasingly intense training regimens, while the safe limits of such athletic participation in growing children is unknown. It is unclear, too, if training schedules and anticipated adaptations in mature athletes can be appropriately transferred to young competitors. At the other end of the exercise scale, concern grows that youth are becoming increasingly sedentary, and that a lifestyle of physical inactivity, persisting into the adult years, may pose a serious long-term health risk (Chapters 17.1 and 28). Attention has been focused, then, on the salutary role that regular exercise in children might play in preventive health efforts. In addition, there is growing interest in the potential therapeutic effects of exercise in children with chronic cardiac, pulmonary and musculoskeletal disease.

Beyond these pragmatic issues, insights into the mechanisms surrounding changes in physical performance, as children grow, might increase our understanding of the physiological bases of physical performance. Children progressively improve in all areas of endurance, strength and short-burst fitness as they grow. It follows that the determinants of exercise performance must evolve in parallel with these trends. Developmental exercise physiology in youth, then, may serve as a model by which the nature of these basic factors can be clarified.

This chapter will examine the physiological changes that accompany the development of physical performance in children and adolescents. The discussion will focus on healthy youth, and features of athletic youth, for the most part, will not be considered. The influence of gender on these characteristics will be addressed, as well as the effect of endocrinological changes surrounding puberty (see also Chapter 11).

In this discussion, it is important that the reader appreciate certain unique issues and caveats involving children that have both limited and challenged our understanding of developmental exercise physiology. Ethical constraints in minors preclude invasive procedures, exposure to environmental extremes and pharmacological interventions (Chapters 19 and 20, Section 6 Introduction). Consequently, the paediatric exercise physiologist cannot utilise techniques or methods that could add valuable insights (e.g. muscle biopsies, hyperthermia). Cause-and-effect issues become complicated, as many variables that rise in close relationship over time are independently associated with the growth process itself. Similarly, the proper means for adjusting physiological variables for increases in body size (a critical issue for understanding exercise physiology in growing subjects) continues to be debated (Nevill 1997, Welsman & Armstrong 2000).

What is clear is that the hallmark of exercise physiology during childhood is change. As children grow, their physical, physiological and performance outcome markers continuously evolve towards the mature state. It will become apparent in the discussions that follow that the patterns of these changes differ over time. Some factors progressively increase during the childhood years (e.g. muscle strength), while others remain relatively stable during the preadolescent years, but then demonstrate sudden changes at puberty (e.g. haemoglobin concentration contributing to a rise in maximal aerobic power in males). Some developmentally related physiological changes are largely the result of increases in body organ size with whole-body growth (e.g. maximal stroke volume). Others are independent of growth (e.g. increases in anaerobic metabolic capacity). Understanding the nature and mechanisms underlying these various developmental curves is a principal challenge of paediatric exercise physiology.

1 ENDURANCE FITNESS

By any marker one wishes to consider, endurance performance improves progressively during the course of childhood. In a traditional model, fixed-distance run times in boys and girls progressively decline from age 5 to age 14 years. The average 14-year-old boy, for example, can cover a 1.6 km (1 mile) in half the time (~7.00 min) that it took him when he was 5 (~14.00 min; American Alliance for Health, Physical Education, Recreation and Dance 1980; Figure 15.1). In the laboratory, a progressive, 30% rise in endurance time is also observed in children between ages 5 and 12 years, using a standardised treadmill protocol (Cumming et al. 1978). Furthermore, on a progressive cycling test, exercise time to exhaustion steadily increases with age (Washington et al. 1988).

Which anatomical and physiological factors might account for this dramatic rise in the threshold for endurance exercise fatigue as children grow? The answer might well be enlightening to exercise physiologists, for whom identifying the critical factors limiting endurance performance at any age remains a central enigma (MacLaren et al. 1989). Unfortunately, few of the many possible physiological determinants of improvements in endurance

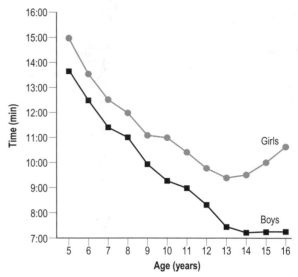

Figure 15.1 One-mile run times in American children and adolescents based on mean values for over 12,000 subjects. Data from the American Alliance for Health, Physical Education, Recreation and Dance (1980).

performance during childhood have been investigated, largely due to ethical constraints. That is, whilst our knowledge concerning central fatigue (Chapters 5 and 10.1), failure of neuromuscular transmission (Chapter 5) or metabolite depletion at exhaustive exercise (Chapters 6 and 7) is well advanced for adults, virtually nothing is known regarding possible developmental changes in these factors. A number of considerations regarding the role of maximal oxygen delivery, as well as running economy, however, may be pertinent.

In any marker of endurance fitness, mean values of performance are consistently better in boys than girls at all ages (Figure 15.1). For example, average finish times in a 1.6 km (1 mile) run at 8 years are 11.00 and 12.00 min for boys and girls, respectively, and at 12 years, 8.00 and 9.30 min (American Alliance for Health, Physical Education, Recreation and Dance 1980). A number of factors may account for this gender difference (e.g. girls have a lower maximal aerobic power, less habitual physical activity, greater body fat content). It is important to note, however, that the rate of improvement in endurance performance over time in this data set is similar in boys and girls. That is, between ages 5 and 12 years, boys shorten these run times by ~42% and girls by ~37%. This observation would suggest that the mechanisms for developmental changes in endurance fitness during childhood are independent of gender.

1.1 Maximal oxygen uptake

Not surprisingly, the maximal ability of a child to utilise oxygen during a progressive exercise test steadily improves

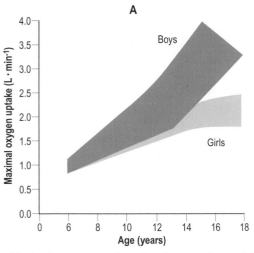

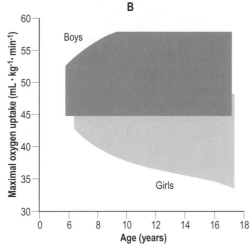

Figure 15.2 Maximal oxygen uptake related to age in youth in absolute values (A) and related to body mass (B). Shaded areas represent data from 1730 girls and 2180 boys as reported in multiple studies. From Bar-Or & Rowland (2004), reprinted with permission.

with age. This attribute is called the maximal (peak) oxygen uptake (consumption) or aerobic power ($\dot{V}_{O_{2max}}$ or $\dot{V}_{O_{2peak}}$), and is largely dependent on size-related variables (cardiac stroke volume, active muscle mass) which are expected to enlarge with growth. Average values for absolute peak aerobic power during treadmill testing in boys increase from about 1.0 L·min^{-1} at age 6 years to 2.8 L·min^{-1} at age 15 (Krahenbuhl et al. 1985). Respective values in females of the same age are slightly less, but can differ by up to 30% in adults (Chapter 11). When expressed relative to body mass (normalised), peak aerobic power does not change in boys during childhood, with a stable average value of approximately 50 mL·kg^{-1}·min^{-1}, while values in girls decline from about 50 mL·kg^{-1}·min^{-1} at age 8 years to 40 mL·kg^{-1}·min^{-1} at age 16 (Figure 15.2). However, expressing oxygen uptake relative to body mass (the ratio standard) may provide spurious values, and normalising to body size using allometric scaling is preferred (Welsman & Armstrong 2000). Although trends in size-normalised maximal oxygen uptake may be somewhat altered by this approach, the overall picture is that it does not change appreciably in either gender over the course of childhood.

Mathematically, the improvements in absolute maximal oxygen uptake during childhood are an expression of increases in maximal cardiac stroke volume, as this is the only component of the Fick Equation (oxygen uptake = stroke volume · heart rate · arteriovenous oxygen difference; Chapter 1) that is influenced by growth (Rowland 2000). Maximal stroke volume reflects resting stroke volume, which in turn is related to left ventricular volume (Nottin et al. 2002, Rowland & Blum 2000). There is no indication of changes in myocardial contractile responses to exercise with growth.

Maximal heart rate during exercise testing remains stable in both boys and girls until the mid-teen years (average ~200 and 195 beats·min^{-1} on treadmill and cycle testing, respectively; Bailey et al. 1978). Thus, formulae used for predicting maximal rate in adults (such as 220–age) are not applicable in this age group. Maximal arterial venous oxygen difference does not change during childhood (Yamaji & Miyashita 1977), but an increase (and surge in absolute $\dot{V}_{O_{2max}}$) is seen with the androgen-stimulated rise in haemoglobin concentration in males at puberty (Rowland et al. 1997). Since absolute maximal oxygen uptake, measured over time in the prepubertal years, is affected only by changes in organ (i.e. heart) size, it is not surprising that, when adjusted for body size, it does not change with age (at least in boys) in the preadolescent years.

1.1.1 Maximal oxygen uptake and endurance performance

In any group of adult subjects with heterogeneous levels of fitness, endurance performance is closely linked with maximal oxygen uptake. This observation supports a model of fatigue in which the limits of circulatory oxygen delivery constrain exercise performance (Chapter 10.1), and provides a laboratory marker of aerobic or endurance fitness (also see debate in Chapter 10.2). The same findings are seen in children. For example, Rowland et al. (1999) reported a correlation of 0.77 between a time distance run and maximal oxygen uptake normalised to body mass in 12-year-old boys, with the latter typically being 40–50% higher in highly trained prepubertal endurance athletes than in non-athletes (Rowland 1997).

While the importance of oxygen delivery in endurance fitness in children is thereby supported, it is intriguing to observe that change in maximal oxygen uptake appears to have no role in the development of endurance fitness over time, during childhood. As noted above, normalised maximal oxygen uptake (mL·kg⁻¹·min⁻¹) remains stable in boys until at least age 16 years, while values in females actually slowly decline from age 8 onwards. The average American 5-year-old boy can run 1.6 km (1 mile) in 13.46 min and 10 years later, his finish time will be 7.14 (Figure 15.1). During this time, however, his maximal oxygen uptake will remain unchanged at ~50 mL·kg⁻¹·min⁻¹. Changes in maximal aerobic power, then, clearly cannot explain the dramatic improvements occurring at the same time in endurance fitness (Chapter 10.2).

1.1.2 Gender differences

Among adults, men generally demonstrate a 30% higher maximal oxygen uptake compared to women and this gender difference can be explained largely by differences in body composition and haemoglobin content that occur at the time of puberty (Chapter 11). Among prepubertal children, the gender difference in mean absolute maximal aerobic power is already evident, but the gap is narrower, about 12–15% (Krahenbuhl et al. 1985). This difference can be accounted for by the greater development of muscle mass in boys and body fat in the girls, as no significant differences in blood haemoglobin concentration are seen before the age of puberty. Once body composition is considered, physiological aerobic fitness is not substantially different between prepubertal boys and girls (Welsman et al. 1977).

1.2 Submaximal exercise economy

While maximal oxygen uptake does not contribute to the development of endurance performance during childhood, changes in submaximal oxygen utilisation over time may be more pertinent. Most particularly, during running or walking, the metabolic (oxygen uptake) demands of a given level of work, expressed relative to body mass, gradually fall as a child ages (Kanaley et al. 1989). As indicated in Figure 15.3, these maturational differences in exercise economy are far from trivial. Among a group of 10-year-old boys, the energy requirement of running on a treadmill, at four submaximal speeds, was 15–20% greater than that in young adult men (Unnithan & Eston 1990). This improvement in metabolic demand of weight-bearing activities has been linked to developmental gains in endurance performance since, as a result, the relative intensity (percent $\dot{V}_{O_{2max}}$) of a given level of work falls as the child ages (Figure 15.4).

Whether gender differences exist in submaximal exercise economy among children is an unsolved issue. Quite puzzling is the observation that approximately half of the studies have concluded that girls, in general, are more economical than boys, while the other half reveal no gender difference; none, however, has described superior economy in boys. Several explanations have been offered for a greater

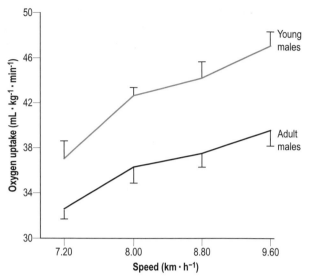

Figure 15.3 Submaximal oxygen uptake at four different treadmill speeds in 10-year-old boys and young adult men. From Unnithan & Eston (1990), reprinted with permission.

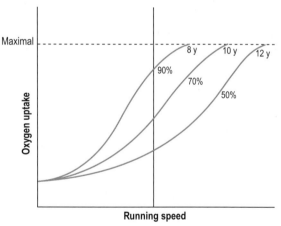

Figure 15.4 As children age, improvements in running economy cause them to exercise at a relatively lower intensity (percent maximal oxygen uptake) at the same treadmill speed. From Rowland (2005), reprinted with permission.

economy in young females: girls have a lower resting metabolic rate than boys, carry more body fat and may possess different biomechanical characteristics. At present, however, the question of possible gender differences in exercise economy among children remains unresolved.

Changes in economy, then, are clearly associated with developmental improvements in endurance performance. The above observations, however, beg the question of why submaximal energy demands decline throughout childhood. The issue has received considerable research attention, since the answer would help clarify possible mechanisms behind increasing endurance fitness during childhood. As a result, the potential roles of the many contributors to energy demands during exercise have come under scrutiny.

1.2.1 Muscular efficiency

As will be reviewed below (cellular metabolic determinants), certain biochemical differences distinguish children from adults (glycolytic capacity, aerobic enzyme activity). Could these processes in some way affect the efficiency of energy transfer or contraction coupling in the muscle cell? Muscular energy efficiency has been compared in children and adults by assessing delta efficiency (difference between energy demand for work achieved at two different workloads), as well as net efficiency (comparison of efficiency at a given work load compared to that at rest). These have not revealed significant differences between children and adults.

Cooper et al. (1984) reported average values of delta efficiency of 28% and 29% in 6- and 18-year-old boys, respectively, during cycle exercise. Rowland et al. (1990) found that, above a cycling intensity of 50% maximal oxygen uptake, mean net efficiency in prepubertal boys and young men was almost identical (~19%). It appears, then, that differences in exercise economy in children and adults cannot be explained by maturational variations in the energy efficiency of the muscle contractile process itself.

1.2.2 Stride frequency

Biologists have long recognised that the metabolic cost of running or walking in mature animals progressively declines as the animal increases in size. While running at $2 \, km \cdot h^{-1}$, the oxygen consumption (expressed relative to body mass) of a squirrel is three times that of a pony, yet only half that of a mouse (Taylor et al. 1984). This observation has traditionally been explained on the basis of differences in animal stride frequency. That is, energy demands relative to body size during locomotion should be expressed per stride, and when doing so, these energy requirements become similar regardless of the size of the animal.

For paediatric exercise physiologists, these observations in animals suggest that improvements in running economy during growth are related to increases in body size itself (rather than some other aspect of biological maturation), and that differences in stride frequency, based on leg length, might explain the decline in energy demands of locomotion as children grow. Research evidence has supported these concepts. Stride frequency in prepubertal boys, during treadmill running, is approximately 17% greater than young adults (Rowland et al. 1987). In cross-sectional studies, the energy cost of running at a given speed, when normalised to body mass and stride frequency, is similar in children and adults, and independent of biological maturation (Ebbeling et al. 1992, Rowland et al. 1987, Unnithan & Eston

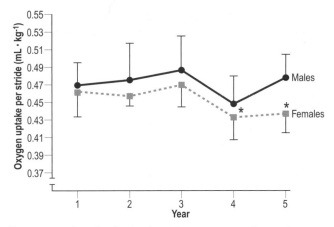

Figure 15.5 Longitudinal values for oxygen uptake per kg per stride at a given treadmill speed in boys and girls. From Rowland (1996), reprinted with permission.

1990). In a longitudinal study, Rowland & Cunningham (unpublished data) found that oxygen uptake per kg per stride during treadmill walking did not change in children between the ages of 9 and 13 years, while economy improved progressively (Figure 15.5).

Maliszewski & Freedson (1996) compared the oxygen cost of treadmill running at the same speed, and then at a speed adjusted for body size (leg length), in 9–11-year-old children and young adults. As expected, at an identical treadmill speed ($9.6 \, km \cdot h^{-1}$), energy demands were greater in the children ($40.6 \pm 2.6 \, mL \cdot kg^{-1} \cdot min^{-1}$ versus $34.9 \pm 3.2 \, mL \cdot kg^{-1} \cdot min^{-1}$). However, no significant difference in economy was observed when exercising at a speed adjusted for body size (37.7 ± 2.8 (children) versus $39.0 \pm 3.5 \, mL \cdot kg^{-1} \cdot min^{-1}$).

These findings would suggest that developmental changes in energy economy during weight-bearing exercise can largely be explained by anatomical differences in leg length and stride frequency. When the exercise task is adjusted for body size, children and adults appear to demonstrate no differences in running or walking economy. As a corollary, then, it may be suggested that improvements in endurance performance as children grow may be explained primarily on an anatomical rather than on physiological, biochemical or biomechanical bases.

1.2.3 Biomechanical factors

By common observation, the running style of children is less fluid than that of adults. In fact, a number of specific differences in the gait of children have been documented: young children demonstrate a greater vertical displacement, increased leg joint extension at take-off, greater time in the non-support phase of the stride and smaller relative distance of the support foot ahead of the centre of gravity (Foley et al. 1979, Wickstrom 1983). Differences in linear displacements, velocities and acceleration of body segments, as well as high peak vertical ground forces, have also been described in very young children (2–6 years).

Documenting the extent to which these differences might affect energy utilisation during exercise in children has been difficult. However, Ebbeling et al. (1992) examined biomechanical features (joint angles at touchdown, maximum flexion, total range of motion) during treadmill exercise in 8–10-year-old boys and young men, who demonstrated the expected differences in economy (mean oxygen uptake 19.7 and 15.0 mL·kg^{-1}·min^{-1}, respectively). They concluded that the magnitude of differences in biomechanical features in the two groups was insufficient to explain variations in exercise economy.

Findings of Frost and colleagues (1997) indicated that developmental differences in muscle co-contraction might help explain changes in exercise economy. Co-contraction, the activation of an antagonist muscle to maintain joint stability, was found to be 30% greater in 7–8 year olds compared to 10–12 year old subjects, at different treadmill speeds. This corresponded to an energy cost of locomotion that was ~20% greater in the former group. The explanation for the greater degree of co-contraction in the younger children remains uncertain.

1.2.4 Other determinants

Other factors have been examined that might alter energy requirements during exercise in children versus adults. The magnitude of the contribution of any of these determinants to the overall differences observed in exercise economy during childhood is uncertain, but would seem to be small.

Elastic elements in the limbs can alter the muscular force and therefore the energy demand of locomotion. It has been suggested, then, that elastic recoil forces could contribute to interindividual differences in exercise economy. Some evidence exists that such forces might be less developed in children than adults, but any maturational differences have yet to be quantified (Schepens et al. 1998).

Resting energy expenditure, relative to body size, falls throughout the course of childhood. It is tempting, then, to suggest that the decline in submaximal energy requirements, as children grow, is only a parallel reflection of trends in resting values. Unfortunately, this simple explanation does not hold up after mathematical analysis. When resting oxygen uptake is subtracted from submaximal values, the gap in energy demands of exercise between adults and children is diminished, but significant differences remain (Robinson 1938).

Efficiency of ventilation is less in children than adults. Prepubertal subjects ventilate more than adults for each litre of oxygen consumed during exercise; that is, they have a higher ventilatory equivalent for oxygen (Andersen et al. 1974). The extra energy cost of this inefficiency is small at low levels of exercise but increases as intensity rises. At maximal levels of exercise, the added energy demands might be substantial, as ventilation may account for 14–19% of maximal oxygen uptake.

1.3 Cellular metabolic determinants

The cellular metabolic *milieu* within the contracting muscle is recognised to be a critical determinant of exercise endurance performance. Several lines of evidence indicate that some biochemical features differ in children compared to adults, and that these variations evolve as the child grows. The extent to which such changes might influence development of endurance performance capabilities, however, remains problematic.

1.3.1 Aerobic enzyme activity

Energy production for endurance activity relies on aerobic (oxygen-dependent) metabolic processes within the cell, most particularly the rate of oxidative phosphorylation in the Krebs cycle and the electron transport chain. In adults, biopsy studies indicate that endurance fitness can be linked to aerobic enzyme activity within these metabolic pathways.

Information in children is limited because of ethical barriers to invasive muscle measurement techniques. However, the small window provided by available data suggests that cellular aerobic enzyme activity decreases with increasing age. Haralambie (1980) reported citrate synthase activity in vastus lateralis muscle of 30 U·g^{-1} and 20 U·g^{-1} in 5–7-year-old children and mature adults, respectively. Berg et al. (1986) described an inverse relationship between cellular fumerase activity and age in children 6–17 years old. In that study, mean citrate synthetase activity was 22% lower in the oldest compared to youngest group.

These scant findings in children mimic those previously described in animals. An inverse relationship has clearly been indicated between body mass of adult animals and mitochondrial aerobic enzyme activity (Kunkel et al. 1956). Again, this is a matter of body size rather than biological maturation; cells from larger animals consume less oxygen and have lower aerobic enzyme activity than cells from smaller animals. The explanation for a lower size-specific metabolic rate with greater body size has been a matter of extensive unresolved debate for biologists. The same phenomenon appears to be evident in human children, but the implications of these characteristics of the resting muscle cell to energy production with exercise and endurance performance remain to be clarified.

1.3.2 Substrate utilisation

The means by which carbohydrates and lipids are utilised as energy substrate during exercise has also been considered a central factor to the limits of physical endurance (Chapter 7). In particular, traditional tenets hold that depletion of glycogen stores, the primary fuel for muscle contraction, leads to fatigue and defines one's endurance exercise capacity. Consequently, factors that would increase carbohydrate stores and spare glycogen utilisation during exercise are expected to enhance endurance fitness.

There is reason to believe that children rely more on fatty acid oxidation than glycogen for energy during endurance exercise. But, once again, how this might cause immature subjects to differ in endurance performance compared to adults is not known. As will be outlined further in the discussion below on short-burst activities, considerable evidence indicates that the capacity for glycolysis is inferior in children. As a result, some but not all research findings indicate that children may shift to the alternative means of fatty acid oxidation for metabolic fuel during exercise.

Riddell et al. reported (2000, 2001), for example, that in 10–14 and 14–17-year-old subjects, fats contributed to 50% and 30%, respectively, of the energy requirements of submaximal cycling. Martinez & Haymes (1991) found that values for the respiratory exchange ratio, a marker of substrate utilisation, indicated lower carbohydrate utilisation in 8–10-year-old girls compared to adult women. However, some observations during exercise must be interpreted cautiously, since the respiratory exchange ratio only reflects cellular metabolism under steady-state conditions, due to the effect of breathing pattern on carbon dioxide production (when measured at the mouth).

1.3.3 Are children metabolic non-specialists?

Bar-Or (1983) was the first to suggest that, when it comes to sports performance, children may be metabolic non-specialists compared to adults. He noted that during the childhood years, the youngster who is the star athlete in a particular sport (e.g. basketball) often excels in many other types of sports (such as swimming, tennis, baseball). This is in distinction to adults, who tend to be specialists in certain types of activities. That is, an Olympic marathon runner would not be expected to function very well in full-contact sports. Bar-Or suggested that before puberty, lack of aerobic or anaerobic metabolic differentiation might account for this phenomenon.

The studies examining this issue have provided conflicting results and the issue is not yet resolved. Correlations between absolute measures of oxygen uptake, muscle strength and anaerobic testing in children have generally been high (Docherty & Gaul 1991, Falk & Bar-Or 1993, Suei et al. 1998), but these associations could be accounted for by parallel increases in body size alone. When values are expressed relative to body size, such correlations often disappear. Murphy (2000) found correlation coefficients of 0.40–0.56 between maximal oxygen uptake and anaerobic power (Wingate testing) normalised (adjusted allometrically) for body size in both untrained 10-year-old girls and 22-year-old women. This indicated that metabolic non-specialisation was equally evident in children and adults who were not trained athletes.

The latter study suggests that observations of specialisation by sport type, in adults compared to children, might reflect variations in trainability, rather than maturational metabolic differences. That is, what has been interpreted as metabolic specialisation in adults might indicate the greater ability of the mature individual to improve in a certain sport with training. Alternatively, greater sport specialisation in adults might reflect somatotypic differentiation that occurs at the time of puberty. Many of the features that permit sport specialisation, such as large muscle mass in the weight lifter, occur at puberty. What appears to be metabolic specialisation in the adult, then, might be an expression of somatotype specialisation.

1.4 Responses to endurance training

Previously sedentary adults who are placed in a programme of regular (three times a week) endurance exercise, performed at least 20–30 minutes at a moderately high intensity, will be expected to improve their maximal oxygen uptake by ~15–30%. Such people are high responders to adaptation stimuli for this physiological attribute (Chapter 21). This endurance training effect represents the collective adaptation of the multiple determinants of oxygen delivery and utilisation, including increases in plasma volume, ventricular diastolic size, maximal stroke volume, cellular enzyme activity and muscle capillarisation.

In prepubertal children, however, such responses of maximal aerobic power to identical endurance training programmes are dampened, and a number of studies have failed to reveal significant increases (see Rowland 2005). On average, a rise in maximal oxygen uptake of approximately 5% is expected in this age group (Payne & Morrow 1993) and there appears to be no gender difference in this response.

The explanation for this maturational difference in aerobic trainability remains elusive. However, examining this issue might pay dividends in a better understanding of factors that influence physiological adaptations to endurance training in general.

There is some evidence to suggest that children might require a longer period of training to effect changes in maximal oxygen uptake. For example, most studies in this age group involve training programmes of no more than 12 weeks in duration, but the three longest (15 weeks, 28 weeks, 18 months) also reported the greatest change (10.3%, 12.2% and 18.9%, respectively; Mobert et al. 1997, Williford et al. 1996, Yoshizawa et al. 1997). It has been suggested, too, that the higher intrinsic daily activity levels of children might provide a training stimulus and thus, there is a less pronounced response to formal endurance training programmes. This has been deemed unlikely, however, since the daily, short-burst activities of children are not the type expected to stimulate changes in aerobic fitness (Bailey et al. 1995), and little or no relationship has been observed between levels of habitual physical activity and maximal oxygen uptake in this age group (Morrow & Freedson 1994).

A physiological explanation for the dampened maximal aerobic power response to training in children is plausible but the component of the cardiovascular response to training that is blunted in children, and why this might be so, remains conjectural. Although not formally documented, the limited training response in young subjects is presumed to be demarcated by puberty. Thus, endocrinological changes during adolescence that might affect training influences need to be considered. For example, both testosterone and oestrogen are recognised to increase blood volume; thus, maturational differences in blood volume response to training might be important. Also, there is evidence from animal studies that the degree of increase in muscle aerobic enzyme activity with training may be inversely related to body size (Lewis & Haller, cited by Simoneau et al. 1990).

It is unclear whether or not the limited physiological response to aerobic training in prepubertal children can be translated into a diminished capacity for improving endurance performance with training. Studies addressing this issue have been confounded by the many influences on endurance performance, such as learning effects, growth, motivation, strategising and environmental conditions. An answer to this question would be most useful, however, for structuring age-appropriate training schedules for young endurance athletes.

2 SHORT–BURST (ANAEROBIC) FITNESS

In contrast to endurance exercise, which is unusual in the daily lives of children, youngsters typically engage in short-burst activities, lasting from a few seconds to not more than a minute or two. This type of exercise has received less research attention in the paediatric age group, probably because it has not been linked specifically to health outcomes. However, energy for short-burst activities is derived largely from anaerobic metabolism, and the available research regarding short-burst activities has provided insights into the evolution of anaerobic fitness as children grow.

2.1 Sprint performance

Sprinting is the most commonly used field performance marker of anaerobic fitness, as a 40 m or 50 m dash can be expected to rely principally on glycolytic energy metabolism. As the child grows, performance in such events steadily improves, although changes in sprint performance are more marked in boys than girls. The average finish time in a 50 yard dash in 10-year-old boys, of about 8.5 s, shortens to 6.8 s at age 16 years. Respective times for girls are 8.6 s and 8.0 s (American Alliance for Health, Physical Education, Recreation and Dance 1980).

A host of anthropometric, anatomical, neural, biomechanical and metabolic factors might contribute to this improvement in short-burst fitness. Interestingly, current data appear to indicate that glycolytic metabolic capacity is not a central determinant of changes in sprint performance during childhood. Instead, most of this improvement can

be accounted for by increases in body size per se: longer stride length with greater force applied per stride, as a result of increasing muscle mass.

Sprint performance during childhood has been closely linked to body height (and presumably leg length) in both cross-sectional (Mero 1998) and longitudinal studies (Shephard et al. 1980). On the other hand, sprint times expressed relative to body mass steadily decline as a child grows. This is of interest, since markers of metabolic anaerobic capacity (see below) increase with respect to body mass, over the same time. This conforms to findings in adults that sprints do not exhaust anaerobic metabolic capacity (Weyand et al. 1999). Leg muscle force production rises as children grow in direct proportion to the mass that needs to be moved in the sprint (Shephard et al. 1980). Patterns of motor unit recruitment as children age, and how this might affect sprint performance, have not been investigated. Nerve conduction speed does not appear to be affected by biological maturation (Garcia et al. 2000).

Information on muscle fibre types and their relationship to sports performance in children is necessarily limited. Mero and colleagues (1990) reported that 11–13-year-old athletic boys who were sprinters, weightlifters or tennis players had a greater number of fast-twitch (type II) muscle fibres than a group of endurance runners. This conforms to concepts developed in adult athletes. However, whether changes in muscle fibre type distribution as children age might affect the development of athletic performance has not been fully clarified. Indeed, fibre composition may, through self-selection, dictate sports participation.

Muscle fibre type populations are generally considered genetically fixed early in life, but some studies have suggested developmental changes (Lexell et al. 1992). Of course, muscle fibre types are determined by the innervating motor unit and, while the histochemical properties are responsive to training stimuli, the fibres themselves can only change type following reinnervation.

2.2 Laboratory (Wingate) testing

The Wingate test, which measures power production during a 30 s all-out cycling bout, has been considered the best laboratory indicator of anaerobic fitness. Extensive normative data are available in children, providing a developmental picture of anaerobic capacity, and a number of correlative studies have been performed with both biochemical and performance markers of anaerobic fitness (Bar-Or 1987).

During childhood, absolute measures of anaerobic power rise progressively in both boys and girls (Bar-Or 1983). Mean power at age 8 years is approximately 160 W, rising to 275 W at age 12. Values are similar in boys and girls until puberty, when a spurt is seen in the males. When these values are adjusted for body mass, the increase is less dramatic but still persists (Figure 15.6). From this information, it can be concluded that anaerobic power, as estimated by Wingate testing, improves at a faster rate than can be

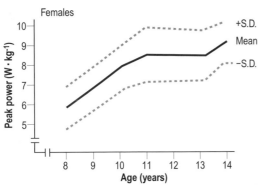
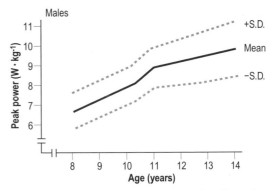

Figure 15.6 Peak anaerobic power expressed relative to body mass in boys and girls during Wingate anaerobic testing. From Bar-Or & Rowland (2004), reprinted with permission.

explained by gains in body size and muscle mass alone. This conclusion is consistent with other data (see below) suggesting that size-independent factors that might contribute to anaerobic fitness, particularly glycolytic capacity, improve during the course of childhood.

Power measured on Wingate testing has been associated with field sprint performance, with varying correlation coefficients ranging from 0.23 to 0.84 (Almuzaini 2000, Van Praagh et al. 1989, 1990). From this information, Bar-Or (1987, p. 388) noted that 'one may conclude that the correlation between the Wingate anaerobic test power indices and anaerobic performance is quite high but not high enough for using the Wingate anaerobic test as a predictor of success in these specific tasks'.

2.3 Biochemical markers

Unlike the maximal oxygen uptake test, there exists no simple and universally applied laboratory measure of anaerobic fitness. However, if the child's capacity for anaerobic metabolic output during exercise changes with growth, one would expect to observe parallel developmental variations in biochemical markers of anaerobic metabolism. Indeed, evidence from serum lactate concentrations and anaerobic enzyme activity with muscle biopsies supports improvements in anaerobic function with age, although the literature is limited.

2.3.1 Serum lactate concentrations

As lactic acid is a byproduct of glycolytic metabolism, serum lactate levels during exercise have been used as an indicator of anaerobic metabolic capacity. This is not without detractors: serum lactate levels can be influenced by not only cellular production but also blood clearance, rate of muscle cell release, rate of utilisation by other organs and volume of distribution. Moreover, there exist a number of methodological issues, including timing and mode of blood sampling (see Chapters 6, 7 and 10.3 for detailed

discussion). Accordingly, such observations need to be interpreted cautiously, particularly if neither lactate production nor its removal is quantified.

Notwithstanding these caveats, a number of studies have indicated that blood lactate concentration at maximal exercise rises significantly over the course of childhood and equivalently in both boys and girls. A summary of six such cross-sectional studies indicated a rise from 6 mmol·L^{-1} at age 6 years in boys to 10 mmol·L^{-1} at age 15 (Rowland 2005). Similar findings were observed by Paterson et al. (1986) in a 5-year longitudinal study. Corresponding to this trend, blood pH at the end of exercise decreases as children grow (Bar-Or 1983).

The consistency of these lactate data supports the concept that anaerobic metabolic capacity improves during childhood. As noted above, though, the influence of this metabolic trend on physical performance of children remains to be demonstrated.

2.3.2 Anaerobic enzyme activity

If metabolic anaerobic fitness improves during childhood, one would expect to find evidence of lower glycolytic enzymatic activity in children compared to adults. In fact, the meagre amount of research data supports this concept. Most frequently cited is the vastus lateralis biopsy study of five boys by Eriksson et al. (1973). This indicated an average activity of phosphofructokinase, a possible rate-limiting enzyme in the glycolytic cascade, of 8.4 μmol·g^{-1}·min^{-1}, which was about half that observed in other studies of adults.

Berg et al. (1986) described a direct correlation of activity of both pyruvate kinase and aldolase with age (0.45 and 0.35, respectively) in vastus lateralis specimens in children aged 4–18 years. This trend in anaerobic enzyme activity was confirmed by Haralambie (1980), who reported that activities of these two enzymes in 5–9-year-old children were approximately half that of adults. It has been pointed out, however, that this information describes glycolytic metabolic function at rest and provides no insights regarding responses to exercise (Van Praagh 2000).

2.4 Ventilatory anaerobic threshold

The anaerobic threshold defines the intensity, during a progressive exercise test, at which blood lactate concentration begins to rise. While the interpretation and physiological significance of this measure remain highly debated (Chapters 6 and 10.3), the anaerobic threshold has been viewed by many as a general indicator of the balance of aerobic and anaerobic fitness in this testing model. The anaerobic threshold can be estimated non-invasively by the point of divergence of the rise in oxygen uptake and minute ventilation (Owles point, ventilatory threshold); that is, the point beyond which ventilation starts to rise disproportionately faster than oxygen uptake. While the physiological mechanisms that explain this point, and even its derivation, are vigorously debated (Chapter 10.3), it does appear to be quite reproducible.

In a study of 6–12-year-old children, Hebestreit et al. (2000) reported a correlation of 0.92 between the ventilatory threshold, and peak oxygen uptake. In children, as in adults, this threshold may thus be used as a submaximal marker of aerobic fitness. Interestingly, the ventilatory threshold, as a percentage of maximal oxygen uptake, is higher in children than adults, and a 6-year longitudinal study of children surrounding the age of peak height velocity (Vanden Eynde & Van Gerven 1989) found that the threshold fell from 68% to 59% of maximal oxygen uptake. This observation has been interpreted as indicating improvements in anaerobic capacity as children grow.

2.5 Responses to anaerobic training

Whether a period of training with intense, short-burst activities will affect the various markers of anaerobic fitness in children is not altogether clear. One is left with a number of methodological problems in performing such investigations. For instance, what constitutes an appropriate training stimulus (type, duration, frequency and intensity of exercise)? How can one separate out responses purely of an anaerobic nature (e.g. improved glycolytic capacity) from those of strength, neural input and aerobic fitness? In field tests such as sprints, how does one account for a learning effect of improved strategy, skill and motivation?

These issues notwithstanding, some information is available regarding metabolic, laboratory and field performance responses of children to a period of anaerobic training. Eriksson et al. (1973) reported a rise in muscle phosphofructokinase activity from 8.4 ±1.5 to 15.4 ±1.6 $\mu mol\ g^{-1} \cdot min^{-1}$ after 6 weeks of endurance cycle training in 11-year-old boys. Similar endurance training regimens have failed to indicate any change in maximal blood lactate concentration. For example, Prado (1997) studied the effects of a 6-week

anaerobic swim training programme of repeated sprints in 11-year-old boys and young adult males. The adults improved their performance on a 100 m sprint, but no changes in performance were seen in the children. No increases in maximal blood lactate were seen in either group.

Improvements in sprint times were reported following training in one study of prepubertal male soccer players (Diallo et al. 1999) but not in another (Mosher et al. 1985). Several studies have indicated small but significant improvements in peak and mean power during Wingate testing in children following anaerobic training (Grodjinovsky et al. 1980, Rotstein et al. 1986, Sargeant et al. 1985). Taken together, these data do not provide a clear picture of the plasticity of markers of anaerobic fitness to training in children.

3 MUSCLE STRENGTH

Absolute measures of muscle strength improve steadily during the course of childhood (Figure 15.7). This trend is observed regardless of muscle group or mode of testing (isometric or isokinetic). Strength in boys and girls is similar until the preadolescent years, when the improvement curve begins to become accentuated in males (Blimkie 1989). By age 17, the pubertal effects of testosterone in males account for their twofold greater strength compared to females (Chapter 11).

Increase in muscle mass is the most obvious explanation for this developmental rise in strength, as cross-sectional muscle area is closely linked to force production. However, factors independent of changes in body size and composi-

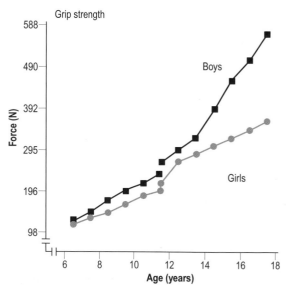

Figure 15.7 Grip strength in children relative to age. From Malina & Bouchard (1991), reprinted with permission.

tion appear to also contribute to improvements in skeletal muscle strength that occur during the childhood years.

3.1 Muscle size

Muscle cell (myocyte) number is fixed at birth or during early infancy and subsequent growth of muscle mass during childhood involves fibre hypertrophy. The curves of estimated muscle mass for boys and girls mimic almost exactly those of increases in various measures of muscle strength (Malina & Bouchard 1991). Before puberty, gender differences in muscle development are small, with mean values for boys consistently, albeit not dramatically, greater than girls. At puberty, males demonstrate an accelerated growth of muscle mass in response to androgenic stimulation, with average muscle mass, relative to total body mass, rising from 42% at 5 years to 53% at 17 years. A similar trend is not observed in females.

As expected, a close relationship has been observed between measures of muscle strength and muscle cross-sectional area, as children grow. In studies involving young subjects in a wide age range, correlation coefficients as high as 0.90 are typical (Blimkie 1989, Malina 1975). There is evidence, however, that development of skeletal muscle mass in children cannot fully explain improvements in muscle strength with growth. For example, according to dimensionality theory, muscle strength should relate to both muscle cross-sectional area and the square of body height. However, studies indicate that empirically measured strength gains during childhood are greater than can be explained by height squared. For example, Carron & Bailey (1974) reported a 22.7% increase in the annual rise in strength in 10–16-year-old boys, while the rise expected from changes in height squared was only 12.1%.

These observations suggest that other, size-independent factors, besides changes in muscle size, contribute to the development of muscle strength in children. This idea is further supported by the observation that improvements in muscle strength with resistance training in prepubertal children are not typically accompanied by increases in muscle size.

3.2 Neural influences

The contractile force of muscle is influenced by its innervation characteristics and developmental changes in neurological influences could contribute to the development of strength during childhood. Insights are limited, however, by the technical difficulty of measuring innervation characteristics of exercising muscle, particularly in children.

Most studies of nerve conduction velocity have indicated that maximal values do increase during childhood, with adult levels being approached at an early age (4–5 years; Garcia et al. 2000). Thus, it would appear unlikely that conduction velocity contributes to improvements in muscle strength across the paediatric years. Little is known

regarding other potential neurological variables. Motoneuron firing rate and pattern of recruitment of motor units during exercise remain unexplored in the childhood age group.

At present, technical limitations preclude any conclusion regarding the presumed role of neurological factors in the development of strength in children. Limited information in children undergoing resistance training outlined below does, however, provide some supportive evidence.

3.3 Muscle fibre characteristics

Developmental changes in the intrinsic contractile function of skeletal muscle could help explain improvements in strength over time. However, studies addressing the question of whether or not muscle function in children is qualitatively different from adults have provided conflicting results. It does appear that the metabolic recovery of skeletal muscle is faster in children than adults (Hebestreit et al. 1996), and this is reflected in a slower decline in strength with repeat activations (Kanehisa et al. 1995).

Possible changes in muscle fibre architecture with growth have also been examined. The angle of pennation in skeletal muscle affects strength production, and some evidence suggests that this angle may change as children grow. Using ultrasound measurements, Fukunga & Kawakami (cited by Blimkie & Sale 1998) reported that the pennation angle in the vastus lateralis muscle increases by 35% over the childhood and adolescent years. However, a comparison of strength in children and adults related to ultrasound measurements by Kanehisa et al. (1994) suggested that pennation angle did not play a significant role in developmental changes in muscle strength.

Maturational changes in central inhibition or the limitation of peripheral muscle contractile force by the central nervous system could help explain strength changes with growth. Studies utilising the interpolated twitch technique, where supramaximal electrical stimuli are applied beyond that of voluntary muscle activation, have provide limited support for this idea (Belanger & McComas 1989, Blimkie 1989).

3.4 Response to resistance training

Historically, prepubertal children were considered incapable of achieving gains in skeletal muscle strength from resistance training, due to a lack of circulating testosterone. Weight training in youth was further discouraged because of concerns of potential damage to growth tissues, in particular the ephiphyseal plates. Research performed over the past two decades has dramatically altered this picture, indicating that both prepubertal boys and girls are, in fact, capable of improving muscle strength with resistance training. Gains from such training have been quantitatively equivalent to those observed in adults. Moreover, the safety of strength training by youth in properly supervised programmes has been documented. Consequently, resistance training has been advocated for injury prevention, improved athletic performance and health outcomes (bone health, obesity treatment) in the prepubertal age group.

3.4.1 Strength gains

In a metaanalysis of 28 studies, Payne et al. (1997) reported an overall improvement in strength training in children and adolescents ranging from 30–40% over an 8–12-week period. No relationship to quantitative strength response to training and age was observed. In a similar analysis of studies involving only children under age 12–13 years, the mean response was 13–30% (Falk & Tenenbaum 1996). The magnitude of these improvements was considered equivalent to those expected in studies of young adults. No training difference was observed between boys and girls, and this challenges the notion that strength development requires the presence of high circulating concentrations of testosterone. Importantly, too, no injuries were reported, supporting the safety of resistance training in youth, at least in supervised settings.

3.4.2 Mechanisms

In virtually all of these studies, the observed improvements in strength with resistance training in prepubertal subjects were not accompanied by increases in skeletal muscle mass. Thus, at least one aspect of historical dogma appears to have been true: before the age of androgen stimulation at puberty, children cannot be expected to improve muscle bulk with resistance training. This phenomenon does raise an interesting question with mechanistic implications. Lacking increases in muscle cross-sectional area, what accounts for the improvements in strength with resistance training in prepubertal subjects?

In adults, supportive evidence exists for the role of neural adaptations in strength responses to a period of resistance training. Increased electromyographic activity, maximal motoneuron firing rate, velocity of force production and a reduction in muscle co-contraction have all been reported in responses to weight training programmes. These same mechanisms have been presumed to account for the size-independent strength responses to training in children. However, experimental evidence to implicate neural mechanisms in this age group is scant.

Ozmun et al. (1994) reported a 17% increase in electromyographic amplitude after 8 weeks of resistance training in eight prepubertal children. In that programme (dumbbell biceps curls), isometric and isokinetic arm strength rose by 23% and 28%, respectively. Ramsay et al. (1990) demonstrated a 22–35% increase in strength but no change in muscle cross-sectional area, after 20 weeks of training in 13 prepubertal boys. A trend was observed for changes in motor unit recruitment in the elbow flexors and knee extensors, but it did not reach statistical significance.

4 CONCLUSION

During the growing years, progressive improvements are witnessed in virtually all measures of physical performance. These changes are observed regardless of testing modality, duration or expected metabolic demand. Deciphering the determinants of these developmental changes offers an important opportunity for understanding basic mechanisms underlying human muscle performance.

A review of the information provided in this chapter suggests that the progressive improvements in physical performance during childhood are principally the consequence of parallel increases in body dimensions. Improvements in endurance performance are linked to changes in stride frequency, sprint performance is associated with leg length and power production, and muscle strength is most prominently influenced by muscle cross-sectional size. At the same time, there exist intriguing clues that size-independent factors may also contribute to developmental changes in all these forms of fitness.

Average differences in physical performance between boys and girls are evident throughout childhood. Generally, before the preteen years, these mean differences are small, but as puberty is achieved, significant advantages are seen in males compared to females (Chapters 11 and 14.2). Most evidence indicates that gender differences in performance in children are related to variations in body size and composition. Once these are accounted for, little variability between the genders is observed.

References

Almuzaini KS 2000 Optimal peak and mean power on the Wingate test: relationship with sprint ability, vertical jump and standing long jump in boys. Pediatric Exercise Science 12:349–359

American Alliance for Health, Physical Education, Recreation and Dance 1980 Youth fitness testing manual. Washington, DC

Andersen KL, Seliger V, Rutenfranz J, Messel S 1974 Physical performance capacity of children in Norway. Part III. Respiratory responses to graded exercise loadings-population parameters in a rural community. European Journal of Applied Physiology 33:265–274

Armstrong N, Van Mechelen W (eds) 2000 Paediatric exercise science and medicine. Oxford University Press, Oxford

Bailey DA, Ross WD, Mirwald RL, Weese C 1978 Size dissociation of maximal aerobic power during growth in boys. Medicine in Sport 11:140–151

Bailey RC, Olson J, Pepper SL, Porszasz J, Barstow TJ, Cooper DM 1995 The level and tempo of children's physical activities: an observational study. Medicine and Science in Sports and Exercise 27:1033–1041

Bar-Or O 1983 Sports medicine for the practitioner. Springer Verlag, New York, 311–314

Bar-Or O 1987 The Wingate anaerobic test. Update on methodology, reliability and validity. Sports Medicine 4:381–394

Bar-Or O, Rowland TW 2004 Pediatric exercise medicine. From physiological principles to health care application. Human Kinetics, Champaign, IL

Belanger AY, McComas AJ 1989 Contractile properties of human skeletal muscle in childhood and adolescence. European Journal of Applied Physiology 58:563–567

Berg A, Kim SS, Keul J 1986 Skeletal muscle enzyme activities in healthy young subjects. International Journal of Sports Medicine 7:236–239

Blimkie CJR 1989 Age- and sex-associated variation in strength during childhood: anthropometric, morphological, neurologic, biochemical, endocrinologic, genetic and physical activity correlates. In: Gisolfi CV, Lamb DR (eds) Youth, exercise and sport. Benchmark Press, Indianapolis, 133–166

Blimkie CJR, Sale DG 1998 Strength development and trainability during childhood. In: Van Praagh E (ed) Pediatric anaerobic performance. Human Kinetics, Champaign, IL, 193–224

Carron AV, Bailey DA 1974 Strength development in boys from 10 to 16 years. Journal of the Society for Research in Child Development 39:1–37

Cooper DM, Weiler-Ravell D, Whipp BJ, Wasserman K 1984 Aerobic parameters of exercise as a function of body size during growth in children. Journal of Applied Physiology 56:628–634

Cumming GR, Everatt D, Hastman L 1978 Bruce treadmill test in children: normal values in a clinic population. American Journal of Cardiology 41:69–75

Diallo O, Doré E, Hautier C, Duche P, Van Praagh E 1999 Effect of jump and sprint training on athletic performance in prepubescent boys (abstract). Medicine and Science in Sports and Exercise 31 (Suppl):S317

Docherty D, Gaul CA 1991 Relationship of body size, physique and composition to physical performance in young boys and girls. International Journal of Sports Medicine 12:525–532

Ebbeling CJ, Hamill J, Freedson PS, Rowland TW 1992 An examination of efficiency during walking in children and adults. Pediatric Exercise Science 4:36–49

Eriksson BO, Gollnick PD, Saltin B. 1973 Muscle metabolism and enzyme activities after training in boys 11–13 years old. Acta Physiologica Scandinavica 87:485–497

Falk B, Bar-Or O 1993 Longitudinal changes in peak aerobic and anaerobic mechanical power of circumpubertal boys. Pediatric Exercise Science 5:318–331

Falk B, Tenenbaum G 1996 The effectiveness of resistance training in children: a meta-analysis. Sports Medicine 22:176–186

Foley CD, Quanbury AO, Steinke T 1979 Kinematics of normal child locomotion – a statistical study based on TV data. Biomechanics 12:1–6

Frost G, Dowling J, Dyson K, Bar-Or O 1997 Cocontraction in three age groups of children during treadmill locomotion. Journal of Electromyography and Kinesiology 7:179–186

García A, Calleja J, Antolín FM, Berciano J 2000 Peripheral motor and sensory nerve conduction studies in normal infants and children. Clinical Neurophysiology 111:513–520

Grodjinowsky A, Inbar O, Dotan R, Bar-Or O 1980 Training effect on the anaerobic performance of children as measured by the Wingate anaerobic test. In: Berg K, Eriksson BO (eds) Children and exercise IX. University Park Press, Baltimore, MD, 139–145

Haralambie G 1980 Activites enzmatiques dans le muscle squelettique des enfants de divers ages (Enzymatic activity in the skeletal muscle of children of various ages). In: Le sports et l'enfant. Euromed, Montpelier, 243–258

Hebestreit H, Meyer F, Htay-Htay, Heigenhauser GJ, Bar-Or O 1996 Plasma metabolites, volume and electrolytes following 30-s high intensity exercise in boys and men. European Journal of Applied Physiology 72:563–569

Hebestreit H, Staschen B, Hebestreit A 2000 Ventilatory threshold: a useful method to determine aerobic fitness in children? Medicine and Science in Sports and Exercise 32:1964–1969

Kanaley JA, Boileau RA, Massey BH, Misner JE 1989 Muscular efficiency during treadmill walking: the effects of age and workload. Pediatric Exercise Science 1:155–162

Kanehisa H, Ikegawa S, Tsunoda N, Fukunaga T 1994 Strength and cross-sectional area of knee extensor muscles in children. European Journal of Applied Physiology 68:402–405

Kanehisa H, Okuyama H, Ikegawa S, Fukunaga T 1995 Fatigability during repetitive maximal knee extensions in 14-year old boys. European Journal of Applied Physiology 72:170–174

Krahenbuhl GS, Skinner JS, Kohrt WM 1985 Developmental aspects of maximal aerobic power in children. Exercise and Sport Science Reviews 13:503–538

Kunkel HO, Spalding JF, de Francisis G, Futrell MF 1956 Cytochrome oxidase activity and body weight in rats and in three species of larger animals. American Journal of Physiology 186:203–206

Lexell J, Sjöström M, Nordlund AS, Taylor CC 1992 Growth and development of human muscle: a quantitative morphological study of whole vastus lateralis from childhood to adult age. Muscle and Nerve 15:404–409

Maclaren DP, Gibson H, Parry-Billings M, Edwards RH 1989 A review of metabolic and physiological factors in fatigue. Exercise and Sport Science Reviews 17:29–66

Malina RM 1975 Anthropometric correlates to performance. Exercise and Sport Science Reviews 3:249–274

Malina RM, Bouchard C 1991 Growth, maturation and physical activity. Human Kinetics, Champaign, IL, 111–131

Maliszewski AF, Freedson PS 1996 Is running economy different between children and adults? Pediatric Exercise Science 8:351–360

Martinez LR, Haymes EM 1991 Substrate utilization during treadmill running in prepubertal girls and women. Medicine and Science in Sports and Exercise 24:976–983

Mero A 1998 Power and speed training in childhood. In: Van Praagh E (ed) Pediatric anaerobic performance. Human Kinetics, Champaign, IL, 241–267

Mero A, Kauhanen H, Peltola E, Vuorimaa T, Komi PV 1990 Physiological performance capacity in different prepubescent athletic groups. Journal of Sports Medicine and Physical Fitness 30:57–66

Mobert J, Koch G, Humplik O, Oyen EM 1997 Cardiovascular adjustment to supine and seated postures: effect of physical training. In: Armstrong N, Kirby BJ, Welsman JR (eds) Children and exercise XIX. Spon, London, 429–433

Morrow JR, Freedson PS 1994 Relationship between habitual physical activity and aerobic fitness in adolescents. Pediatric Exercise Science 6:315–329

Mosher RE, Rhodes EC, Wenger HA, Filsinger B 1985 Interval training: the effects of a 12-week programme on elite prepubertal male soccer players. Journal of Sports Medicine 25:5–9

Murphy SE 2000 The relationship between aerobic and anaerobic power in untrained pre- and post-menarcheal females. Unpublished Master's thesis, University of Massachusetts, Amherst, MA

Nevill AM 1997 The appropriate use of scaling techniques in exercise physiology. Pediatric Exercise Science 9:295–298

Nottin S, Vinet A, Stecken F, Nguyen LD, Ounissi F, Lecoq AM, Obert P 2002 Central and peripheral cardiovascular adaptations during maximal cycle exercise in boys and men. Medicine and Science in Sports and Exercise 33:456–463

Ozmun JC, Mikesky AE, Surburg PR 1994 Neuromuscular adaptations following prepubescent strength training. Medicine and Science in Sports and Exercise 26:510–514

Paterson DH, Cunningham DA, Bumstead LA 1986 Recovery O_2 and blood acid: longitudinal analysis in boys aged 11 to 15 years. European Journal of Applied Physiology 55:93–99

Payne VG, Morrow JR 1993 The effect of physical training on prepubescent VO$_2$max: a meta-analysis. Research Quarterly for Exercise and Sport 64:305–313

Payne VG, Morrow JR Jr, Johnson L, Dalton SN 1997 Resistance training in children and youth: a meta-analysis. Research Quarterly for Exercise and Sport 68:80–88

Prado LS 1997 Lactate, ammonia and catecholamine metabolism after anaerobic training. In: Armstrong N, Kirby B, Welsman J (eds) Children and exercise XIX. Human Kinetics, Champaign, IL, 306–312

Ramsay JA, Blimkie CJ, Smith K, Garner S, MacDougall JD, Sale DG 1990 Strength training effects in prepubescent boys. Medicine and Science in Sport and Exercise 22:605–614

Riddell MC, Bar-Or O, Schwarcz HP, Heigenhauser GJ 2000 Substrate utilization in boys during exercise with [13C]-glucose ingestion. European Journal of Applied Physiology and Occupational Physiology 83:441–448

Riddell MC, Bar-Or O, Wilk B, Parolin ML, Heigenhauser GJ 2001 Substrate utilization during exercise with glucose and glucose plus fructose ingestion in boys ages 10–14 yr. Journal of Applied Physiology 90:903–911

Robinson S 1938 Experimental studies of physical fitness in relation to age. Arbeitsphysiologie 10:251–323

Rotstein A, Dotan R, Bar-Or O, Tenenbaum G 1986 Effects of training on anaerobic threshold, maximal aerobic power and anaerobic performance of preadolescent boys. International Journal of Sports Medicine 7:281–286

Rowland TW 1996 Development exercise physiology. Human Kinetics, Champaign, IL, 178

Rowland TW 1997 The aerobic trainability of athletic and non-athletic children. In: Froberg K, Lammert O, St Hansen H, Blimkie CJR (eds) Exercise and fitness. Odense University Press, Odense, 183–192

Rowland TW 2000 Cardiovascular function. In: Armstrong N, Van Mechelen W (eds) Paediatric exercise science and medicine. Oxford University Press, Oxford, 163–171

Rowland TW 2005 Children's exercise physiology. Human Kinetics, Champaign, IL

Rowland T, Blum JW 2000 Cardiac dynamics during upright cycle exercise in boys. American Journal of Human Biology 12:749–759

Rowland TW, Auchinachie JA, Keenan TJ, Green GM 1987 Submaximal running economy and treadmill performance in prepubertal boys. International Journal of Sports Medicine 9:187–194

Rowland TW, Staab JS, Unnithan VB, Rambusch JM, Siconolfi SF 1990 Mechanical efficiency during cycling in prepubertal and adult males. International Journal of Sports Medicine 11:452–455

Rowland TW, Popowski B, Ferrone L 1997 Cardiac responses to maximal upright cycle exercise in healthy boys and men. Medicine and Science in Sports and Exercise 29:1146–1151

Rowland T, Kline G, Goff D, Martel L, Ferrone L 1999 One-mile run performance and cardiovascular fitness in children. Archives of Pediatric and Adolescent Medicine 153:845–849

Sargeant AJ, Dolan P, Thorne A 1985 Effects of supplementary physical activity on body composition, aerobic and anaerobic power in 13-year old boys. In: Binkhorst RA, Kemper HCG, Saris WH (eds) Children and exercise XI. Human Kinetics, Champaign, IL, 140–150

Schepens B, Willems PA, Cavagna GA 1998 The mechanics of running in children. Journal of Physiology 509:927–940

Shephard RJ, Lavallee H, LaBarre R 1980 On the basis of data standardization in prepubescent children. In: Ostyn M (ed) Kinanthropometry II. Karger, Basel, 306–316

Simoneau J-A, Hood DA, Pette D 1990 Species-specific response in enzyme activities of anaerobic and aerobic energy metabolism to increased contractile activity. In: Taylor AW, Gollnick PD, Green HJ, Ianuzzo CD, Noble EG, Metivier G, Sutton JR (eds) Biochemistry of exercise VII. Human Kinetics, Champaign, IL, 95–104

Suei K, McGillis R, Calvert R, Bar-Or O 1998 Relationships among muscle endurance, explosiveness and strength in circumpubertal boys. Pediatric Exercise Science 10:48–56

Taylor CR, Heglund NC, Maloiy GMO 1984 Energetics and mechanics of terrestrial locomotion. I. Metabolic energy consumption as a function of speed and body size in birds and mammals. Journal of Experimental Biology 97:1–21

Unnithan VB, Eston RG 1990 Stride frequency and submaximal running economy in adults and children. Pediatric Exercise Science 2:149–155

Van Praagh E 2000 Development of anaerobic function during childhood and adolescence. Pediatric Exercise Science 12:150–173

Van Praagh E, Falgairette G, Bedu M, Fellmann N, Coudert J 1989 Laboratory and field test in 7-year old boys. In: Oseid S, Carlsen K-H (eds) Children and exercise XIII. Human Kinetics, Champaign, IL, 11–17

Van Praagh E, Fellmann N, Bedu M, Falgariette G, Coudert J 1990 Gender differences in the relationship of anaerobic power output to body composition in children. Pediatric Exercise Science 2:336–348

Vanden Eynde B, Van Gerven D 1989 Endurance fitness and peak height velocity in Belgian boys. In: Oseid S, Carlson K-H (eds) Children and exercise XIII. Human Kinetics, Champaign, IL, 19–26

Washington RL, van Gundy JC, Cohen C, Sondheimer HM, Wolfe RR 1988 Normal aerobic and anaerobic exercise data for North American school-age children. Journal of Pediatrics 112:223–233

Welsman JR, Armstrong N 2000 Statistical techniques for interpreting body size-related exercise performance during growth. Pediatric Exercise Science 12:112–127

Welsman JR, Armstrong N, Kirby BJ, Winsley RJ, Parsons G, Sharpe P 1997 Exercise performance and magnetic resonance imaging-determined thigh muscle volume in children. European Journal of Applied Physiology 76:92–97

Weyand PG, Lee CS, Martinez-Ruiz R, Bundle MW, Bellizzi MJ, Wright S 1999 High-speed running performance is largely unaffected by hypoxic reductions in aerobic power. Journal of Applied Physiology 86:2059–2064

Wickstrom RL 1983 Fundamental motor patterns. Lea and Febiger, Philadelphia

Williford HN, Blessing DL, Duey WJ 1996 Exercise training in black adolescents: change in blood lipids and VO$_2$max. Ethnicity and Disease 6:279–285

Yamaji K, Miyashita M 1977 Oxygen transport system during exhaustive exercise in Japanese boys. European Journal of Applied Physiology 36:93–99

Yoshizawa S, Honda H, Nakamura N, Itoh K, Watanabe N 1997 Effects of an 18-month endurance run training program on maximal aerobic power in 4- to 6-year old girls. Pediatric Exercise Science 9:33–43

Chapter 16

The physiology of ageing in active and sedentary humans

Herbert Groeller

1 WHAT IS AGEING?

In its broadest sense, ageing refers to all time-related events that occur in the life of a human or organism. Ageing affects all organisms and inanimate objects. Consider a bridge. Immediately it is erected, some ageing or deterioration of the structure will commence. The maintenance workers on the bridge are analogous to the repair processes within an organism. Should the number or productivity of the workers decline, or the inherent properties of the structural elements decrease, deterioration of the bridge will result. In most cases, ageing of inanimate objects results in adverse changes. However, human ageing is not always associated with a decline in structural or functional integrity. Indeed, ageing in the adolescent results in significant growth and marked improvements in a broad range of physiological functions (Chapter 15), and this may be somewhat analogous to new and more advanced materials being added to the bridge. In contrast, tissue damage outstrips repair activity in the older individual, leading to physical decline.

While both adolescents and older individuals are characterised as ageing, in this chapter, the principal focus will be upon the physiological adaptations that occur exclusively to the older individual (>65 years), or during senescence. Ageing is also covered in other chapters within this text, including Chapters 13 (postmenopausal women), 17.1 (daily exercise requirements), 17.2 (maximal aerobic power), 28 (lifestyle and disease) and 31.1 (penalties of physical inactivity). Therefore, topics covered within those chapters are not discussed in this chapter.

1.1 The demographic dimension of ageing

An understanding of the dynamics of population-based changes in ageing allows for an appreciation of the magnitude of ageing-related shifts within the community. Too often, the focus of our efforts in physiology can be upon discrete biological changes that occur with age, without serious consideration of population-based impacts. This section provides a broad introductory overview of population-based shifts due to ageing in the global community, and how these shifts in population can be measured and interpreted.

The changing demographics of ageing are highlighted by the following statistics. The ten nations with the most people aged 65 years and older, were estimated to have a cumulative ageing population of 147 million in 1975 (WHO 1998). By 2050, these nations are predicted to have a total ageing population in excess of 915 million, representing a sixfold increase within just 75 years, with China and India accounting for 63% of this number (WHO 1998). The upward shift in population age is made starker in light of the predicted reduction in world population growth from 2050. Indeed, the number of people older than 70 years will accelerate between 2025 and 2050, growing in excess of 50% (WHO 1998).

One variable that has powerfully influenced the rise in the mean population age is the increase in average life expectancy of humans, which has risen 66% and 71% for males and females respectively since the 1900s. In 1970, the average life expectancy in developed countries was estimated to be 74 years, and by 2025 this is anticipated to rise to 82 years (WHO 1998). Eastern Mediterranean and South East Asian countries are predicted to have a 20-year increase in average life expectancy over this period (WHO 1998).

These data highlight the significant rise in the proportion of ageing individuals in the world and it is against this background that we will explore ageing populations. While these data are helpful to understanding the shift in ageing populations, they provide no indication of when ageing (senescence) actually begins. For instance, chronological age is the conventional means of measuring age of a population or individual. But a significant increase in average lifespan has also increased the time during which individuals are healthy, and living and working independently (Arking 2006). Thus, chronological age on its own can be misleading, and it has been suggested that a better way to consider ageing in a population is not via the calculation of average chronological age but by estimating the years remaining until death (Sanderson & Scherbov 2005). For example, a 30-year-old in 2040 may have a life expectancy of 60 years while in 1990 a 20-year-old may have had the same life expectancy. Both individuals would be given the same standardised age. Using this type of analysis, Sanderson & Scherbov (2005) predicted that the standardised median age would decline slightly, representing an increase in youthfulness and functional capacity of the population. Thus, the average person aged 65 years in 1950 would be likely to have a lower health status and level of independence than the average person aged 65 years in 2050. How then can ageing be represented to give an indication of the commencement of senescence? One way is to calculate the standard mortality rate for ageing cohorts within different age bands.

Survival curves are a graphical representation of life tables, and these allow one to understand shifts in the

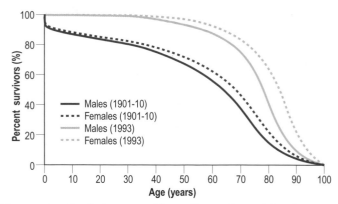

Figure 16.1 Survival curves of Australian males and females during 1901–10 and 1993. Modified from Australian Bureau of Statistics (1995) with permission.

population survival (longevity) over time. Figure 16.1 shows the survival curves for Australian males and females in 1901–10 and in 1993. These data reflect those found in many countries, and they show that in the early 1900s, 10–15% of the population died in the first 5 years of life (infant mortality), as represented by a significant downward displacement of the gender-specific survival curves. The primary impact during the 20th century on these curves was a significant attenuation of premature death (Arking 2006). By 1993, significant gains in survival were made both in the middle-aged and older adults. Thus, the 1993 survival curves were higher and extended further to the right, before showing more rapid increases in mortality. These trends are real but do they reflect changes in the biological rate of ageing during this period?

It has long been known that the death rate is exponentially related to age (Arking 2006). However, there are periods during which the mortality rate of certain groups deviates from this relationship, and these are illustrated in Figure 16.2. For instance, there is initially a high mortality rate in infants, which reaches its lowest point at 10 years. This point may be representative of the population being at its healthiest, with the mortality increase beyond this age possibly marking the onset and continuation of ageing (Arking 2006). A second increase in mortality is observed among teenagers and adults up to 30 years, with a possible overrepresentation among males, and this change is associated with an increased probability of risk-taking behaviours.

Figure 16.2 (logarithmic scale) shows the rise in age-specific mortality until advanced old age. It has been proposed that the linear portion of this relationship provides evidence of senescence (Finch et al. 1990), from which was developed an index of ageing: the mortality rate doubling time. This index defines the duration over which it takes

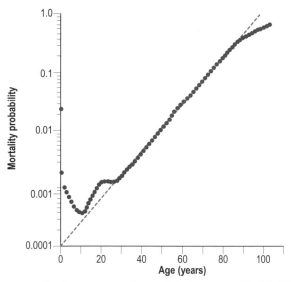

Figure 16.2 The human mortality probability curve. Modified from Arking (2006) with permission.

the mortality rate to increase twofold, such that a higher mortality rate doubling time may signify slower ageing within and across species. For example, humans are estimated to have a mortality rate doubling time of 8.0 years, a horse 4 years and a mouse 1.2 years. This index is of considerable interest for the investigation of human ageing. For instance, Masoro (1995) compared the mortality rate doubling time for US women in 1997 (8.0 years) with that of female prisoners of war in 1945 (7.7 years). Despite the prisoners having a 100-fold greater mortality rate, the mortality rate doubling time between the two cohorts was very similar. This indicates that the actual rates of ageing did not vary between the groups (Masoro 1995).

2 THE MEASUREMENT OF AGE–RELATED PHYSIOLOGICAL CHANGES

Ageing appears to result in significant changes to a wide range of physiological variables but, in a population which has a life expectancy of approximately 80 years, how should these variables be investigated? The choices that investigators make when considering this question will have a marked impact upon how the experimental observations should be interpreted. Indeed, one may need to apply filters to the available literature, such that a clear and valid understanding of human ageing can be obtained. In this section, some aspects of this filtration process are examined.

2.1 Experimental design

The most common experimental design used to investigate the effects of ageing is the cross-sectional design. In this design, researchers simultaneously obtain population samples from several different age groups, thereby providing a snapshot or point of time analysis of age effects. This design does not allow for the direct measurement of the effects of ageing per se, as would be the case if a sample was studied over many years (longitudinal design). Instead, researchers using this design must infer the effects of ageing on the basis of responses and observations obtained from the different cohorts.

Consider for a moment differences in the life experiences of two relatives, one 90 years old and the other 30 years old, both of whom may be recruited to participate in such an investigation. The dietary practices, both in quality and quantity, of the older individual are likely to have varied significantly over the life of that person. Since diet affects stature, and since stature co-varies with several physiological functions (e.g. static lung volumes), then age-related comparisons of such functions can be influenced by factors that are unrelated to ageing, causing apparent ageing to be masked or even exaggerated. Such age-specific experiences that relate only to one subject group are termed cohort effects, and these can confound the interpretation of ageing trends.

A second challenge is to consider the impact of selective mortality. Let us say there are two age groups in a cross-sectional investigation: an 85-year-old and 20-year-old cohort. The elderly group contains individuals who are older than the average human life expectancy, and are therefore clearly well adapted for life. In contrast, the younger group contains individuals who may die at a relatively young age or who may survive to an older age. Therefore, this latter group may be considered to be more representative of the human population while the former, through subject attrition, contains only those individuals possessing superior survival traits. Comparisons between two such samples are not necessarily going to elucidate physiological ageing.

A third challenge is to ensure that an appropriate age range is used for cross-sectional sampling. For example, if one investigator selects subjects from people in the range 20–50 years old, while another chooses subjects in the 20–90 years range, then two different impressions of ageing may be obtained (Lakatta 1993).

Therefore, whilst cross-sectional designs are frequently the pragmatic option, it must be recognised that observations of ageing inferred from discrete groups across a broad age range may not necessarily reflect the way that individuals age. To make such an inference, a longitudinal experimental design is required. In this design, repeated observations are made on the same group of subjects. However, subjects in a longitudinal investigation may, for a variety of reasons, including improved interest in their own health due to participating in such research, modify lifestyle habits (e.g. nutrition and exercise) during the course of the investigation. This type of experimental design is relatively costly to conduct and is susceptible to subject drop-out. The repeated assessment of some effort- or skill-related variables may see practice effects becoming apparent, thus changes may not necessarily be due to an ageing effect, but may reflect enhanced skill in performing the assessment task.

From this discussion, it becomes clear that the robustness of an experimental design hinges significantly on the composition of the cohorts recruited for the investigation. Inappropriate cohort selection and recruitment can reduce the validity of the experimental data and their applicability for inferring changes due to the ageing process.

2.2 Cohort selection

An 80-year-old person has aged 20 years more than a 60-year-old individual. This is a straightforward and accurate assumption. However, chronological age does not necessarily provide an indication of how ageing has affected the body structures and regulatory systems, and how it has interacted with the effects of the environment. The former group of changes are known as primary ageing and these describe the gradual process of bodily deterioration throughout life. On top of this process are the influences of disease and environmental exposures. Consider the pulmonary function of two individuals aged 60 years. One has spent 40 years working in a highly toxic environment, for which adequate respiratory protection only became available 15 years before retirement. The other worked in a physically demanding trade and successfully competed as an endurance athlete from 15 years to 60 years. It would not be unreasonable to expect to observe differences in pulmonary function between these individuals. However, such differences may not necessarily reflect primary ageing, but the impact of disease and environmental influences in addition to ageing. Such an impact is called secondary ageing (Masoro & Austad 2006).

The difficulty in separating subjects who are diseased from those who are ageing in the absence of disease is immense. For example, of the 60% of males who die over the age of 60 years from heart disease, only 15–20% have obvious clinical symptoms (Lakatta 1993). Furthermore, as screening technology develops and standards change, so do the definitions of disease. For instance, the definition of hypertension has changed in relation to the level of systolic blood pressure and its classification as a disease. Similarly, bone loss, which is a common and progressive occurrence with increasing age, is classified as a pathological state (osteoporosis) when it reaches a critical point. Screening procedures are increasingly more sensitive in the detection of pathological conditions. However, if one wishes to investigate primary ageing, in the absence of secondary ageing affects, then such screening significantly limits subject participation, and will result in the selection of subjects who are atypical of contemporary human health (Chapters 28 and 30). Primary ageing does not acknowledge disease processes that are age dependent such as osteoporosis, atherosclerosis and degenerative joint diseases. Thus, any definition of ageing should include age-dependent disease processes, as ageing in the absence of disease is very rare (Masoro & Austad 2006).

Consideration of these points goes to the very centre of ageing research. In whom do we wish to investigate ageing: people with our evolutionary phenotype (physically active hunters and gatherers) or chronically sedentary people in whom secondary ageing affects may be prevalent? Sedentary behaviour is associated with a significant elevation in the risk of developing chronic diseases (Chapters 28 and 31.1), such as diabetes (Manson et al. 1992), hypertension (Blair et al. 1984) and cardiovascular disease (Manson et al. 2002, Tanasescu et al. 2002). Furthermore, the relative risk of all-cause mortality is significantly elevated in men and women of low physical fitness (Blair et al. 1996). In contrast, moderate and higher levels of cardiorespiratory fitness are associated with a considerably lower death rate (Blair et al. 1996).

With these considerations in mind, it has been suggested that experimental designs should be modified to use physically active subject groups as the experimental control group (Booth & Lees 2006, Booth et al. 2000). Physical activity should be treated as the normal state, with physical inactivity as an abnormal manifestation of human physiology. The rationale of this suggestion is based on evidence that indicates that certain human genes require a minimal level of physical activity to prevent the occurrence of abnormal phenotypic expression (Booth et al. 2000, Rowe & Kahn 1987). Thus, using physically active cohorts may significantly reduce the influence of secondary ageing, and the associated loss of physical function, on experimental observations, thereby allowing greater insight into successful ageing and the development of age-dependent diseases (Rowe & Kahn 1987). For instance, Tanaka & Seals (1997) examined the effects of ageing on physiological functional capacity in masters swimming athletes, and the use of highly trained, older athletes has been suggested as a possible model with which to examine normal and successful ageing (Bortz & Bortz 1996, Hawkins et al. 2003).

In addition, one must also consider how best to study a particular physiological system. To illustrate this, we shall briefly consider the cardiovascular system. The resting human cardiovascular system functions at approximately one-fifth to one-tenth of its maximal capacity (Chapter 1). Therefore, investigations of the resting cardiovascular system do not adequately describe the function of this system, and differences with ageing may also fail to be revealed (Lakatta 1995). When people are physically stressed, differences between younger and older individuals may become increasingly more apparent. However, physical stress tests for older subjects may affect a wider range of physical, physiological and psychological factors. For instance, during a progressive (graded) exercise test, exercise termination may be due to non-cardiovascular factors, and the capacity of the cardiovascular system in the aged individual may therefore be grossly underestimated.

3 CARDIOVASCULAR FUNCTION

3.1 Myocardial structure and function

Ageing of the myocardium is associated with a small and gradual increase in cardiac mass from the third to the ninth decades. This increase in myocardial mass and left ventricular wall thickness appears to occur independently of factors known to increase the work of the heart, such as hypertension with its associated increase in afterload (Gerstenblith et al. 1977), or a decrease in work of the heart as a consequence of declining levels of physical activity. The origin of this myocardial hypertrophy appears to be related to an increase in cardiomyocyte size, while the cardiomyocyte number is decreased. However, by the ninth decade, a decrease in heart mass has been observed (Olivetti et al. 1995). Despite these age-related structural changes, there appears to be a minimal impact on resting cardiac performance.

3.1.1 Systolic function

At rest, healthy older persons appear to have a left ventricular ejection fraction (an index of systolic performance) similar to that of younger individuals (Fleg et al. 1995). However, during exhaustive exercise, younger subjects are able to increase ejection fraction to a level that is more than 20% higher than observed in the healthy aged, as illustrated in Figure 16.3 (Fleg et al. 1995). Thus, the end-systolic blood volume is significantly lower in the young heart during exercise.

Despite an apparent failure of the aged heart to fully utilise the end-diastolic volume, stroke volume index (mL·m^2) does not significantly decline with ageing. During

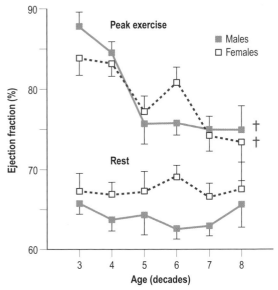

Figure 16.3 Changes in resting and peak exercise left ventricular ejection fraction in males and females with ageing. Modified from Fleg et al. (1995) with permission.

submaximal exercise, end-diastolic volume index is maintained similarly in younger and older cohorts, but during exhaustive exercise, disparate responses are observed. For example, the end-diastolic volume index in a young cohort will drop slightly below resting levels, but in aged adults, there is a net increase in diastolic volumes compared to the resting state, suggesting that diastolic filling must be greater during exhaustive exercise in the aged, and this appears to be the case (Fleg et al. 1995).

3.1.2 Diastolic function

Diastolic performance of the ageing myocardium changes significantly. Although left ventricular diastolic volume during supine rest does not necessarily change in the aged heart, the manner in which the heart is filled is altered. For example, the early-phase diastolic filling in an 80-year-old left ventricle is reduced by approximately half, as indicated by a decline in early phase ventricular to atrial filling ratio. However, this decrement is compensated by a more vigorous atrial contraction and greater ventricular filling (preloading). The end-diastolic volume index increases similarly in the young and aged during submaximal exercise. In contrast, during exhaustive exercise, a diminishing end-diastolic volume index is observed in the young but not healthy aged. This is contrary to a popular belief that diastolic filling is not compromised in the aged during intense exercise (Lakatta & Levy 2003b).

3.1.3 Arterial structure and function

Blood vessels contain various proportions of elastic (elastin) and inelastic (collagen) connective tissue, as well as vascular smooth muscle. These components participate actively and passively in the modulation of blood vessel diameter (Chapters 1 and 3). With ageing, there is a loss of elastin, a fragmentation of existing elastin and an increased collagen production, and these changes lead to a cascade of modifications to the ageing vascular structures. For example, ageing arteries have an increased vessel stiffness (reduced compliance), diameter, wall thickness and vessel length (Lakatta 1993, Learoyd & Taylor 1966, Reneman et al. 1985). These modifications are marked, with a two–threefold increase in the thickness of the inner membrane of the carotid arteries occurring between 20 and 90 years (Lakatta & Levy 2003a). The increase in vessel diameter shifts the aortic pressure volume curve to higher volumes, and the concomitant decline in aortic compliance (dispensability) increases the pulse pressure for a given change in volume. Changes in arterial compliance are not uniform throughout the arterial tree, and depend on gender and anatomical location (Van der Heijden-Spek et al. 2000).

This age-related change in arterial compliance has a number of consequences. First, it exposes the left ventricle to higher peak arterial pressures during systole. Thus, for a fixed stroke volume and systemic resistance, left ventricular afterload will increase significantly, causing adaptive structural changes within the cardiac tissue. Second, the reduced contractility of the myocardium with ageing, when exposed to elevated peak systolic blood pressures, lengthens systolic time at the expense of the diastolic phase, thereby increasing the likelihood of compromising coronary circulation (Folkow & Svanborg 1993). In contrast, younger individuals primarily influence systemic blood pressure via autonomically driven changes in peripheral vascular resistance. However, structural changes to the arterial tree are not the only means by which arterial stiffness is increased with age.

A healthy endothelium is important for regulating vascular tone via the release of a variety of vasoactive substances (Dinenno 2004). Ageing is associated with a decline in endothelium-dependent vasodilatation (Taddei et al. 1995). A decline in endothelial vasodilators, such as nitric oxide, increases vascular stiffness and the risk of developing atherosclerosis (Taddei et al. 1995). An age-related impairment of endothelial function during exercise has also been well documented (Schrage et al. 2007, Taddei et al. 2000, Thijssen et al. 2006). Such functional changes may be related to an observed 20% decline in exercise hyperaemia in older individuals. Flow-mediated dilatation, a marker of endothelial function, is also impaired (Thijssen et al. 2006). The contribution of nitric oxide to exercise hyperaemia declines approximately 45% in older individuals during exercise (Schrage et al. 2007). Furthermore, Schrage et al. (2007) have suggested that ageing results in the loss of prostaglandin-mediated vasodilatation during exercise.

3.1.4 Cardiac pump dynamics

Resting heart rate (Craft & Schwartz 1995, Levy et al. 1998, Schulman et al. 1992), stroke volume (Schulman et al. 1992), cardiac output (Fleg et al. 1995, Rodeheffer et al. 1984) and total vascular resistance (Fleg et al. 1995) remain similar across the ageing spectrum. In contrast, under exercise stress, a marked divergence in cardiac responsiveness (20–30%) becomes evident. Blunted chronotropic and inotropic responses to submaximal and peak exercise are apparent with age (Fleg et al. 1995, Taylor et al. 1992). However, despite a reduction in peak heart rate and ejection fraction, stroke volume is maintained via elevations in end-diastolic and systolic volumes. These changes in ventricular volumes increase reliance on the Frank–Starling mechanism during exercise, but this is not sufficient to prevent a 30% reduction in maximal cardiac output due to a similar decline in peak heart rate (Ferrari et al. 2003).

What is the cause of this reduction in the cardiac responsiveness of the ageing heart during exercise? Insight into the possible mechanism of reduced cardiac responsiveness during exercise can be obtained from pharmacological blockade of cardiac sympathetic modulation. For example, simultaneous β-adrenergic and muscarinic receptor blockade allows the investigation of the intrinsic control of heart rate – heart rate free from autonomic influences (Jose 1966). Using this technique, Craft & Schwartz (1995) observed a significant reduction in the intrinsic heart rate in 60-year-old males compared to 20–40-year-old individuals. The

findings suggest that parasympathetic and sympathetic influences do not explain the observed age-related change in intrinsic heart rate at rest. Furthermore, Conway et al. (1971) observed that younger subjects, under β-adrenergic blockade, had similar heart rates and cardiac outputs to unblocked older subjects. Thus, the older heart could, in many ways, be seen as being representative of a younger β-blocked heart (Ferrari et al. 2003). Therefore, the possibility exists that the cardiac changes observed during exercise in the aged may be due to changes in autonomic nervous system activity, and this is explored in the next section.

3.2 Autonomic control of cardiovascular function

The sympathetic branch of the autonomic nervous system has primary control over myocardial contractility, cardiac output and regional vascular conductance at rest and during exercise (Christensen & Galbo 1983, Seals & Esler 2000). However, at rest, the parasympathetic arm largely dictates heart rate (Chapter 1), by slowing depolarisation frequency of the sinoatrial node.

There are a number of experimental methods that may be used to assess autonomic nervous system activity. For example, these may involve direct measurement of sympathetic neural activity, the measurement of the neurohumoral responses (reuptake, spillover and clearance) or target organ responses (e.g. heart rate variability). For instance, beat-to-beat fluctuations in heart rhythm may allow one to infer changes in the autonomic modulation of cardiac function. Rapid fluctuations in heart rhythm (>0.15 Hz) are associated with parasympathetic modulation, while slower fluctuations (0.04–0.15 Hz) are associated with both sympathetic and parasympathetic modulation (European Society of Cardiology and the North American Society of Pacing and Electrophysiology 1996).

The age-related modification of cardiovascular responsiveness to exercise may originate from alterations within sympathetic nervous function (Conway et al. 1971), rather than from structural cardiovascular limitations (Julius et al. 1967). Younger subjects were observed to have a greater attenuation of submaximal exercise cardiac output, relative to older individuals, when a β-adrenergic antagonist (propranolol) was applied. This blunting of the cardiovascular response is indicative of diminished sympathetic outflow during exercise (Conway et al. 1971).

Ageing results in a significant reduction in beat-to-beat variation of heart rate (Gregoire et al. 1996, Levy et al. 1998, Lipsitz et al. 1990). A reduction in parasympathetic nervous system activity, and therefore a relative increase in sympathetic predominance, has been suggested as the primary reason for this reduced heart rate variation. Although a reduction in heart rate variability has strong correlations with increased risk of cardiovascular mortality (Dekker et al. 2000, Kikuya et al. 2000, Kleiger et al. 1987, Tsuji et al. 1994), sudden death (Algra et al. 1993, Billman et al. 1984) and diabetic neuropathy (Stein & Kleiger 1999), discrimination of sympathetic and parasympathetic nervous system modulation on the basis of heart rate variability, time- and frequency-domain indices remains contentious (European Society of Cardiology and the North American Society of Pacing and Electrophysiology 1996).

In contrast, the resting plasma norepinephrine concentration has been observed to increase with age (Goldstein et al. 1983, Ziegler et al. 1976), or remain the same as healthy young adults (Fleg et al. 1985, Ng et al. 1993, Taylor et al. 1992). Similar results have been reported during exercise (Taylor et al. 1991). Interpreting these data presents some significant challenges, since plasma concentrations are merely the algebraic sum of catecholamine production (autonomic and adrenal cortex) and its removal (sympathetic nerve ending reuptake and metabolic clearance). Thus, plasma norepinephrine concentrations are merely turnover indices (as is the case for many blood-borne substances), and changes may not be directly representative of altered sympathetic activity (Esler et al. 1995a). However, determination of catecholamine production (spillover) using radioisotope dilution methods has supported an increase in sympathetic nervous activity with ageing during rest, but not during acute stress (Esler et al. 1995b, Seals & Esler 2000), although catecholamine secretion varies among the organs of the body.

Sympathetic flow to resting muscle increases markedly with age (Dinenno et al. 1999, Kingwell et al. 1994, Ng et al. 1993), effectively doubling between 25 and 65 years (Seals & Esler 2000). In contrast, no age effect was observed during acute sympathetic provocation activities, such as the cold pressor test and isometric handgrip exercise (Ng et al. 1994). Ng and colleagues (1994) did, however, observe higher resting levels of muscle sympathetic nerve activity with age.

From a distillation of these observations drawn from experiments using different methods, it can be determined that ageing results in a modification of autonomic nervous system activity, and a reduction in cardiovascular responsiveness. This can impact unfavourably upon other regulatory systems, for example temperature regulation (Chapters 19 and 20). However, the modification of cardiovascular responsiveness appears to occur in an environment of increased resting sympathetic activity and possibly during acute stress. This apparent incongruence between heightened sympathetic efferent activity, yet blunted cardiovascular response with age, may imply that there may be reduced end-organ sensitivity (gain; Chapter 18) to the elevated level of sympathetic activity (Lakatta 1993). In the next section, we will explore cardiac and vascular responsiveness with age.

3.3 Cardiac and vascular responsiveness

Isoproterenol is a β-adrenergic receptor agonist that has been shown to elicit a diminished exercise-related increase in cardiac output, left ventricular ejection fraction and heart rate in older, relative to younger, individuals. An increase in parasympathetic activity could account for this attenuation of β-adrenergic receptor sensitivity to isoproterenol. In contrast, a reduction in high-frequency heart rate oscillations is commonly observed with ageing, and this is suggestive of a reduction, rather than an increase, in cardiac parasympathetic activity, and it is therefore unlikely that altered parasympathetic states attenuate the responsiveness of β-adrenergic receptors (Lipsitz et al. 1990).

Elevated sympathetic nervous system activity with age is known to have a marked effect on peripheral vasoconstrictor responsiveness, skin blood flow (Chapters 1 and 19) and blood flow to resting and active skeletal muscle. Basal whole-limb (skeletal muscle, skin, subcutaneous tissue, bone) blood flow and vascular conductance to the legs are reduced with ageing (Dinenno et al. 1999). In contrast to younger individuals, Dinenno and colleagues (1999) observed a 30% reduction in femoral vascular conductance, a 45% increase in femoral vascular resistance, and a 75% increase in peroneal muscle sympathetic nerve activity in older subjects. However, after taking into account differences in skeletal muscle sympathetic nerve activity, the authors reported these age-related differences were no longer apparent. Thus, increased tonic vasoconstriction with age is largely mediated by elevations in α-adrenergic sympathetic tone (Dinenno et al. 2001). α-Adrenergic receptors in older individuals appear to be somewhat desensitised, and this may therefore be responsible for the reduction in sympathetic vasoconstrictor responsiveness in older individuals (Hogikyan & Supiano 1994, Seals & Dinenno 2004).

Neural control of the vasculature is critical to the regulation of mean arterial pressure (Chapter 18) and body temperature (Chapter 19), and also to the maintenance of ventricular filling pressure (preload) and cardiac output, both at rest and during dynamic exercise. Sympathetic vasoconstriction of splanchnic (visceral) vascular beds and non-active muscle permits redistribution of blood flow (Rowell 2004). However, the maximal vascular conductance of skeletal muscle far exceeds the maximal cardiac output available from the heart (Chapters 1, 10.1 and 10.2). Therefore, without vasoconstriction of skeletal muscle, systemic blood pressure could not be elevated or even maintained during exercise and heat stresses. Dynamic exercise appears to modulate intramuscular vasoconstrictor tone, with an attenuation of tone within active skeletal muscle (functional sympatholysis; Dinenno et al. 2005, Koch et al. 2003, Parker et al. 2007). Thus, despite an elevated systemic blood pressure, blood flow to aged active skeletal muscle is reduced, contributing to impaired exercise capacity (Dinenno et al. 2005).

3.4 Cardiovascular reflex control

3.4.1 Arterial baroreflex
The arterial baroreflex provides short-term reflex regulation of blood pressure to ensure adequate tissue perfusion, particularly during postural and exercise transitions. Stretch

receptors in the aortic arch and carotid sinuses are essential components of this cardiovascular reflex, with an elevation in arterial blood pressure increasing baroreceptor discharge, and eliciting a rapid (within one heart beat) slowing of the heart rate. This is predominantly a parasympathetically mediated response, which reduces cardiac output and the mean arterial pressure. A decrease in arterial pressure reduces receptor discharge and elicits a slower, sympathetically mediated response aimed at increasing vascular resistance and central venous pressure. Heart rate and cardiac output are therefore interim reflex adjustments to defend against a fall in arterial pressure (Rowell 1993).

The arterial baroreflex responses of healthy older individuals have been assessed using a variety of methods. For example, the use of vasoactive agents, such as α-receptor agonists (phenylephrine) or hypotensive agents (nitroprusside), has consistently resulted in the observation of a decline in the chronotropic responsiveness to a modification of systemic blood pressure with age (Gribbin et al. 1971, Hogikyan & Supiano 1994, Hunt et al. 2001, Jones et al. 2003, Matsukawa et al. 1996, Monahan et al. 2004). Similarly, baroreflex sensitivity, determined from spontaneous or provoked (Valsalva manoeuvre) systolic blood pressure and heart rate variations, has also revealed an attenuated baroreflex responsiveness (Bowman et al. 1997, Monahan et al. 2000, 2001, Parati et al. 1995).

However, not all techniques have resulted in such changes being observed in older individuals. For example, carotid baroreflex sensitivity, determined using direct stimulation of the carotid sinus via randomly applied negative or positive pressure pulses, was observed to be similar between younger and older individuals, despite a reduced range of heart rate response in the older subjects (Shi et al. 1996).

Precise identification of the factors that may be contributing to a reduction in cardiovascular reflex responsiveness is presently unclear. However, several investigations have focused on tissue compliance surrounding the mechanosensitive afferents of the carotid sinus. Ageing, and some disease states, cause significant structural changes to the large elastic arterial vessels, and these changes may attenuate baroreceptor sensitivity (Labrova et al. 2005). Researchers have suggested that the reduced arterial compliance is a significant cause of baroreflex attenuation with ageing. The logic of this suggestion is based upon the notion that, with a lower arterial compliance, there will also be reduced arterial expansion and baroreceptor activation for a given blood pressure change. However, despite its strong correlation, the decline in arterial compliance does not fully explain the 30–50% loss of baroreflex sensitivity (Hunt et al. 2001, Monahan et al. 2001). Indeed, Hunt et al. (2001) found no difference in the arterial compliance or baroreflex sensitivity between physically active older and sedentary younger subjects.

3.4.2 Cardiopulmonary baroreflex

The cardiopulmonary baroreceptors are located in the vena cavae, the chambers of the heart and the pulmonary artery and veins. These receptors are not stimulated by the same pressures that modulate arterial baroreceptor firing. These baroreceptors are thought to be responsible for the regulation of cardiac filling pressure and plasma volume (Raven et al. 2000). They not only function as independent pressure-sensing (stretch) receptors, but have an interaction with the carotid baroreceptors during low-pressure orthostatic challenges (Pawelczyk & Raven 1989). Thus, modification of cardiopulmonary baroreceptor sensitivity with ageing may also influence arterial baroreceptor responsiveness.

Experimentally, lower-body negative pressure has been used to decrease central venous pressure without altering mean arterial blood pressure, thereby selectively unloading the cardiopulmonary baroreceptors. Cleroux et al. (1989) used this experimental design, observing a similar decrease in central venous pressure in young, middle and old subjects, but with a diminished forearm vascular resistance, plasma renin and norepinephrine response in the old individuals. This diminished cardiopulmonary responsiveness was also observed in the sensitivity of the carotid baroreflex. Maximal gain of the carotid-cardiac and carotid-vasomotor stimulus–response relationship was augmented during lower-body negative pressure in younger but not older males, indicating that the cardiopulmonary baroreceptor interaction with the carotid baroreflex may be diminished within older individuals (Shi et al. 1996).

4   ENERGY EXPENDITURE

A gradual but persistent increase in adiposity is commonly observed from the second to the seventh decades in many ageing individuals (Vaughan et al. 1991). Conversely, a decline in lean body mass intensifies the shift in body composition which tends, with sedentary ageing, to move towards a greater percentage of body fat (Janssen et al. 2000, Vaughan et al. 1991). Whilst the loss of lean body mass relates to muscle mass and fibre fibre loss (section 6, sarcopenia), which can be attributed to the death of motoneurons (Holloszy & Kohrt 1995), the precise reasons for this change in body composition have not been fully elucidated. Nevertheless, such a change may impact upon whole-body metabolic rate, since adipose tissue and skeletal muscle vary markedly in both their basal and peak metabolic rates. Accordingly, in this section, we will explore the impact of ageing on energy balance, energy storage and energy expenditure, but with a primary focus on changes to energy expenditure.

Whole-body, 24-h energy expenditure has been estimated using respirometers (calorimetry chambers) or the double-labelled water technique. Such measures need to be very sensitive to small changes in energy metabolism to provide meaningful results. For example, if we consider that a 1% change in energy metabolism over a decade is all that is required to lead to significant changes in body composition (Wilson & Morley 2003), then one can appreciate that the signal-to-noise ratio for this method is very low indeed. Therefore, until more sensitive techniques are developed, readers in this area should interpret scientific findings with some caution (Wilson & Morley 2003).

The total, 24-h energy expenditure is made up of three components: basal metabolic rate (60–70%), diet-induced thermogenesis (8–12%) and physical activity (15–30%; see Figure 32.1). The last component is heavily dependent upon sustaining a life-long exercise habit (Chapters 17.2, 31.1 and 32), and its twofold variation reflects differences in exercise habits among people. Typically, ageing is associated with reduced habitual exercise and such reductions are associated with a greater incidence of disease (Chapters 29 and 30). Currently, there are limited data on the effect of ageing on diet-induced thermogenesis, though some have reported a decline with age in males but not in females (Wilson & Morley 2003).

The most significant portion of 24-h human energy utilisation consists of the basal (resting) metabolic energy expenditure. The basal metabolic rate is the lowest standardised metabolic rate for an individual, and is measured under conditions of significant subject constraint (e.g. fasting 12–14 h with no physical activity). These conditions do not reflect the typical human resting state, but provide a measurement of the lowest (basal) awake metabolic rate of the subject.

Many investigations have reported a reduction in basal and resting energy expenditures in ageing individuals (Keys et al. 1973, Poehlman 1992, Vaughan et al. 1991). Indeed, most texts cite this apparent ageing trend. For instance, Vaughan et al. (1991) studied >100 men and women aged 18–85 years, noting a significant reduction in resting, whole-body energy expenditure in older subjects. When these data were normalised to the estimated fat-free mass, since adipose tissue has a low metabolic rate, there still remained a small but statistically significant decrease in energy expenditure in the aged (Vaughan et al. 1991). Despite this normalisation of resting metabolic rate accounting for a significant proportion of the variation in expenditure, there still remained evidence that indicates an age-related decline in metabolism (Alfonzo-Gonzalez et al. 2006, Hunter et al. 2001, Piers et al. 1998). It appeared that older subjects (50–77 years) have a 600 kJ·day^{-1} lower basal metabolic rate, after normalisation for fat-free mass, than younger individuals (Alfonzo-Gonzalez et al. 2006, Piers et al. 1998).

However, normalising energy expenditure on the basis of the fat-free mass does not account for the significant proportion of the body mass that consists of elements that do not expend energy, such as body water and mineral content. Gallagher and colleagues (1996) observed that normalisation to the body cell or fat-free masses did not provide equivalent measures of metabolic activity, suggesting that the interpretation of normalised energy expenditure data should be applied with restraint. Indeed, a fat-free normalisation does not differentiate between tissues of varying metabolic activity.

Changes in fat-free mass have been estimated to account for over 50% of the observed interindividual variation in resting metabolic rate, with age-related sarcopenia proposed as the primary explanation of this observation (Wilson & Morley 2003). Despite skeletal muscle representing approximately 40% of total body mass, it only represents about 22% of the total metabolic energy expenditure. The brain and liver account for more than 40% of metabolic energy expenditure, despite representing <5% of the total body mass (McCarter 1995). Indeed, the summed mass of the most metabolically active organs (heart, kidney, brain and liver) remains relatively unchanged through to the seventh decade of life. In contrast, skeletal muscle mass declines considerably with age. Therefore, the interpretation of whole-body metabolic rate measures can vary considerably, depending upon how these data are normalised, and evidence based upon changes in the four most metabolically active tissues indicates that age-related changes in the metabolic rates of these tissues do not occur (McCarter 1995). Thus, the reduction in whole-body basal metabolism can primarily be explained on the basis of a differential change in body composition, rather changes in tissue metabolism per se.

Nevertheless, many mechanisms have been proposed to explain the apparent decline in resting metabolic rate, and these include a decline in sodium-potassium-ATPase activity, reduced tissue and organ oxygen consumption, decreased protein turnover in the skeletal muscle and changes to the mitochondrial membrane proton permeability (Piers et al. 1998, Wilson & Morley 2003), as explained in the next section.

4.1 Mitochondrial metabolism

Mitochondria are the powerhouses for cellular oxidative phosphorylation, and these organelles contain their own DNA, making them crucial components in the shaping and creation of the energy transduction system (Ozawa 1997). Modifications to mitochondrial structure or function can have a significant impact on whole-body energy expenditure, and on this basis, we will explore some of the possible age-related effects on mitochondrial function.

Mitochondrial DNA is susceptible to a higher mutation rate than nuclear DNA, due to inefficient repair systems, its more rapid turnover, a lack of protective histones and its location close to sites of reactive oxygen species (free radical) generation that increase the likelihood of damage and progression to mutation (Brierley et al. 1997b, McCarter 1995). Indeed, an accumulation of mutated mitochondrial DNA has been proposed as a mechanism of ageing and disease (Conley et al. 2007, McCarter 1995), and a recent investigation using genetically engineered mice, carrying a mutated enzyme responsible for mitochondrial DNA metabolism, reported significant ageing effects in the animals (Trifunovic et al. 2004). The mutation in the mice significantly increased replication errors of the mitochondrial DNA, distributing these errors into the synthesis of new mitochondria, thus accelerating apparent ageing effects in the mice, such as mass loss, shortened lifespan, curvature of the spine and hair loss (Trifunovic et al. 2004). The findings from this investigation add support to the theory of mitochondrial involvement in age-related physical deterioration.

Mitochondrial DNA damage from reactive oxygen species leads to defects in the mitochondrial inner membrane, and these can directly affect the electron transport chain, reducing energy transduction capability (Masoro & Austad 2006). A reduction in energy transduction has been proposed via the uncoupling of oxidative phosphorylation, reducing ATP synthesis per unit of oxygen consumed and thereby significantly lowering metabolic efficiency (Conley et al. 2007). Uncoupling of oxidative phosphorylation and a reduction in cytochrome C oxidase have been proposed as an explanation for the reduced exercise efficiency in the elderly (Conley et al. 2000a, 2007, Woo et al. 2006).

Woo et al. (2006) observed an 8% decline in exercise efficiency in 65–75-year-old sedentary men and women. However, the most interesting finding of the investigation was not the attenuation in exercise efficiency, but changes in efficiency observed upon completion of an endurance training programme. At the completion of 6 months of endurance running, Woo and colleagues (2006) observed a reversal of age-related decrements in the excess postexercise oxygen uptake, recovery and exercise efficiency. Observations such as these reinforce the difficulties of investigating primary ageing using a sedentary sample.

Observations from in vivo investigations have shown a marked attenuation of mitochondrial quantity and quality with ageing, leading to compromised energy transduction (Conley et al. 2000b, Petersen et al. 2003). Conley et al. (2000b) observed a 50% lowering of oxidative capacity and a 20% decrease in mitochondrial content in subjects aged 20–80 years, thereby reducing oxidative capacity of individual mitochondria by approximately 30% (Figure 16.4). Phosphocreatine recovery following dynamic exercise is a marker of oxidative capacity, and this has been observed to be 100% higher in younger than older individuals. However, the extrapolation of these data to assess mitochondrial number to intra- and interindividual ageing responses is tenuous.

Declines in mitochondrial function, such as those described above, have not been shown consistently within the literature (Brierley et al. 1997b, Kent-Braun & Ng 2000, Nair 2005). Mitochondria are highly plastic, markedly increasing proliferation in tissues with elevations in aerobic metabolism. It is possible, therefore, that these age-related changes in mitochondrial function, although convincing, represent modifications in habitual physical activity that accompany ageing, rather than ageing per se. Indeed, when habitual physical activity was characterised in elderly and younger highly trained individuals, no difference was observed in respiratory chain function (Brierley et al. 1997a). We know that mitochondrial adaptations are specific to the type of physical training stimulus, with resistance training increasing mitochondrial density and oxidative capacity, whilst endurance training increases only oxidative capacity (Jubrias et al. 2001).

When taken together, the results from Brierley et al. (1997b) and Woo et al. (2006) indicate that secondary ageing, accompanying more sedentary behaviours, may be responsible for the decline in mitochondrial oxidative capacity, rather than a direct primary ageing effect upon mitochondrial function. Interestingly, Conley et al. (2000b) concurred with this interpretation, observing that the attenuation in mitochondrial oxidative capacity with ageing may be due to insufficient endurance exercise in their older sample, having recruited recreationally active older individuals for their project.

4.2 Fat deposition and carbohydrate metabolism

The World Health Organisation predicts that, by 2015, approximately 2.3 billion adults will be overweight (body mass index ≥25) and more than 700 million will be classified as obese (body mass index ≥30; (WHO 2006). The fattening of the world population is endemic, due to combined influences of reduced physical activity and an excess consumption of easily available food. This worrying trend places a

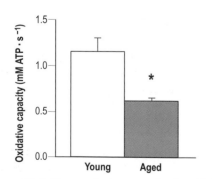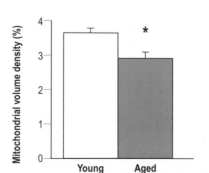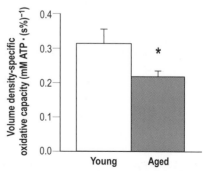

Figure 16.4 Changes in human mitochondrial oxidative function with ageing. Modified from Conley et al. (2000b) with permission.

significant and progressively increasing medical burden on the global community, increasing the risk of cardiovascular disease, diabetes, cancers and musculoskeletal disorders (Chapters 28 and 30). With this background in mind, we will now proceed, with some caution, to differentiate between the environmental and primary ageing effects on fat deposition and carbohydrate metabolism.

Increased fat mass, and in particular fat located in the peritoneal cavity between the internal organs (visceral fat), is known to increase with age, typically between the third and seventh decades. However, in cohorts that have maintained high levels of endurance fitness, increased visceral fat deposits may not occur. For example, masters athletes (49–73 years) were observed to have no significant elevation in central adiposity compared to matched younger athletes (Van Pelt et al. 1998). In contrast, sedentary older women, when compared to younger individuals who were matched for physical activity habits, possessed a significant increase in fat mass, waist circumference and central adiposity, and a decline in the fat-free mass (Van Pelt et al. 1998). Ryan et al. (1996) noted no difference in body fat and fat-free mass with age but an increase in visceral fat in older female masters athletes. Interestingly, the trunk fat mass in the 40–49-year-old (5.5 kg) and 50–69-year-old athletes (5.8 kg) was only significantly higher when compared to that of 30–39-year-old athletes (3.8 kg), but not 18–29-year-old athletes (5.1 kg; Ryan et al. 1996). When compared to sedentary women of a similar age, 40–49-year-old athletes had over 50% less visceral fat, indicating the substantial effect that habitual physical activity has on the size of the central adipose mass (Kohrt 2002).

The study of visceral fat levels is important, due to its strong association with insulin resistance, impaired glucose tolerance and increased risk of cardiovascular disease (Chapter 30). This link was clearly established by Ronnemaa et al. (1997), who investigated monozygotic twins with markedly different body masses. Despite an average inter-twin difference in body mass of 18 kg, it was only those twins who differed most in visceral fat that were observed to have impaired glucose and insulin control. This clear association between localised deposits of fat and insulin resistance was further reinforced by the observation that the ratio of the waist and hip girths accounted for most of the variance in peripheral tissue-specific insulin action, whereas age explained only a minor fraction of the total variance (Cefalu et al. 1995).

It has been proposed that the mechanism by which visceral fat influences insulin action may be via an increased flow of free fatty acids to the liver and systemic circulation, leading to increased tissue metabolism of fat rather than glucose (Cefalu et al. 1995, Gabriely et al. 2002). This direct effect of localised abdominal fat deposits on glucose metabolism was most clearly seen when the visceral (epididymal and perinephric) fat deposits of rats were surgically removed (Gabriely et al. 2002). This fat accounted for about 18% of the total body fat, and its removal returned the peripheral and hepatic insulin activity to levels observed within younger rats (Gabriely et al. 2002). This change was only observed when the visceral fat deposits were excised, with the removal of the same relative magnitude of subcutaneous fat tissue from a second group of rats failing to change insulin control (Gabriely et al. 2002). When rats used as an animal model of type 2 diabetes (Zucker diabetic fatty rats) had visceral fat deposits removed, two effects were noted. First, there was a delay in the development of diabetes. Second, the rate of decline in insulin action was reduced (Gabriely et al. 2002). In summary, the visceral fat depot appears to play an important role in glucose metabolism, and the size of the depot is influenced primarily by secondary environmental factors (exercise and surplus nutrition) rather than primary ageing.

A reduced ability to regulate blood glucose concentration, in combination with a progressive impairment of insulin secretion and sensitivity, is often observed with ageing. Initially, insulin resistance occurs, and this is overcome by an elevated insulin secretion to maintain blood glucose levels (Chapter 30). However, hypersecretion does not appear to be maintained as insulin resistance progresses and glucose intolerance and type 2 diabetes mellitus gradually develop. While this cascade in glucose dysfunction is present in many older adults, it is not necessarily the result of primary ageing. Indeed, cross-sectional investigations of highly trained athletes across a broad age spectrum have shown that exercise habit, and not ageing, has the most profound effect on glucose tolerance (Manetta et al. 2001, 2003, Pratley et al. 1995, Rogers et al. 1990, Seals et al. 1984, Yamanouchi et al. 1992).

5 PULMONARY FUNCTION

Optimal pulmonary function is realised at approximately 20 and 25 years for females and males (respectively), followed by a period of relative stability, and eventually an age-related progressive decline is observed (Janssens et al. 1999). Despite this decline in pulmonary performance, adequate gas exchange is maintained over the human lifespan. Nevertheless, three primary age-related changes affect the mechanical properties of the respiratory system: a decrease in respiratory muscle strength, reduced chest wall compliance and a decrease in static elastic recoil.

The development of maximal static inspiratory and expiratory pressures is used as an index of respiratory muscle strength (Chapter 2), which decreases with ageing. Some of this decline is a part of the normal ageing process that occurs in all skeletal muscles (Janssen et al. 1993). However, since the upper and lower limits of the total lung capacity are largely determined by the ability of the respiratory muscles to expand or compress the thorax, then changes in muscle strength will impact upon the static lung volumes. Accordingly, significant falls in the maximal expiratory (at functional residual capacity and residual volume) and maximal inspiratory pressures (developed at functional residual capacity and total lung capacity) are known to occur with ageing (Chen & Ku 1989, Enright et al. 1994). Furthermore, the ability to sustain breathing against a fixed inspiratory load, a measure of inspiratory muscle endurance, is reduced by 75% and 47% in older women and men, respectively (Chen & Ku 1989). Some of this change, while influenced by muscle function, can be attributed to an increased rigidity (reduced compliance) of the chest wall.

Chest wall compliance progressively decreases in older individuals, due to calcification of costal rib joint cartilage directly affecting the mobility of the rib cage (Estenne et al. 1985, Mittman et al. 1965, Rizzato & Marazzini 1970). This stiffening of the chest wall increases the static work of breathing, and this change is comparable to a restrictive pulmonary disorder or chest strapping (Chaunchaiyakul et al. 2004, O'Donnell et al. 2000). In contrast, lung tissue compliance is increased, with the parenchyma losing its elasticity and becoming more distensible and easier to expand, particularly at the higher lung volumes (Knudson et al. 1977, Turner et al. 1968). Thus, with age the natural tendency of the chest wall to pull the thoracic cage outward is diminished, and the natural tendency of the lung parenchyma to recoil inward or collapse is also reduced.

These structural changes have been estimated to significantly increase the elastic work of breathing at rest and also during exercise (Chaunchaiyakul et al. 2004, Turner et al. 1968). For example, the resting lung tissue elastic work has been found to decrease 46% while chest wall elastic work increased by 110% in healthy older individuals, when compared to a young healthy group (Chaunchaiyakul et al. 2004). The elastic recoil of the chest wall (negative elastic work) assists lung inflation, but this stored elastic energy is reduced in the older person, who must perform additional inspiratory muscle work during lung inflation. The problem is minimal at rest but it is compounded during exercise, significantly increasing the amount of additional work required to inflate the lung. In fact, the absolute chest wall elastic work has been shown to increase fivefold and the relative work by 175%, when older subjects are exercising at 60% of the cardiac reserve (Chaunchaiyakul et al. 2004).

The change in tissue properties of the chest wall and lung tissue modifies the dynamic interaction between the lungs and chest wall, therefore changing both lung volumes and respiratory air flows. Despite this, the increased elastic load on the chest wall is counterbalanced by diminished lung elastic recoil, leaving the total lung capacity essentially unchanged with age (Janssens et al. 1999, Knudson et al. 1977, Sparrow & Weiss 1995). However, the residual volume increases significantly. Thus, given the relative stability in total lung capacity, vital capacity is reduced (Cohn & Donso 1963, Janssens et al. 1999, Sparrow & Weiss 1995) and functional residual capacity increases slightly with age (Cohn & Donso 1963, Janssens et al. 1999, Sparrow & Weiss 1995).

An age-related increase in lung compliance facilitates a significant elevation in closing volume, the volume at which the small airways begin to collapse during expiration, markedly affecting air flow and gas exchange, due to a loss of some of the peripheral airways (Janssens et al. 1999). The forced vital capacity and the forced expiratory volume in 1 second diminish significantly with age, with the greatest decline observed in forced expiratory flow at 25–75% of vital capacity (Chen & Ku 1989, Sparrow & Weiss 1995).

The distribution of ventilation in the older lung, during a resting tidal volume, is located increasingly in the apical regions. In comparison with younger individuals, such a ventilatory distribution is only observed when ventilation approaches residual volume (Holland et al. 1968). However, the regional distribution of blood flow remains the same, leading to a lowered ventilation to perfusion ratio, which reduces the arterial oxygen partial pressure by approximately 0.7 kPa per decade (Mansell et al. 1972, Sparrow & Weiss 1995). In contrast, alveolar oxygen partial pressure remains relatively constant with age, due to an increase in alveolar-arterial oxygen difference (Janssens et al. 1999). The ageing of the alveoli and related structures reduces the effective size of the lung, the available surface area for gas exchange and the diffusion capacity of the aged lungs (Sparrow & Weiss 1995, Viegi et al. 2001).

The control of respiration, via chemoreceptor afferents, appears to be compromised in older individuals. For instance, the ventilatory responses (sensitivity) to hypoxia and hypercapnia are both reported to be attenuated with age (Kronenberg & Drage 1973). However, the attenuated response to hypoxia is less certain (Sparrow & Weiss 1995).

6 SARCOPENIA

Skeletal muscle mass gradually decreases from 30 years, with a noticeable decrease at 50 years, and a more rapid decline beyond 60 years (Holloszy & Kohrt 1995, Janssen et al. 2000). Similarly, muscle cross-sectional area decreases approximately 40% between 20–60 years (Doherty 2003), with one longitudinal investigation of subjects aged 65 years estimating that muscle cross-sectional area declines approximately 1.4% per year after the age of 50 (Frontera et al. 2000). Over the 12-year span of that investigation, lower-limb muscle cross-sectional area decreased approximately 12–16%. Furthermore, the loss of muscle cross-sectional area was estimated to account for about 90% of the variation in strength (Frontera et al. 2000).

The term sarcopenia, which is derived from Greek origins ('sacro' denoting flesh, 'penia' meaning deficiency), is used to describe the significant loss of muscle mass that generally occurs with advancing age and some pathologies. Sarcopenia is used to describe not only the loss of mass but also reduced skeletal muscle function (Baumgartner et al. 1998), and its effects within the community are substantial. For example, age-related sarcopenia was estimated to cost the US health-care system $18.5 billion dollars in 2000 (Janssen et al. 2004).

The prevalence of such losses in muscle mass was investigated in 883 Hispanic and non-Hispanic white men and women: the New Mexico Elder Health Survey (Baumgartner et al. 1998). From this sample, 199 participants were assessed for appendicular skeletal muscle mass (dual-energy X-ray absorptiometry). Sarcopenia was defined as a muscle mass two standard deviations away from the reference population of young adults, and it was observed in 13–24% of individuals under the age of 70 years and in over 50% in subjects over 80 years. Importantly, these investigators observed that sarcopenia was also associated with a three–fourfold increase in the likelihood of a disability in the elderly. This relationship was primarily a function of muscle mass changes, and was largely independent of age, gender, obesity, ethnicity, socio-economic status, chronic morbidity and health behaviours (Baumgartner et al. 1998). More recently, Janssen et al. (2004) estimated that a 10% reduction in the incidence of sarcopenia in the US would result in health-care savings of $1.1 billion. Thus, sarcopenia is a significant health problem for ageing global communities.

Regular participation in resistance training is the most effective means of reversing (and preventing) the effects of sarcopenia, particularly in the oldest and most frail individuals (Doherty 2003). The remarkable plasticity of skeletal muscle in this frail population was demonstrated in 100 residents aged 72–98 years, who participated in a high-intensity resistance exercise programme for 10 weeks (Fiatarone et al. 1994). In these aged subjects, a 100% improvement in single repetition maximum strength, a 30% increase in physical activity and a 12% improvement in gait velocity were observed. Such changes emphasise the value of reversing senile sarcopenia to improve physical function (Baumgartner et al. 1998, Kraemer et al. 2002, Sowers et al. 2005), and these changes are likely to be primarily influenced by secondary environmental effects, such as positive changes in physical activity habits, rather than a potentiation of the responsiveness to resistance exercise.

6.1 Development of muscle force

The loss of muscular strength with increasing age appears to affect all muscles of the body similarly. Thus, the smaller muscles of the hand display similar rates of loss with age as the large locomotive muscles of the lower limb. Isometric strength has been shown to decline at approximately 60 years, and by the seventh and eighth decades, muscle strength has declined by 20–40% in healthy elderly compared to young individuals (Vandervoort & McComas 1986). By the ninth decade, strength declines of 50% have been reported (Doherty 2003). In a 20-year longitudinal study of older athletes, Pollock et al. (1997) observed a strength decline of 54% from 60 years to 90 years, in both single repetition maximum leg and chest press. Interestingly, this fall in concentric strength was primarily confined to subjects over the age of 90 years, whereas between the ages of 60 and 80 years, only a minimal decline in force production was observed.

When strength scores are normalised to muscle cross-sectional area, a measure of voluntary force development per unit of muscle mass is obtained. This is called muscle quality or specific strength. Age comparisons now reveal a slightly different picture, with some studies revealing a decline in specific strength (Lindle et al. 1997, Lynch et al. 1999, Petralla et al. 2004) and others showing no change (Kent-Braun & Ng 1999). Thus, the data at this stage are difficult to interpret, primarily because of differences in the methods used to estimate muscle size, which may account for the equivocal results. Nevertheless, these data appear to indicate that there is an age-related decline in muscle quality or specific strength (Narci & Maganaris 2006, Petralla et al. 2004).

Muscle power is critical for most daily activities (walking, stair climbing, standing from a chair) and it appears to decline significantly more with ageing than does muscle strength (Petralla et al. 2004). The rate of muscle power loss is approximately 3–4% per annum, with losses occurring earlier than strength-related declines (Petralla et al. 2004).

The early decline in muscle power was confirmed via retrospective analyses of age-group records for weightlifting and power lifting (Anton et al. 2004). These researchers had previously used this approach to assess physiological functional capacity during swimming and running championships, in an attempt to understand the effects of normal ageing (Tanaka et al. 1997). Reductions in muscle power commenced at an earlier age, and were most prominent in tasks requiring very rapid and highly coordinated movements (Anton et al. 2004). A decline in the development of muscle force with ageing appears to occur regardless of movement speed, physical fitness or muscle activation; a modification of muscle structure or neural activation may account for this change.

6.2 Muscle structure and neuromuscular alterations with age

On the basis of muscle biopsy samples, often vastus lateralis, estimates of fibre type and muscle fibre cross-sectional area have been determined. Clearly, this is a difficult task and it has possibly led to some increase in data variability. Nevertheless, ageing studies have revealed a decrease in muscle fibre numbers, a 20–30% reduction in the average size of type II fibres, an increased co-expression of myosin heavy chain isoforms within muscle fibres, and possibly a slight reduction in the cross-sectional area of type I fibres (Doherty 2003, Masoro & Austad 2006). Therefore, through the loss of muscle fibres and selective atrophy of type II fibres, the aged muscle has shifted toward a slower myosin heavy chain isoform profile (Doherty 2003), and this isoform profile transition appears to result from primary ageing. This displacement directly affects the force generation capability of the muscle, which is even evident in trained individuals. For example, highly trained masters sprint athletes have also displayed this transition, despite extensive physical training (Kornhonen et al. 2006).

Although the precise mechanism that triggers the loss of muscle fibres has not been elucidated, it is believed satellite cells may play a significant role in tissue ageing (Verdijk et al. 2007). The number of satellite cells in type I fibres is similar in healthy younger and older persons. However, the number of satellite cells per type II fibre is reduced by approximately 50% in elderly subjects (Figure 16.5), suggesting satellite cell number may have an important link to age-related muscle atrophy in type II muscle fibres (Verdijk et al. 2007).

The co-expression of myosin heavy chain isoforms within the same fibre, and a preferential atrophy of type II fibres, highlights a process of denervation and reinnervation occurring within the muscle. It has long been known that fibre transitions only occur with changes in innervation. In ageing muscle, this may be due to the loss of motor units (Doherty & Brown 1997, Vandervoort 2002), which leads to reinnervation and an expansion of the number of fibres innervated by the remaining motor units. The nett result is fewer motor units, but with a greater motor unit size and reduced activation and relaxation speeds, and a slower development of twitch tension (Doherty & Brown 1997). These adaptations may have a number of functional implications for ageing individuals, such as the loss of steadiness during slow, low-load actions (Knight & Kamen 2007, Laidlaw et al. 1999) and the slowing down of muscle twitch activation times (Vandervoort & McComas 1986).

7 CONCLUSION

Ageing has a significant impact upon a number of body systems, causing a reduction in system efficiency and

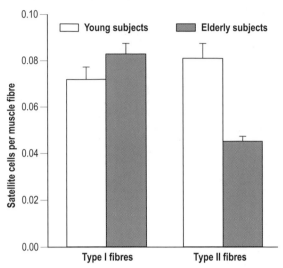

Figure 16.5 Satellite cell content in type I and II muscle fibres of young and aged subjects. Satellite cell content in the type II fibres of the elderly individuals are significantly lower than observed in type I fibres of the same subjects, and in type II of the younger individuals. Modified from Verdijk et al. (2007) with permission.

homeostatic regulation, reduced tissue compliance, lowered reflex sensitivity and control, and a marked decline in muscle mass. Healthy humans have a significant surplus in physiological capacity when resting. However, this state may conceal many age-related changes that act to slowly erode the physiological functional capacity, and these deficiencies do not become apparent until the system is placed under a significant physical stress. The challenge will be to continue the study of normal ageing, but now using physically fit volunteers, who perhaps best represent our evolutionary phenotype.

References

Alfonzo-Gonzalez G, Doucet E, Bouchard C, Tremblay A 2006 Greater than predicted decrease in resting energy expenditure with age: cross sectional and longitudinal evidence. European Journal of Clinical Nutrition 60:18–24

Algra A, Tijssen JG, Roelandt JR, Pool J, Lubsen J 1993 Heart rate variability from 24-hour electrocardiography and the 2-year risk for sudden death. Circulation 88(1):180–185

Anton M, Spirduso WW, Tanaka H 2004 Age-related declines in anaerobic muscular performance: weightlifting and powerlifting. Medicine and Science in Sports 36(1):143–147

Arking R 2006 The biology of aging: observations and principles. Oxford University Press, Oxford

Australian Bureau of Statistics 1995 Australian social trends 1995. ABS Catalogue No 4102.0. Australian Bureau of Statistics, Canberra

Baumgartner RN, Koehler KM, Gallagher D, Romero L, Heymsfield SB, Ross RR, Garry PJ, Lindeman RD 1998 Epidemiology of sarcopenia among the elderly in New Mexico. American Journal of Epidemiology 147(8):755–763

Billman GE, Schwartz PJ, Stone HL 1984 The effects of daily exercise on susceptibility to sudden cardiac death. Circulation 69(6):1182–1189

Blair SN, Goodyear NN, Gibbons LW, Cooper KH 1984 Physical fitness and incidence of hypertension in healthy normotensive men and women. Journal of the American Medical Association 252:487–490

Blair SN, Kampert JB, Kohl HW 3rd, Barlow CE, Macera CA, Paffenbarger RS Jr, Gibbons LW 1996 Influences of cardiorespiratory fitness and other precursors on cardiovascular disease and all-cause mortality in men and women. Journal of the American Medical Association 276(3):205–210

Booth FW, Lees SJ 2006 Physically active subjects should be the control group. Medicine and Science in Sports and Exercise 38(3):405–406

Booth FW, Gordon SE, Carlson CJ, Hamilton MT 2000 Waging war on modern chronic diseases: primary prevention through exercise biology. Journal of Applied Physiology 88(2):774–787

Bortz WM, Bortz WM 1996 How fast do we age? Exercise performance over time as a biomarker. Journal of Gerentology: Medical Science 51A(5):M223–M225

Bowman AJ, Clayton RH, Murray A, Reed JW, Subhan MF, Ford GA 1997 Baroreflex function in sedentary and endurance-trained elderly people. Age and Ageing 26:289–294

Brierley EJ, Johnson MA, Bowman AJ, Ford G, James OFW, Turnbull DM 1997a Mitochondrial respiratory chain function does not deteriorate with age in people who exercise regularly. Annals of Neurology 41:117–120

Brierley EJ, Johnson MA, James OFW, Turnbill DM 1997b Mitochondrial involvement in the ageing process. Facts and controversies. Molecular and Cellular Biochemistry 174:325–328

Cefalu WT, Wang ZQ, Werbel S, Bell-Farrow A, Crouse JR 3rd, Hinson WH, Terry JG, Anderson R 1995 Contribution of visceral fat mass to insulin resistance in aging. Metabolism 44(7):954–959

Chaunchaiyakul R, Groeller H, Clarke JR, Taylor NAS 2004 The impact of aging and habitual physical activity on static respiratory work at rest and during exercise. American Journal of Physiology. Lung Cell Molecular Physiology 287:L1098–L1106

Chen H, Ku C 1989 Relationship between respiratory muscle function and age, sex and other factors. Journal of Applied Physiology 66(2):943–948

Christensen NJ, Galbo H 1983 Sympathetic nervous activity during exercise. Annual Review of Physiology 45:139–153

Cléroux J, Giannattasio C, Bolla G, Cuspidi C, Grassi G, Mazzola C, Sampieri L, Seravalle G, Valsecchi M, Mancia G 1989 Decreased cardiopulmonary reflexes with aging in normotensive humans. American Journal of Physiology. 257:H961–H968

Cohn JE, Donso HD 1963 Mechanical properties of lung in normal men over 60 years old. Journal of Clinical Investigation 42(9):1406–1410

Conley KE, Esselman PC, Jubrias SA, Cress ME, Inglin B, Mogadam C, Schoene RB 2000a Ageing, muscle properties and maximal O2 uptake rate in humans. Journal of Physiology 526(1):211–217

Conley KE, Jubrias SA, Esselman PC 2000b Oxidative capacity and ageing in human muscle. Journal of Physiology 526(1):203–210

Conley KE, Jubrias SA, Amara CE, Marcinek D 2007 Mitochondrial dysfunction: impact on exercise performance and cellular aging. Exercise and Sport Science Reviews 35(2):43–49

Conway J, Wheeler R, Sannerstedt R 1971 Sympathetic nervous activity during exercise in relation to age. Cardiovascular Research 5(4):577–581

Craft N, Schwartz J 1995 Effects of age on intrinsic heart rate, heart rate variability and AV conduction in healthy humans. American Journal of Physiology. Heart and Circulatory Physiology 268 (4 Pt 2):H1441–H1452

Dekker JM, Crow RS, Folsom AR, Hannan PJ, Liao D, Swenne CA, Schouten EG 2000 Low heart rate variability in a 2-minute rhythm strip predicts risk of coronary heart disease and mortality from several causes: the ARIC Study. Atherosclerosis Risk In Communities. Circulation 102(11):1239–1244

Dinenno FA 2004 Ageing, exercise training and resistance vessels: more than just no NO. Journal of Physiology 563(3):673

Dinenno FA, Jones P, Seals DR, Tanaka H 1999 Limb blood flow and vascular conductance are reduced with age in healthy humans: relation to elevations in sympathetic nerve activity and declines in oxygen demand. Circulation 100:164–170

Dinenno FA, Tanaka H, Stauffer BL, Seals DR 2001 Reductions in basal limb blood flow and vascular conductance with human ageing: role for augmented a-adrenergic vasoconstriction. Journal of Physiology 536(3):977–983

Dinenno FA, Masuki S, Joyner M 2005 Impaired modulation of sympathetic a-adrenergic vasoconstriction in contracting forearm muscle of ageing men. Journal of Physiology 567(1):301–321

Doherty TJ 2003 Invited review: aging and sarcopenia. Journal of Applied Physiology 95:1717–1727

Doherty TJ, Brown WF 1997 Age-related changes in the twitch contractile properties of human thenar motor units. Journal of Applied Physiology 82(1):93–101

Enright PL, Kronmal RA, Manolio TA, Schenker MB, Hyatt RE 1994 Respiratory muscle strength in the elderly. Correlates and reference values. Cardiovascular Health Study Research Group. American Journal of Respiratory and Critical Care Medicine 149:430–438

Esler MD, Turner AG, Kaye DM, Thompson JM, Kingwell BA, Morris M, Lambert GW, Jennings GL, Cox HS, Seals DR 1995a Aging effects on human sympathetic neuronal function. American Journal of Physiology. 268:R278–285

Esler M, Kaye D, Thompson J, Jennings G, Cox H, Turner A, Lambert G, Seals D 1995b Effects of aging on epinephrine secretion and regional release of epinephrine for the human heart. Journal of Clinical Endocrinology and Metabolism 80:435–442

Estenne M, Yernault JC, De Troyer A 1985 Rib cage and diaphragm-abdomen compliance in humans: effects of age and posture. Journal of Applied Physiology 59(6):1842–1848

European Society of Cardiology and the North American Society of Pacing and Electrophysiology 1996 Heart rate variability: standards of measurement, physiological interpretation and clinical use. Circulation 93:1043–1065

Ferrari AU, Radaelli A, Centola M 2003 Invited review: aging and the cardiovascular system. Journal of Applied Physiology 95(6):2591–2597

Fiatarone MA, O'Neill EF, Ryan ND 1994 Exercise training and nutritional supplementation for physical frailty in very elderly people. New England Journal of Medicine 330(25):1769–1775

Finch CE, Pike MC, Witten M 1990 Slow mortality rate accelerations during aging in some animals approximate that of humans. Science 249:902–905

Fleg JL, Tzankoff P, Lakatta EG 1985 Age-related augmentation of plasma catecholamines during dynamic exercise in healthy males. Journal of Applied Physiology 59(4):1003–1039

Fleg JL, O'Connor F, Gerstenblith G, Becker LC, Clulow J, Schulman SP, Lakatta EG 1995 Impact of age on the cardiovascular response to dynamic upright exercise in healthy men and women. Journal of Applied Physiology 78(3):890–900

Folkow B, Svanborg A 1993 Physiology of cardiovascular aging. Physiological Reviews 73(4):725–764

Frontera WR, Hughes VA, Fielding RA, Fiatarone MA, Evans WJ, Roubenoff R 2000 Aging of skeletal muscle: a 12-yr longitudinal study. Journal of Applied Physiology 88:1321–1326

Gabriely I, Ma XH, Yang XM, Atzmon G, Rajala MW, Berg AH, Scherer P, Rossetti L, Barzilai N 2002 Removal of visceral fat prevents insulin resistance and glucose intolerance of aging. Diabetes 51:2951–2958

Gallagher D, Visser M, Wang Z, Harris T, Pierson RN, Heymsfield SB 1996 Metabolically active component of fat-free body mass: influences of age adiposity and gender. Metabolism 45(8):992–997

Gerstenblith G, Frederiksen J, Yin FC, Fortuin NJ, Lakatta EG, Weisfeldt ML 1977 Echocardiographic assessment of a normal adult aging population. Circulation 57:273–278

Goldstein DS, Lake CR, Chernow B, Ziegler MG, Coleman MD, Taylor AA, Mitchell JR, Kopin IJ, Keiser HR 1983 Age-dependence of hypertensive-normotensive differences in plasma norepinephrine. Hypertension 5:100–104

Gregoire J, Tuck S, Yamamoto Y, Hughson RL 1996 Heart rate variability at rest and exercise: influence of age, gender and physical training. Canadian Journal of Applied Physiology 21(6):455–470

Gribbin B, Pickering TG, Sleight P, Peto R 1971 Effect of age and high blood pressure on baroreflex sensitivity in man. Circulation Research 29(4):424–431

Hawkins SA, Wiswell RA, Marcell TJ 2003 Exercise and the master athlete – a model of successful aging. Journal of Gerentology: Medical Sciences 58A(11):1009–1011

Hogikyan RV, Supiano MA 1994 Arterial a-adrenergic responsiveness is decreased and SNS activity is increased in older humans. American Journal of Physiology. Endocrine Metabolism 266:E717–E724

Holland J, Milic-Emili J, Macklem PT, Bates DV 1968 Regional distribution of pulmonary ventilation in elderly subjets. Journal of Clinical Investigation 47:81–92

Holloszy JO, Kohrt WM 1995 Exercise. In: Masoro EJ (ed) Handbook of physiology: section 11 aging: a critical, comprehensive presentation of physiological knowledge and concepts. Oxford University Press, Oxford, 633–655

Hunt BE, Farquhar WB, Taylor A 2001 Does reduced vascular stiffening fully explain preserved cardiovagal baroreflex function in older physically active men? Circulation 103:2424–2427

Hunter GR, Weisner RL, Gower BA, Wetzstein C 2001 Age-related decrease in resting energy expenditure in sedentary white women: effects of regional differences in lean and fat mass. American Journal of Clinical Nutrition 73:333–337

Janssen MJ, de Bie J, Swenne CA, Oudhof J 1993 Supine and standing sympathovagal balance in athletes and controls. European Journal of Applied Physiology 67(2):164–167

Janssen I, Heymsfield S, Wang ZM, Ross RR 2000 Skeletal muscle mass and distribution in 468 men and women aged 18-88 yr. Journal of Applied Physiology 89:81–88

Janssen I, Shephard DS, Katzmarzyk PT, Roubenoff R 2004 The healthcare costs of sarcopenia in the United States. Journal of the American Geriatrics Society 52(1):80–85

Janssens JP, Pache JC, Nicod LP 1999 Physiological changes in respiratory function associated with ageing. European Respiratory Journal 13:197–205

Jones PP, Demetra CD, Jordan J, Seals D 2003 Baroreflex buffering is reduced with age in health men. Circulation 107:1770–1774

Jose AD 1966 Effect of combined sympathetic and parasympathetic blockade on heart rate and cardiac function in man. American Journal of Cardiology 18(3):476–478

Jubrias SA, Esselman PC, Price LB, Cress EM, Coney HD 2001 Large energetic adaptations of elderly muscle to resistance and endurance training. Journal of Applied Physiology 90:1663–1670

Julius S, Amery A, Whitlock LS, Conway J 1967 Influence of age on the hemodynamic response to exercise. Circulation 36(2):222–230

Kent-Braun JA, Ng AV 1999 Specific strength and voluntary muscle activation in young and elderly women and men. Journal of Applied Physiology 87(1):22–29

Kent-Braun JA, Ng AV 2000 Skeletal muscle oxidative capacity in young and older women and men. Journal of Applied Physiology 89:1072–1078

Keys A, Taylor HL, Grande F 1973 Basal metabolism and age of adult man. Metabolism 22(4):579–587

Kikuya M, Hozawa A, Ohokubo T, Tsuji I, Michimata M, Matsubara M, Ota M, Nagai K, Araki T, Satoh H, Ito S, Hisamichi S, Imai Y 2000 Prognostic significance of blood pressure and heart rate variabilities: the Ohasama study. Hypertension 36(5):901–906

Kingwell BA, Thompson JM, Kaye DM, McPherson GA, Jennings GL, Esler MD 1994 Heart rate spectral analysis, cardiac norepinephrine spillover and muscle sympathetic nerve activity during human sympathetic nervous activation and failure. Circulation 90(1):234–240

Kleiger RE, Miller JP, Bigger JT Jr, Moss AJ 1987 Decreased heart rate variability and its association with increased mortality after acute myocardial infarction. American Journal of Cardiology 59(4):256–262

Knight CA, Kamen G 2007 Modulation of motor unit firing rates during a complex sinusoidal force task in young and older adults. Journal of Applied Physiology 102:122

Knudson RJ, Clark DF, Kennedy TC, Knudson DE 1977 Effect of ageing alone on mechanical properties of the normal adult human lung. Journal of Applied Physiology 43(6):1054–1062

Koch DW, Leuenberger UA, Proctor DN 2003 Augmented leg vasoconstriction in dynamically exercising older men during acute sympathetic stimulation. Journal of Physiology 551(1):337–344

Kohrt WM 2002 Aging, obesity and metabolic regulation: influence of gender and physical activity. In: Shephard RJ (ed) Gender, physical activity and aging. CRC Press, London

Korhonen MT, Cristea A, Alén M, Häkkinen K, Sipilä S, Mero A, Viitasalo JT, Larsson L, Suominen H 2006 Aging, muscle fibre type and contractile function in sprint-trained athletes. Journal of Applied Physiology 101:906–917

Kraemer WJ, Adams K, Cafarelli E 2002 American College of Sports Medicine position stand. Progression models in resistance training for healthy adults. Medicine and Science in Sports and Exercise 34(2):364–380

Kronenberg RS, Drage CW 1973 Attenuation of the ventilatory and heart responses to hypoxia and hypercapnia with aging in normal men. Journal of Clinical Investigation 52:1812–1819

Lábrová R, Honzíková N, Maderová E, Vysocanová P, Nováková Z, Závodná E, Fiser B, Semrád B 2005 Age-dependent relationship between the carotid intima-media thickness, baroreflex sensitivity and the inter-beat interval in normotensive and hypertensive subjects. Physiological Research 54:593–600

Laidlaw DH, Kornatz KW, Keen DA, Suzuki S, Enoka RM 1999 Strength training improves the steadiness of slow lengthening contractions performed by old adults. Journal of Applied Physiology 87(5):1786–1795

Lakatta EG 1993 Cardiovascular regulatory mechanisms in advanced age. Physiological Reviews 73(2):413–467

Lakatta EG 1995 Cardiovascular system. In: Masro EJ (ed) Handbook of physiology. Section II: Aging–organ system and organismic aging. Oxford University Press, Oxford, 413–474

Lakatta EG, Levy D 2003a Arterial and cardiac aging: major shareholders in cardiovascular disease enterprises: Part I: aging arteries: a 'set up' for vascular disease. Circulation 107(1):139–146

Lakatta EG, Levy D 2003b Arterial and cardiac aging: major shareholders in cardiovascular disease enterprises: Part II: the aging heart in health: links to heart disease. Circulation 107(2):346–354

Learoyd BM, Taylor MG 1966 Alterations with age in the viscoelastic properties of human arterials walls. Circulation Research 18:278–292

Levy WC, Cerqueira MD, Harp GD, Johannessen KA, Abrass IB, Schwartz RS, Stratton JR 1998 Effect of endurance exercise training on heart rate variability at rest in healthy young and older men. American Journal of Cardiology 82(10):1236–1241

Lindle RS, Metter EJ, Lynch NA, Fleg JL, Fozard JL, Tobin J, Roy TA, Hurley BF 1997 Age and gender comparisons of muscle strength in 654 women and men aged 20-93 yr. Journal of Applied Physiology 83(5):1581–1587

Lipsitz LA, Mietus J, Moody GB, Goldberger AL 1990 Spectral characteristics of heart rate variability before and during postural tilt. Relations to aging and risk of syncope. Circulation 81(6):1803–1810

Lynch NA, Metter EJ, Lindle RS, Fozard JL, Tobin JD, Roy TA, Fleg JL, Hurley BF 1999 Muscle quality. I. Age-associated differences between arm and leg muscle groups. Journal of Applied Physiology 86(1):188–194

Manetta J, Brun JF, Callis A, Mercier J, Prefaut C 2001 Insulin and non-insulin-dependent glucose disposal in middle-aged and young athletes versus sedentary men. Metabolism 50(3):349–354

Manetta J, Brun JF, Maimoun L, Prefaut C, Mercier J 2003 Serum levels of insulin-like growth factor-I (IGF-I) and IGF-binding proteins-1 and -3 in middle-aged and young athletes versus sedentary men: relationship with glucose disposal. Metabolism 52(7):821–826

Mansell AC, Bryan C, Levison H 1972 Airway closure in children. Journal of Applied Physiology 33:711–714

Manson JE, Nathan DM, Krolewski AS, Stampfer MJ, Willett WC, Hennekens CH 1992 A prospective study of exercise and incidence of diabetes among US male physicians. Journal of the American Medical Association 268:63–67

Manson JE, Greenland P, LaCroix AZ, Stefanick ML, Mouton CP, Oberman A, Perri MG, Sheps DS, Pettinger MB, Siscovick DS 2002 Walking compared with vigorous exercise for the prevention of cardiovascular events in women. New England Journal of Medicine 347(10):716–725

Masoro EJ 1995 Aging: current concepts. In: Handbook of physiology: a critical, comprehensive presentation of physiological knowledge and concepts: section 11: aging. Oxford University Press, Oxford

Masoro EJ, Austad SN 2006 Handbook of the biology of aging, 6th edn. Elsevier, Boston, MA

Matsukawa T, Sugiyama Y, Mano T 1996 Age-related changes in baroreflex control of heart rate and sympathetic nerve activity in healthy humans. Journal of the Autonomic Nervous System 60(3):209–212

McCarter R 1995 Energy utilisation. In: Masoro EJ (ed) Handbook of physiology: a critical, comprehensive presentation of physiological knowledge and concepts: section 11: aging. Oxford University Press, Oxford

Mittman C, Edelman H, Norris AH, Shock NW 1965 Relationship between chest wall and pulmonary compliance and age. Journal of Applied Physiology 20(6):1211–1216

Monahan KD, Dinenno FA, Seals DR, Clevenger CM, Desouza CA, Tanaka H 2001 Age-associated changes in cardiovagal baroreflex sensitivity are related to central arterial compliance. American Journal of Physiology. Heart and Circulatory Physiology 281(1): H284–H289

Monahan KD, Dinenno FA, Tanaka H, Clevenger CM, DeSouza CA, Seals DR 2000 Regular aerobic exercise modulates age-associated declines in cardiovagal baroreflex sensitivity in healthy men. Journal of Physiology 529(Pt 1):263–271

Monahan KD, Eskurza I, Seals DR 2004 Ascorbic acid increases cardiovagal baroreflex sensitivity in healthy older men. American Journal of Physiology. Heart and Circulatory Physiology 286(6): H2113–H2117

Nair SK 2005 Aging muscle. American Journal of Clinical Nutrition 81:953–963

Narci MV, Maganaris CN 2006 Adaptability of elderly human muscles and tendons to increased loading. Journal of Anatomy 208:433–443

Ng AV, Callister R, Johnson DG, Seals DR 1993 Age and gender influence muscle sympathetic nerve activity at rest in healthy humans. Hypertension 21:498–503

Ng AV, Callister R, Johnson DG, Seals DR 1994 Sympathetic neural reactivity to stress does not increase with age in healthy humans. American Journal of Physiology. Heart and Circulatory Physiology 267:H344–H353

O'Donnell DE, Hong HH, Webb KA 2000 Respiratory sensation during chest wall restriction and dead space loading in exercising men. Journal of Applied Physiology 88(5):1859–1869

Olivetti G, Giordano G, Corradi D, Melissari M, Lagrasta C, Gambert SR, Anversa P 1995 Gender differences and aging: effects on the human heart. Journal of the American College of Cardiology 26:1068–1079

Ozawa T 1997 Genetic and functional changes in mitochondria associated with aging. Physiological Reviews 77(2):425–464

Parati G, Frattola A, Di Rienzo M, Castiglioni P, Pedotti A, Mancia G 1995 Effects of aging on 24-h dynamic baroreceptor control of heart rate in ambulant subjects. American Journal of Physiology 268(4 Pt 2):H1606–1612

Parker BA, Smithmyer SL, Jarvis SS, Ridout SJ, Pawelczyk JA, Proctor DN 1997 Evidence for reduced sympatholysis in leg resistance vasculature of healthy older woman. American Journal of Physiology. Heart and Circulatory Physiology 292:H1148–H1156

Pawelczyk JA, Raven PB 1989 Reductions in central venous pressure improve carotid baroreflex responses in conscious men. American Journal of Physiology 257(5 Pt 2):H1389–1395

Petersen KF, Befroy D, Dufour S, Dziura J, Ariyan C, Rothman DL, DiPietro L, Cline GW, Shulman GI 2003 Mitochondrial dysfunction in the elderly: possible role in insulin resistance. Science 300:1140–1141

Petralla JK, Kim J, Tuggle CS. Hall SR, Bamman MM 2004 Age differences in knee extension power, contractile velocity and fatigability. Journal of Applied Physiology 98:211–220

Piers LS, Soares MJ, McCormak LM, O'Dea K 1998 Is there evidence for an age related reduction in metoblic rate. Journal of Applied Physiology 85(6):2196–2204

Poehlman ET 1992 Energy expenditure and requirements in aging humans. Journal of Nutrition 122:2057–2065

Pollock ML, Mengelkoch LJ, Graves JE, Lowenthal DT, Limacher MC, Foster C, Wilmore JH 1997 Twenty-year follow-up of aerobic power and body composition of older track athletes. Journal of Applied Physiology 82(5):1508–1516

Pratley RE, Hagberg JM, Rogus EM, Goldberg AP 1995 Enhanced insulin sensitivity and lower waist-to-hip ratio in master athletes. American Journal of Physiology. Endocrine Metabolism 268(31):484–490

Raven PB, Potts JT, Shi X, Pawelczyk J 2000 Baroreceptor-mediated reflex regulation of blood pressure during exercise. In: Saltin B, Boushel R, Secher NH, Mitchell JH (eds) Exercise and circulation in health and disease. Human Kinetics, Champaign, IL

Reneman RS, Van Merode T, Hick P, Hoeks APG 1985 Flow velocity patterns in and distensibility of the carotid artery bulb in subjects of various ages. Circulation 71:500–509

Rizzato G, Marazzini L 1970 Thoracoabdominal mechanics in elderly men. Journal of Applied Physiology 28(4):457–460

Rodeheffer RJ, Gerstenblith G, Becker LC, Fleg JL, Weisfeldt ML, Lakatta EG 1984 Exercise cardiac output is maintained with advancing age in healthy human subjects: cardiac dilatation and increased stroke volume compensation for a diminished heart rate. Circulation 69(2):203–213

Rogers MA, King DS, Hagberg JM, Ehsani AA, Holloszy JO 1990 Effect of 10 days of physical inactivity on glucose tolerance in master athletes. Journal of Applied Physiology 68(5):1833–1837

Ronnemaa T, Koskenvuo M, Marniemi J, Koivunen T, Sajantila A, Rissanen A, Kaitsaari M, Bouchard C, Kaprio J 1997 Glucose metabolism in identical twins discordant for obesity. The critical role of visceral fat. Journal of Clinical Endocrinology and Metabolism 82(2):383–387

Rowe JW, Kahn RL 1987 Human aging: usual and successful (physiological changes associated with aging). Science 237: 143–147

Rowell LB 1993 Human cardiovascular control. Oxford University Press, New York

Rowell LB 2004 Ideas about control of skeletal and cardiac muscle blood flow (1876–2003): cycles of revision and new vision. Journal of Applied Physiology 97:384–392

Ryan AS. Nicklas BJ, Elahi D 1996 A cross-sectional study on body composition and energy expenditure in women athletes during aging. American Journal of Physiology 271(5 Pt 1):E916–921

Sanderson WC, Scherbov S 2005 Average remaining lifetimes can increase as human populations age. Nature 435:811–813

Schrage WG, Eisenach JH, Joyner MJ 2007 Ageing reduces nitric-oxide- and prostaglandin-mediated vasodilation in exercise humans. Journal of Physiology 579(1):227–236

Schulman SP, Lakatta EG, Fleg JL, Lakatta L, Becker LC, Gerstenblith G 1992 Age-related decline in left ventricular filling at rest and exercise. American Journal of Physiology 263(32):H1932–H1938

Seals DR, Dinenno FA 2004 Collateral damage: cardiovascular consequences of chronic sympathetic activation with human aging. American Journal of Physiology. Heart and Circulatory Physiology, 287:H1875–H1905

Seals DR, Esler MD 2000 Human ageing and the sympathoadrenal system. Journal of Physiology 528(3):407–417

Seals DR, Hagberg JM, Allen WK, Hurley BF, Dalsky GP, Ehsani AA, Holloszy JO 1984 Glucose tolerance in young and older athletes and sedentary men. Journal of Applied Physiology 56(6):1521–1525

Shi X, Gallagher K, Welch-O'Connor R, Foresman B 1996 Arterial and cardiopulmonary baroreflexes in 60- to 69- vs 18- to 36-yr-old humans. Journal of Applied Physiology 80(6):1903–1910

Sowers MR, Crutchfield M, Richards K, Wilkin MK, Furniss A, Jannausch M, Zhang D, Gross M 2005 Sarcopenia is related to physical functioning and leg strength in middle-aged women. Journal of Gerentology: Medical Sciences, 60A(4):486–490

Sparrow D, Weiss ST 1995 Respiratory system. In: Masoro EJ (ed) Handbook of physiology: a critical, comprehensive presentation of physiological knowledge and concepts: section 11: aging. Oxford University Press, Oxford

Stein PK, Kleiger RE 1999 Insights from the study of heart rate variability. Annual Review of Medicine 50:249–261

Taddei S, Galetta F, Virdis A, Ghiadoni L, Salvetti G, Franzoni F, Giusti C, Salvetti A 2000 Physical activity prevents age-related impairment in nitric oxide availability in elderly athletes. Circulation 101:2896–2901

Taddei S, Virdis A, Mattei P, Ghiadoni L, Gennari A, Fasolo CB, Sudano I, Salvetti A 1995 Aging and endothelial function in normotensive subjects and patients with essential hypertension. Circulation 91:1981–1987

Tanaka H, Seals DR 1997 Age and gender interactions in physiological functional capacity – insight from swimming performance. Journal of Applied Physiology 82(3):846–851

Tanaka H, Bassett DR Jr, Howley ET, Thompson DL, Ashraf M, Rawson FL 1997 Swimming training lowers the resting blood pressure in individuals with hypertension. Journal of Hypertension, 15(6):651–657

Tanasescu M, Leitzmann MF, Rimm EB, Willett WC, Stampfer MJ, Hu FB 2002 Exercise type and intensity in relation to coronary heart disease in men. Journal of the American Medical Association 288(16):1994–2000

Taylor JA, Hand GA, Johnson DG, Seals DR 1991 Sympathoadrenal-circulatory regulation during sustained isometric exercise in young and older men. American Journal of Physiology 261(5 Pt 2): R1061–1069

Taylor JA, Hand GA, Johnson DG, Seals DR 1992 Augmented forearm vasoconstriction during dynamic exercise in healthy older men. Circulation 86(6):1789–1799

Thijssen DHJ, de Groot P, Kooijman M, Smits P, Hopman M 2006 Sympathetic nervous system contributes to the ag-related impairment of flow-mediated dilation of the superficial femoral artery. American Journal of Physiology. Heart and Circulatory Physiology 291:H3122–H3129

Trifunovic A, Wredenberg A, Falkenberg M, Spelbrink JN, Rovio AT, Bruder CE, Bohlooly-Y M, Gidlöf S, Oldfors A, Wibom R, Törnell J, Jacobs HT, Larsson NG 2004 Premature ageing in mice expressing defective mitochondrial DNA polymerase. Nature 429:417–423

Tsuji H, Venditti FJ Jr, Manders ES, Evans JC, Larson MG, Feldman CL, Levy D 1994 Reduced heart rate variability and mortality risk in an elderly cohort: The Framingham heart study. Circulation 90:878–883

Turner JM, Mead J, Wohl ME 1968 Elasticity of human lungs in relation to age. Journal of Applied Physiology 25(6):664–671

van der Heijden-Spek JJ, Staessen JA, Fagard RH, Hoeks AP, Boudier HA, van Bortel LM 2000 Effect of age on brachial artery wall properties differs from the aorta and is gender dependent: a population study. Hypertension 35:637–642

Van Pelt RE, Davy KP, Stevenson ET, Wilson TM, Jones PP, Desouza CA, Seals DR 1998 Smaller differences in total and regional adiposity with age in women who regularly perform endurance exercise. American Journal of Physiology. Endocrine Metabolism 275(38):E626–E634

Vandervoort AA 2002 Aging of the human neuromuscular system. Muscle and Nerve 25:17–25

Vandervoort AA, McComas AJ 1986 Contractile changes in opposing muscles of the human ankle with aging. Journal of Applied Physiology 61(1):361–367

Vaughan L, Zurlo F, Ravussin E 1991 Aging and energy expenditure. American Journal of Clinical Nutrition 53:821–825

Verdijk LB, Koopman R, Schaart G, Meijer K, Savelberg HH, van Loon LJ 2007 Satellite cell content is specifically reduced in type II skeletal muscle fibres. American Journal of Physiology. Endocrine Metabolism 292:E151–E157

Viegi G, Sherrill DL, Carrozzi L, Di Pede F, Baldacci S, Pistelli F, Enright P 2001 An 8-year follow-up of carbon monoxide diffusing capacity in a general population sample of northern Italy. Chest 120:74–80

Wilson MG, Morley JE 2003 Invited review: aging and energy balance. Journal of Applied Physiology 95:1728–1736

World Health Organisation 1998 World atlas of ageing. World Health Organisation: Centre of Human Development, Kobe

World Health Organisation 2006 Obesity and overweight. Fact Sheet No 311. World Health Organisation, Geneva

Woo SJ, Derleth C, Stratton JR, Levy WC 2006 The influence of age, gender and training on exercise efficiency. Journal of the American College of Cardiology 47(5):1049–1057

Yamanouchi K, Nakajima H, Shinozaki T, Chikada K, Kato K, Oshida Y, Osawa I, Sato J, Sato Y, Higuchi M, Kobayashi S 1992 Effects of daily physical activity on insulin action in the elderly. Journal of Applied Physiology 73(6):2241–2245

Ziegler MG, Lake CR, Kopin IJ 1976 Plasma norepinephrine increases with age. Nature 261:333–345

Chapter 17

Topical discussions

Chapter **17.1**

Thirty minutes of exercise: is it sufficient for better health?

Hidde P. van der Ploeg   Adrian E. Bauman

There has been a growing interest in physical activity and population health in recent decades (Chapter 28), with concomitant debate concerning the amount of physical activity required for health, and whether it should be structured as habitual exercise or just any large muscle movement (physical activity). This chapter summarises the current epidemiological debate on the minimum amount of daily physical activity required for health maintenance, compared to the benefits of habitual exercise alone. Habitual exercise is defined as deliberate regular exercise (training) and is one of the subdomains of physical activity.

1 EXERCISE FOR FITNESS RECOMMENDATIONS

It has long been recognised that frequent vigorous aerobic exercise improves physical fitness (American College of Sports Medicine 1978). The training effects of improved cardiorespiratory fitness can be achieved through vigorous intensity activities, performed three times a week for ≥ 20 min. This would represent exercising at an intensity >6 metabolic equivalents (METs: the ratio of work to a standard resting metabolic rate of ~4.2 $kJ \cdot kg^{-1} \cdot h^{-1}$ (3.5 $mL \cdot kg^{-1} \cdot min^{-1}$)). Improved physical fitness influences physiological changes that contribute to better health, e.g. lower blood pressure, higher maximal oxygen uptake, better blood lipid profiles and increased muscle with reduced fat masses.

2 PHYSICAL ACTIVITY FOR HEALTH RECOMMENDATIONS

By the late 1980s, the accumulated epidemiological evidence suggested that moderate-intensity physical activity (3–6 MET) had a beneficial effect on all-cause mortality and cardiovascular disease risk (Blair et al. 1989, Powell et al. 1987). The distillation of this evidence resulted in a health-directed physical activity recommendation – that adults undertake 30 min of at least moderate-intensity physical activity, accumulated in bouts of at least 10 minutes on ≥ 5 $d \cdot wk^{-1}$ (Pate et al. 1995, US Department of Health and Human Services 1996). The major innovation of the health-related recommendation was targeting high-risk sedentary people, aiming for moderate energy expenditures rather than aerobic training levels. This led to a substantial change in physical activity recommendations, with a change from the low-population prevalence, vigorous activities, to more moderate-intensity activities, including walking.

3 CURRENT EPIDEMIOLOGICAL EVIDENCE

This section explores the recent epidemiological evidence about physical activity and health, and examines whether it has changed since the 1996 physical activity for health recommendation. First, it is important to know whether the relationship between physical activity and health is of a curvilinear dose–response form, as it appears to be for fitness and health (Blair et al. 2001). This curvilinear dose–response relationship means that improving fitness by the same amount will have higher health benefits for an unfit than a fit person (who was already at a higher level of health). In other words, the benefits of fitness for health will level off or even plateau as an individual gets fitter. It seems that the same curvilinear relationship also applies for physical activity in general, with the maximum risk reduction occurring in moving the sedentary to become at least moderately active (Bauman 2004).

A review of observational studies showed that meeting the physical activity for health recommendation reduced all-cause mortality risk by 20–30% in European and US samples (Lee & Skerrett 2001). A recent study in a large representative cohort from China showed a 17% risk reduction in all-cause mortality from regular work-related physical activity alone (He et al. 2005). Most of the effects on all-cause mortality can be assigned to the positive effects of physical activity on cardiovascular disease and cancer, the leading causes of mortality and morbidity in developed and most developing countries (World Health Organisation 2002; Chapter 28).

3.1 Cardiovascular disease

The protective effects of physical activity on cardiovascular disease risk have been recognised for two decades (Berlin & Colditz 1990, Powell et al. 1987). A recent metaanalysis suggests some protective effects of physical activity in reducing stroke risk (Lee et al. 2003). A consensus conference of leading scientists supported a causal and inverse dose–response relationship between physical activity and the risk of cardiovascular disease (Kohl 2001). It seems that both the amount and the intensity of physical activity follow a dose–response relationship.

Another epidemiological review suggested a curvilinear dose–response relationship between physical activity and cardiovascular disease (Bauman 2004). This relationship was illustrated by a descriptive summary of studies published in 2000–2003, revealing that the largest risk reduction

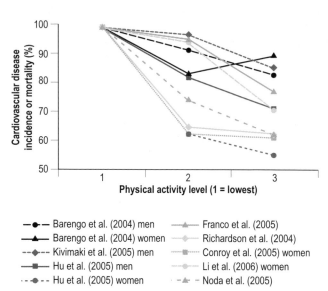

Figure **17.1.1** Risk reduction estimates of the relationship between physical activity and cardiovascular disease, from epidemiological studies published from 2003 to 2006.

in cardiovascular disease was from the first quintile (lowest 20%) to the second and third quintiles of self-reported physical activity. That is, the most sedentary, high-responding people would gain the greatest health benefit from increasing their physical activity level.

For this chapter, an extension of this review was carried out (2003–2006), with eight prospective epidemiological studies identified. Figure 17.1.1 shows that the most recent data support the dose–response relationship between physical activity and the risks of cardiovascular disease (incidence or mortality) for three physical activity groups, as reported in these studies. This figure reinforces earlier notions that the largest risk reduction in cardiovascular disease is from the sedentary to the mid-level physical activity group, showing an average decrease of 20%, compared to a further 9% risk reduction from the mid-level to the high-level group. This finding is supported by the metaanalysis of cohort studies on physical activity and stroke (Lee et al. 2003). Moderately active individuals had a 17% lower risk on stroke incidence or mortality than sedentary people, while highly active individuals showed a further 8% risk reduction compared to the moderately active individuals.

3.2 Cancer

Physical activity reduces overall all-cause cancer risk (Thune & Furberg 2001). The benefit is mostly due to the protective effects of physical activity on colon and breast cancer. The strongest evidence has been reported for colon cancer, with a metaanalysis of 19 cohort studies showing that habitually physically active people had a 20–30% reduction in colon cancer risk compared with sedentary people (Samad et al. 2005). However, there is no consensus on the required dose. For example, one review suggested that 30–60 min·d^{-1} of moderate- to vigorous-intensity physical activity is needed to decrease colon cancer risk (Lee 2003), another suggested that only 3.5–4.0 h·wk^{-1} of vigorous activity may be needed to optimise protection (Slattery 2004), whilst a third review suggested that a dose–response relationship was strongest for moderate-intensity physical activity (>4.5 METs; Thune & Furberg 2001). Although there is still a lack of consensus here, it seems that the current 30 min daily physical activity for health recommendations might be insufficient to reduce colon cancer risk.

Physical activity reduces the risk of breast cancer in women by 20–30% (Lee 2003, Thune & Furberg 2001). Even though there seems to be a dose–response relationship, the evidence is less clear on the volume or intensity required, leaving it unclear if the current physical activity for health recommendation is sufficient to reduce breast cancer risk.

3.3 Metabolic conditions

Physical activity reduces the risk of obesity, diabetes and other metabolic conditions (Chapter 30). Obesity results from disturbances in energy balance, due to sedentary lifestyles and excessive caloric intake. The current physical activity for health recommendation appears to be insufficient to prevent body mass gain or reduce body mass among those already obese. However, achieving the physical activity for health recommendation protects against all-cause, cardiovascular and cancer mortality, regardless of body mass (Hu et al. 2005). Indeed, habitual physical activity and obesity, whilst related, are independent risk factors. Thus, obese but physically active people have lower risks on all-cause, cardiovascular and cancer mortality than sedentary people with normal body mass. The message is that meeting the physical activity for health recommendation is also beneficial for people with continuing obesity.

A consensus statement suggests that 45–60 min·d^{-1} of at least moderate-intensity physical activity is required to prevent a transition to overweight and obesity (Institute of Medicine 2002, Saris et al. 2003), with others suggesting even more, recommending 60–80 min·d^{-1} of moderate-intensity physical activity for body mass loss or maintenance (Bensimhon et al. 2006, Fogelholm & Kukkonen-Harjula 2000; see also Chapter 13). This variation centres on the different requirements for body mass maintenance and reduction.

Obesity is also a risk factor for diabetes mellitus (Chapter 30). Apart from the effects of physical activity on body mass loss and maintenance, there may be a direct beneficial effect of physical activity on diabetes (LaMonte et al. 2005), possibly independent of body mass loss (Ramachandran 2006). However, combined body mass loss and habitual, moderate-intensity physical activity seems an optimal recommendation to reduce diabetes incidence in at-risk populations with impaired glucose tolerance (Knowler 2002).

4 THIRTY MINUTES OF EXERCISE: IS IT SUFFICIENT FOR BETTER HEALTH?

The current evidence indicates that the recommended 30 min·d^{-1} of at least moderate-intensity physical activity, performed 5 d·wk^{-1}, is important in the prevention of cardiovascular disease, colon and breast cancer and diabetes. However, it seems that a greater volume and intensity are needed to optimise the protective effect against colon and breast cancer. For body mass maintenance and loss, the 30 min·d^{-1} prescription appears to be insufficient.

Do moderate-intensity physical activities benefit health? This appears to be the case, especially for cardiovascular disease prevention and reducing blood pressure, even though vigorous physical activities might still be more effective in cancer prevention and body mass loss. Unfortunately, only ~15% of the population habitually participates in vigorous aerobic exercise. Moderate-intensity activities are more achievable by most people. This level is already prevalent and is associated with lower adverse effects (e.g. injury incidence, risk of cardiovascular events for sedentary people who trial vigorous activities too early). Moderate activities are easily integrated and maintained into everyday life, including walking, cycling, moderate gardening, vacuum cleaning and stair climbing.

The exercise for fitness and physical activity for health recommendations have different objectives, and co-exist perfectly. From the public health point of view, initial efforts should focus on the physical activity for health recommendation, since this has the highest potential to get as many people as possible to become sufficiently physically active, reducing morbidity, mortality and, as a consequence, health-care costs in the population (Chapter 31.1). The main focus should be to encourage sedentary people (~40–50% of the population) to meet physical activity for health recommendations. If, for example, all sedentary people met the physical activity for health recommendation, around 20% of all cardiovascular deaths might be prevented (Bauman & Miller 2004).

In conclusion, 30 min·d^{-1} of at least moderate-intensity physical activity, performed 5 d·wk^{-1}, is a good, but minimal start for adults to significantly reduce non-communicable disease risk. More specific recommendations should also be formulated for some specific conditions (Pedersen & Saltin 2006) and for secondary and tertiary prevention goals among those already with chronic disease.

References

American College of Sports Medicine 1978 American College of Sports Medicine position statement on the recommended quantity and quality of exercise for developing and maintaining fitness in healthy adults. Medicine and Science in Sports 10(3):vii–x

Barengo NC, Hu G, Lakka TA, Pekkarinen H, Nissinen A, Tuomilehto J 2004 Low physical activity as a predictor for total and cardiovascular disease mortality in middle-aged men and women in Finland. European Heart Journal 25(24):2204–2211

Bauman AE 2004 Updating the evidence that physical activity is good for health: an epidemiological review 2000–2003. Journal of Science and Medicine in Sport 7(suppl 1):6–19

Bauman AE, Miller Y 2004 The public health potential of health enhancing physical activity. In: Oja P, Borms J (eds) Health enhancing physical activity. Meyer and Meyer Sport, Oxford, 125–147

Bensimhon DR, Kraus WE, Donahue MP 2006 Obesity and physical activity: a review. American Heart Journal 151(3):598–603

Berlin J, Colditz GA 1990 A meta analysis of physical activity in the prevention of coronary heart disease. American Journal of Epidemiology 132(4):612–628

Blair SN, Cheng Y, Holder JS 2001 Is physical activity or physical fitness more important in defining health benefits? Medicine and Science in Sports and Exercise 33(suppl 6):S379–399

Blair SN, Kohl HW 3rd, Paffenbarger RS Jr, Clark DG, Cooper KH, Gibbons LW 1989 Physical fitness and all-cause mortality. A prospective study of healthy men and women. Journal of the American Medical Association 262(17):2395–2401

Conroy MB, Cook NR, Manson JE, Buring JE, Lee IM 2005 Past physical activity, current physical activity and risk of coronary heart disease. Medicine and Science in Sports and Exercise 37(8):1251–1256

Fogelholm M, Kukkonen-Harjula K 2000 Does physical activity prevent weight gain – a systematic review. Obesity Reviews 1(2):95–111

Franco OH, de Laet C, Peeters A, Jonker J, Mackenbach J, Nusselder W 2005 Effects of physical activity on life expectancy with cardiovascular disease. Archives of Internal Medicine 165(20):2355–2360

He J, Gu D, Wu X 2005 Major causes of death among men and women in China. New England Journal of Medicine 353(11):1124–1134

Hu G, Tuomilehto J, Silventoinen K, Barengo NC, Peltonen M, Jousilahti P 2005 The effects of physical activity and body mass index on cardiovascular, cancer and all-cause mortality among 47 212 middle-aged Finnish men and women. International Journal of Obesity 29(8):894–902

Institute of Medicine 2002 Dietary reference intakes: energy, carbohydrates, fiber, fat, protein and amino acids. National Academy Press, Washington, DC

Kivimäki M, Ferrie JE, Brunner E, Head J, Shipley MJ, Vahtera J, Marmot MG 2005 Justice at work and reduced risk of coronary heart disease among employees: the Whitehall II Study. Archives of Internal Medicine 165(19):2245–2251

Knowler WC, Barrett-Connor E, Fowler SE, Hamman RF, Lachin JM, Walker EA, Nathan DM 2002 Reduction in the incidence of type 2 diabetes with lifestyle intervention or metformin. New England Journal of Medicine 346(6):393–403

Kohl HW 2001 Physical activity and cardiovascular disease: evidence for a dose response. Medicine and Science in Sports and Exercise 33(suppl 6):S472-S483

LaMonte MJ, Blair SN, Church TS 2005 Physical activity and diabetes prevention. Journal of Applied Physiology 99(3):1205–1213

Lee CD, Folsom AR, Blair SN 2003 Physical activity and stroke risk: a meta-analysis. Stroke 34(10):2475–2481

Lee IM 2003 Physical activity and cancer prevention – data from epidemiologic studies. Medicine and Science in Sports and Exercise 35(11):1823–1827

Lee IM, Skerrett PJ 2001 Physical activity and all-cause mortality: what is the dose response relation? Medicine and Science in Sports and Exercise 33(suppl 6):S459–471

Li TY, Rana JS, Manson JE, Willett WC, Stampfer MJ, Colditz GA, Rexrode KM, Hu FB 2006 Obesity as compared with physical activity in predicting risk of coronary heart disease in women. Circulation 113(4):499–506

Noda H, Iso H, Toyoshima H, Date C, Yamamoto A, Kikuchi S, Koizumi A, Kondo T, Watanabe Y, Wada Y, Inaba Y, Tamakoshi A 2005 Walking and sports participation and mortality from coronary heart disease and stroke. Journal of the American College of Cardiology 46(9):1761–1767

Pate R, Pratt M, Blair SN, Haskell WL, Macera CA, Bouchard C, Buchner D, Ettinger W, Heath GW, King AC, Kriska A, Leon AS, Marcus BH, Morris J, Paffenbarger RS, Patrick K, Pollock ML, Rippe JM, Sallis J, Wilmore JH 1995 Physical activity and public health. A recommendation from the Centers for Disease Control and Prevention and the American College of Sports Medicine. Journal of the American Medical Association 273(5):402–407

Pedersen BK, Saltin B 2006 Evidence for prescribing exercise as therapy in chronic disease. Scandinavian Journal of Medicine and Science in Sports 16(suppl 1):3–63

Powell KE, Thompson PD, Caspersen CJ, Kendrick JS 1987 Physical activity and the incidence of coronary heart disease. Annual Review of Public Health 8:253–287

Ramachandran A, Snehalatha C, Mary S, Mukesh B, Bhaskar AD, Vijay V 2006 The Indian Diabetes Prevention Programme shows that lifestyle modification and metformin prevent type 2 diabetes in Asian Indian subjects with impaired glucose tolerance (IDPP-1). Diabetologia 49:289–297

Richardson CR, Kriska AM, Lantz PM, Hayward RA 2004 Physical activity and mortality across cardiovascular disease risk groups. Medicine and Science in Sports and Exercise 36(11):1923–1929

Samad AK, Taylor RS, Marshall T, Chapman MA 2005 A meta-analysis of the association of physical activity with reduced risk of colorectal cancer. Colorectal Disease 7(3):204–213

Saris WH, Blair SN, Van Baak MA Eaton SB, Davies PSW, Di Pietro L, Fogelholm M, Rissanen A, Schoeller D, Swinburn B, Tremblay A, Westerterp KR, Wyatt H 2003 How much physical activity is enough to prevent unhealthy weight gain? Outcome of the IASO 1st Stock Conference and consensus statement. Obesity Reviews 4(2):101–114

Slattery ML 2004 Physical activity and colorectal cancer. Sports Medicine 34(4):239–252

Thune I, Furberg A 2001 Physical activity and cancer risk: dose–response and cancer, all sites and site-specific. Medicine and Science in Sports and Exercise 33(suppl 6):S530-S550

US Department of Health and Human Services 1996 Physical activity and health: a report of the Surgeon General. US Department of Health and Human Services, Centers of Disease Control and Prevention, National Center for Chronic Disease Prevention and Health Promotion, Atlanta, GA

World Health Organisation 2002 World health report. World Health Organisation, Geneva

Chapter 17.2

Exercise and ageing: can the biological clock be stopped?

David N. Proctor   Michael J. Joyner

CHAPTER CONTENTS

1 INTRODUCTION

Starting at ~30 years, sedentary adults begin to lose 5–10% of their ability to exercise maximally each decade (peak aerobic power, peak or maximal oxygen uptake; Buskirk & Hodgson 1987, Holloszy & Kohrt 1995). In sedentary 60–70-year-old individuals (high responders), 4–6 months of endurance training can increase maximal oxygen uptake ~20%, reversing nearly two decades of loss (Huang et al. 2005). Beyond ~50 years, sedentary individuals start losing an average of 10–15% of their muscle strength and 6% of their muscle mass each decade (Janssen et al. 2000, Kallman et al. 1990, Lindle et al. 1997). Again, 2–3 months of resistance training in 65–75-year-old individuals can increase muscle strength by almost one-third, making up for nearly three decades of functional decay (Lemmer et al. 2000, Roth et al. 2001). These results are impressive and support the premise that exercise training can, from a physiological functional standpoint, turn back the biological clock.

Equally impressive are the effects of exercise on health maintenance and longevity (Chapters 17.1 and 28). It is now generally accepted that physically active individuals tend to live longer than their sedentary peers (Blair et al. 1996, Lee & Skerrett 2001). A recent analysis of 44 observational studies shows that adults expending at least 4.2 MJ·wk^{-1} (1000 kcal·wk^{-1}) in leisure physical activities reduce their overall risk of premature death by 20–30% (Lee & Skerrett 2001, Oguma et al. 2002). Death rates and risk factors for cardiovascular diseases, which increase steeply with advancing age (Lakatta & Levy 2003), are also substantially lower in moderately active adults (Kohl 2001). Regular exercise appears to induce these cardioprotective effects not only by favourably modifying established coronary disease risk factors, but also by exerting direct effects on the functional properties of vascular endothelial and smooth muscle cells (Hambrecht et al. 2000, Laughlin 2004). The benefits of exercise, however, extend beyond just a reduction in premature mortality.

Regular exercise can also increase active life expectancy or the number of years spent living independently and free of disability (Shephard 1997, Spirduso et al. 2005, Wang

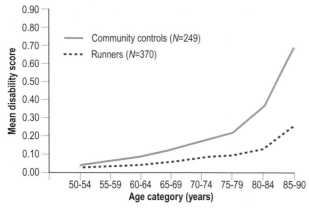

Figure 17.2.1 Physical disability score, derived from an annual health assessment questionnaire, for running club members and non-runners (community control subjects) based on the longitudinal study of Wang et al. (2002). Running club members experienced significantly (P < 0.001) lower mean disability scores relative to controls within any age category, and exhibited a delay in the time to reach a given level of disability, consistent with the compression of morbidity hypothesis.

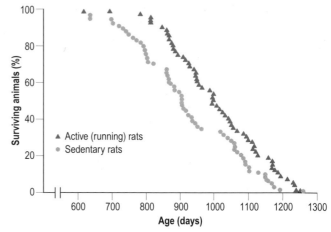

Figure 17.2.2 Survival curves of female rats either having free access to voluntary running wheels, starting at the age of 4 months (runners), or kept inactive and housed in individual cages (sedentary). Results indicate that wheel running initiated early in life can improve average life expectancy in rats, but does not increase maximal lifespan. Graph redrawn from Holloszy (1993) with permission.

et al. 2002). The postponement of disability as close to the age of natural death as possible, through exercise and other healthy lifestyle habits, is graphically depicted in Figure 17.2.1, and conforms to the concept originally termed the compression of morbidity (Fries 1980). Collectively, the epidemiological literature supports the widely held belief that regular exercise is broadly protective against the premature development of chronic diseases, and can positively influence both the quantity and quality of life.

While the above results clearly demonstrate the potential benefits of regular exercise for restoring physical function and protecting against the negative health consequences of a sedentary lifestyle (minimising the effects of secondary ageing), these data do not directly address the more basic question of whether exercise can slow, or possibly reverse, the primary ageing process. To change ageing processes would require changing the rate of ageing, thereby increasing the maximal lifespan.

Investigations of rats given voluntary access to running wheels at an early age has provided a well-controlled experimental model for addressing this question, in a relatively short-lived species. In these studies, maximal lifespan (age at 100% mortality) was similar in rats given free access to running wheels compared with sedentary rats in adjacent cages that had no access to running wheels (Holloszy 1993, Holloszy & Kohrt 1995). However, a higher percentage of the runners lived to an older age compared to the non-runners, as illustrated in Figure 17.2.2 as a rightward shift of survival curve in the runners, but with a similar maximal lifespan (~1250 days). These findings suggest that lifelong exercise does not slow the primary ageing process in rats, but it can increase average lifespan, presumably by slowing the rate of secondary ageing (Chapter 16).

Determining if and how exercise affects the primary ageing process in humans is extremely difficult. First, it is necessary to rigorously exclude subjects with underlying pathology from research. This allows the investigation of age-related changes in physiological function in the absence of age-related diseases, such as atherosclerosis, hypertension, neurological disease, etc. There is also the normal tendency for both the total amount and intensity of daily physical activity to decline as people grow older (Donato et al. 2003, Goldspink 2005, Holloszy & Kohrt 1995, Saltin 1986, Shephard 1997). Since many of the physiological changes typically attributed to advancing age mimic those observed during periods of reduced physical activity (e.g. deconditioning, bed rest; Chapter 9), it has been difficult to separate the adaptations associated with a sedentary lifestyle from the intrinsic changes associated with ageing. Much of the early research on ageing and physiological function was not adequately controlled to differentiate between the effects of ageing, disuse, disease or even gender differences. Fortunately, contemporary research in this area has acknowledged these issues by studying carefully screened (healthy) human subjects in well-defined subgroups, or by using study designs and statistical techniques to take physical activity and other lifestyle factors into account.

In the remainder of this chapter, we critically review the literature that has examined the influence of habitual physical exercise on the physiological ageing process in healthy humans. We have focused on the age-related decline in maximal aerobic power and muscle function because the influence of habitual exercise on these age-associated changes remains unclear, and in some cases highly controversial; there are extensive cross-sectional and longitudinal data for these variables and their physiological determinants (e.g. muscle mass and quality); and maintenance of an adequate level of these functional attributes is critical to physical independence and quality of life.

2 MAXIMAL AEROBIC POWER

Arguably the most widely studied physiological change in the human ageing and exercise literature is the age-related decline in maximal oxygen uptake, a change that reflects a reduced cardiovascular and skeletal muscle functional reserve. This decline means that older individuals work closer to maximum effort when performing a standardised submaximal task, as compared to themselves when younger. Peak aerobic power is also an independent risk factor for cardiovascular and all-cause mortality (Blair et al. 1996), and favourably influences changes in cognitive function and other quality of life indicators with advancing age (Laurin et al. 2001).

Despite decades of research on maximal oxygen uptake and ageing, there remain several unresolved issues. Experimental studies in this area have attempted to address the following questions. Does exercise slow the rate of decline in maximal oxygen uptake with age? To what extent are central (cardiac) and peripheral (skeletal muscle) factors responsible for its decline in physically active and sedentary populations? Are these age-associated reductions gender dependent?

The first question has typically been probed by examining the average slopes of the age-related decline in peak aerobic power, derived from habitually active populations, and comparing these to the decline in maximal oxygen uptake reported for sedentary populations, which averages 0.4–0.5 mL·kg^{-1}·min^{-1}·y^{-1} or approximately 9% per decade. Early longitudinal studies often reported that the largest declines in maximal oxygen uptake were among endurance athletes, with relatively high values, who subsequently became less active or stopped training (0.9–1.3 mL·kg^{-1}·min^{-1}·y^{-1} or 12–15% per decade). In effect, these studies revealed the combined effects of ageing and a reduced training stimulus (Holloszy & Kohrt 1995).

More contemporary investigations, focusing on endurance-trained male athletes who had continued to train and compete over many years, reported age-associated declines that were roughly half the rates seen in sedentary subjects (5% versus 9% per decade; Hagberg et al. 1985, Heath et al. 1981, Trappe et al. 1996). Longitudinal studies by Pollock et al. (1987), Rogers et al. (1990) and Kasch et al. (1993) further showed that maximal oxygen uptake could be maintained over 10–20-year periods in middle-aged men who maintained absolute training intensity and did not gain mass. These findings, primarily based on longitudinal studies in a relatively small number of elite older males, are in keeping with the premise that vigorous endurance exercise slows the loss of maximal aerobic power with ageing.

However, recent studies involving larger numbers of subjects from a broader age range, including women, have begun to challenge the generality of this concept. Two metaanalyses, one involving men (Wilson & Tanaka 2000) and the other women (Fitzgerald et al. 1997), show no clear difference in the relative rates of maximal oxygen uptake decline (% per decade) between sedentary and habitually endurance-trained populations over a broad age range (18–89 years). Furthermore, Ezkurza et al. (2002) reported that the longitudinal reduction in maximal oxygen uptake for ~50–60-year-old competitive women distance runners, who maintained or increased training volume, was not different from that of sedentary women, in contrast to previous findings in men (Kasch et al. 1993, Pollock et al. 1987, Rogers et al. 1990). Finally, Fleg et al. (2005) recently published peak oxygen uptake data (treadmill) from 375 healthy women and 435 men (Baltimore Longitudinal Study on Aging), and observed no alteration in the peak aerobic power decline across six decades (in either gender), after adjusting for self-reported habitual physical activity. Furthermore, the accelerated rate of decline after age 70 was not influenced by habitual physical activity in either gender.

Collectively, these studies suggest that habitual physical activity among the general population, and prolonged vigorous endurance exercise among older women, does not markedly slow the age-related decline in maximal oxygen uptake. Similar conclusions are reached when examining average rates of change in age group world records for endurance events that are significantly influenced by aerobic power (Holloszy & Kohrt 1995, Joyner 1993). In these events, the average rate of decline, as a function of age (~10% per decade), is not much different from that observed for maximal oxygen uptake in the sedentary population.

To summarise, the current state of knowledge suggests that habitual exercise does not markedly slow the age-related decline in maximal oxygen uptake in healthy adults; the possible exception is middle-aged men who maintain a high volume and intensity of endurance exercise. However, even the most highly fit individuals inevitably experience a reduction in the absolute intensity of their training, particularly after ~60 years (Ezkurza et al. 2002, Pollock et al. 1987, Rogers et al. 1990, Saltin 1986, Trappe et al. 1996). This more rapid decline is also observed, although at a slightly older age threshold (~70 years), in non-weight bearing endurance activities such as swimming, in which orthopaedic injury rates are low (Tanaka & Seals 2003). A final point to emphasise is that, although endurance-trained individuals show similar rates of decline in mass-adjusted maximal oxygen uptake as sedentary individuals, they are on a much higher slope; at any age, trained individuals have a higher absolute peak aerobic power. In this respect, they retain a considerable functional advantage over their healthy but less active peers.

2.1 Physiological determinants of maximal oxygen uptake

The relative contributions of central (cardiac) and peripheral (muscle mass, muscle blood flow, oxidative capacity, oxygen extraction) factors to the age-related decline in maximal oxygen uptake have long been debated. Indeed, these contributions are debated with respect to their importance in determining maximal oxygen uptake in young adults (Chapter 10.1). The most consistent central circulatory change with age is the decrease in maximal heart rate: 0.7 beats·min^{-1}·y^{-1} (Tanaka et al. 2001). This reduction typically accounts for 30–50% of the age-associated decrease in peak aerobic power in sedentary adults, and is not generally influenced by exercise habit (Robinson 1938, Saltin 1986, Strandell 1976).

By contrast, there is considerable variability among studies in the contribution of maximal stroke volume to the age-related decline in maximal oxygen uptake. Maximal stroke volume during exhaustive upright exercise has been shown to be higher (Rodeheffer et al. 1984), lower (Ogawa et al. 1992, Proctor et al. 2004) or not different (Beere et al. 1999, Fleg et al. 1995) in older compared to younger sedentary adults. These variable results are possibly due to between-study differences in cardiac output measurement techniques, exercise modes, the rigour of subject screening and the extent to which subjects are encouraged to reach a true maximal effort. Consequently, the extent to which habitual endurance exercise can modify any age-related alteration in maximal stroke volume has been difficult to ascertain. Nonetheless, there is now general agreement among cross-sectional studies that overall cardiac performance during maximal exertion (maximal cardiac output) is diminished across the adult lifespan in healthy sedentary men and women (Fleg et al. 1995, Weiss et al. 2006). Depending on the age range studied and the mode of exercise, reductions in maximal cardiac output have accounted for 50% to as much as 90% of the age-related difference in peak aerobic power (Beere et al. 1999, Fleg et al. 1995, Ogawa et al. 1992, Proctor et al. 2004, Weiss et al. 2006).

Until recently, there was very little information available regarding the effects of ageing on blood flow or oxygen extraction within the active muscles during exercise. Our studies of healthy, recreationally active adults indicate that reduced blood flow to the leg muscles is a major determinant of the age-associated reduction in peak oxygen uptake during exhaustive cycling (Proctor et al. 2004). Peak arteriovenous oxygen differences across the exercising legs tend to be lower in older adults at maximal exertion, but these differences were small (<1 mL·dL^{-1} in men (Beere et al. 1999, Proctor et al. 2003) or not significant (women; Proctor et al. 2004). This is in general agreement with the small reductions observed in leg muscle capillarity with ageing in non-endurance trained adults (Coggan et al. 1992, Harris 2005, Proctor et al. 1995). Little is known about possible reductions in peripheral oxygen extraction in older age groups (>70 years), when there is an accelerated loss of muscle mass.

The role of declining muscle mass per se in the age-related decline in maximal oxygen uptake has been seldom studied. Fleg & Lakatta (1988) were the first to explicitly address this issue, finding the age-associated decline in peak aerobic power (mL·kg^{-1}·min^{-1}) of sedentary men and women (21–87 years) was blunted by ~50% when normalised to urinary creatinine excretion, an index of whole-body muscle mass. We also observed a nearly 50% reduction in the age-associated difference in aerobic power when we normalised the treadmill maximal oxygen uptake values of younger and older endurance-trained athletes to a more precise measure of their active muscle mass (arm plus leg muscle mass; Proctor & Joyner 1997). Because maximal oxygen uptake indexed to muscle mass essentially factors out the influence of adipose tissue, these data could be interpreted to suggest that body fat accumulation, and not muscle loss, contributed to the decline in whole-body aerobic power with age in these studies. Regardless, it is unlikely that reduced muscle mass plays a major role in this decline, because most healthy older adults have sufficient muscle mass to reach maximal oxygen uptake (Day et al. 2003, Holloszy & Kohrt 1995, Proctor & Joyner 1997). It is likely that the normalisation of aerobic power to estimates of muscle mass (including fat-free or lean body mass) will continue to be most useful when comparing the performance of the cardiorespiratory system between populations that differ widely in body size or composition (e.g. men versus women, children versus adults), and in subjects who exhibit the greatest degree of muscle loss.

Does the peripheral capacity for oxygen consumption decline with advancing age? Although not traditionally considered a limiting factor to aerobic performance (Chapter 10.1), there are emerging data from both the human and animal literature indicating that a reduction in the oxidative capacity of the locomotor muscles is an important determinant of reduced maximal oxygen uptake in sedentary older individuals (Conley et al. 2000a).

Mitochondrial volume densities and the maximal activities of several oxidative enzymes are lower in leg muscle biopsy samples taken from untrained older men and women compared to younger controls (Coggan et al. 1992, Short et al. 2003); this age-related reduction in muscle oxidative potential also extends to the individual fibre types (Proctor et al. 1995). Conley and colleagues (2000b) reported that in vivo estimates of oxidative capacity, per unit volume of quadriceps muscle, were also reduced in sedentary older adults and linearly correlated with the age-related decline in cycling peak oxygen uptake. Finally, in an isolated pump-perfused, distal hindlimb preparation, designed to avoid age-associated reductions in systemic blood delivery, Hepple et al. (2003) demonstrated reduced muscle peak oxygen uptake in 28–30-month-old versus 8-month-old rats, at matched rates of oxygen delivery. Collectively, these recent human and animal data indicate that capacity for skeletal muscle oxygen uptake is reduced with sedentary ageing, and contributes to the reduction in whole-body oxygen uptake during maximal exertion.

3 SKELETAL MUSCLE SIZE AND FUNCTION

Peak isometric and dynamic muscle strength in most normally active adults does not generally decline to a significant extent until ~50 years of age, with accelerated losses occurring after age 70 (Hurley 1995, Lindle et al. 1997). The rate of decline in leg strength is quite similar in men and women (Chapter 16), but women have lower initial levels (Chapters 11, 13, 14.1), thus reaching minimum strength thresholds needed to perform ambulatory daily tasks at earlier ages (Guralnick et al. 1995, Hurley 1995, Lynch et al. 1999, Shephard 1997). A major determinant underlying the age-associated declines in peak strength appears to be the reduction in muscle cross-sectional area and volume (Doherty 2003, Holloszy & Kohrt 1995, Janssen et al. 2000), which results from reductions in total fibre number (Lexell et al. 1988) and preferential atrophy of the remaining fast-twitch (type II) fibres (Coggan et al. 1992, Lexell et al. 1988, Proctor et al. 1995). Sedentary individuals lose significant amounts of muscle during the course of the adult lifespan, particularly in the lower body (30–40% by 70–80 years; Janssen et al. 2000).

Muscle mass and strength usually cannot be preserved well into old age unless a sufficient intensity of muscular loading is maintained. Regular endurance exercise training within the general population, or by competitive master athletes does not augment maximum voluntary strength or contraction velocity (Goldspink 2005, Harridge et al. 1997, Klitgaard et al. 1990), nor does it preserve fat-free mass (Klitgaard et al. 1990, Pollock et al. 1987). Additionally, we have reported both cross-sectional and longitudinal evidence for fast-twitch fibre atrophy in the quadriceps of older compared to younger endurance-trained athletes, despite indications that these fibres were regularly recruited (i.e. fibres exhibited elevated succinate dehydrogenase activities and high capillary-fibre ratios; Proctor et al. 1995). Collectively, these results suggest that endurance exercise is not a sufficient stimulus to counteract the age-associated atrophy of fast-twitch muscle fibres, at least in men. It appears that overloading the muscles regularly with resistance training exercises is necessary to augment muscle size and strength in older adults (Doherty 2003). However, it is interesting to note that even strength-trained older athletes (Klitgaard et al. 1990) do not exhibit the muscle size and strength characteristics of younger athletes. Perhaps this is because these older athletes did not initiate strength training until after age 50, after some irreversible loss of muscle fibre number had already probably occurred.

Can regular participation in strength training slow the loss of peak muscular strength with advancing age? The information available to address this question is very limited because the number of laboratory-based physiological comparisons of strength-trained athletes at various ages is small, by comparison with the literature on ageing endurance athletes (Spirduso et al. 2005). Cross-sectional studies indicate that elite masters weightlifters experience similar average rates of decline in peak isometric strength with age as healthy sedentary individuals (Klitgaard et al. 1990, Pearson et al. 2002, Spirduso et al. 2005). Similar conclusions are reached when examining average rates of change in age group world records for weightlifting events (e.g. Shephard 1997, Spirduso et al. 2005). That is, the average rates of change for weightlifting records, as a function of age, are not much less than the rates of strength loss in the general sedentary population. However, strength-trained athletes are stronger and more powerful at any given age, providing a significantly higher functional reserve.

In addition to its critical function in bodily movement, skeletal muscle plays a central role in several metabolic processes (protein, carbohydrate, lipid metabolism), and is a major determinant of basal metabolic rate. Because of changes in skeletal muscle composition with advancing age, in particular increased lipid content (Janssen & Ross 2005), there has been growing interest in determining the cause of intramuscular lipid accumulation in older adults, and how this may be linked to adverse metabolic consequences in ageing humans, such as decreased insulin sensitivity and mitochondrial dysfunction. To this end, increased intramuscular lipid accumulation has been linked to variation in dietary fat intake, relative obesity and decreased habitual physical activity in older adults (Janssen & Ross 2005). Therefore, it is quite possible that the increased intramuscular lipid deposition within aged muscles is due, at least in part, to lifestyle factors (Chapters 28 and 30).

4 CONCLUSION

Can the biological clock be stopped? From a functional standpoint, the evidence is very supportive. However, there appear to be limits to the retention of maximal cardiovascular and skeletal muscle functioning in older humans via exercise. For example, long-term participation in endurance exercise training can augment cardiac function in older men, but this type of activity appears to do little to restore peak cardiac function in older women, or protect against the atrophy of fast-twitch muscle fibres in either gender. Resistance training, by contrast, has beneficial effects on muscle size, but this type of activity does not generally increase maximal oxygen uptake or fully protect against the loss of muscle power. Several lines of evidence also point to an age threshold (~70 years) beyond which many age-related changes, including functional changes discussed herein, appear to undergo an exponential decline, regardless of the amount or type of exercise undertaken. This deterioration pattern is seen with reductions in peak aerobic power, muscle strength, age group world record times for distance running and swimming, and reductions in preferred walking speed (Donato et al. 2003, Tanaka & Seals 2003). Collectively, these findings indicate that exercise can delay, but not prevent, the deleterious effects of biological ageing. This information is of more than theoretical interest; it has implications for the optimal timing and specificity of activity-based, preventive health interventions in our rapidly expanding older population (Chapters 16, 17.1, 28 and 31.1).

References

Beere PA, Russell SD, Morey MC, Kitzman DW, Higginbotham MB 1999 Aerobic exercise training can reverse age-related peripheral circulatory changes in healthy older men. Circulation 100:1085–1094

Blair SN, Kampert JB, Kohl HW 3rd, Barlow CE, Macera CA, Paffenbarger RS Jr, Gibbons LW 1996 Influences of cardiorespiratory fitness and other precursors on cardiovascular disease and all-cause mortality in men and women. Journal of the American Medical Association 276:205–210

Buskirk ER, Hodgson JL 1987 Age and aerobic power: the rate of change in men and women. Federal Proceedings 46:1824–1829

Coggan AR, Spina RJ, King DS, Rogers MA, Brown M, Nemeth PM, Holloszy JO 1992 Histochemical and enzymatic comparison of the gastrocnemius muscle of young and elderly men and women. Journal of Gerontology 47:B71–76

Conley KE, Esselman PC, Jubrias SA, Cress ME, Inglin B, Mogadam C, Schoene RB 2000a Ageing, muscle properties and maximal O2 uptake rate in humans. Journal of Physiology 526 Pt 2:211–217

Conley KE, Jubrias SA, Esselman PC 2000b Oxidative capacity and ageing in human muscle. Journal of Physiology 526 Pt 1:203–210

Day JR, Rossiter HB, Coats EM, Skasick A, Whipp BJ 2003 The maximally attainable VO2 during exercise in humans: the peak vs. maximum issue. Journal of Applied Physiology 95:1901–1907

Doherty TJ 2003 Invited review: aging and sarcopenia. Journal of Applied Physiology 95:1717–1727

Donato AJ, Tench K, Glueck DH, Seals DR, Eskurza I, Tanaka H 2003 Declines in physiological functional capacity with age: a longitudinal study in peak swimming performance. Journal of Applied Physiology 94:764–769

Eskurza I, Donato AJ, Moreau KL, Seals DR, Tanaka H 2002 Changes in maximal aerobic capacity with age in endurance-trained women: 7-yr follow-up. Journal of Applied Physiology 92:2303–2308

Fitzgerald MD, Tanaka H, Tran ZV, Seals DR 1997 Age-related declines in maximal aerobic capacity in regularly exercising vs. sedentary women: a meta-analysis. Journal of Applied Physiology 83:160–165

Fleg JL, Lakatta EG 1988 Role of muscle loss in the age-associated reduction in VO2 max. Journal of Applied Physiology 65:1147–1151

Fleg JL, Morrell CH, Bos AG, Brant LJ, Talbot LA, Wright JG, Lakatta EG 2005 Accelerated longitudinal decline of aerobic capacity in healthy older adults. Circulation 112:674–682

Fleg JL, O'Connor F, Gerstenblith G, Becker LC, Clulow J, Schulman SP, Lakatta EG 1995 Impact of age on the cardiovascular response to dynamic upright exercise in healthy men and women. Journal of Applied Physiology 78:890–900

Fries JF 1980 Aging, natural death and the compression of morbidity. New England Journal of Medicine 303:130–135

Goldspink DF 2005 Ageing and activity: their effects on the functional reserve capacities of the heart and vascular smooth and skeletal muscles. Ergonomics 48:1334–1351

Guralnik JM, Ferrucci L, Simonsick EM, Salive ME, Wallace RB 1995 Lower-extremity function in persons over the age of 70 years as a predictor of subsequent disability. New England Journal of Medicine 332:556–561

Hagberg JM, Allen WK, Seals DR, Hurley BF, Ehsani AA, Holloszy JO 1985 A hemodynamic comparison of young and older endurance athletes during exercise. Journal of Applied Physiology 58:2041–2046

Hambrecht R, Wolf A, Gielen S, Linke A, Hofer J, Erbs S, Schoene N, Schuler G 2000 Effect of exercise on coronary endothelial function in patients with coronary artery disease. New England Journal of Medicine 342:454–460

Harridge S, Magnusson G, Saltin B 1997 Life-long endurance-trained elderly men have high aerobic power, but have similar muscle strength to non-active elderly men. Aging (Milano) 9:80–87

Harris BA 2005 The influence of endurance and resistance exercise on muscle capillarization in the elderly: a review. Acta Physiologica Scandinavica 185:89–97

Heath GW, Hagberg JM, Ehsani AA, Holloszy JO 1981 A physiological comparison of young and older endurance athletes. Journal of Applied Physiology 51:634–640

Hepple RT, Hagen JL, Krause DJ, Jackson CC 2003 Aerobic power declines with aging in rat skeletal muscles perfused at matched convective O2 delivery. Journal of Applied Physiology 94:744–751

Holloszy JO 1993 Exercise increases average longevity of female rats despite increased food intake and no growth retardation. Journal of Gerontology 48:B97–100

Holloszy JO, Kohrt WM 1995 Exercise. In: Masoro EJ (ed) Handbook of physiology: aging. Oxford University Press, New York, 633–666

Huang G, Gibson CA, Tran ZV, Osness WH 2005 Controlled endurance exercise training and VO2max changes in older adults: a meta-analysis. Preventive Cardiology 8:217–225

Hurley BF 1995 Age, gender and muscular strength. Journal of Gerontology Series A. Biological Sciences and Medical Sciences 50:41–44

Janssen I, Heymsfield SB, Wang ZM, Ross R 2000 Skeletal muscle mass and distribution in 468 men and women aged 18–88 yr. Journal of Applied Physiology 89:81–88

Janssen I, Ross R 2005 Linking age-related changes in skeletal muscle mass and composition with metabolism and disease. Journal of Nutrition, Health and Aging 9:408–419

Joyner MJ 1993 Physiological limiting factors and distance running: influence of gender and age on record performances. Exercise and Sport Sciences Reviews 21:103–133

Kallman DA, Plato CC, Tobin JD 1990 The role of muscle loss in the age-related decline of grip strength: cross-sectional and longitudinal perspectives. Journal of Gerontology 45:M82–88

Kasch FW, Boyer JL, Van Camp SP, Verity LS, Wallace JP 1993 Effect of exercise on cardiovascular ageing. Age and Ageing 22:5–10

Klitgaard H, Mantoni M, Schiaffino S, Ausoni S, Gorza L, Laurent-Winter C, Schnohr P, Saltin B 1990 Function, morphology and protein expression of ageing skeletal muscle: a cross-sectional study of elderly men with different training backgrounds. Acta Physiologica Scandinavica 140:41–54

Kohl HW 3rd 2001 Physical activity and cardiovascular disease: evidence for a dose response. Medicine and Science in Sports and Exercise 33:S472–483; discussion S493–474

Lakatta EG, Levy D 2003 Arterial and cardiac aging: major shareholders in cardiovascular disease enterprises: Part I: aging arteries: a "set up" for vascular disease. Circulation 107:139–146

Laughlin MH, Joseph B 2004 Wolfe memorial lecture. Physical activity in prevention and treatment of coronary disease: the battle line is in exercise vascular cell biology. Medicine and Science in Sports and Exercise 36:352–362

Laurin D, Verreault R, Lindsay J, MacPherson K, Rockwood K 2001 Physical activity and risk of cognitive impairment and dementia in elderly persons. Archives of Neurology 58:498–504

Lee IM, Skerrett PJ 2001 Physical activity and all-cause mortality: what is the dose-response relation? Medicine and Science in Sports and Exercise 33:S459–471; discussion S493–494

Lemmer JT, Hurlbut DE, Martel GF, Tracy BL, Ivey FM, Metter EJ, Fozard JL, Fleg JL, Hurley BF 2000 Age and gender responses to strength training and detraining. Medicine and Science in Sports and Exercise 32:1505–1512

Lexell J, Taylor CC, Sjostrom M 1988 What is the cause of the ageing atrophy? Total number, size and proportion of different fiber types studied in whole vastus lateralis muscle from 15- to 83-year-old men. Journal of the Neurological Sciences 84:275–294

Lindle RS, Metter EJ, Lynch NA, Fleg JL, Fozard JL, Tobin J, Roy TA, Hurley BF 1997 Age and gender comparisons of muscle strength in 654 women and men aged 20–93 yr. Journal of Applied Physiology 83:1581–1587

Lynch NA, Metter EJ, Lindle RS, Fozard JL, Tobin JD, Roy TA, Fleg JL, Hurley BF 1999 Muscle quality. I. Age-associated differences between arm and leg muscle groups. Journal of Applied Physiology 86:188–194

Ogawa T, Spina RJ, Martin WH 3rd, Kohrt WM, Schechtman KB, Holloszy JO, Ehsani AA 1992 Effects of aging, sex and physical training on cardiovascular responses to exercise. Circulation 86:494–503

Oguma Y, Sesso HD, Paffenbarger RS Jr, Lee IM 2002 Physical activity and all cause mortality in women: a review of the evidence. British Journal of Sports Medicine 36:162–172

Pearson SJ, Young A, Macaluso A, Devito G, Nimmo MA, Cobbold M, Harridge SD 2002 Muscle function in elite master weightlifters. Medicine and Science in Sports and Exercise 34:1199–1206

Pollock ML, Foster C, Knapp D, Rod JL, Schmidt DH 1987 Effect of age and training on aerobic capacity and body composition of master athletes. Journal of Applied Physiology 62:725–731

Proctor DN, Joyner MJ 1997 Skeletal muscle mass and the reduction of VO2max in trained older subjects. Journal of Applied Physiology 82:1411–1415

Proctor DN, Koch DW, Newcomer SC, Le KU, Smithmyer SL, Leuenberger UA 2004 Leg blood flow and VO2 during peak cycle exercise in younger and older women. Medicine and Science in Sports and Exercise 36:623–631

Proctor DN, Newcomer SC, Koch DW, Le KU, MacLean DA, Leuenberger UA 2003 Leg blood flow during submaximal cycle ergometry is not reduced in healthy older normally active men. Journal of Applied Physiology 94:1859–1869

Proctor DN, Sinning WE, Walro JM, Sieck GC, Lemon PW 1995 Oxidative capacity of human muscle fiber types: effects of age and training status. Journal of Applied Physiology 78:2033–2038

Robinson S 1938 Experimental studies of physical fitness in relation to age. Arbeitsphysiologie 10:251–323

Rodeheffer RJ, Gerstenblith G, Becker LC, Fleg JL, Weisfeldt ML, Lakatta EG 1984 Exercise cardiac output is maintained with advancing age in healthy human subjects: cardiac dilatation and increased stroke volume compensate for a diminished heart rate. Circulation 69:203–213

Rogers MA, Hagberg JM, Martin WH 3rd, Ehsani AA, Holloszy JO 1990 Decline in VO2max with aging in master athletes and sedentary men. Journal of Applied Physiology 68:2195–2199

Roth SM, Ivey FM, Martel GF, Lemmer JT, Hurlbut DE, Siegel EL, Metter EJ, Fleg JL, Fozard JL, Kostek MC, Wernick DM, Hurley BF 2001 Muscle size responses to strength training in young and older men and women. Journal of the American Geriatric Society 49:1428–1433

Saltin B 1986 The aging endurance athlete. In: Sutton JB (ed) Sports medicine for the mature athlete. Benchmark Press, Indianapolis, 59–80

Shephard RJ 1997 Aging, physical activity and health. Human Kinetics, Champaign, IL

Short KR, Vittone JL, Bigelow ML, Proctor DN, Rizza RA, Coenen-Schimke JM, Nair KS 2003 Impact of aerobic exercise training on age-related changes in insulin sensitivity and muscle oxidative capacity. Diabetes 52:1888–1896

Spirduso WW, Francis KL, MacRae PG 2005 Physical dimensions of aging. Human Kinetics, Champaign, IL

Strandell T 1976 Cardiac output in old age. In: Caird FI, Dall JLC, Kennedy RD (eds) Cardiology in old age. Plenum Press, New York, 81–100

Tanaka H, Monahan KD, Seals DR 2001 Age-predicted maximal heart rate revisited. Journal of the American College of Cardiology 37:153–156

Tanaka H, Seals DR 2003 Invited review: dynamic exercise performance in Masters athletes: insight into the effects of primary human aging on physiological functional capacity. Journal of Applied Physiology 95:2152–2162

Trappe SW, Costill DL, Vukovich MD, Jones J, Melham T 1996 Aging among elite distance runners: a 22-yr longitudinal study. Journal of Applied Physiology 80:285–290

Wang BW, Ramey DR, Schettler JD, Hubert HB, Fries JF 2002 Postponed development of disability in elderly runners: a 13-year longitudinal study. Archives of Internal Medicine 162:2285–2294

Weiss EP, Spina RJ, Holloszy JO, Ehsani AA 2006 Gender differences in the decline in aerobic capacity and its physiologic determinants during the later decades of life. Journal of Applied Physiology 101(3):938–944

Wilson TM, Tanaka H 2000 Meta-analysis of the age-associated decline in maximal aerobic capacity in men: relation to training status. American Journal of Physiology. Heart and Circulation Physiology 278:H829–834

SECTION 4

Environmental physiology

SECTION CONTENTS

Section introduction: Human performance from the ocean floor to deep space

Nigel A.S. Taylor

Humans live, work and play in a wide range of hostile environments. At the Earth's surface, for example, air temperatures can range from 56.7°C (134°F) in Death Valley (USA) through to −89.6°C (−129°F), recorded at Vostok Station (Antarctica). Survival at these extremes for unprotected individuals is transient (Chapters 19, 20 and 21).

Oxygen is absolutely essential for life, yet, while the composition of air remains constant up to altitudes over 100 km above the Earth's surface (the Kármán line), the driving force that is essential for oxygen to pass from the lungs into the bloodstream (inspired oxygen partial pressure) is a function of barometric pressure. This pressure changes as one moves above, and below, sea level. With the surface of the Earth extending from 8848 m above sea level (Mount Everest) to 10,911 m in our deepest oceans (Challenger Deep, Mariana Trench), the barometric pressure range that one may encounter far exceeds the range of air temperatures.

At sea level, the mean atmospheric pressure is about 101 kPa (760 mmHg), representing the effect of gravity on all the molecules in a column of air above that location. However, this pressure decreases to 33.4 kPa at Mount Everest, where the partial pressure of oxygen is only just sufficient to support life (Chapters 24 and 25). Below the ocean surface, atmospheric and hydrostatic pressures combine, such that a descent of only 10 m adds the equivalent of another full atmosphere to the pressure load, due to the much greater density of water. Thus, the pressure change that one experiences when going to the top of Mount Everest from sea level can be experienced simply by submerging just slightly deeper than 6.5 m. Therefore, even a head-out immersion exposes the body to a large pressure gradient over the skin surface, which has a significant impact upon physiological function (Chapter 22). But as one descends deeper, the inspired oxygen partial pressure is increased and when it approaches or exceeds 160 kPa, oxygen becomes highly toxic (Chapter 23). In the Challenger Deep, the atmospheric pressure increases to almost 110,800 kPa, so it is both the absolute pressure and the oxygen partial pressure that challenge life.

There is no doubt that unprotected human survival at this depth is impossible. Yet in 1960, Jacques Piccard and Don Walsh descended to the bottom of the Challenger Deep in the bathyscaph *Trieste* (a deep submergence vehicle). A steel sphere allowed its occupants to remain at sea level pressure as the *Trieste* descended. While cold (the air temperature was 7°C), neither man was unduly challenged by this 8.5 h journey (Bathyscaph *Trieste* Alumni Association: www.bathyscaphtrieste.com/). Slightly less than 15 months later, the Russian cosmonaut Yuri Gagarin became the first man to leave the Earth's atmosphere, orbiting the Earth in the Vostok 3KA-2 spacecraft.

While the ocean depths represent our closest unexplored realm, many look towards space travel, with 16 nations currently involved in assembling the International Space Station (NASA: http://spaceflight.nasa.gov/station/). This artificial habitat, which has a living area slightly larger than 425 m², will orbit the Earth at an altitude of approximately 400 km (within the thermosphere), travelling at speeds in excess of 25,000 km·h⁻¹. At this altitude, the gravitational force is still about 85% of that which is present on Earth. However, since the space station is in a constant state of free fall, being locked into orbit by the Earth's gravitational pull, then its residents experience a constant state of weightlessness (Chapter 26). Outside the station, the gas molecules of the thermosphere absorb solar radiation and can increase in temperature to 2000°C, though the very low gas density largely prevents unprotected skin from sensing this temperature.

Survival in each of these environmental extremes is wholly dependent upon human ingenuity, which, through the development of protective clothing, portable life-support apparatus and mobile habitats, has allowed exploration to regions once considered beyond the reach of humans. Accordingly, through such man-made protective equipment, the lethal characteristics of these uninhabitable environments have been modified so that life can be sustained, and such strategies are collectively referred to as behavioural responses to environmental extremes. Indeed, those travelling in deep submergence vehicles experience very little of the external environment, as do the crew of nuclear-powered submarines, which typically remain at sea for up to 90 days.

In 1943, Emile Gagnan and Jacques-Yves Cousteau invented the demand-valve (regulator) for use in self-contained underwater breathing apparatus (SCUBA). This now allowed divers to stay underwater for extended durations without relying upon surface air supplies, and such diving, as it had for centuries before, exposed divers to more powerful changes within the surrounding environment. In such conditions, the behavioural and autonomic responses combine to determine human performance, and even survival. Now, the longer a diver stayed at depth, the more nitrogen was absorbed into the tissues. Beyond a critical duration, rapid resurfacing invariably resulted in decompression sickness (the bends; Chapter 23). This condition was first encountered in the mid-19th century, when labourers who were working in pressurised retaining structures (caissons) returned to the surface (caisson disease).

To prevent decompression sickness, divers would slowly decompress, gradually allowing nitrogen to leave the tissues and return to the lungs. This proved tedious and inefficient for working divers so, in 1942, the concept of the saturation dive was developed by Al Benhke (1942) and in 1957 George Bond, a US naval surgeon, undertook a series of animal experiments to further explore saturation and decompression (Vorosmarti 1997). Bond proposed that divers could remain under pressure for extended periods once complete inert gas saturation had occurred. From this state, a standardised decompression profile would be followed, regardless of how long the diver stayed at depth. The principles of saturation diving were, however, described some 50 years earlier by John Haldane (1907). Saturation diving is now less common, but it was extensively used for offshore oil and natural gas exploration and recovery.

Between these pressure extremes, men and women push the physiological boundaries, some with and some without the help of protective equipment. The great ocean explorers Christopher Columbus, Ferdinand Magellan and James Cook, along with their crews, sailed into vast and unknown oceans in search of new lands, with little in the way of support. However, it is the exploits of those who conquered the polar regions (Fridtjof Nansen, Roald Amundsen, Ranulph Fiennes) and the great mountaineers (Tenzing Norgay, Edmund Hillary, Reinhold Messner) who inspire the adventurous and bewilder those who are not so inclined. Each has overcome extremes of physiological and psychological strain to achieve feats that are universally recognised as falling outside that which is achievable by most people.

With most of our planet explored, surveyed and constantly photographed via networks of satellites, those seeking adventure often turn their attention to feats that require great physiological and mental strength, and adaptation. In many such cases, there is a complete reliance upon the autonomic regulation of the internal environment (Chapter 18), for when these regulatory mechanisms fall short of sustaining homeostasis by failing to compensate for changes in the external environment, performance declines, eventually leading to life-threatening states. Consider these examples. The current records for the 'no limits' breath-hold diving discipline, where divers may use any means of breath-hold descent, are 160 m (women: Tanya Streeter) and 183 m (men: Herbert Nitsch; International Association for the Development of Freediving: www.aida-international. org/). Whilst a descent to these depths on a single breath is difficult for most humans to imagine, it is well inside the depths routinely achieved by diving mammals, with the northern elephant seal capable of diving to approximately 1500 m. English Channel swimming (England to France) exemplifies endurance in cold water, and often with strong tidal currents. Matthew Webb made the first unassisted swim in 1875, with Alison Streeter making the most crossings (>40: Channel Swimming Association: www. channelswimmingassociation.com/). On land, the 254 km ultra-marathon across the Moroccan desert is considered to be the most demanding foot race on Earth (Marathon des Sables: www.marathondessables.com/index_uk.php). This region forms part of the Sahara desert and, although the race is held in the spring, it is often run under very hot and windy conditions, sometimes with dust storms. In each of these examples, homeostasis is challenged well beyond the experiences of modern man. How is it possible for such feats of endurance to be accomplished?

Much of the contemporary research interest in the physiology of environmental extremes can trace its origins to military medicine, which was driven by military commanders and their need for new knowledge in times of war. For example, many military institutes of aviation, naval and army medicine came into existence during and following World War II. The impetus for this growth in environmental physiology was frequently the rate of technological advancement, which resulted in people being exposed to increasingly more challenging and unfamiliar environments. Indeed, most authors of the chapters within this section have either worked for or are currently employed by such research institutes.

There are nine chapters in this section, and three topical discussions. In Chapter 18, readers are introduced to the critical concepts of physiological regulation, with human thermoregulation being the central focus. Autonomic thermoregulation is then developed to show how humans fiercely defend deep tissue (body core) temperatures during both hot and cold exposures (Chapters 19 and 20). In the latter case, readers are introduced to cold water immersion, which is tightly linked with physiological changes described in Chapters 22–25. For example, the summit air temperature

of Mount Everest averages about −36°C. While this is not surprising, Mount Kilimanjaro, which is situated close to the equator, has a mean temperature of approximately −10°C.

Before leaving thermal physiology, Chapter 21 describes how chronic exposures to both cold and hot climates can result in physiological adaptation (acclimatisation). The authors of several chapters discuss physiological adaptation (e.g. section 1, Introduction, Chapters 3, 4, 9 and 25), so readers are introduced to the principles of adaptation theory. One may conclude from Chapter 21 that the behavioural thermoregulatory capabilities of humans far exceed our autonomic capabilities to generate and lose heat. Thus, if humans had to rely solely upon shivering and sweating to maintain body temperature, we would not have ventured far from our equatorial origins.

Water immersion elicits a wide range of physiological responses, but it primarily affects cardiovascular and body fluid regulation (Chapters 1, 27.3 and 33). For instance, upright immersion increases the central blood volume and simulates microgravity. Thus, water immersion has been used to investigate space physiology (Chapters 9 and 26), and it is also a very important consideration for both thermal and diving physiologists (Chapters 20 and 23). In addition, the diving physiology chapter covers breath-hold diving, nitrogen narcosis, decompression sickness, barotrauma, underwater breathing apparatus and oxygen toxicity.

The final collection of chapters (24–26) within this section may broadly be classified as topics in aerospace physiology. The first two deal with the acute and chronic (adaptation) consequences of repeated altitude exposure, both in lowlanders and indigenous highlanders. With about 4 million people residing permanently above 4500 m, such indigenes provide scientists with a population in whom phenotypic and genotypic adaptation may be investigated. In a sense, altitude exposure (hypobaric hypoxia) can be used as a model for the other forms of hypoxia, since many of the physiological responses are common to the different forms of hypoxia. These chapters also deal with the physiological impact of changes in the density, viscosity and humidity of air, which affect the mechanics of ventilation and tissue dehydration. Such topics are also a common theme in Chapters 19, 20 and 23. In space, the impact of these physical changes is so strong that an entirely artificial habitat is essential for survival. Furthermore, the effects of weightlessness must now be tolerated and, where possible, minimised (Chapters 9 and 26).

References

Behnke A 1942 Effects of high pressures: prevention and treatment of compressed gas illness. Medical Clinics of North America. July:1212–1237

Haldane JS 1907 Deep water diving. Report of a Committee appointed by the Lords Commissioners of the Admiralty. Parliamentary Paper CN1549

Vorosmarti J 1997 A very short history of saturation diving. Historical Diving Times 20

Chapter **18**

Concepts in physiological regulation: a thermoregulatory perspective

Jürgen Werner Igor B. Mekjavic Nigel A.S. Taylor

1 INTRODUCING PHYSIOLOGICAL REGULATION

Tissue temperature is one of the qualities of the mammalian internal environment that, according to Bernard (1865), needs to be maintained or fixed within a range that is compatible with life. Throughout this book, a number of physiological variables have been identified as being regulated, including mean arterial and central venous blood pressures (Chapters 1 and 3), blood gas partial pressures (Chapters 2 and 3), plasma osmolality (Chapters 19 and 34.2) and blood glucose concentration (Chapter 30). Indeed, within this chapter, the fundamentals of physiological regulation are developed but using temperature regulation as a working example, since it is embedded within and shares common effector mechanisms with the regulatory systems for respiratory, cardiovascular, body fluid and osmoregulation.

Bernard was the first to introduce the concept of physiological regulation of the qualities and quantities of the internal environment at set (or fixed) levels. It was later realised that this type of rigid control of a physiological variable was not typically observed within physiological systems. This is why Cannon (1929) suggested a modification of Bernard's initial proposition and coined the phrase 'homeostasis of the internal environment'. The word 'homeostasis' is derived from the Greek words *homeo* meaning similar and *stasis* meaning stabilisation or regulation. Thus, homeostasis of a physiological variable implies regulation at a similar level, allowing for some degree of variability in the regulated level. Accordingly, throughout this volume, physiological regulation is the phrase of choice, in preference to physiological control, when referring to mechanisms that maintain the body's internal environment. In section 2.2.3, however, it is shown that some degree of variability in the regulated level is indeed a basic and inherent property of what the control engineer calls proportional feedback control.

Regulation of the entire internal environment requires the concerted action of a multitude of physiological regulating systems. Regulation of physical quantities at a desired level, or within a given range, occurs at the molecular,

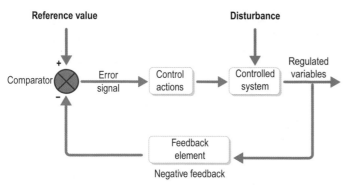

Figure 18.1 A negative feedback control systems model. Such models are used to represent the regulation in physiological systems.

cellular and systems levels. However, within this chapter, we will limit discussion to physiological regulation at a systems level. Common to all attempts at fitting a numerical model to a physiological system is the representation of the system as a negative feedback control model. Such models are frequently used in engineering (cybernetics) and one such physical model is depicted in Figure 18.1. This approach is contrary to that which may be expected, based on Cannon's thesis. However, taking body temperature regulation as an example, due to the convenience of representing body temperature regulation as a simple thermostat, these types of models became the historical tools of choice in the development of physiological models in general.

A fundamental knowledge of how such control models were developed is a necessary prerequisite for understanding most regulatory systems. However, it is necessary to further elaborate on the differentiation between physiological regulation and control, since both occur within the body and these terms are not physiological synonyms. Control is frequently used ambiguously in the lay literature and applied to the description of different concepts that scientists do not consider to be synonymous. First, it simply means to modify a variable or quantity in such a way as to achieve a defined goal (e.g. increasing skin blood flow, sweating or shivering). In fact, in control theory, this action is referred to as feedforward; the term 'central command' is also used to describe this process, particularly when it originates from higher (cortical) regions. Most commonly, control is also used with reference to feedback control, implying a sensory device that provides feedback of information to a controller, as depicted in Figure 18.1. Both feedforward and feedback controls occur within the body.

Let us continue this elaboration, but using the cardiovascular system as a working example. Blood pressure is the regulated variable since, without an adequate pressure gradient, blood flow cannot occur, and without blood flow to deliver essential molecules and to remove metabolic wastes, cells will die. Blood pressure is created by the cardiac pump and influenced by downstream flow resistance within the tubes through which the blood travels. Thus, one can

modulate (control) heart rate and stroke volume (the product of which is cardiac output) and also vasomotor and venomotor tone (tubular or vascular resistance). Using subtle combinations of neural and humoral stimulation, the body controls cardiac output and vascular resistance so that mean arterial blood pressures can be regulated within the physiological range necessary to ensure adequate tissue perfusion (Chapters 1 and 10.1). The sensors for this system are the high-pressure baroreceptors, which provide feedback to a central integrator or controller. These central neural mechanisms then control cardiac output and vascular resistance to ensure that mean arterial blood pressure is regulated at a level that will ensure adequate tissue perfusion for the circumstance in question. In fact, structures that actively control such physiological functions shall herein be referred to as effector controllers. Within every physiological regulatory system, there exist variables that are modified by way of feedforward control generated by effector controllers, which themselves are subservient to the needs of one or more regulated variables.

Now consider a disturbance that is presented to the engineering model in Figure 18.1. This can be of internal or external origin and it causes a change in the regulated variable, which is sensed by appropriate sensors. Information regarding the impact (magnitude) of this disturbance is fed to a comparator, which compares the prevailing value with a reference or set value, also referred to as the set-point value (the flaws in the reference signal concept, as it relates to physiological regulation, are discussed in sections 2.2.3 and 2.3). The algebraic difference is an error signal, sometimes called the load error or load signal, which initiates actions that modulate the function of one or more controlled variables. This modulation is aimed at restoring the value of the regulated variable, such that the error signal is minimised.

The aim of this chapter is not to provide a catalogue of models for all physiological regulatory systems but to present an overview of the manner in which physiological modelling has progressed, and how this has helped us to better understand physiological regulation, using human temperature regulation as the working example.

1.1 Why regulate body temperature?

Endothermic species, including humans, evolved from beings that acquired the capacity to produce an excess of thermal energy during metabolic processes, which ran at rates beyond that found in co-existing species (tachymetabolism). It has been hypothesised that the natural selection of some species may be explained on the basis of possessing an ability to regulate an elevated body temperature. Whilst this is clearly advantageous, it is perhaps more probable that this attribute may have co-existed with other favourable characteristics. Indeed, Ruben (1995) hypothesised that species possessing a greater maximal aerobic power would have been well suited to survival, due to a superior ability to hunt and evade predators. Such selected species may also have possessed an elevated resting metabolic rate, with the corresponding endogenous heat production necessitating the presence of mechanisms that prevented excessive heat storage, since this impairs physiological and cognitive functions and eventually leads to more catastrophic events, such as tissue damage and death (Chapter 19). Similarly, the prevention of excessive heat loss also became essential (Chapter 20). Indeed, in mammals, the efficiency of many biochemical and physiological processes appears optimal within just a very narrow body temperature range. Thus, these species evolved with the anatomical structures and control mechanisms that enabled and required the regulation of body temperature.

2 INTRODUCING REGULATORY MODELS

For any given regulatory system, one can identify the appropriate sensors, a comparator and corresponding control actions or effector mechanisms. This basic model can generally be applied, with minimal modification, to all forms of physiological regulation and one can readily identify the regulated variable(s), the sensors and feedback (afferent) elements, the comparator(s) (sometimes residing in more than one location), the effector controller(s), the controlling (efferent) pathways and the controlled (effector) structures and variables. However, within any regulated, physiological system, the information travelling along the sensor-to-effector pathways is most likely to be modified centrally, such that a transfer function needs to be determined for each such system. This transfer function defines the input-to-output relations of the regulatory system.

The thermoregulatory system has been the focus of extensive modelling efforts, due to the need to predict human performance in a wide range of thermal extremes. The resultant models can be classified using different strategies. For the purpose of this chapter, these strategies will be classified as didactic, control engineering and neuro-humoral models.

2.1 Didactic models

As the name implies, these models are primarily teaching tools. They serve to demonstrate simple regulatory mechanisms (Chapters 1 and 10.1). As such, the range of didactic models for a given physiological system is by far the greatest among the different categories of models. The most general and most applied didactic model was introduced in Figure 18.1. Other didactic models use a variety of electrical and mechanical examples to represent the concept of regulation. A frequently used didactic model of feedforward control is shown in Figure 18.2, where the level of water in a tank is determined by controlling two valves, each of which is connected to a float. One valve controls the inflowing water and the other the outflowing water. This model has also been used for the purpose of explaining the

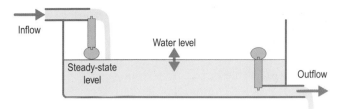

Figure 18.2 A didactic (feedforward control) model of physiological regulation.

regulation of body temperature, using the analogy of inflow to represent heat gain and of outflow for heat loss. However, as it is a feedforward model, it explains in terms of attaining a steady state the aim of the regulatory system, but it cannot be used to predict physiological responses, let alone simulate the manner in which, for example, body temperature is actually regulated (Werner 1980).

Most modelling research has focused on the development of models that enable solving the heat balance equation (Equation 1), which is a specific application of the First Law of Thermodynamics. This law is more fully described within Chapter 19 but, in essence, it dictates that stored thermal energy (S) results from the balance among evaporative (E: condensation on the skin will result in heat gain), radiative (R), convective (C) and conductive (K) thermal exchanges, and heat produced through metabolic energy transformations (M) and exchanged when performing mechanical work (W; IUPS Thermal Commission 2001). This law is expressed mathematically below and control engineering models are ideally suited to solving this equation, and, by so doing, providing an analysis of the regulated system:

Equation 1: $S = M - (\pm W) - E \pm R \pm K \pm C$ [W.m^{-2}]

2.1.1 Electrical engineering models

Some of the first control engineering models, which have also served didactic purposes, used electric circuits to model temperature regulation. This approach was convenient due to its applicability to thermal analysis, with Ohm's Law providing a suitable analogue: electrical current (I) = potential difference (U) / resistance (R). Heat flow is analogous to current, thermal conductivity to the inverse of resistance and the temperature gradient is analogous to the potential difference. Thus, the basic definition of heat flow becomes:

Equation 2:   Heat flow = thermal conductivity .
temperature gradient

We can extend the analogy by taking into account the capacity of the body to store heat, such that heat loss may be represented by a simple resistance-capacitor electrical circuit. The supply voltage in such a model would represent the thermal load to the body and the time constant of the capacitive element would be related to some physical traits of the human body, determining its ability to store and lose heat. To a student of engineering, such a simple engineering model could also represent a didactic model, which could also be used to make certain predictions, by applying fundamental equations of electrical theory to represent the heat exchange process between the body and its environment. It therefore comes as no surprise that control engineering models became the preferred choice for model development. However, electrical analogues did not offer the elegance of representing body temperature regulation, as did control systems models.

2.2 Control systems models

Presently, control engineering models are the most useful models for predicting the effector responses and thus quantifying the consequences of these responses. The control systems modelling approach to temperature regulation usually incorporates a complex control loop that consists of two subsystems: the passive system and the active or controlling system (Figure 18.3). The passive system includes all anatomical structures of the body, and can be represented as a passive heat transfer system that exchanges thermal energy with its surroundings. In a purely passive system, there is no neural control of physiological functions with reference to the status of a regulated variable and, in terms of thermal physiology, such a system would simply track changes in the surrounding environment or internal metabolic disturbances. That is, this system is an open loop and is characterised by the biophysics of heat transfer. The body's composition (i.e. muscle, fat, bone, etc.) and its physical dimensions (i.e. mass, height, surface area) determine the manner in which heat is stored or dissipated. These characteristics will also determine the manner in which an exogenous thermal load will affect the thermal status of the body. These heat exchanges occur from one tissue to another and between the body and the external environment.

The regulated variable is an integrated (or mean) temperature of the body, which is affected by heat transfer within the passive system and is supported also by the active system, that modulates the appropriate effector responses aimed at defending the regulated temperature.

Active control is achieved by a controlling system, which is composed of sensors (thermoreceptors) that appear to be heterogeneously distributed throughout the body, the ascending and descending neural pathways and the spatially distributed effector mechanisms (Werner 1998, 2005). For simplicity, we shall consider the active system to be composed of three parts: sensors that detect changes in the thermal status of the passive system, an effector controller and one or more effectors. The thermoregulatory effector mechanisms include both behavioural changes (e.g. posture, clothing, physical activity and climate control) and autonomic responses, with the latter involving blood vessels of the skin (vasomotion and venomotion), the sweat glands (sudomotion) and the skeletal muscles (thermogenesis). Collectively, this system represents a control loop with negative feedback, which can compensate for unfavourable changes in environmental influences (host factors) such as ambient temperature, water vapour pressure, radiation and air/water velocity, or cope with additional heat produced by muscular work. In situations where the effector capacities are overwhelmed, the body temperature will deviate substantially from the desired regulated level, resulting in either hyper- or hypothermia. In several sections below, we shall refer to closed and open control loops. The term 'closed control loop' is used to describe a controlling system in which all its afferent and efferent connections are intact and operating normally. When the normal operation of one or more parts of a control loop is prevented due to neural damage (e.g. spinal cord injury) or the thermal clamping of specific tissue temperatures (Cotter & Taylor 2005, Jessen 1981), the control loop is said to have been opened. In these 'open-loop' states, one can investigate the characteristics of the central controller without thermoafferent feedback from selected regions.

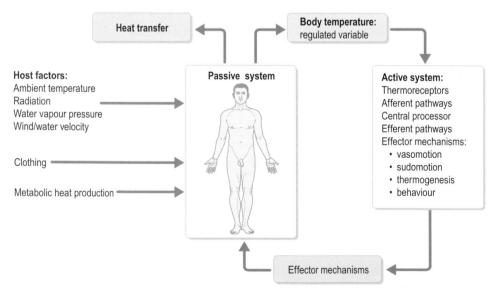

Figure 18.3 A simplified control systems model of human thermoregulation.

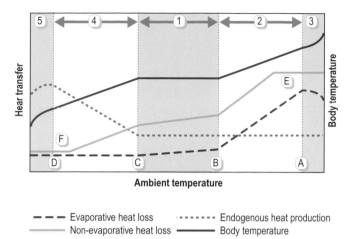

Figure 18.4 A qualitative overview of thermoeffector and body temperature responses across a wide range of air temperatures. Five zones are defined: 1 interthreshold, vasomotor, comfort, thermoneutral, indifference or null zone (Mekjavic & Eiken 2006); 2 sudomotor regulatory zone; 3 upper thermoregulatory failure (incompensable) zone; 4 metabolic regulatory zone; 5 lower thermoregulatory failure (incompensable) zone. The dashed lines correspond to peak sweat secretion (A) and maximal shivering thermogenesis (D). Thermoeffector thresholds are illustrated by points B and C (the upper and lower critical temperatures), with maximal vasodilatation at point E and maximal vasoconstriction at point F. Drawn using ideas presented by Stanier et al. (1984), Bligh (1987) and Mekjavic et al. (2003).

The controlled mechanisms for the regulation of body temperature, and the manner in which they respond to environmental disturbances are illustrated in Figure 18.4. Body temperature can be regulated over a wide range of ambient temperatures, with this range defining the thermoregulatory zone (zones 1, 2 and 4), since temperature regulation is achieved by the actions of the thermoregulatory effector mechanisms identified above. Fine regulation of heat loss is provided by vasomotor activity which, in neutral thermal environments, can maintain a constant body temperature in a narrow temperature range (zone 1: the interthreshold zone), bound by the lower and upper critical temperatures (lines C and B, respectively). These are essentially the threshold temperatures at which the effectors of endogenous heat production (thermogenesis), non-evaporative heat loss (vasomotion) and evaporative heat loss (sudomotion) are activated. As ambient temperature increases, vasodilatation and sweating are activated, though not necessarily simultaneously. Conversely, reductions in the surrounding temperature elicit first vasoconstriction and then thermogenesis. When maximal sweating and vasodilatation are obtained in the heat (line A and point E) or when maximal thermogenesis and vasoconstriction occur in the cold (point F and line D), further increments in thermal strain will overwhelm the effector responses, such that the body loses its capacity to defend body temperature.

Accordingly, one then enters the incompensable zones of incipient hyperthermia (zone 3) or hypothermia (zone 5). Between these thermoeffector thresholds and the upper regulatory limits, body temperature is still regulated (zones 2 and 4) but at temperatures that may be as much as 2°C away from that which occurs in thermoneutrality (zone 1; also known at the comfort or indifference zone).

The regulated body temperature may change periodically (e.g. circadian rhythm) or temporarily, due to the interference of non-thermal factors in the regulatory processes (Chapter 19), the interaction of pathological states (e.g. fever) and the processes of thermal adaptation (Chapter 21). Such changes are thought to be due to altered thermoregulatory thresholds or gains (sensitivities) of the thermoeffector responses which, in engineering language, means changes in the characteristics of the effector controller (Andres et al. 1999, Roberts et al. 1977; Chapter 21).

In the following subsections, the characteristics of both the passive and active components of the thermoregulatory system will be developed. However, whilst the focus will be on temperature regulation, it should be remembered that similar processes apply to other homeostatic mechanisms that regulate the internal environment. Of particular relevance across regulatory systems is the gain (or sensitivity) of the central controlling mechanism, which is a function of the change in effector function relative to the size of the change in the regulated variable. Readers not requiring this level of detail may choose to move directly to section 2.2.3.

2.2.1 Characteristics of the passive system

A passive thermal system, in the absence of temperature regulation, behaves as an open-loop control system into and from which thermal energy will continually flow, according to the dictates of shifting temperature gradients. The characteristics that determine the thermodynamics of such a passive system are illustrated in Figure 18.5 and are described qualitatively and mathematically below.

Since the body is very inefficient, approximately 80% of the energy liberated during metabolism will appear as thermal energy. Some of this heat must be transported to the skin surface for dissipation to the environment. Therefore, when wishing to describe the biophysics of the passive system, it is reasonable, and in most cases sufficient, to formulate the heat balance equation for just two tissue compartments: the core (central nervous system, bones, muscles, viscera) and the shell or skin tissues (dermal tissues, subcutaneous fat). The summation of the temperatures of these compartments (core temperature and (mean) skin temperature), as performed by the central nervous system, identifies the regulated variable of interest in mammalian thermoregulation: mean body temperature (Jessen 1996). It should be noted, however, that the integrated thermoafferent signal is not identical to the mean body temperature obtained from the weighted sum

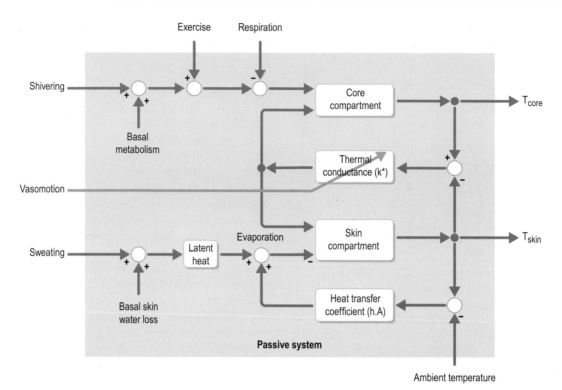

Figure 18.5 A signal flow diagram of the passive thermal system, with the body as an uncontrolled, open-loop heat transfer system. A thermal generator provides heat: basal metabolism. System outputs are core (T_{core}) and skin temperatures (T_{skin}). A disturbance to the thermal energy content of the system may be created by changes in ambient temperature ($\pm$) and exercise (concentric (positive) or eccentric (negative): Equation 1). Three physiological variables provide the means by which a control system could modulate heat loss (gain or conservation): vasomotion, shivering and sweating. Heat flows are affected by changes in tissue conductance (k^*) and the heat transfer coefficient (h: A = surface area).

of the heat capacity of the body compartments (the thermal energy content of the body: IUPS Thermal Commission 2001).

Thermal energy (heat) storage (S) or loss, is the product of tissue mass (m), its specific heat (c) and the change in tissue temperature with respect to time (dT/dt). The heat balance equation (Equation 1) states that the overall heat flow is equal to the difference between heat gain and heat loss. For the core compartment, heat gain may be derived from the basal metabolic heat production (M) minus mechanical power (W), when positive external work is performed (or negative for eccentric work), plus any heat production due to shivering (thermogenesis). Some of this endogenous heat (H_i) is transferred to the shell (skin) compartment, which is generally cooler, via intercellular conductive and vascular convective pathways. Thermal energy from the core is also transferred to the environment as evaporative heat loss from the respiratory tract (E_R). Note that several terms, introduced here as heat loss components, may change their sign (i.e. turn into heat gains) when the mean skin temperature exceeds body core temperature. These energy exchanges are summarised in the following expression.

Equation 3: $\quad m_{core}c_{core}\dfrac{dT_{core}}{dt} = M - W - H_i - E$

The skin compartment exchanges thermal energy with both the core tissues and the surrounding environment. The latter represent heat losses in ambient conditions that are cooler than mean skin temperature and occur in the form of convective (C), conductive (K), and radiative (R) transfers. When ambient temperature exceeds mean skin temperature, these environmental heat flows are reversed (i.e. signs become positive), forcing the skin to rely wholly upon the evaporation of sweat (E) for heat loss, which itself is determined by multiplying the evaporated sweat by the latent heat of vaporisation. These heat transfers are explained in more detail in Chapter 19 and may be summarised as:

Equation 4: $\quad m_{skin}c_{skin}\dfrac{dT_{skin}}{dt} = H_i - C - K - R - E$

Heat transfer between the core and skin compartments is proportional to the temperature gradient, taking into account the ease with which thermal energy can pass through the intervening tissues (tissue conductance: k^*). Heat loss from the skin to the environment via conduction, convection and radiation is also proportional to the corresponding temperature gradient, but will be influenced by the surface area (A) and the dry heat transfer coefficient (h; Figure 18.5). Thus, Equations 3 and 4 can be modified to account for the heat transfer between the core and skin, and between the skin and the environment.

Equation 5: $m_{core}c_{core}\dfrac{dT_{core}}{dt} = M - W - k*(T_{core} - T_{skin}) - E$

Equation 6: $m_{skin}c_{skin}\dfrac{dT_{skin}}{dt} = k*(T_{core} - T_{skin}) - E - $
$$h.A\ (T_{skin} - T_{ambient})$$

If this passive system is in a steady state, there are no further net temperature changes and the two equations above are equal to zero. However, by solving these equations for the core and skin temperatures, we may obtain the following steady-state characteristics of the passive system.

Equation 7: $T_{core} = \dfrac{k*+h.A}{k*h.A}(M - W - E_R) - \dfrac{1}{h.A}E + T_{ambient}$

Equation 8: $T_{skin} = \dfrac{1}{h.A}(M - W - E - E_R) + T_{ambient}$

2.2.2 Characteristics of the active (controlling) system, negative feedback and proportional control

To regulate body temperature, core and shell tissue temperatures are sensed by thermoreceptors that provide information to the central nervous system pertaining not only to local temperature but also to its rate of change (Chapter 19). This information is fed as afferent action potential trains to the active system, as illustrated in Figure 18.6 and described mathematically below.

The simplest algorithm, for which much experimental evidence has been gathered, assumes that the essential integrated signal is formed using the weighted summation of core and skin temperatures. That is, whilst feedback concerning tissue temperatures is provided from the core and shell compartments, this information is not necessarily given equal importance. For example, in most circumstances, a change in core temperature is more heavily weighted (g = 0.9) than is an equivalent change in skin temperature (g = 0.1). Nevertheless, a thermal input signal (*a*) is derived, as represented in the following equation, and this signal has been interpreted as representing the mean body temperature.

Equation 9: $a = gT_{core} + (1 - g)T_{skin}$

If this weighted signal (*a*) differs from an effector-specific threshold value (a_0: i.e. $a-a_0 \neq 0$), the corresponding effector mechanism will be activated. The extent to which an effector is stimulated will be a function of its response gain (sensitivity; Equation 10), from which it becomes evident that effector activation is also proportional to the load error ($a-a_0$). Each effector system has its own gain and threshold (a_0) values (Figure 18.6). These concepts are

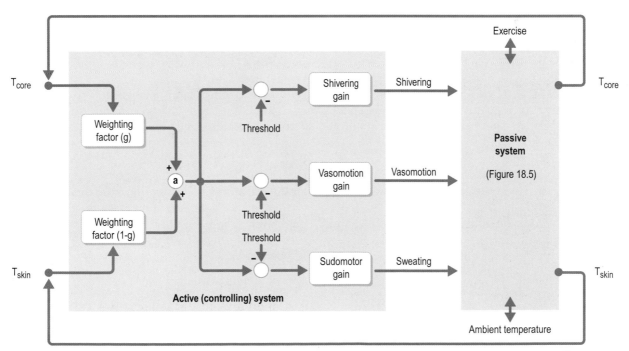

Figure 18.6 A signal flow diagram combining the passive system from Figure 18.5 via negative feedback to the controlling systems. This guarantees that the body temperature is regulated close to the thernoneutral zone (Figure 18.4). Negative feedback informs the central nervous system about the thermal status of the core (T_{core}) and shell tissues (T_{core}) and these inputs are weighted centrally (g) to derive an integrated temperature (T_{body} or *a*): Equation 9. Efferent flows to effectors (right) are a function of separate effector response thresholds (a_0) and gains (sensitivities): Equation 10.

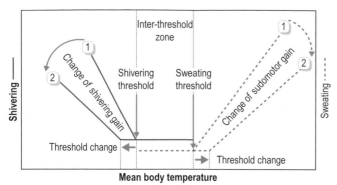

Figure 18.7 Mean body temperature is regulated within the range of temperatures bound by the threshold temperatures for shivering and sweating. This region is the interthreshold zone and is also known as the vasomotor, null or thermoeffector threshold zone. The responses of sweating and shivering are characterised by the body temperatures at which these effectors are activated and the response gain (sensitivity) of each effector: Equation 10. Various thermal and non-thermal factors can influence both of these characteristics (Chapter 19). Changes in the former would alter the magnitude of the interthreshold zone, whereas changes in the latter alter the intensity of the response. Adapted from Figure 18.4 and from Mekjavic & Eiken (2006).

demonstrated graphically in Figure 18.7 for the thermoeffectors of sweating and shivering, as a function of mean body temperature.

Equation 10: $\quad Activation = Gain \cdot (a - a_0)$

Under normal circumstances, body temperature is maintained within the interthreshold (vasomotor or comfort) zone (Figure 18.4), bound by the thresholds for initiating shivering and sweating, which are similar but not equivalent to those associated with vasoconstriction and vasodilatation, respectively. As indicated above, the regulated level of body temperature can change due to a variety of thermal and non-thermal factors influencing the effector responses. These effects may be expressed either as a displacement of the threshold temperature at which an effector is initiated or as a change in the effector gain of the response (Figure 18.7). In the examples illustrated, the thresholds are shifted, such that the interthreshold zone is expanded and the gains are reduced, resulting in delayed and less powerful thermoeffector responses for a given body temperature change. However, thermal and non-thermal factors may also selectively influence one effector mechanism and may limit this effect to either the threshold temperature or to the gain, but do not necessarily simultaneously alter both characteristics (Mekjavic & Eiken 2006).

The above effector responses now need to be incorporated into the active (controlling) system of the thermoregulatory model. Thus, the difference between a given body temperature and the threshold temperature ($a-a_0$) for a given

response will provide the error signal (load error) for that effector response. These error signals for shivering, vasomotor changes and sudomotion are forms of negative feedback and their independent gains are illustrated conceptually in Figure 18.6, with each effector mechanism possessing its own threshold and gain characteristics. Thus, this figure illustrates a negative feedback control system that is able to compensate, to a large extent, for disturbances in its regulated variable: mean body temperature. This model also implies that the weighting factors for the core and skin temperatures may also vary for each effector. Unfortunately, current knowledge concerning these weightings is rudimentary.

Most physiological effector (controlled) responses are modulated in proportion to the load error or body temperature deviation in this working example. For a better understanding of the manner in which proportional control is achieved, an example of the defence of body temperature via sweating, during exposure to a hot environment (Chapter 19), will be developed.

We have established above that body temperature can be affected by changes in ambient temperature ($\Delta T_{ambient}$) and various biophysical functions (Equation 1). For example, sitting in a sufficiently hot bath will eventually elicit sweating, by first increasing skin (ΔT_{skin}) and eventually core temperature (ΔT_{core}). Let us now consider an individual exercising in a heated room. The initial heat exposure may not immediately induce a load error but when exercise commences, sweating will be initiated soon after, and transcutaneous evaporative rate (ΔE) will rise. If one uses appropriately sensitive measuring devices, one can observe a transient body core temperature (ΔT_{body}) fall in response to this sudden increase in evaporative heat loss, before it eventually rises again. Thus, changes in both ambient temperature and evaporative rate can evoke changes in body temperature.

By considering just the changes in body temperature and evaporation, it is possible to combine and solve Equations 7 and 8 for these deviations (Equation 11). From this solution, it is evident that all components from Equations 7 and 8 that do not change will disappear from the computation (M, W, E_R). These are still present from a physiological perspective but are not changing, so do not account for the change in body temperature. Hence, the solution is an extremely simple equation, valid not only for changes in core and skin temperatures but also for changes in body temperature:

Equation 11: $\quad \Delta T_{body} = -(1/h.A) \cdot \Delta E + \Delta T_{ambient}$

The generic effector equation presented above (Equation 10) can now be solved for the specific example of the proportional control of sweating (ΔSweating) and hence also for changes in the rate of sweat evaporation (ΔE). This solution also incorporates both the relevant biophysical (latent heat of vaporisation) and physiological properties (the gain factor for the sweat controller). The control loop represented

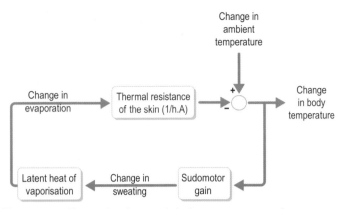

Figure 18.8 Proportional control during exposure to a hot environment. The example shows the manner in which the defence of body temperature is achieved following a change in ambient temperature that elicits an elevation in body temperature. The minus sign in the control loop guarantees feedback control. However, proportional control implies that body temperature load errors are minimised but not eliminated.

by the two resulting equations (12a) and (12b) is shown in Figure 18.8.

Equation 12a: $\Delta E = LatentHeat \cdot \Delta Sweating$

Equation 12b: $\Delta E = LatentHeat \cdot Gain \cdot \Delta T_{body}$

By substituting Equation 12a, which describes the control system, into Equation 11, which describes the passive system, we derive one equation for the closed control loop (Equation 13a). The resulting expression relates the output (body temperature change: ΔT_{body}) to the input signal (ambient temperature change: $\Delta T_{ambient}$). The quantities for the heat transfer coefficient (h), area (A), latent heat of vaporisation and effector gain may be combined into a single value (α), which is known as the control factor, and Equation 13a can be simplified (Equation 13b):

Equation 13a: $\Delta T_{body} = \dfrac{1}{1+(1/h.A) \cdot LatentHeat \cdot Gain} \cdot$
$\Delta T_{ambient}$

Equation 13b: $\Delta T_{body} = \alpha \cdot \Delta T_{ambient}$

Thus, a disturbance in ambient temperature would be expected to cause a deviation in body temperature (load error) from the interthreshold zone. This load error is inevitable, since it is inherent in the concept of proportional control (Equation 10). However, the magnitude of the body temperature change would depend upon the control factor (α) and this change would be low if the effector (controller) gain is high (i.e. gain is a denominator in Equation 13a). Hence, a large effector gain infers a small change in body temperature, and a high degree of effector responsiveness serves to reduce the effect of the original ambient temperature disturbance on the body temperature. Therefore, only in the purely theoretical case, where effector gain is raised to infinity, would the control factor (α), and hence the load

error, become zero. In technical control systems (e.g. precisely controlled climatic chambers), a constancy of the controlled variable (load error is zero) is achieved by using the so-called integral controllers. These controllers do not react proportionally to the input, as is the case with the proportional controller described above, but sum up (integrate) the input signals. Such controller types do not seem to act within physiological regulatory systems in which the autonomic nervous system is used to modulate effector mechanisms. However, the human motor control system, which exerts much more precise effector control, does appear to approximate this type of controller action.

The above discussion has focused wholly upon thermoregulation which, as noted in the opening to this chapter, shares effectors with respiratory, cardiovascular, body fluid regulation and osmoregulatory mechanisms. These interrelationships are illustrated in Figure 18.9, which demonstrates that a modulation of one effector response, and in particular the peripheral vascular resistance, has physiological consequences for several other regulatory processes. A discussion of these interactions is beyond the scope of this chapter but some interactions are explored within other chapters (e.g. Chapter 19). However, it is imperative that those investigating physiological regulation do not forget these interdependent effects.

2.2.3 How does the active (controlling) system obtain its reference and error signals?

Thus far, we have spoken about the mean body temperature and load error (a-a_0), without describing how such information is obtained by the central controller. Neural afferents provide information concerning the thermal status of both the body core and shell compartments. These signals are centrally evaluated, presumably in the form of a weighted summation (mean body temperature; Equation 9, Figure 18.6), within the preoptic anterior hypothalamus. So there exists a means through which the central controller can obtain information concerning the thermal status of the passive system. But is there some preprogrammed reference temperature to which this mean body temperature is compared, so that a load error may be derived? This topic will also be explored in detail in section 2.3, with respect to the neurohumoral models of thermoregulation. However, since many control system models of physiological regulation are reliant upon the concept of a reference signal or set-point (Figure 18.1), then this topic will also be covered under this category of models, again using thermoregulation as an example.

In the following, the concept of attaining a steady state in the thermoregulatory control loop is explained and so too is the reason why a higher thermal load, whether evoked by environmental conditions, by heavy work or by the use of thermal protective clothing, must result in a higher deviation of body temperature, in spite of negative feedback control. For the moment, let us assume there is no feedback, and thus we consider just the properties of the passive and

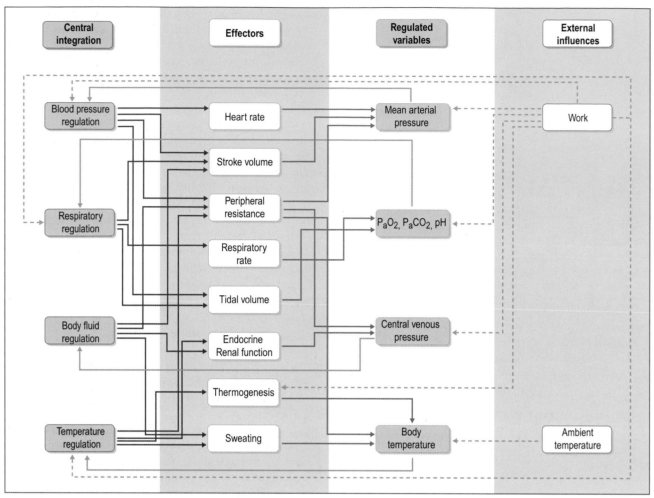

Figure 18.9 An overview of human thermoregulation as embedded within other physiological regulatory systems. The input from external influences are shown as dotted lines.

active (controlling) system, as if each was an isolated open-loop system in which feedback is not present or the feedback control loop has been opened (artificially or surgically ablated). This means that the controlling system receives no afferent information concerning heat gain/loss or tissue temperatures and thus these are free to vary across a very broad range.

The input to the passive (controlled) system is, in addition to changes in ambient temperature, the sum of effector mechanisms in terms of net heat gain, and the output is a change in body temperature (T_{body}), as outlined in Figure 18.10A. Thus, the passive system responds like an inanimate object or a dead animal, which may be heated or cooled simply by changing the internal or external thermal environment.

Note that, for the sake of simplicity, in the coordinate axes of Figure 18.10, we consider only deviations from the state where the effector activities tending to counteract alterations of body temperature (particularly metabolic heat production and evaporative heat loss) are minimal. In the closed-loop state, we describe the resulting body

temperature as being within the interthreshold zone (Figures 18.4 and 18.7). In this zone, the sympathetic vasoconstrictor arm controls skin blood flow (Chapter 19), with an increase in vasomotor tone (vasoconstriction) resulting in heat conservation and reduced vasomotor tone (vasodilatation) resulting in heat loss, when ambient temperature remains constant. As a consequence, in the interthreshold zone (represented in Figure 18.10A by the circle in the coordinate origin), the resultant body temperature will depend primarily on vasomotor status.

However, in the open-loop state, other effector mechanisms (sweating, shivering) may be activated. Therefore, in Figure 18.10A we also consider input from additional effector mechanisms. To the right of the coordinate origin, heat is gained and to the left, heat is lost but these changes in the thermal energy content are not controlled through any form of feedback. As a result of these changes, the temperature of the passive system moves along the diagonal lines illustrated. These lines are the so-called biophysical 'characteristics' of the passive system and may be computed using Equations 7–9. For neutral ambient tempera-

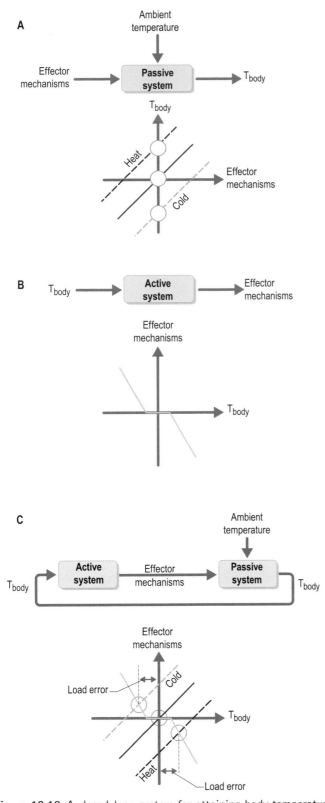

Figure 18.10 A closed-loop system for attaining body temperature steady states during heat and cold exposures (see text for details). (A) The open-loop characteristics of the passive system. (B) The open-loop characteristics of the active (controlling) system. (C) Body temperature steady states (circles) attained in the closed control loop. Modified from Werner (2005).

ture, the diagonal passes through the origin. For this line, the point at which vasoconstrictor tone elicits a fairly steady-state body temperature for a resting, thermoneutral (comfortable) person is indicated by the circle at the origin of both axes. As shown in Figure 18.10A, for such an open-loop (passive) system, there are two inputs (changes in the effector mechanisms and ambient temperature) and one output (body temperature change: T_{body}). For altered input in terms of ambient temperature, the body temperature will move vertically within the diagram to the broken lines that correspond to the hot or cold conditions. Without further effector input in terms of heat gain or loss, the circles indicated in Figure 18.10A represent the corresponding steady states. These states are substantial deviations in body temperature. With additional heat gain or loss, more severe displacements along either of the broken diagonal lines could be observed in the open-loop system.

Consider now the active system (Figure 18.10B) as an open-loop system, with its input being body temperature change (T_{body}) and its effector mechanism output driving changes in the three effector responses (Figure 18.6: vasomotion, shivering, sweating). In the corresponding graph, the abscissa and ordinate have been changed, since a body temperature alteration drives changes in the effector mechanisms. Thus, an increasing body temperature will decrease vasomotor tone and activate sweating to counteract disturbances to the passive system. With cooling, there is vasoconstriction and the initiation of shivering. In both instances, the changes in the effector responses are proportional to that change in body temperature (Equation 10). Note also that the effector mechanisms are not activated until the body temperature reaches the effector-specific threshold values (a_0: Equation 9; a-$a_0 \neq 0$). As a consequence, the typical interthreshold zone can be observed (Figure 18.4).

By combining the flow diagrams from Figures 18.10A and B and adding a feedback loop, a closed-loop system is obtained (Figure 18.10C). In all physiological regulatory systems, the passive (controlled) and active (controlling) systems have to interact and the output of the first becomes the input of the second, and vice versa. Thus, a thermal steady state must be compatible with the characteristics shown in Figures 18.10A and B, which are now unified within Figure 18.10C. This figure demonstrates that steady states only exist at the intersections of the lines that define the characteristics of the passive and active systems. These are indicated by the three circles, which correspond with steady states for thermoneutral (middle), cold (upper) and warm (lower) conditions. These deviations of body temperature in the cold and the heat (load errors: Equation 10: a-a_0) are an inherent property of a proportional feedback control system. These different steady-state points become the new regulated temperatures (sometimes called setpoints) for this regulatory system. If the effector mechanisms were not activated, the body temperature would have moved along the abscissa until it met one of the diagonal broken lines. It can easily be seen that, with thermoeffector activation, the body temperature is regulated significantly closer to its thermoneutral steady state.

During hyperthermia and hypothermia, the body temperature deviates substantially from these regulated temperatures, mostly because the capacity of effector mechanisms is insufficient to defend body temperature, and becomes overwhelmed by the prevailing environmental conditions (Chapters 19 and 20). These regulated temperatures may change periodically (e.g. circadian rhythm) or temporarily, due to interference from the regulation of non-thermal variables or due to pathological, non-thermal influences (e.g. fever). In addition, the processes of acclimatisation can also change these regulated temperatures. These changes are thought to be due to alterations to the characteristics of the thermal controller (active system), in particular, changes to the thermoeffector activation threshold or the gain (sensitivity) of the thermoeffector to a given neural drive (Figure 18.7; Chapter 21).

Unfortunately, the term 'set-point' is frequently used in the literature pertaining to physiological regulation, and is used to describe the concept of some innate or predetermined value for the regulated variable (e.g. body temperature). In fact, its use has evoked much confusion, since it has been used to refer to and to describe various phenomena, many of which are different from those defined above (IUPS Thermal Commission 2001). For instance, it has been used for the steady-state body temperature for which there is neither positive nor negative heat storage. The body temperatures reached in a steady state depend on the extent of external or internal thermal load. If the thermoeffector capacities are exceeded due to excessive load or pathological processes, a steady state will not be reached, leading to severe hypo- or hyperthermia. It has also been used to describe a central reference signal which, obviously, does not explicitly exist for the thermoregulatory system. Furthermore, it has been used to describe and define the interthreshold zone (Figures 18.4 and 18.7); within this zone is the state that may be called the set-point. However, this is not correct in acclimated, febrile (fever) and other states. For example, during a fever or following thermal adaptation, the characteristics of the thermocontroller change, particularly the effector thresholds. A threshold reduction or an increased effector gain that accompany heat adaptation (Chapter 21) means that the regulated temperature is now brought closer the thermoneutral steady state.

The analysis above has shown that, to satisfy the demands of thermoregulation, such a regulatory system has no need for an explicit reference signal with which to compare mean body temperature. According to this concept, a balance of the passive and active processes within the system is all that is necessary to regulate body temperature (Werner 1990). Similar analyses may be applied to other physiological regulatory systems.

2.3 Neurohumoral models

Control theory has contributed immensely to the development of practical models of various physiological systems. These models have served a didactic as well as a predictive role. In the field of temperature regulation, the main trait of many control systems models is the presence of a reference signal (Figure 18.1) which has been used to suggest that this is the manner in which the physiological regulation of body temperature is achieved (Hammel 1968, Hammel et al. 1963). To account for situations where body temperature is regulated at a higher (i.e. fever) or lower (i.e. hibernation) level, the reference signal was suggested to be adjustable (Hammel et al. 1963). This approach has also been applied to the modelling of regulation within other physiological systems and, prior to 1970, this was a common feature in all thermoregulation models. However, as illustrated above, it is not an essential requirement for body temperature regulation. Indeed, there is not even any evidence for the existence of a reference signal.

The set-point theory of mammalian temperature regulation initiated the search for the components of the control model. The sensors, afferent and efferent pathways and effector mechanisms were easily defined. The problem became identifying the set-point and explaining the manner in which it was adjusted. No neuroanatomical structure could be found that could provide the manner of control described by the control models. It became apparent that, in order to gain further insight into the physiological mechanisms, another modelling approach was needed. This was the impetus for the development of neurohumoral models.

In contrast to engineering models, neurohumoral models do not have the ability to provide numerical predictions of the magnitude of a particular response and how this will affect body temperature. However, they do provide a physiological diagram of the neurohumoral pathways and mechanisms involved in any given effector response. Based on the evidence provided by a multitude of neuroanatomical studies, it was established almost a century ago that two main neural foci in the hypothalamus were involved in temperature regulation, one responsible for heat production, the other for heat loss. Physiological experiments seemed to indicate that these two centres mutually inhibited each other (Bazett 1949). Based on this evidence in the thermoregulatory system, and the prior demonstration of Sherrington of the importance of reciprocal inhibition of agonist and antagonist muscles during voluntary muscle actions, Bligh (1998) suggested that the principle of reciprocal inhibition may be the unifying theory for all regulatory processes in the body. The reciprocal inhibition theory of temperature regulation states that the cold- and warm-sensitive sensor-to-effector pathways provide reciprocal cross-inhibition (Figure 18.11). In this manner, activation of the cold sensor-to-effector pathway, which ultimately increases heat production, would simultaneously inhibit the

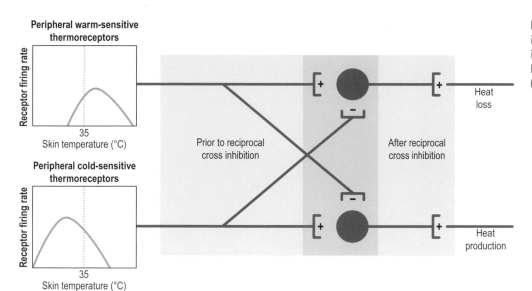

Figure 18.11 A schematic illustration of the reciprocal cross inhibition theory. Modified from Bligh (1998) and Mekjavic & Eiken (2006).

heat loss responses of sweating and vasodilatation. Conversely, excitatory signals in the warm sensor-to-effector pathway initiate sweating and vasodilatation, whilst exerting an inhibitory effect on the cold sensor-to-effector pathway, inhibiting the heat production response. In this manner, the overlapping activity and temperature characteristics of the peripheral cold- and warm-sensitive thermoreceptors could establish a regulated body temperature.

The notion that one mechanism of regulation, namely reciprocal cross-inhibition, may perhaps be the neurohumoral building block of all regulatory systems (Bligh 1998) was quite elegant. Unfortunately, as pointed out by Wilkie (1954): 'Facts and theories are natural enemies. A theory may succeed for a time in domesticating some facts but sooner or later inevitably the facts revert to their predatory ways'. Thus, many beautiful and elegant theories were destroyed by one ugly fact. That different sensor-to-effector pathways communicate with each other is well established. However, whether or not such reciprocal inhibition is essential for physiological regulation is questionable. In fact, studies investigating the effect of some of the non-thermal factors described in preceding sections, and in Chapter 19, do not, at least at the systems level, seem to provide unequivocal support of the importance of reciprocal cross-inhibition in the regulation of body temperature (Mekjavic & Eiken 2006). Certainly, the effects of non-thermal factors appear to act after the site of reciprocal cross-inhibition.

Nevertheless, this reciprocal cross-inhibition theory provided an explanation as to how two different types of sensors (warm- and cold-sensitive), with overlapping bell-shaped characteristics, could provide for the regulation of an internal temperature. The zone of overlap for these thermoreceptors coincided with the regulated level of the internal body temperature. Thus, decreasing temperature would provide an excitatory stimulus to heat production and, due to the reciprocal inhibition, a concomitant inhibitory stimulus to reduced heat loss. Similarly, an elevation in temperature would enhance the excitatory stimulus for heat loss and act to inhibit heat production. This represents the second means through which the thermoregulatory system can regulate body temperature without requiring a reference signal or set-point.

Any neurohumoral model of temperature regulation should also include knowledge of the characteristics of the central thermosensitive neurons which, in essence, modulate the information emanating from peripheral cold- and warm-sensitive receptors. One such model is that proposed by Boulant (1981) and presented in Figure 18.12. This model summarises the observations of neuroanatomical studies and confirms many of the results reported at the systems level. This model reveals how thermoafferent information from cold- and warm-sensitive thermoreceptors is modulated by central thermosensitive neurons to establish the characteristics of heat production and heat loss.

Using this thermoregulatory perspective, it is obvious that neurohumoral models of physiological regulation must attempt to establish the central pathways and their interconnections. This will help to explain how many different factors may affect the manner in which a physiological variable is regulated. For example, the fact that some of the central warm-sensitive receptors are osmosensitive and some of the cold sensors glucosensitive explains why dehydration attenuates sweating (Chapters 19, 33 and 34.2), and hypoglycaemia (Chapters 20 and 30) attenuates heat production.

The model in Figure 18.12 incorporates four types of central thermosensitive neurons (three warm- and one cold-sensitive), each with specific response characteristics (inset panels). Thermoafferent drive emanating from the peripheral warm- and cold-sensitive sensors, and converging on the central thermoreceptors, is integrated and modified by these sensors and thereby provides the neural drive

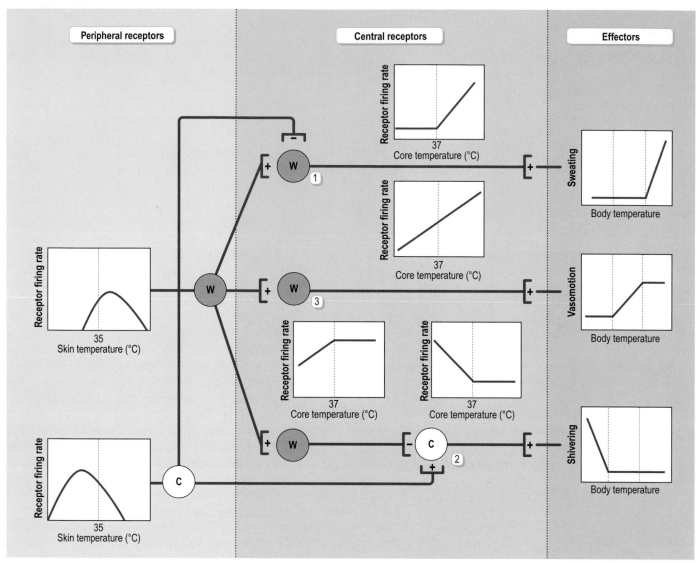

Figure 18.12 Neuronal model illustrating possible mechanisms by which the central cold-sensitive (C) and warm-sensitive (W) sensors of the preoptic anterior hypothalamus integrate thermoafferent information from the peripheral thermoreceptors and activate the thermoregulatory effectors responses (shivering, vasomotor tone, sweating). The inset graphs illustrate the input/output characteristics of each component. The numbers correspond with the possible sites of interaction by non-thermal factors: increased plasma osmolality (1), reduced plasma glucose concentration (2) and motion sickness (3). Adapted from Boulant (1981) and Mekjavic & Eiken (2006) with permission.

for the effector responses of sweating, vasomotor activity and shivering. Based on the studies conducted by Boulant and co-workers (Boulant 1981, Silva & Boulant 1984), Mekjavic & Eiken (2006) have proposed that the observed physiological effects of several non-thermal factors (e.g. increased plasma osmolality (Figure 18.12, point 1), decreased plasma glucose concentration (point 2) and motion illness (point 3)) may be appropriately explained through interactions with thermoregulation, on the basis of this neurohumoral model.

A final important feature of any physiological regulatory system is the ability of that system to regulate a variable at different levels, rather than inexorably striving to restore the same steady state, regardless of the stress applied to

the system. For example, during exercise, there is a metabolically driven increase in body temperature. For low-intensity exercise, the available autonomic and behavioural thermoregulatory mechanisms would be capable of dissipating the heat that is produced, thus regulating body temperature at normal levels. While vasomotor tone is altered, as it is within the resting state (Figure 18.4), sweating is not activated.

Consider now the application of a square-wave, moderate- to high-intensity exercise function from rest. At the instant that exercise commences, convectional heat loss from almost the entire body surface is suddenly increased. Whilst heat production from the active skeletal muscles is also instantaneously elevated, there is a significant phase delay between the onset of heat production and its central appearance. As a consequence, body temperature transiently declines (Figure 18.13). Thus, there is an absence of a thermally mediated neuronal drive for heat dissipation, though feedforward drive will activate primed thermoeffectors (Chapter 19). In this state, there occurs a sudden mismatch between the acute elevation in heat production and heat loss. This mismatch results in an elevation of heat storage and an increase in body temperature, which then stabilises at a new but higher operating level (Figure 18.13). This body temperature increase is illustrated in zone 2 of Figure 18.4. Notwithstanding this elevation, temperature regulation is still functioning, albeit with a higher operating level, and can be explained using the models presented in section 2.2.3.

The thermal descriptions above are entirely logical. However, during exercise at moderate levels, where heat production could easily be countered by heat loss, this is frequently not observed (Figure 18.13). Certainly, the regulation of body temperature during exercise, at the level observed when resting, would be physiologically costly and perhaps even unnecessary, since moderate elevations in body temperature are well tolerated and could even be advantageous. Thus, one must ask: is the new operating level a regulated temperature or is it merely a consequence of the imbalance between heat production and loss? In the event of the former, how does exercise, as a non-thermal factor, initiate the regulation of body temperature at a new level? Some would suggest that the elevation of this regulated temperature may be interpreted merely as a consequence of proportional control described in section 2.2 (Werner 2005). Others would suggest

that the answers to these questions are not yet available (Mekjavic & Eiken 2006).

The observation of an exercise-induced elevation can easily be incorporated into the control systems model. This, however, will not fully explain the physiological mechanisms underlying this effect. We must look towards neurohumoral models to provide this information. Future developments in physiological modelling are likely to see the marriage of engineering and neurohumoral models. These models will be capable of representing the physiological mechanisms involved in the regulation (qualitative features) but will also allow prediction of the responses or rather the consequences of the responses (quantitative features).

The regulation of body temperature is not achieved solely by autonomic responses. The first line of defence of body temperature is achieved by behavioural changes (Chapters 19 and 20). Thus, a complete thermoregulatory model should include both autonomic and behavioural thermoregulatory responses. The latter are a consequence of the cortical integration of thermoafferent information, providing the perception of thermal states. How thermal sensation is then translated into individual assignments of thermal comfort/discomfort, which ultimately drives the behavioural responses, is largely unknown. Many physiological systems involve both types of regulation but despite the obvious importance of behavioural actions in maintaining not only body temperature but also other qualities and quantities of the internal environment (e.g. hydration (Chapters 33 and 34.2), plasma glucose concentration (Chapter 30)), modelling behavioural regulation of such factors is lacking. The incorporation of autonomic and behavioural regulation into common models of physiological regulation will no doubt be one of the avenues research in this field will follow.

3 CONCLUSION

Attempts at representing the functional characteristics of other physiological systems mirror the progress in thermoregulatory modelling presented in this chapter. Users of such models should be aware of their limitations and use the most appropriate model for the task at hand. Engineering models allow quantitative predictions, whereas neurohumoral models provide a method with which to build a diagram of the known mechanisms involved in the regulation of any physiological variable.

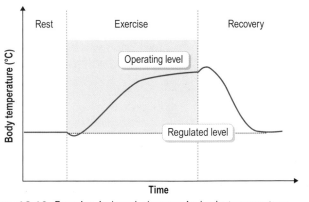

Figure 18.13 Exercise-induced changes in body temperature during a square-wave function from rest to a moderate–high work level, and during post-exercise recovery.

References

Andres T, Hexamer M, Werner J 1999 Heat acclimation of humans: hot environment versus physical exercise. Journal of Thermal Biology 25:139–142

Bazett HC 1949 The regulation of body temperature. In: Newburgh LH (ed) Physiology of heat regulation and the science of clothing. Saunders, Philadelphia, PA, 109–192

Bernard C 1865 Introduction á l'Etude de la Médicine experimentale. Baillière et Fils, Paris

Bligh J 1987 Human cold exposure and the circumstances of hypothermia. In: Mekjavic IB, Banister EW, Morrison JB (eds) Environmental ergonomics. Taylor and Francis, London

Bligh J 1998 Mammalian homeothermy: an integrative thesis. Journal of Thermal Biology 23:143–258

Boulant JA 1981 Hypothalamic mechanisms in thermoregulation. Federation Proceedings 40:2843–2850

Cannon WB 1929 Organisation for physiological homeostasis. Physiological Reviews 9:399

Cotter JD, Taylor NAS 2005 Distribution of cutaneous sudomotor and alliesthesial thermosensitivity in mildly heat-stressed humans: an open-loop approach. Journal of Physiology (London) 565(1):335–345

Hammel HT 1968 Regulation of internal body temperature. Annual Reviews of Physiology 30:641–710

Hammel HT, Jackson DC, Stolwijk JAJ, Hardy JD, Stromme SB 1963 Temperature regulation by hypothalamic proportional control with an adjustable set-point. Journal of Applied Physiology 18:1146–1154

IUPS Thermal Commission: Commission for Thermal Physiology of the International Union of Physiological Sciences 2001 Glossary of terms for thermal physiology. Japanese Journal of Physiology 51(2):245–280

Jessen C 1981 Independent clamps of peripheral and central temperatures and their effects on heat production in the goat. Journal of Physiology 311:11–22

Jessen C 1996 Interaction of body temperatures in control of thermoregulatory effector mechanisms. In: Fregly MJ, Blatteis CM (eds) Environmental physiology. Handbook of physiology, volume 1. Oxford University Press, New York, 127–138

Mekjavic IB, Eiken O 2006 Contribution of thermal and nonthermal factors to the regulation of body temperature in humans. Journal of Applied Physiology 100:2065–2072

Mekjavic IB, Tipton MJ, Eiken O 2003 Thermal considerations in diving. In: Brubakk AO, Neumann TS (eds) Bennett and Elliott's physiology and medicine of diving, 5th edn. Saunders, Edinburgh, 115–152

Roberts MF, Wenger, CB, Stolwijk JAJ, Nadel ER 1977 Skin blood flow and sweating changes following exercise and heat acclimation. Journal of Applied Physiology 43:133–137

Ruben JA 1995 The evolution of endothermy in mammals and birds: from physiology to fossils. Annual Review of Physiology 57:69–95

Silva LN, Boulant AJ 1984 Effects of osmotic pressure, glucose and temperature on neurons in preoptic tissue slices. American Journal of Physiology 247:R335–R345

Stanier MW, Mount LE, Bligh J 1984 Energy balance and temperature regulation. Cambridge texts in physiological sciences 4. Cambridge University Press, Cambridge

Werner J 1980 The concept of regulation for human body temperature. Journal of Thermal Biology 5:75–82

Werner J 1990 Functional mechanisms of temperature regulation, adaptation and fever: complementary system theoretical and experimental evidence. In: Schonbaum E, Lomax P (eds) Thermoregulation: physiology and biochemistry. Pergamon Press, New York, 185–208

Werner J 1998 Biophysics of heat exchange between body and environment. In: Blatteis M (ed) Physiology and pathophysiology of temperature regulation. World Scientific Publications, Singapore, 23–45

Werner J 2005 Regulatory processes of the human body during thermal and work strain. In: Tochihara Y, Ohnaka T (eds) Environmental ergonomics. Elsevier, Tokyo, 3–9

Wilkie DR 1954 Facts and theories about muscle. Progress in Biophysics 4:288–324

Chapter 19

The physiology of acute heat exposure, with implications for human performance in the heat

Nigel A.S. Taylor   Narihiko Kondo   W. Larry Kenney

CHAPTER CONTENTS

1 INTRODUCTION

Humans evolved over millions of years from species that acquired the capacity to produce an abundance of metabolic heat. Approximately 250,000 years ago, unusually rapid, global climatic changes resulted in the African climate changing from being very cold to tropical within just one century (Gowlett 2001). Such rapid changes, in combination with other selective pressures, can result in extinctions. Speciation of *Homo sapiens* possibly occurred at this time (Balter 2002), with survivors capable of avoiding, tolerating or adapting to extremes of cold and heat (Chapters 20 and 21). These behavioural and thermoregulatory characteristics facilitated the migration of hominids extending from the Arctic Circle to the Equator.

Whilst capable of tolerating a wide range of climates, we live within a very narrow and fiercely protected range of deep tissue (body core) temperatures (thermal homeostasis; Chapter 18), with resting core (deep body) temperatures normally being between 36.5–37°C (97.7–98.6°F). The maximal tolerance limits for cells ranges from ~0°C (ice crystal formation) to ~45°C (coagulation of intracellular proteins). However, in humans, the lowest recorded accidental and survivable core temperature is 13.7°C (56.7°F: Gilbert et al. 2000). At the other extreme, survival has been reported for a man with a core temperature of 46.5°C (115.7°F: Slovis et al. 1989). In the heat, if sweating and evaporation are unlimited, most people can withstand extreme heat for short periods, if protected from contact with hot surfaces (e.g. oven temperatures >200°C). Nevertheless, we can tolerate core temperatures outside the range of 35–41°C for only very brief periods (Table 19.1). Yet, even within this regulatory zone (Figure 18.4), tissue temperatures vary markedly throughout the body (Eichna et al. 1951), particularly at the skin surface (Werner & Reents 1980).

This variation is created by the constant exchange of thermal energy within the body and with the environment, even under steady-state conditions (dynamic equilibrium). Indeed, this variability is essential for life and results from differences in local metabolic rate (or metabolic energy transformation), the temperature and flow of blood through

Table 19.1 Clinically significant core and skin temperatures (°C).

Core temperatures	
>45	Possible death without treatment
>40.5	Profound clinical hyperthermia (heatstroke)
>39.5	Profound hyperthermia
38.5–39.5	Moderate hyperthermia (heat exhaustion)
37.2–38.5	Mild hyperthermia
36.5–37	Normothermia
Skin temperatures	
>50	Second-degree burn
>45	Tissue damage
41–43	Burning pain
39–41	Pain
33–39	Skin warmth through to discomfort (hot)
28–33	Thermal comfort

tissues and heat transfer (exchange) among the surrounding tissues and objects. Acute changes in thermal stress, of either external (exogenous) or internal (endogenous) origin, disturb thermal homeostasis. Heat storage elevates the mean body temperature (weighted sum of core and skin (shell) temperatures) and sets into motion a series of physiological adjustments to eliminate body heat, through the finely controlled coordination of several body systems. In Chapter 18, the concepts of body temperature regulation were explored, and the glossary developed by the IUPS Thermal Commission (2001) supplements this chapter, as well as providing detailed descriptions of the language used in thermal physiology. Both should be consulted when reading this chapter, which focuses upon the physiological impact of heat storage, through changes in either the environment or metabolic rate. Before discussing these changes, we will first elaborate upon the thermodynamics of heat transfer and the neurophysiological components that enable the sensing of tissue temperatures and the autonomic and behavioural responses to changes in these temperatures.

2 BIOPHYSICS OF HEAT TRANSFER

2.1 Introduction to thermodynamics

Humans are open energy systems, constantly exchanging energy with our surroundings. The biophysics of thermal energy exchanges is known as thermodynamics – a cornerstone of human thermoregulation. Thermal energy exchanged between man and the environment may be quantified using the general heat balance equation; a specific application of the First Law of Thermodynamics. This law dictates that stored thermal energy (S) results from the balance among evaporative (E: condensation on this skin surface will result in heat gain), radiative (R), convective (C) and conductive (K) thermal exchanges and heat produced through metabolic energy transformations (M) and exchanged when performing mechanical work (W;

IUPS Thermal Commission 2001). It may be expressed mathematically as:

Equation 1: $\quad S = M - (\pm W) - E \pm R \pm K \pm C \; [\text{W} \cdot \text{m}^{-2}]$

These avenues for energy exchange are affected by the magnitude of the water vapour pressure and thermal gradients that dictate heat flow (Second Law of Thermodynamics). For an elaboration of these avenues of heat transfer, readers are directed to Gagge & Gonzales (1996) and the IUPS Thermal Commission (2001). However, several key points are summarised below, with Equation 1 defining the balance between heat gains and losses. In the heat, this balance is tipped in favour of heat storage and the body must dissipate this heat. In the cold (Chapter 20), heat loss is favoured and heat conservation becomes the primary focus.

Evaporative heat transfer and condensation occur within gaseous media. During vaporisation, thermal energy is transferred to liquid molecules until a critical temperature is achieved. At this point, further heat does not raise water temperature but alters its state from a liquid to a gaseous phase, resulting in heat dissipation at approximating 2.43 kJ·g^{-1} (0.58 kcal·mL^{-1}). This energy remains within the molecules until they cool, permitting condensation back into a liquid, releasing energy. Such evaporation occurs from all moist surfaces, with respiratory evaporation accounting for ~10% of resting heat loss (Burton & Edholm 1955).

The radiative, conductive and convective thermal exchanges constitute dry heat transfers. During cold-water immersions, where skin temperature approximates water temperature, convective heat losses dominate (Rapp 1971). However, for most resting air exposures, radiation generally dominates (Mitchell et al. 1968). For example, at 10°C, radiation accounts for ~57% and convection ~42% of heat loss, with negligible evaporative cooling (<1%). At 21°C, these relationships are retained: radiation (57%) and convection (40%). As air temperature increases, the role of evaporative cooling is elevated, such that at 30°C, the following heat losses would exist: radiation (30%), convection (15%) and evaporation (55%). If the air is hot enough, dry heat transfer will be impeded, even being reversed, leading to heat influx and the relative contributions become more variable, especially when exposed to powerful radiant heat sources. For instance, at 40°C, radiation (80%) and convection (20%) both result in heat gains, with evaporation being the only avenue available for heat loss. The critical air temperature at which radiative and convective heat losses cease is about 35°C, where the skin–air thermal gradient approaches 0°C. This can also occur during heavy exercise in still hotter conditions, even though the mean skin temperature can reach 36–37°C.

Thermal radiation (photons) is emitted by all objects possessing thermal energy and is frequently the dominant source of heat loss or gain. A person standing in snow on a clear day will not only emit thermal radiation to surrounding cold objects but will absorb solar radiation. When working on a hot day in the sun, the effect of solar radiation can be extremely powerful (800 $W \cdot m^{-2}$; watts).

Thermal conduction is generally small, though pertinent to many ergonomic applications, and occurring when objects at different temperatures come into contact. Energy is exchanged between the molecules and this exchange is dependent upon the contact surface areas, temperature gradient, thermal conductivity and specific heat capacity of each object, and the distance through which heat is conducted.

Convectional heat transfer occurs between the skin and the surrounding medium. Under comfortable (thermoneutral) conditions, skin temperature averages 31–33°C. When the medium is cooler than the skin, heat transfer creates thermal currents, resulting in the bulk movement of molecules away from the skin, due to heat-induced changes in the density of the medium. Cooler water/air moves into this space, ensuring continued heat loss. The rate of convective heat transfer is dependent upon the thermal conductivity, specific heat capacity and density of the medium, the temperature gradient and the exposed skin surface area. In situations where a cooler medium is moving across the skin (relative motion: wind, current) or where the body is moving through a stationary medium (absolute motion), forced convectional heat transfer occurs. This is a function of the relative or absolute velocity. A physiological source of convective heat transfer occurs in the form of blood flow through tissues, where heat delivery (or removal) is modified through neurally mediated changes in vasomotor tone.

Let us now consider metabolism. When stored chemical energy fuels metabolic processes (cellular respiration), the chemical bonds joining carbohydrates, fats and proteins are broken. This releases thermal energy: metabolic energy transformation. However, the inefficiency of cellular respiration results in heat production being about four times greater than the liberation of useful energy; humans are only ~20% efficient. This metabolic heat is initially stored within the body but heat storage can present a challenge to thermal homeostasis.

Finally, energy leaves the body when performing (positive, concentric) work (W). Conversely, energy can enter when (negative, eccentric) work is performed on the body by an external energy source. The combination of these metabolic and mechanical energy exchanges $(M - (\pm W))$ is termed metabolic heat production (H; IUPS Thermal Commission 2001). During heavy exercise, this can be very extensive. Thus, while air temperature is strongly associated with heat illness, it is frequently not the most important factor (Goldman 2001). Indeed, for most healthy adults, the risk of heat illness is more likely to originate from an excessive metabolic heat production (exertional heat illness) than from climatic extremes (classic heat illness).

To illustrate this, let us consider a 70 kg person (generic male-female) performing 200 W (~1200 $kg \cdot m \cdot min^{-1}$) of external work. This person has a metabolic heat production

of ~1000 $J \cdot s^{-1}$, with ~800 $J \cdot s^{-1}$ (800 W) being converted into thermal energy. The retention of 3.47 kJ (0.83 kcal) of thermal energy within 1 kg of tissue results in an average tissue (mean body) temperature elevation of 1°C (Burton 1935). If thermal energy neither enters nor leaves the body (the adiabatic state), then heat storage at 800 $J \cdot s^{-1}$ will cause the average body temperature to rise 1°C in ~5 min. The capacity to continue this metabolic heat production, without a progressive elevation in mean body temperature, is now dictated by the thermal compensability of the environment.

2.2 Predicting problems in heat balance

Thermal compensability refers to the interaction of physiological functions, clothing and environmental conditions. Of course, given the appropriate selection of behavioural choices (i.e. protective clothing, thermal insulation, air conditioning plants), there is virtually no environment in which humans cannot comfortably survive. Indeed, it is often much more efficient to recruit behavioural than autonomic regulatory mechanisms. Thus, within this chapter and the next, thermal compensability will be used to refer exclusively to the autonomic regulation of body temperature, and it defines a range of heat transfer beyond which the body will move inexorably towards either hypothermia (35°C; 95°F) or hyperthermia (39°C; 102°F). In hot environments, thermal (autonomic) compensability is dictated by the ratio of the required evaporative heat loss (E_{req}) to the maximal evaporative cooling (E_{max}) that the environment, including clothing, will permit. The derivation of each function (Belding & Hatch 1955) provides a first-principles method for evaluating combinations of environmental and physiological states. If E_{req} is greater than E_{max}, then the conditions are uncompensable (Figure 18.4, zone 3).

$$\text{Equation 2:} \quad E_{req} = H - E_{resp} \pm R \pm C \text{ [walts, W]}$$

where:

E_{req} = required evaporative cooling [W]
H = metabolic heat production $(M - (\pm W))$ [W]
E_{resp} = evaporation accompanying ventilation [W]
R and C = heat transfer via radiation and convection [W]

$$\text{Equation 3:} \quad E_{max} = 6.45 \cdot A_D \cdot i_m / I_{TOT} \cdot 2.2 \cdot \\ (P_{sk} - (RH_a \cdot P_a)) \text{ [W]}$$

where:

E_{max} = maximal attainable evaporative cooling for environmental and clothing combinations [W]
A_D = body surface area (DuBois equation) [m^2]
i_m = moisture permeability index (0.45 if unknown: dimensionless)
I_{TOT} = total insulation (1 clo = 0.155 $m^2 \cdot K \cdot W^{-1}$), including the trapped boundary layer air and clothing insulation [$m^2 \cdot K \cdot W^{-1}$]
RH_a = relative humidity of the air [%]

P_a = water vapour pressure of the air [kPa]
P_{sk} = water vapour pressure at the skin surface [kPa]
6.45 and 2.2 = constants.

The concept of the body temperature operating level was introduced in Chapter 18. At rest, body temperature is regulated but it moves outside this operating level when heat balance is disturbed. During light–moderate exercise in a cool environment, an increase in body temperature is not usually evident, since the autonomic heat loss responses (vasodilatation and sweating) should be capable of defending this regulated temperature. However, when the same exercise is performed in warmer conditions, a body temperature rise occurs, but this is often simply to a new steady state or operating level. This new body temperature is either regulated or is simply a consequence of a change in the balance between heat production and heat loss. When environmental conditions are uncompensable, the body temperature will rise inexorably, eventually leading to heat illness or the failure of cardiovascular regulation.

3 NEUROPHYSIOLOGY OF THERMORECEPTION

Chapter 18 covered primary concepts of temperature regulation in detail. Herein, we highlight the essential neurophysiological background to the behavioural and autonomic regulation of mean body temperature.

The conventional, though not unequivocal (Webb 1995), understanding is that humans regulate an integrated composite of body core and superficial (skin) temperatures: mean body temperature (Jessen 1996). One may conceptually view the body as a two-compartment system, in which the temperature of the passive system is affected by the balance of heat transfer within the system and between that system and the surrounding environment. Simultaneously, the temperature of this system is regulated by an active (thermoregulatory) system through the modulation of physiological (effector) functions, that modify heat gain and loss. If mean body temperature was faithfully regulated, this would imply a homogeneous distribution of thermoreceptors. Since we know that such homogeneity does not occur, it can be assumed that humans regulate some integrated body temperature, the form of which varies among different thermal stresses.

3.1 Thermoreceptors

Humans possess many different receptors through which the internal (interoceptors) and the surrounding (exteroceptors) environmental conditions are monitored. Some tissues respond to perturbations in thermal energy content (temperature-responsive tissues), while others transduce a neural response that correlates with this change (thermosensitive tissues). However, thermosensitivity does not imply functional significance, as some neurons are influenced by changes in tissue temperature but do not

participate in temperature regulation (Boulant 1996). Other thermosensitive tissues (neurons) give rise to an awareness of a thermal stimulation, and the initiation of appropriate autonomic and behavioural responses. These are the thermoreceptors located in the skin, viscera, spinal cord, brain stem and hypothalamus (Boulant 1996, Pierau 1996).

Within the skin, cold- and warm-sensitive thermoreceptors provide our first source of thermal awareness. These receptors are not uniformly distributed, with some sites responding to warm stimuli but not cool, while others react to cool but not warmth. Indeed, the cutaneous thermoreceptive fields reveal a mosaic of thermosensitivity, with considerable overlap. Most receptors in the skin are excited by a variety of stimuli. However, regardless of the mode of activation, the resultant neural response always elicits the same general sensation. For instance, stimulation of a cold receptor by noxious heat will elicit the paradoxical sensation of coldness. Cutaneous thermoreceptors produce a constant (static), temperature-dependent neural discharge when held at a stable temperature, and a dynamic response when the rate of local temperature change is modified. This is characterised by either a discharge frequency overshoot, when receptor-specific stimulation is applied, or an inhibition with the opposite stimulation (Figure 19.1). Thus, during a sudden cold-water immersion, the simultaneous powerful stimulation of cold-sensitive receptors, and the inhibition of warm-sensitive receptor, largely accounts for the intensity of the cold-shock response (Chapter 20).

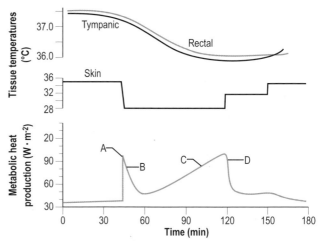

Figure 19.1 Thermal and metabolic responses elicited from square-wave changes in skin temperature (water immersion) and illustrating dynamic thermoreceptor properties. Abbreviations: **A** dynamic response overshoot due to powerful cutaneous stimulation; **B** gradual decay as overshoot response subsides; **C** slow rise as core temperature falls; **D** dynamic (peripheral) inhibition with skin warming. Redrawn from Brown & Brenglemann (1970) with permission.

To date, only cutaneous cold receptors have been isolated, existing as a three-dimensional array of free nerve endings within the lower epidermis. Experimental evidence indicates their density is several-fold that of warm-sensitive receptors (Hensel 1952), with multiple receptors arising from a single myelinated fibre, that branches into several unmyelinated terminals (Pierau 1996). Cold-sensitive receptors respond to temperatures between −5° and 43°C and demonstrate maximal discharge rates in the temperature range 25–30°C. Warm-sensitive receptors are thought to be free nerve endings, emanating from unmyelinated C-fibres (Darian-Smith et al. 1979). These receptors respond maximally at ~40°C but operate over the range 28–48°C. The wider temperature response range, in combination with the greater density of the cold-sensitive receptors, is of considerable functional significance during cold exposure and defence, which can be driven by cutaneous thermoreceptors.

Regional differences in cutaneous thermosensitivity have been demonstrated for animals (Hales & Hutchinson 1971). Recently, Cotter & Taylor (2005) investigated local cutaneous warm and cool sensitivities for sweating and whole-body thermal discomfort in humans, under open-loop conditions. The face displayed a greater thermosensitivity than other skin surfaces to cooling and, to a lesser extent, to warming. Thus, facial cooling elicited a two-to-fivefold more powerful suppression of sweating and thermal discomfort than did equivalent cooling of an equal skin area from any other body segment. In addition, the torso displayed high warmth sensitivity for sudomotor control.

The spinal cord relays thermoafferent signals and performs some central integration. However, it is also thermosensitive, containing warm- and cold-sensitive neurons in a 3:1 ratio, with the intersection of their static response curves occurring at approximately 37°C (Simon et al. 1998).

The thermosensitivity of the hypothalamus has been known for more than 60 years, with thermosensitive neurons identified in the preoptic anterior, posterior, lateral and dorsal areas. Of these regions, the posterior hypothalamus appears to modulate behavioural responses, with autonomic responses elicited from the preoptic and posterior hypothalamus (Kanosue et al. 1998). Approximately 40% of the preoptic neurons are thermosensitive, with the ratio of warm- to cold-sensitive neurons being about 3:1. However, these sites also receive thermoafferent flow from other structures.

3.2 Central integration

To regulate body temperature, a centrally integrated signal from both deep body (core: central nervous system, muscle, viscera) and superficial (shell or skin: dermal tissues, subcutaneous adipose tissues) thermosensitive structures is evaluated at the hypothalamus (Chapter 18). For most circumstances, when both core and skin temperatures can freely fluctuate, experimental evidence supports a dominant role of body core thermoreceptive flow in mammalian thermoregulation in the heat, in an approximate 9:1 (core: shell) ratio. However, this ratio is not evident under all experimental conditions and should be considered as a generalised simplification, rather than a precise scientific fact (Bligh 1973).

While we are not certain how these signals interact during integration, it is currently believed that some form of reciprocal cross-inhibition exists between warm- and cold-sensitive thermoafferents and the preoptic hypothalamic foci responsible for initiating an increase in metabolic rate (thermogenesis) or sweating (Chapter 18). That is, while sweating is driven primarily by central warm-sensitive signals, cold-sensitive signals from the shell will, at least transiently, suppress sweating. Furthermore, it is highly probable that the preoptic foci also interact, perhaps also in a reciprocal, inhibitory manner (Boulant 1981). Such a regulatory mechanism is inconsistent with the historically based view of some cybernetic modellers, who have suggested the existence of a discrete reference signal or an operational set-point. Unfortunately, these older concepts do not conform to more recent experimental observations (Mekjavic & Eiken 2006).

In neutral and comfortable conditions, afferent flow is continuously reaching the hypothalamus but these signals do not evoke either behavioural or autonomic responses. However, when exposed to conditions on either side of this zone, a deviation in mean body or skin temperature occurs and thermoeffector mechanisms are activated. The body temperatures at which this activation occurs are known as the thermoregulatory thresholds (see Figure 18.4: points B and C), with the interthreshold zone separating these thresholds defining the thermoneutral zone (see Figure 18.4: zone 1), in which neither a greater metabolic rate (energy transformation; thermogenesis) nor evaporative cooling is activated. Thus, instead of set-point regulation, mammalian thermoregulation is more likely to be based on keeping mean body temperature within an interthreshold zone, the size of which is affected by both adaptive (Chapter 21) and non-thermal influences (Mekjavic & Eiken 2006; Chapter 18).

Once centrally initiated, the effector responses will be proportional to the deviation in mean body temperature, as indicated by the positive and negative slopes for sweating, thermogenesis and skin blood flow (see Figure 18.4). These slopes describe the gain (sensitivity) of the thermoeffectors and can themselves be modified by thermal adaptation and various non-thermal factors (Mekjavic & Eiken 2006).

4 AUTONOMIC REGULATION

Humans can survive long-term exposure to extreme cold and intense heat but such thermal tolerance is only possible due to our technological capacities, permitting the modification of the local environment. During daily life, we regulate body temperature via behavioural and physiological means, permitting thermal energy exchanges between the environment and body without protracted changes in body temperature. However, this does not always occur.

Consider our 70 kg person, now wearing athletic clothing, exercising at 200 W and producing thermal energy (~800 J·s^{-1}). If this person is immersed in water at 10°C, all of this heat would be lost and core temperature would not be elevated. If the water temperature was 37°C (thereby establishing an adiabatic state), all heat would be retained, with core temperature rapidly rising. Between these states occur conditions encountered by most exercising people, where some, but not all heat is dissipated. For instance, when exercising in air at 25°C (50% relative humidity), the required evaporative cooling (E_{req}) would be 330 W (4.7 kcal·min^{-1}). However, athletic clothing and the environment only support a maximal evaporative cooling (E_{max}) of 150 W (2.2 kcal·min^{-1}). Thus, the physiological demand for heat loss is more than twice the capacity for it to occur, and heat will be stored at the rate of ~180 J·s^{-1} (2.6 kcal·min^{-1}) and body tissue temperatures will rise at a rate of about 1°C every 20–25 min. It is universally accepted that such core temperature increases are proportional to the intensity of the exercise forcing function (Saltin & Hermansen 1966).

An elevation in tissue temperatures during exercise should not necessarily be considered problematic. While there does exist the notion of a critical and limiting core temperature (Chapter 27.2), we must recall that, for heat to flow to the skin, we must sustain a favourable thermal gradient. During exercise in the heat, this can only occur if the core temperature is allowed to rise. This is somewhat analogous to the elevation in mean arterial pressure during exercise. That is, regulated variables are not always held constant. Instead, regulation sometimes results in an elevation to a higher, yet relatively stable level.

Behavioural interventions (e.g. clothing and climate control) modify the microclimate, and are aimed at reducing heat storage. Physiologically, we modulate (control) cutaneous vascular resistance, thermogenesis and evaporative cooling to enable successful exposure to a broad range of thermal environments. The resulting heat transfers are proportional, not just to neural drive but to the thermal conductivity and temperature of the surrounding medium, tissue insulation and the temperature, evaporation rate and the size of the exposed skin surface. Our technological, behavioural and physiological characteristics collectively define the outer limits of thermal compensability.

4.1 Cardiovascular modulation

4.1.1 Control of skin blood flow

When exposed to hot conditions, peripheral heterothermy is replaced by more uniform skin temperatures (Werner & Reents 1980), reflecting generalised cutaneous vasodilatation and facilitating heat transport to the periphery. Thermal energy reaches the skin via conduction but this is a slow process. It is much faster to transport heat in the blood: convective exchange. Since blood has a high volume specific heat (3.85 kJ·L^{-1}·°C^{-1}; 0.92 kcal·L^{-1}·°C^{-1}), it is ideally suited for heat transport, and changes in skin blood flow represent the first of our heat dissipation responses. Indeed, a primary function of skin blood flow, once it has satisfied local metabolic requirements, is to modulate the internal heat transfer, through either cutaneous vasodilatation or vasoconstriction.

The delivery of heat to the skin is a function of skin blood flow, the core–skin temperature gradient and the volume specific heat of blood. At rest in a thermoneutral (comfortable) environment, skin blood flow is approximately 200–500 mL·min^{-1}, or about 5–10% of the cardiac output (Rowell 1974). Because there exists a 4°C core–skin gradient under these conditions, metabolic heat is constantly delivered in the blood (convected) to the skin for dissipation. With skin blood flow averaging ~350 mL·min^{-1}, convective heat transfer may approximate 5.4 kJ·min^{-1} (3.85 kJ·L^{-1}·°C^{-1} * 0.35 L·min^{-1} * 4°C: 1.3 kcal·min^{-1}). In fact, at rest, thermal homeostasis can be achieved entirely through subtle changes in skin blood flow, particularly to the hands, face and feet (if exposed). The upper and lower ambient temperatures within which this vasomotor-mediated heat loss dominates are dependent upon the thermal conductivity and specific heat of the surrounding medium and clothing worn: the thermoneutral zone (Chapter 18 and Figure 18.4). Under cooler conditions, cutaneous vasoconstriction increases tissue insulation, causing skin temperatures to fall, sacrificing peripheral heat to regulate body temperature.

In contrast, under a maximal, externally applied heat stress at rest (e.g. water-perfusion suit), skin blood flow can reach 7–8 L·min^{-1}: >50% of the cardiac output (Rowell 1974). For a 1°C core–skin temperature gradient, this blood flow is capable of a core–skin convective heat transfer of 28.9 kJ·min^{-1} (3.85 kJ·L^{-1}·°C^{-1} * 7.5 L·min^{-1} * 1°C: 6.9 kcal·min^{-1}). This extreme cutaneous perfusion is attained through a chronotropically driven elevation of cardiac output, and 25–40% reductions in splanchnic, renal and muscle blood flow. Such a progressively rising skin blood flow, in combination with heat gained from the environment, drives skin temperatures upwards, for which there are three immediate consequences. First, it buffers further exogenous heat gains. Second, it increases cutaneous water vapour pressure, increasing evaporation (E_{max}); we shall return to this point later. Third, an increasing skin temperature gradually reduces heat flow from the core.

The example above represents the upper limit of cutaneous vasodilatation. Maximal thermogenesis (shivering) defines the lower limit of the thermoregulatory zone (see Figure 18.4 point D), whilst peak sweat secretion marks the upper boundary (point A). Within this zone may be found points of maximal vasoconstriction (insulation; point F) and vasodilatation (point E). Since our focus lies to the right of the thermoneutral zone, we shall first track changes in skin blood flow within two, independently controlled arms of the cutaneous vasculature.

Skin blood flow is primarily responsive to increases in core temperature and, to a lesser extent, skin temperature. Blood flow to the acral skin regions (nose, ears, lips, palms and soles) is modulated via adrenergic vasoconstrictor fibres. In the thermoneutral state, constrictor tone is powerful and these regions have a very low blood flow. Passive cooling will elicit near-maximal vasoconstriction, whilst heating gradually abolishes constrictor tone, leading to passive vasodilatation (Kellogg 2006, Kenney & Johnson 1992, Roddie 1983, 2003). This results in a pressure-driven elevation in skin blood flow (Figure 19.2A).

At the remaining non-acral skin surfaces, blood flow is controlled via two separate sympathetic pathways. Adrenergic vasoconstrictor fibres also exist in this region, but 80–95% of the skin blood flow increase is mediated via an active vasodilator system. However, the neurotransmitter mechanisms for active vasodilatation have not been fully elucidated (Kellogg 2006, Kenney & Johnson 1992, Roddie 2003). In the thermoneutral state, adrenergic constrictor tone is present and active dilatory influences are minimal.

Cooling induces further adrenergic and noradrenergic constriction, without affecting the vasodilatory mechanism. Heating results in a biphasic elevation in skin blood flow (Figure 19.2B curves 1 and 2). The first phase is associated with the abolition of constrictor tone, while the second results from active vasodilatation.

The onset of active vasodilatation is called the vasodilatory threshold. It is dictated by events within the hypothalamus and is usually defined in terms of the mean body temperature beyond which progressive vasodilatation is evident. This threshold is generally 0.2–0.5°C greater than the mean body temperature of a thermoneutral, resting person. Beyond this threshold, the rise in skin blood flow can be tracked against mean body temperature increments, with the ratio of these changes (mL·100 min^{-1}·°C^{-1}) describing the sensitivity of vasomotor control (Chapter 18). Both the vasodilatory threshold and sensitivity are subject to modification through heat adaptation, the preexercise body temperature (Chapter 21) and a range of non-thermal factors, such as endurance fitness, hydration state and illness.

Cutaneous blood returns to the heart via either superficial or deep venous beds. These beds are interconnected. The former are relatively well innervated and both core and skin cooling elevates venoconstrictor tone, allowing blood to return via the well-insulated deeper venous beds, thus reducing heat loss. Relaxation of the superficial venoconstrictor tone accompanies skin heating. Since these veins are very compliant, a significant portion of the circulating volume pools in these vessels, particularly within dependent regions (below heart level). This aids in heat transfer by slowing capillary circulation and increasing the blood transit time. However, this venous pooling, coupled with fluid losses from sweating, may also decrease central venous return.

4.1.2 Integrated cardiovascular responses

The relationships described above do not occur in isolation. Thus far, we have described how skin blood flow facilitates heat loss. However, we must not lose sight of the fact that vasomotor function more specifically subserves blood pressure regulation and critically influences body fluid regulation. The former is discussed in detail in Chapter 1. Therefore, skin blood flow modulations will also be affected by other non-thermal, autonomic functions. This second layer of blood flow control is critical, in that it modifies skin blood flow when cardiovascular stability is threatened (e.g. reduced mean arterial pressure). This becomes evident during extended-duration exercise, particularly in an upright posture and when dehydration occurs.

Habitual exercise is arguably the greatest provocation to cardiovascular regulation, especially when the intensity is ramped towards maximal. During exercise in hot conditions, the core-to-skin thermal gradient is smaller and the necessary convective heat transfer requires a large increase in skin blood flow. However, blood flow to the exercising

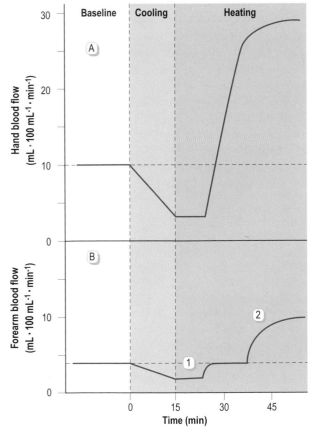

Figure 19.2 Skin blood flow in acral (A) and non-acral regions (B) in the thermoneutral state, followed by cooling (15 min) and heating (60 min). Modified from Roddie (1983) with permission.

muscles is simultaneously elevated. Indeed, these requirements can become competitive. Since vasomotor function is critical to blood pressure regulation, and since this takes precedence over thermoregulation when the former is compromised, then exercise- and heat-induced reductions in either body fluid volumes or central venous pressure have a powerful impact on skin blood flow. This impact occurs through reflexes activated when cardiac filling pressure is decreased and the cardiopulmonary (low-pressure) baroreceptors, located in the large veins and right atrium, are unloaded. These reflexes function to maintain mean arterial pressure and, in the case of exercise, adequate blood flow to active muscles. This occurs through a coordinated response of the entire cardiovascular system, with skin blood flow possibly being sacrificed. Thus, skin blood flow at any given time represents the aggregated effects of thermoregulatory and non-thermoregulatory reflexes, with thermal homeostasis possibly being threatened (Kenney & Johnson 1992, Rowell 1974).

Early investigators noted that, when skin temperature was increased, heart rate and cardiac output increased appreciably. These changes can be produced experimentally using heated, water-perfused suits, with heat transferred to the blood via conduction and to the core by convection. The rise in skin temperature induces an immediate increase in heart rate, with minimal change in stroke volume, resulting in a greater cardiac output and skin blood flow (Table 19.2). However, the skin blood flow elevation exceeds that provided via changes in cardiac output.

The additional blood is obtained from that which is translocated from visceral structures (e.g. renal and splanchnic regions) and inactive muscles, as part of the integrated cardiovascular response. A lower renal blood flow is accompanied by reduced glomerular filtration, which has significant water conservation outcomes. Since many organs receive blood well in excess of their metabolic requirement,

such flow reductions are well tolerated. Exceptions include a constant cerebral and metabolically driven coronary blood flow. Most of this redistributed blood is pumped to the skin. Central blood volume falls transiently, then increases as blood is passively displaced from preventricular sumps, including the splanchnic veins. The fact that stroke volume increases from the initiation of heating implies that ventricular contractility has experienced a temperature-mediated increase. This inotropic effect is sympathetically driven, with a simultaneous withdrawal of parasympathetic activity. Thus, a doubling of the cardiac output has been achieved via an increase in ventricular work and without the addition of energy from the venous system.

Exercise in the heat exacerbates competition for a limited cardiac output, as working muscle places a significant further demand on the cardiovascular system. This is illustrated in Figure 19.3; the cardiovascular responses to an increasing (graded) exercise forcing function, performed at 25°C and 43°C (air temperatures). During light-to-moderate exercise, the requisite increase in cardiac output was unaffected by air or core temperature, as cardiac output was well supported by the elevation in heart rate; note that stroke volume increases very little at exercise intensities >40% of maximum work rate. Indeed, with a simultaneously elevated demand for blood flow at the skin and exercising muscles, venous return can be reduced. The combined effects of an elevated cardiac contractility, increased mean arterial pressure, skeletal muscle pumping and increased respiration enhance venous return, at least during short-term exercise in comfortable conditions. However, in the heat and particularly during long-duration exercise, a significant blood volume pools in the vaso- and venodilated skin and exercising limbs. Pooling is most pronounced in dependent regions, reducing venous return and the central blood volume. This lowers ventricular preloading, with a consequent reduction in stroke volume. Thus, in the heat,

Table 19.2 Integrated cardiovascular responses during passive heating (water-perfusion suit) of the skin to 40°C (45 min) in supine, resting subjects. As blood temperature increases, skin blood flow and cardiac output also increase. The changes in cardiac output, splanchnic blood flow, renal blood flow and inactive muscle blood flow combine to meet the demands of the increased cutaneous flow (7.8 L·mim^{-1}; data extracted from Rowell 1974)

Variable	Control	Heating	Change
Skin blood flow (mL·min^{-1})	200–500	7800	+2130%
Cardiac output (mL·min^{-1})	6400	13,000	+103%
Heart rate (beats·min^{-1})	64	120	+88%
Stroke volume (mL)	100	108	+8%
Splanchnic blood flow (mL·min^{-1})	1500	900	−40%
Renal blood flow (mL·min^{-1})	1300	900	−31%
Muscle blood flow (mL·100 min^{-1}·min^{-1})	2.8	2.1	−25%
Mean arterial pressure (mmHg)	90	86	−4%
Mean right atrial pressure (mmHg)	5.4	0.5	−91%

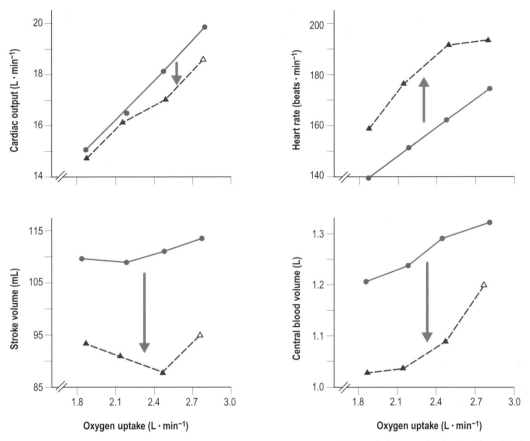

Figure 19.3 Cardiovascular responses relative to absolute oxygen uptake, during graded, upright exercise in hot (43°C: triangles) and neutral conditions (25°C: circles). Arrows highlight the direction of change for each variable affected by the heat. Redrawn from Rowell (1974) with permission.

the heart rate is higher at any given exercise intensity, to sustain cardiac output, and to compensate for the reduced central blood volume and stroke volume. Indeed, this relative tachycardia serves as a useful measure of thermally induced cardiovascular strain.

When light-to-moderate exercise is continued for an extended duration, venous pooling becomes greater. This is driven, at least to some extent, by the gradual elevation in core temperature. Continued sweating results in a progressive reduction in blood volume and these combine to further reduce central blood volume and stroke volume. If the same work rate is to be maintained, then cardiac output and the supply of oxygen to the working muscle must also be maintained. For this to occur, the heart rate must slowly creep upwards. This phenomenon is known as the cardiovascular drift.

At higher exercise intensities, the demand for elevated skin and muscle blood flows is again supported by redistributing blood flow away from the visceral organs (spleen, liver, kidneys, intestines, gonads). These flow reductions can be quite extensive and protracted and are sometimes thought to cause adverse outcomes, such as endotoxaemia

(associated with extended intestinal blood flow reductions). While this redistribution helps offset the detrimental effects of peripheral blood pooling, maximal heart rate is approached and the person slowly becomes incapable of sustaining the necessary cardiac output. Skin blood flow will now be reduced as the low-pressure baroreceptors are activated and blood pressure regulation takes precedence over thermoregulation. In this state, tissue temperatures rapidly rise. Maximal heart rate is now attained at significantly lower exercise intensities. When this occurs, increments in exercise intensity cannot be supported through increased oxygen supply, and the cessation of exercise is imminent.

4.2 Sudomotor control

Water is continually lost through the skin, even when no apparent sweat secretion is evident. Such transpiration occurs at a rate of approximately $0.3 \ mL \cdot kg^{-1} \cdot h^{-1}$, accounting for ~20% of the daily water loss in a resting person, and shown as a non-zero baseline flow in Figure 18.4. This is not a thermal secretion.

Thermoregulatory sweating occurs when mean body temperature exceeds the sweating (sudomotor) threshold, usually 0.2–0.5°C above its thermoneutral state (Chapter 18). It is controlled by the hypothalamus and displays an initial proportional (positive) relationship with changes in mean body temperature. However, over its full secretory range, the sweating response is best described as curvilinear, rising asymptotically towards peak secretion. The upper limit of the (sudomotor) thermoregulatory zone is bordered by this secretion peak (see Figure 18.4), a point marking the boundary above which man loses the physiological capacity to dissipate more heat. In this section, we will describe events that occur between the sudomotor threshold and peak sweating. These points are dictated by hypothalamic control and the functional sudomotor capacity and, along with sudomotor sensitivity ($mg \cdot cm^{-2} \cdot min^{-1} \cdot °C^{-1}$), are subject to modification through various physiological and pathophysiological changes, including morphological and functional adaptations (Chapter 21).

Blood-borne heat is convected from the core to the shell. The evaporation of sweat provides an extremely effective means for cooling the skin, permitting the blood to unload some of its thermal energy, prior to returning to the deep tissues. This increases peripheral tissue temperatures, with further elevations accompanying vasodilatation, enhancing evaporation by increasing water vapour pressure at the skin surface (E_{max}), independently of sudomotor function. However, not all sweat secretion is advantageous. For instance, sweating is energetically wasteful, it may result in a potentially excessive water loss, and it will occur even in conditions where evaporation is impossible. In a Turkish bath, for example, the relative humidity approaches 100% and evaporative cooling may be impossible (E_{max}). Indeed, when one first enters the bath, the cool skin results in condensation of water droplets on the skin surface and thermal energy is exchanged from these water molecules to the skin. This extreme example serves to highlight the point that, unless the water vapour pressure gradient favours evaporation, then sweating will not cool the skin. Whenever clothing is worn, and in particular vapour barrier-protective ensembles, or the relative humidity of the surrounding air increases, the skin–air water vapour pressure gradient is reduced, compromising evaporation.

The capacity of this thermoeffector mechanism is determined by the number of active glands and the ability to optimally activate these glands (sustainable sweat rate). Humans possess two types of sweat glands, the secretions of which target the skin surface (exocrine glands). The apocrine sweat glands are generally larger glands clustered around the axilla, auditory canal, eyelid, areola, genital and circumanal regions, and secrete into hair follicles. In many such glands, a thicker secretion is produced, containing part of the cellular cytoplasm. Thus, a recovery period must occur before further secretion is possible. From a thermal perspective, it is the eccrine sweat glands that are the principal functional units. These glands are merocrine in nature,

Table 19.3 Regional sweat gland counts ($glands \cdot cm^{-2}$) obtained from African, European and Korean males. Thompson (1954) counted glands in exercise-heat stressed subjects, while Szabo (1962) and Hwang & Baik (1997) used cadaveric tissue samples. The former technique generally fails to activate 5–10% of sweat glands

Region	Thompson (1954)		Szabo (1962)	Hwang & Baik (1997)
	African	European	European	Korean
Forehead	254	215	360	–
Chest	86	81	175	86
Back	94	88	160	96
Arm	119	111	150	98
Forearm	109	114	225	86
Thigh	84	86	120	118
Leg	78	87	150	104
Dorsal foot	175	194	250	144

in that their secretory product (sweat) does not contain cellular material, permitting continuous secretion, directly onto the skin surface.

Humans have 2–5 million eccrine sweat glands, scattered over the body surface, with a mean glandular density of 120–200 $glands \cdot cm^{-2}$ and with regional densities being inversely related to local surface areas (Szabo 1962, Thompson 1954). While not verified through longitudinal investigation, gland counts seem to be fixed at birth or within the first few years, with subsequent differences in regional surface area growth resulting in variations in gland density (Kuno 1956). Thus, glandular distribution is non-uniform (Table 19.3), but there is little substantive evidence for racial differences in eccrine gland counts (Taylor 2006), with perhaps one exception (Hwang & Baik 1997).

In addition to this surface–area relationship, some sites have much greater gland counts, with the highest densities being on the palms and the soles of the feet. Presumably, these anomalies form part of our evolutionary heritage, where sweat secretion was important for increasing friction between the skin and contact surfaces, elevating tactile and thermal sensitivity and reducing the probability of tissue damage. For example, the dorsal foot surface has about 175 $glands \cdot cm^{-2}$ (range 145–250), with the plantar surface having approximately 460 $glands \cdot cm^{-2}$ (range 300–620; Taylor et al. 2006).

The second aspect of the sudomotor capacity is the ability to optimally activate the eccrine sweat glands. Not all glands are active during thermoregulatory sweating; in fact, some 5–10% of these glands always remain inactive (non-functional). Moreover, it appears that short-term heat adaptation does not alter the number of active sweat glands (Inoue et al. 1999). This activation trend accounts for some of the regional differences presented in Table 19.3.

Eccrine sweat glands consist of a coiled secretory portion, 2–5 mm in length and 60–80 μm in diameter, a reabsorptive duct of approximately the same length but slightly smaller in diameter, and a skin pore. Three cell types are found in the epithelium of the secretory coil: clear (secretory) cells; myoepithelial cells (possibly specialised smooth muscle cells), wound in longitudinal spirals around the tubule, that expel sweat when stimulated; and dark cells of an unknown function. Primary sweat is produced within the secretory coils. This is an ultrafiltrate of plasma, coming directly from the interstitial space, with various solutes (sodium, chloride, potassium, bicarbonate) diffusing directly into the secretory duct. The reabsorptive ducts contain basal lamina cells with a high mitochondrial density, facilitating active ion transport across the duct wall and back to the interstitial space. This is principally an anaerobic process, resulting in sweat having a lactate concentration of approximately 9.2 mmol·L^{-1} and a pH of about 5.6 (Patterson et al. 2000).

Much like selective reabsorption within renal nephrons, ions are actively reabsorbed in the downstream portion of the sweat duct. Sodium, chloride and bicarbonate ions are the primary reabsorbed solutes. The sodium concentration in the reabsorptive duct cells is kept low by the continuous action of sodium-potassium pumps within the cell membranes. These pumps exchange interstitial potassium for sodium, which is redistributed throughout the body via the extracellular (interstitial and plasma) fluid. The resulting intracellular electronegativity of these ductal cells allows sodium ions to passively enter from the sweat gland lumen, with chloride ions following passively. This process can be modulated hormonally, primarily by aldosterone, displaying an inverse and gender-independent relationship with sweat rate (Buono et al. 2007, van den Heuvel et al. 2007). Water is reabsorbed as a passive (obligatory) consequence of ion reabsorption, though electrolyte reabsorption is proportionately greater, resulting in an odourless, colourless and relatively dilute (hypotonic) secretion. When analysed across different skin surfaces, sweat electrolyte concentrations average: sodium 36.3 mmol·L^{-1}, chloride 31.3 mmol·L^{-1}, potassium 4.8 mmol·L^{-1} and bicarbonate 1.3 mmol·L^{-1} (Patterson et al. 2000).

Like vasomotor signals, the sympathetic impulses that activate eccrine sweat glands originate in the hypothalamus and descend through the brain stem, from whence they join peripheral mixed nerves, before reaching the sweat glands. These fibres are sympathetic, postganglionic and unmyelinated C-fibres, with acetylcholine the primary neurotransmitter. However, their innervation was originally adrenergic but these fibres gradually transformed into cholinergic neurons. This metamorphosis occurs within the early postnatal developmental stage, at least in mice (Guidry & Landis 1998), and is believed to also occur in man. Identification of the chemical agent(s) that drives this transformation has not yet been achieved. However, the process is believed to involve two steps, activated when the

neuron first comes into close proximity with its target gland. This triggers adrenergic sweat gland stimulation, followed by a retrograde neuronal response to agent(s) produced by the sweat glands. This second, target-derived signal causes a previously adrenergic neuron to become cholinergic. It then retains that phenotype, but this may perhaps explain why eccrine sweat glands also respond to adrenergic transmitters. This metamorphosis may also help explain the descriptions of Kuno (1956), who believed that active eccrine gland counts were determined within the first few years of life.

Thermoefferent signals reach the sweat glands in waves, resulting in pulsatile sweat secretion, synchronised across regions, and generally ranging between 5 and 30 sweat expulsions per minute. The volume of sweat produced is dependent upon gland size, with up to fivefold variations observed among people, and upon physiological and environmental influences. Regional variations in sweat rate depend on both gland recruitment (functional gland density) and glandular flow, with daily, whole-body sweat losses for people working or exercising under hot conditions approaching 10–15 L. Such secretion rates have significant logistical implications for those planning such activities away from a ready water source.

In Chapter 21, the impact of heat adaptation on sudomotor function is described. These morphological and functional effects combine to dictate maximal glandular flow, which varies from 2 to >20 nL·min^{-1}. During a moderate exercise-heat stress, whole-body sweat rates typically range between 1 and 1.5 L·h^{-1}, with these rates doubling following heat adaptation and long-term endurance training. Indeed, the highest reported sweat rate (3.7 L·h^{-1}) was observed for a heat-adapted marathoner (Armstrong et al. 1986).

The high latent heat of vaporisation (2.43 kJ·mL^{-1}) makes the evaporation of sweat ideally suited for cooling the skin. If one assumes complete evaporation, then a sweat rate of 1 L·h^{-1} could potentially dissipate 2430 kJ of thermal energy over 60 min (2.43 kJ·mL^{-1} * 1000 mL: 580 kcal). Let us again consider our 70 kg, clothed person, exercising at 200 W (25°C, 50% relative humidity). Recall that the required evaporative cooling (E_{req}) was 330 W (1188 kJ·h^{-1}; 285 kcal·h^{-1}). Over 60 min, 1188 kJ of heat needed to be dissipated via evaporative cooling. This is physiologically attainable, requiring the complete evaporation of only 490 mL of sweat over that time. However, these clothing and environmental conditions limit evaporative cooling (E_{max}) to 150 W (540 kJ·h^{-1}; 130 kcal·h^{-1}). This is a key concept to appreciate: evaporation is not determined by sweat rate but the maximal evaporative cooling permitted by the environment and clothing. In this example, while the required sweat rate was 490 mL·h^{-1}, conditions dictated that evaporation would only occur at the rate 225 mL·h^{-1}. Thus, sweat rates in excess of that represent wasteful fluid losses that may subsequently challenge body fluid regulation. As we shall see in Chapter 21, much of the additional sweat secretion that accompanies heat and endurance adaptation is extravagant. While this additional secretion may have a negligible affect upon evaporation and heat loss, it can have a significant impact upon plasma volume and osmolality, the topic of our next subsection.

Before leaving this topic, we shall briefly describe the suppression of sweat output accompanying an elevated skin wettedness: hidromeiosis. This occurs in very humid environments, following extended-duration sweating, or on skin surfaces constantly covered by wet clothing. The most widely accepted theory to explain this phenomenon is mechanically based, and attributed to a pore blockage following the absorption of water into the stratum corneum or the reabsorption of water by deeper skin layers. Both could lead to an accumulation of fluid within the tissues, inducing swelling and blockage of the sweat duct. It has also been hypothesised that sweat gland fatigue leads to a progressive reduction in sweat secretion. Both theories have been contested within the literature and the precise mechanism remains elusive. Nevertheless, hidromeiosis can be considered to serve as a protective mechanism against progressive dehydration, since sweat secretion at a rate that exceeds evaporating fails to cool the skin.

5 BODY FLUID REGULATION

The fluid replacement requirement for a sedentary person is about $1.6 mL \cdot kg^{-1} \cdot h^{-1}$ or $110 mL \cdot h^{-1}$ for our 70 kg person. Approximately 5% of water loss is faecal, ~55% appears in the urine, and equal proportions come from respiratory and cutaneus transpiration losses ($0.3 mL \cdot kg^{-1} \cdot h^{-1}$ each). The combined effects of heat and exercise modify both the respiratory and sweat losses. In the former instance, this increases approximately linearly with the elevation in minute ventilation. In the case of thermal sweating, even a modest fluid loss ($1 L \cdot h^{-1}$ or $12–15 mL \cdot kg^{-1} \cdot h^{-1}$) will dramatically affect the relative magnitudes of these fluid losses. For example, even without the powerful exercise heat-induced suppression of glomerular filtration rate, the contribution of the urinary flow would decrease to ~5%, with transcutaneous water losses increasing from 20% to 90% of the total body fluid reduction. This can significantly challenge body fluid homeostasis and cardiovascular stability, particularly during prolonged exercise, when dehydration may become a critical determinant of performance (Chapter 33).

Humans are about 60% water, having a total body water content of $500–600 mL \cdot kg^{-1}$ (female–male), distributed across both intracellular and extracellular compartments ($300–340 mL \cdot kg^{-1}$ and $200–260 mL \cdot kg^{-1}$, respectively). Much of the intersubject variability (range: 45–80%) is due to differences in adiposity, with considerable variability also evident among tissues. For example, renal tissues contain the most (~85%) and adipose tissue the least water (~10%). The membranes that separate these fluid compartments are selectively permeable and contain mechanisms ensuring a predominant, unidirectional flow of ions. Thus, trans-membrane ion concentrations are not identical. In the extracellular space, the predominant cation is sodium, while chloride and bicarbonate ions dominate the anion composition, therefore determining the composition of primary sweat.

During a resting heat exposure, humans experience a blood volume expansion (Harrison 1985, Maw et al. 2000). However, when exercise is initiated, there is a rapid (within 10 min) 5–10% shift of fluid from the plasma to the interstitial space of the active muscles (Maw et al. 1998). This exercise-induced phenomenon occurs independently of ambient temperature, it is proportional to exercise intensity and it results from a rapid and generalised cutaneous venodilatation. Venodilatation affects the Starling forces acting across all vascular membranes, particularly capillary hydrostatic pressure and also the capillary surface area, resulting in haemoconcentration. This fluid is not lost but it transiently leaves the vascular space, returning within about 30 min during continued exercise under cool-temperate conditions. However, during an exercise-heat exposure, this plasma fluid displacement is both larger, being associated also with sweating, and more protracted, returning only when exercise ceases. It appears that such body fluid losses are drawn primarily from the extracellular reserves, with intracellular fluid remaining relatively stable (Maw et al. 1998).

The plasma volume represents <10% of total body water or $40 mL \cdot kg^{-1}$ in either gender. Therefore, its contribution to evaporative heat loss (sweating) is relatively small. Nevertheless, since fluid moves easily between the vascular and the interstitial spaces and since proportionately more water is lost, sweating invariably increases plasma tonicity. The ensuing exercise- and heat-induced increase in plasma oncotic (protein) pressure minimises further plasma losses. However, plasma hyperosmolality (hypertonicity) dehydrates the hypothalamic osmoreceptors, and the plasma volume reduction, in combination with other vascular changes, may now activate the low-pressure baroreceptors. Since it is the volume and osmolality of the plasma that are regulated, then signals from both the osmoreceptors and baroreceptors now result in a centrally mediated defence of the circulating blood volume. The osmoreceptor pathway is more sensitive and is activated earlier, while baroreceptor-driven regulation exerts a more powerful influence.

Volume-defence mechanisms involve both neural and humoral factors. Prior to the commencement of, and just after commencing exercise, there is a sustained and generalised increase in sympathetic nervous system outflow (feedforward or central command). This activity affects many functions. At the kidney, it reduces renal blood flow and glomerular filtration rate. These changes are dependent upon hydration state and exercise intensity, but defend plasma volume by decreasing urine production. During the course of extended exercise in the heat, negative feedback from the osmoreceptors stimulates thirst and antidiuretic hormone (arginine vasopressin) secretion. The latter, along with negative feedback from low-pressure baroreceptors, increases the permeability of the distal and collecting tubules of the kidney to water. In addition, a plasma volume reduction stimulates cells located near the glomeruli to secrete renin, leading eventually to increased thirst and aldosterone secretion. This hormone increases sodium and (indirectly) water reabsorption in the distal and collecting tubules. When exercise is performed in a hypohydrated state, these changes are magnified to preserve the existing plasma volume.

6 AGE AND GENDER DIFFERENCES

Experimental evidence has shown that the elderly often have diminished autonomic function (Collins et al. 1980; Chapter 16), a reduced skin blood flow responsiveness to thermal stress (Collins et al. 1985, Richardson & Shepherd 1991), a generally lower sweating reaction (Kenney & Fowler 1988) and less stable body temperature regulation (Marion et al. 1991). Furthermore, it is not uncommon for the elderly to be taking a variety of prescription drugs that may interact with both thermoreceptor sensitivity and effector function. Collectively, such functional changes can result in a diminished ability to generate, conserve and dissipate thermal energy, and may predispose this group to thermoregulatory insufficiency when placed under thermal strain.

However, there is contradictory evidence in the literature about whether older individuals are less heat tolerant, experiencing more rapid elevations in core temperature than younger subjects, particularly during exercise. Much of the older literature has reported greater physiological strain in exercising older men and women. This observation is valid for the general population of older men and women, whose lower average maximal aerobic power (oxygen uptake; Chapters 16 and 17.2) predetermines that a given absolute exercise intensity (W) will correspond to a greater relative workload. However, when older and younger subjects are matched for maximal oxygen uptake, with both exercising at the same absolute and relative intensities, there are seldom differences in either core temperature or heat storage (Kenney & Anderson 1988, Kenney & Ho 1995, Kenney et al. 1990).

Havenith et al. (1994) tested a large number of subjects (20–73 years) in a standard heat challenge (35°C), then used multiple regression analyses to evaluate the relative influence of individual characteristics on thermoregulatory responses, including age and maximal aerobic power. After 1 h of low-intensity (60 W), steady-state exercise, core temperature and heat storage were both significantly correlated with aerobic power. After inclusion of the aerobic power effect into prediction models, age had no significant influence, implying that once natural variation in physical fitness was considered, the effect of chronological age per se appeared to be negligible.

Do older men and women sweat less when exposed to exercise and heat stress? While there is a large variability in sweat gland responses to stimulation by either heat or pharmacological agents, some clear effects of ageing are evident. Local sweating rates are lower in older subjects for a given pharmacological stimulus, an effect that can be attributed to a smaller sweat output per activated gland (Kenney & Fowler 1988), though the density of activated glands appears to be unaffected by age. This decline probably relates to a combination of structural and functional alterations that accompany the ageing process and long-term exposure to ultraviolet radiation and other environmental factors.

However, this age-related deficit in sweat gland flow does not necessarily translate into lower sweat rates or evaporative heat loss during exercise in the heat. Sweat rates not only depend upon genetic and physiological factors but are strongly influenced by thermal adaptation, physical fitness, hydration state and various prescription drugs, resulting in quite large interindividual variability. While peak sweat rates are usually lower in older men and women, it is still possible for heat-adapted or endurance-trained individuals to produce adequate sweat secretion, even during quite strenuous exercise. Indeed, within more humid conditions, where evaporation is limited, a lower peak sweat rate may not adversely affect evaporative cooling.

One response characteristic that does appear to be universally altered by ageing is the skin blood flow response to heat stress. The maximal ability of the skin blood vessels to dilate declines progressively from childhood through to old age (Martin & Kenney 1995). When blood flow responses of older fit and healthy men and women (60–85 years) were compared with a sample of 20–30-year-old subjects with similar physical and physiological characteristics, the older individuals responded to exercise with a lower skin blood flow at a given core temperature (Kenney 1988, Kenney et al. 1990, 1991). Above the vasodilatory threshold temperature, the sensitivity of the cutaneous blood flow response of older men and women was greatly attenuated. Thus, on average, cutaneous blood flow for exercising older subjects is 25–50% lower than for younger people, matched for maximal aerobic power.

Finally, there is evidence indicative of localised reductions in sweating and skin blood flow with ageing. Inoue et al. (2002) observed an age-related decrement in heat loss (effector) functions, such that a successive decrement in cutaneous vasodilatation, sweat output per gland and the density of active sweat glands may occur, commencing at the lower limbs and proceeding to the back, chest, torso and finally to the head.

During heat exposures, while gender differences do appear to influence physiological responses, particularly during the luteal phase of the menstrual cycle, the majority of experimental evidence demonstrates that heat tolerance is more closely related to cardiovascular function and hydration state than it is to gender. However, differences in morphological configuration and the sweat response mean that women are better suited to vasomotor thermal adjustments, being more reliant upon convective and conductive rather than upon evaporative cooling. The typically higher skin temperature of the woman reduces dry heat transfer from a hotter environment to the skin whilst simultaneously increasing cutaneous water vapour pressure and enhancing evaporative cooling.

Women almost universally display a lower sweating response to equivalent thermal loads, during both resting and exercising heat exposures. Whilst some of this difference may be explained on the basis of morphological variations, women show a lower sweat threshold for the initiation of sweating when stimulated via the intradermal injection of acetylcholine (Janowitz & Grossman 1950), and a lower sweat gland recruitment than males following the injection of equal concentrations of acetylcholine.

Women also appear better able to adjust sweat secretion to increments in skin wettedness and so display greater sweating efficiency. The combination of these factors results in the tendency for women to be better able to tolerate hot-humid conditions than men. However, both genders adapt equally well to the heat and women with equivalent endurance and heat acclimation histories appear to tolerate the combined effects of exercise and heat at least as well as men.

7 NON-THERMAL FACTORS

Thus far, we have focused on the well-known changes in sweating and skin blood flow, controlled by the hypothalamus to regulate mean body temperature (thermal factors). However, these thermoeffectors, their activation thresholds and their sensitivities can be modified by non-thermal factors (see Figure 18.4 and Chapter 18; Mekjavic & Eiken 2006). For instance, various pharmacological agents, febrile states, changes in plasma tonicity and glucose concentration, and altered hydration state can modify the size of the interthreshold zone and thermoeffector sensitivity. In addition, there are several exercise-dependent, non-thermal factors that influence sweating and skin blood flow, including feedforward (central command) and feedback from mechanoreceptors and metaboreceptors from exercising muscles, and from baroreceptors, osmoreceptors and mental stress (Kondo et al. 1999). Moreover, it has been found that exercise modifies the threshold for skin vasodilatation and induces changes in the sensitivity of the sudomotor and vasodilatory responses (Kellogg et al. 1991, Kondo et al. 1998, Taylor et al. 1988). In this subsection, we focus on the contribution of these non-thermal factors during exercise, finishing with an integrated overview of these interactions.

7.1 Central feedforward

The central motor command (feedforward) signal emanates from the rostral brain and radiates to autonomic circuits in the brain stem, causing parallel activation of motor and sympathetic neurons (Chapters 1 and 18). Evidence for this is found in the instantaneous elevation in heart rate at the onset of volitional exercise. In heated humans, the commencement of exercise is invariably associated with a reduction in skin blood flow and frequently with increased sweating (Christensen & Nielsen 1942, Van Beaumont & Bullard 1963). These non-thermal effects are intensity dependent, resulting from feedforward modulation of thermoeffector function. Indeed, when partial neuromuscular blockade is used to reduce force generation, the resultant increase in effort necessary to sustain a target force results in greater sympathetic outflow to the skin. Effort sense, an index of central command, also increases during such an experimental manipulation, with that change occurring in proportion to the increase in sweat secretion. Thus, central command is a major mechanism stimulating sympathetic outflow to the sweat glands (Shibasaki et al. 2003).

7.2 Feedback

Sweating can also be influenced by afferents arising from within the exercising muscles: mechanoreceptors (Chapters 1, 2 and 18). Such feedback is initiated within a few seconds of an elevation in muscle tension. In sweating humans, secretion similarly increases and without a change in body temperature, but such feedback appears not to affect skin blood flow. These changes are evident even during passive limb movement, indicating that mechanoreceptor feedback is significant, although its overall sudomotor impact is relatively small (Kondo et al. 1997).

In addition to mechanoreceptors, muscles also contain metabosensitive elements (Chapters 1 and 2). Postexercise ischaemia has been used to elevate intramuscular metabolite concentrations, resulting in greater sweat secretion. Since metaboreceptor afferents are not activated during ischaemia, with muscle relaxation eliminating both feedforward and feedback, then sweating is modulated by intramuscular metaboreceptor activity (Kondo et al. 1999). In contrast, metaboreceptor activation appears to inhibit active vasodilatation (Crandall et al. 1998). The bulk of this research was focused upon isometric exercise. However, recent work by Eiken & Mekjavic (2004) and Kacin et al. (2005) has supported these observations during dynamic exercise.

7.3 Other non-thermal factors

We have described above the sweating and skin blood flow responses during exercise in the heat, and the modulation of cardiovascular and hormonal functions via negative feedback from the baroreceptors and osmoreceptors. This interaction also affects sweating and skin blood flow. For

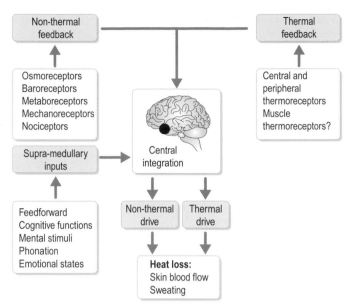

Figure 19.4 An overview of the thermal and non-thermal factors affecting heat loss responses during exercise. Details of the thermoregulatory mechanisms involved in heat loss are described in detail in Chapter 18.

example, unloading the cardiopulmonary baroreceptors and increasing plasma osmolality reduces both the sudomotor and skin blood flow responses. It appears that a plasma volume decrease will reduce the sensitivity of both thermoeffectors, while an increase in plasma osmolality alters the sudomotor and vasodilatory thresholds (Takamata et al. 1998).

7.4 Interaction of thermal and non–thermal factors

The thermal and non-thermal interactions for the control of sweating and skin blood flow are illustrated in Figure 19.4. During dynamic exercise, sweating and skin blood flow are modulated through an integration of these non-thermal factors and the interaction of thermal and non-thermal factors. The latter can affect skin blood flow under thermo-neutral conditions. However, the non-thermal effects on sudomotor function only become evident after sweating has been initiated. Thus, these non-thermal factors appear to dominate during low-level, steady-state thermal loading, whilst thermal factors primarily control heat loss when mean body temperature displacement is sufficiently large (Kondo et al. 2002).

8 PATHOPHYSIOLOGICAL CONSIDERATIONS

As a general clinical guideline, core temperature variations greater than 2°C either side of 37°C are associated with either thermoregulatory failure or a regulatory system overload (Tables 19.1 and 20.1). However, core temperatures >39°C are routinely encountered during endurance

exercise, even under temperate conditions (Pugh et al. 1967), due to very high metabolic heat productions. Indeed, such temperature elevations are a perfectly normal regulatory responses (Chapter 18), much like an elevated heart rate, and are well tolerated in most healthy individuals. Nevertheless, excessive core temperature increases can result in heat illnesses which form a continuum of pathophysiological disorders ranging from mild and transient hypotension through to heatstroke, which may be accompanied by cellular damage and even death. Skin temperatures generally increase with an elevation in core temperature, but high skin temperatures can also occur in the absence of a change in core temperature, due to brief exposures to hot objects and high radiant heat sources. Local temperatures >45°C are accompanied by tissue damage and skin burns (Table 19.1; Moritz & Henriques 1947).

Heat illnesses are classified according to the predominant heat source. For instance, exertional heat illness results from an excessive or overwhelming metabolic heat production, and is the most common cause of hyperthermia in healthy adults. Classical (non-exertional) heat illness results from climatic extremes that often challenge individuals with impaired thermoregulation or compromised cardiovascular function. This is most evident at both age extremes, in the infirmed and in those taking medication that may impair sweating (e.g. antihypertensives, antidepressants, antihistimines, anticholinergics; Cheshire & Fealey 2008). In various emergency services and military trades, exertional heat illness is not uncommon, but can occur in individuals working at moderate metabolic rates whilst wearing thermal and other forms of protective clothing. Thus, this metabolic heat, which would normally escape, is trapped, leading to hyperthermia.

8.1 Heat cramps

Skeletal muscle cramps occur in those who have been sweating profusely, and are often present before heat acclimatisation has been satisfactorily achieved. Thus, limb and abdominal cramping may accompany strenuous physical activity in the heat. While the aetiology of is unresolved, many believe that a sodium deficit is involved. These cramps occur in ~1% of workers, and have been classified clinically on an occupational rather than a mechanistic basis: cane-cutter's cramp, fireman's cramp, miner's cramp and stoker's cramp.

8.2 Heat exhaustion

The most common form of heat illness is heat exhaustion, which is another form of fatigue, but is associated with the additional physiological strain accompanying protracted work in the heat. It is frequently seen among the elderly, but will occur in all who drive themselves to the point of physiological failure. The affected person is unable to continue working or exercising at the same intensity, and must either cease work (totally or temporarily) or dramatically reduce the work intensity. Heat exhaustion may develop over several days in those working hard, but not excessively. In most cases, fatigue is due to an inadequate cardiovascular response to the combined metabolic and thermal loads, resulting in impaired blood pressure regulation. That is, the initial increased skin blood flow to dissipate heat is not compensated by a simultaneous increase in blood volume, an adequate vasoconstriction in other vascular beds or a sufficiently large cardiac output response. These factors are exacerbated by progressive dehydration.

Heat exhausted individuals still sweat profusely, and will generally have normal mental function, albeit slightly degraded. The symptoms of heat exhaustion include: a sense of depression or gloom (pallor), headache, vomiting, postural syncope, urge to defaecate, giddiness and loss of coordination, fatigue, hyperventilation, tachycardia and profuse sweating.

8.3 Heatstroke

An excessive core temperature elevation (hyperpyrexia) is due to either a relative or absolute thermoregulatory failure. That is, effective temperature regulation has been compromised, and such an individual enters an uncompensable state (Figure 18.4, zone 3) where the core temperature will continue to rise unless external assistance is provided. This form of heat illness must be treated as a medical emergency, for which rapid whole-body cooling is absolutely essential, since the time that an individual remains within this hyperpyrexic state directly influences the prognosis.

Heatstroke is diagnosed when a core temperature of 40.5°C or greater is observed in the presence of cognitive function impairment and an absence of sweating (anhidrosis). This qualification is essential since high core tempera-tures in workers and athletes are not uncommon. Indeed, some consider anhidrosis to be the single most important diagnostic factor, since it signifies central thermoregulatory failure, possibly due to impaired hypothalamic function. In addition, patients will present with an increased respiratory rate and depth (hyperpnoea), varying degrees of consciousness (lethargy, stupor, coma), convulsions may occur and there may be an elevation in blood urea nitrogen concentration (e.g. 20–40 mg·100 mL^{-1} is common). The pathophysiology of heatstroke is covered in detail elsewhere (e.g. Hales 1996), but it is frequently accompanied by the denaturation of proteins, blood coagulation, skin haemorrhages, a decreased ability to form and pass urine, gastrointestinal bleeding (severe cases), the possibility of extensive muscle damage (rhabdomyolysis), muscle and neural necroses, myoglobin in the urine and inflammation of the myocardium.

8.4 Individual variations

There is considerable variation among individuals in their susceptibility to heat illness and their tolerance of hyperthermia. For instance, while case studies indicate that well-motivated, non-elite distance runners will routinely complete a marathon race with a core temperature >41°C, deaths have been reported in patients with core temperatures <40°C, with gross rhabdomyolysis, organ failure and death being reported in some who have run <10 km in comfortable climatic conditions. Notwithstanding certain clinical states and drug interactions, high risk individuals are those who may be described as being overweight, of poor physical fitness, having impaired cardiovascular function or a concurrent illness, using some prescription drugs, heavy alcohol or drug use, having a previous heat illness, dehydrated, poorly acclimatised, fatigued or of advanced age.

References

Armstrong LE, Hubbard RW, Jones BH, Daniels JT 1986 Preparing Alberto Salazar for the heat of the 1984 Olympic Games. Physician and Sportsmedicine 14:73–81

Balter M 2002 Why get smart? Science 295:1225

Belding HS, Hatch TF 1955 Index for evaluating heat stress in terms of resulting physiological strain. Heating, Piping and Air Conditioning 27:129–136

Bligh J 1973 Temperature regulation in mammals and other vertebrates. North-Holland Publishing Company, Amsterdam

Boulant JA 1981 Hypothalamic mechanisms in thermoregulation. Federation Proceedings 40:2843–2850

Boulant JA 1996 Hypothalamic neurons regulating body temperature. In: Fregly MJ, Blatteis CM (eds) Environmental physiology. Handbook of physiology, volume 1. Oxford University Press, New York, 105–126

Brown AC, Brenglemann GL 1970 The interaction of peripheral and central inputs in the temperature regulation system. In: Hardy JD, Gagge AP, Stolwijk JAJ (eds) Physiological and behavioral temperature regulation. C.C. Thomas, Springfield, IL, 684–702

Buono MJ, Ball KD, Kolkhorst FW 2007 Sodium ion concentration vs. sweat rate relationship in humans. Journal of Applied Physiology 103:990–994

Burton AC 1935 Human calorimetry. II. The average temperature of the tissues of the body. Journal of Nutrition 9:261–280

Burton AC, Edholm OG 1955 Man in a cold environment: physiological and pathological effects of exposure to low temperatures. Edward Arnold, London

Cheshire WP, Fealey RD 2008 Drug-induced hyperhidrosis. Incidence, prevention and management. Drug Safety 31:109–126

Christensen EH, Nielsen M 1942 Investigation of the circulation in the skin at the beginning of muscular work. Acta Physiologica Scandinavica 4:162–170

Collins KJ, Exton-Smith AN, James, MH, Oliver DJ 1980 Functional changes in autonomic nervous responses with ageing. Age and Ageing 9:17–24

Collins KJ, Easton JC, Belfield-Smith H, Exton-Smith AN, Pluck RA 1985 Effects of age on body temperature and blood pressure in cold environments. Clinical Science 69:465–470

Cotter JD, Taylor NAS 2005 Distribution of cutaneous sudomotor and alliesthesial thermosensitivity in mildly heat-stressed humans: an open-loop approach. Journal of Physiology (London) 565(1):335–345

Crandall CG, Stephens DP, Johnson JM 1998 Muscle metaboreceptor modulation of cutaneous active vasodilation. Medicine and Science in Sports and Exercise 30:490–496

Darian-Smith I, Johnson KO, LaMotte C, Shigenaga Y, Kennis P, Champness P 1979 Warm fibres innervating palmar and digital skin of the monkey: response to thermal stimuli. Journal of Neurophysiology 42:1297–1315

Eichna LW, Berger AR, Rader B, Becker WH 1951 Comparison of intracardiac and intravascular temperatures with rectal temperatures in man. Journal of Clinical Investigation 30:353–359

Eiken O, Mekjavic IB 2004 Ischaemia in working muscle potentiates the exercise-induced sweating response in man. Acta Physiologica Scandinavica 181:305–311

Gagge AP, Gonzales RR 1996 Mechanisms of heat exchange: biophysics and physiology. In: Fregly MJ, Blatteis CM (eds) Environmental physiology. Handbook of physiology, volume 1. Oxford University Press, New York, 45–84

Gilbert M, Busund R, Skagseth A, Nilsen PA, Solbø JP 2000 Resuscitation from accidental hypothermia of 13.7°C with circulatory arrest. Lancet 355:375–376

Goldman RF 2001 Introduction to heat-related problems in military operations. In: Pandolf KB, Burr RE, Wenger CB, Pozos RS (eds) Medical aspects of harsh environments. Volume 1. Department of the Army, Office of the Surgeon General and Borden Institute, Washington, DC, 3–49

Gowlett JAJ 2001 Out in the cold. Nature 413:33–34

Guidry G, Landis SC 1998 Developmental regulation of neurotransmitter in sympathetic neurons. Advances in Pharmacology 42:895–898

Hales JRS 1996 Limitations to heat tolerance. In: Fregly MJ, Blatteis CM (eds) Environmental physiology. Handbook of Physiology, volume 1. Oxford University Press, New York, 285–355

Hales JRS, Hutchinson JCD 1971 Metabolic, respiratory and vasomotor responses to heating the scrotum of the ram. Journal of Physiology (London) 212:353–375

Harrison MH 1985 Effects of thermal stress and exercise on blood volume in humans. Physiological Reviews 65:149–209

Havenith G, Inoue Y, Luttikholt V, Kenney WL 1994 Age predicts cardiovascular but not thermoregulatory, responses to humid heat stress. European Journal of Applied Physiology 70:88–96

Hensel H 1952 Physiologie der thermoreception. Ergebnisse der Physiologie 47:166–368

Hwang K, Baik SH 1997 Distribution of hairs and sweat glands on the bodies of Korean adults: a morphometric study. Acta Anatomica 158:112–120

Inoue Y, Havenith G, Kenney WL, Loomis JL, Buskirk ER 1999 Exercise- and methylcholine-induced sweating responses in older and younger men: effect of heat acclimation and aerobic fitness. International Journal of Biometeorology 42:210–216

Inoue Y, Shibasaki M, Araki T 2002 Strategy for preventing heat illness in children and in the elderly. In: Nose H, Spriet LL, Imaizumi K, Copper PG (eds) Exercise, nutrition and environmental stress, vol 2. GSSI Sports Science Network Forum 2000

IUPS Thermal Commission: Commission for Thermal Physiology of the International Union of Physiological Sciences 2001 Glossary of terms for thermal physiology. Japanese Journal of Physiology 51(2):245–280

Janowitz HD, Grossman MI 1950 The response of the sweat glands to some locally acting agents in human subjects. Journal of Investigative Dermatology 14:453–458

Jessen C 1996 Interaction of body temperatures in control of thermoregulatory effector mechanisms. In: Fregly MJ, Blatteis CM (eds) Environmental physiology. Handbook of physiology, volume 1. Oxford University Press, New York, 127–138

Kacin A, Golja P, Eiken O, Tipton MJ, Gorjanc J, Mekjavic IB 2005 Human temperature regulation during cycling with moderate leg ischaemia. European Journal of Applied Physiology 95:213–220

Kanosue K, Hosonso T, Zhang Y-H, Chen XM 1998 Neuronal networks controlling thermoregulatory effectors. In: Sharma HS, Westman J (eds) Progress in brain research, vol 115. Elsevier, Amsterdam, 50 62

Kellogg DL 2006 In vivo mechanisms of cutaneous vasodilation and vasoconstriction in humans during thermoregulatory challenges. Journal of Applied Physiology 100:1709–1718

Kellogg DL, Johnson JM, Kosiba WA 1991 Control of internal temperature threshold for active cutaneous vasodilation by dynamic exercise. Journal of Applied Physiology 71:2476–2483

Kenney WL 1988 Control of heat-induced vasodilation in relation to age. European Journal of Applied Physiology 57:120–125

Kenney WL, Anderson RK 1988 Responses of older and younger women to exercise in dry and humid heat without fluid replacement. Medicine and Science in Sports and Exercise 20:155–160

Kenney WL, Fowler SR 1988 Methylcholine-activated eccrine sweat gland density and output as a function of age. Journal of Applied Physiology 65:1082–1086

Kenney WL, Ho CW 1995 Age alters regional distribution of blood flow during moderate intensity exercise. Journal of Applied Physiology 79:1112–1119

Kenney WL, Johnson JM 1992 Control of skin blood flow during exercise. Medicine and Science in Sports and Exercise 24:303–312

Kenney WL, Tankersley CG, Newswanger DL, Hyde DE, Puhl SM 1990 Age and hypohydration independently influence the peripheral vascular response to heat stress. Journal of Applied Physiology 68:1902–1908

Kenney WL, Tankersley CG, Newswanger DL, Puhl SM 1991 a_1-adrenergic blockade does not alter control of skin blood flow during exercise. American Journal of Physiology 260:H855–H861

Kondo N, Tominaga H, Shiojiri T, Aoki K, Takano S, Shibasaki M, Koga S 1997 Sweating responses to passive and active limb movements. Journal of Thermal Biology 22:351–356

Kondo N, Takano S, Aoki K, Shibasaki M, Tominaga H, Inoue Y 1998 Regional differences in the effect of exercise intensity on thermoregulatory sweating and cutaneous vasodilation. Acta Physiologica Scandinavica 164:71–78

Kondo N, Tominaga H, Shibasaki M, Aoki K, Koga S, Nishiyasu T 1999 Modulation of the thermoregulatory sweating response to mild hyperthermia during activation of the muscle metaboreflex in humans. Journal of Physiology (London) 515:591–598

Kondo N, Horikawa N, Aoki K, Shibasaki M, Inoue Y, Nishiyasu T, Crandall CG 2002 Sweating responses to a sustained static exercise is dependent on thermal load in humans. Acta Physiologica Scandinavica 175:289–295

Kuno Y 1956. Human perspiration. C.C. Thomas, Springfield, IL

Marion GS, McGann KP, Camp DL 1991 Core temperature in the elderly and factors which influence its measurement. Gerontology 37:225–232

Martin HS, Kenney WL 1995 Maximal skin vascular conductance in subjects aged 5 to 85 yr. Journal of Applied Physiology 79:297–301

Maw GJ, Mackenzie IL, Taylor NAS 1998 Body-fluid distribution during exercise in hot and cool environments. Acta Physiologica Scandinavica 163(3):297–304

Maw GJ, Mackenzie IL, Taylor NAS 2000 Can skin temperature manipulation, with minimal core temperature change, influence plasma volume in resting humans? European Journal of Applied Physiology 81:159–162

Mekjavic IB, Eiken O 2006 Contribution of thermal and nonthermal factors to the regulation of body temperature in humans. Journal of Applied Physiology 100:2065–2072

Mitchell D, Wyndham CH, Atkins AR, Vermeulen AJ, Hofmeyr HS, Strydom NB, Hodgson T 1968 Direct measurement of the thermal responses of nude resting men in dry environments. Pflugers Archives 303:324–343

Moritz AR, Henriques FC 1947 Studies of thermal injury II: relative importance of time and surface temperature in the cutaneous burns. American Journal of Pathology 23:695–720

Patterson MJ, Galloway SD, Nimmo MA 2000 Variations in regional sweat composition in normal human males. Experimental Physiology 85:869–875

Pierau F-K 1996 Peripheral thermosensors. In: Fregly MJ, Blatteis CM (eds) Environmental physiology. Handbook of physiology, volume 1. Oxford University Press, New York, 85–104

Pugh LGCE, Corbett JL, Johnson RH 1967 Rectal temperatures, weight losses, and sweat rates in marathon running. Journal of Applied Physiology 23:347–352

Rapp GM 1971 Convection coefficients of man in a forensic area of thermal physiology: heat transfer in underwater exercise. Journal of Physiology (Paris) 63:392–396

Richardson D, Shepherd S 1991 The cutaneous microcirculation of the forearm in young and old subjects. Microvascular Research 41:84–91

Roddie IC 1983 Circulation to skin and adipose tissue. In: Shepherd JT, Abboud FM (eds) The cardiovascular system. Volume III. Peripheral circulation and organ blood flow. Part 1. Handbook of physiology. American Physiological Society. Bethesda, MD, 285–317

Roddie IC 2003 Sympathetic vasodilatation in human skin. Journal of Physiology (London) 548:336–337

Rowell LB 1974 Human cardiovascular adjustments to exercise and thermal stress. Physiological Reviews 54:75:159

Saltin B, Hermansen L 1966 Esophageal, rectal and muscle temperature during exercise. Journal of Applied Physiology 21:1757–1762

Shibasaki M, Kondo N, Crandall CG 2003 Non-thermoregulatory modulation of sweating in humans. Exercise and Sport Science Reviews 31:34–39

Simon E, Schmid HA, Pehl U 1998 Spinal neuronal thermosensitivity in vivo and in vitro in relation to hypothalamic neuronal thermosensitivity. In: Sharma HS, Westman J (eds) Progress in brain research, vol 115. Elsevier, Amsterdam, 25–47

Slovis CM, Anderson GF, Casolaro A 1989 Survival in a heat stroke victim with a core temperature in excess of 46.5°C. Annals of Emergency Medicine 11:269–271

Szabo G 1962 The number of eccrine sweat glands in human skin. Advances in Biology of Skin 3:1–5

Takamata A, Nagashima K, Nose H, Morimoto T 1998 Role of plasma osmolality in the delayed onset of thermal cutaneous vasodilation during exercise in humans. American Journal of Physiology 275: R286–290

Taylor NAS 2006 Ethnic differences in thermoregulation: genotypic versus phenotypic heat adaptation. Journal of Thermal Biology 31:90–104

Taylor WF, Johnson JM, Kosiba WA, Kwan CM 1988 Graded cutaneous vascular responses to dynamic leg exercise. Journal of Applied Physiology 64:1803–1809

Taylor NAS, Caldwell JN, Mekjavic IB 2006 A closer examination of the sweating foot during exercise-induced hyperthermia. Aviation, Space and Environmental Medicine 77:1020–1027

Thompson ML 1954 A comparison between the number and distribution of functioning eccrine glands in Europeans and Africans. Journal of Physiology (London) 123:225–233

Van Beaumont W, Bullard RW 1963 Sweating: its rapid response to muscular work. Science 141:643–646

van den Heuvel AMJ, van den Wijngaart L, Taylor NAS 2007 Absence of a gender affect on the flow-dependent nature of sweat sodium loss. In: Mekjavic IB, Kounalakis SN, Taylor NAS (eds) Environmental ergonomics XII. Biomed d.o.o., Ljubljana, Slovenia, 298–300

Webb P 1995 The physiology of heat regulation. American Journal of Physiology 268:R838–R850

Werner J, Reents T 1980 A contribution to the topography of temperature regulation in man. European Journal of Applied Physiology 45:87–94

Chapter **20**

The physiology of acute cold exposure, with particular reference to human performance in the cold

Nigel A.S. Taylor   Igor B. Mekjavic   Michael J. Tipton

1 INTRODUCTION

Modern man is of African descent (Ray et al. 2005), with northern migrations from the African and Asian continents (Piazza et al. 1981) right up to the Arctic Circle occurring about 40,000 years ago. These warm-climate hominids, who possessed behavioural and thermoregulatory characteristics that enabled survival in the cold, now found themselves in frequently inhospitable climates. Indeed, almost half of the landmass above 40° north latitude is above the freezing line (0°C). In the south, this region is restricted to the Antarctic Continent whilst in the north, the freezing line crosses through the US, Europe (Norway, Denmark, Germany, Italy, Romania, Turkey) and Asia (India, China, Japan; Bates and Bilello 1966).

Air temperatures more than 20°C below skin temperature are very stressful for unprotected humans. However, cold-water immersion at equivalent temperatures can rapidly become life threatening, even for people wearing clothing. This occurs for two reasons. First, water displaces air, which is a very good insulator. Indeed, most of the protective insulation provided by thermal protective clothing is derived from the ability of the clothing to trap and retain a sufficiently large volume of air between the skin surface and the surrounding air. This trapped air is rapidly warmed, thereby providing a thermal buffer and reducing transcutaneous heat loss. Immersion removes this protection. Second, the thermal conductivity of water (37°C) is 24 times greater than that of air (630.5 versus 26.2 mW·m^{-1}·K^{-1}). This means that, for the same thermal gradient, the potential for heat loss is elevated 24-fold during water immersion. In addition, the specific heat capacity of water is four times higher (4.179 versus 1.007 J·g^{-1}·K^{-1}), and its density is 827 times greater than air (0.9922 versus 0.0012 g·cm^{-3}). The product of specific heat capacity and density yields a volume-specific heat capacity, which quantifies the amount of heat required to raise the temperature of a given volume of water by 1 K. For water, this value is 3431 times that of air at 37°C, and increasing by <0.01% at 15°C. Water not just has a greater capacity to accept thermal energy, but this energy transfer will proceed at a much greater rate, thus placing the body under far greater physiological strain.

Our thermal considerations thus far relate to sea-level exposures. However, cold exposures can occur at almost any latitude, since air temperature varies as a function of altitude, and water (sea) temperature declines with depth. Air close to the Earth's surface is heated by reflected solar radiation. Since this effect decreases with altitude, the air temperature change in the troposphere is −1.98°C for each 305 m. Thus, at the top of the troposphere (18,000 m), the air temperature approaches −100°C; beyond the ozone layer, ambient temperature increases as one moves towards the sun. While these data pertain primarily to aviators and altitudes above sea level (standard atmosphere), they also impact upon mountaineers (Chapter 24), with the summit air temperature of Mount Everest (8848 m; 27° north) averaging about −36°C, and that for Mount Kilimanjaro (5895 m), situated close to the equator (3° south), being approximately −10°C. Conversely, with increasing water depth, the solar heating of oceans and lakes is reduced and divers can be exposed to very stressful conditions. For example, while the majority of diving takes place at water temperatures between 8 and 14°C (Bowen 1968), the temperature of northern waters may be 4–6°C (Mekjavic et al. 2001), and as low as −2°C in Arctic waters (Morrison and Zander 2007; Chapter 23). Beyond the surface layer, and regardless of its temperature, deep water temperatures approach 5°C at 1000 m, with a seabed temperature of approximately 3°C.

In addition to decreasing air temperature with altitude, and water temperature with depth, many non-thermal factors associated with the hypo- and hyperbaric environments modulate thermoregulatory responses, further impairing thermal homeostasis. For example, decreasing partial pressure of oxygen with altitude (Golja et al. 2004) and increasing the partial pressure of nitrogen with depth (Mekjavic et al. 1995) will affect the heat loss and heat production effectors, respectively.

Each of these exposure categories challenges thermal homeostasis, with the resultant thermal gradient favouring heat loss. Human body temperatures are normally regulated (Chapter 18) such that the resting core (deep body) temperature is typically between 36.5 and 37°C (97.7–98.6°F). In fact, we can only tolerate core temperatures outside 35–41°C (95–105°F) for very short periods (Table 20.1). Nevertheless, some individuals have survived remarkable core temperature extremes, as a result of either incredible physiological resilience or fortuitous circumstances. The lowest recorded survivable (accidental) core temperature is 13.7°C (56.7°F: Gilbert et al. 2000), with the highest being 46.5°C (115.7°F: Slovis et al. 1989). When skin temperatures drop below 20°C, there is an impairment of manual dexterity, with greater cooling leading to pain (<15°C) and eventually to tissue damage (Table 20.1). In this Chapter, the focus is upon the physiological responses elicited by acute cold-air and cold-water exposures. Chapter 21 describes how chronic

Table 20.1 Clinically significant core and skin temperatures (°C)

Core temperatures	
36.5–37.0	Normothermia
36–33	Mild hypothermia
33–25	Moderate hypothermia
<25	Profound hypothermia
<24	Possible death without rewarming
<22	Profound clinical hypothermia
Skin temperatures	
28–33	Thermal comfort
25–28	Cool through to discomfort (cold)
20	Impaired dexterity
15	Pain
10	Loss of skin sensation
5	Non-freezing cold injury (time dependent)
<0.55	Freezing cold injury (frostbite)

exposures to both cold and hot climates can result in physiological adaptation (acclimatisation).

2 BIOPHYSICS OF HEAT TRANSFER

2.1 Heat balance

This topic has been covered in some detail within Chapters 18 and 19 and readers should consult those Chapters for the necessary background information. However, it is important to briefly elaborate on the biophysics of thermal energy exchanges (thermodynamics) as it relates to coldair and -water exposures. The heat balance equation again provides a basis for this description. The primary emphasis in the cold is dry heat transfer (R, K, C), which is dictated by the thermal gradient between the body and the surrounding air, water or contact surfaces. This gradient dictates heat flow which, in the cold, favours heat loss, and to ensure survival, the body must conserve heat, through either autonomic regulation or behavioural strategies.

Equation 1: $S = M - (\pm W) - E \pm R \pm K \pm C$ [W·m^{-2}]

where:

S = stored thermal energy [W·m^{-2}]
M = metabolic rate or energy transformation [W·m^{-2}]
W = mechanical work [W·m^{-2}]
E, R, K and C = evaporative (condensation results in heat gain), radiative, conductive and convective heat transfer [W·m^{-2}].

During cold-water immersions, where skin temperature approximates water temperature, convective heat losses dominate (Rapp 1971). However, for most resting exposures in still air, radiation generally dominates (Mitchell et al. 1968). For example, in air at 10°C, radiation accounts for ~57% and convection ~42% of heat loss, with negligible evaporative cooling (<1%). Thermal conduction is generally small, though pertinent to many ergonomic applications. This can become particularly important when people are handling very cold objects with bare hands. It can also be relevant during accidental hypothermia, where a collapsed individual may lie on the cold ground for some hours.

The heating of cool air or water close to the body surface creates thermal (convectional) currents, resulting in the bulk movement of molecules away from the skin, with cooler water/air moving into this space. When the cooler medium is moving across the skin or where the body is moving through a stationary medium, forced convectional heat transfer occurs. This is a function of both relative and absolute velocity. In most survival situations, when it is often windy and wet, radiation can become irrelevant, with convectional heat losses dominating.

2.2 The interaction of body composition and morphology

Skin, adipose tissue and vasoconstricted skeletal muscle act as thermal insulators arranged in series, with heat flux being proportional to the reciprocal of their combined thickness. Most heat loss in subjects resting in water at 15°C will occur primarily via the torso (Hayward et al. 1973), with skin and adipose tissue primarily determining tissue insulation in these regions. Adipose tissue is relatively poorly perfused and contains less water than muscle. Accordingly, its thermal conductivity is ~35% that of blood and <50% that of skeletal muscle (Ducharme & Tikuisis 1991), and behaves as a fixed insulator. This insulative nature of subcutaneous adipose tissue has long been known (Pugh & Edholm 1955), and appears critical for cold-tolerant swimmers.

However, less than 50% of the tissue insulation of the limbs can be attributed to skin and adipose tissue, with poorly perfused muscle providing a large proportion of the total insulation. Of particular importance is the regional distribution of adipose tissue in relation to the active muscle mass, which can modify heat loss significantly (Wade et al. 1979). For example, individuals having a greater limb adiposity (most women) should possess a thermal advantage during cold-water exercise, due to greater insulation of active and vasodilated muscle (Tipton et al. 1999). Unfortunately, when exercise commences and muscle blood flow is elevated, much of the limb insulation is lost (Veicsteinas et al. 1982).

Due to the fact that the subcutaneous tissue has a low thermal conductivity and constitutes the outer layer of the body, it is considered to play a dominant role in the amount of heat lost from the body. Specifically, it is generally considered to determine the rate of core temperature cooling during cold exposure. This relation between subcutaneous adipose tissue, as represented by skinfold thickness, and core temperature cooling rate was demonstrated by Keatinge (1960), and is shown in Figure 20.1. This study seemingly proved the obvious, that heat loss is a simple function of subcutaneous insulation, a fact that is absolutely valid for

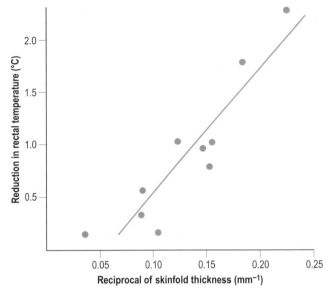

Figure 20.1 The apparent effect of subcutaneous adipose tissue thickness on core temperature cooling during cold-water immersion. Modified from Keatinge (1960) with permission.

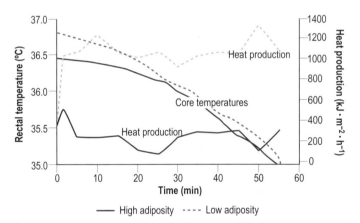

Figure 20.2 Core temperature cooling and shivering thermogenesis during a cold-water immersion (10°C) of a lean and moderately obese subject. Data taken from Mekjavic et al. (1987a).

inanimate objects. However, this figure has inadvertently oversimplified physiological heat loss. That this relation is more an exception than the rule can be demonstrated from data obtained from two subjects of widely variable adiposity (8% versus 38% body fat) and shivering responses, during a cold-water immersion (10°C; Mekjavic et al. 1987a), and illustrated in Figure 20.2. Both subjects experienced an almost identical core temperature cooling rate from 36°C to 35°C, despite their substantially different adiposity. Thus, physiological function has modified the impact of tissue insulation on heat loss. Certainly, the leaner individual had less inherent thermal protection (resistance) and would lose heat faster. However, this individual demonstrated a substantially more powerful shivering response (endogenous heat production or thermogenesis). Thus, whilst heat loss was probably greater, as predicted in Figure 20.1, heat storage, the net result of heat loss and production (Equation 1), as reflected in body core temperature, remained very similar between these subjects. That is, a greater heat loss in the leaner individual was offset by a greater heat production. Thus, these observations lead one to conclude that, during cold-water immersion, skinfold thickness is not the sole determinant of the core temperature cooling rate. Indeed, the relationship presented in Figure 20.1 would hold for all individuals if endogenous heat production (shivering) was simply a function of skinfold thickness, or if endogenous heat production for a given decrement in body temperature was always the same, and independent of the core temperature cooling rate. Since neither of these assumptions has been proven, the relationship proposed by Keatinge (1960) has its limitations and should be applied with some caution.

The examples provided above indicate that the range of thickness of the subcutaneous fat layer in a normal population is not sufficient to impact upon core temperature cooling rate. Thermal balance during cold exposure will be a consequence of the combined influences of the biophysics of heat exchange and the physiology of temperature regulation. Relating subcutaneous fat thickness directly to cooling rate not only ignores the relevance of the thermoregulatory responses but also dismisses the contribution of other tissues to the amount of heat retained in the body. As demonstrated by the heat balance equation, overall thermal energy balance is a consequence of heat production, heat loss and heat retention. Rather than trying to equate heat loss to single components of body composition, it may be simpler, and more appropriate, to equate the amount of heat retained to the overall composition of the body.

The difficulty with this approach is the accurate quantification of the composition of the body. Algorithms have been developed based on human cadaver dissections to predict body composition (Clarys et al. 1999), and these have been used to correlate components of body composition with core temperature cooling rate during immersion in 28°C water (White et al. 1992). This correlation was conducted for the range of core temperatures within the thermoneutral or interthreshold zone (see Figures 18.4 and 18.7), and bound by the thresholds for shivering and sweating. In this manner, the contribution of sweating and shivering to core temperature cooling rate was eliminated and the only physical characteristics of the subjects that correlated significantly to core temperature cooling rate were body mass and the body surface area. Since the latter is predicted from the mass and length (DuBois & DuBois 1916), the significance of surface area may be due to its correlation with mass. This further demonstrates that during cold exposure, the variation in the components of body composition anticipated in a population is not sufficient to significantly affect cooling rate. The overall mass (specific heat capacity of the body; Chapter 19) and endogenous heat production of shivering are therefore the most important factors determining thermal balance during cold exposure.

The discussion so far has demonstrated that core temperature cooling rate cannot be conveniently correlated to any single tissue compartment. Adipose tissue is not only found within the subcutaneous layer but is also distributed throughout the core. Thus, rather than considering the insulative characteristics of a given tissue compartment, it is preferable to consider the ability of the tissue to retain or store heat. This may be defined as the net result of the heat balance equation, but it can also be determined as the product of the specific heat of the body, body mass and the change in body temperature. To accommodate body composition, the specific heat of the body can be defined to represent the proportions of the different tissues in the body (Kakitsuba & Mekjavic 1987).

Notwithstanding the need to consider specific heat capacity and the intensity of the thermogenic response, it has been shown that, when resting in cool-temperate water (20°, 24°, 28°C), men with a greater body fat content are able to attain thermal homeostasis without shivering (McArdle et al. 1984), while leaner men were unable to defend core temperature. This divergence was not apparent in women, who experienced a greater core temperature reduction than men of a similar adiposity. This difference may have been due to gender-based variations in the body surface area to mass ratio, with the larger ratio of women increasing the available surface area for heat loss.

The body surface area to mass ratio can have a significant influence on body cooling rate and this ratio is generally larger for smaller individuals. Some people are best described as being of a more linear (height·mass^{-3}) body shape, and such a somatotype facilitates heat loss (Morrison et al. 1980). Consequently, for a given rate of endogenous heat production, adolescents, women with an adiposity equivalent to that of men, and tall, lean people tend to cool more rapidly. In addition, women and children tend to have a relatively smaller muscle mass, which is a major contributor to resting insulation.

The loss of 3.47 kJ (0.83 kcal) of thermal energy from 1 kg of tissue will result in an average body tissue temperature reduction of 1°C (Burton 1935). The capacity of an individual to support this heat loss through an elevated metabolic rate, without a progressive fall in body temperature, is dictated not only by the magnitude of the shivering response, and thus the endogenous heat produced by shivering, but also by the thermal compensability of the environment.

2.3 Predicting problems in heat balance

The interaction of physiological functions, clothing and environmental conditions modifies the exchange of thermal energy between the body and the surrounding environment. Our capacity to modify the impact of almost any environment via behavioural strategies (protective clothing, air conditioning, portable life support) means that we need rarely experience uncompensable environmental conditions. However, when such strategies are not available, then we must rely upon autonomic temperature regulation, and the autonomic compensability of a cold exposure defines a range of heat transfer beyond which the thermal energy content of the body progressively moves towards hypothermia (35°C; 95°F). This is dictated by the heat balance equation and, by using an analogue of the required evaporative heat loss (E_{req}; Chapter 19), can be evaluated from the required metabolic heat production (H_{req}). Since external work is not usually performed on the body (eccentric exercise), then the required metabolic heat production will be a function of the total heat production that can be achieved through either exercise or shivering.

Equation 2: $H_{req} = -E \pm R \pm K \pm C$ [watts, W]

where:

H_{req} = metabolic heat production ($M - (\pm W)$) [W]
E = evaporative cooling [W]
R, K and C = heat transfer via radiation, conduction and convection [W].

An average adult can work for 3–5 h at an intensity of approximately 40–45% of maximal. A 70 kg person with an above average physical fitness ($50\ mL \cdot kg^{-1} \cdot min^{-1}$) will have a resting metabolic energy transformation (or metabolic rate: IUPS Thermal Commission 2001) of ~105 W ($1.5\ W \cdot kg^{-1}$), and could sustain an external work rate of ~120 W for more than 1 h. The total metabolic heat production of this person would be ~585 W ($M + W \cdot 5 - W$ or $105 + 120 \cdot 5 - 120$). During intense shivering, metabolic rate can be elevated to 5–6 times that observed at rest (Glickman et al. 1967, Iampietro et al. 1960). However, Tikuisis et al. (1999) reported that only a threefold increase in the resting oxygen uptake is sustained when lightly clothed subjects are exposed to cold-wet conditions (4 h, 10°C air, 10°C water spray, wind velocity $1.7\ m \cdot s^{-1}$). If the required metabolic heat production is greater than the sustainable shivering thermogenesis at rest (350 W), the sustainable total metabolic heat production during exercise (585 W) or their combined thermal effects, then the conditions are deemed to be autonomically uncompensable (Figure 18.4, zone 5). This thermal compensability is illustrated within predicted survival curves developed from data obtained during wholebody, cold-water immersion (Figure 20.3). These curves indicate that a safe 6 h exposure occurs in water at 19°C, and that death is almost certain within 1 h when water temperature approaches 0°C.

In Chapter 18, the concept of the body temperature operating level was introduced and it was explained using the example of exercise-induced increments in body temperature. During light-moderate exercise in a cool–cold environment, an increase in body temperature from its normal resting (regulated) level is not always evident, since the autonomic heat loss responses (vasodilatation and sweat-

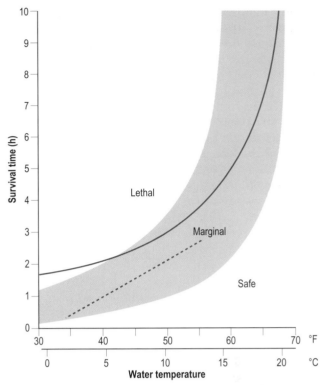

Figure 20.3 Predicted survival times during cool–cold water immersions, indicating safe, 50% mortality (marginal) and 99% (lethal) mortality zones. Redrawn from Hayward et al. (1975) with permission.

ing) should be capable of providing the required heat loss to eliminate the heat produced during exercise, thus defending body temperature. However, when the same exercise is performed in warmer conditions, a body temperature rise does occur, but this is often simply to a new steady state or operating level (Chapter 18). This new body temperature is either regulated or is simply a consequence of a change in the balance between heat production and heat loss. This same example can now be applied to exposure to a cold environment.

The activation of any autonomic response is proportional to the magnitude of thermoafferent feedback (Chapter 18). Thus, a mild cold exposure does not maximally activate shivering. Nevertheless, in some circumstance, it may be metabolically wasteful to activate shivering thermogenesis every time one experiences cold stress. In such instances, slight decrements in body temperature are tolerated. Thus, even in thermally compensable environments, the autonomic responses are not always activated to precisely match the required heat loss or heat production, presumably placing some reliance for this on the behavioural responses, which are more efficient. This topic is again covered in Chapter 21, where adaptation to chronic cold exposure is discussed across a range of ethnic groups.

Most researchers focus on either the autonomic or behavioural components of temperature regulation, but rarely do they simultaneously investigate these mechanisms. Consequently, the interaction of these defence mechanisms in regulating body temperature during either cold or warm exposure, in a thermally compensable environment, remains unresolved.

However, since behavioural responses are extremely powerful, it is worth introducing readers to the concept of required insulation. During cold exposures, added layers of clothing reduce heat loss to the surrounding air. This is achieved by increasing the resistance to heat transfer through garments. Materials vary in their inherent thermal resistance, with those having a high resistance being good insulators. Since air is one of the best known insulators, the insulation provided by any garment will largely be a function of its ability to trap air within its layers and prevent it from moving and escaping. Not surprisingly, thicker garments trap more air, as do garments and clothing ensembles with a greater number of layers. Indeed, it is possible to quantify the thermal insulation (resistance) of fabrics and garments. If one knows the insulation provided by a garment and the rate at which heat is lost, then one may derive the insulation necessary to prevent heat loss. Thus, just as one may compute the required metabolic heat production (Equation 2) for a person to remain at the same body temperature (autonomic thermoregulation), one can also derive the total insulation required to keep the body temperature constant for resting and exercising steady states, without the need to recruit physiological regulatory mechanism (behavioural thermoregulation). This concept is known as the required insulation (I_{req}), and was developed by Holmér (1984).

3 NEUROPHYSIOLOGY OF THERMORECEPTION

The essential neurophysiological background to the behavioural and autonomic regulation of body temperature is contained in Chapters 18 and 19, with a brief summary set out below. In the latter case, the emphasis was upon heat dissipation by modulating skin blood flow (vasodilatation and venodilatation) and sweat secretion. Herein, heat production (thermogenesis) and conservation (vasoconstriction and venoconstriction) form the primary focus, thereby completing a detailed discussion of the thermoeffectors within the human temperature regulation system (Chapter 18).

Humans regulate a composite of body core and skin temperatures (mean body temperature; Jessen 1996; Chapter 18) through the modulation of physiological (effector) functions that modify heat gain and loss. Cold- and warm-sensitive thermoreceptors located in the skin, viscera, spinal cord, brain stem and hypothalamus (Boulant 1996, Pierau 1996) provide feedback to the central integrator within the hypothalamus concerning the thermal energy content of local tissues. In some cases, this feedback is very powerful. For example, during a sudden cold-water immersion, the simultaneous powerful stimulation of cold-sensitive receptors results in the cold-shock response (section 7.1), which can be lethal. In addition, it is believed that some reciprocal cross-inhibition exists between warm- and cold-sensitive thermoafferents (Chapter 18). That is, while shivering is driven by cold-sensitive signals, warm-sensitive signals will, at least transiently, suppress shivering.

When exposed to conditions on either side of the thermoneutral zone (see Figure 18.4: zone 1), the resultant deviation in mean body temperature leads to the activation of one or more thermoeffector mechanisms, and defines their thermoregulatory thresholds (Figure 18.4: point C). These effector responses will be proportional to the deviation in mean body temperature, with the slope of this relationship describing the gain (sensitivity) of the thermoeffectors (Chapter 18).

Thus, while the absolute temperature that one encounters, or the magnitude of the deviation in mean body temperature, dictates the nature and magnitude of the thermoeffector responses, the rate of change in mean body temperature is also a very potent stimulus. It has been demonstrated, for example, that the cold-shock response to cold-water immersion is a function of the rate of change of skin temperature (Mekjavic et al. 1987b), whereas an increase in the rate of core temperature cooling will enhance the shivering response.

It should also be emphasised that, although there is evidence that the static and dynamic temperature profiles of the core and skin compartments affect the thermoregulatory responses, the effector responses may not always reflect neurogenic drive. This point is best illustrated with the example of the cold-shock response, which is characterised by the increase in minute ventilation corresponding to the decrease in skin temperature change, both in terms of the magnitude (static) and rate (dynamic) of these changes. The respiratory drive during the cold-shock response was quantified using the mouth occlusion pressure method, in which measures of the inspiratory pressure were recorded at the mouth during the initial 100 ms of an airway occlusion. Mekjavic et al. (1987b) showed that occlusion pressure reflected thermogenic drive. Although respiratory drive increases linearly with increasing rates of skin temperature cooling, presumably due to a greater neurogenic feedback from the cold receptors, this linear increase is not observed in the minute ventilation, which eventually attains asymptotic values. Thus, although the neurogenic drive for respiration increases with decreasing skin temperature, the minute ventilation response, which is an outcome measure influenced by the mechanics of the respiratory system, does not completely reflect this increasing drive.

A similar situation may also exist for the other effector responses, such as shivering, vasomotor tone and sweating. It is therefore not only the sensitivity of a response that may vary from one individual to the next but also the asymptotic values of the effector responses. This may be misinterpreted as a reduced sensitivity, when it is really a limited range of activity. Thus, the shivering response for a given decrease in temperature may be the same in two individuals but the final maximal levels may differ.

4 AUTONOMIC REGULATION

In the thermoneutral state, heat transfer is controlled and temperature is regulated via subtle changes in cutaneous vascular tone. In thermally stressful environments, behavioural interventions (e.g. clothing changes) can be used to modify the microclimate, and we can further modulate (control) cutaneous vascular resistance and recruit thermogenesis and evaporation to modify heat transfer. Collectively, these physiological processes form the effector limb of the thermoregulatory system.

4.1 Cardiovascular modulation

4.1.1 Control of skin blood flow

A principal function of skin blood flow, after serving the metabolic requirements of cutaneous tissues, is to modulate heat transfer from the body core to the periphery. At rest in a thermoneutral (comfortable) environment, skin blood flow averages ~ 350 mL·min^{-1}, with the skin receiving approximately 5–10% of the cardiac output (Rowell 1974). Since blood has a high volume-specific heat (3.85 kJ·L^{-1}·°C^{-1}), and since there exists a 4°C core–skin thermal gradient under these conditions, metabolic heat is constantly being delivered to the skin for removal. In fact, at rest, thermal homeostasis can be achieved within the thermoneutral zone (see Chapter 18, Figure 18.4) entirely through changes in skin blood flow, particularly in the hands, face and feet (if exposed).

Changes in skin blood flow represent the first line of heat conservation, with cold-induced cutaneous vasoconstriction causing skin temperatures to fall, thereby reducing the thermal gradient between the skin and the surrounding medium. Thus, cold exposure cools the skin, which reduces skin blood flow, resulting in further skin cooling. The more uniform skin temperatures observed in the heat (Chapter 19) are now replaced with a peripheral heterothermy that is designed to conserve heat, and the point corresponding to maximal vasoconstriction (insulation; Figure 18.4 point F) represents the upper limit of this physiological heat conservation. This is a metabolically efficient mechanism. While local skin temperature reductions elicit both regional and generalised vasoconstriction, the magnitude of this local response is, in part, core temperature dependent.

Not surprisingly, the first result of cold exposure is an immediate and generalised reduction in skin temperature, leading to cutaneous veno- and vasoconstriction (Stocks et al. 2004b). These elevations in vascular tone are elicited via adrenergic receptor activation (Granberg et al. 1971, Lennquist et al. 1974), through a direct effect of the lower skin temperature on blood vessel diameter, and also by an elevation in plasma noradrenaline concentration (Rowell 1986). Venoconstriction occurs more rapidly since the cutaneous veins have a greater thermal sensitivity (Webb & Shepard 1968), and increased tone in these capacitance vessels reduces the volume of blood at the periphery. These vascular changes displace blood from the superficial cutaneous vessels into deeper veins, and from the periphery to the core (Rowell 1986). The nett result is a rise in mean arterial pressure, cardiac output and stroke volume, with a consequent reduction in heart rate (Leppaluoto et al. 1988, Raven et al. 1970).

Cold-induced vasoconstriction is maximal even in moderate air temperatures (Bittel et al. 1988), and its activation can almost instantaneously reduce heat loss during an acute cold exposure. This delays the cooling of deeper peripheral tissues, and the establishment of convective (vascular) pathways for heat loss from the core, and it increases tissue insulation. Cutaneous vasoconstriction in the cold, and vasodilatation in the heat, transiently alter heat balance and account, for the paradoxical changes in core temperature often seen in resting subjects during the early phase of cold and heat exposures (Hardy 1954). This paradox is a nice example of the temporal difference between a physical change (slower conductive heat transfer) and the immediate physiological responses (principally vasomotion or blood-borne convective heat transfer). Thus, during an acute cold exposure, deep body heat storage will initially be positive (heat gain) until the cutaneous conductive heat losses result in a lowering of the peripheral tissue temperatures, to the extent that deep body heat storage is reversed (heat loss).

The cutaneous blood flow response to cold varies across body regions (Hensel 1981), due largely to local variations in vasoconstrictor control, with major differences between the acral and non-acral regions. In the acral skin regions (nose, ears, lips, palms and soles), blood flow is modulated via adrenergic vasoconstrictor fibres. In the thermoneutral state, constrictor tone in these regions is powerful and blood flow is very low. Passive cooling elicits almost maximal vasoconstriction (see Figure 19.2A; Kellogg 2006, Roddie 1983). Ducharme et al. (1999) have demonstrated that skin blood flow to the fingers, while generally modified by both local skin and deep body temperatures, can be substantially maintained by core heating, even when the hands are exposed to very cold air. Using passive torso heating to 42°C, during clothed, whole-body cold exposure (−23°C, 3 h), including bare hands, they observed that both finger blood flow and manual dexterity could be preserved, whereas neither was sustained when hand heating (31°C) alone was used.

The extremities, particularly the hands, feet and ears, contain networks of arteriovenous anastomoses that supply blood to the venous plexus directly from small arteries. These structures play an important role in temperature regulation in the cold since their synchronised closing, caused by efferent sympathetic impulse bursts (Bini et al. 1980), is linked to heat balance. During thermoneutral exposures, anastomoses constrict up to three times a minute

(Lossius et al. 1993), causing rapid blood velocity fluctuations. These anastomoses remain closed during cold stress, but open during heating, producing stable, low-velocity blood flow.

Such vascular changes can, in very cold conditions, lead to dangerously low tissue temperatures, and may result in tissue damage (section 7.3). The risk of this is reduced by cold-induced vasodilatation (CIVD): cyclic changes in skin blood flow, perhaps driven centrally (Lindblad et al. 1990). When the core temperature is normal, cold-induced vasodilatation periodically warms the skin by transferring warmer blood from the core to the periphery.

Unlike the extremities, the head displays only a minimal constrictor response to cold, having a high sympathetic tone even under thermoneutral conditions. Therefore, skin blood flow responses of the head do not form part of the generalised peripheral vasoconstriction response (Stocks et al. 2004b).

Blood flow to the non-acral surfaces is controlled via two separate sympathetic pathways (Chapter 19), with vasoconstrictor fibres dominating during cold exposure by adrenergic and noradrenergic elevation of their mild constrictor tone present under thermoneutral conditions (Kellogg 2006). As with heat-induced vasodilatation, the onset of this more powerful vasoconstriction is known as the vasoconstriction threshold, which is driven by changes in both skin and core temperatures. Thus, cutaneous vasoconstriction is influenced by local thermal changes and hypothalamic control, with the reduction in skin blood flow, relative to changes in mean body temperature ($mL \cdot 100\ min^{-1} \cdot {}^{\circ}C^{-1}$), providing an index of the sensitivity of such vasomotor control (Chapter 18). These threshold and sensitivity measures may be modified by cold adaptation, the preexercise body temperature (Chapter 21) and a range of non-thermal factors, such as endurance fitness, hydration state and illness.

Core and skin cooling both elevate venoconstrictor tone, which occurs quite rapidly, changing the path of venous return to the heart from the superficial cutaneous to the deeper veins (Rowell 1986). Since these vascular beds are interconnected, with the superficial vessels being relatively well innervated, this rerouting allows the blood to return via the well-insulated deeper venous beds, thus reducing heat loss. Furthermore, the proximity of smaller blood vessels carrying blood in opposite directions has been suggested to provide an avenue for countercurrent heat transfer between these blood vessels (Pennes 1948). The nett result was proposed to be a direct transfer of thermal energy between vessels of different temperatures, such that heat is retained centrally. More recently, Brink & Werner (1994a,b) have shown that such heat transfer takes place mainly from smaller arteries (radius: 0.6–0.02 mm), and such vascular networks are predominantly located in muscles found close to the skin. From vessels larger and smaller than these, there will be almost no such heat transfer, since the combination of blood vessel diameter and local flow will largely exclude

the possibility of countercurrent heat transfer (Brink & Werner 1994a,b).

4.1.2 Integrated cardiovascular responses

In Chapter 19, the interrelationships between skin blood flow changes and blood pressure (Chapter 1) and body fluid regulation (Chapter 33) were described. These integrated responses are again relevant to cold exposures, particularly when immersion is involved, since thermoneutral immersion has separate and independent cardiovascular implications (Chapter 22). The translocation of blood from the peripheral to the central vascular spaces during cold exposure stimulates changes in water balance (section 5.2), and the increase in thoracic blood volume has a significant physiological impact during cold-water immersion (Arborelius et al. 1972, Epstein 1978).

Cold-induced peripheral vasoconstriction elevates total peripheral resistance and blood pressure, and modifies capillary fluid and ion exchange between the intravascular and interstitial spaces (Vogelaere et al. 1992). During cold-water immersion, the combined effects of thermal and hydrostatic stimuli result in a significant displacement of peripheral blood into the central venous volume (Arborelius et al. 1972), producing a rise in mean arterial pressure, stroke volume and cardiac output (Raven et al. 1970). The elevation in stroke volume is largely attributable to right ventricular preloading accompanying the increase in central blood volume, and elicits a cardiac output elevation varying between 30% and 60%, depending on immersion depth, posture and water temperature (Krasney 1996). These are inotropic responses associated with the Frank–Starling mechanism (Chapters 1 and 22), with the simultaneous stimulation of the high- and low-pressure baroreceptors (stretch receptors) leading to a reduction in heart rate (Raven et al. 1970) and increased secretion of atrial natriuretic peptide (Stocks et al. 2004a).

Since this central vascular loading affects both sides of the heart, pulmonary artery pressure and blood volume will increase. The lungs are well suited to accommodate this blood (Chapter 2), but it does impact upon respiratory mechanics, reducing lung volumes and increasing the work of breathing (Hajduczok et al. 1987, Taylor & Morrison 1991, 1999). There is also an increase in blood flow to the respiratory muscles and the myocardium (Hajduczok et al. 1987).

Muscle blood flow is low during resting cold exposures and becomes even lower, particularly within dependent regions, when combined with immersion. Consequently, Veicsteinas et al. (1982) found that skeletal muscle accounted for ~80% of total body insulation in subjects resting in water held just above the shivering threshold (the lower critical temperature). This is particularly so for the limbs, in which muscle provides a large proportion of the total insulation. However, exercise elevates muscle blood flow, with the associated hyperaemia resulting in more rapid heat loss (Nadel et al. 1974, Veicsteinas et al. 1982), even though exercise also increases the metabolic energy transformation.

This is why exercise can accelerate the rate of heat loss in cold water, while simultaneously suppressing shivering (Hong & Nadel 1979). Thus, while the variable insulation of muscle plays a principal role at rest, this role is reduced progressively with increments in exercise intensity, and is negligible when metabolic heat production reaches ~180 W·m^{-2} (Rennie 1988). This combination of conditions maximises tissue thermal conductance, and if maximal metabolic heat production is less than heat loss, thermal homeostasis is unachievable. When this occurs, the resting and exercise metabolic energy transformations must be supplemented with shivering thermogenesis to prevent a progressive core temperature decline.

4.2 Shivering thermogenesis

At rest, the ambient temperature for thermoneutrality varies as a function of the physical characteristics of the surrounding medium (air: 23–26°C; water: 34–36°C; helium: 31–32°C; Chapter 23). The lower critical temperature defines the lower end of thermoneutrality and corresponds with the ambient temperature below which shivering thermogenesis is initiated. Whilst succeeding the vascular responses, shivering commences very rapidly following either an acute cold-air or cold-water exposure (Tikuisis et al. 1991) and is driven primarily via the motor pathways, aided by catecholamine release (Banet et al. 1978).

Shivering is a form of involuntary skeletal muscle activation (oscillation; Pozos et al. 1986), with the contractile force generated being about 15–20% of that achieved during maximal voluntary muscle activation. While peak shivering will increase metabolic rate 5–6 times above that observed at rest (Glickman et al. 1967, Iampietro et al. 1960), a three-fold increase is more realistic for sustained shivering (Tikuisis et al. 1999). Given the inefficiency of all metabolic pathways (Chapter 19), with shivering serving only to increase heat production, this has a significant impact on heat balance. For instance, an additional oxygen uptake of 1 L·min^{-1} (or 3–4 times resting oxygen uptake), in combination with a respiratory exchange ratio of 0.9, will provide an additional 16.8 kJ·min^{-1} to the metabolic energy transformation.

Once initiated, the shivering intensity is dependent upon several factors. The first stimulus for shivering comes from an elevated activity of the cutaneous cold-sensitive receptors, accompanying the decline in skin temperature. Indeed, in normothermic and mildly hyperthermic people, shivering can be initiated by an acute cold stimulus (see Figure 19.1). If heat loss exceeds the combined effects of cutaneous vasoconstriction and thermogenesis to sustain body heat content, then the central thermoreceptors will be stimulated by the ensuing fall in core temperature, thus inducing a more pronounced thermogenesis (see Chapter 18). In humans, shivering is more sensitive to temperature changes acting on the core than the skin, although heat production is proportional to the magnitude of the change in mean body temperature.

However, there is a multiplicative interaction of skin and core temperatures on shivering intensity (Benzinger 1970), such that when the core temperature is elevated before a standardised skin-cooling stimulus, the shivering response will be smaller. Conversely, a lower preexposure core temperature enhances thermogenesis. Finally, while the absolute skin temperature is an important static influence, the rate of skin temperature change also affects shivering, being most pronounced when skin-cooling rates are both large and rapid. This highlights the powerful dynamic influence of cutaneous thermoreceptors (see Chapter 19).

An acute cold exposure will stimulate sympathoadrenal secretion (Frank et al. 1997) with potent effects on energy utilisation, as catecholamines stimulate lipolysis, hepatic glycogenolysis and gluconeogenesis. Glucagon secretion is also elevated, promoting hepatic glycogenolysis and gluconeogenesis, as well as lipolysis and hepatic ketone production. These changes elevate the blood-borne concentrations of substrates for lipid and carbohydrate metabolism. Insulin secretion is inhibited during more severe cold stress, therefore reducing glucose uptake from all tissues and conserving blood glucose, perhaps for the central nervous system.

Carbohydrate oxidation is increased during more intense shivering, with its contribution to the total energy consumption increasing to equal that of lipid metabolism (Vallerand & Jacobs 1989). In this situation, it is the decrease in blood glucose concentration, and the corresponding central effects of hypoglycaemia, that may limit shivering (Beckman & Reeves 1966, Gale et al. 1981, Passias et al. 1996), rather than muscle glycogen per se.

First, hypoglycaemia will elicit vasodilatation in the muscle and cutaneous vascular beds (Allwood et al. 1959), facilitating heat loss by reducing the variable (tissue) insulation. Second, Gale et al. (1981) demonstrated that the hypoglycaemic effect on shivering was centrally mediated. Using insulin-induced hypoglycaemia, they confirmed the heavy reliance of shivering on carbohydrate metabolism. They observed a suppression of the metabolic energy transformation in shivering subjects to basal levels, when plasma glucose concentration fell to <2.5 mmol·L^{-1}. A systemic glucose infusion restored shivering and the rapidity of this effect, along with the fact that shivering was also restored within an arterially occluded leg, into which normoglycaemic blood could not perfuse, indicated that hypoglycaemia was acting on the central nervous system.

Furthermore, Passias et al. (1996) demonstrated that a 50% reduction of the plasma glucose concentration could abolish shivering, resulting in a marked increase in core temperature cooling rate. They attributed these observations to the dual modality of some of the central thermosensitive neurons in the cold-sensor-to-heat production pathway. Silva & Boulant (1984) reported that a substantial portion of the cold-sensitive neurons in the hypothalamus were also glucosensitive. Thus, for a given body temperature, the activity of such neurons would also be modulated by changes in plasma glucose concentration, and this effect is shown diagrammatically in Chapter 18 (Figure 18.12; point 2). A non-thermal factor, such as hypoglycaemia, may not only influence the autonomic response of shivering, but has also been demonstrated to attenuate the perception of temperature and of thermal comfort (Passias et al. 1996), implying that behavioural thermoregulatory responses might also be impaired in the presence of hypoglycaemia.

Since carbohydrate oxidation is increased during cold stress, and shivering is heavily reliant upon carbohydrate metabolism, then intramuscular or hepatic glycogen availability may also represent a metabolic limit to shivering (Jacobs et al. 1994). However, while muscle glycogen depletion results in fatigue during moderate- to high-intensity exercise, this may not occur during shivering. Indeed, dietary manipulations have not supported this, with carbohydrate loading not appearing to improve cold tolerance. Furthermore, when muscle glycogen was depleted prior to a resting cold-water exposure (18°C), thermoregulation was not impaired, with perhaps a greater reliance upon lipid oxidation supporting shivering (Young et al. 1989). It is likely that the metabolic pathways supporting shivering are modified as subjects become fatigued (Weller et al. 1998), particularly when subjects are also food deprived (5 h) prior to cold exposure (Tikuisis et al. 1999). It appears that, in the non-fatigued state, shivering may rely upon carbohydrates to a greater extent, with a shift towards lipid metabolism as fatigue develops within an extended cold exposure (4 h). This metabolic shift occurs without significantly altering either the metabolic energy transformation or thermal homeostasis. Thus, it seems that the central neural influence of hypoglycaemia is more important than the intramuscular changes. Accordingly, hypoglycaemia is considered to be a useful predictor of imminent hypothermia (Passias et al. 1996, Thompson & Hayward 1996).

5 HORMONAL AND BODY FLUID RESPONSES

5.1 Hormonal changes

Sudden and powerful cold stimuli, particularly water immersions, stimulate intense sympathoadrenal activity, resulting in increased noradrenaline, adrenaline and cortisol secretion (Wilkerson et al. 1974). The catecholamine responses are very rapid and will invariably precede core temperature changes. For example, the circulating noradrenaline concentration can increase to about 180% of its basal concentration within the first 2 min of cold-water immersion. Indeed, it falls rapidly on leaving the water, even though the core temperature is still depressed (Johnson et al. 1977). Thus, this catecholamine response is mediated peripherally by the rapid and intense cooling of the skin. More recently, Frank et al. (1997), using cold-saline infusion, demonstrated that the noradrenaline response, but not adrenaline secretion, could be induced by central circulatory cooling, and without simultaneous skin cooling. It is

concluded that, while intense skin cooling elicits a generalised catecholamine release, mild core cooling only stimulates noradrenaline release.

5.2 Body fluid regulation

The independent, but often simultaneous, influences of thermal, hydrostatic (immersion) and exercise loading on the cardiovascular system also affect body fluid regulation, with volume defence mechanisms involving both neural and humoral factors (Chapters 19 and 22). When exercise is initiated, there is a rapid and temperature-independent reduction of the plasma volume (Maw et al. 1998). Similarly, cold stress in resting subjects can reduce plasma volume by 7–15% in air and by 15–20% in water (Young et al. 1987). However, a thermoneutral immersion will elevate the plasma volume (Stocks et al. 2004a). While these influences on body fluid balance are driven by different causes, they activate similar physiological mechanisms.

The mechanisms underlying the elevation in plasma volume during a thermoneutral immersion are described in detail in Chapter 22 (see Figure 22.4). In short, the Starling forces acting across all capillary membranes are altered in favour of reabsorption, but only within the immersed body regions, and primarily through an elevation in interstitial pressure relative to the capillary hydrostatic pressure. Most of the fluid shift originates from the intracellular compartment, with renal water removal minimising the rise in plasma volume.

Each of the other changes acts to increase the plasma osmolality and sodium concentration (haemoconcentration). In the case of exercise, there is a transient fluid displacement into the interstitial space of the active muscles (Chapter 19). The hydrostatically and cold-induced plasma volume reductions have been attributed to diuresis, which can increase fluid loss almost twofold. However, the exact mechanism of cold-induced diuresis remains unclear. One hypothesis, which remains unsubstantiated, is that the increase in central blood volume, which stimulates low- and high-pressure baroreceptors, inhibits antidiuretic hormone (arginine vasopressin) secretion, leading to diuresis and hypovolaemia (Raven et al. 1970). However, a suppression of antidiuretic hormone secretion leads to a free-water diuresis (Gauer & Henry 1963), while cold-induced diuresis is associated with an elevated osmotic clearance, but not a free-water clearance (Knight & Horvath 1985). Therefore, other fluid-regulatory hormones appear to be involved in this diuresis. One candidate is atrial natriuretic peptide, because its secretion is increased during cold stress (section 4.1.2) in response to atrial stretching, and it enhances both sodium and water excretion.

While the physiological mechanisms behind the cold-induced diuresis have not been resolved, it is apparent that diuresis is not the only mechanism responsible for the reduction in plasma volume, since the plasma volume change usually exceeds that which can be explained by diuresis. Since cold-induced cutaneous vasoconstriction elevates total peripheral resistance and blood pressure, as well as modifying capillary fluid and ion exchanges between the intravascular and interstitial fluid compartments (Vogelaere et al. 1992), then hypovolaemia during cold stress may be due to both an increased urine production, accompanied by a reduced renal water reabsorption which occurs during hypothermia, and a relocation of fluid to the interstitium. Whilst these combined mechanisms are plausible, Young et al. (1987) failed to find a significant correlation between the reduction in plasma volume and the thermogenic, diuretic or tissue temperature responses.

Notwithstanding the uncertainties above, there is no doubt that both hydrostatically and thermally mediated vascular factors are involved in fluid regulation during immersion, with each influence sometimes opposing the other. For example, Janský et al. (1996) observed a 50% reduction in plasma renin activity, but no change in plasma aldosterone concentration, during cold immersion (14°C). Since equivalent suppression of renin and aldosterone has been reported during thermoneutral immersion (Epstein et al. 1975), the changes in plasma renin activity were interpreted to reflect a hydrostatic, rather than a thermal effect. However, Janský et al. (1996) suggested that the stability of the plasma aldosterone concentration may have resulted from a cold-induced suppression of the hydrostatic influence on aldosterone secretion. It was suggested that atrial natriuretic peptide, released during atrial distension (section 5.1), may have counteracted the hydrostatic inhibition of aldosterone secretion. This hypothesis is at least partially supported by more recent evidence showing that atrial natriuretic peptide secretion, which may not occur during a thermoneutral immersion, is induced during cold-water immersion, when the combined affects of thermal and hydrostatic stimuli result in a significant displacement of peripheral blood into the central venous volume (Stocks et al. 2004a).

6 INTERACTIONS OF AGE, GENDER, PHYSICAL FITNESS AND EXERCISE WITH THE COLD RESPONSES

6.1 Age and cold stress

People at either end of the age spectrum have a higher risk of both hyper- and hypothermia. Indeed, neonates and the aged may be considered to be morphologically (e.g. subcutaneous adipose tissue) and functionally different from young adults, particularly with respect to thermoregulation, with many of these differences helping to explain trends within the epidemiological data. However, the aged are a generally more frail group and, as such, are more susceptible to a wider range of pathological conditions. Thus, the aged are not at greater risk of heat- or cold-related illness than they are of other diseases and disorders; instead, they are simply a broadly high-risk group (Taylor et al. 1994).

Neonates do not shiver, but, like almost all neonatal mammals they can produce heat via non-shivering thermogenesis. This is a form of heat production that exceeds the basal metabolic rate and exists only for the purpose of regulating body temperature. It is modulated via noradrenaline secretion from sympathetic fibres that stimulate brown adipose tissue, resulting in the activation of the uncoupling protein thermogenin (Cannon & Nedergaard 2004). While human neonates generally have small subcutaneous adipose tissue deposits (less fixed insulation), it is the interscapular and perirenal brown adipose depots that facilitate thermal balance. However, the human morphological configuration means that smaller people will invariably have a greater surface area to mass ratio. This does not favour thermal homeostasis, and in neonates, this ratio may be twice that of an adult. In children 6–8 years old and those around puberty, subcutaneous adipose tissue deposits are generally smaller than in healthy young adults. These children also have a significantly greater surface area, with ratios ~140% of those observed in adults. Thus, Keatinge & Sloan (1972) attributed the high incidence of hypothermia in adolescents during recreational swimming (e.g. exposure to 20°C for 40 min) to these morphological differences.

The size of the subcutaneous adipose tissue deposits in adults tends to increase as one moves through life (Chapter 31), generally reflecting poor lifestyle choices (Chapters 28 and 30). However, this trend is reversed in the aged (>65 y), with the elderly generally having less subcutaneous adipose than younger adults. In addition, ageing adults often display diminished autonomic function (Collins et al. 1980), reduced skin blood flow responsiveness to both hot and cold stresses (Collins et al. 1985, Richardson & Shepherd 1991), and less stable body temperature regulation (Marion et al. 1991). Prolonged skin cooling will increase erythrocyte counts, blood pressure and blood viscosity, and these changes may help explain the increased incidence of coronary and cerebral thromboses during the winter months (Keatinge et al. 1984). Complicating these states is the high probability that many elderly will be using prescription drugs, some of which may interact with thermoreceptor sensitivity and effector function. Collectively, such functional changes can result in a diminished ability to generate and conserve thermal energy, and may predispose this group to thermoregulatory insufficiency during a cold stress.

The effect of ageing on the regulation of body temperature can be considered as a transition from a fine to a coarser type of regulation, as a consequence of age-related changes in functional characteristics of both the autonomic and behavioural thermoregulatory responses. Compared to children, adults have a wider interthreshold zone, which is even greater in the elderly (Anderson & Mekjavic 1996). Thus, heat production is activated at a lower body temperature and heat loss responses are initiated at a higher temperature. In addition, the gains (sensitivity) for these responses are also attenuated in the elderly. The reduced heat production can be due to a decreased neurogenic drive to the muscles for shivering, a reduction in the proportion of muscles activated or a reduction of muscle mass (atrophy).

Apart from these functional differences, greater cold intolerance may also be attributed to the less precise recognition of, and response to, stressful thermal challenges. For example, when similarly clothed young and older subjects were asked to control room temperature at a comfortable state, the older subjects made fewer temperature adjustments, and allowed air temperature to reach hotter and cooler limits before responding (Collins et al. 1981). This experiment was repeated more recently, with a similar outcome (Taylor et al. 1995). However, the latter group was also able to show that, at points where low air temperatures prompted a response, the elderly had significantly cooler calf, thigh, chest and hand temperatures, but they reported being significantly more comfortable at these air temperatures. If one assumes that thermal discomfort drives behaviour, then the elderly subjects seemed to require a stronger thermal stimulus to evoke the appropriate behavioural response. Such a behavioural delay may help explain the overrepresentation of the elderly within hypothermia morbidity and mortality statistics. Indeed, given the interaction of hypoglycaemia and behavioural thermoregulation, and the increased prevalence of impaired blood glucose regulation in sedentary and overweight people (Chapter 28 and 30), one wonders whether some part of these observations can be ascribed to some interactive influences.

6.2 Gender differences

Interactions between the menstrual cycle and other regulatory hormones modify body fluid and electrolyte regulation, thermal comfort and the thermoregulatory thresholds (De Souza et al. 1989, Hessemer & Brück 1985). In fact, the thermosensitivity of many hypothalamic neurons shows some degree of plasticity, due to the influence of oestrogen cycling (Silva & Boulant 1986). In addition to the menstrual cycle, circadian changes can give rise to between-phase fluctuations in core temperature of >0.7°C. Such oscillations can have a significant impact upon vasomotor control. Consequently, between-gender comparisons require careful control to ensure that the experimental design matches the hypothesis testing requirements of each investigation. A philosophical reflection on decisions related to sample selection for research involving women is contained within the introduction to Section 2 of this book.

Unlike the heat, very few investigators have endeavoured to compare the genders in the cold, much less attempting to control for phases of the menstrual cycle. Accordingly, we have a relatively poor understanding of female thermoregulation during cold stress, with most of the gender-based differences being attributable to either morphological or body composition differences. However, these variations do not adequately explain every observation.

During cool-air exposures, women universally have lower skin temperatures (Cunningham et al. 1978), which are sustained during exercise. This is the opposite of what is observed in the heat, with women generally showing higher skin temperatures (Chapter 19). Lower skin temperatures in the cold are most notable where subcutaneous adipose tissue provides a greater tissue insulation from the conductive transfer of central heat (i.e. the trunk and proximal limb segments). In addition, some of this temperature difference can be attributable to a lower skin blood flow (Fox et al. 1969). Consequently, women display a greater resistance to cutaneous heat loss, and the skin–environment temperature gradient is generally smaller in the cold.

Women also report a greater subjective sensitivity to skin cooling, particularly during the luteal phase, and generally prefer a warmer skin temperature (Cunningham & Cabanac 1971). While most couples can provide anecdotal evidence to support this, it does have a sound physiological basis. The highest density of cold-sensitive thermoreceptors is located in the skin. Due to the more even distribution of subcutaneous adipose tissue in women, cutaneous vasoconstriction, in combination with a greater fixed insulation, results in greater skin temperature decline during skin cooling. Thus, one would expect a greater afferent flow from the cooler cutaneous thermoreceptors of women during an equivalent thermal stress, and a stronger thermal sensation.

Grucza et al. (1999) have shown that women have a significantly lower sensitivity of the shivering response during both the luteal and follicular phases of the menstrual cycle. That is, for an equivalent reduction in core (rectal) temperature, the women studied in this project shivered less than their male counterparts. This observation is consistent with the early data of Rennie et al. (1962), who, using immersion water temperatures at the lower critical temperature, found that men were better able to tolerate cooler water than women. However, these trends may be partially related to the adiposity of the female sample, since others have shown that women with more subcutaneous adipose tissue, in particular cold-adapted diving women (e.g. Korean Ama), were better able to withstand cooler water than less fat males (Hong 1963), although some part of this latter difference could be ascribed to a greater cold habituation in the diving women (Chapter 21). Confirming that adiposity does not fully explain these data, Kollias et al. (1974) observed that women with a greater adiposity (22%), who were immersed in 20°C water, cooled at much the same rate as leaner men (15% fat). Clearly, some gender-related variations are a function of differences in body composition and morphology, while others await elucidation.

6.3 Physical fitness

Since habitual physical exercise affects the fixed (adipose tissue) and variable insulation (muscle mass and its vascularisation), as well as metabolic activity, it is probable that endurance training may influence cold resistance. During short-term cold air exposures, where exercise-induced heat production is likely to be most beneficial, the ability to work at high intensities increases with physical fitness, thereby supporting thermal homeostasis. However, Keatinge (1961) found that cold-immersed subjects displayed a reduced metabolic response within the first 30 min of an extended exposure, following endurance training. Others have similarly found that cold-exposed, endurance-trained subjects displayed a reduced thermogenic threshold (Dressendorfer et al. 1977, Kollias et al. 1972), while other investigators have reported improved cold tolerance (Jacobs et al. 1984) and an elevated thermoregulatory sensitivity (Bittel et al. 1988). Notwithstanding these disparate outcomes, it may be argued that endurance training increases metabolic efficiency during the early stages of cold exposure and, like some cold-adapted ethnic populations, may facilitate enhanced energy conservation during the more stressful stages of exposure. However, little is known about how improved physical endurance influences cold tolerance when subjects are fatigued, and taken to the point of thermoregulatory failure.

Fatigue is delayed in endurance-trained people (Chapters 6 and 7) and since fatigue might predispose to thermoregulatory insufficiency, it is assumed that increased physical fitness may improve cold tolerance. Unquestionably, the combination of chronic exercise-induced fatigue, food restriction and sleep deprivation lowers cold tolerance due to both an absolute mass (tissue insulation) reduction and a lower thermogenic responsiveness (Young et al. 1998). However, acute fatigue per se has little effect upon either shivering or body cooling, even when evaluated during a 4-h cold-stress test following 5 h of demanding exercise (Tikuisis et al. 1999).

6.4 Exercise and work in the cold

There is abundant evidence that apparently healthy, strong hikers and swimmers can perish when exercising in the cold (Stocks et al. 2004b, Tipton et al. 1999). During exercise, the exposed skin surface area of unclothed subjects is increased, most notably at the joints of active limbs. This is most evident during swimming, and is in marked contrast to the shielding associated with body hunching seen during resting cold stress. In addition, forced convectional currents (absolute or relative) are increased, disturbing the insulating boundary layer and decreasing skin temperature. Muscle blood flow is increased, reducing limb insulation and exacerbating heat loss (sections 2.2 and 4.1.2). These conditions maximise thermal conductance, and if maximal metabolic heat production is less than heat loss, thermal homeostasis is unachievable.

The metabolic cost of exercise increases linearly with work rate during running, cycling and flume swimming. However, oxygen uptake, at a fixed swimming velocity, also varies inversely with water temperature (Nadel et al. 1974),

due to the superimposition of shivering thermogenesis, rather than physical changes in the water. When resting in still water, shivering may be detrimental to heat balance, since it increases muscle blood flow and disturbs the boundary layer of warm water close to the skin surface, thereby increasing (forced) convective heat transfer. However, during swimming, these factors are already maximised and shivering may now facilitate thermal homeostasis by supporting exercise-induced heat production. Indeed, Holmér & Bergh (1974) found a negative linear relationship between core temperature and oxygen uptake during cold-water swimming. That is, as subjects cooled, oxygen uptake (and metabolic heat production) was elevated through shivering, just as it is in resting cold-exposed subjects, although as shivering progresses, the capacity to swim regresses. Recently, it has been shown that, during non-immersed exercise, as subjects become fatigued or food deprived during cold exposure, shivering was unable to prevent heat loss, and there was a metabolic shift towards greater lipid oxidation (Tikuisis et al. 1999, Weller et al. 1998).

Not only does exercise accelerate heat loss but cold exposure may also impair the ability to exercise (Tipton et al. 1999). Several investigators have found that maximal exercise is attenuated when immersed in cool water, following the first observations of Pugh & Edholm (1955). However, Åstrand & Saltin (1961) found that peak aerobic power was not influenced by air temperatures within the range from −5°C to 20°C, although this may not be so under more extreme conditions. For example, Horvath & Freedman (1947) observed static muscle strength reductions of >50% following 3 h at −23°C. Bergh & Ekblom (1979) confirmed this, finding that dynamic strength and power were similarly affected. Since these power reductions during cold immersion were due to decreasing body temperature, it appears that neither maximal exercise nor shivering is obtainable during even mild hypothermic states.

Since the metabolic energy transformation during shivering is added to that associated with exercise, it is of critical importance to know how much heat can be produced via shivering. Several groups have addressed this issue, and two pieces of information are required: the peak and the sustainable shivering rates. Iampietro et al. (1960) found the peak oxygen uptake (shivering thermogenesis) of resting subjects to be five times greater than baseline. More recently, Tikuisis et al. (1999) reported that only a threefold increase in resting oxygen uptake could be sustained during a 4-h, cold-wet air exposure (10°C air, 10°C water spray, wind velocity 1.7 m·s^{-1}). Thus, in the absence of physical activity, maximal shivering will always fall short of the upper limit of peak metabolic heat production, and will rarely exceed 50% of maximal oxygen uptake.

Therefore, thermal homeostasis may be difficult, if not impossible, to attain during moderately stressful resting cold exposures or during exercise (even at peak intensities) at the lower temperature extreme. Indeed, there are even circumstances in which exercise may actually be detrimental to thermal homeostasis. For example, Keatinge (1972) showed that low-intensity exercise may prove disadvantageous for someone immersed in water too cool to achieve thermal equilibrium. At 25°C, exercise failed to retard the core temperature decline, and at 5°C and 15°C, exercise always elevated the rate of heat loss, with core temperatures decreasing faster than at rest. Another key consideration is the mode of exercise. Since the arms are a major site for heat loss, due to a small muscle mass and a larger segmental surface area to mass ratio, some forms of exercise may predispose to more rapid heat loss than others.

In each of the experiments described above, subjects were cooled from a thermoneutral state. Such observations provide little information concerning the sudden cooling of heated people, such as may occur under some occupational settings. Let us first consider this from a theoretical perspective, as it relates to any inanimate object. Preheating acts to modify only the rate of heat loss and not the thermal energy content at the point of thermal equilibrium, or the time it takes to attain this state. That is, if one immerses two bowling balls in cold water (one of which is preheated), they will each attain the same terminal temperature at the same time. The difference is that the heated ball simply loses heat faster. Engineers regard this as self-evident, yet physiologists have not always recognised this fact. These physical principles also apply to humans, with muscle and core temperatures tracking these expectations when both preheated and precooled subjects are exercised in the heat (Booth et al. 2004). Following the removal from cold water, the core temperature of a hypothermic individual will continue to fall, with this thermal afterdrop being elegantly demonstrated using a dead pig model (Golden & Hervey 1977). However, humans also have the capacity to alter insulation and heat loss by changing blood flow to the skin and muscles.

Castellani et al. (1999) exercised and passively heated subjects to the same core temperature, and then rested each in cold air (4.6°C) for 120 min. They found that the exercised subjects cooled more rapidly, presumably via the relatively vasodilated legs, with these subjects experiencing a greater reduction in core temperature. Both of these observations are consistent with the discussion in the paragraph above. It is the final core temperature that is critical, not its rate of change. If heat is lost more rapidly, core temperature will change rapidly. But the same terminal core temperature will eventually be achieved. These observations indicate that the blood volume redistribution towards the cutaneous blood vessels accelerates heat loss, supporting earlier observations of Windle et al. (1994) in subjects immersed in cold water following passive (hot bath) and active warming (exercise).

Two conclusions may be drawn from this section. First, with adequate adipose tissue and the appropriate exercise intensity, body temperature defence is possible, at least within the short term. Second, for adult men immersed in water temperatures <25°C, whole-body exercise is often detrimental to thermal homeostasis. However, the validity of this latter conclusion for people of varying body composition, or women, has not yet been verified.

7 PATHOPHYSIOLOGICAL CONSIDERATIONS

Situations that diminish the ability to generate or conserve thermal energy can lead to thermoregulatory insufficiency, frank hypothermia and tissue damage (Tables 20.1 and 20.2). Excessively cold exposures result in primary (acute) hypothermia, while pathological states and physiological impediments can precipitate secondary (chronic) hypothermia. Epidemiological evidence shows that, between 1979 and 1990, hypothermia caused >9300 deaths in the US (Morbidity and Mortality Weekly Report 1993), while over a similar period hypothermia led to 176 deaths in New Zealand (Taylor et al. 1994). Approximately 65% of UK hospital admissions in winter involve hypothermia (Prescott et al. 1962), whilst in New Zealand (1979–86), people diagnosed with hypothermia accounted for <0.001% of all hospitalisations (Taylor et al. 1994). The very young dominated these data, yet they seldom died from hypothermia. The elderly accounted for almost 70% of all hypothermia-related deaths, with the hypothermia mortality rate being equivalent to that associated with other factors affecting health. Nevertheless, the case–fatality ratio (deaths following hospitalisation) in the aged was three times greater than reported for other medical conditions. Thus, the prognosis for elderly hypothermia patients is less favourable.

The above sections provide a background of knowledge around which one may identify the agents and host factors likely to precipitate accidental hypothermia: age, environment and fatigue. As children are amongst the most susceptible to cooling, they have the greatest risk. They have a high surface area to mass ratio, a low body fat content, a relatively small muscle mass and a low absolute metabolic rate. From an environmental perspective, if the initial exposure is to cold and dry conditions, with a low wind velocity, and people dress accordingly, then such people may well be unprepared for deteriorating weather conditions. A reduction in air temperature combined with rain

Table 20.2 Symptoms and physiological consequences of hypothermia (°C)

Core temperatures	
35–33	Confusion, disorientation, amnesia
33–30	Cardiac arrhythmia, unconsciousness
28–27	Inability to respond to verbal commands, loss of voluntary movement, possible ventricular fibrillation
26–24	Loss of pupillary light reaction and deep tendon reflexes, loss of superficial skin responses and the gag reflex, death or failure to revive
<17	Cerebral electrical activity ceases in some individuals at this temperature

and an increase in wind speed significantly increase the thermal and physical demands of the environment. Exercising into the wind can increase work demand by as much as 40%. Furthermore, the insulative properties of clothing may be degraded under these conditions. Clothing that is not windproof experiences an insulation reduction of ~30% in a wind of 14.5 km·h^{-1}, with a 50% reduction via wetting (if not waterproof), and an 85% decrease in the combination of wind, wetting and locomotion (Pugh 1966). Fatigue is the next host factor. Wind and wet clothing increase the work necessary for locomotion, hastening the onset of exhaustion and hypoglycaemia, and impairing metabolic heat production. Muscle cooling will also decrease muscle performance and metabolic efficiency. Thus, heat production by exercise or shivering is impaired. The inevitable consequence is body cooling, with the strong possibility of hypothermia. These factors have come together on many occasions, often resulting in death from hypothermia, with perhaps the best described being the deaths during the 1964 Four Inns Walk in the UK (Pugh 1964).

7.1 Cold shock

Sudden cold-water immersion provides both severe and immediate stimulation of the cutaneous cold-sensitive thermoreceptors which, in turn, initiate powerful cardiovascular and respiratory changes (Tipton 1989). These responses constitute 'cold shock', and include a gasp response, uncontrollable hyperventilation, hypertension and tachycardia. Cold shock, by acting as a precursor to drowning and cardiac problems, is probably responsible for a large percentage of cold immersion-related deaths.

7.2 Peripheral incapacitation

Skin cooling can result in a series of clinical problems ranging from peripheral pain and loss of tactility to non-freezing and freezing cold injury (section 7.3). As the exposure time increases, the superficial muscles and distal joints become affected, as these tissues cool very quickly due to their relatively large surface area, small muscle mass and minimal heat content. In fact, the principal heat source for these tissues is the blood, with its flow being rapidly reduced, particularly in the acral skin regions, with potentially debilitating consequences.

Cuteneous receptors sensitive to temperature, pressure and touch can lose sensitivity at a local skin temperature of ~5°C. Neural transmission speed of the ulnar nerve is reduced by ~15 m·s^{-1} for every 10°C fall in local temperature, with neural impulses being blocked within 1–15 min when tissue temperatures fall to 5–15°C (Douglas & Malcolm 1955).

Subcutaneous temperatures fall very rapidly during cold immersion, decreasing from 32.9°C to 23.3°C after 10 min in water at 18°C (Zeyl et al. 2004). Forearm muscle temperature falls rapidly at rest, reaching 27°C during a 20-min cold-water immersion (12°C), and in 40 min in water at 20°C (Barcroft & Edholm 1946). Maximal muscle power falls by ~3% for each 1°C fall in tissue temperature, with mechanical efficiency being similarly reduced (Bergh & Ekblom 1979). These changes may be explained on the basis of a contractility impairment due to decreased enzyme activity, decreased perfusion, decreased electrical responses, decreased acetylcholine and calcium release, and increased intramuscular viscosity (Vincent & Tipton 1988).

These muscle and peripheral nerve cooling patterns result in a neuromuscular dysfunction equivalent to peripheral paralysis. Muscle rigidity makes movement difficult. Hands take on a semi-rigid and claw-like appearance. Thus, before hypothermia becomes a generalised problem, peripheral cooling can adversely affect activities involving the hands (dexterity), as well as those that require muscle force generation, such as walking and swimming. In water, these factors may be precursors to drowning.

7.3 Freezing and non–freezing cold injuries

Pathological states associated with peripheral cold injury occur as one approaches the lower limit of thermal homeostasis. These states are due entirely to the protracted exposure to very low tissue temperatures, in the presence of maximal vasoconstriction. Localised peripheral cold injuries are intensity dependent and vary from mild non-freezing tissue damage to tissue freezing, and may occur in the absence of frank hypothermia.

Non-freezing cold injury occurs when tissue temperatures remain below about 17°C for a protracted period, thereby inducing neurovascular damage, but without ice-crystal formation (Bangs & Hamlet 1983). Immobility, posture, dehydration, low physical fitness, inadequate nutrition, constricting footwear, fatigue, stress or anxiety, concurrent illness and physical injuries can all increase the likelihood of developing this form of cold injury. Classically, the condition occurs in the feet (immersion foot, trench foot). It is believed that exposure to a tissue temperature <5°C (41°F) for a period in excess of 30–45 min will produce the requisite conditions for injury to occur. At higher ambient temperatures, the exposure time required to produce injury is proportionately longer, but little information is available to define the risk of injury more precisely.

It is usually on rewarming that the initial indications of injury become apparent. On presentation, there is typically a history of a digit, hand or foot being very cold, ischaemic, numb and pain free for a long period of exposure. Moderate to severe cases present in four stages:

1. during cold exposure (1 day to 1 week): loss of sensation, extremities initially bright red then paler

2. following cold exposure (hours to days): small increase in peripheral blood flow, the extremities become mottled blue, and the injured area is cold and numb with the loss of sensory and motor function, oedema and a weak peripheral pulse

3. postexposure hyperaemia (days to weeks, usually 6–10 weeks): the injured part is hot and flushed with a full peripheral pulse but sluggish microcirculation; there is intense pain as well as oedema and blistering

4. post hyperaemia (weeks to lifelong): the patient has protracted cold-induced vasoconstriction following a cold stimulus, and hyperhidrosis (local increased sweating); both of these can accentuate local cooling (increasing the risk of future cold injury), and there is often also persistent pain.

The majority of those suffering from non-freezing injuries are likely to be symptomatic 6 months after the time of injury, and 10% will still suffer symptoms 5 years after injury. A smaller percentage continue to be symptomatic for the rest of their lives.

The pathogenesis of non-freezing cold injury is unclear but appears to involve prolonged cooling, local ischaemia, hypoxia in the nerves and the liberation of reactive oxygen species during reperfusion. The threshold for injury is more easily achieved if individuals are dehydrated. These factors often co-exist on exposure to cold. In addition, the pathology of non-freezing cold injury is also obscure. Injury to unmyelinated nerve fibres would be most consistent with the clinical symptoms but experimental evidence also indicates that myelinated fibres sustain the greatest damage. The most common observation with regard to the circulation is cold-induced endothelial injury.

The prevention of these cold injuries may be achieved by limiting exposure to cold and maintaining adequate peripheral blood flow. In some scenarios, this may be difficult. During scientific studies at the Institute of Naval Medicine in the UK, the medical withdrawal criterion used to avoid non-freezing cold injury during experiments in the cold is the observation of a local tissue temperature of 8°C for ≥15 minutes, or 6°C at any time. During long-duration exposures to the cold, subjects are withdrawn and slowly rewarmed if any skin temperature falls below 15°C for more than 12 hours.

Freezing injuries (frostnip and frostbite) occur when ice crystals form within cells or the interstitial space. Such freezing is a function of the rate of heat loss, the biophysics of which is dictated by local surface area and mass relationships. However, skin cells are very resistant to freezing and, once frozen, can return to normal function with the appropriate rewarming procedures.

The first symptom of freezing cold injury is numbness. As the superficial tissues freeze they become white, hard and waxy in appearance. Superficial and reversible freezing is called frostnip. It can be identified early by exposed individuals watching out for each other, and can be treated by placing the affected part against a warm area of skin (usually that of someone else). Human tissue freezes at around −0.55°C and, depending on the rate of freezing, intracellular crystals may form (rapid cooling), causing direct mechanical disruption of the tissues. The more common slow cooling and freezing results in predominantly extracellular water crystallisation, and this increases plasma and interstitial fluid osmotic pressure. The resulting osmotic outflow of intracellular fluid raises intracellular osmotic pressure and can cause damage to the capillary walls. This, along with the local reduction in plasma volume, causes oedema and reduced local blood flow, and encourages capillary sludging. These changes can produce thromboses and a gangrenous extremity. The risk of frostbite is low above air temperatures of −7°C, irrespective of wind speed, and can become quite pronounced when ambient temperature is below −25°C, even at low wind speeds.

When the core temperature is still within its normal range, cold-induced vasodilatation may occur within some skin regions. These blood flow oscillations periodically warm the skin by transferring warmer blood from the core to the periphery, minimising the probability of frostbite. Wilson & Goldman (1970) found that, when cold-induced vasodilatation occurred, freezing did not occur, even when one subject experienced local skin temperatures <0°C for 60 min. However, without cold-induced vasodilatation, they found that air temperature, but not wind speed, was the main factor determining the possibility of skin freezing.

References

Allwood MJ, Hensel H, Papenburg J 1959 Muscle and skin blood flow in the forearm during insulin hypoglycaemia. Journal of Physiology (London) 147:269–273

Anderson GS Mekjavic IB 1996 Thermoregulatory responses of circumpubertal children. European Journal of Applied Physiology 74:404–410

Arborelius M, Balldin UI, Lilja B, Lundgren CEG 1972 Hemodynamic changes in man during immersion with the head above water. Aerospace Medicine 43:592–598

Åstrand P-O, Saltin B 1961 Maximal oxygen uptake and heart rate in various types of muscular activity. Journal of Applied Physiology 16:977–981

Banet M, Hensel H, Liebermann H 1978 The central control of shivering and non-shivering thermogenesis in the rat. Journal of Physiology (London) 283:569–584

Bangs C, Hamlet MP 1983 Hypothermia and cold injuries. In: Auerbach PS, Geehr EC (eds) Management of wilderness and environmental emergencies. Macmillan, New York, 27–63

Barcroft H, Edholm O 1946 Temperature and blood flow in human forearm. Journal of Physiology (London)104:366

Bates RE, Bilello MA 1966 Defining the cold regions of the Northern Hemisphere. Technical Report 178. US Army Cold Regions Research and Engineering Laboratory, Hanover, NH

Beckman EL, Reeves E 1966 Physiological implications as to survival during immersion in water at 75°F. Aerospace Medicine 37:1136–1142

Benzinger TH 1970 Peripheral cold reception and central warm reception, sensory mechanisms of behavioral and autonomic thermostasis. In: Hardy JD, Gagge AP, Stolwijk JAJ (eds) Physiological and behavioral temperature regulation. C.C. Thomas, Springfield, IL, 831–855

Bergh U, Ekblom B 1979 Influence of muscle temperature on maximal muscle strength and power output in human skeletal muscles. Acta Physiologica Scandinavica 107:33–37

Bini G, Hagbarth KE, Hynninen P, Wallin BG 1980 Thermoregulatory and rhythm-generating mechanisms governing the sudomotor and vasomotor outflow in human cutaneous nerves. Journal of Physiology (London) 306:537–552

Bittel JHM, Nonotte-Varly C, Livecchi-Gonnot GH, Savourey GLMJ, Hanniquet AM 1988 Physical fitness and thermoregulatory reactions in a cold environment in men. Journal of Applied Physiology 65:1984–1989

Booth JD, Wilsmore BR, MacDonald AD, Zeyl A, Storlien LH, Taylor NAS 2004 Intramuscular temperatures during exercise in the heat following pre-cooling and pre-heating. Journal of Thermal Biology 29(7–8):709–715

Boulant JA 1996 Hypothalamic neurons regulating body temperature. In: Fregly MJ, Blatteis CM (eds) Environmental physiology. Handbook of physiology. Volume 1. Oxford University Press, New York, 105–126

Bowen S 1968 Diver performance and effects of cold. Human Factors 10:445–463

Brink H, Werner J 1994a Estimation of the thermal effect of blood flow in a branching countercurrent network using a three-dimensional vascular model. Journal of Biomechanical Engineering 116:324–330

Brink H, Werner J 1994b Efficiency function: improvement of classical bioheat approach. Journal of Applied Physiology 77:1617–1622

Burton AC 1935 Human calorimetry. II. The average temperature of the tissues of the body. Journal of Nutrition 9:261–280

Cannon B, Nedergaard J 2004 Brown adipose tissue: function and physiological significance. Physiological Reviews 84:277–359

Castellani JW, Young AJ, Kain JE, Rouse A, Sawka MN 1999 Thermoregulation during cold exposure: effects of prior exercise. Journal of Applied Physiology 87:247–252

Clarys JP, Martin AD, Marfell-Jones MJ, Janssens V, Caboor D, Drinkwater DT 1999 Human body composition: a review of adult dissection data. American Journal of Human Biology 11:167–174

Collins KJ, Exton-Smith AN, James MH, Oliver DJ 1980 Functional changes in autonomic nervous responses with ageing. Age and Ageing 9:17–24

Collins KJ, Exton-Smith AN, Dore C 1981 Urban hypothermia: preferred temperature and thermal perception in old age. British Medical Journal 282:175–177

Collins KJ, Easton JC, Belfield-Smith H, Exton-Smith AN, Pluck RA 1985 Effects of age on body temperature and blood pressure in cold environments. Clinical Science 69:465–470

Cunningham DJ, Cabanac M 1971 Evidence from behavioral thermoregulatory responses of a shift in setpoint temperature related to the menstrual cycle. Journal of Physiology (Paris) 63:236–238

Cunningham DJ, Stolwijk JAJ, Wenger CB 1978 Comparative thermoregulatory responses of resting men and women. Journal of Applied Physiology 45:908–915

De Souza MJ, Maresh CM, Maguire MS, Kraemer WJ, Flora-Ginter G, Goetz KL 1989 Menstrual status and plasma vasopressin, renin activity, and aldosterone exercise responses. Journal of Applied Physiology 67:736–743

Douglas WW, Malcolm JL 1955 The effect of localised cooling on conduction in cat nerves. Journal of Physiology (London) 130:53–71

Dressendorfer RM, Smith RM, Baker DG, Hong SK 1977 Cold tolerance of long-distance runners and swimmers in Hawaii. International Journal of Biometeorology 21:51–63

DuBois D, DuBois ER 1916 Clinical calorimeter. A formula to estimate the approximate surface if height and weight be known. Archives of Internal Medicine 17:863–871

Ducharme MB, Tikuisis P 1991 In vivo thermal conductivity of the human forearm tissues. Journal of Applied Physiology 70:2682–2690

Ducharme MB, Brajkovic D, Frim J 1999 The effect of direct and indirect hand heating on finger blood flow and dexterity during cold exposure. Journal of Thermal Biology 24:391–396

Epstein M 1978 Renal effects of head-out water immersion in man: implications for an understanding of volume homeostasis. Physiological Reviews 58:529–581

Epstein M, Pins DS, Sancho J, Haber E 1975 Suppression of plasma renin and plasma aldosterone during water immersion in normal man. Journal of Clinical Endocrinology and Metabolism 41:618–625

Fox RH, Löfstedt BE, Woodward PM, Eriksson E, Werkstrom B 1969 Comparison of thermoregulatory function in men and women. Journal of Applied Physiology 26:444–453

Frank SM, Higgins MS, Fleisher LA, Sitzmann JV, Raff H, Breslow MJ 1997 Adrenergic, respiratory, and cardiovascular effects of core cooling in humans. American Journal of Physiology 272:R557–562

Gale EAM, Bennett T, Green JH, MacDonald IA 1981 Hypoglycaemia, hypothermia and shivering in man. Clinical Science 61:463–469

Gauer OH, Henry JP 1963 Circulatory basis of fluid volume control. Physiological Reviews 43:423–481

Gilbert M, Busund R, Skagseth A, Nilsen PA, Solbø JP 2000 Resuscitation from accidental hypothermia of 13.7°C with circulatory arrest. Lancet 355:375–376

Glickman N, Mitchell HH, Keeton RW, Lambert EH 1967 Shivering and heat production in men exposed to intense cold. Journal of Applied Physiology 22:1–8

Golden FStC, Hervey GR 1977 The mechanism of the afterdrop following immersion hypothermia in pigs. Journal of Physiology 272:26–27

Golja P, Kacin A, Tipton MJ, Mekjavic IB 2004 Hypoxia increases the cutaneous threshold for the sensation of cold. European Journal of Applied Physiology 92:62–68

Granberg PO, Lennquist S, Low H, Werner S 1971 Hormonal changes during cold diuresis. Swedish Journal of Defence Medicine 7:191–202

Grucza R, Pekkarinen H, Hänninen O 1999 Different thermal sensitivity to exercise and cold in men and women. Journal of Thermal Biology 24:397–401

Hajduczok G, Miki K, Claybaugh JR, Hong SK, Krasney JA 1987 Regional circulatory responses to head-out water immersion in conscious dogs. American Journal of Physiology 253:R254–R263

Hardy JD 1954 Control of heat loss and heat production in physiologic temperature regulation. Harvey Lecture 49:242–270

Hayward JS, Collis M, Eckerson JD 1973 Thermographic evaluation of relative heat loss areas of man during cold water immersion. Aerospace Medicine 44:708–711.

Hayward JS, Eckerson JD, Collis ML 1975 Thermal balance and survival time prediction of man in cold water. Canadian Journal of Physiology and Pharmacology 53:21–32

Hensel H 1981 Thermoreception and temperature regulation. Monographs of the Physiological Society number 38. Academic Press, London

Hessemer V, Brück K 1985 Influence of menstrual cycle on shivering, skin blood flow, and sweating responses measured at night. Journal of Applied Physiology 59:1902–1910

Holmér I 1984 Required clothing insulation (IREQ) as an analytical index of cold stress. ASHRAE Transactions 90:1116–1128

Holmér I, Bergh U 1974 Metabolic and thermal response to swimming in water at varying temperatures. Journal of Applied Physiology 37:702–705

Hong SK 1963 Comparison of diving and nondiving women of Korea. Federation Proceedings 28:831–833

Hong SI, Nadel ER 1979 Thermogenic control during exercise in cold environment. Journal of Applied Physiology 47:1084–1089

Horvath SM, Freedman A 1947 The influence of cold upon the efficiency of man. Journal of Aviation Medicine 18:158–164

Iampietro PF, Vaughan JA, Goldman RF, Kreider MB, Masucci F, Bass DE 1960 Heat production from shivering. Journal of Applied Physiology 15:632–634

IUPS Thermal Commission: Commission for Thermal Physiology of the International Union of Physiological Sciences 2001 Glossary of terms for thermal physiology. Japanese Journal of Physiology 51(2):245–280

Jacobs I, Romet T, Frim J, Hynes A 1984 Effects of endurance fitness on responses to cold water immersion. Aviation, Space and Environmental Medicine 55:715–720

Jacobs I, Martineau L, Vallerand AL 1994 Thermoregulatory thermogenesis in humans during cold stress. Exercise and Sports Science Reviews 22:221–250

Janský L, Srámek P, Savlíková J, Ulicný B, Janáková H, Horký K 1996 Changes in sympathetic activity, cardiovascular functions and plasma hormone concentrations due to cold water immersion in men. European Journal of Applied Physiology 74:148–152

Jessen C 1996 Interaction of body temperatures in control of thermoregulatory effector mechanisms. In: Fregly MJ, Blatteis CM (eds) Environmental physiology. Handbook of physiology. Volume 1. Oxford University Press, New York, 127–138

Johnson DG, Hayward JS, Jacobs TP, Collis ML, Eckerson JD, Williams RH 1977 Plasma norepinephrine responses of man in cold water. Journal of Applied Physiology 43:216–220

Kakitsuba N, Mekjavic IB 1987 Determining the rate of body heat storage by incorporating body composition. Aviation, Space and Environmental Medicine 58:301–307

Keatinge WR 1960 The effects of subcutaneous fat and of previous exposure to cold on the body temperature, peripheral blood flow and metabolic rate of men in cold water. Journal of Physiology 153:166–178

Keatinge WR 1961 The effect of repeated daily exposure to cold and of improved physical fitness on the metabolic and vascular responses to cold air. Journal of Physiology (London) 157:209–220

Keatinge WR 1972 Cold immersion and swimming. Journal of the Royal Navy Medical Service 58:171–176

Keatinge WR, Sloan REG 1972 Effect of swimming in cold water on body temperatures of children. Journal of Physiology (London) 226:55–56

Keatinge WR, Coleshaw SRK, Cotter F, Mattock M, Murphy M, Chelliah R 1984 Increases in platelet and red cell counts, blood viscosity and arterial pressure during mild surface cooling: factors in mortality from coronary and cerebral thrombosis in winter. British Medical Journal 289:1405–1408

Kellogg DL 2006 In vivo mechanisms of cutaneous vasodilation and vasoconstriction in humans during thermoregulatory challenges. Journal of Applied Physiology 100:1709–1718

Knight DR, Horvath SM 1985 Urinary responses to cold temperature during water immersion. American Journal of Physiology 248:R560–R566

Kollias J, Boileau R, Buskirk ER 1972 Effects of physical conditioning in man on thermal responses to cold air. International Journal of Biometeorology 16:389–402

Kollias J, Barlett L, Bergsteinová V, Skinner JS, Buskirk ER, Nicholas WC 1974 Metabolic and thermal responses of women during cooling in water. Journal of Applied Physiology 36:577–580

Krasney JA 1996 Physiological responses to head-out water immersion: animal studies. In: Fregly MJ, Blatteis C (eds) Handbook of physiology. Environmental physiology. Volume II. Oxford University Press, New York, 855–888

Lennquist S, Grandberg PO, Wedin B 1974 Fluid balance and physical work capacity in humans exposed to cold. Archives of Environmental Health 29:241–249

Leppäluoto J, Korhonen I, Huttunen P, Hassi J 1988 Serum levels of thyroid and adrenal hormones, testosterone, TSH, LH, GH and prolactin in men after a 2-h stay in a cold room. Acta Physiologica Scandinavica 132:543–548

Lindblad LE, Ekenvall L, Klingstedt C 1990 Neural regulation of vascular tone and cold induced vasoconstriction in human finger skin. Journal of the Autonomic Nervous System 30:169–174

Lossius K, Eriksen M, Walløe L 1993 Fluctuations in blood flow to acral skin in humans: connection with heart rate and blood pressure variability. Journal of Physiology (London) 460:641–655

McArdle WD, Magel JR, Gergley TJ, Spina RJ, Toner MM 1984 Thermal adjustment to cold-water exposure in resting men and women. Journal of Applied Physiology 56:1565–1571

Marion GS, McGann KP, Camp DL 1991 Core temperature in the elderly and factors which influence its measurement. Gerontology 37:225–232

Maw GJ, Mackenzie IL, Taylor NAS 1998 Body-fluid distribution during exercise in hot and cool environments. Acta Physiologica Scandinavica 163(3):297–304

Mekjavic IB, Mittleman KD, Kakitsuba N 1987a The role of shivering thermogenesis and total body insulation in core cooling rate. Annals of Physiology and Anthropology 6:61–68

Mekjavic IB, La Prairie A, Burke W, Lindborg B 1987b Respiratory drive during sudden cold water immersion. Respiratory Physiology 70:121–130

Mekjavic IB, Savic SA, Eiken O 1995 Nitrogen narcosis attenuates shivering thermogenesis. Journal of Applied Physiology 78:2241–2244

Mekjavic IB, Golden FStC, Eglin CM, Tipton MJ 2001 Thermal status of saturation divers during operational dives in the North Sea. Undersea Hyperbaric Medicine 28:149–155

Mekjavic IB, Tipton MJ, Eiken O 2003 Thermal considerations in diving. In: Brubakk AO, Neuman TS (eds) Physiology and medicine of diving, 5th edn. Saunders, New York, 323–357

Mitchell D, Wyndham CH, Atkins AR, Vermeulen AJ, Hofmeyr HS, Strydom NB, Hodgson T 1968 Direct measurement of the thermal responses of nude resting men in dry environments. Pflugers Archives 303:324–343

Morbidity and Mortality Weekly Report 1993 Hypothermia-related deaths: Cook County, Illinois, November 1992–March. Morbidity and Mortality Weekly Report 42:558–560

Morrison JB, Zander JK 2007 The effects of exposure time, pressure and cold on hand skin temperature and manual performance when wearing 3-fingered neoprene gloves. Report CR-2007-164, Defence Research and Development Canada - Toronto

Morrison JB, Conn ML, Hayward JS 1980 Accidental hypothermia: the effect of initial body temperatures and physique on the rate of rewarming. Aviation, Space and Environmental Medicine 51:1095–1099

Nadel ER, Holmér I, Bergh U, Åstrand P-O, Stolwijk JAJ 1974 Energy exchanges of swimming man. Journal of Applied Physiology 36:465–471

Passias TC, Meneilly GS, Mekjavic IB 1996 Effect of hypoglycemia on thermoregulatory responses. Journal of Applied Physiology 80:1021–1032

Pennes HH 1948 Analysis of tissue and arterial blood temperatures in resting forearm. Journal of Applied Physiology 1:93–122

Piazza A, Menozzi P, Cavalli-Sforza LL 1981 Synthetic gene frequency maps of man and selective effects of climate. Proceedings of the National Academy of Science 78:2638–2642

Pierau F-K 1996 Peripheral thermosensors. In: Fregly MJ, Blatteis CM (eds) Environmental physiology. Handbook of physiology. Volume 1. Oxford University Press, New York, 85–104

Pozos RS, Stauffer EK, Iaizzo PA, Mills WJ, Howard D, Israel D 1986 Shivering and other forms of tremor. In: Heller HC, Musacchia XJ, Wang LCH (eds) Living in the cold: physiological and biochemical adaptations. Elsevier, New York, 531–537

Prescott LF, Peard MC, Wallace IR 1962 Accidental hypothermia: a common condition. British Medical Journal 2:1367–1370

Pugh LGCE 1964 Deaths from exposure on Four Inns Walking Competition, March 14–15. Lancet 1:1210–1212

Pugh LGCE 1966 Clothing insulation and accidental hypothermia in youth. Nature 209:1281–1286

Pugh LGCE, Edholm OG 1955 The physiology of channel swimmers. Lancet 2:761–768

Rapp GM 1971 Convection coefficients of man in a forensic area of thermal physiology: heat transfer in underwater exercise. Journal of Physiology (Paris) 63:392–396

Raven PB, Niki I, Dahms TE, Horvath SM 1970 Compensatory cardiovascular responses during an environmental cold stress, 5°C. Journal of Applied Physiology 29:417–421

Ray N, Currat M, Berthier P, Excoffier L 2005 Recovering the geographic origin of early modern humans by realistic and spatially explicit simulations. Genome Research 15:1161–1167

Rennie DW 1988 Tissue heat transfer in water: lessons from the Korean divers. Medicine and Science in Sports and Exercise 20:S177–S184

Rennie DW, Covino BG, Howell BJ, Song SH, Kang BS, Hong SK 1962 Physical insulation of Korean diving women. Journal of Applied Physiology 17:961–966

Richardson D, Shepherd S 1991 The cutaneous microcirculation of the forearm in young and old subjects. Microvascular Research 41:84–91

Roddie IC 1983 Circulation to skin and adipose tissue. In: Shepherd JT, Abboud FM (eds) The cardiovascular system. Volume III. Peripheral circulation and organ blood flow Part 1. Handbook of physiology. American Physiological Society, Bethesda, MD, 285–317

Rowell LB 1974 Human cardiovascular adjustments to exercise and thermal stress. Physiological Reviews 54:75–159

Rowell LB 1986 Human circulation: regulation during physical stress. Oxford University Press, New York

Silva NL, Boulant JA 1984 Effects of osmotic pressure, glucose, and temperature on neurons in preoptic tissue slices. American Journal of Physiology 247:R335–R345

Silva NL, Boulant JA 1986 Effects of testosterone, estradiol, and temperature on neurons in preoptic tissue slices. American Journal of Physiology 250:R625–R632

Slovis CM, Anderson GF, Casolaro A 1989 Survival in a heat stroke victim with a core temperature in excess of 46.5°C. Annals of Emergency Medicine 11:269–271

Stocks JM, Patterson MJ, Hyde DE, Jenkins AB, Mittleman KD, Taylor NAS 2004a Effects of immersion water temperature on whole-body fluid distribution in humans. Acta Physiologica Scandinavica 182(1):3–10

Stocks JM, Taylor NAS, Tipton MJ, Greenleaf JE 2004b Human physiological responses to cold exposure. Aviation, Space and Environmental Medicine 75(5):444–457

Taylor NAS, Morrison JB 1991 Lung volume changes in response to altered breathing gas pressure during upright immersion. European Journal of Applied Physiology 62(2):122–129

Taylor NAS, Morrison JB 1999 Static respiratory muscle work during immersion with positive and negative respiratory loading. Journal of Applied Physiology 87(4):1397–1403

Taylor NAS, Griffiths RF, Cotter JD 1994 Epidemiology of hypothermia: fatalities and hospitalisations in New Zealand. Australian and New Zealand Journal of Medicine 24:705–710

Taylor NAS, Allsopp NK, Parkes DG 1995 Preferred room temperature of young versus aged males: the influence of thermal sensation, thermal comfort, and affect. Journal of Gerontology A: Biological Science and Medical Science 50:M216–M221

Thompson RL, Hayward JS 1996 Wet-cold exposure and hypothermia: thermal and metabolic responses to prolonged exercise in rain. Journal of Applied Physiology 81:1128–1137

Tikuisis P, Bell DG, Jacobs I 1991 Shivering onset, metabolic response, and convective heat transfer during cold air exposure. Journal of Applied Physiology 70:1996–2002

Tikuisis P, Ducharme MB, Moroz D, Jacobs I 1999 Physiological responses of exercised-fatigued individuals exposed to wet-cold conditions. Journal of Applied Physiology 86:1319–1328

Tipton MJ 1989 The initial responses to cold-water immersion in man. Clinical Science 77:581–588

Tipton M, Eglin C, Gennser M, Golden FStC 1999 Immersion deaths and deterioration in swim performance in cold water. Lancet 354:626–629

Vallerand AL, Jacobs I 1989 Rates of energy substrates utilization during human cold exposure. European Journal of Applied Physiology 58:873–878

Veicsteinas A, Ferretti G, Rennie DW 1982 Superficial shell insulation in resting and exercising men in cold water. Journal of Applied Physiology 52:1557–1564

Vincent MJ, Tipton MJ 1988 The effects of cold immersion and hand protection on grip strength. Aviation, Space and Environmental Medicine 59:738–741

Vogelaere P, Savourey G, Deklunder G, Lecroart J, Brasseur M, Bekaert S, Bittel J 1992 Reversal of cold induced haemoconcentration. European Journal of Applied Physiology 64:244–249

Wade CE, Dacanay S, Smith RM 1979 Regional heat loss in resting man during immersion in 25.2°C water. Aviation, Space and Environmental Medicine 50:590–593

Webb PM, Shepard JT 1968 Responses of superficial limb veins of the dog to changes in temperature. Circulation Research 22:737–746

Weller AC, Greenhaff P, MacDonald IA 1998 Physiological responses to moderate cold stress in man and the influence of prior prolonged exhaustive exercise. Experimental Physiology 83:679–695

White MD, Ross WD, Mekjavic IB 1992 Relationship between physique and rectal temperature cooling rate. Undersea Biomedicine Research 19:121–130

Wilkerson JE, Raven PB, Bolduan NW, Horvath SM 1974 Adaptations in man's adrenal function in response to acute cold stress. Journal of Applied Physiology 36:183–189

Wilson O, Goldman RF 1970 Role of air temperature and wind in the time necessary for a finger to freeze. Journal of Applied Physiology 29:658–664

Windle CM, Hampton IFG, Hardcastle P, Tipton MJ 1994 The effects of warming by active and passive means on the subsequent responses to cold water immersion. European Journal of Applied Physiology 68:194–199

Young AJ, Muza SR, Sawka MN, Pandolf KB 1987 Human vascular fluid responses to cold stress are not altered by cold acclimation. Undersea Biomedical Research 14:215–228

Young AJ, Sawka MN, Neufer PD, Muza SR, Askew EW, Pandolf KB 1989 Thermoregulation during cold water immersion is unimpaired by low muscle glycogen levels. Journal of Applied Physiology 66:1809–1816

Young AJ, Castellani JW, O'Brien C, Shippee RL, Tikuisis P, Meyer LG, Blanchard LA, Kain JE, Cadarette BS, Sawka MN 1998 Exertional fatigue, sleep loss, and negative energy balance increase susceptibility to hypothermia. Journal of Applied Physiology 85:1210–1217

Zeyl A, Stocks JM, Taylor NAS, Jenkins AB 2004 Interactions between temperature and human leptin physiology in vivo and in vitro. European Journal of Applied Physiology 92(4–5):571–578

Chapter 21

Physiological adaptation to hot and cold environments

Michael J. Tipton   Kent B. Pandolf   Michael N. Sawka
Jürgen Werner   Nigel A.S. Taylor

1 INTRODUCTION

The 3–4 million-year evolution of humans has been influenced and determined by the environment. The colonisation of the planet from man's origins as a tropical animal of the African or Asian plains was largely complete by 30,000–15,000 BC. These migrations were dependent on the ability to adapt behaviourally and physiologically to the environmental extremes experienced by humans as they moved further from their equatorial origins.

The term adaptation can be defined as changes or adjustments, often hereditary, in the structure or habits of a species or individual that improve its condition in relationship to its environment. In its broadest sense, adaptation can influence all the systems and states of a living organism and, in so doing, is fundamental to survival and prosperity. In this chapter, we focus on human adaptation to hot and cold environments and the integrated physiological responses that accompany these adaptations, resulting in a more effective defence of body temperature in the presence of thermal challenges.

As described in Chapters 18 and 19, humans possess regulatory mechanisms that ensure the stability of the internal environment (homeostasis). The thermoregulatory system contains sensors, signal integrators, effector organs and a communication network designed to regulate body temperature within a narrow range. Significant perturbations in body temperature evoke corrective responses in this system to restore normality. Repeated perturbations evoke adaptations. These minimise the impact of an acute stimulus, enabling the body to cope more effectively with thermal stresses. Humans have a large capacity to adapt anatomically, biochemically, physiologically and psychologically to a broad range of thermal environments. They also possess the intellect to employ technology to modify the thermal environment, returning it to an acceptable (stress-free) state. For example, the oldest building made by homonids (Tanzania) was a windbreak constructed by *Australopithecus* ~3.25 million years ago. Over a million years ago, *Homo erectus* was building huts from stones, branches and furs. The earliest evidence for the use of fire, a source of light and radiant heat, comes from China (600,000 BC), whilst the oldest clothed body yet discovered was that of man who died in Russia about 35,000 years ago (Tipton 1986).

Two conclusions can be drawn. First, the behavioural thermoregulatory capabilities of humans far exceed their physiological capacity to generate and lose heat. If humans had to rely solely on shivering and sweating to maintain body temperature, we would not have ventured far from our equatorial origins. Second, the ability to control the thermal environment removes the stimulus to adapt. So it is that humans in all parts of the globe use clothing and buildings to maintain their mean skin temperature at ~33°C, a temperature we find comfortable (Fanger 1973), recreating our equatorial thermal profile. This ability to manipulate the macro- and microclimate has had a greater impact on the perceived potential for humans to adapt to cold compared to heat. Because it is easier and cheaper to stay warm (wear clothing, build a fire) than cool (air conditioning), there is no debate about the existence of a physiological adaptation to heat in humans; it has been well researched and consistently described. In contrast, debate still abounds concerning the nature, and even the existence, of human adaptation to the cold.

2   PRINCIPLES OF ADAPTATION

2.1   Phenotypic and genotypic adaptation

Physiological adaptations may take the form of inherited (genotypic) or acquired (phenotypic) variations in the morphological (anatomical) and functional (physiological) status of the individual. The former is invariably indistinguishable from the latter (Lagerspetz 2006), yet both result in advantageous variations in physiological functions (polymorphism). The emphasis in this chapter is upon thermally induced phenotypic adaptation, expressed through the reversible modifications of the morphological configuration (e.g. sweat gland size, thickness of subcutaneous adipose tissue) or functional changes in effector organ control that occur (e.g. the threshold and gain of the shivering response). These thermal adaptations can occur in response to the naturally occurring, broad spectrum of environmental changes (acclimatisation), to deliberate artificial thermal exposures (acclimation) or to changes in body temperature, induced through changes in metabolic heat production (the sum of metabolic rate and external work, e.g. endurance training; Chapter 19; IUPS Thermal Commission 2001).

Positive and negative forms of adaptation may be observed, such that the acute responses to a stress application can appear to be either potentiated or blunted (habituated). A classic example of a negative adaptation is evident in the blunted metabolic reaction of Australian Aborigines to cold stress (Hicks & Matters 1933), where shivering thermogenesis was found to be less pronounced than observed in non-adapted Europeans, during an equivalent cold exposure. It is often thought that heat adaptation elicits only positive phenotypic trends (Duncan & Horvath 1988, Wyndham et al. 1964), as evident in the amplification of the sweating response. However, this is not necessarily correct, with many years of heat exposure producing an habituated sweat response (Taylor 2006).

There are two causes for the confusion that abounds within the field of human cold adaptation. First, the interchangeable and imprecise use of the terms acclimation, acclimatisation, habituation and their translations. Second is the requirement, in some definitions, for the changes in physiological function to be beneficial in order to qualify as an adaptation. The problem here is that some adaptations can be beneficial in one context, but detrimental in another. Again, an example is the habituation of the shivering response seen with repeated exposure to cold. This is beneficial, in that it decreases substrate utilisation and improves thermal comfort and the ability to perform fine motor skills, but detrimental in that it can accelerate the rate at which deep body (core) temperature declines during cold exposure. Thus, the same response may be regarded as an adaptation or maladaptation, depending on the circumstance.

2.2   Functional and morphological adaptation

The components of the body that passively accept thermal changes induced by the environment and muscle activity, as described by the physical laws of heat transfer (Werner 1998), are called the passive (thermal or controlled) system (Figure 21.1). When the core temperature is ~37°C, there is no functional activation of the thermoregulatory effector mechanisms (Chapters 19 and 20). However, thermal disturbances (exogenous or endogenous) transfer the thermal energy of this passive system from one steady state to another. This new state is detected by spatially distributed thermosensitive tissues (thermoreceptors; Chapter 19), providing feedback to parts of the central nervous system that play an active role in the regulation of mean body temperature. Collectively, these structures make up the active (regulatory) system (Figure 21.1), since they activate and control thermoeffector mechanisms (metabolic rate (or energy transformation), sweating, vasomotor activity) to reduce mean body temperature deviations (cold and heat defence mechanisms). Thus, we regulate body temperature by controlling (modulating) thermoeffector function.

The neuronal outputs of the regulatory system, in response to a thermal disturbance, are transformed into heat gains or heat losses within the passive system, compensating, at least partially, for the disturbing thermal inputs from the environment and muscle. This compensation is achieved through a regulatory loop, in which the mean thermal energy content of the passive system (mean body temperature) is regulated via the modulation of thermoeffectors, under the influence of the active system; the acute thermoregulatory responses (Werner 2005; Chapter 18).

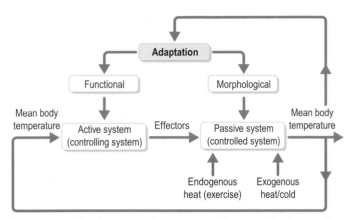

Figure 21.1 The thermoregulatory control loop and its interaction with long-term thermal adaptation.

A higher level of thermoregulatory system performance is evident within longer-term thermal adaptations (Figure 21.1) which, as a consequence of persistent or repetitive stresses, alter either the physical properties of the passive system (morphological adaptation) or the operational characteristics of the active system (functional adaptation). Such adaptations, in general, increase the efficiency of the regulatory system, with acclimatisation being strongly determined by behavioural mechanisms and acclimation relying more or less exclusively on adjustments of physiological (autonomic) control. The remaining discussion in this section is confined to the acclimation processes.

Morphological adjustments typically affect the properties of the passive system, and alter heat exchanges between the body core, body shell (skin) and the environment. For example, long-term adjustments of the peripheral circulatory system, development of the fat layer and (in many animals) a change of fur insulation are all forms of morphological adaptation. In addition, adaptive changes in the basal metabolic or evaporative rates (e.g. sweat gland hypertrophy) and of heat capacity should also be attributed to morphological alterations, since they are present even if the regulatory mechanisms are not activated.

The most commonly demonstrated functional effect of acclimation is a change in the effector threshold (Chapter 18), meaning that the body temperature at which an effector mechanism is activated is shifted down or upwards. This adaptation seems to play a dominant role during adaptation. However, another functional adaptation is a change of the gain (sensitivity) factor transforming the overall sensory input into an effector signal (Chapter 18). That is, for a given thermal stimulus, acclimated individuals frequently display increased thermoeffector gain, e.g. a greater sweating response (slope) for an equivalent change in body temperature. Another possible functional adjustment could result from a change in the weightings of the core and cutaneous sensory inputs. It is generally considered that the decisive input signal to the central temperature regulator is a composite of core and skin thermoafferent signals,

weighted in an approximately 9:1 (up to 8:2) ratio. However, an adjustment of the impact of the core relative to peripheral signals during acclimation has not been clearly demonstrated to date.

Analyses such as those described above take place at the macroscopic system level, and many efforts have been devoted to the question of their neurophysiological and pharmacological correlates (Werner 1994). These may be found at the sensory, central integrative or thermoeffector levels. Some evidence has been gathered that threshold and gain (sensitivity) changes may be traced back to ionic and transmitter processes of central neuronal networks. This analysis has been restricted to the effects demonstrated in adult humans, so the problems of non-shivering thermogenesis in brown adipose tissue, which are of great importance for the neonate human and also for some adult animal species, cannot be taken into account.

The phenomenology of adaptive effects covers an extremely wide spectrum, with many observations revealing real or apparent discrepancies, leading sometimes to confusion and debate. One reason for this is that experimental procedures used for adaptation may be widely variable. As thermal adaptation is a long-term process, it is difficult to precisely determine when the postadaptive steady state occurs. Thus, studies demonstrating postadaptation differences may refer to very different phases of the adaptation process (continuum), which themselves depend strongly on variations in the acclimation protocol such as: the form and combination of stresses (e.g. external temperature, humidity, wind speed, exercise, posture, clothing), the intensity of stresses, the time course and duration of stresses (continuous, intermittent, constant, variable) and a wide range of individual factors (responsiveness), not to mention the many problems induced by using different or inadequate measuring techniques. Some of these issues are discussed in the next two sections.

2.3 Adaptation theory

The capacity of any stress to induce adaptation is a function of its application frequency, duration, intensity and variability (Adolph 1964), superimposed upon the genetic, phenotypic and physiological status of the individual (section 1, Introduction). These variables can be combined to quantify the tendency for a series of stimulus applications to elicit an adaptation: the cumulative adaptation impulse (stress volume; Equation 1). This derivation is a modification of the training impulse model (Banister & Calvert 1980), and can be viewed as the sum of the products of the changes in body temperature and the corresponding exposure duration of each stimulus. This concept provides a very useful, albeit simplistic way in which one may compare variations in stimuli and their presentation.

Equation 1:   Adaptation impulse $= ((T_{b-1} - T_{b-0}) \cdot t_1) + ((T_{b-2} - T_{b-0}) \cdot t_2) + ((T_{b-i} - T_{b-0}) \cdot t_i)$ [°C·min]

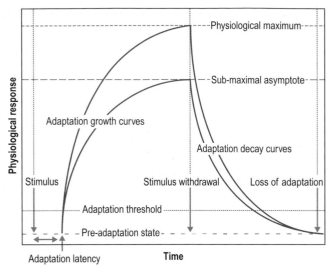

Figure 21.2 Adaptation theory: physiological changes following the application and withdrawal of an adaptation stimulus. From Taylor & Cotter (2006), reproduced with permission.

where:

T_{b-N} = mean body temperature at time N [°C]
T_{b-0} = initial (time zero) mean body temperature [°C]
t_N = duration of each stimulus [min].

Since humans contain numerous interdependent regulatory systems, often sharing common effector organs, physiological adaptations will vary across stimuli, and even within an adaptation stimulus. For example, repeated exposure to hot-dry or hot-humid conditions will elicit similar, but not identical adaptation trends.

The time course of adaptation may be described using a combination of curvilinear growth and decay curves (Figure 21.2), from which six general characteristics may be identified (Adolph 1964). First, a stimulus must exceed a critical threshold before adaptation can be induced. For instance, stimuli that fail to disturb homeostasis also fail to evoke either acute corrective adjustments or physiological adaptation. Second, while acutely applied stimuli evoke immediate responses, a phase delay (latency) always occurs before physiological adaptations become evident. Third, for each effector organ affected by the stimulus, there is a physiological and possibly a genetically determined maximum, beyond which there is considerable adaptation resistance. Fourth, the speed of tissue, organ or systemic adaptations varies broadly within (Armstrong & Maresh 1991) and among individuals. Fifth, optimal adaptation results when the cumulative adaptation impulse is maximised, whilst simultaneously ensuring that the overall physiological strain remains within tolerance limits. It is well established that people respond at different rates to equivalent adaptation stimuli (i.e. low, moderate and high responders). Typically, the higher the background adaptation of the individual, the lower will be the adaptation response. Sixth, once repeated application of the adaptation stimulus ends, there is the gradual reversal (decay) of the morphological and functional adaptations.

2.4 Physiological forcing functions

All organisms are in a state of dynamic equilibrium, with the thermal environment constantly undergoing energy exchanges. Acute changes in thermal stress, of either external (exogenous) or internal (endogenous) origin, can disturb the body surface and internal environments. Such disturbances are called forcing functions, and can vary in form (e.g. steady state, square-wave (step), ramp (linear), sinusoidal), size, frequency and duration.

It is well established that the dynamics of physiological responses do not match that of the stimulating forcing function. This provides an opportunity for researchers to investigate regulatory mechanisms that modulate effector structures. Just as acute physiological responses are dictated by the characteristics of the forcing function, physiological adaptations are also tightly linked with characteristics of the adaptation stimulus. For example, conventional acclimation regimens involve moderate-to-heavy exercise in a temperature- and humidity-controlled chamber. However, the cumulative adaptation impulse can be modified independently of climatic conditions, by changing the external work rate. Three exercise forcing functions are typically used (Taylor 2000): (a) constant work-rate regimens (Pandolf et al. 1988), (b) self-regulated exercise regimens (Armstrong et al. 1986b) and (c) controlled-hyperthermia regimens (Fox et al. 1961). Each method induces heat adaptation and each affects the same physiological systems. However, the nature of these adaptations varies, and the reason for this variability lies within the thermal potency of the different methods.

To illustrate the potential impact of thermal forcing function differences, consider two 12-day adaptation regimens (constant work-rate regimens and controlled-hyperthermia), both of which used exercise in the heat (90 min·d⁻¹). Each method aimed to elevate core temperature to 38.5°C. Constant work-rate regimens achieve this by setting the required work rate on day 1; this is then held constant for 12 days. Such regimens produce a gradual rise towards the target core temperature (Figure 21.3A; Taylor & Cotter 2006), since the initial exercise intensity is then sustained for 90 min. However, since adaptation, by definition, progressively reduces the physiological impact of the forcing function, then the adaptation stimulus decreases over successive exposures, as indicated by the fall in the cumulative core temperature (inset). The controlled-hyperthermia protocol rapidly elevates body temperature using higher intensity exercise, where it is then clamped. This is repeated during successive exposures (Figure 21.3B). Thus, as adaptation progresses, the external work rate used to clamp core temperature is increased, resulting in the adaptation stimulus being higher and more stable (Figure 21.3A versus 21.3B inset).

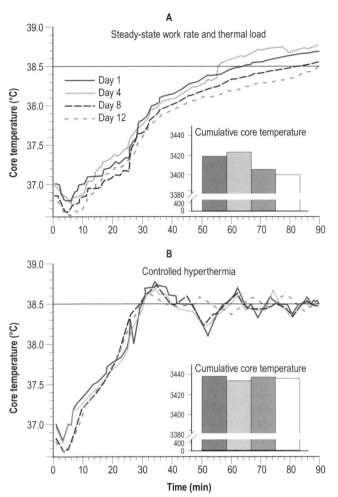

Figure 21.3 Core temperature changes accompanying two, 12-day heat acclimation regimens using the constant work rate (A) and controlled-hyperthermia methods (B). Insets show daily integrated core temperature data. From Taylor & Cotter (2006), reproduced with permission.

Both of these regimens result in physiological adaptation and both have useful applications. One method targets a specific work rate, while the other targets a thermal load. However, since physiological systems adapt to the specific nature of the adaptation stimulus, both regimens can invoke qualitatively similar, yet quantitatively different adaptations. These differences can be illustrated by comparing acclimation-induced expansions of the plasma volume. This is an early adaptive response, mediated either by reduced plasma protein loss (Harrison 1985, Senay 1972) or greater extracellular electrolyte retention (Patterson et al. 1999). Plasma volume enlargement is generally considered to wane with repeated heat exposures (Bass et al. 1955, Wyndham et al. 1968). However, this tendency is only evident when constant work rate functions are used. When a controlled-hyperthermia function is used, this expansion can be sustained along with the entire extracellular fluid volume, for at least 3 weeks (Patterson et al. 2004a). If one considers that this adaptation facilitates cardiovascular sta-

bility and the maintenance of the osmotic potential of the blood, then these divergent trends may conceivably impact upon other simultaneously occurring adaptations, and therein lies the significance of understanding the forcing function driving adaptation.

3 ADAPTATION TO COLD

3.1 An overview of cold–adaptive response patterns

One of the criticisms of the definitions of acclimatisation and acclimation is that they refer to the stimuli to which an individual is exposed, rather than the adaptive responses. As a consequence, some authors have included reference to adaptive responses in their definitions of the cold-adapted state. Scholander (1960), for example, emphasised the ability to sleep in a cold environment as a defining characteristic of cold adaptation. Eide (1973) concluded that the most precise and meaningful way of defining adaptation is in terms of thermoregulatory homeostasis, seeing adaptation as the process securing or facilitating homeostatic regulations.

Based on the heat balance equation, Hammel (1964) suggested that humans could, in theory, adapt to cold in three ways. Body temperature could be allowed to fall (hypothermic adaptation), insulation could be increased (insulative adaptation) or heat production could be elevated (metabolic adaptation). Thus, hypothermic acclimatisation would be obtained in the field and characterised by a greater fall in body core temperature on subsequent cold exposures. This approach therefore describes both the stimulus to adapt and the response.

A striking feature of cold adaptation research is that one can find examples of each of Hammel's adaptation options within the literature. The reasons for this are probably more methodological than physiological, since the ability of humans to avoid the cold means that studies investigating human cold adaptation have, by necessity, been somewhat fragmented and diverse. These have included field- and laboratory-based experiments involving a broad spectrum of subjects (e.g. ethnic populations, athletes, military personnel, explorers). They have used seasonal variations in the response to cold as well as long- and short-term exposures to air and water (Figure 21.4). Studies in the field have not always been confined to cold exposure, but have often been accompanied by alterations in diet, physical fitness and light/dark cycles, all of which can influence the thermoregulatory response to cold. The problem is that increases in fitness or protein content in the diet can mimic metabolic adaptation changes (Adams & Heberling 1958). Increased fitness can also mimic hypothermic adaptation (Baum et al. 1976). Loss of circadian cues can mimic hypothermic adaptation (Moore-Ede 1983), and non-freezing cold injury and sleep deprivation can mimic peripheral adaptation to cold (Brown et al. 1954).

It is therefore impossible to reach a definitive characterisation of human cold adaptation merely on the basis of observations from studies investigating that condition. An alternative possibility, and one that avoids the confusion or masking of the adaptive response created by the variety of the methods employed to induce adaptation, is that the nature of the adaptation itself varies depending on other factors pertaining at the time (e.g. nutritional, metabolic).

In addition to the confusion surrounding these definitions, there is also the uncertainty that arises from the separate examination of the functional compared to morphological adaptations. Let us look at the two apparently incompatible, but not unrealistic observations: cold adaptation evokes a lower metabolic rate and (consequently) a lower mean body temperature; and cold adaptation evokes a lower metabolic rate but (nevertheless) a higher mean body temperature. Both apparently contradictory statements are true, if the first refers to functional adaptive effects, and the second to morphological effects.

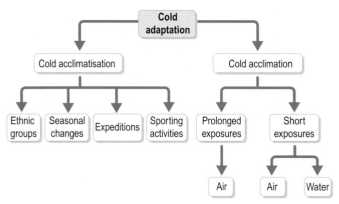

Figure 21.4 The range and types of experiments conducted within the field of human cold adaptation.

This paradox can be explained using Figure 21.5, and may require an understanding of the principles detailed within Chapter 18. In an open-loop thermoregulatory system, where heat loss is prevented, mean body temperature would increase with increments in metabolic heat production. This is illustrated in Figures 21.5A and B by unbroken lines with positive slopes that describe the relationship between metabolic heat production and mean body temperature (passive system), although these relationships are not necessarily linear. The thermoregulatory (active) system responds to falling body temperatures by increasing heat production, represented by unbroken lines with negative slopes (and horizontal tails). These interrelationships (positive and negative lines) are the only necessary requirement for negative feedback control, and the only metabolic and thermal steady state possible under these conditions, for closed-loop operation, is determined by the points of intersection of these unbroken lines and shown by the horizontal and vertical lines that are extended to each axis (Figures 21.5A and B). This is because it is the only state that fulfils the requirements of both subsystems.

Figure 21.5A deals exclusively with morphological adaptation, in the form of a better insulation, represented by a right and downward shift (I) of the positive sloping line to the position occupied by the broken line. If metabolic rate did not change (broken horizontal line), the temperature of the passive system would rise. However, a steady state can now only be achieved if the regulating system reduces metabolism (M) as dictated by the point of intersection between the unchanged characteristic of the regulatory (active) system and the changed (broken) characteristic of the passive system. Thus, the new state (after morphological adaptation) is inevitably characterised by a higher body temperature (T) in spite of decreasing metabolic rate.

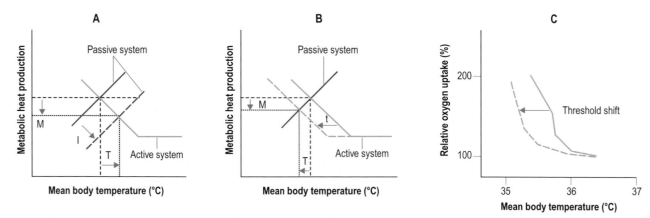

Figure 21.5 The consequences of morphological (A) and functional (B) cold adaptation on the relationship between metabolic heat production and mean body temperature. Reduced heat production is accompanied in case A (morphological adaptation increasing tissue insulation) by a higher body temperature. In case B, following the functional adaptation in graph C, reduced heat production produces a lower body temperature. Unbroken lines are applicable to the preadaptation state and broken lines to the postadaptation state. Graph C shows a cold-acclimated subject (6 d), before and after acclimation: 100% = initial resting level. Data extracted from Bruck et al. (1976).

On the other hand, if there was only a functional adaptation (Figure 21.5B), in the form of a reduced body temperature shivering threshold (t), the characteristics of the regulating system move to the broken line, and the new state would necessarily mean a lower body temperature (T) because of a lower metabolic rate (*M*).

Finally, if both morphological and functional adaptations are simultaneously present, there may be no change of body temperature at all. So, a class of very different observations may be explained by variations in the proportional contributions of the morphological and functional adaptations within a person, following repeated cold exposures.

3.2 Cold adaptation: evidence from ethnic groups

Australia is the hottest continent, yet inland night temperatures fall to <5°C (frequently <0°C) in winter. This environment imposed a significant thermal stress upon the traditional inhabitants (Aborigines), who slept unclothed between small fires. Under such conditions, unadapted Caucasians elevate metabolic rate and reduce skin blood flow. However, the Aborigines were observed to rely more heavily upon energy-efficient vasomotor changes, appearing to defend body temperature primarily by increasing peripheral tissue insulation (Hammel et al. 1959, Hicks & Matters 1933, Scholander et al. 1958). These classic responses are illustrated in Figure 21.6.

The Aboriginal lifestyle was characterised by cycles of feast and famine, possibly favouring those who possessed a relatively low metabolic rate (Neel 1962). People with this genotype have a propensity to store fat, using it during periods of famine. It is possible that protracted geographic isolation, in combination with lifestyle and a unique environment, may have resulted in the natural selection of those possessing a metabolically efficient genotype, and a less intense shivering response. That is, the metabolically conservative cold response may constitute a characteristic of a thrifty genotype (Chapter 28).

The literature contains many examples of cold adaptation across indigenous populations (Eskimos: Rodahl 1952; Kalahari Bushmen: Wyndham & Morrison 1958; Negroes: Adams & Covino 1958; Andean Indians: Elsner 1963), yet two groups appear unique (Australian Aborigines: Hicks & Matters 1933; Alacaluf Indians: Hammel 1961), both of which are believed to possess the thrifty gene(s). When compared with similarly stimulated, non-adapted Caucasians, the metabolic rate of the Aborigine was found to remain relatively constant, while skin temperatures decreased and core temperature slowly declined (Figure 21.6; Hammel et al. 1959, Hicks & Matters 1933). These responses were consistent with an habituated metabolic response (negative adaptation) and a sustained cutaneous vasoconstrictor reaction (hypothermic-insulative adaptation).

However, an acute cold challenge to traditional Kalahari Bushmen was found to elicit a metabolic response similar

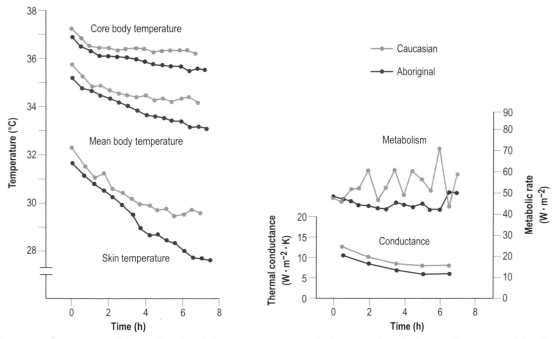

Figure 21.6 The thermal responses of Australian Aborigines and Caucasians during an 8-h, naked cold-air exposure (sleeping; 5°C). Modified from Hammel et al. (1959) with permission.

to that of Caucasians (Ward et al. 1960), yet their lifestyle and thermal environment were very similar to those of the Australian Aborigines. These divergent observations have been interpreted to reveal a possible genetic interaction with these cold-induced responses. However, such an explanation is not totally convincing. The fact that habituated metabolic response, once believed unique to Australian Aborigines, can readily be induced in Caucasians (Golden & Tipton 1988, Stocks et al. 2001) suggests that it may simply be attributable to physiological adaptation, and not necessarily to phylogenetic differences.

Mammals increase insulation at the skin surface during winter by increasing subcutaneous adipose tissue deposits or thickening the fur. Humans modify peripheral insulation behaviourally using clothing. Insulation may also be modulated morphologically (adipose tissue) and physiologically, through changes in skin blood flow. However, there is no evidence for a greater subcutaneous adiposity in traditional Australian Aborigines (Webster 1974). Thus, reduced skin temperatures and thermal conductance observed during cold stress (Hammel et al. 1959) are consistent with a more powerful cutaneous vasoconstriction. Such a vascular response supports nicely the habituated metabolic response by facilitating heat conservation. However, it is inconsistent with vasomotor habituation. Indeed, repeated local and whole-body cold exposures may result in an habituated vasoconstrictor response (LeBlanc 1978, Radomski & Boutelier 1982). The failure to observe such a vascular habituation in Aborigines may imply a genetic interaction, which Hammel (1964) suggested was 'a characteristic of the . . . race'.

Three lines of evidence support this proposition. First, there are no apparent seasonal differences in the thermoregulation of Aborigines (Scholander et al. 1958). Second, significant differences in thermal homeostasis were not apparent between coastal (tropical) and central (desert) groups (Hammel et al. 1959). Finally, individuals who were studied years after adopting the European lifestyle still displayed a powerful insulative (vascular) response (Scholander et al. 1958). Collectively, these observations led Hammel (1964) to conclude that the thermal responses of Aborigines were a function of race and attributable to a separate evolutionary development; this view has remained largely unchallenged.

Whilst these racial differences in thermoregulation are consistent with this hypothesis, they do not implicitly substantiate the case for genetic divergence, and should perhaps be viewed with caution. When these classical studies were performed, limited experimental control and standardisation procedures were used. For example, none of these studies controlled for, or matched the current or past nutritional status of the subjects. Only limited standardisation was attempted for preexperimental differences in morphological or functional adaptation. Furthermore, the observation of a reduced cutaneous thermal conductance in Aborigines (Hammel et al. 1959) has been challenged. Young (1996) postulated that these differences may simply have been due to a lower core temperature, associated with an habituated metabolic response, and may not necessarily represent a true vascular response.

It is entirely possible that the Australian Aborigines only differed in their thermoregulatory responses because they were well adapted to their environment. That is, a genetically determined insulative response may not have existed. Instead, they, like the Alacaluf Indians, may have acquired a metabolic, phenotypic adaptation in response to their unique lifestyle and environment.

3.3 The nature of human adaptation to cold

The response that has been reported most frequently in studies involving humans and animals without significant brown adipose tissue is a hypothermic adaptation, characterised by an habituated metabolic response, a faster fall in deep body temperature and, in humans, increased thermal comfort (Bittel 1987, Brück et al. 1976, Golden & Tipton 1988). In most of these studies there is also evidence of a reduction in skin blood flow.

The change observed in the thermogenic response appears to be a downward shift in the shivering threshold, rather than a change in its sensitivity (Brück et al. 1976, Rees et al. 2002). It also appears that the adaptation of this response is specific to the core temperatures experienced during adaptation (Rees et al. 2002). That is, when an acute cold stress causes core temperature to fall to a lower level than experienced during adaptation, then the metabolic response returns to that evident when unacclimated. This applies regardless of whether the greater decline in core temperature results from a longer exposure (Rees et al. 2002) or the absence of exercise (Golden & Tipton 1987). Interestingly, this recent finding now supports the previously unsupported hypothesis of Hicks & O'Connor (1938), proposed following their work with Australian Aborigines. Thus, it may be concluded that the blunted (habituated) shivering response accompanying hypothermic adaptation would not remain attenuated once core temperature fell beyond that experienced during adaptation, and would certainly not be sustained to the point of death.

One special environment is worthy of note, and that is cold water. Because of the cooling power of water, skin temperature is rapidly reduced and clamped close to water temperature. With immersion, this rapid skin temperature reduction produces a set of responses collectively known as the cold-shock response (Tipton 1989) that is not seen on sudden exposure to cold air. The response includes an immediate, yet transient loss of respiratory control, evidenced by a reduced breath-hold time and hyperventilation (hypocapnia), as well as tachycardia and hypertension. Interestingly, as few as five 2-min immersions in cold water are sufficient to reduce the respiratory and cardiac responses by about 50%, with the responses still being reduced by 25% 14 months after the initial period of acclimation (Tipton et al. 1998b, 2000). It appears that the site of this habituation is central to the cutaneous cold receptors (Tipton et al. 1998a).

4 ADAPTATION TO HEAT

Humans have a remarkable ability to adapt to heat, both morphologically and functionally, and given adequate water and solar protection, a heat-acclimated person can tolerate extended exposure to virtually any naturally occurring hot-weather condition (Sawka et al. 1996, Wenger 1988). These adaptations involve integrated changes in cardiovascular, body fluid and thermal regulation. Throughout this section, the terms heat acclimation and heat acclimatisation will be used interchangeably; both methods elicit similar biological adaptations (Wenger 1988). Historically, however, more scientific effort has been focused on the time course and mechanisms for the acquisition of human heat acclimation than its retention or decay (Pandolf 1998).

4.1 Heat adaptation: evidence from ethnic groups

In hot climates, air temperature approaches and exceeds skin temperature (~33°C), thus minimising or reversing dry heat loss (Chapter 19) and leaving evaporative cooling as the principal avenue for heat dissipation. Adaptation to such climates is classically associated with a reduction in physiological strain (core temperature and heart rate) during heat exposure and a greater sweat secretion. Our focus will be directed towards possible differences in sweat gland (sudomotor) function and skin blood flow in indigenes from hot climates.

Sweating, particularly in hot dry climates, may challenge fluid homeostasis. Since natural selection generally favours adaptations that optimise efficiency, we shall first explore the possibility that a reduction in metabolic rate is a more effective way to help maintain thermal balance. Such a change could result from a frank reduction in basal metabolic rate or merely accompany a lower body mass.

Since dry heat exchanges are the most efficient manner through which to dissipate heat, then morphological configurations that maximise the surface area for a given mass are well suited to heat tolerance. For humans, this equates with a lower body mass. Bergmann (1847) observed that some species show an inverse relationship between body mass and environmental temperature. While many species do not conform to this principle (Feist & White 1989), due to morphological adaptations (Scholander et al. 1950), Roberts (1953) found evidence consistent with this generalisation in humans across 116 indigenous groups (18,000 individuals) from ten geographical regions (six continents). Of course, whilst such differences could result from natural selection, gross seasonal changes within an individual would not occur. However, it is possible, across ethnic groups, that genetic factors dictate morphological configurations, with some groups varying markedly from others. Indeed, energy-efficient configurations may have favoured selection and heat tolerance, and in such groups, the predominant ethnic adaptation to heat may have been morphological rather than functional. With this possibility in mind, the data of Roberts (1953) were reanalysed (Table 21.1; Taylor 2006), and are presented now as surface areas and surface area to mass ratios, normalised to that of the regional group with the largest values. Notwithstanding the impact of diet on mass, it is clear that indigenes from the hottest regions also had the largest surface area to body mass ratios.

There is some evidence that humans experience seasonal changes in basal metabolism (Mason & Jacob 1972, Vallery-Masson et al. 1980, Wilson 1956). However, we do not have a clear understanding of the differences among ethnic groups. Whilst a 5% reduction in basal metabolic rate would really only be of benefit under resting conditions, such a change could result in a reduced mean body temperature.

Table 21.1 Morphometric characteristics of indigenous people from 10 different geographical regions, derived using data from Roberts (1953) (from Taylor 2006 with permission)

Region	Mass (kg)	Height (m)	Surface area (m^2)	Surface area (%)	SA/Mass (m^2·kg^{-1})	SA/Mass (%)
South Asia	46.1	1.57	1.43	76	0.031	100
Africa	51.6	1.62	1.53	81	0.030	96
America	59.6	1.53	1.54	82	0.026	84
East Mongolia	53.8	1.62	1.56	83	0.029	94
Melanesia	55.6	1.60	1.57	84	0.028	91
India	54.1	1.68	1.60	85	0.030	95
Australia	55.0	1.69	1.62	87	0.030	95
Central Asia	64.7	1.64	1.70	91	0.026	85
Europe	66.1	1.71	1.77	94	0.027	86
Polynesia	75.9	1.71	1.88	100	0.025	80

SA, surface area. *Note:* America includes indigenous South American and Eskimo people.

Such temperature reductions accompany heat acclimation (Buguet et al. 1988, Patterson et al. 2004b, Vallery-Masson et al. 1980), but the underlying mechanisms have not been determined and very little support exists for ethnic differences. For instance, Buguet et al. (1988) reported no apparent difference when Negroid subjects and Caucasians were compared, whilst Rising et al. (1995), in a very well-controlled investigation, showed that the sleeping core temperature of Pima Indians was significantly lower than that of matched Caucasians.

Since physical activity can elevate metabolism several-fold, then differences in metabolic efficiency could have a powerful effect upon heat production, and adaptation-induced changes in muscle metabolism may be of considerable benefit. Enhanced efficiency of muscle metabolism appears to accompany exercise-heat adaptation (Jooste & Strydom 1979, Sawka et al. 1983a), with substrate metabolism apparently favouring greater lipid oxidation (King et al. 1985). Very few investigations have focused on ethnic differences in muscle metabolism during exercise. Nevertheless, Coetzer et al. (1993) observed a greater fatigue resistance, while Weston et al. (2000) found a greater metabolic efficiency in Negroid endurance athletes. The observation of a greater skeletal muscle oxidative capacity in an untrained Negroid sample (Suminski et al. 2000) is consistent with the possibility of ethnic differences in muscle metabolism, but a large part of this puzzle is missing.

Once body temperature crosses the sudomotor threshold, sweating commences (Chapter 18). Heat adaptation lowers this threshold (Collins et al. 1965, Roberts et al. 1977), reflecting a centrally mediated regulatory modification (Armstrong & Stoppani 2002). Indeed, both basal and threshold temperatures appear to be equally reduced following adaptation (Patterson et al. 2004b). However, only one report has adequately addressed racial differences in this threshold (Fox et al. 1974). This group studied two New Guinean ethnic groups, from hot-humid and cool-dry climates, in comparison with two Caucasian samples (heat acclimatised and unacclimatised). Sudomotor threshold differences were not observed among the acclimatised groups, but were significantly lower in both indigenous groups, relative to the unacclimatised Caucasians. Thus, while this topic remains largely unexplored, it appears that the central control of sweating does not differ between indigenes from New Guinea and Caucasians.

The capacity of the sweat system is a function of the number of eccrine sweat glands and the ability to optimally activate these glands over time (sustainable sweat rate), with morphological and functional adaptations independently affecting sweat capacity. While short-term heat adaptation does not elevate the number of active sweat glands (Inoue et al. 1999), genetically determined differences in gland numbers could provide a thermoregulatory advantage in hot climates. However, with the exception of two studies using Asian samples (Hwang & Baik 1997, Toda 1967), the literature does not support the existence of racial differences in sweat gland counts (Taylor 2006).

Heat adaptation enhances individual sweat gland flow, yet evaporative cooling is only slightly increased, particularly in Caucasian males (Mitchell et al. 1976). Nevertheless, low sweat rates during heat stress are reported indicators of incomplete heat adaptation (Duncan & Horvath 1988, Wyndham et al. 1964). This may represent a misinterpretation of the literature, since there is ample evidence to show that indigenous people from hotter climates are actually conservative sweaters (e.g. Edholm et al. 1964, Fox et al. 1974, McCance & Purohit 1969, Thompson 1954). Indeed, lower sweat rates may represent thermoregulatory habituation and perhaps indicate superior adaptation.

This phenomenon was postulated by Glaser & Whittow (1953), then observed by Thompson (1954) and Fox et al. (1974), with Hori et al. (1976) suggesting that long-term heat exposure, at least within Asians, may result in sudomotor habituation. Candas (1987) proposed that sudomotor habituation represents the third (longer-term) phase of heat adaptation. This may occur through a time-dependent attenuation of the sudomotor response, or it may be an adaptation that optimises efficiency, thus relying more heavily upon heat dissipation via the most efficient means. The latter would be more evident in people with a greater surface area to mass ratio, and perhaps occurs independently of race. Recently, Bae et al. (2006) have provided evidence to show an increased sudomotor efficiency in Asians during prolonged heat adaptation.

Consider the morphological configurations in Table 21.1 and the apparent relationship with climate. Indigenes from the hottest regions had the largest surface area to body mass ratios. This configuration is well suited to dry heat exchanges, permitting a reduced need for evaporative cooling. First-principles calculations to derive the required evaporative heat loss (E_{req}: Chapter 19), enable prediction of the physiological impact of these morphological differences. When resting in air at 35°C (70% relative humidity) with a skin temperature of 33°C, the required evaporative cooling for the Asian sample is about 205 watts; for Caucasians, it is 265 watts. This is a 22% lower reliance upon evaporative cooling.

In the heat, skin temperatures become more uniform, first reflecting heat gain from the environment, then cutaneous vasodilatation. This temperature change reduces exogenous heat gain, while simultaneously increasing water vapour pressure at the skin surface and enhancing evaporation. In a resting person (air temperature 35°C, 70% relative humidity), a rise of 1°C in skin temperature (33–34°C) reduces the required evaporative heat loss by about 35%, independently of morphological configuration.

Thompson (1954) reported significantly higher skin temperatures and lower sweat rates in Negroid subjects relative to Caucasians, when exercising in the heat; both groups had almost identical surface area to mass ratios. Fox et al. (1974) measured skin (hand) blood flow in two groups of indigenous New Guineans, in comparison with two Caucasian samples (as described above). They found the indigenes to have an approximately 50% lower skin blood flow than the unacclimatised Caucasians. More recently, Katsuura et al. (1993) observed that Japanese people born and raised in the tropics had a significantly lower forearm blood flow during heated exercise than native Japanese from the same ethnic group. These independent observations follow an energy-efficient insulative response. The reduction in skin blood flow allows the skin temperature to rise, buffering heat gains and elevating evaporation. This represents an ideal physiological adaptation to the hot-humid environment in which they live.

4.2 Heat acclimation: its induction, retention and decay

4.2.1 Inducing heat acclimation

Pioneering work in the 1940s advanced our early understanding of the heat acclimation process and its retention or decay. From three classical publications (Bean & Eichna 1943, Eichna et al. 1945, Robinson et al. 1943), descriptive conclusions were made concerning the time course of heat acclimation and the incidence of heat syncope. The acquisition time course for heat acclimation was about the same for hot-dry and hot-humid conditions (Eichna et al. 1945, Robinson et al. 1943), with ~80% of the adaptive responses and improvements in performance occurring during the first 7 days of a 23-day acclimation period (Robinson et al. 1943). Heat acclimation began on the initial day of exposure, progressed rapidly during the next 2–4 exposure days, and was virtually complete after 7–10 days (Eichna et al. 1945). Brief periods of physical exercise were necessary (60–90 min·d^{-1}), but some acclimation occurred during rest in the heat (Eichna et al. 1945, Robinson et al. 1943). Physically fit men acclimated faster than less fit men, in both dry and humid heat (Bean & Eichna 1943, Eichna et al. 1945, Robinson et al. 1943). Cardiovascular adaptations from heat acclimation resulted in a decreased incidence of heat syncope after the first day of exposure (Bean & Eichna 1943). The classical adjustments during heat acclimation involving exercise were a lowered heart rate, reduced skin and core temperatures and sometimes a potentiated sweating response, while tolerance to exercise in the heat was markedly improved (Bean & Eichna 1943, Eichna et al. 1945, Robinson et al. 1943).

The more recent literature has refined our understanding of human heat acclimation, while focusing on the underlying mechanisms (Pandolf & Young, 2000, Sawka et al. 1996, Wenger 1988). These functional adaptations depend largely on the severity, duration, frequency and number of heat exposures (section 2.3). Physical exercise in the heat is still the most effective method for developing heat acclimation.

However, even resting in the heat can result in limited acclimation (Taylor 2000, Taylor & Cotter 2006). Full development of exercise-heat acclimation need not involve daily 24-h exposure. A continuous, daily, 100-min exposure appears to produce optimal heat acclimation in dry heat (Lind & Bass 1963). Studies examining heat acclimation have generally used daily heat exposures; however, this is not necessary to produce heat acclimation. For example, Fein et al. (1975) studied the time course of adaptation to a total of 10 days of heat exposure, with subjects exposed either daily (10 days) or every third day (27 days). Both programmes were equally effective.

During the first heat exposure, physiological strain peaks, with large elevations in core temperature and heart rate. Strain gradually abates with each day of acclimation. Through daily exercise in the heat, most of the improvements in heart rate, skin and core temperatures and sweat rate are achieved during the first 7 days of exposure (Sawka et al. 1996). The reduction in heart rate develops most rapidly (4–5 days) as cardiovascular stability improves, being virtually complete after 7 days. Most of the improvements in skin and core temperature also occur during this time, with the thermoregulatory benefits from heat acclimation being ~75% developed after the first week, and are generally thought to be complete after 10–14 days of exposure (Sawka et al. 1996, Wenger 1988). However, other authors (Pandolf 1998, Pandolf & Young 2000) suggest that nearly complete exercise-heat acclimation for hot-dry or hot-humid conditions occurs after 7–10 days of exposure. Some authors further suggest that competitive athletes who expect to take part in an event involving heat stress should train in the hot condition for at least 5 days prior to the event to help maximise their performance (Taylor & Cotter 2006).

These observations largely represent functional adaptations, and can be described using Figure 21.7. As for Figure 21.5, the mean body temperature and evaporative heat loss before adaptation are defined by the intersection of the unbroken lines of the passive and regulating systems. The broken line for the regulating system represents the downward (leftward) shift of the body temperature sweating threshold (t). A reduction in skin blood flow is represented by an upward and rightward shift of the passive system characteristics (B). Following acclimation, a lower skin blood flow is frequently, though not always, reported, in spite of a downward shift of the vasodilatation threshold, due to the reduction in body temperature with acclimation. A lower blood flow without a sweat threshold change would result in a higher body temperature. However, when a lower skin blood flow occurs concomitantly with a sweat threshold reduction, mean body temperature is reduced (T). Thus, the point of intersection of the two broken lines is consistent with most experimental results: higher evaporative heat loss (E) and lower body temperature. The overall benefit is a lower body heat content and reduced cardiovascular strain.

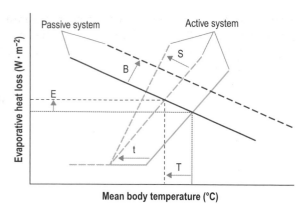

Figure 21.7 Functional heat adaptation in humans: relationships for the active (regulating) and passive (controlled) systems. Unbroken lines are for the preadaptation state and broken lines for the postadaptation state. The two adaptive effects result in greater evaporative heat loss (E) and a lower mean body temperature (T_b).

4.2.2 Retention/decay of heat acclimation

Between 1943 and 1963, eight publications exist on heat acclimation retention or decay, of which half examined hot-dry exposure (range 40–49°C, 15–25% relative humidity; Bean & Eichna 1943, Henschel et al. 1943, Lind & Bass 1963, Robinson et al. 1943) and half examined hot-humid exposure (range 33–42°C, 50–96% relative humidity; Adam et al. 1960, Eichna et al. 1945, Stein et al. 1949, Wyndham & Jacobs 1957). Unfortunately, most of this research is flawed by very small samples, inappropriate heat acclimation procedures or poor measurement techniques (Pandolf 1998). Nevertheless, the collective observations from these early publications are pioneering, indicating that retention/decay differs dramatically among individuals and between hot-dry or hot-humid conditions (Pandolf 1998). For instance, retention of the benefits of heat acclimation seem to remain longer for physically fit individuals and for those exposed to hot-dry conditions (Pandolf 1998).

Heat acclimation is transient and gradually decays or disappears if not maintained by additional exercise-heat exposures (Sawka et al. 1996). The heart rate improvement, which develops most rapidly, is also lost most rapidly (Pandolf et al. 1977, Williams et al. 1967). However, there is little agreement concerning the rate of decay or loss of heat acclimation (Pandolf 1998, Sawka et al. 1996).

For example, Lind (1964) believed that heat acclimation might be retained for 2 weeks after the last heat exposure, and then rapidly lost over the next 2 weeks. In contrast, Williams and colleagues (1967) report significant loss of hot-humid acclimation in sedentary men after 1 week, with the percentage loss being greater with increasing time. By 3 weeks, losses of 92% for heart rate and 45% for core temperature were observed. However, following dry-heat accli-

mation, Pandolf et al. (1977) observed non-significant losses in fit young men for both heart rate and core temperature, with decay periods of 6, 12 and 18 days in cool conditions.

These last two studies seem to further support the possibility that the retention of heat acclimation benefits remains longer for dry compared to humid heat. Williams et al. (1967) did not evaluate the aerobic fitness of their subjects, while Pandolf et al. (1977) concluded that aerobic fitness was a major factor explaining the slight decay, even after 18 days. Thus, physically trained and aerobically fit persons may retain heat acclimation benefits longer than relatively unfit counterparts (Pandolf et al. 1977). Recently, Saat and colleagues (2005) exercise-heat acclimated fit young men to hot-humid conditions, evaluated acclimation retention after 14 days in cool conditions, and reported apparent non-significant losses for both heart rate and core temperature. The mean maximal oxygen uptake of both subject groups was identical (49.5 mL·kg^{-1}·min^{-1}; Saat et al. 2005, Pandolf et al. 1977), providing further support for the importance of aerobic fitness in acclimation retention. Based on the collective literature, competitive athletes should expect to retain the benefits of exercise-heat acclimation for at least 1 week, but probably less than 1 month after being heat acclimated (Pandolf 1998). This is presumably due to the benefits associated with repeated core temperature elevation accompanying endurance exercise, even under cool conditions (section 4.3).

4.2.3 Reinduction of heat acclimation

Much less has been published about the reinduction of heat acclimation, as compared to its initial acquisition or its retention and decay. Wyndham & Jacobs (1957) acclimated 73 men for 12 days to humid heat, observing that core (oral) temperature was elevated after 6 days in cool conditions (acclimation decay). However, after just one reacclimation day, core temperature was significantly reduced towards its final acclimation value. Williams and colleagues (1967) concluded that the practical implication of this was that 1 day of reacclimation was necessary for individuals who had not exercised in hot-humid conditions for 1 week.

Pichan and colleagues (1985) studied reinduction of heat acclimation in 12 young men after 21 days in cool conditions, preceded by 8 days of dry-heat acclimation, while Saat et al. (2005) evaluated reinduction of eight young men after 14 days in cool conditions, preceded by 14 days of humid-heat acclimation. Both groups reported that 3 days of reacclimation were necessary to regain full heat acclimation status.

Finally, Strydom et al. (1975) acclimated 21 men for 8 days to hot-humid conditions, with subjects then placed in cool conditions for 4 weeks, except for 4 h of exercise-heat exposure every seventh day. These authors concluded that, after these 4 weeks, subjects were still adequately heat acclimated. Even though core temperatures and heart rates were significantly higher, sweat rates did not differ from, final acclimation values.

4.3 Impact of aerobic fitness

Endurance training in temperate climates reduces physiological strain and increases exercise capabilities in the heat, with endurance-trained individuals showing many of the characteristics of heat-acclimated individuals (Armstrong & Pandolf 1988, Sawka et al. 1996). Also, aerobically fit persons seem to develop heat acclimation more rapidly than less fit persons, and high aerobic fitness might reduce susceptibility to heat illness (Gardner et al. 1996). Figure 21.8 displays observations from different hot climates (hot-humid (A); hot-dry (B)) and shows that maximal oxygen uptake (aerobic power) can explain ~42–46% of the variability in core temperature after 3 h of exercise in the heat (A), or the acclimatisation day at which a plateau is attained for core temperature (Armstrong & Pandolf 1988).

Figure 21.9 contrasts the impact of an endurance-training programme with heat acclimation on physiological strain (core temperature and heart rate) during an exercise-heat stress (4 h at ~30–35% maximal oxygen uptake; Cohen & Gisolfi 1982). After an initial (pretraining) exercise-heat test,

six women completed an interval training programme in temperate conditions (22°C) and then repeated the exercise-heat test. Finally, subjects were exercise-heat acclimated for 8 days. Endurance training lowered physiological strain and increased endurance time, but these improvements were modest compared to those achieved through heat acclimation, which facilitated core temperature stability. Thus, high aerobic fitness, achieved through endurance

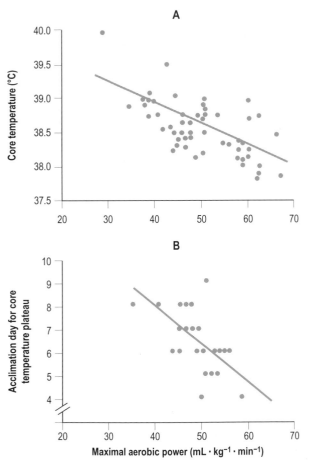

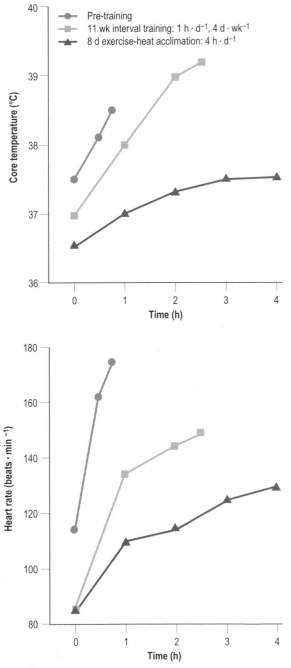

Figure 21.8 The relationship between maximal aerobic power and core temperature in a hot–humid environment (A), and between maximal aerobic power and the acclimation day at which a plateau in core temperature was attained during a dry–heat exposure (B). Adapted from Armstrong & Pandolf (1988) with permission.

Figure 21.9 Core (rectal) temperature and heart rate responses of young women during a standardised exercise-heat exposure (45°C, 33% relative humidity), in three states: untrained and unacclimated; interval trained; heat acclimated. Redrawn from Cohen & Gisolfi (1982).

training, only partially acclimatises individuals to the heat (Armstrong & Pandolf 1988, Pandolf 1998).

For endurance training to improve thermoregulatory responses during exercise in the heat, training must first produce a substantial increase in core temperature and sweating rate (Hessemer et al. 1986). Henane and colleagues (1977) compared thermoregulatory responses of aerobically fit skiers with those of equally fit swimmers, finding the former were more heat tolerant and better acclimatised. Differences were attributed to a smaller increase in the swimmers' core temperature and negligible sweating during training. In support, Avellini et al. (1982) observed that 4 weeks of cycle-exercise training in 20°C water increased aerobic power by 15% but did not improve thermoregulation during exercise-heat stress. Thus, high aerobic power per se is not always associated with improved exercise-heat tolerance.

4.4 Adaptive actions and physiological mechanisms

Table 21.2 and Figure 21.10 summarise the adaptive actions of human heat acclimation, improving thermal comfort and submaximal exercise performance in the heat. The benefits of heat acclimation are achieved by a reduced core temperature, improved sweating and, in some cases, an increased skin blood flow, better fluid balance and improved cardiovascular stability, and a lower metabolic rate. No single mechanism can explain this adaptive process, as heat acclimation results from the interplay of many physiological mechanisms (Pandolf & Young 2000).

4.4.1 Exercise performance
Heat-induced reductions in maximal aerobic power are not affected by heat acclimation (Sawka et al. 1985). Furthermore, heat acclimation does not change the maximal core temperature a person can tolerate during exercise in the heat (Nielsen et al. 1993, 1997). However, persons who live and train over many weeks in the heat may be better able to tolerate higher maximal core temperatures (Sawka et al. 2001). In addition, athletes who excel in hot-weather competition may also be able to tolerate higher core temperatures (González-Alonso et al. 1999, Pugh et al. 1967).

In contrast, heat acclimation markedly improves submaximal exercise-heat performance, with acclimated subjects easily completing tasks that were previously difficult or impossible. Figure 21.11 illustrates this improvement in subjects attempting 100 min of treadmill walking (49°C, 20% relative humidity) on 7 consecutive days (Pandolf & Young 1992). No subjects completed the task on the first day, 40% were successful by day 3, 80% by day 5 and all but one was successful by the seventh acclimation day.

It is worth noting that a psychological component (mental preparation) of improved performance in the heat has recently been reported by Barwood et al. (2006). These authors found that subjects were able to run >1 km further (8% increase) in the heat over 90 min following psychological skills training, but in the absence of heat adaptation.

4.4.2 Sweating
Eccrine sweat rate is usually increased by the second day of heat acclimation (Eichna et al. 1950, Nielsen et al. 1997, Strydom et al. 1966), with earlier and greater sweat rates generally improving evaporative cooling. Such increases result from a rise in the steady-state sweat rate (Libert et al. 1983), increased sudomotor sensitivity and a reduced mean body temperature threshold for sweating (sudomotor threshold; Figure 21.10; Nadel et al. 1974, Patterson et al. 2004b). However, whilst such increases are advantageous for sedentary people with a low maximal sweat rate (high responders), it is rarely so for endurance-trained people, who typically possess very high sweat rates. Indeed, evaporative cooling is not determined by sweat rate, but the maximal evaporation permitted by the environment and clothing (microclimate; Chapter 19), with sweat rates in excess of ~500 mL·h⁻¹ representing wasteful fluid loss even

---

Table 21.2 Actions of exercise-heat acclimation (adapted from Sawka & Young 2000)

Thermal comfort – improved	Exercise performance – improved
Core temperature – reduced	Cardiovascular stability – improved
Sweating – improved Earlier onset Higher rate Hidromeiosis resistance (tropical)	Heart rate – lowered Stroke volume – increased Blood pressure – better defended Myocardial compliance - improved
Skin blood flow – increased Earlier onset Higher flow	Fluid balance – improved Thirst – improved Electrolyte loss – reduced Total body water – increased
Metabolic rate – lowered	Plasma volume – increased and better defended

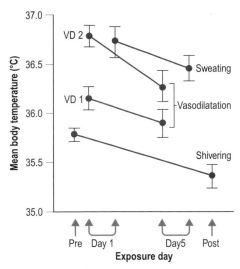

Figure 21.10 Concurrent threshold temperature shifts for all thermoregulatory effector reactions, during a 5-day heat adaptation stimulus ($N = 7$). The shivering threshold was determined 1 d before and 1 d after acclimation. Two vasodilatory relationships are indicated: sympathetic release (VD 1) and active vasodilatation (VD 2). Modified after Hessemer et al. (1986) with permission.

in warm, moderately humid conditions. Mitchell et al. (1976) described much of this additional secretion as extravagant, finding that a 30% elevation in sweat rate increased evaporation by only ~10%.

Heat adaptation also produces morphological changes, in the form of eccrine sweat gland hypertrophy (Sato & Sato 1983). In Figure 21.7, this is illustrated by an upward shift of the passive system characteristic (B; previously used to illustrate a change in skin blood flow). Now, for a given body temperature, there is greater sweat secretion and potentially superior evaporative cooling.

It was once considered that heat adaptation universally resulted in a redistribution of sweat secretion towards the limbs (Höfler 1968). Recently, using five simultaneously measured local sweat rates, Patterson et al. (2004b) demonstrated that this was not correct, at least for hot-humid conditions. Whilst whole-body sweat rate increased significantly over 22 days, not all skin regions exhibited equivalent sweat rate elevations. For instance, forearm sweat rate increased 117%, far exceeding changes at the forehead (47%) and thigh (42%), but was equivalent to changes observed at the scapula (85%) and chest (106%). Thus, these data did not support the hypothesis of a generalised and preferential trunk-to-limb sweat redistribution following heat acclimation.

Functional changes can also occur at the glandular level, increasing cholinergic sensitivity and sweat secretion (Chapters 18 and 19; Sato et al. 1990), and shown as a shift

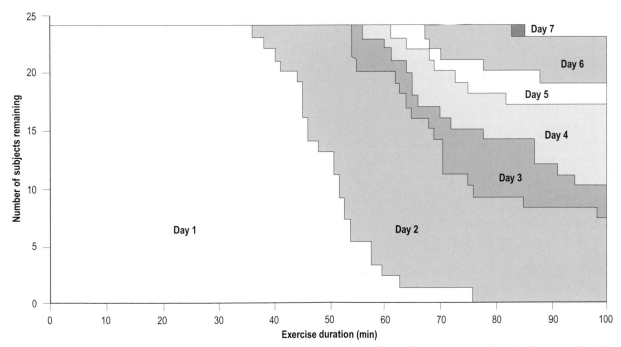

Figure 21.11 Day-to-day improvements in exercise-heat tolerance of young men ($N = 24$) participating in a dry-heat acclimation programme (49°C, 20% relative humidity). Adapted from Pandolf & Young (1992) with permission.

to the unbroken, steeper positive line (S; Figure 21.7). This occurs without recruiting more sweat glands (Inoue et al. 1999, Peter & Wyndham 1966, Sargent et al. 1965); however, these glands now reabsorb more sodium and chloride (Allan & Wilson 1971).

As a result of these morphological and functional changes, the non-adapted sweat rate (1–1.5 L·h^{-1}) can be doubled, with quite prolific sweating observed in some elite athletes (3.5 L·h^{-1}; Armstrong et al. 1986a). The sweat glands also become resistant to hidromeiosis (water accumulation on the skin; Candas 1987) and fatigue, particularly in tropical conditions, so that higher sweat rates can be sustained. These changes reduce body heat storage and skin temperature. Indeed, the resting, thermoneutral mean body temperature is lower following acclimation (Patterson et al. 2004b). Many of these adaptations also accompany endurance training, even in cool-temperate climates, but are less evident than those elicited through similar training in the heat.

Lower skin temperatures decrease the cutaneous blood flow needed for heat balance, due to a greater core-to-skin temperature gradient. Thus, a greater blood volume is redistributed from the peripheral to central circulation. All of these factors help reduce cardiovascular strain and enhance exercise-heat tolerance (Sawka et al. 1996, Wenger 1988).

4.4.3 Cardiovascular stability

On the first day of exercise-heat acclimation, heart rate is much higher and stroke volume is lower than in temperate conditions at the same exercise intensity (Sawka et al. 1996, Wenger 1988). Thereafter, the heart rate elevation during exercise-heat stress begins to abate. These changes are initially rapid but continue more slowly for about 5 days. Many mechanisms are involved during acclimation and their relative contributions will vary, both during acclimation and among individuals (Sawka et al. 1996, Wenger 1988). These mechanisms include improved skin cooling and a more effective redistribution of blood volume (Sawka & Coyle 1999); plasma volume expansion (Patterson et al. 2004a, Senay et al. 1976); increased venous tone from cutaneous and non-cutaneous beds (Wood & Bass 1960); and reduced body temperature (Patterson et al. 2004b, Sawka et al. 1996). Myocardial adaptations observed in rats include increased myocardial compliance (Horowitz et al. 1986b) and isoenzyme transitions, both of which reduce myocardial energy cost (Horowitz et al. 1986a).

Heat acclimation effects on stroke volume and cardiac output responses to exercise-heat stress are less clear. Two studies (Rowell et al. 1967, Wyndham et al. 1968) show increased stroke volume with little change in cardiac output, as heart rate decreased with heat acclimation. Wyndham (1951) reported a less pronounced elevation in exercising cardiac output, as heart rate decreased with little change in stroke volume. Another study (Wyndham et al. 1976) reported a mixed response pattern, with two subjects showing a steady increase in stroke volume, one subject a

transient increase, reversing after the sixth day, and another no increase with heat acclimation. The reasons for these differences are not immediately evident. One possibility might be that Rowell et al. (1967) used dry-heat acclimation, while Wyndham (1951) and Wyndham et al. (1968, 1976) used humid-heat acclimation. For an equivalent metabolic demand and air temperature, humid heat represents a greater thermal load (forcing function), since less heat can be dissipated via evaporation.

Nielson and colleagues (1993, 1997) studied stroke volume responses during exercise before and after heat acclimation. In one study (Nielsen et al. 1993), they acclimated subjects for 9–12 days to hot-dry conditions during cycling exercise. Exercise-heat acclimation increased stroke volume and cardiac output (~1.8 L·min^{-1}). In another study, Nielsen et al. (1997) acclimated subjects for 8–13 days to hot-humid conditions (cycling). Acclimation did not alter stroke volume or cardiac output, yet both studies showed a plasma volume expansion of 9–13% with acclimation. It seems possible that dry- and humid-heat acclimation can increase stroke volume, but that an improved cardiac output is more likely with dry-heat acclimation.

4.4.4 Metabolism

Heat acclimation can alter both whole-body (Sawka et al. 1996) and muscle metabolism (Young 1990), with some evidence demonstrating seasonal changes in basal metabolism (Hori 1995, Mason & Jacob 1972, Vallery-Masson et al. 1980, Wilson 1956). Oxygen uptake responses to submaximal exercise are reduced (greater efficiency) following exercise-heat acclimation (Jooste & Strydom 1979, Sawka et al. 1983a), with substrate metabolism apparently favouring greater lipid oxidation (King et al. 1985). For example, both King et al. (1985) and Kirwan et al. (1987) observed 40–50% reduction in exercise-related muscle glycogen utilisation following acclimation. Similarly, Young et al. (1985) have shown a significant glycogen-sparing effect; this was small and seen only during exercise in cool conditions. Such changes are consistent with a lower lactate accumulation in blood and muscle during submaximal exercise after heat acclimation (Febbraio et al. 1994).

4.4.5 Fluid balance and blood volume

Heat acclimation improves fluid balance due to a better matching of fluid consumption to body water needs, reduced sweat sodium losses, increased total body water and increased blood volume (Mack & Nadel 1996, Sawka & Coyle 1999). Heat acclimation improves the relationship of fluid consumption to body water needs so that voluntary dehydration is markedly (~30%) reduced (Bean & Eichna 1943, Eichna et al. 1950). Thus, heat-acclimated persons are able to maintain hydration state during exercise in the heat, provided that access to fluids is not restricted. This is an important adaptation since heat acclimation increases sweating, thereby elevating fluid replacement requirements to sustain euhydration.

An unacclimated person may secrete sweat with a sodium concentration of ~60 meq·L^{-1} or higher and, if sweating profusely, can lose large amounts of sodium. With acclimation, sodium is conserved, and sweat concentration can be as low as 10 meq·L^{-1}. This salt-conserving effect depends upon aldosterone, which is secreted in response to exercise-heat exposure and sodium depletion. The conservation of salt also helps maintain the number of osmotically active particles in the extracellular fluid, and sustaining or increasing extracellular fluid volume (Nose et al. 1988).

Most studies report that heat acclimation increases total body water (range 2–3 L or ~5–7% of total body water; Sawka & Coyle 1999). However, the relative contribution of the intracellular fluid and extracellular fluid volumes to this elevation varies among studies. The plasma volume is also expanded (Patterson et al. 2004a, Sawka & Coyle 1999), with increments ranging up to 30% being related to the adaptation stimulus (rest versus exercise), the acclimation day and hydration state (Sawka 1988). For example, this expansion seems to be greatest during upright exercise on about the fifth day of heat acclimation, and when fully hydrated (Sawka & Coyle 1999). As a result, heat-acclimated persons show a more stable plasma volume and a more consistent intracellular fluid response during an exercise-heat stress than unacclimated individuals (Sawka 1988).

It is generally considered that this plasma volume expansion will subside as adaptation proceeds (Bass et al. 1955, Wyndham et al. 1968), primarily representing an early adaptation phase that is not sustained (Senay et al. 1976). However, such observations are more a function of the adaptation stimulus, in this case a constant work-rate forcing function, than they are a description of a physiological adaptation. As discussed in section 2.4, this rise and fall in plasma volume does not occur when the controlled-hyperthermia protocol is used. Patterson et al. (2004a) measured intra- and extravascular body fluid compartments in 12 resting males before, during (day 8) and after a 3-week (day 22) exercise-heat acclimation stimulus. On days 8 and 22, the extracellular fluid and plasma volumes were expanded and maintained. These data illustrate that acclimation-induced plasma volume expansion can be sustained using small but progressive increments in the adaptation stimulus. In addition, this volume expansion was not selective, but represented a general expansion of the entire extracellular compartment.

The total body water increase can be attributed, at least in part, to an elevated aldosterone secretion or renal sensitivity to aldosterone. Francesconi et al. (1983) reported that, while an exercise-heat exposure elevates plasma aldosterone concentration, this elevation is abated by heat acclimation. This observation is consistent with an increased renal sensitivity, since sodium retention is enhanced at both the kidneys and sweat glands (Allan & Wilson 1971, Finberg & Berlyne 1977). However, it may also be explained on the basis of a plasma volume expansion, reduced physiological strain associated with a constant-load forcing function or a lower sensitivity of the adrenal cortex to its stimulating hormone.

Similarly, the mechanism(s) responsible for hypervolaemia also remain unresolved, but may include expansion of the extracellular fluid compartment, mediated by either increased crystalloid retention (mainly sodium chloride) and an increase in plasma volume, selectively mediated by the oncotic effect of intravascular protein (Mack & Nadel 1996, Mack et al. 1997). Recent evidence contests the latter possibility, showing that both the interstitial fluid and vascular compartments are equivalently expanded following heat adaptation (Patterson et al. 2004a).

4.5 Dry–heat versus humid–heat comparisons and cross–acclimation

Although dry-heat acclimation confers an advantage in humid heat, the biophysical differences between dry and humid conditions (Chapter 19) lead one to expect that the more stressful humid-heat acclimation would produce different physiological adaptations from dry-heat acclimation (Sawka et al. 1996). There is, however, a paucity of research that has focused on this topic.

To achieve high evaporative cooling rates in humid conditions, it is essential to overcome the high ambient water vapour pressure, either by elevating cutaneous water vapour pressure (requiring a higher skin temperature; Chapter 19) or increasing the wetted skin surface area. Unless core temperature is allowed to rise with skin temperature, a high skin temperature must be reached by increasing core-to-skin thermal conductance, which requires a greater skin blood flow. Thus, one difference between humid-heat and dry-heat acclimation is that the former involves greater circulatory adaptations to support high skin blood flow with minimal circulatory strain.

Fox et al. (1967) compared the effects of dry- and humid-heat acclimation on local sweat inhibition (hidromeiosis). They acclimated resting subjects using controlled hyperthermia, maintaining core temperature at ~38.2°C, 2 h·d^{-1} for 12 days, using dry heat for one group and humid heat for another. Both groups had their left arms covered with plastic bags to collect sweat, creating a locally warm-humid microclimate. After acclimation, both groups showed similar decreases in heart rate, core and skin temperatures, with similar increases in sweating during an exercise-heat test. That is, both groups demonstrated acclimation-induced changes. In a 2-h, controlled-hyperthermia test with subjects resting in humid heat, both groups had similar whole-body sweat rates. The arms exposed to humid heat during acclimation showed similar increases in local sweat production, but sweating became inhibited as time progressed, although this hidromeiotic effect occurred more slowly after acclimation than before. However, the right arms of the dry-heat group, which had not been exposed to high humidity during acclimation, also revealed an elevated local sweat rate, but now sweating declined just as rapidly as it did before acclimation. Thus, humid-heat acclimation was associated with diminished hidromeiosis, enabling subjects to sustain a greater sweat flow.

Another possible difference between humid- and dry-heat acclimation is that the former may allow more efficient use of the skin as an evaporating surface. In humid heat, the wetted skin surface area may increase, due to reduced hidromeiosis, thus increasing potential, if not actual evaporation. This may reduce the extent to which sweating in some regions is in excess of the rate at which it can be evaporated. Humid-heat adaptation was also believed to result in greater sweat production on the limbs. However, recent research does not support this possibility (Patterson et al. 2004b).

The magnitude of cross-adaptation that exercise combined with either dry or humid heat confers during exercise in the other hot climate has not been fully evaluated (Sawka et al. 1996). However, several reports show some adaptation transfer between humid-heat and dry-heat exposure. Passive-dry heat or passive-humid heat acclimation elicit similar core temperature changes during exercise in both hot-dry and hot-humid climates (Fox et al. 1967). Exercise-dry heat acclimation confers an advantage (compared to no acclimation) during exercise in humid heat (Bean & Eichna 1943, Fox et al. 1967) and vice versa (Eichna et al. 1945). However, Shapiro et al. (1980) reported that exercise-dry heat acclimation resulted in equal or greater core temperatures during subsequent exercise in humid heat, than a matched dry-heat climate (wet bulb globe temperature (WBGT) = 34°C). Unfortunately, this paper did not show the preacclimation data, it employed only dry-heat acclimation and thermal matching based upon the WBGT index, which does not equate physiological strain. Subsequently, Sawka et al. (1983b) reported similar core temperatures during exercise in matched hot-dry and hot-wet conditions (WBGT = 32°C), both before and after a heat acclimation programme consisting of daily, alternating dry-heat and humid-heat exposures.

Griefahn (1997) contrasted the time course of a 15-day acclimation to either humid heat, dry heat or radiant heat, each at an equivalent WBGT (33°C). Whilst an unknown number of subjects participated in two or more acclimation programmes, separated by at least 52 days, it was observed that humid heat elicited a more rapid acclimation and lower physiological strain (core temperature, heart rate, sweating rate) than dry-heat exposure. Unfortunately, the experimental design did not allow cross-acclimation effects to be evaluated.

To our knowledge, no study has directly compared the retention of heat acclimation for matched groups after either humid-heat or dry-heat acclimation. However, individual reports mostly indicate that the retention of heat acclimation benefits seem to persist longer and decay slower for dry heat (Pandolf 1998, Pandolf & Young 2000).

5 THE RELATIONSHIP BETWEEN ADAPTATION TO COLD AND HEAT

Thermal adaptation of physiological (autonomic) regulation of body temperature improves the ability to cope with persisting thermal stresses. Cold adaptation results primarily in greater homeostatic economy, with a preservation of energy, often at the cost of a lower mean body temperature (and peripheral heterothermy) during cold stress. Heat adaptation, whether achieved by exposure to a hot environment or by endogenous heat produced during exercise, often brings about a greater regulatory efficiency; a lower mean body temperature during heat stress, but at the cost of a higher water loss.

A question that is frequently asked concerns the possible detrimental effects of heat acclimation on cold exposure and vice versa. Significant morphological effects of heat adaptation, in terms of a reduction of insulation, that may be detrimental in the cold, have not been reported. When considering the detrimental effects of cold adaptation, we should look primarily at its influences on the heat defence mechanisms. It is possible that morphological cold adaptation, in terms of improved insulation, may be detrimental during heat exposure. This is also the case if peripheral blood flow is reduced. There may also be an upward shift of evaporation heat loss (Werner & Graener 1986), an effect that would be detrimental to efficient heat defence.

In summary, while thermal adaptation increases tolerance to the kind of stress that induced adaptation, with some degree of thermal specificity, it may be detrimental when exposed to stresses at the opposite end of the thermal spectrum.

US Government disclaimer

References

Adam JM, Fox RH, Grimby G, Kidd DJ, Wolff HS 1960 Acclimatization to heat and its rate of decay in man. Journal of Physiology (London) 152:26–27

Adams T, Covino BG 1958 Racial variations to a standardized cold stress. Journal of Applied Physiology 12:9–12

Adams T, Heberling EJ 1958 Human physiological responses to a standardized cold stress as modified by physical fitness. Journal of Applied Physiology 13(2):226–230

Adolph EF 1964 Perspectives of adaptation: some general properties. In: Dill DB, Adolph EF (eds) Handbook of physiology. Section 4.

Adaptation to the environment. American Physiological Society, Washington, DC, 27–35

Allan JR, Wilson CG 1971 Influence of acclimatization on sweat sodium concentration. Journal of Applied Physiology 30:708–712

Armstrong LE, Maresh CM 1991 The induction and decay of heat acclimatisation in trained athletes. Sports Medicine 12:302–312

Armstrong LE, Pandolf KB 1988 Physical training, cardiorespiratory physical fitness and exercise-heat tolerance. In: Pandolf KB, Sawka MN, Gonzalez RR (eds) Human performance physiology and environmental medicine at terrestrial extremes. Benchmark Press, Indianapolis, 199–226

Armstrong LE, Stoppani J 2002 Central nervous system control of heat acclimation adaptations: an emerging paradigm. Reviews in the Neurosciences 13:271–285

Armstrong LE, Hubbard RW, Jones BH, Daniels JT 1986a Preparing Alberto Salazar for the heat of the 1984 Olympic Games. Physician and Sportsmedicine 14:73–81

Armstrong LE, Hubbard RW, DeLuca, JP, Christensen EL 1986b Self-paced heat acclimation procedures. Technical report number T8/86. US Army Research Institute of Environmental Medicine, Natick, MA

Avellini BA, ShapiroY, Fortney SM, Wenger CB, Pandolf KB 1982 Effects on heat tolerance of physical training in water and on land. Journal of Applied Physiology 53:1291–1298

Bae J-S, Lee J-B, Matsumoto T, Othman T, Min Y-K, Yang H-M 2006 Prolonged residence of temperate natives in the tropics produces a suppression of sweating. Pflugers Archiv European Journal of Physiology 453:67–72

Banister EW, Calvert TW 1980 Planning for future performance: implications for long term training. Canadian Journal of Applied Sport Science 5:170–176

Barwood MJ, Datta A, Thelwel R, Tipton MJ 2006 Psychological skills training improves exercise performance in the heat. In: Proceedings of the Physiological Society: Main Meeting. University College London, London, 24–25

Bass DE, Kleeman DR, Quinn M, Henschel A, Hegnauer AH 1955 Mechanisms of acclimatization to heat in man. Medicine 34:323–380

Baum E, Brück K, Schwennicke HP 1976 Adaptive modifications in the thermo-regulatory system in long-distance runners. Journal of Applied Physiology 40:404–410

Bean WB, Eichna LW 1943 Performance in relation to environmental temperature. Reactions of normal young men to simulated desert environment. Federation Proceedings 2:144–158

Bergmann C 1847 Ueber die verhaeltnisse der waermeoekonomie der tiere zu ihrer groesse. Goettinger Studien, 595–708

Bittel JHM 1987 Heat debt as an index for cold adaptation in men. Journal of Applied Physiology 62:1627–1634

Brown GM, Bird GS, Boag LM, Delahaye DJ, Green JE, Hatcher JD, Page J 1954 Blood volume and basal metabolic rate of Eskimos. Metabolism 3:247–254

Brück K, Baum E, Schwennicke HP 1976 Cold-adaptive modifications in man induced by repeated short-term cold-exposures and during a 10-day and -night cold-exposure. Pflugers Archiv European Journal of Physiology 363:125–133

Buguet A, Gati R, Soubiran G, Straboni JP, Hanniquet AM, Livecchi-Gonnot G, Bittel J 1988 Seasonal changes in circadian rhythms of body temperatures in humans living in a dry tropical climate. European Journal of Applied Physiology 58:334–339

Candas V 1987 Adaptation to extreme environments. Thermophysiological changes in man during humid heat acclimation. In: Dejours P (ed) Comparative physiology of environmental adaptations. Volume 2. Karger, Basel, 76–93

Coetzer P, Noakes TD, Sanders B, Lambert MI, Bosch AN, Wiggins T, Dennis SC 1993 Superior fatigue resistance of elite black South African distance runners. Journal of Applied Physiology 75:1822–1827

Cohen JS, Gisolfi CV 1982 Effects of interval training on work-heat tolerance of young women. Medicine and Science in Sports and Exercise 14:46–52

Collins KJ, Crockford GW, Weiner JS 1965 Sweat-gland training by drugs and thermal stress. Archives of Environmental Health 11:407–422

Duncan MT, Horvath SM 1988 Physiological adaptations to thermal stress in tropical Asians. European Journal of Applied Physiology 57:540–544

Edholm OG, Fox RH, Goldsmith R, Hampton IFG, Pillai KV 1964 A comparison of heat acclimatization in Indians and Europeans. Journal of Physiology (London) 117:15P–16P

Eichna LW, Bean WB, Ashe WF, Nelson N 1945 Performance in relation to environmental temperature. Reactions of normal young men to hot, humid (simulated jungle) environment. Bulletin of the Johns Hopkins Hospital 76:25–58

Eichna LW, Park CR, Nelson N, Horvath SM, Palmes ED 1950 Thermal regulation during acclimatization in a hot, dry (desert type) environment. American Journal of Physiology 163:585–597

Eide R 1973 The conceptual framework of cold adaptation. In: Edholm OG, Gunderson EKE (eds) Polar human biology. The Proceedings of the SCAR/IUPS/IUBS Symposium on Human Biology and Medicine in the Antarctic. Heinemann Medical Books, London, 290–296

Elsner RW 1963 Comparison of Australian Aborigines, Alacaluf Indians and Andean Indians. Federation Proceedings 22:840–842

Fanger PO 1973 The variability of man's preferred ambient temperature from day to day. Archive of Science and Physiology (Paris) 27:403–407

Febbraio MA, Snow RJ, Stathis CG, Hargreaves M, Carey MF 1994 Effect of heat stress on muscle energy metabolism during exercise. Journal of Applied Physiology 77:2827–2831

Fein JT, Haymes EM, Buskirk ER 1975 Effects of daily and intermittent exposures on heat acclimation of women. International Journal of Biometeorology 19:41–52

Feist DD, White RG 1989 Terrestrial mammals in cold. In: Wang LCH (ed) Advances in comparative and environmental physiology. Springer Verlag, Berlin, 327–360

Finberg JPM, Berlyne GM 1977 Modification of renin and aldosterone response to heat acclimatization in man. Journal of Applied Physiology 42:554–558

Fox RH, Goldsmith R, Kidd DJ, Lewis HE 1961 Acclimatization of the sweating mechanism in man. Journal of Physiology (London) 157:56–57

Fox RH, Goldsmith R, Hampton IFG, Hunt TJ 1967 Heat acclimatization by controlled hyperthermia in hot-dry and hot-wet climates. Journal of Applied Physiology 22:39–46

Fox RH, Budd GM, Woodward PM, Hackett AJ, Hendrie AL 1974 A study of temperature regulation in New Guinea people. Philosophical Transactions of the Royal Society of London. Series B 268:375–391

Francesconi RP, Sawka MN, Pandolf KB 1983 Hypohydration and heat acclimation: plasma renin and aldosterone during exercise. Journal of Applied Physiology 55:1790–1794

Gardner JW, Kark JA, Karnei K, Sanborn JS, Gastaldo E, Burr P, Wenger CB 1996 Risk factors predicting exertional heat illness in male Marine Corps recuits. Medicine and Science in Sports and Exercise 28:939–944

Glaser EM, Whittow GC 1953 Evidence for a non-specific mechanism of habituation. Journal of Physiology (London) 122:3P–4P

Golden FStC, Tipton MJ 1987 Human thermal responses during leg-only exercise in cold water. Journal of Physiology (London) 391:399–405

Golden FStC, Tipton MJ 1988. Human adaptation to repeated cold immersions. Journal of Physiology (London) 396:349–363

González-Alonso J, Teller C, Anderson SL, Jensen FB, Hyldig T, Nielsen B 1999 Influence of body temperature on the development of fatigue during prolonged exercise in the heat. Journal of Applied Physiology 86:1032–1039

Griefahn B 1997 Acclimation to three different hot climates with equivalent wet bulb globe temperatures. Ergonomics 40:223–234

Hammel HT 1961 Thermal and metabolic responses of the Alacaluf Indians to moderate cold exposure. Wright Air Development Technical Report 60–633. US Air Force

Hammel HT 1964 Terrestrial animal in cold: recent studies of primitive man. In: Dill DB, Adolph EF (eds) Handbook of physiology. Section 4. Adaptation to the environment. American Physiology Society, Washington, DC, 413–434

Hammel HT, Elsner RW, LeMessurier DH, Anderson HT, Milan FA 1959 Thermal and metabolic responses of the Australian Aborigine exposed to moderate cold in summer. Journal of Applied Physiology 14:605–615

Harrison MH 1985 Effects of thermal stress and exercise on blood volume in humans. Physiological Reviews 65:149–209

Henane R, Flandrois R, Charbonnier JP 1977 Increase in sweating sensitivity by endurance conditioning in man. Journal of Applied Physiology 43:822–828

Henschel A, Taylor HL, Keys A 1943 The persistence of heat acclimatization in man. American Journal of Physiology 140:321–325.

Hessemer V, Zeh A, Brück K 1986 Comparison of the effects of passive heat adaptation and moderate sweatless conditioning on responses to cold and heat. European Journal of Applied Physiology 55:281–289

Hicks CS, Matters RF 1933 The standard metabolism of the Australian Aborigines. Australian Journal of Experimental Biology and Medical Science 11:177–183

Hicks CS, O'Connor WJ 1938 Skin temperature of Australian Aboriginals under varying atmospheric conditions. Australian Journal of Experimental Biology and Medical Science 16:1–18

Höfler W 1968 Changes in regional distribution of sweating during acclimatization to heat. Journal of Applied Physiology 25:503–505

Hori S 1995 Adaptation to heat. Japanese Journal of Physiology 45:921–946

Hori S, Ihzuka H, Nakamura M 1976 Studies on physiological responses of residents in Okinawa to a hot environment. Japanese Journal of Physiology 26:235–244

Horowitz M, Peyser YM, Muhlrad A 1986a Alterations in cardiac myosin isoenzymes distribution as an adaptation to chronic environmental heat stress in the rat. Journal of Molecular and Cellular Cardiology 18:511–515

Horowitz M, Shimoni Y, Parnes S, Gotsman MS, Hasin Y 1986b Heat acclimation: cardiac performance of isolated rat heart. Journal of Applied Physiology 60:9–13

Hwang K, Baik SH 1997 Distribution of hairs and sweat glands on the bodies of Korean adults: a morphometric study. Acta Anatomica 158:112–120

Inoue Y, Havenith G, Kenney WL, Loomis JL, Buskirk ER 1999 Exercise- and methylcholine-induced sweating responses in older and younger men: effect of heat acclimation and aerobic fitness. International Journal of Biometeorology 42:210–216

IUPS Thermal Commission: Commission for Thermal Physiology of the International Union of Physiological Sciences 2001 Glossary of terms for thermal physiology. Japanese Journal of Physiology 51:245–280

Jooste PL, Strydom NB 1979 Improved mechanical efficiency derived from heat acclimation. South African Journal of Research in Sport, Physical Education and Recreation 2:45–53

Katsuura T, Tachibana ME, Okada A, Kikuchi Y 1993 Comparison of thermoregulatory responses of heat between Japanese Brazilians and Japanese. Journal of Thermal Biology 18:299–302

King DS, Costill DL, Fink WJ, Hargreaves M, Fielding RA 1985 Muscle metabolism during exercise in the heat in unacclimatized and acclimatized humans. Journal of Applied Physiology 59:1350–1354

Kirwan JP, Costill DL, Kuipers H, Burrell MJ, Fink WJ, Kovaleski JE, Fielding RA 1987 Substrate utilization in leg muscle of men after heat acclimation. Journal of Applied Physiology 63:31–35

Lagerspetz KYH 2006 What is thermal acclimation? Journal of Thermal Biology 31:332–336

LeBlanc J 1978 Adaptation of man to cold. In: Wang LCH, Hudson JW (eds) Strategies in cold: natural torpidity and thermogenesis. Academic Press, New York, 695–715

Libert JP, Candas V, Vogt JJ 1983 Modifications of sweating responses to thermal transients following heat acclimation. European Journal of Applied Physiology 50:235–246

Lind AR 1964 Physiologic responses to heat. In: Licht S (ed) Medical climatology. Waverly Press, Baltimore, MD, 164–195

Lind AR, Bass DE 1963 Optimal exposure time for development of acclimatization to heat. Federation Proceedings 22:704–708

McCance RA, Purohit G 1969 Ethnic differences in the response of the sweat glands to pilocarpine. Nature 221:378–379

Mack GW, Nadel ER 1996 Body fluid balance during heat stress in humans. In: Fregly MJ, Blatteis CM (eds) Environmental physiology. Oxford University Press, New York, 187–214

Mack GW, Nagashima K, Haskell A, Nadel E 1997 The role of albumin in the hypervolemia of exercise. In: Nose H, Nadel ER, Morimoto T (eds) The 1997 Nagano symposium on sports sciences. Cooper Publishing, Carmel, CA, 375–383

Mason ED, Jacob M 1972 Variations in metabolic rate responses to change between tropical and temperate climate. Human Biology 44:141–172

Mitchell D, Senay LC, Wyndham CH, Van Rensburg AJ, Rogers GG, Strydom NB 1976 Acclimatization in a hot, humid environment: energy exchange, body temperature and sweating. Journal of Applied Physiology 40:768–778

Moore-Ede MC 1983 Hypothermia: A timing disorder of circadian thermoregulatory rhythms? In: Pozos RS, Wittmers LE (eds) The nature and treatment of hypothermia. University of Minnesota Press, Minneapolis, 69–80

Nadel ER, Pandolf KB, Roberts MF, Stolwijk JAJ 1974 Mechanisms of thermal acclimation to exercise and heat. Journal of Applied Physiology 37:515–520

Neel JV 1962 Diabetes mellitus a 'thrifty' genotype rendered detrimental by 'progress'? American Journal of Human Genetics 14:352–353

Nielsen B, Hales JRS, Strange S, Christensen NJ, Warberg J, Saltin B 1993 Human circulatory and thermoregulatory adaptations with heat acclimation and exercise in a hot, dry environment. Journal of Physiology (London) 460:467–485

Nielsen B, Strange S, Christensen NJ, Warberg J, Saltin B 1997 Acute and adaptive responses in humans to exercise in a warm, humid environment. Pflugers Archiv European Journal of Physiology 1997:49–56

Nose H, Mack GW, Shi X, Nadel ER 1988 Shift in body fluid compartments after dehydration in humans. Journal of Applied Physiology 65:318–324

Pandolf KB 1998 Time course of heat acclimation and its decay. International Journal of Sports Medicine 19:S157–S160

Pandolf KB, Young AJ 1992 Environmental extremes and endurance performance. In: Astrand PO, Shephard RJ (eds) Endurance in sport. Blackwell Scientific Publications, Oxford, 270–282

Pandolf KB, Young AJ 2000 Assessment of environmental extremes and competitive strategies. In: Shephard RJ, Astrand PO (eds) Endurance in sport. Blackwell Scientific Publications, Oxford, 287–300

Pandolf KB, Burse RL, Goldman RF 1977 Role of physical fitness in heat acclimatization, decay and reinduction. Ergonomics 20:399–408

Pandolf KB, Cadarette BS, Sawka MN, Young AJ, Francesconi RP, Gonzalez RR 1988 Thermoregulatory responses of middle-aged and young men during dry-heat acclimation. Journal of Applied Physiology 65:65–71

Patterson MJ, Stocks JM, Taylor NAS 1999 Heat acclimation-induced plasma volume expansion: the role of electrolyte retention. Journal of Physiology (London) 521:102

Patterson MJ, Stocks JM, Taylor NAS 2004a Sustained and generalised extracellular fluid expansion following heat acclimation. Journal of Physiology (London) 559:327–334

Patterson MJ, Stocks JM, Taylor NAS 2004b Humid heat acclimation does not elicit a preferential sweat redistribution towards the limbs. American Journal of Physiology 286:R512–R518

Peter J, Wyndham CH 1966 Activity of the human eccrine sweat gland during exercise in a hot humid environment before and after acclimatization. Journal of Physiology (London) 187:583–594

Pichan G, Sridharan K, Swamy YV, Joseph S, Gautam RK 1985 Physiological acclimatization to heat after a spell of cold conditioning in tropical subjects. Aviation, Space and Environmental Medicine 56:436–440

Pugh LGCE, Corbett JL, Johnson RH 1967 Rectal temperatures, weight losses and sweat rates in marathon running. Journal of Applied Physiology 23:347–352

Radomski MW, Boutelier C 1982 Hormone response of normal and intermittent cold-preadapted humans to continuous cold. Journal of Applied Physiology 53:610–616

Rees A, Eglin C, Taylor NAS, Hetherington M, Mekjavic IB, Tipton MJ 2002 The nature of human adaptation to cold. Proceedings of the 10th International Conference on Environmental Ergonomics, Fukuoka, Japan 23–27 September, 143–146

Rising R, Fontvieille AM, Larson DE, Spraul M, Bogardus C, Ravussin E 1995 Racial difference in body core temperature between Pima Indian and Caucasian men. International Journal of Obesity 19:1–5

Roberts DF 1953 Body weight, race and climate. American Journal of Physical Anthropology 11:533–558

Roberts MF, Wenger CB, Stolwijk JAJ, Nadel ER 1977 Skin blood flow and sweating changes following exercise and heat acclimation. Journal of Applied Physiology 43:133–137

Robinson S, Turrell ES, Belding HS, Horvath SM 1943 Rapid acclimatization to work in hot environments. American Journal of Physiology 140:168–176

Rodahl K 1952 Basal metabolism of the Eskimo. Journal of Nutrition 48:359–368

Rowell LB, Kraning KK II, Kennedy JW, Evans TO 1967 Central circulatory responses to work in dry heat before and after acclimatization. Journal of Applied Physiology 22:509–518

Saat M, Sirisinghe RG, Singh R, Tochihara Y 2005 Decay of heat acclimation during exercise in cold and exposure to cold environment. European Journal of Applied Physiology 95:313–320

Sargent F, Smith CR, Batterton DL 1965 Eccrine sweat gland activity in heat acclimation. International Journal of Biometeorology 9:229–231

Sato K, Sato F 1983 Individual variations in structure and function of human eccrine sweat gland. American Journal of Physiology 245:R203–R208

Sato F, Owen M, Matthes R, Sato K, Gisolfi CV 1990 Functional and morphological changes in the eccrine sweat gland with heat acclimation. Journal of Applied Physiology 69:232–236

Sawka MN 1988 Body fluid responses and hypohydration during exercise-heat stress. In: Pandolf KB, Sawka MN, Gonzalez RR (eds) Human performance physiology and environmental medicine at terrestrial extremes. Cooper Publishing, Indianapolis, 227–266

Sawka MN, Coyle EF 1999 Influence of body water and blood volume on thermoregulation and exercise performance in the heat. In: Hollozsy JO (ed) Exercise and sport sciences reviews. Williams and Wilkins, Baltimore, MD, 167–218

Sawka MN, Young AJ 2000 Exercise in hot and cold climates. In: Garrett WE, Kirkendell DT (eds) Exercise and sport science. Williams and Wilkins, Philadelphia, 385–400

Sawka MN, Pandolf KB, Avellini BA, Shapiro Y 1983a Does heat acclimation lower the rate of metabolism elicited by muscular exercise? Aviation, Space and Environmental Medicine 4:27–31

Sawka MN, Toner MM, Francesconi RP, Pandolf KB 1983b Hypohydration and exercise: effects of heat acclimation, gender and environment. Journal of Applied Physiology 55:1147–1153

Sawka MN, Young AJ, Cadarette BS, Levine L, Pandolf KB 1985 Influence of heat stress and acclimation on maximal aerobic power. European Journal of Applied Physiology 53:294–298

Sawka MN, Wenger CB, Pandolf KB 1996 Thermoregulatory responses to acute exercise-heat stress and heat acclimation. In: Fregly MJ, Blatteis CM (eds) Handbook of physiology, section 4, environmental physiology. Oxford University Press, New York, 157–185

Sawka MN, Latzka WA, Montain SJ, Cadarette BS, Kolka MA, Kraning KK, Gonzalez RR 2001 Physiologic tolerance to uncompensable heat: intermittent exercise, field vs laboratory. Medicine and Science in Sports and Exercise 33:422–430

Scholander T 1960 Habituation of autonomic response elements under two conditions of alertness. Acta Physiologica Scandinavica 50:259–68

Scholander PF, Hock R, Walters V, Irving L 1950 Adaptation to cold in arctic and tropical mammals and birds in relation to body temperature, insulation and basal metabolic rate. Biological Bulletin 99:259–271

Scholander PF, Hammel HT, Hart JS, LeMessurier DH, Steen J 1958 Cold adaptation in Australian Aborigines. Journal of Applied Physiology 13:211–218

Senay LC 1972 Changes in plasma volume and protein content during exposures of working men to various temperatures before and after acclimatization to heat: separation of the roles of cutaneous and skeletal muscle circulation. Journal of Physiology (London) 224:61–81

Senay LC, Mitchell D, Wyndham CH 1976 Acclimatization in a hot, humid environment: body fluid adjustments. Journal of Applied Physiology 40:786–796

Shapiro Y, Pandolf KB, Avellini BA, Pimental NA, Goldman RF 1980 Physiological responses of men and women to humid and dry heat. Journal of Applied Physiology 49:1–8

Stein HJ, Eliot JW, Bader RA 1949 Physiological reactions to cold and their effects on the retention of acclimatization to heat. Journal of Applied Physiology 1:575–585

Stocks JM, Patterson MJ, Hyde DE, Mittleman KD, Taylor NAS 2001 Metabolic habituation following repeated resting cold-water immersion is not apparent during low-intensity cold-water exercise. Journal of Physiological Anthropology 20:263–267

Strydom NB, Wyndham CH, Williams CG, Morrison JF, Bredell GAG, Benade AJS, Rahden M 1966 Acclimatization to humid heat and the role of physical conditioning. Journal of Applied Physiology 21:636–642

Strydom NB, Kok R, Jooste PL, Van Der Walt WH 1975 Intermittent exposure to heat, and the retention of heat acclimatization. Journal of the South African Institute of Mining and Metallurgy 75:315–318

Suminski RR, Robertson RJ, Goss FL, Arslanian S 2000 Peak oxygen consumption and skeletal muscle bioenergetics in African-American and Caucasian men. Medicine and Science in Sports and Exercise 32:2059–2066

Taylor NAS 2000 Principles and practices of heat adaptation. Journal of the Human-Environment System 4:11–22

Taylor NAS 2006 Ethnic differences in thermoregulation: genotypic versus phenotypic heat adaptation. Journal of Thermal Biology 31:90–104

Taylor NAS, Cotter JD 2006 Heat adaptation: guidelines for the optimisation of human performance. International SportMed Journal 7:33–57

Thompson ML 1954 A comparison between the number and distribution of functioning eccrine glands in Europeans and Africans. Journal of Physiology (London) 123:225–233

Tipton MJ 1986 Human adaptation to cold. PhD thesis, University of London

Tipton MJ 1989 The initial responses to cold-water immersion in man. Clinical Science 77:581–588

Tipton MJ, Franks CM, Golden FStC 1998a Habituation of the initial responses to cold water immersion in humans: a central or peripheral mechanism? Journal of Physiology (London) 512:621–628

Tipton MJ, Golden FStC, Mekjavic IB, Franks CM 1998b Temperature dependence of habituation of the initial responses to cold water immersion. European Journal of Applied Physiology 78:253–257

Tipton MJ, Mekjavic IB, Eglin CM 2000 Permanence of the habituation of the initial responses to cold-water immersion. European Journal of Applied Physiology 83:17–21

Toda Y 1967 Measurement and regional distribution of active sweat glands in Indonesians. Kobe Journal of Medical Science 13:157–164

Vallery-Masson J, Boulière J, Poitrenaud J 1980 Can a protracted stay in the tropics permanently lower basal metabolic rates in European expatriates? Annals of Human Biology 7:267–271

Ward JS, Bredell CAC, Wenzel HG 1960 Responses of Bushmen and Europeans on exposure to winter night temperatures in the Kalahari. Journal of Applied Physiology 15:667–670

Webster AJF 1974 Physiological effect of cold exposure. In: Robertshaw D (ed) Environmental physiology. Physiology series one, volume 7. Butterworths, London, 33–69

Wenger CB 1988 Human heat acclimatization. In: Pandolf KB, Sawka MN, Gonzalez RR (eds) Human performance physiology and environmental medicine at terrestrial extremes. Benchmark Press, Indianapolis, 153–197

Werner J 1994 Beneficial and detrimental effects of thermal adaptation. In: Zeisberger E, Schönbaum E, Lomax P (eds) Thermal balance in health and disease. Birkhäuser, Basel, 141–154

Werner J 1998 Biophysics of heat exchange between body and environment. In: Blatteis M (ed) Physiology and pathophysiology of temperature regulation. World Scientific Publishers, Singapore, 23–45

Werner J 2005 Regulatory processes of the human body during thermal and work strain. In: Tochihara Y, Ohnaka T (eds) Environmental ergonomics. Elsevier, Tokyo, 3–9

Werner J, Graener R 1986 Thermoregulatory responses to cold during a 7 week acclimatization process in rabbits. Pflugers Archiv European Journal of Physiology 406:547–551

Weston AR, Mbambo Z, Myburgh KH 2000 Running economy of African and Caucasian distance runners. Medicine and Science in Sports and Exercise 32:1130–1134

Williams GG, Wyndham CH, Morrison JF 1967 Rate of loss of acclimatization in summer and winter. Journal of Applied Physiology 22:21–26

Wilson O 1956 Adaptation of the basal metabolic rate of man to climate – a review. Metabolism 5:531–542

Wood JE, Bass DE 1960 Responses of the veins and arterioles of the forearm to walking during acclimatization to heat in man. Journal of Clinical Investigation 39:825–833

Wyndham CH 1951 Effect of acclimatization on circulatory responses to high environmental temperatures. Journal of Applied Physiology 4:383–395

Wyndham CH, Jacobs GE 1957 Loss of acclimatization after six days of work in cool conditions on the surface of a mine. Journal of Applied Physiology 11:197–198

Wyndham CH, Morrison JF 1958 Adjustment to cold of Bushmen in the Kalahari Desert. Journal of Applied Physiology 13:219–225

Wyndham CH, Metz B, Munro A 1964 Reactions to heat of Arabs and Caucasians. Journal of Applied Physiology 19:1051–1054

Wyndham CH, Benade AJA, Williams CG, Strydom NB, Goldin A, Heyns AJA 1968 Changes in central circulation and body fluid spaces during acclimatization to heat. Journal of Applied Physiology 25:586–593

Wyndham CH, Rogers GG, Senay LC, Mitchell D 1976 Acclimatization in a hot, humid environment: cardiovascular adjustments. Journal of Applied Physiology 40:779–785

Young AJ 1990 Energy substrate utilization during exercise in extreme environments. In: Pandolf KB, Hollozsy JO (eds) Exercise and sport sciences reviews. Williams and Wilkins, Baltimore, MD, 65–117

Young AJ 1996 Homeostatic responses to prolonged cold exposure: human cold acclimatization. In: Fregly MJ, Blatteis CM (eds) Environmental physiology. Handbook of physiology. Volume 1. Oxford University Press, New York, 419–438

Young AJ, Sawka MN, Levine L, Cadarette BS, Pandolf KB 1985 Skeletal muscle metabolism during exercise is influenced by heat acclimation. Journal of Applied Physiology 59:1929–1935

Chapter 22

The physiology of water immersion

John A. Krasney David R. Pendergast

1 INTRODUCTION

Head-out (upright) water immersion is a simple, non-invasive manoeuvre that increases central blood volume and elicits buoyancy effects that lead to a microgravity-like state. Thus, water immersion has been used to study the regulation of blood volume and to simulate space physiology (Chapter 26), it is also relevant to diving and thermal physiology (Chapters 20 and 23) and is a useful non-pharmacological method for the treatment of fluid retention disorders. Since the hydrostatic pressure gradient acting upon the body surface during immersion means that postural changes can have pronounced effects upon physiological function, in this chapter, the focus will be primarily upon upright immersion, unless noted otherwise. Furthermore, since for humans, the thermoneutral temperature is considered to be 34–35°C for water immersions of 3–6 h, then this chapter will deal predominantly with thermoneutral immersions, leaving Chapter 20 to describe the physiology of cold water immersion.

The physiological responses to head-out immersion are not simply due to the removal of gravity since, during immersion, there is a unique set of stimuli that is not present in true microgravity. Consistent with greater antigravity challenges, mechanisms of physiological regulation during water immersion in bipedal humans differ somewhat from those observed in quadrupeds. The overall physiological responses during water immersion regulate systemic and regional delivery of oxygen.

2 CARDIAC-RENAL RESPONSES

Gauer & Henry (1951) provided the first evidence that stretching the cardiac atria causes a reflex diuresis (increased renal water loss). In anaesthetised dogs, obstruction of the mitral valve, by inflating a balloon in the left atrium, caused a reduction of vasopressin (antidiuretic hormone) secretion and an increase in renal free-water clearance. These responses were abolished by cutting the cervical vagus nerves, indicating that blood volume is regulated by intrathoracic stretch receptors via a cardiac-renal link (Figure 22.1).

During thermoneutral water immersion in humans, there is an increase in the cardiopulmonary volume (Epstein 1992, Krasney et al. 1989) that augments the cardiac output via the length-tension response. Since systemic oxygen uptake does not change in a thermoneutral immersion, an unusual situation develops where systemic oxygen delivery exceeds systemic tissue requirements. Normally, blood flow is autoregulated to meet the metabolic demands of peripheral tissues (Chapter 1; Guyton & Coleman 1980). Figure 22.2 indicates that autoregulation of blood flow is modified during immersion to allow for an increased systemic blood flow (Christie et al. 1990, Hajduczok et al. 1987b).

Originally, Gauer & Henry (1976) postulated that the increased fluid output by the kidneys during immersion would lead to a reduction of plasma volume. However, this view was later modified, because there is a major transcapillary fluid shift from the extravascular compartments (Figure 22.3). External hydrostatic pressure decreases the capacity of the venous compartment, primarily the splanchnic veins, shifting blood into the thorax (Johansen et al. 1997). In addition, the autotransfusion or transcapillary shift of fluid from the extravascular compartment into the vascular compartment is derived primarily from the capillaries of the legs, and augments plasma volume and reduces

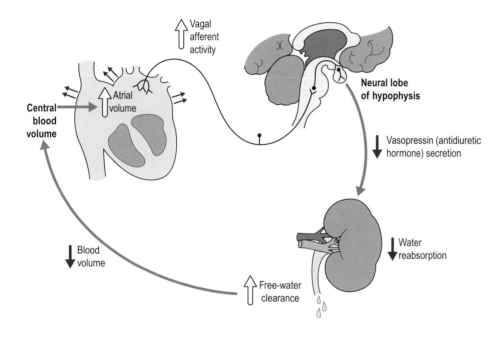

Figure 22.1 An early version of the Gauer–Henry hypothesis. Dashed arrows indicate an increase or stimulation of the variable, darkened arrows indicate a decrease or inhibition of the variable. Redrawn from Krasney (1996) with permission.

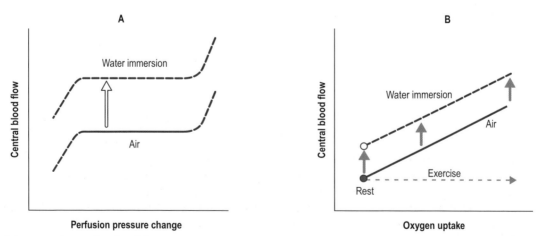

Figure 22.2 Upright water immersion (rest) increases central blood flow, both absolutely and relative to metabolism (oxygen uptake; A), where oxygen uptake is constant. Autoregulation of blood flow occurs but the level at which systemic flow is held constant over a range of perfusion pressures is shifted upwards. As exercise elevates oxygen uptake (B), the level of systemic flow is elevated for any oxygen uptake during immersion. Redrawn from Krasney (1996) with permission.

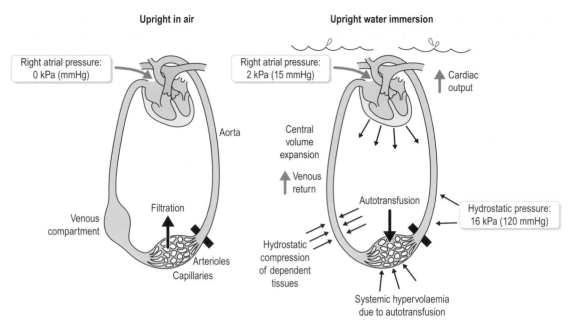

Figure 22.3 While standing in air (A), right atrial pressure is low, (gravity) dependent veins are distended and net plasma filtration occurs in the limb capillaries. During upright water immersion (B), central volume expansion occurs with increased right atrial pressure and cardiac output. These result from hydrostatic compression of the dependent tissues and capillary reabsorption or an autotransfusion in dependent limbs.

plasma oncotic pressure (Johansen et al. 1995). This fluid shift results from the impact of hydrostatic compression of the dependent tissues on the Starling forces that dictate transcapillary plasma movements. When upright in air for short periods, this is generally an efflux at the arterial ends of peripheral capillaries, with an approximately equivalent influx at the venous ends. With upright immersion, there is a net increase in capillary reabsorption (autotransfusion) in the dependent limbs. The fluid is derived from the intracellular compartment and the role of the kidney during water immersion is to minimise the increase in plasma volume, which would otherwise approximate +40% (Krasney 1996, Miki et al. 1986a, 1987). Plasma volume continues to be elevated during 6–12 h immersions, suggesting that the intracellular reservoir is not exhausted (Johansen et al. 1992).

The immersion responses are temperature dependent (Pendergast 1988) and, therefore, the study of water immersion requires the elimination of thermal stress. In humans, this is achieved by using water temperatures of 34–35°C for exposure <6 h. For measurements of haemodynamics, it is important to determine the hydrostatic indifference point – the point in the vasculature at which pressure is independent of posture. This is a transition zone at which intravascular pressure remains constant and as such represents a center of gravity for the cardiovascular system. (Gauer & Thron 1965, Rowell 1986). In humans, this point is usually considered to be at the level of the right atrium (Rowell 1986). However, during immersion it is very likely

to shift, but it is inappropriate to reference pressures to the surface level of the water. It is better to insert a reference catheter in the oesophagus for estimation of pleural and transmural pressures across the heart and great vessels (Arborelius et al. 1972, Miki et al. 1989b).

Since water immersion is non-invasive, Gauer & Henry (1976) considered it to be the investigative tool of choice for studying responses to volume expansion. Nevertheless, immersion cannot be strictly compared to true volume expansion, microgravity or head-down tilt, since there are unique characteristics associated with each manoeuvre. Compared to true volume expansion, the magnitude of the diuresis and natriuresis (increased renal sodium loss) caused by water immersion is equivalent to the infusion of 2 L of 0.9% saline (sodium chloride) solution (Epstein 1992).

3 CARDIOVASCULAR REGULATION

Circulatory and renal responses to water immersion are elicited reflexly by mechanical loading of cardiovascular stretch receptors. In humans, immersion to the midcervical level causes cardiac output to increase from 32–62%, with the magnitude of this change depending upon the method and subjects used (Krasney 1996). Stroke volume increases in spite of a decrease in heart rate, while mean arterial pressure generally does not change, indicating that total peripheral resistance to blood flow declines. Arterial pulse pressure increases consistently, secondary to the rise in stroke volume (Norsk et al. 1990). Cardiac output increases according to the depth of immersion, increasing progressively from leg (only) immersion through to head-out immersion, and is sustained for several hours. This is a cardiac length-tension response due to the Frank–Starling mechanism. That is, an increased central blood volume stretches (preloads) cardiac muscle fibres, resulting in more forceful pumping.

Pulmonary artery pressure and vascular volume increase with a decline of vital capacity (Taylor & Morrison 1991). Hydrostatic compression leads to elastic loading of the chest wall and negative pressure breathing (Hong et al. 1969). There are increases in blood flow to the respiratory muscles, reflecting the increased work of breathing (Hajduczok et al. 1987b, Taylor & Morrison 1999). Prefaut et al. (1979) observed mild hypoxaemia in humans with increased lung closing volume. However, there is increased perfusion of the apical portions of the lung, which are normally less well perfused when upright in air, with improved matching of ventilation–perfusion relationships (Arborelius et al. 1972).

Von Diringshofen (1948) postulated a shift of fluid into the plasma compartment during water immersion. This hypothesis was validated in dog studies by Davis & DuBois (1977) and Miki et al. (1986a, 1987, 1989b), with increases of ~7% following 100 min of immersion. Interstitial pressure rises above the estimated capillary hydrostatic pressure, favouring capillary reabsorption. As immersion depth increases, there is a linear coupling of tissue pressure, capillary pressure and central venous pressure. While plasma osmolarity does not change, there is a decline of plasma oncotic pressure leading to haemodilution. Interstitial fluid volume and lymph flow do not change and amino acids and potassium concentrations rise in the plasma, indicating that most of the fluid shifts out of the intracellular compartment (Davis and DuBois 1977, Krasney 1996). The kidneys minimise the rise in plasma volume, since evidence from immersed, anaesthetised and nephrectomised dogs has shown plasma volume to increase by 40% instead of the 7% increase observed in dogs with intact kidneys.

Figure 22.4 indicates the transcellular, transcapillary and renal fluid shifts that occur during water immersion. There are several possible mechanisms for the dramatic fluid shift out of the cellular compartment. First, a primary movement of isotonic fluid out of the interstitium would leave behind osmotically active proteins that could in turn draw water out of the cells. Second, relative differences in compliances between cells, the interstitial compartment and the capillary could decrease cell volume more than the interstitial volume, leading to an increase in interstitial pressure that could in turn increase capillary reabsorption. Third, if cells perceive hydrostatic compression as an increase in cell volume, then this would activate cellular volume regulatory decreases via solute efflux; cells can detect and respond to volume changes of <3%. The rise in plasma potassium content during water immersion is com-

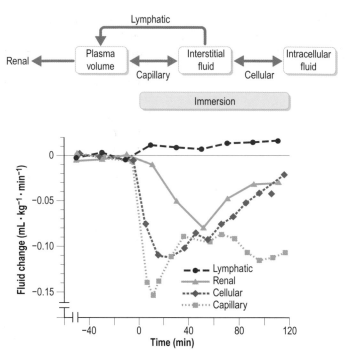

Figure 22.4 There are three major fluid shifts that occur during water immersion (upper flow diagram): across the capillary, across the cell wall and across the kidney. The lymphatic fluid shift is minor. These compartmental fluid changes are then illustrated (graph) for a 120-min upright, thermoneutral immersion. Redrawn from Krasney (1996) with permission.

patible with cellular regulatory volume decreases due to loss of potassium chloride, caused by activation of separate cell membrane potassium and chloride channels, and potassium-chloride co-transporters (Strange 2004). Johansen et al. (1997) suggested that the fluid shift occurs mainly from the lower extremities.

Along with increased blood flow to the respiratory muscles (diaphragm and intercostals), coronary blood flow increases commensurate with the increase in cardiac work during immersion (Hajduczok et al. 1987b). Blood flow to the cerebellum also increases, reflecting altered vestibular and proprioceptive inputs secondary to buoyancy and the microgravity state. However, total cerebral blood flow is not changed, implying vasoconstriction in some regions. While core temperature is unchanged, the transition from air to thermoneutral water heats up the integument, since there is an 8–10°C difference in the temperature of thermoneutral air (lower) and water. Accordingly, blood flow to skin and subcutaneous fat rises in the order of several hundred percent. Increased cutaneous blood flow could account for the common observation that the cutaneous veins on the dorsum of the feet remain distended while standing in water.

The mechanisms for other regional flow adjustments during water immersion are less certain. While renal blood flow is unchanged, there are early increases in flows to the gastrointestinal tract, liver, pancreas and spleen. These increases are proportional to the change in cardiac output. After about 30 min of immersion, the visceral flows decline to preimmersion levels, and the increased cardiac output is now redirected into non-respiratory skeletal muscles. These regional hyperaemias imply that water immersion is potentially useful for the treatment of decompression sickness (Chapter 23), muscle injury and for increasing drug delivery to specific organs, such as the liver. Perhaps theses regional hyperaemias offset tendencies for fluid to shift out of the cells in some tissues.

4 VASOPRESSIN (ANTIDIURETIC HORMONE)

Hydration state and physical fitness influence the renal response to water immersion. After 20–40 min of immersion in euhydrated individuals, diuresis, natriuresis, kaliuresis (increased renal potassium loss) and an increased renal free-water clearance all ensue (Epstein 1978, 1992). The kaliuresis reflects tubular washout of potassium due to the high urine flow. In subjects who are well hydrated prior to immersion but then are not allowed to drink, the renal responses persist for 2–4 h, whilst in euhydrated subjects, these renal responses are partially sustained for the duration of the immersion. In dehydrated subjects, there is a smaller diuresis with an increase of osmolar clearance (Behn et al. 1969). Similar observations have been made in repleted and non-repleted awake dogs (Sondeen et al. 1990). There have been many studies of the renal response to head-out immersion in anaestheised dogs. However, anaesthesia markedly impairs the canine natriuretic response, so conclusions about kidney regulatory mechanisms from anaesthetised studies are not valid (Krasney 1996). The level of physical training also influences the character of the immersion diuresis. For example, Claybaugh et al. (1986) found in humans that both diuresis and natriuresis were reduced significantly in trained runners and swimmers compared to sedentary individuals, despite larger and more persistent increases in cardiac output.

Water immersion does not alter glomerular filtration rate. Hence, the dramatic kidney responses are due to tubular mechanisms. Vasopressin (antidiuretic hormone) mediates the regulation of the total body fluid and plasma osmolarity. Since plasma osmolarity does not change during immersion, the control of vasopressin secretion depends upon stimulation of volume receptors. Norsk & Epstein (1988) have indicated that a reduction in plasma vasopressin concentration is responsible for the increase in renal free-water clearance in humans during immersion. However, vasopressin levels are quite low in euhydrated subjects and it has been difficult to detect reductions in circulating vasopressin, although recent studies with improved vasopressin assays report consistently small but significant reductions

in such subjects (Gabrielsen et al. 2000a). By contrast, vasopressin concentrations are high in dehydrated subjects and decrease during immersion, but renal water clearance does not increase. However, the kidney is quite sensitive to small changes in plasma vasopressin (Bie et al. 1984), and the renal free-water clearance response is abolished when subjects are pretreated with vasopressin (Epstein et al. 1981).

Hajduczok et al. (1987a) found a diuresis and natriuresis in awake dogs during water immersion but no change in either vasopressin or renal water clearance, despite large increments in atrial pressure. By contrast, after total cardiac denervation, immersion led to a decline of vasopressin concentration, with diuresis now due to an increase in water clearance. The Bainbridge reflex increases heart rate and cardiac output in the intact dog during water immersion, due to increased venous return and stimulation of the low-pressure baroreceptors, while arterial pulse pressure does not change. However, after cardiac denervation, the increase in heart rate is abolished, since it was driven autonomically, but an identical increase in cardiac output occurs due to a preload-induced elevation in stroke volume. Arterial pulse pressure now increases. These observations indicate that, in the dog, the decline in circulating vasopressin was due to increased arterial baroreceptor loading, unmasked by cardiac denervation. Furthermore, the natriuresis was dependent upon intact cardiac nerves.

It is therefore evident that considerable redundancy exists within the control systems for body fluid regulation, as is evident for other regulatory systems (Chapter 18). In awake dogs, monkeys and humans, the primary mechano-receptors modulating vasopressin secretion appear to be the arterial baroreceptors (Krasney 1996, Rowell 1993), although graded distension of central cardiac receptors modulates vasopressin secretion in humans (Gabrielsen et al. 2000a).

5 RENIN–ANGIOTENSIN II–ALDOSTERONE SYSTEM, RENAL SYMPATHETIC NERVES AND ATRIAL NATRIURETIC PEPTIDE

The renin-angiotensin-aldosterone system and the renal sympathetic nerves are antinatriuretic in action, and interact with the atrial natriuretic peptide (ANP) to regulate extracellular fluid volume and plasma sodium content. In immersed humans, plasma renin activity and aldosterone concentrations decline in a more consistent manner than plasma vasopressin, and appear to be less related to the degree of hydration (Epstein 1992, Krasney 1996). However, the diuretic and natriuretic responses are present after 40 min of immersion and are too rapid in onset to be due primarily to suppression of aldosterone secretion. Indeed, Hajduczok et al. (1987a) and Sondeen et al. (1990) found that renal responses of immersed awake dogs were poorly correlated with plasma renin activity.

Distension of the atria stimulates ANP release, eliciting diuresis, natriuresis, vasodilatation and a fluid shift out of the vascular compartment. Water immersion elevates ANP in plasma rapidly in humans, dogs and rats (Krasney 1996). However, the relative time courses of the ANP and renal responses during immersion differ. For example, although circulating ANP concentration rises rapidly, the diuresis and natriuresis are not evident until 40 min.

In fact, it is uncertain whether these renal responses can actually be elicited by the levels of ANP that are attained during water immersion (Goetz et al. 1986), and the renal responses are poorly correlated with plasma ANP concentrations (Miki et al. 1986b, Sondeen et al. 1990). Metzler & Ramsay (1989) showed that the renal responses to ANP were greatly augmented in hypervolaemic (but not haemodiluted) awake dogs. Subsequently, Krasney et al. (1991) demonstrated that the renal sensitivity to two doses of ANP was greatly augmented in conscious dogs during volume-replete water immersion. Therefore, it can be speculated that ANP is only effective when the plasma volume is expanded.

Atrial natriuretic peptide reduces plasma volume and increases haematocrit by causing a transcapillary fluid shift (Rutlen et al. 1990). Krasney et al. (1991) found in awake dogs that ANP infusion caused a haemoconcentration in air. During water immersion, there was an expected haemodilution, and this was attenuated in a graded fashion by increasing doses of ANP. Thus, ANP modulates and opposes the autotransfusion during water immersion, possibly by raising capillary hydrostatic pressure (Krasney 1996).

DiBona & Kopp (1997) and others have demonstrated that renal sympathetic neural activity can elicit important changes in kidney function, in the absence of renal haemodynamic responses. For example, sympathetic activation at intensities that do not alter renal blood flow or glomerular filtration rate causes antinatriuresis, whereas suppression of neural activity evokes a natriuresis. Mechanical stretch of atrial or arterial baroreceptors causes striking reductions in renal sympathetic activity, increasing urine flow and sodium excretion. In addition to this suppression, Epstein et al. (1983) and Norsk et al. (1990) have reported that plasma norepinephrine concentration declines by as much as 50% during water immersion.

Hajduczok et al. (1987a) found in dogs with denervated hearts that the natriuresis of water immersion was entirely due to the presence of the cardiac nerves, although a water diuresis persisted in the cardiac-denervated dogs, due to a decline of vasopressin levels. Thus, the reflex suppression of adrenergic systems in water immersion is dependent upon the stimulation of cardiac afferent nerves, and major alterations in vasopressin do not occur in neurally intact animals. The decline in plasma renin activity usually observed during water immersion is therefore likely to be related to a decline in renal sympathetic neural activity.

Miki et al. (1989a) recorded renal sympathetic activity in awake dogs, providing the first direct evidence that this activity is suppressed during water immersion. The magnitude of this neural activity suppression was ~50% below preimmersion levels, and the renal response in these dogs consisted of diuresis and natriuresis, with no change in renal free-water clearance. After chronic, bilateral renal denervation, the diuresis and natriuresis to water immersion were abolished. Miki et al. (1989a) also provided strong evidence that immersion elicits a reflex neurogenic natriuresis, since this natriuresis was also abolished by denervation of the heart.

The dramatic effects of renal denervation emphasise the important role of reflex suppression of renal sympathetic activity in the renal response to water immersion, and imply that the roles of vasopressin, aldosterone and ANP are less important. This concept was emphasised by studies showing a significant circadian influence on the renal response to immersion. For instance, Krishna & Danovitch (1983) demonstrated that these renal responses were attenuated at night. Subsequently, Shiraki et al. (1986) confirmed these observations and further showed that the increases in cardiac output and the decreases in plasma renin activity, aldosterone and vasopressin were similar during the day and night. Later, Miki et al. (1988) reported that elevations of ANP during water immersion at night were similar to those during the day, despite nocturnal suppression of the diuretic and natriuretic responses. Since the day versus night hormonal responses were similar, by exclusion, these circadian studies imply that a reduced reflex suppression of renal sympathetic activity at night is responsible for the attenuated diuresis and natriuresis during water immersion.

It has been well documented that the kidneys respond to a rise in arterial pressure with a rise in interstitial pressure, and this causes pressure-induced diuresis and natriuresis (Cowley 1992). However, Hajduczok et al. (1987a) indicated that the immersion-induced natriuresis was abolished after cardiac denervation, despite similar elevations in arterial pressure, and Miki et al. (1989a) showed abolition of the natriuresis and diuresis following renal denervation, despite similar elevations in arterial pressure. Thus, increased arterial pressure does not appear to contribute in a major way to the water immersion natriuresis.

Autotransfusion during upright immersion causes a hypervolaemic haemodilution and a decline of plasma colloid oncotic pressure. The latter would diminish the tubular reabsorptive capacity for sodium, contributing to natriuresis. Using graded immersions in humans and the application of thigh cuffs to reduce fluid shifts from the legs, Johansen et al. (1998) postulated the decline in plasma colloid oncotic pressure could account for a significant portion of the increase in sodium excretion observed during water immersion. On the other hand, as indicated above, the haemodilution responses in humans during water immersion reveal minimal circadian influences, yet the natriuretic responses are suppressed at night, reinforcing the primary role of renal sympathetic neural activity in mediating immersion-induced natriuresis and diuresis.

6 MODULATING FACTORS

6.1 Time

The cardiac-renal responses to water immersion described above are time dependent. The central shift of vascular fluid and the resulting increases in stroke volume and cardiac output occur rapidly (Krasney 1996), and are sustained at elevated levels for hours (Begin et al. 1976, Claybaugh et al. 1986, Krasney 1996, Pendergast et al. 1987). In fact, during space flight, stroke volume and cardiac output remain elevated for up to 15 days (Shykoff et al. 1996). The autotransfusion of intracellular fluid into the vascular compartment is slower to develop than the shift of blood from dependent to central regions, but there is a significant haemodilution by 20 min and the plasma volume remains elevated for 6–12 h (Johansen et al. 1992).

By contrast, the renal responses to water immersion are slower to develop and subside sooner than the cardiac responses, with peak natriuretic and diuretic responses developing within 1–2 h but returning to preimmersion levels by 4 h.

The apparent dissociation between cardiac and renal responses in the time domain, in terms of their relative on-set and off-set times, emphasises that control of the cardiac-renal systems involves multifactorial and redundant components.

6.2 Fluid supplementation

Various fluid supplementation protocols have been applied during extended water immersion, with the idea of helping to sustain the blood volume and based on the assumption that the plasma volume declines (Gauer & Henry 1976). Protocols have included hourly boluses of water and replacement of fluid losses with saline, resulting in a water diuresis. However, due to immersion-induced autotransfusion, this assumption is incorrect, and the rationale for particular hydration protocols has never been entirely clear (Krasney 1996).

Notwithstanding, upon exiting the water, the fluid shifts experienced during immersion are reversed, causing reductions of cardiac output and plasma volume, and favouring orthostatic intolerance. However, this would be more likely with longer immersions, as is the case with sojourns in space (Rowell 1993).

6.3 Gender

When differences in body size are considered there are no gender-based differences in the cardiovascular or renal responses to thermoneutral water immersion (Watenpaugh et al. 2000). During immersion in cold water, there are also no gender differences, after correction for body fatness and surface area, in either the physiological or metabolic responses (Tikuisis et al. 2000). Thus, the above description of responses to water immersion can be causally applied to both men and women (Glickman-Weiss et al. 2000).

6.4 Ageing

Although the renal responses to water immersion are attenuated at night (Krishna & Danovitch 1983, Shiraki et al. 1986), this may not be the case in elderly subjects. Nocturnal urine production increases with age after 50 years, with increased urination frequency being reported (Blanker et al. 2002). Although the increase in cardiac output observed in young persons is blunted in the elderly (Pendergast et al. 1993), natriuretic responses to water immersion are augmented, with increases in glomerular filtration rate (Tajima et al. 1988) despite a decline in pressure-dependent sodium and water excretion with age (Vargas et al. 1997).

6.5 Exercise

When subjects exercise in water, the cardiovascular system's baseline is altered, with increased cardiac output and stroke volume, perfusion to non-muscle tissues, reduced heart rate and total peripheral resistance. However, blood pressures are similar to those observed in air. In spite of this difference in resting cardiovascular baseline, the cardiopulmonary responses to increased metabolism are similar in both thermoneutral water and air, after attaining an oxygen uptake of about 1.0 L·min^{-1} and up to ~80% of maximal oxygen uptake (Pendergast 1988, Perini et al. 1998). At low exercise intensities, cardiac output and stroke volume do not increase from rest as oxygen consumption increases, while muscle blood flow, ventilation and oxygen transport are elevated. Maximal cardiac output, heart rate, blood flow, oxygen transport and power output are about 15% lower during water immersion than air, even in thermoneutral water (Pendergast 1988).

The potential for pulmonary oedema increases during exercise in water (Slade et al. 2001). This appears to be due to increased pulmonary blood flow and pressure, combined with reduced resting lung volumes, followed by the additional exercise-induced increase in blood flow and pressure, resulting in pulmonary capillary engorgement, increased transmural pressures and plasma efflux into the interstitium.

6.6 Changes in water temperature

Cold water immersion, relative to thermoneutral water immersion, elicits similar reductions in intracellular fluid, although the increase in plasma volume is reduced with

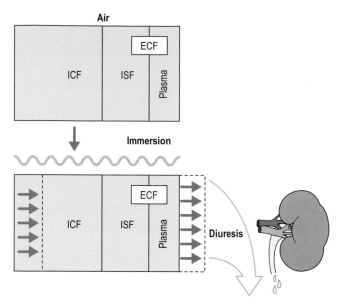

Figure 22.5 Upright immersion expands the plasma volume, primarily from the intravascular compartment (ICF) and via the interstitial (ISF) and extracellular spaces (ECF). The role of the kidney is to minimise this hypervolaemia by increasing renal free-water clearance. Redrawn from Krasney (1996) with permission.

cold water immersion (Stocks et al. 2004). Exercise performance is impaired by brief exposures to cold water, even in elite athletes, and the impairment is magnified by prolonged exposure (Pendergast 1988, Schniepp et al. 2002). Most cold-induced physiological changes are due to increased sympathetic nerve activity (Sramek et al. 2000).

Cardiac output is generally similar for both cold and thermoneutral immersion but the heart rate is depressed (diving reflex), such that stroke volume is elevated. Arterial blood pressure is not elevated because the vasoconstriction in skin, subcutaneous tissues and muscle is offset by vasodilatation in other areas, and total peripheral resistance remains unchanged (Pendergast 1988). In cold water, cutaneous vasoconstriction is initiated by decreased skin temperature. However, a gradual reduction in core temperature greatly augments sympathetic activity with further vasoconstriction during sustained cold exposure and cold acclimation (O'Brien et al. 2000). Cooling the skin, but not the core, reduces thermal strain during exercise and may improve performance in warm air environments (Kay et al. 1999), and postexercise cooling may facilitate subsequent performance and tissue repair.

7 CONCLUSION

The physiological response to water immersion is geared toward readjustment of blood flow to metabolic demand. The primary end-organ for this readjustment is the kidney, which increases urine flow and sodium excretion to minimise the immersion-induced increase in plasma volume, resulting from a major fluid shift out of the intracellular compartment (Figure 22.5). Figure 22.6 summarises the circulatory, hormonal and renal responses to thermoneutral water immersion, and emphasises the redundancy in the several control systems and the primary role of the renal sympathetic nerves in mediating the renal responses.

The physiological adjustments that occur during water immersion offset the primary changes caused by the hydrostatic pressure difference (increased venous return and autotransfusion), establish a new homeostasis and do not appear to limit performance during immersion. However, the reversal of these adjustments on emersion may cause orthostatic intolerance and reduced performance. Water immersion appears to be especially useful for treatment of fluid retention disorders such as hypertension of pregnancy, cirrhosis of the liver and the nephrotic syndrome (Rascher et al. 1986). Water immersion elicits a diuresis and natriuresis in patients with congestive heart failure; however, these responses are attenuated compared to control subjects due to higher plasma levels of angiotensin II and aldosterone in the heart failure patients (Gabrielsen et al. 2000b). The weightlessness caused by immersion is also a useful tool for postinjury rehabilitation of both humans and animals, as well as for improving the physical fitness of patients and elderly persons.

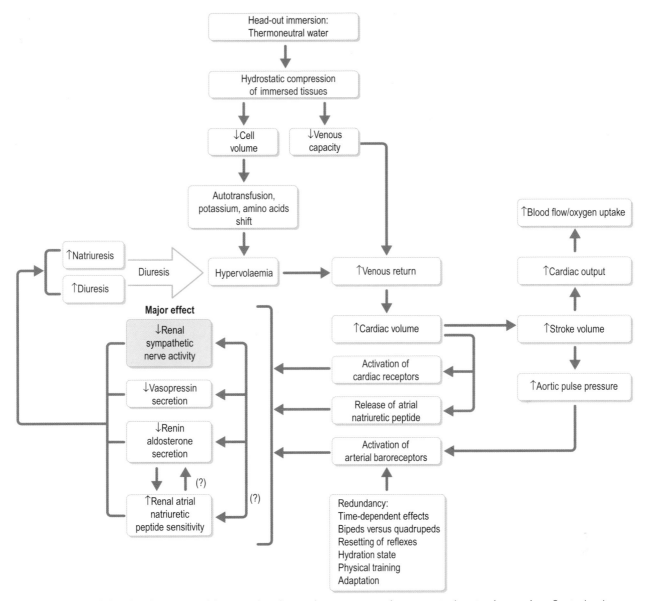

Figure 22.6 Summary of the circulatory, renal hormonal and neural responses to thermoneutral water immersion. Central volume expansion and elevated cardiac output are caused by compression of dependent veins and autotransfusion. The rise in cardiac output exceeds the metabolic demand at rest and during exercise. Activation of cardiovascular mechanoreceptors and increased atrial natriuretic peptide secretion sets into motion neural and hormonal mechanisms that promote sodium and fluid loss, thus minimising hypervolaemia and theoretically readjusting blood flow to the prevailing oxygen uptake. The most powerful efferent mechanism affecting the kidney appears to be the sympathetic nerves. The associated hormonal responses appear to modulate the primary renal response, with many additional factors modulating the basic renal neurohumoral response to immersion. Redrawn from Krasney (1996) with permission.

References

Arborelius MJ, Balldin UI, Lilja B, Lundgren CEG 1972 Hemodynamic changes in man with head above water. Aerospace Medicine 43:592–598

Begin R, Epstein M, Sackner MA, Levinson R, Dougherty R, Duncan D 1976 Effects of water immersion to the neck on pulmonary circulation and tissue volume in man. Journal of Applied Physiology 40:293–299

Behn C, Gauer OH, Kirsch K, Eckert P 1969 Effects of sustained intrathoracic vascular distention on body fluid distribution and renal excretion in man. Pflugers Archiv 313:123–135

Bie P, Mumksdorf M, Warburg J 1984 Renal effects of over-hydration during vasopressin infusion in conscious dogs. American Journal of Physiology 247:F103–F109

Blanker MH, Bernsen RM, Bosch JL, Thomas S, Groeneveld FP, Prins A, Bohnen AM 2002 Relations between nocturnal voiding frequency and nocturnal urine production in older men: a population-based study. Urology 60:612–616

Christie JL, Sheldahl LM, Tristani FE, Wann LS, Sagar KB, Levandoski SG, Ptacin MJ, Sobocinski KA, Morris RD 1990 Cardiovascular regulation during head-out water immersion exercise. Journal of Applied Physiology 69:657–664

Claybaugh JR, Pendergast DR, Davis JE, Akiba C, Pazik M, Hong SK 1986 Fluid conservation in athletes: responses to water intake, supine posture and immersion. Journal of Applied Physiology 61:7–15

Cowley AW 1992 Long-term control of arterial pressure. Physiological Reviews 72:231–300

Davis JT, DuBois 1977 Immersion diuresis in dogs. Journal of Applied Physiology 42:915–922

DiBona GF, Kopp UG 1997 Neural control of renal function. Physiological Reviews 77:76–197

Epstein M 1978 Renal effects of head-out water immersion in man: implications for an understanding of volume homeostasis. Physiological Reviews 58:529–581

Epstein M 1992 Renal effects of head-out water immersion in humans: a 15 year update. Physiological Reviews 72:563–621

Epstein M, DeNunzio AG, Loutzenheiser RD 1981 Effects of vasopressin administration on the diuresis of water immersion in normal humans. Journal of Applied Physiology 51:1384–1387

Epstein M, Johnson M, DeNunzio AG 1983 Effects of water immersion on plasma catecholamines in normal humans. Journal of Applied Physiology 54:244–248

Gabrielsen A, Warberg J, Christensen NJ, Bie P, Stadeager C, Pump B, Norsk P 2000a Arterial pulse pressure and vasopressin release during graded water immersion in humans. American Journal of Physiology 278:R1583–R1588

Gabrielsen A, Sørensen VB, Pump B, Galatius S, Videbaek R, Bie P, Warberg J, Christensen NJ, Wroblewski H, Kastrup J, Norsk P 2000b Cardiovascular and neuroendocrine responses to water immersion in compensated heart failure. American Journal of Physiology 279: H1931–H1940

Gauer OH, Henry JP 1976 Neurohumoral control of plasma volume. In: Guyton AC, Cowley AW (eds) Cardiovascular physiology II. University Park Press, Baltimore, MD, 145–189

Gauer OH, Thron HL 1965 Postural changes in the circulation. In: Hamilton WF, Dow P (eds) Handbook of physiology. Circulation. section 2, volume III. American Physiological Society, Washington, DC, 2409–2439

Gauer OH, Henry JP, Sieker HO, Wendt WE 1951 Heart and lungs as a receptor region controlling blood volume. American Journal of Physiology 167:786–794

Glickman-Weiss EL, Cheatham C, Caine M, Blegen M, Marcinkiewicz J, Mittleman KD 2000 The influence of gender and menstrual phase on thermosensitivity during cold water immersion. Aviation, Space and Environmental Medicine 71:715–722

Goetz, KL, Wang BC, Geer PG, Lendly RJ Jr, Reinhardt HW 1986 Atrial stretch increases sodium excretion independently of release of atrial peptides. American Journal of Physiology 250:R946–R950

Guyton AC, Coleman TG 1980 Quantitative analysis of the pathophysiology of hypertension. Circulation Research 24:1–12

Hajduczok G, Hong SK, Claybaugh JR, Krasney JA 1987a The role of the cardiac nerves in the hemodynamic and renal responses to head-out water immersion in conscious dogs. American Journal of Physiology 253:R242–R253

Hajduczok G, Miki K, Claybaugh JR, Hong SK, Krasney JA 1987b Regional circulatory responses to head-out water immersion in conscious dogs. American Journal of Physiology 253:R254–R263

Hong SK, Ceretelli P, Cruz JC, Rahn H 1969 Mechanisms of respiration during submersion under water. Journal of Applied Physiology 27:535–538

Johansen LB, Foldager N, Stadeager C, Kristensen MS, Bie P, Warberg J, Kamegai M, Norsk P 1992 Plasma volume, fluid shifts and renal responses in humans during 12 h of head-out water immersion. Journal of Applied Physiology 73:539–544

Johansen LB, Bie P, Warberg J, Christensen NJ, Norsk P 1995 Role of hemodilution on renal responses to water immersion in humans. American Journal of Physiology 269:R1068–R1076

Johansen LB, Jensen TU, Pump B, Norsk P 1997 Contribution of abdomen and legs to central blood volume expansion in humans during immersion. Journal of Applied Physiology 83:695–699

Johansen LB, Pump B, Warburg J, Christensen NJ, Norsk P 1998 Preventing hemodilution abolishes natriuresis of water immersion in humans. American Journal of Physiology 275:R879–R888

Kay D, Taaffe DR, Marino FE 1999 Whole-body core-cooling and heat storage during self-paced cycling performance in warm humid environment. Journal of Sports Sciences 17:937–944

Krasney JA 1996 Physiological responses to head-out water immersion: animal studies. In: Fregly MJ, Blatteis C (eds) Handbook of physiology: environmental physiology, volume II. Oxford University Press, New York, 855–888

Krasney JA, Hajduczok G, Miki K, Claybaugh JR, Sondeen JL, Pendergast DR, and Hong SK 1989 Head-out water immersion: a critical evaluation of the Gauer–Henry hypothesis. In: Claybaugh JR, Wade CE (eds) Hormonal regulation of fluids and electrolytes. Plenum, New York, 147–185

Krasney JA, Carroll M, Krasney E, Iwamoto J, Claybaugh JR, Hong SK 1991 Renal, hormonal and fluid shift responses to ANP during head-out water immersion in awake dogs. American Journal of Physiology 261:R188–R197

Krishna GG, Danovitch GM 1983 Renal response to central volume expansion in humans is attenuated at night. American Journal of Physiology 244:R48–R486

Metzler CJ, Ramsay DJ 1989 Atrial peptide potentiates renal responses to volume expansion in conscious dogs. American Journal of Physiology 256:R284–R289

Miki K, Hajduczok G, Hong SK, Krasney JA 1986a Plasma volume changes during head-out water immersion in the conscious dog. American Journal of Physiology 251:R284–R289

Miki K, Hajduczok G, Klocke MJ, Krasney JA, Hong SK, DeBold AJ 1986b Atrial natriuretic factor and renal function during head-out water immersion in conscious dogs. American Journal of Physiology 251:R1000–R1008

Miki K, Hajduczok G, Hong SK, Krasney JA 1987 Extracellular fluid and plasma volumes during water immersion in nephrectomized dogs. American Journal of Physiology 252:R972–R978

Miki K, Shiraki K, Sagawa S, DeBold AJ, Hong SK 1988 Atrial natriuretic factor during head-out immersion at night. American Journal of Physiology 254:R235–R241

Miki K, Hayashida Y, Sagawa S, Shiraki K 1989a Renal sympathetic nerve activity and natriuresis during water immersion in conscious dogs. American Journal of Physiology 256:R299–R305

Miki K, Klocke MR, Hong SK, Krasney JA 1989b Interstitial and intravascular pressures in conscious dogs during head-out water immersion. American Journal of Physiology 256:R358–R364

Norsk P, Epstein M 1988 Effects of water immersion on arginine vasopressin release in humans. Journal of Applied Physiology 64:1–10

Norsk P, Bonde-Peterson F, Christensen NJ 1990 Catecholamines, circulation and the kidney during head-out water immersion in humans. Journal of Applied Physiology 69:479–484

O'Brien C, Young AJ, Lee DT, Shitzer A, Sawka MN, Pandolf KB 2000 Role of core temperature as a stimulus for cold acclimation during repeated immersion in 20 degrees C water. Journal of Applied Physiology 89:242–250

Pendergast DR 1988 The effect of body cooling on oxygen transport during exercise. Medicine and Science in Sports and Exercise 20(suppl):S171–S176

Pendergast DR, DeBold AJ, Pazik M, Hong SK 1987 Effect of head-out immersion on plasma atrial natriuretic factor in man. Proceedings of the Society for Experimental Biology and Medicine 184:429–435

Pendergast DR, Fisher NM, Calkins E 1993 Cardiovascular, neuromuscular and metabolic alterations with age leading to frailty. Journals of Gerontology. Series A, Biological Sciences and Medical Sciences 48(Special Issue):61–67

Perini R, S Milesi, Biancardi L, Pendergast DR, Veicsteinas A 1998 Heart rate variability in exercising humans: effect of water immersion. European Journal of Applied Physiology 77:326–332

Prefaut C, Dubois F, Roussos C, Amaral-Marque R, Macklem PT, Ruff F 1979 Influence of immersion to the neck in water on airway closure and distribution of perfusion in man. Respiration Physiology 37:313–323

Rascher W, Tulassay T, Sevberth HW, Himbert U, Lang U, Scharer K 1986 Diuretic and hormonal responses to head-out water immersion in nephrotic syndrome. Journal of Pediatrics 109:609–614

Rowell LB 1986 Human circulation regulation during physical stress. Oxford University Press, New York

Rowell LB 1993 Human cardiovascular control. Oxford University Press, New York

Rutlen DL, Christensen G, Helgesen KG, Ilebekk A 1990 Influence of atrial natriuretic factor on intravascular volume displacement in pigs. American Journal of Physiology 259:H1595–H1600

Schniepp J, Campbell TS, Powell KL, Pincivero DM 2002 The effects of cold-water immersion on power output and heart rate in elite cyclists. Journal of Strength and Conditioning Research 16:561–566

Shiraki K, Konda N, Sagawa S, Claybaugh JR, Hong SK 1986 Cardiorenal-endocrine responses to head-out immersion at night. Journal of Applied Physiology 60:176–183

Shykoff BE, Farhi LE, Olszowka AJ, Pendergast DR, Rokitka MA, Eisenhardt CG, Morin RA 1996 Cardiovascular responses to submaximal exercise in sustained microgravity. Journal of Applied Physiology 81(1):26–32

Slade JB Jr, Hattori T, Ray CS, Bove AA, Cianci P 2001 Pulmonary edema associated with scuba diving: case reports and review. Chest 120:1686–1694

Sondeen JL, Hong SK, Claybaugh JR, Krasney JA 1990 Effect of hydration state on renal responses to head-out water immersion in conscious dogs. Undersea Biomedical Research 17:395–411

Sramek P, Simeckova M, Jansky L, Savlikova J, Vybiral S 2000 Human physiological responses to immersion into water of different temperatures. European Journal of Applied Physiology 81:436–442

Stocks JM, Patterson MJ, Hyde DE, Jenkins AB, Mittleman KD, Taylor NAS 2004 Effects of immersion water temperature on whole-body fluid distribution in humans. Acta Physiologica Scandinavica 182:3–10

Strange K 2004 Cellular volume homeostasis. Advances in Physiology Education 28:155–159

Tajima F, Sagawa S, Iwamoto J, Miki K, Claybaugh JR, Shiraki K 1988 Renal and endocrine responses in the elderly during head-out water immersion. American Journal of Physiology 254:R977–R983

Taylor NAS, Morrison JB 1991 Lung volume changes in response to altered breathing gas pressures during upright immersion. European Journal of Applied Physiology 62:122–129

Taylor NAS, Morrison JB 1999 Static respiratory muscle work during immersion with positive and negative respiratory loading. Journal of Applied Physiology 87:1397–1403

Tikuisis, P, Jacobs I, Moroz D, Vallerand AL, Martineau L 2000 Comparison of thermoregulatory responses between men and women in cold water. Journal of Applied Physiology 89:1403–1411

Vargas F, Ortiz MC, Fortepiani LA, Atucha NM, Garcia-Estan J 1997 Age-elated changes in the pressure diuresis and natriuresis response. American Journal of Physiology 273:R578–R582

Von Diringshofen H 1948 Die Wirkungen des hydrostatischen druckes des wasserbades auf den blutdruck in den kapillaren un die bindegewebsentwasserung 7. Kreislaufforschung 37:382–390

Watenpaugh, DE, Pump B, Bie P, Norsk P 2000 Does gender influence human cardiovascular and renal responses to water immersion? Journal of Applied Physiology 89:621–628

Chapter 23

Diving physiology: free diving, breathing apparatus, saturation diving

James B. Morrison John R. Clarke

1 OVERVIEW

Underwater diving is one of the few earth-bound activities where people must carry their own gas supply or have it delivered through a hose. It is certainly the only activity where a human routinely breathes gas other than air or oxygen. Although divers usually breathe compressed air, they can also breathe mixtures of nitrogen and oxygen (nitrox), helium and oxygen (heliox) or nitrogen, helium and oxygen (trimix; section 6). In deep experimental dives to depths in the order of 500 metres of seawater (5.1 MPa), mixtures of hydrogen, helium and oxygen have been breathed (hydreliox). In shallow experimental trials, divers have breathed oxygenated mixtures of neon and argon.

As we will see in this chapter, all the gases entering a diver's body exert an influence upon the body. The purpose of those gases is to make sure that the pressure of water outside the human body is counterbalanced by the pressure of gas in air spaces inside the body. Without a proper counterbalancing of internal and external pressure, the body could be crushed, as purportedly happened during the early years of hardhat diving when shipboard gas compressors failed, allowing the pressure in diving helmets to drop below that of the surrounding seawater (Davis 1981). Although this problem has been overcome with improved breathing systems, divers still experience injuries due to sudden pressure changes (barotrauma), through expansion or contraction of gases in air spaces (lungs or sinuses; section 2.2).

The breathing gas supplied to a diver is first pressurised, stored in gas storage bottles and then regulated by the diver's underwater breathing apparatus to match the surrounding pressure of the water column (hydrostatic pressure). This process increases the number of molecules compressed into a given volume and therefore increases the gas density, which makes it more difficult for a diver to move air through the airways and breathing apparatus. Fortunately, density increases can be partially offset with breathing gases like helium and hydrogen that are considerably less dense than air. Normally, ventilation of the diver's lungs is measured in $L \cdot min^{-1}$ at body temperature

Table 23.1 Commonly used units of pressure and their equivalence to a standard atmosphere (atm)

Unit	atm	pascal	bar	psi	msw	fsw	mmHg
Equivalence	1.0	101,325	1.01325	14.696	10.13	33.08	760

psi, pounds per square inch; msw, metres of seawater; fsw, feet of seawater, mmHg, millimetres of mercury.

(37°C) and pressure saturated conditions (BTPS), whereas oxygen uptake and carbon dioxide production are measured in L·min^{-1} at standard temperature (0°C) and pressure (101.3 kPa) dry conditions (STPD).

The energy a diver must expend to breathe is a major concern, since an insufficiency of gas flow results in a feeling of suffocation or breathlessness (dyspnoea). When assessing the ease of breathing through breathing apparatus at depth, various terms are used, such as the work of breathing or resistive effort. The physical units associated with these measures vary. For instance, the physical work of breathing is often expressed in joules (J). However, more often, work is normalised for tidal volume and thus may have units of J·L^{-1} (and simplified to kilopascals (kPa)).[1] Physiological pressures are commonly measured in kPa or mmHg. However, ambient seawater pressure (depth) is measured in metres (or feet) of seawater (msw, fsw), kPa, atmospheres or bar (100 kPa), whilst gas storage is measured in MPa or pounds per square inch (psi). Common units of pressure and their equivalence to a standard atmosphere (CGPM 1954) and SI units (pascal or N·m^{-2}), are shown in Table 23.1. We mention this in the overview to clarify the interchangeability of terminology used both in the diving literature and elsewhere in this chapter.

2 PHYSIOLOGICAL AND PHYSICAL STRESSES OF DIVING

2.1 Decompression disorders

As a diver descends, the absolute pressure of gases in the lungs increases, creating gas partial pressure gradients between the alveoli and the pulmonary circulation. Oxygen and inert gas will diffuse from the alveoli and dissolve in the bloodstream until a new equilibrium pressure (saturation) is reached. This process is repeated at the tissue level where gases diffuse from the systemic capillaries into the surrounding tissues. While oxygen is metabolised, the volume of inert gas (e.g. nitrogen, helium, hydrogen) dissolved in these tissues will continue to rise until saturation is reached or the diver ascends. As the diver ascends, the

process is reversed, and inert gas diffuses from the tissues to the circulation and is released via the alveoli. In an orderly ascent, inert gas will be released from the tissue and circulation mainly by diffusion. However, if the ambient pressure drops below that of tissue inert gas pressure, inert gas will be released from the tissue and circulation in the form of bubbles.

If the diver ascends too quickly, gas bubbles will form, and may grow in size to cause decompression disorders in the form of pain in tissues or blockage of the circulation. In its most common form, decompression illness presents as pain in the region of a synovial joint that may vary in focus and intensity, and is known as 'the bends'. Other forms of decompression illness include oedema due to lymphatic blockage, transient itching (skin bends) and loss of balance due to inner ear disturbance (the staggers). In more serious decompression disorders, bubbles may cause blockage of the pulmonary circulation (respiratory decompression illness or the chokes), peripheral sensory and motor disorders that may develop rapidly into temporary or permanent paralysis (spinal bend) and visual blurring, headaches and confusion that, in serious cases, will lead to paralysis or coma (central nervous system bend). In all cases, the recognised treatment is immediate recompression to reduce bubble size and also to reduce or reverse tissue supersaturation, accompanied by pure oxygen breathing to enhance the tissue to capillary inert gas partial pressure gradient, thereby accelerating inert gas elimination (US Navy Diving Manual 2005).

In practice, divers will decompress in accordance with carefully tested decompression tables that have been developed using theoretical models of inert gas elimination, based on theories of inert gas diffusion, tissue perfusion or bubble dynamics (Tikuisis & Gerth 2003). Provided recreational air divers operate within the bounds of recognised decompression tables, decompression illness amongst this group should be rare. Although decompression illness cannot be ruled out entirely, the main causes of serious decompression illness among scuba divers are overconfidence, recklessness and human error.

2.2 Barotrauma

Barotrauma does not result from the release of inert gas from solution, but is caused by the expansion or contraction of gases in an existing air space. If an air space is transiently

---

[1]The simplest of these units is kPa, the units left when dividing joules by litres. However, to avoid confusion when using kPa, authors must differentiate between normalised measures of work and measures of peak or mean respiratory pressures.

occluded during compression or decompression, a pressure difference is developed across the tissue enclosing that space, causing tissue stress and pain. Common sites of barotrauma include the middle ear, sinuses, teeth, lungs, mask, helmet and diving suit.

Normally air spaces within the body have an opening to the atmosphere. For example, air passes to and from the middle ear via the eustachian tube. Generally, the eustachian tube vents air from the middle ear as air pressure within this cavity rises during decompression (e.g. ears 'pop' when driving up a mountain). This action equalises pressure between the surrounding air and this cavity. However, difficulties can occur during compression. Failure to equalise can result in a ruptured tympanic membrane at relatively shallow water depths (e.g. 5 metres of seawater). If a diver has a cold, the middle ear or sinus may be blocked, creating low pressure in these spaces during compression. Alternatively, air spaces may equalise during compression, but become blocked on the return to surface, causing pain from overpressure. The sinuses or dental cavities may cause severe pain during decompression. Similarly, a diver must constantly adjust mask, helmet and dry suit pressure during descent. Failure to do so can cause severe squeezing during compression (e.g. face squeeze occurs from an unvented mask).

The most hazardous form of this phenomenon is pulmonary barotrauma or burst lung. It occurs due to the rapid expansion of alveolar gas volume during decompression. As barotrauma is independent of dive time, and the greatest expansion of gas occurs during the last 10 metres before surfacing, it can occur even in short, shallow dives. Although the most likely cause is failure to exhale sufficiently during ascent, it may also occur when a diver exhales properly, but can result from a partial blockage of the airway, due to lung disease or congestion. The alveolar membranes are damaged and gas may escape into the pleural space, causing pneumothorax, or enter the circulation, causing arterial gas embolism. A typical symptom is loss of consciousness on arrival at the surface. However, the symptoms can be less catastrophic, such as chest pain, irregular breathing, weakness or paralysis, impaired vision and confusion, and can be difficult to differentiate from other forms of decompression illness (Neuman 2003). Pulmonary barotrauma is a potentially fatal disorder and treatment requires immediate recompression, with an emphasis on reduction of gas emboli, followed by a period of oxygen breathing (US Navy Diving Manual 2005).

2.3 Narcosis

There are two types of narcosis encountered in diving: inert gas (nitrogen or helium) and carbon dioxide narcosis. By far the most common is nitrogen narcosis, which is likely to be experienced to varying degrees when breathing air deeper than 30 metres of seawater (401 kPa). Symptoms of narcosis include euphoria, excitement and mental impairment and at extremes, confusion, disorientation and loss of consciousness. Nitrogen narcosis has been shown to slow mental activity, increase errors in cognitive and fine motor tasks, increase response time to stimuli and impair short-term memory (Bennett & Rostain 2003a).

When breathing air, there are no noticeable narcotic effects at depths shallower than 20 metres of seawater (301 kPa). At 30 metres of seawater, divers display mild euphoria and significant but small decrements in cognitive function. At 60 metres of seawater, symptoms become more noticeable and resemble intoxication, with marked impairment of mental and motor functions, and increasing errors in tasks. At 90–120 metres of seawater (1.0–1.3 MPa), divers breathing air experience severe narcosis, including an inability to perform complex tasks or respond to instructions, and may suffer from confusion and impending loss of consciousness. The effects of narcosis are not alleviated with time at pressure and are reported to be aggravated by fatigue, hard work and anxiety. For these reasons, air diving is generally not recommended beyond 50 metres of seawater.

Although the mechanism of inert gas narcosis is not well understood, it has been shown that the narcotic potency of a gas has a strong correlation with its solubility in lipids (Bennett & Rostain 2003a). Different gases will display similar narcotic effects when they reach the same molar concentration in lipids. Thus, the more soluble the inert gas, the lower the partial pressure required to achieve narcosis. As helium has a low solubility in lipids and is also less dense than nitrogen, replacing nitrogen with helium in the diver's breathing gas eliminates inert gas narcosis, and considerably reduces the work of breathing at depth. In most military and commercial diving operations, divers will switch to a heliox or trimix breathing gas mixture when diving beyond 40 or 50 metres of seawater.

The effects of nitrogen narcosis can be further exacerbated by the presence of carbon dioxide narcosis. Military divers use closed-circuit breathing apparatus for covert operations, and divers rebreathe the same gas but with the carbon dioxide removed (scrubbed). When scrubbers near the end of their life expectancy, carbon dioxide partial pressures of up to 5 kPa (~5% of 1 atmosphere) can occur in the breathing gas. Such carbon dioxide levels can disrupt physiological gas exchange and lead eventually to disorientation and unconsciousness. Even without a build-up of carbon dioxide in breathing apparatus, it is not uncommon for divers to experience elevated end-tidal carbon dioxide partial pressures that can exceed 8 kPa (60 mmHg) during underwater work (sections 2.3 and 3.3), compared with normal surface levels of approximately 5.3 kPa (40 mmHg). Carbon dioxide is an extremely potent narcotic, and an end-tidal carbon dioxide partial pressure increase of 2.7 kPa (20 mmHg) can have a synergistic effect that transforms the diver from a state of moderate narcosis to a state of confusion, disorientation, amnesia and possible loss of consciousness (sections 3.3 and 3.4).

A carbon dioxide concentration of a few percent is a strong respiratory stimulant, via chemoreceptor feedback. However, at concentrations exceeding 10%, it is a respiratory depressant. In the medical arena, concentrations of as much as 30% carbon dioxide in oxygen found clinical application in the 1950s and 1960s as a treatment for psychoneuroses. Psychiatric patients were given 20–30 breaths of the so-called Meduna mixture (Meduna 1950). Reportedly, the carbon dioxide narcosis treatment, a type of shock therapy, had a palliative effect on psychoses, but was replaced when safer and more convenient drug therapies became available.

2.4 Oxygen toxicity

A fact of diving that is rarely known by non-divers is that oxygen is toxic. Oxygen in the air we breathe daily is not poisonous only because we have evolved biochemical defences against it. However, when air is compressed as a diver descends, the number of molecules of oxygen breathed in with each breath increases to the point of overwhelming our innate protection. This is especially important for divers who breathe pure oxygen (section 5.3.2).

When planning working dives with gas mixtures using elevated partial pressures of oxygen, divers must take into account the two forms of oxygen toxicity: pulmonary and central nervous system. The first causes chest discomfort, cough and a burning sensation on inspiration. In extreme cases, pulmonary oxygen toxicity can cause fluid formation in the lungs (pulmonary oedema). Due to these pulmonary effects, critical care patients cannot be maintained on 100% oxygen for extended periods since, after only 6 h of breathing 100% oxygen, healthy subjects experience symptoms similar to those of tracheobronchitis (Ryerson & Block 1991).

Central nervous system oxygen toxicity can cause the sudden onset of seizures. There may be prodromal symptoms (precursor indicators), like a metallic taste, visual symptoms or fingertip tingling. However, these premonitory symptoms are not reliable, and the first sign of central nervous system toxicity may well be grand mal seizures. Of course, if a diver seizes while underwater and breathing from a mouthpiece, the mouthpiece will be displaced and the diver will drown.

Whereas pulmonary effects begin to develop over several hours and whenever oxygen pressure exceeds 1 atmosphere (101.3 kPa), central nervous system effects can occur within minutes when oxygen partial pressure approaches or exceeds 160 kPa (~1.6 atmospheres) during mixed gas diving. Symptoms seem to occur in a dose–response manner: the higher the dose, the faster their onset. Onset is also aggravated by other confounding factors such as physical work, gas density and elevated carbon dioxide partial pressure. Thus, although pure oxygen may be breathed for up to 100 min (with 5-min air breaks every 20 min) at an ambient pressure of 285 kPa during recompression therapy in a hyperbaric chamber, the inspired pressure of oxygen is limited to 178 kPa for 240 min when breathing pure oxygen underwater, and to 130 kPa for 120 min when breathing mixed gas during deeper dives (US Navy Diving Manual 2005).

2.5 Carbon dioxide sensitivity

Our ventilatory system is designed not only to participate in oxygen delivery but to facilitate carbon dioxide elimination. Carbon dioxide dissolved in blood stimulates central and peripheral chemoreceptors, driving ventilation. On average, divers ventilate an additional 3 L·min^{-1} for each 0.13 kPa (1 mmHg) increase in arterial carbon dioxide partial pressure.

However, divers have varying sensitivities to carbon dioxide. Some divers (high responders) increase ventilation by 5 L·min^{-1} for the same (1 mmHg) change in carbon dioxide partial pressure, while others (low responders) increase their ventilation by less than 2 L·min^{-1} (Pendergast et al. 2006). As arterial carbon dioxide rises, high responders ventilate considerably more than low responders, but are prone to ventilation-induced dyspnoea (breathlessness). In contrast, low responders remain comfortable in their breathing, even to the point of becoming disoriented or unconscious due to inadequate ventilation in the face of a rising arterial carbon dioxide tension.

Why would arterial carbon dioxide rise? First, in rebreathing apparatus, as the carbon dioxide absorbent becomes depleted, the carbon dioxide content begins to rise and can go up to dangerous levels.

Second, in the face of high breathing resistance, divers tend to slow breathing, occasionally to the point of hypoventilation, resulting in carbon dioxide accumulation within the blood (hypercapnia).

Respiratory muscles can be trained (Chapter 3) and interestingly, it appears that respiratory muscle training can help low responders (hypoventilators) attain a more normal ventilatory response to carbon dioxide (Pendergast et al. 2006). Curiously, high responders seem to become less sensitive to carbon dioxide, also approaching normality, countering the notion that response to carbon dioxide is purely determined by chemoreceptors.

2.6 Carbon dioxide and oxygen interaction

One of the more dangerous aspects of hypercapnia is that cerebral blood flow is increased (Brian 1998, Kety & Schmidt 1948, Patterson et al. 1955). While that is not dangerous by itself, when that blood is carrying larger than normal quantities of oxygen, the high blood flow exposes the brain to a greater dose of oxygen, increasing the diver's susceptibility to central nervous system oxygen toxicity.

A worst-case scenario for a deleterious interaction between carbon dioxide and oxygen would be the following: a diver working hard using a high-resistance, closed-circuit rebreather is prone to hypoventilation, causing a rise in arterial carbon dioxide. If the carbon dioxide scrubbing canister becomes depleted, then inspired carbon dioxide will begin to rise, further exacerbating hypercapnia. If the rebreather is a pure oxygen rig that is being dived too deeply (to avoid detection), then the blood and brain become hyperoxic. This combination of factors conspires against the diver, increasing the probability of an oxygen-induced seizure.

2.7 Cold

Exposure to cold water is an important issue in diving (Chapter 20). Although recreational divers may prefer warm climates, a great deal of recreational, military and commercial diving takes place in cold waters. It has been estimated that the majority of diving takes place in water temperatures of 8–14°C (Bowen 1968), but temperatures may be 4–6°C in northern waters (Mekjavic et al. 2001), and as low as –2°C in arctic waters (Morrison & Zander 2005a). Thus, without proper protection, divers are prone to hypothermia. The physiology of temperature regulation (Chapter 18) and adverse effects of cold exposure (Chapter 20) are covered in detail elsewhere. An extensive review of thermal considerations in diving can also be found in Mekjavic et al. (2003).

Rates of core cooling in water vary widely and are dependent on body composition, the body surface area to mass ratio and physiological responses. In 10–12°C water, a person of low body fat and without clothing can cool at $8°C \cdot h^{-1}$, whereas an endomorph may cool at $0.5°C \cdot h^{-1}$ and typical rates are $2–5°C \cdot h^{-1}$ (Morrison & Conn 1980). In the same conditions, wearing a 6 mm wetsuit, the average core cooling rate will be approximately $0.2–0.3°C \cdot h^{-1}$ (Hayward et al. 1978). Thus, provided divers wear appropriate thermal protection, hypothermia should not present a serious problem. For air diving in water >10°C, a neoprene wetsuit is generally adequate, provided the suit fits closely to the skin surface. However, the wetsuit insulation depends on gas bubbles trapped within the neoprene and as the diver descends the insulation diminishes. When diving at depths >20 metres in cold water, a wetsuit may prove inadequate due to loss of suit thickness, and the lower water temperature at depth. In these conditions, a dry suit will provide superior thermal protection, as the insulative layer of air inside the suit can be replenished from the diver's air supply. In heliox diving, the protective qualities of air within the dry suit are lost due to the higher thermal conductivity of helium, and in cold water, a heated suit (generally hot water) is essential. In these circumstances, the breathing gas delivered to the diver must also be heated to prevent severe respiratory cooling.

Peripheral cooling also presents a problem to the cold-water diver due to the large surface area of the fingers and hands. When wearing neoprene gloves in cold water, divers are likely to suffer peripheral cooling, with loss of tactile sensitivity, manual dexterity and grip strength (Morrison & Zander 2007a,b). This can place the diver in a hazardous situation if unable to operate equipment controls or use hand strength to execute essential tasks.

2.8 Buoyancy

If you have ever taken a deep breath and dived to the bottom of a pool, you have noticed that, when not actively pulling yourself down, you float to the surface. That is the result of positive buoyancy caused by the displacement of water by your body, including the air in your lungs. If you empty your lungs, you are likely to sink.

As every boat builder knows, as long as the mass of water displaced by a vessel exceeds the mass of the vessel, then the boat will float. The same goes for divers, with one important exception. If a diver continues to dive deeper in a lake or the ocean while breath-holding, the increasing water pressure will compress the gas in the lungs, making the lungs and chest smaller. This will decrease body buoyancy. Thus, at some depth, the diver will no longer have the buoyancy required to return to the surface unassisted, and will have to either swim to the surface or use some buoyancy aid.

Divers using underwater breathing apparatus often wear neoprene foam thermal clothing to keep warm. To counteract the natural buoyancy of this clothing, divers wear lead weighted belts. An incorrectly chosen lead mass causes unwanted sinking or flotation, causing the diver to work hard to maintain the desired depth. This wasted work increases gas consumption, leading to a shortened dive.

Modern buoyancy compensators help solve the problem caused by water pressure increasing with depth. Compensators are partly inflated using air from the diver's air supply, compensating for the loss of wet suit buoyancy. Unfortunately, the bulk caused by an inflated buoyancy compensator adds drag, increasing the work required for swimming.

Novice divers often work harder, and consume more air, than experienced divers because they are incorrectly weighted and suffer buoyancy control problems, leading to either overinflated buoyancy compensators or a struggle to avoid sinking. Divers who are too buoyant have been known to pick up rocks, an inefficient way to control buoyancy, but better than unexpectedly bobbing to the surface.

3 BREATH-HOLD DIVING

Man's earliest attempts at diving emulated the breath-hold diving of birds and mammals (Butler 1982). But, as anyone who has held their breath on land can attest, the ability to breath-hold is limited. It is logical to assume that breath-holding limits are due to the inexorable consumption of oxygen in the limited volume of the lungs and blood. But what in fact causes us to break our breath-hold is the accumulation of carbon dioxide in arterial blood (partial pressure >7.3 kPa (55 mmHg)). Our sensitivity to carbon dioxide is a protective mechanism keeping us from becoming unconscious from, among other things, childhood temper tantrums during which breath-holding is relatively common. Unfortunately, the protective effect of carbon dioxide is not fully developed in some young children, who develop relatively harmless breath-hold spells, leading to cyanosis and unconsciousness. Fortunately, the event is self-limiting; unconsciousness quickly leads to resumption of breathing. Underwater, however, syncope from breath-holding may not be self-limiting.

3.1 What is possible?

The oldest group of professional breath-hold divers are the Japanese and Korean Ama divers, mostly women, who reportedly have been breath-hold diving for >2000 years. The object of their diving is shellfish (abalone) or edible seaweed. Modern Ama routinely and repeatedly dive to 20 metres of seawater for typically 60–90 s (Hong et al. 1963). Pearl divers in Indonesia and the South Pacific (mostly male) are currently diving to depths of 50 metres of seawater (601 kPa), although they occasionally suffer decompression sickness. Even the shallow-diving Ama have reported transient neurological symptoms, suggestive of decompression sickness (Kohshi et al. 2005).

The records set by competitive free divers are remarkable (Table 23.2). However, these records have been set at great loss (Clarey 2002). Fatalities in breath-hold diving are a matter of concern. Pollock (2006) reported 128 known fatalities from 1994 to 2003. Divers Alert Network reported 22 fatalities in nine countries in 2004 (Vann et al. 2006). Edmonds & Walker (1999) reported 60 fatalities in Australia over a 10-year period, with drowning, cardiac events and hypoxia the main causes of death. Using data from eight countries, Mass (2007) reported 52 fatalities per year from shallow-water blackout. Breath-hold divers succumb all too frequently to the insidious effects of hypoxia and shallow-water blackout, for reasons described below.

Table 23.2 International free diving records (as of 2006)

CNF m		Dynamic m		Static apnoea min (s)		No limit m	
80	55	212	200	8 (58)	7 (30)	172	160
♂	♀	♂	♀	♂	♀	♂	♀

Notes: ♂ = male, ♀ = female. CNF: constant mass without fins (diver wears no fins, must not touch the rope during the dive, usually uses breaststroke to descend and ascend). Dynamic: with fins (divers swims horizontally not >1 m underwater in a swimming pool). Static apnoea: diver holds breath floating face down in a swimming pool. No limit: diver descends on a weighted sled and returns using a lift bag inflated at depth.

3.2 Physiological effects

It has been known for over a century that diving animals reduce their heart rate when submerged (Bert 1870). This bradycardia, part of the diving reflex, is elicited in humans by breath-holding during facial immersion in cool water. It is usually muted compared to that of animals, but is nevertheless effective at conserving oxygen. In the work of Andersson et al. (2002, 2004), apnoeas with facial immersion resulted in heart rate reductions of 33%, blood pressure increases of 42% and a reduction of arterial oxygen saturation of 5.2%. Apnoea without facial immersion led to a statistically greater desaturation (6.8%). Oxygen uptake decreased by 25% and plasma lactate concentration increased up to 20%, possibly indicating increased anaerobic metabolism during the breath-hold (see Chapters 6 and 10.3). It was concluded that the diving reflex had an oxygen-conserving effect.

The most remarkable combination of features of human breath-hold diving are seemingly unique to humans. Ferrigno et al. (1997) studied three elite breath-hold divers as they made simulated dives to 40–55 metres of seawater, finding that heart rates dropped to 20–30 beats·min^{-1}, but, surprisingly, blood pressure rose as high as 280/200 mmHg (systolic/diastolic). What was most alarming, however, was the remarkable arrhythmias, with R-R intervals of as much as 7.2 s, corresponding to a heart rate of as low as 8 beats·min^{-1} during descent in cool water (25°C; Figure 23.1).

In studies of arterial gas partial pressures (or tensions), made in Ama during and after dives of ~60 s to 4–5 metres of seawater, arterial oxygen tension rose at depth to 18.8 kPa

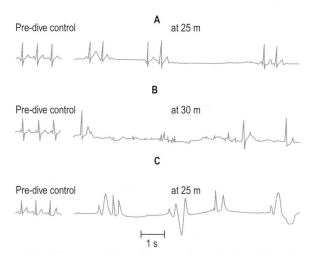

Figure 23.1 Electrocardiographic recordings obtained from three breath-hold divers (A, B, C) before and during the descent phases of breath-hold dives to 40 and 50 m of seawater (25°C) in a hyperbaric chamber. Redrawn from Ferrigno et al. (1997) with permission.

(141 mmHg), and arterial carbon dioxide tension rose to 6.2 kPa (46.6 mmHg; Qvist et al. 1993). Near the end of the dives, arterial oxygen tension dropped to 8.3 kPa (62.6 mmHg) and arterial carbon dioxide tension rose to 6.7 kPa (50 mmHg). Ferretti et al. (1991) found that, in three elite breath-hold divers, arterial oxygen tension dropped as low as 4.1 kPa after dives to 40–70 metres of seawater for durations of 88–151 s. It is generally believed that 3.3–4.0 kPa (25–30 mmHg) is the minimum arterial oxygen tension for supporting consciousness (Åstrand 1960, Åstrand & Rodahl 1970). In control subjects with dry breath-holds, arterial oxygen tension dropped to 6.0 kPa. In both elite divers and controls, arterial carbon dioxide tension climbed to about 6.7 kPa.

Schagatay et al. (2001) noted that, in response to breath-holding during facial immersion, the emptying of red blood cells from the spleen extended breath-holding time an average of 17 s. This was inferred from an average of 30% (17 s) longer breath-hold in normal subjects than in splenectomised subjects.

3.3 Hypoxia and shallow–water blackout

Humans are ill equipped for detecting hypoxia. Signs of hypoxia are subtle and indeed, some signs may be nothing more than feeling too good. As evidenced by repeated high-altitude aviation accidents, hypoxia can quickly disable with no warning signs and without eliciting alarm. In diving, the drop of oxygen pressure as gas expands in the lungs near the surface can lead to a feeling of euphoria, similar to the effects of alcohol. When arterial blood desaturates to a sufficiently low level, consciousness may be lost. Of course, when that occurs underwater, drowning is almost inevitable.

Hypoxic syncope during breath-holding is aggravated by predive hyperventilation (Åstrand 1960, Åstrand & Rodahl 1970). Hyperventilation lowers carbon dioxide partial pressure, and thus delays the increase in respiratory drive from carbon dioxide accumulation that normally forces the diver to surface before hypoxia reaches dangerous levels. However, extensive periods of endurance exercise prior to the breath-hold can also lead to syncope due to the depression of carbon dioxide production for a given oxygen uptake. In other words, heavy exercise causes less carbon dioxide to be produced for a given oxygen uptake, with the respiratory exchange ratio shifting to lower values leading to an increased likelihood of hypoxic syncope (Lindholm & Gennser 2005). For further details consult *Bove and Davis's Diving Medicine* (Ferrigno 2004).

4 UNDERWATER WORK

4.1 Ventilation limitation

One of the most noticeable effects of diving on pulmonary function is the increased work of breathing. This is due principally to the increase in breathing gas density, and hence airflow resistance, in proportion to absolute pressure. Increased work of breathing progressively limits maximal ventilation. A useful index of maximal exercise ventilation is maximal voluntary ventilation: the maximal ventilation rate achieved in 15 s by voluntary hyperventilation. This index has been measured by various researchers (Maio & Fahri 1967, Seusing & Drube 1960, Wood 1963) and their results suggest a relationship of the form:

Equation 1: $MVV = MVV_O \cdot (\rho/\rho_O)^{-k}$

where:

MVV_O = maximal voluntary ventilation in air at surface
ρ/ρ_O = ratio of gas density to air density at the surface
k = constant (~0.4).

Thus, the maximal voluntary ventilation reduces from ~175 L·min^{-1} at the surface (101 kPa), to ~100 L·min^{-1} at 404 kPa (30 metres of seawater) and ~76 L·min^{-1} at 808 kPa (71 metres of seawater).

The values above were measured in dry conditions and do not include the additional respiratory work of underwater breathing apparatus, which can reduce maximal voluntary ventilation by ≥10% (Morrison & Butt 1972). Also, Fagraeus & Linnarsson (1973) found that when breathing air at 601 kPa (50 metres of seawater), the maximal exercise ventilation of divers was ~80% of maximal voluntary ventilation. These data indicate that, when working underwater, a diver might achieve a sustained maximal exercise ventilation that is 70% of their maximal voluntary ventilation measured at the same depth in a dry hyperbaric chamber. Therefore, in air diving beyond 30 metres of seawater, or breathing at gas densities greater than four times surface air, divers can expect to experience a ventilatory limitation during heavy exercise which is not evident at sea level (Chapter 2).

4.2 Immersion, lung volumes and pulmonary resistance

Although measures of exercise under pressure are often made in dry hyperbaric chambers, the effects of immersion may seriously limit the pulmonary function and work capacity of divers. During upright immersion breathing at mouth pressure, there is a hydrostatic difference between the mouth pressure and the mean pressure surrounding the chest (lung centroid pressure). The lung centroid pressure has been estimated at 0.14 metre inferior (upright) and 0.07 metre posterior (prone) to the sternal notch (Taylor & Morrison 1989). When a diver in an upright posture inspires air from a source regulated to mouth pressure, the hydrostatic loading on the chest wall will cause a shift to a lower lung relaxation volume, resulting in a lower pulmonary compliance and an increase in pulmonary resistance (Dahlback 1978, Hong et al. 1969, Lollgen et al. 1980, Sterk 1973). The diver will compensate to an extent for the changes in compliance and airway resistance by maintaining an expiratory reserve volume greater than the relaxation volume, at the expense of increased inspiratory muscular effort. Taylor & Morrison (1991) measured a reduction of lung relaxation volume from 2.06 L (in air) to 0.25 L above residual volume when immersed and breathing at mouth pressure. Although end-expiratory lung volume was maintained at 0.84 L, pulmonary resistance (measured at a flow of 0.5 L·s^{-1}) increased from 0.18 to 0.44 kPa·L^{-1}·s and flow-resistive pulmonary work increased from 0.2 to 0.75 J·L^{-1} (Morrison & Taylor 1990).

Although air flows are dependent on muscular effort over the normal range of ventilation and lung volumes, maximal expiratory flow is effort independent (Chapter 2). Fry (1958) and Mead et al. (1967) proposed that maximum expiratory flow is limited by dynamic airway compression. As pressure drops along the airway, a point is reached at which the pleural pressure created by muscular effort equals the airway pressure (equal pressure point). At high flow rates, this point will occur within the thorax and at some point downstream, airway compression will occur due to the pressure gradient across the airway causing the airway to close. At this point, flow becomes effort independent; further increase in muscular effort leads to further airway compression, rather than an increase in flow. An alternative theory of flow limitation due to pressure wave propagation has been proposed by Dawson & Elliott (1977). Although maximal expiratory flow is seldom reached in normal exercise, the effects of immersion and gas density on lung volume and airway resistance are likely to decrease maximal flows sufficiently to cause a ventilatory limitation at depth.

During inspiration, negative pleural pressure created by the inspiratory muscles will act to hold the intrathoracic airways open. However, several studies have reported inspiratory dyspnoea during exercise to be the cause of ventilatory limitation during deep heliox dives (Dwyer et al. 1977, Salzano et al. 1984, Spaur et al. 1977). Flook & Fraser (1992) demonstrated large oscillations in inspiratory flow during heliox saturation dives to 300 and 450 metres of seawater. The authors also measured large increases in resistance to inspiratory flow during air dives to 56 metres of seawater, indicating that maximal inspiratory flow is effort independent at that depth, and proposed these effects were caused by transient tracheal compression due to a negative transmural pressure gradient. The authors also suggest that flow oscillations may be accentuated by development of orifice flow at the vocal cord aperture. Airflow through the compressed aperture may create a Venturi effect that lowers internal airway pressure downstream of the aperture and precipitates further narrowing or closing of the airway. The severity of flow interruption may depend on both gas density and neural control of the aperture.

It is well documented that changes in airflow dynamics can lead to a feeling of dyspnoea in air and heliox diving, particularly at higher gas densities and during exercise. Study of the mechanisms involved suggests that this can be overcome by designing breathing apparatus to provide a degree of pressure compensation of the inspired gas. When the diver wears a helmet, the inspired pressure can be increased to counter the tendency for inspiratory flow limitation, and to partially offset the hydrostatic difference between the mouth pressure and lung centroid pressure. In rebreathing apparatus, the effects of immersion can be largely offset by positioning the counter-lung on the chest. This provides a relatively balanced system during upright immersion and a slight overpressure (positive pressure breathing) in the prone (swimming) position. Conversely, a counter-lung positioned on the diver's back will result in negative pressure breathing in the prone position and is likely to exacerbate flow limitation and sensations of dyspnoea.

4.3 Underwater work capacity

There have been a number of studies of maximal underwater work capacity and aerobic power. Donald & Davidson (1954) measured the oxygen uptake of divers breathing pure oxygen from closed-circuit apparatus. Divers achieved a mean maximal aerobic power of 2.0 L·min^{-1} when wearing boots in mud, and 3.1 L·min^{-1} when fin swimming in shallow water. Using the same technique, Lanphier (1954) measured a maximal aerobic power of 2.5 L·min^{-1} in divers swimming at 1.2 knots. Above this speed, the divers fatigued rapidly. Goff et al. (1956) measured oxygen uptakes of 1.3–2.5 L·min^{-1} in divers swimming distances of 450–1850 metres. Morrison (1973) reported a mean maximal aerobic power of 2.6 L·min^{-1} in six tethered swimmers breathing nitrox from semi-closed circuit breathing apparatus at 2, 23 and 54 metres of seawater. At 54 metres of seawater, two divers failed to complete the exercise and two others experienced headaches. Taylor & Morrison (1990) found no significant difference in the maximal underwater aerobic power of divers breathing from an open-circuit demand valve and performing cycle ergometry at 0.5 and 50 metres of seawater (4.25 versus 4.1 L·min^{-1}), although some divers failed to complete the final increment in workload at depth.

Spaur et al. (1977) measured aerobic power of divers breathing heliox from closed-circuit apparatus at 491 metres of seawater (5.01 MPa). The divers rapidly became exhausted and experienced dyspnoea at an oxygen uptake of 1.9 L·min^{-1}, although ventilation was only 55% of the unloaded maximal voluntary ventilation at that depth. During the *Atlantis* dive series, mild to severe dyspnoea was experienced when breathing heliox and trimix (5–10% nitrogen) at rest and submaximal exercise in dry conditions at 460 and 650 metres of seawater (Salzano et al. 1984). An increase in nitrogen fraction tended to alleviate dyspnoea, despite the higher gas density, indicating that dyspnoea may be partly neural in origin, and a symptom of high-pressure nervous syndrome (section 6.2). During the *Hydra* dive series, Gardette (1989) reported that six divers performed work in open water at 520 metres of seawater (5.3 MPa) while breathing a hydrogen–helium–oxygen mixture, with more comfort and less fatigue than when breathing heliox. Clarke (1992) analysed data from 240 wet dives using combinations of oxygen, nitrogen and helium breathing mixtures. Results showed that the probability of a respiratory event (dyspnoea, respiratory distress, loss of consciousness) was dependent on the inert gas, peak mouth pressure and gas density, with helium having twice the likelihood of causing an event for a given gas density.

These studies imply that, in carefully controlled conditions, divers can achieve work rates similar to surface values at gas densities up to six times normal. However, work rate may be compromised by immersion, respiratory loading of breathing apparatus, or by airway obstruction and dyspnoea associated with high-pressure nervous syndrome.

4.4 Ventilatory response to exercise

Studies of ventilatory responses to exercise reveal a reduction in the ventilatory equivalent for oxygen and increase in the end-tidal carbon dioxide partial pressure when working at depth. As carbon dioxide retention (hypercapnia) is a concern in divers (Lanphier & Camporesi 1982), a number of studies have been directed towards identifying the factors responsible. It has been shown that exercise ventilation decreases and end-tidal carbon dioxide pressure increases in response to increasing inspired oxygen pressure and breathing gas density (Hesser et al. 1968, Lanphier 1963, Salzano et al. 1984), and elevated respiratory loading of breathing apparatus (Lanphier 1963, Morrison et al. 1976, Taylor & Morrison 1990).

The question of why divers hypoventilate can be explained by the manner in which carbon dioxide modulates ventilation. Gas density and external resistance both act to reduce ventilation via changes in the work of breathing. The hypercapnic drive does not relate directly to ventilation, but rather to work performed by the respiratory muscles (Doell et al. 1973). Milic-Emili & Tyler (1963) have shown a linear relationship between end-tidal carbon dioxide pressure and inspiratory work. Thus, as internal or external respiratory resistance increases due to either gas density or breathing apparatus, the same arterial carbon dioxide tension and inspiratory work will elicit progressively lower ventilations.

Lanphier (1963) measured an end-tidal carbon dioxide pressure of 7.3 kPa (55 mmHg) in divers swimming underwater at 30 metres of seawater, reporting individual values as high as 9.3 kPa (70 mmHg). Sterba (1990) reported headache, confusion and amnesia when end-tidal carbon dioxide pressure exceeded 9.3 kPa during underwater work. The effects of depth and work rate on the ventilation and end-tidal carbon dioxide pressure during underwater swimming are illustrated in Figure 23.2. At 0.5 metres of seawater, carbon dioxide pressure followed a typical inverted U rela-

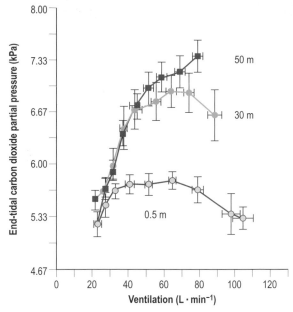

Figure 23.2 Exercise ventilation and end-tidal carbon dioxide partial pressure of divers ($N = 12$) during tethered swimming at three depths. Points represent equivalent increments in forward thrust, up to a maximal load of 130 N at each depth. Data are means with standard errors (Morrison and Wood, unpublished data).

tionship, having a value of 5.3 kPa at a ventilation of 105 L·min⁻¹. At 50 metres of seawater, there was no compensatory drop in end-tidal carbon dioxide pressure, which increased by 40% at maximal work rate whilst maximal ventilation was depressed by 25%.

Taylor & Morrison (1990) measured a mean maximal end-tidal carbon dioxide pressure of 8.4 kPa in 10 divers exercising up to maximal aerobic power during upright immersion at 50 metres of seawater. Again, there was no compensatory drop in carbon dioxide pressure at maximal work rate and divers reported severe narcosis, including visual and mental aberrations and impending loss of consciousness. When breathing pressure was compensated from mouth pressure to mid-thoracic level, exercise ventilation was significantly higher, perceived respiratory discomfort was lower and symptoms of narcosis were judged to be less severe (Taylor & Morrison 1990).

Salzano et al. (1984) found that, in the presence of elevated inspired oxygen pressure, high gas density and a pressure of 6.67 MPa (650 metres of seawater), arterial carbon dioxide tension, hydrogen ion and lactate concentration were higher, with the onset of anaerobic metabolism apparently occurring earlier than when exercising at the surface (see the debate in Chapter 10.3). In these conditions, divers experienced metabolic and respiratory acidosis during heavy exercise, rather than the largely compensated metabolic acidosis normally observed. In addition, Salzano et al. (1984) observed a ventilatory inefficiency at pressure, characterised by an increase in physiological dead space and reduced alveolar ventilation, possibly due to an alveolar ventilation–perfusion mismatch. This led the authors to speculate that inadequate gas exchange may represent a new form of respiratory limitation during deep diving.

4.5 Carbon dioxide retention in divers

It has been noted that trained divers exhibit a lower ventilatory response to exercise (Broussolle et al. 1972, Kerem et al. 1980, Lalley et al. 1974) and to hypercapnia (Florio et al. 1979, Sherman et al. 1980) than non-divers. Lalley et al. (1974) found that divers also have a reduced neurogenic ventilatory drive during exercise, indicating that hypoventilation was not confined to the carbon dioxide response. In these divers (carbon dioxide retainers), hypoventilation appears to be an inherent characteristic, perhaps resulting from a respiratory adaptation to diving (Schaeffer 1965), or from self-selection according to their innate respiratory responsiveness (Kerem et al. 1980). However, the mechanisms and course of development of such respiratory adaptation to diving are unclear.

Carbon dioxide retention has been linked to a number of life-threatening underwater hazards, including oxygen-induced seizures, narcosis, amnesia and loss of consciousness (Fothergill et al. 1991, Lambertsen et al. 1959, Lanphier 1963, Morrison et al. 1978, Sterba 1990). Although some of the evidence is circumstantial, there are physiological grounds to support the onset of these effects in the presence of extreme hypercapnia. It is therefore important that the contributing factors should be carefully controlled by setting strict limits on inspired oxygen pressure, breathing gas density, narcotic potency of breathing gas and design parameters for breathing apparatus (resistance, dead space and hydrostatic imbalance).

5 UNDERWATER BREATHING APPARATUS

Underwater breathing apparatus can be divided into two broad categories: open-circuit and recirculating (semi-closed or closed-circuit) apparatus. Each form takes a different approach to providing the physiological needs of the diver and, at the same time, presents its own unique set of physiological and ergonomic challenges.

5.1 Open–circuit free flow apparatus

Commonly referred to as standard diving dress, this system is used mainly by commercial divers in shallow-water, air diving (<20 metres of seawater). It consists of a one-piece watertight canvas suit, to which is fitted a rigid helmet. Air is supplied from the surface to the diver's helmet via an umbilical hose and exhausted from the helmet through a spring-loaded spindle valve. The diver controls the volume of air in the helmet and suit, and hence buoyancy, by adjusting the back-pressure of the spindle valve.

Although considered an open-circuit design, the diver rebreathes from the helmet–suit atmosphere. Thus, a major limitation of this design is the high airflow required to keep the inspired carbon dioxide pressure below a recommended limit of 2 kPa. The air supply necessary to achieve this depends on the work rate and depth of the diver. However, assuming that the diver's expired carbon dioxide mixes with the air supplied to the helmet and carbon dioxide in the air supply is negligible, the inspired carbon dioxide pressure can be calculated using the helmet gas equilibrium equation (with volumes measured at standard temperature (0°C) and pressure (101.3 kPa), dry conditions):

Equation 2: $P_ICO_2 = [\dot{V}_{CO_2}/\dot{V}H] \cdot P_B$

where:

P_ICO_2 = inspired carbon dioxide partial pressure (kPa)
$\dot{V}CO_2$ = diver's carbon dioxide production (L·min^{-1})
$\dot{V}H$ = helmet airflow (L·min^{-1})
P_B = ambient pressure (kPa)

Assuming a carbon dioxide production ≤2.0 L·min^{-1} for a booted diver, then to limit the inspired carbon dioxide pressure to <2 kPa requires an airflow of up to 100 L·min^{-1} per atmosphere of pressure. Due to the inefficient (wasteful) nature of this system, a surface-supplied open-circuit demand apparatus is now preferred for commercial air diving and for heliox diving.

5.2 Open–circuit demand apparatus

This form of breathing apparatus can be subdivided into two systems: self-contained underwater breathing apparatus (SCUBA or scuba) and surface-supplied demand breathing apparatus. The first open-circuit demand breathing system was developed by Rouquayrol and Denayrouse in 1865 (Davis 1981). It was generally used as a surface-supplied system due to the limited capacity of the air cylinder carried by the diver. In 1943, Cousteau and Gagnan combined the concept of a demand regulator with improved compressed air storage to create the precursor of modern scuba.

5.2.1 Open–circuit demand scuba

The modern scuba consists of a two-stage pressure regulator and air supply. The first stage is attached to an air cylinder on the diver's back, and reduces cylinder air pressure from 20.7 MPa (<3000 psi) to ~965 kPa (~140 psi) above ambient (seawater) pressure. A single hose at intermediate pressure leads to the second-stage regulator (demand valve) attached to the diver's mouthpiece, which supplies air at a pressure equal to that acting on the regulator. Exhaled gas is exhausted from the mouthpiece to the water.

5.2.2 Surface-supplied demand breathing apparatus

In this apparatus, the air (or mixed gas) supply and first-stage regulator are located at the surface (or diving bell) and connected to the diver by an umbilical pressure hose. The umbilical connects, via a manifold, to the second-stage demand regulator. In the event of supply failure, the diver is equipped with an emergency cylinder connected to the manifold via a first-stage regulator.

5.2.3 Physiological limitations of open circuit–demand breathing apparatus

A potential weakness of an open-circuit demand regulator is that once the inlet valve is fully open, it cannot supply a greater flow of air no matter how hard the diver inhales. The deeper the diver ventures, the greater the mass of air inspired per breath and the lower the maximal ventilation available from the demand valve. Thus, the design of the inlet valve orifice and intermediate pressure must be matched to the diver's physiological demands to ensure sufficient air when working at maximum depth.

In surface-supplied apparatus, supply pressure to the demand valve must be increased by an amount equivalent to the depth of the diver, and should also allow for pressure loss in the umbilical, which can exceed 340 kPa (50 psi) at high ventilations (Morrison et al. 1993). A supply (second-stage) pressure of 965 kPa (140 psi), plus 20 kPa·m^{-1} (3 psi·m^{-1}) of depth is recommended. In this apparatus, air is commonly provided by a low-pressure compressor providing an output of 1380 kPa (200 psi). When diving beyond 20 metres of seawater, this configuration will greatly reduce peak flow from the demand valve and may compromise diver safety (Morrison et al. 1993).

Breathing characteristics of demand regulators are generally measured in terms of inhalation and exhalation pressures, and the work of breathing. It is generally accepted that breathing apparatus should enable ventilations up to at least 75 L·min^{-1}, with inhalation and exhalation pressures within the range −1.5 to 1.5 kPa. Figure 23.3 shows the work of breathing from two different scuba regulators (Morrison et al. 1993). The straight lines represent proposed limits of ideal and acceptable breathing effort (Morrison & Reimers 1982). One regulator has excellent breathing characteristics. The other fails to meet physiological needs as depth increases.

5.3 Recirculating underwater breathing apparatus

Although more efficient than free-flow apparatus, open-circuit scuba becomes progressively less efficient as the diver descends. At the surface, the diver's oxygen uptake represents only 4% of the air supplied from the cylinder. However, at 30 metres of seawater, this is reduced to 1%, with the remaining 99% exhausted to the water. This is

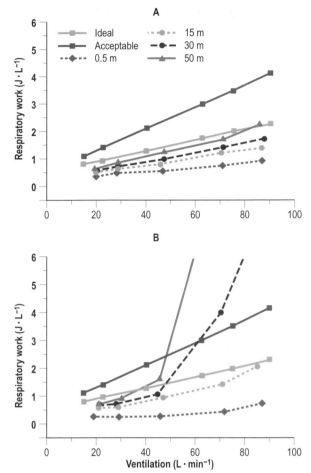

Figure 23.3 Ventilation and the work of breathing at four depths. (A) Demand regulator with ideal breathing characteristics. (B) Demand regulator that limits maximal ventilation beyond 15 metres of seawater due to an inspiratory flow limitation (i.e. points above 'acceptable' line). Redrawn from Morrison et al. (1993) with permission.

because, for the same fractional concentration of oxygen, increments of pressure elevate the inspired oxygen pressure, theoretically increasing the total amount of work that a diver can perform from a fixed volume of air. For scuba diving beyond 30 metres of seawater, open-circuit demand becomes increasingly impractical, and this inefficiency led to the introduction of recirculating (rebreathing) apparatus, in which the gas mixture expired by the diver is recirculated, the expired carbon dioxide removed and the mixture rebreathed. Recirculating apparatus uses semi-closed and closed systems. In a closed-circuit apparatus, an efficiency of almost 100% can be achieved. The dive time of the apparatus is then determined by the capacity and efficiency of carbon dioxide removal (the scrubber duration), rather than the capacity of gas storage.

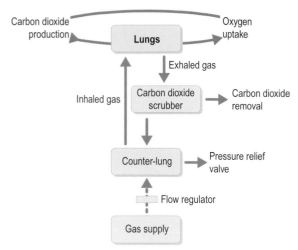

Figure 23.4 Configuration of a semi-closed scuba showing gas flow to (and from) the diver's lung and the counter-lung. Diver consumes oxygen and releases carbon dioxide which is absorbed in the absorbent canister. Gas mixture from supply cylinders is injected to the counter-lung at a controlled flow and excess gas is exhausted from the relief valve.

5.3.1 Semi-closed circuit scuba

Semi-closed circuit apparatus is used extensively by the military, and recently has become popular with research and advanced recreational divers (Bozanic 2002). It consists of gas supply cylinders, a pressure regulator and flow control assembly, a counter-lung from which the diver rebreathes the gas mixture, a carbon dioxide-absorbent canister (scrubber), connecting hoses and a full face mask. Most of the diver's expired gas is recirculated through the carbon dioxide scrubber to the counter-lung, and a small quantity of gas is exhausted to the water through a relief valve (Figure 23.4). The gas mixture can be delivered at a constant mass flow, a constant volume ratio, a constant mass ratio or a constant oxygen pressure (Morrison & Reimers 1982).

In the most common design, a fixed gas mixture is injected into the counter-lung at a constant mass flow. In steady-state conditions, assuming the counter-lung oxygen partial pressure is the same as that exhausted from the relief valve, then the oxygen pressure breathed by the diver can be determined as follows:

Equation 3: $P_IO_2 = (F_{O_2}L - \dot{V}_{O_2}) \cdot P_B/(L - \dot{V}_{O_2})$

where:

L = gas entering the counter-lung (L·min^{-1})
F_{O_2} = oxygen fraction of supply gas mixture
$\dot{V}_{O_2}$ = oxygen uptake (L·min^{-1})
P_B = ambient pressure of diver (kPa).

From the above equation, it can be deduced that the highest inspired oxygen partial pressure will occur at the maximum operating depth at which the apparatus is to be used, with a risk of oxygen toxicity, and the lowest will occur at the surface, with a risk of hypoxia. Therefore, by solving the gas equilibrium equations at surface and at maximum operating depth using defined physiological limits for the inspired pressure of oxygen (20–160 kPa) and oxygen uptake (0.3–3.0 L·min^{-1}), a physiologically safe gas mixture and injection rate can be determined for that particular depth range (Morrison & Reimers 1982).

The major limitations of systems using fixed gas mixtures are that, since oxygen pressure increases with depth, gas mixture and supply flow must be altered depending on the operating depth range, and the required gas flows become excessive beyond 50 metres of seawater when diving from the surface (Morrison & Reimers 1982). In addition, due to the rise in oxygen pressure with depth, bottom time must be carefully controlled within the limits of central nervous system oxygen tolerance.

A more efficient constant oxygen pressure delivery system that more closely reflects the physiological needs of the diver is used by military divers for diving to 80 metres of seawater (901 kPa). Oxygen and the inert gas are supplied from separate cylinders via flow controllers designed to maintain a constant oxygen pressure in the gas mixture supplied to the counter-lung (Morrison & Reimers 1982). This provides a much lower gas use rate and reduces the risk of oxygen toxicity. In addition, the diver can benefit from accelerated in-water decompression by turning off the inert gas supply on ascent to 9 metres of seawater, and breathing pure oxygen.

5.3.2 Closed-circuit scuba

There are two forms of closed-circuit scuba. A pure oxygen system, originally designed by Fleuss in 1876, is used by military divers for shallow-water (covert) operations. This apparatus is limited to <8 metres of seawater (178 kPa) for 240 min due to risks of oxygen toxicity (US Navy Diving Manual 2005). A more sophisticated mixed-gas, closed-circuit apparatus has been developed that uses electronic sensors to control the breathing gas composition. In this apparatus, the pressure of oxygen in the breathing mixture in the counter-lung is sensed by a fuel cell. An electronic module controls the addition of make-up oxygen (via a solenoid valve), replacing oxygen consumed by the diver. Inert gas is injected through a separate valve but only to maintain counter-lung volume as pressure increases during descent (Bozanic 2002).

In mixed-gas constant oxygen pressure systems, when the diver moves quickly from one depth to another, there will be a transient change in counter-lung oxygen pressure, creating a risk of hyperoxia on descent and hypoxia on ascent. These transient characteristics must be taken into account and controlled in the apparatus design.

5.3.3 Closed-circuit station-supplied (push-pull) apparatus

Push-pull apparatus is used in deep heliox diving, where the cost of breathing gas is high. It is similar in concept to surface-supplied, open-circuit demand, except that a back-pressure regulator controls the helmet pressure while allowing expired gas to vent via a return hose to a central processing station (usually a diving bell). Push-pull systems can also operate in a free-flow mode, with gas flowing constantly through the helmet. In this mode, the compliance of the helmet neck dam acts as a form of counter-lung, absorbing fluctuations in air flow into the helmet as the diver breathes in and out. As the breathing gas supply and carbon dioxide absorbent are centrally located, this equipment can operate uninterrupted for long durations. When diving deeper than 200 metres of seawater (2.1MPa), these systems normally require respiratory gas heating to protect the diver from airway cooling and hypothermia, due to low water temperatures and high inspired gas density (Hayes et al. 1981).

6 MIXED-GAS AND SATURATION DIVING

As divers venture deeper into the ocean, the combined effects of nitrogen narcosis, gas density and oxygen toxicity gradually render air breathing impractical. The uptake of inert gas into the tissues results in excessive time for safe decompression of the diver, when returning to the surface. To avoid these hazards, when diving beyond 50 metres of seawater, the nitrogen content of the breathing mixture is generally replaced with helium and the oxygen fraction reduced to provide a partial pressure slightly above normal (usually 30–50 kPa). This provides a lighter gas mixture and eliminates the effects of severe narcosis beyond 60 metres of seawater. However, the use of helium introduces additional problems of speech distortion and thermal comfort. A speech unscrambler is required to communicate with the surface (Bennett et al. 1971), breathing gas requires respiratory heating (Hayes et al. 1981), and in a helium-oxygen atmosphere, thermal balance is restricted to a very narrow temperature range (~2°C) to avoid heat or cold stress (Bennett et al. 1971).

6.1 Saturation diving

To circumvent the problem of lengthy decompression times from dives beyond 50 metres of seawater, the concept of saturation diving was introduced. In pressure exposures lasting more than 8–12 h, divers become saturated with the inert gas (nitrogen, helium, hydrogen). That is, the inert gas dissolved in the body tissues reaches equilibrium with the environment. At this point, there is no further gas uptake, and subsequent decompression becomes independent of the time spent at pressure.

Saturation diving can be conducted from either a habitat placed on the sea floor (Aquarius; Figure 23.5) or from a ship. Habitat diving allows a scientist to live and work for almost unlimited periods in the midst of the ecosystem being studied. Saturation diving from an underwater habitat is most easily accomplished in relatively shallow water

(<30 metres of seawater), although in the 1960s and 1970s the US Navy launched a series of deep-water habitats called Sealab I, II and III (Barth 2000) at depths ranging from 30 to 200 metres of seawater.

In shipboard saturation diving, divers live in a pressure chamber at the water surface, and are transported to the work site on the seabed via a diving bell. The divers live and work at a constant atmospheric pressure for the duration of the underwater task (which may be several days or weeks), and are then decompressed. Saturation diving operations require a surface support vessel or platform, a hyperbaric chamber complex, hyperbaric life support systems, gas storage system and a diving bell. The diving bell must be supplied with communications, heating, lighting and compressed gas via an umbilical cable from the support vessel. Although more efficient in terms of decompression, saturation diving involves a degree of complexity and cost that can only be contemplated by commercial, governmental or military diving operations. The dives described in the following sections took place in a hyperbaric chamber unless otherwise stated.

6.2 High-pressure nervous syndrome

Although the introduction of heliox diving rapidly advanced the depth of human diving beyond 100 metres of seawater (1.1 MPa), it introduced new and previously unseen physiological hazards. Early heliox excursion dives in a hyperbaric chamber to 183 and 244 metres of seawater resulted in symp-

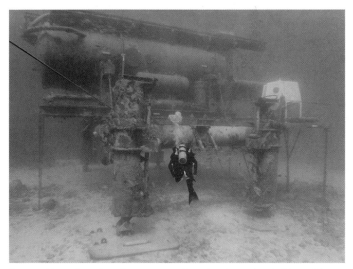

Figure 23.5 A scuba diver approaches the Aquarius habitat, his research home under the sea located on a reef near Key Largo, Florida. Aquarius is owned by the US National Oceanic and Atmospheric Administration (NOAA) and operated by the National Undersea Research Center of the University of North Carolina at Wilmington (UNCW). Aquarius is the world's only research habitat supporting 24-hr a day science missions. From Miller & Cooper (2000) with permission.

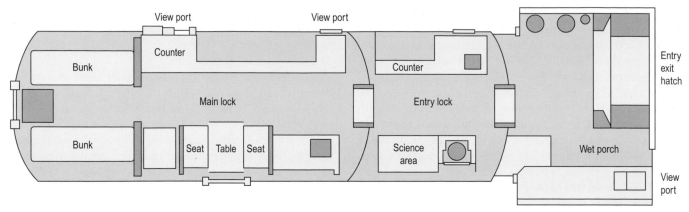

Figure 23.6 National Oceanic and Atmospheric Administration's Aquarius Sea-bed Habitat, situated in 20 metres of seawater off Florida (USA), and used for research and education. From Miller & Cooper (2000) with permission.

toms of dizziness, nausea, vomiting and tremor of hands, arms and torso (Bennett & Dossett 1967). These dives used a rapid compression profile (10–30 m·min^{-1}). In a subsequent series of heliox dives, divers were compressed to increasing depths, down to 363 metres of seawater (3.73 MPa), at a rate of 3 m·min^{-1} (Brauer 1968). In the deepest dive, divers became distressed beyond 330 metres of seawater with progressive symptoms of tremor, motor disturbances, depression of the electroencephalogram and bouts of somnolence (microsleep; Brauer et al. 1969). The dive was stopped at 363 metres of seawater due to the deteriorating condition of the divers. Further dives confirmed these symptoms, termed collectively high-pressure nervous syndrome, and animal experiments revealed that further compression resulted in convulsions of increasing intensity (Brauer 1975).

In contrast, a US Navy saturation dive to 305 metres of seawater for 77 h showed divers to be in good condition with less tremor and no signs of microsleep (Overfeld et al. 1969). In this dive, a slow compression rate was used (12 m·h^{-1}). This was followed by a Swiss/British saturation dive to 305 metres of seawater, with excursions to 350 metres of seawater during which divers swam and worked underwater (Buhlmann et al. 1970).

Concurrent animal studies showed that both the rate of compression and absolute pressure were factors in the onset of high-pressure nervous syndrome. Brauer (1975) demonstrated that the convulsion threshold was dependent on animal species, hydrostatic pressure and compression rate. Albano et al. (1972) reported recovery from symptoms when compression was stopped and animals were maintained at constant pressure.

These findings were confirmed in humans in a dive to 457 metres of seawater (4.67 MPa) for 10 h, using a staged compression profile with 22-h stops at 183, 305, 396 metres of seawater. Divers showed symptoms of finger tremor, involuntary muscle jerks, depression of electroencephalogram activity in the alpha (8–13 Hz) and beta frequencies (13–30 Hz), and increased theta activity (4–8 Hz). Symp-

toms worsened following each compression and showed improvement after 6–10 h at stable pressure (Figure 23.6). Divers were in much better condition at 457 metres of seawater than in the previous dive to 363 metres of seawater, which used a continuous compression profile. There was no decrement in cognitive function, and divers performed moderate exercise with no symptoms of carbon dioxide retention or dyspnoea (Bennett et al. 1971).

Fructus et al. (1976) reported similar results during an excursion dive to 520 metres of seawater (5.3 MPa) using an exponential compression profile, with stages at 350 and 460 metres of seawater. Symptoms of high-pressure nervous syndrome worsened during phases of rapid compression, but no improvement in electroencephalogram was observed during 16-h stages at 350 and 460 metres of seawater. The possibility of pressure adaptation during constant pressure was further studied during a saturation dive to 500 metres of seawater for 100 h. Divers showed symptoms of finger tremor (8–12 Hz), muscle jerks, electroencephalogram changes consisting of reduced alpha and beta activity, and increased theta activity accompanied by drowsiness and sleep disturbance (Fructus et al. 1976). Although the symptoms tended to stabilise at 500 metres of seawater, electroencephalogram changes persisted over the 4-day period at depth, with no evidence of adaptation.

In 1972, using the information acquired from previous dives, two French divers achieved a heliox dive to 610 metres of seawater (6.2 MPa). The dive involved a slow exponential compression, a 2-day stop at 350 metres of seawater to allow symptoms to stabilise, and 14-h stops at 535 and 565 metres of seawater to verify diver status, before proceeding deeper. Although high-pressure nervous syndrome was evident, both divers were in good condition at 610 metres of seawater with similar but less severe symptoms than in the previous dives to 500 metres of seawater. From these dives, it was concluded that slow compression rates and compression stops are equally important factors in combatting this syndrome (Fructus et al. 1976).

Despite these results, other researchers have reported significant problems in divers breathing heliox beyond 300 metres of seawater. US Navy divers experienced severe dyspnoea at 488 metres of seawater when performing moderate work underwater (Spaur et al. 1977), and in a subsequent dive to 549 metres of seawater experienced symptoms of high-pressure nervous syndrome including dyspnoea, dizziness, nausea and fatigue (Bennett & Rostain 2003b). In a series of British heliox dives to progressive depths between 300 and 540 metres of seawater, divers showed symptoms and, in some cases, were clearly distressed, although this was not evident in neurological testing (Hempleman et al. 1978, 1980). At 540 metres of seawater, following 3.5 days of compression, divers experienced dizziness, nausea, vomiting and loss of appetite (Bennett & Rostain 2003b, Torok 1984a). However, in a subsequent dive to 540 metres of seawater with a slower (6 day) compression and different divers, these symptoms were not observed (Torok 1984b).

6.3 Hydrostatic pressure and narcosis

Early research on the effects of hydrostatic pressure on living organisms revealed an antagonism between hydrostatic pressure and anaesthesia (Johnston & Flagler 1950). Miller et al. (1967) and Lever et al. (1971a) showed that narcosis in animals can be reversed by the addition of sufficient hydrostatic pressure. In an extension of the Meyer-Overton hypothesis, relating the narcotic potency of an anaesthetic to its molar concentration in lipid (Bennett & Rostain 2003a), Lever et al. (1971b) calculated that a critical anaesthetic concentration will cause a volume expansion in lipid of 0.4%, and that this expansion would be nullified by application of 10 MPa of pressure. This theory, known as the critical volume hypothesis, was supported by the experimental results obtained in animal studies. A logical extension of this theory is that narcotic agents might be expected to have an antagonistic effect on the adverse effects of hydrostatic pressure. Brauer et al. (1971, 1974) demonstrated that addition of inert gas increased the pressure threshold for tremors and convulsions in animals, and that the effect was closely related to the narcotic potency of the atmosphere.

6.4 The use of trimix in saturation diving

To test the effectiveness of adding nitrogen to the breathing gas to suppress high-pressure nervous syndrome, Bennett et al. (1974) conducted two dives to 305 metres of seawater, with 33 min of compression, in which divers breathed either heliox or trimix (oxygen, helium, nitrogen). The trimix eliminated finger tremor (Figure 23.7), nausea and dizziness seen in the heliox dive, but produced some decrement in cognitive function due to narcosis. Further trimix dives produced similar results (Bennett et al. 1975, Hamilton et al. 1974). However, a rapid trimix dive (6% nitrogen) to 400 metres of seawater in 100 min resulted in tremor, dizziness

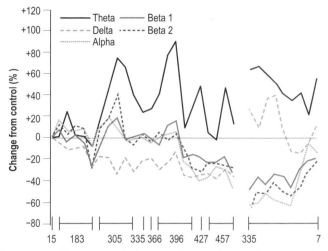

Figure 23.7 Electroencephalogram changes in one diver at various depth (metres) during a heliox dive to 457 metres of seawater (4.67 MPa) and ascent, compared to control data at 15 metres of seawater. Redrawn from Bennett & Towse (1971) with permission from the International Federation of Clinical Neurophysiology.

and confusion, and a subsequent dive to 464 metres of seawater in 4 h was aborted due to the poor condition of the divers (Bennett & Rostain 2003b).

A series of deep saturation dives were conducted to 460 and 650 metres of seawater to establish the optimum compression and fraction of nitrogen in trimix diving (Bennett & McLeod 1984, Bennett et al.1981, 1982). Three divers experienced varying degrees of high-pressure nervous syndrome, including electroencephalogram changes, microsleep, dyspnoea, nausea and fatigue, when breathing 5% nitrogen in helium-oxygen at 460 metres of seawater. These symptoms were suppressed in a dive in which the nitrogen fraction was increased to 10% at 460 metres of seawater (Bennett et al. 1981, Salzano et al. 1984). A further dive to 650 metres of seawater (6.6 MPa) for 4 days, breathing 10% nitrogen, was extended to include an excursion to 686 metres of seawater (6.96 MPa) for 24 h. Divers were in good condition with no dyspnoea and performed exercise up to 240 W at 650 metres of seawater (Bennett et al. 1982). In a comparative dive to 650 metres of seawater breathing 5% nitrogen, divers experienced mild tremor, and although two were in good condition, one diver suffered unique difficulties with symptoms of light headedness, hyperalertness and hallucinations that continued during decompression (Bennett & McLeod 1984).

British, French and Norwegian studies of heliox and trimix diving to depths of 300–660 metres of seawater have produced mixed results, with improvements observed in some but not all trimix dives. Although tremor was suppressed in some trimix dives, electroencephalogram changes were found to persist and, in some cases, divers suffered sleep disturbance, nausea and lassitude similar to that seen in heliox (Rostain et al. 1980, Torok 1984a,b, Vaernes et al. 1985). In addition, cognitive testing during trimix dives indicated that divers experienced symptoms of both narcosis and high-pressure nervous syndrome, particularly beyond 450 metres of seawater. These results suggest that high-pressure nervous syndrome is of heterogeneous origin (Torok 1984b), and that the critical volume hypothesis is insufficient to explain the complexity of the effects of pressure and inert gases on its many symptoms (Rostain et al. 1988).

One problem associated with deep trimix diving is the high density of gas mixtures containing nitrogen. Hydrogen offers the attraction of being less dense than helium while, being more soluble in lipid, it has a greater narcotic potency. A series of progressively deeper dives (*Hydra*) were made in France to test the effects of hydrogen on the symptoms of high-pressure nervous syndrome. During a heliox dive to 300 metres of seawater, divers breathing hydrogen-oxygen (hydrox) on masks experienced narcosis (Fructus 1987), and in a hydrox dive to 300 metres of seawater, two divers experienced psychotic disorders (Rostain et al. 1990). These problems seem to preclude the use of hydrogen alone as the inert gas component. Comparative

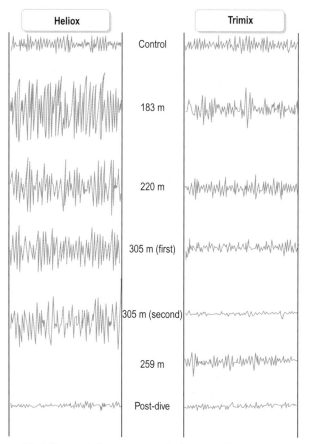

Figure 23.8 Postural finger tremor during two dives to 305 metres of seawater in which divers breathed either heliox or trimix. The tremor was suppressed when nitrogen was added to the gas mixture at 183 metres of seawater and beyond but returned during decompression at 259 metres of seawater, when divers reverted to a heliox mixture. Redrawn from Bennett et al. (1974) with permission.

dives using oxygen-helium-hydrogen (or hydreliox) showed better results (Rostain et al. 1988). These included an off-shore dive to 500 metres of seawater breathing hydreliox containing 49% hydrogen. Divers were in good condition and excursions were made in the open sea to 520 and 530 metres of seawater in which divers performed underwater work. Divers were less tired and more comfortable than when breathing heliox mixture (Gardette 1989).

These dives culminated in *Hydra X* in 1992, with a 3-d stay at 650–675 metres of seawater, during which one diver made an excursion to 701 metres of seawater (7.11 MPa). Compression required 13 days and was approximately exponential, with a series of intermediate stops. At maximum depth, divers breathed a hydreliox mixture containing 28% hydrogen. Divers remained in good condition, although they experienced some tremor and sleep disturbances, and analysis of electroencephalogram showed a decrease of alpha and an increase of theta activity. It was concluded that hydreliox reduced clinical symptoms of high-pressure nervous syndrome and improved the work capabilities of divers at these depths (Bennett & Rostain 2003b, Rostain et al. 1999).

From the above studies, it can be concluded that trained divers can operate safely to depths of 500 metres of seawater in the ocean and 700 metres of seawater (7.1 MPa) in hyperbaric chambers. However, saturation diving beyond 300 metres of seawater requires careful selection of compression rates, compression stops, the fractions of nitrogen or hydrogen to be added to the breathing mixture and vetting of dive personnel, to control and suppress symptoms of high-pressure nervous syndrome.

7 CONCLUSION

Humans have gradually extended their capabilities in the ocean over the past three centuries. Until the advent of the Industrial Revolution, and particularly the invention of compressed air pumps towards the end of the 18th century, humans were limited to brief excursions to about 20–30 metres of seawater in the ocean, accomplished by traditional breath-hold diving, and by using such aids as open diving bells (inverted barrels used as air reservoirs). By the end of the 19th century, compressed air divers were working regularly at 30 metres of seawater but were limited by severe decompression disorders and carbon dioxide narcosis, due to inadequate helmet ventilation. With the introduction of decompression models, improved breathing apparatus and heliox gas mixtures, the frontier of underwater exploration rapidly advanced to 300 metres of seawater (3.1 MPa) in the late 1960s, where a helium barrier due to high-pressure nervous syndrome was confronted.

By the beginning of the 21st century, human capabilities had been extended to a record depth of 701 metres of seawater (7.1 MPa) in an experimental chamber dive. With careful planning and logistical support, humans have been able to work safely at 500 metres of seawater (5.1 MPa) in the ocean. Free diving has reached the remarkable depth of

172 metres of seawater (1.82 MPa). The challenges to further advancement of human underwater excursion are many, including high-pressure nervous syndrome, dyspnoea, breathing gas density, diver heating and temperature regulation. Of these, the most critical factors are the multifaceted symptoms that are collectively referred to as the high-pressure nervous syndrome. Much has been achieved through the careful manipulation of compression rates, staged compression and gas mixtures. However, without a clearer knowledge of the mechanisms underlying muscle tremor, electroencephalogram changes, microsleep, stomach disorders, sleep disturbance and convulsions, and the antagonistic role of protective agents such as inert gas narcosis, it is unlikely that further progress can be made.

Advancements in human capabilities underwater have been achieved through a combination of physiological research and technological developments. As in the advancement of space travel, it may be that the future of human underwater exploration lies in the development of improved atmospheric diving suits that will allow the diver to lock out from a one-atmospheric habitat and work freely on the ocean floor.

References

Albano G, Criscuoli PM, Scaglione GC, La Monaca G, Burruano G 1972 La syndrome da estreme pressioni ambientali. Relievi EEG ed ECG su ratti liberi con elettrodi da dimora. Annali di Medicina Navale 77(1):11–28

Andersson JP, Linér MH, Rünow E, Schagatay EK 2002 Diving response and arterial oxygen saturation during apnea and exercise in breath-hold dives. Journal of Applied Physiology 93:882–886

Andersson JP, Linér MH, Fredsted A, Schagatay EK 2004 Cardiovascular and respiratory responses to apneas with and without face immersion in exercising humans. Journal of Applied Physiology 96:1005–1010

Åstrand P-O 1960 Breath holding during and after muscular exercise. Journal of Applied Physiology 15:220–224

Åstrand P-O, Rodahl K 1970 Textbook of work physiology. McGraw-Hill, New York, 248

Barth B 2000 Sea dwellers: the humor, drama and tragedy of the US Navy Sealab programs. Doyle Publishing Company, Houston, TX

Bennett PB, Dossett AN 1967 Undesirable effects of oxygen helium breathing at great depth. RN Personnel Research Committee, Underwater Physiology Subcommittee Report 260. Medical Research Council, London

Bennett PB, McLeod M 1984 Probing the limits of human deep diving. In: Elliott DH, Smith EB (eds) Diving and life at high pressure. Royal Society, London, 105–117

Bennett PB, Rostain JC 2003a Inert gas narcosis. In: Brubakk AO, Neuman TS (eds) Physiology and medicine of diving, 5th edn. Saunders, New York, 300–322

Bennett PB, Rostain JC 2003b The high pressure nervous syndrome. In: Brubakk AO, Neuman TS (eds) Physiology and medicine of diving, 5th edn. Saunders, New York, 323–357

Bennett PB, Towse EJ 1971 The high pressure nervous syndrome during a simulated oxygen-helium dive to 1500 ft. Electroencephalography and Clinical Neurophysiology 31:383–393

Bennett PB, Morrison JB, Barnard EEP, Eaton WJ, Hempleman HV 1971 Experimental observations on men at pressures between 4 bars (100 ft) and 47 bars (1500 ft). RN Physiological Laboratory Report 1/71, Ministry of Defence (Navy), London

Bennett PB, Blenkarn GD, Roby J, Youngblood D 1974 Suppression of the high pressure nervous syndrome in human deep dives by He-N₂-O₂. Undersea Biomedical Research 1:221–237

Bennett PB, Roby J, Simon RS, Youngblood D 1975 Optimal use of nitrogen to suppress the high pressure nervous syndrome. Aviation, Space and Environmental Medicine 46:37–40

Bennett PB, Coggin R, Roby J 1981 Control of HPNS in humans during rapid compression with trimix to 650 m (2132 ft). Undersea Biomedical Research 8:85–100

Bennett PB, Coggin R, McLeod M 1982 Effect of compression rate on use of trimix to ameliorate HPNS in man to 686 m (2250 ft). Undersea Biomedical Research 9:335–351

Bert P 1870 Lecons sur la physiologie comparee de la respiration. Baillière, Paris, 526–553

Bowen S 1968 Diver performance and effects of cold. Human Factors 10:445–463

Bozanic JE 2002 Mastering rebreathers. Best Publishing, Flagstaff, AZ

Brauer RW 1968 Seeking man's depth level. Ocean Industry 3:28–33

Brauer RW 1975 High pressure nervous syndrome: animals. In: Bennett PB, Elliott DH (eds) The physiology and medicine of diving, 2nd edn. Baillière Tindall, London, 231–247

Brauer RW, Dimor S, Fructus X, Fructus P, Gosset A, Naquet R 1969 Syndrome neurologique et electrographique des hautes pressions. Revue Neurologique 121(3):264–265

Brauer RW, Way RO, Jordan MR 1971 Experimental studies of the high pressure neurological syndrome in various mammalian species. In: Lambertsen CJ (ed) Proceedings of the 4th Symposium on Underwater Physiology. Academic Press, New York, 487–500

Brauer RW, Goldman SM, Beaver RW, Sheehan ME 1974 N₂, H₂ and N₂O antagonism to high pressure neurological syndrome in mice. Undersea Biomedical Research 1:59–72

Brian JE 1998 Carbon dioxide and the cerebral circulation. Anesthesiology 88(5):1365–1386

Broussolle B, Bensimon E, Michaud A, Vegezzi C 1972 Comparaisons des responses ventilatoire et des pressions partielles alveolaires de CO2 de plongeurs sous-marins entraines et de temoins non plongeurs au coeurs du travail musculare en atmosphere hyperbare. In: Fructus X (ed) Les troisiemes journees d'hyperbarie et de physiologie subaquatique. Doin, Paris, 80–87

Bühlmann AA, Matthys H, Overrath G, Bennett PB, Elliott DH, Gray SP 1970 Saturation exposures of 31 ats in an oxygen-helium atmosphere with excursions to 36 ats. Aerospace Medicine 41:394–402

Butler PJ 1982 Respiratory and cardiovascular control during diving in birds and mammals. Journal of Experimental Biology 100:195–221

CGPM 1954 Resolution 4: Comptes Rendus de la 10th Conférence Générale des Poids et Mesures (CGPM). Conférence Générale des Poids et Mesures, Paris, 79

Clarey C 2002 A free-diver's death: tragic plunge to the limits. International Herald Tribune, October 19. Available online at: www.iht.com/articles/2002/10/19/diver_ed3_.php

Clarke JR 1992 Diver tolerance to respiratory loading during wet and dry dives from 0 to 450 m. In: Flook V, Brubakk AO (eds) Lung physiology and divers' breathing apparatus. Sintef Unimed, Aberdeen, 45–61

Dahlback GO 1978 Lung mechanics during immersion in water: with special reference to pulmonary air trapping. PhD thesis, University of Lund, Sweden

Davis RH 1981 Deep diving and submarine operations, 8th edn. Siebe Gorman, Cwmbran, UK

Dawson SV, Elliott EA 1977 Wave-speed limitation on expiratory flow – a unifying concept. Journal of Applied Physiology 43:498–515

Doell D, Zutter M, Anthonisen NR 1973 Ventilatory responses to hypercapnia and hypoxia at 1 and 4 ATA. Respiration Physiology 18:338–346

Donald KW, Davidson WM 1954 Oxygen uptake of 'booted' and 'fin swimming' divers. Journal of Applied Physiology 7:31–37

Dwyer J, Saltzman HA, O'Brian R 1977 Maximal physical work capacity of man at 43.4 ATA. Undersea Biomedical Research 4:359–372

Edmonds CW, Walker DG 1999 Snorkelling deaths in Australia, 1987–1996. Medical Journal of Australia 171:591–594

Fagraeus L, Linnarsson D 1973 Maximal voluntary and exercise ventilation at high ambient air pressures. Forsvarmedicin 9:275–278

Ferretti G, Costa M, Ferrigno M, Grassi B, Marconi C, Lundgren CE, Cerretelli P 1991 Alveolar gas composition and exchange during deep breath-hold diving and dry breath holds in elite divers. Journal of Applied Physiology 70:794–802

Ferrigno M 2004 Breath-hold diving. In: Bove AA (ed) Diving medicine, 4th edn. Saunders, Philadelphia

Ferrigno M, Ferretti G, Ellis A, Warkander D, Costa M, Cerretelli P, Lundgren CE 1997 Cardiovascular changes during deep breath-hold dives in a pressure chamber. Journal of Applied Physiology 83:1282–1290

Flook V, Fraser IM 1992 Resistance to breathing – divers' lungs the main problem? In: Flook V, Brubakk AO (eds) Lung physiology and divers' breathing apparatus. Sintef Unimed, Aberdeen, 45–61

Florio JT, Morrison JB, Butt WS 1979 Breathing pattern and ventilatory response to carbon dioxide in divers. Journal of Applied Physiology 46(6):1076-1080

Fothergill DM, Hedges D, Morrison JB 1991 Effects of CO_2 and N_2 partial pressures on cognitive and psychomotor performance. Undersea Biomedical Research 18:1–19

Fructus XR 1987 Hydrogen, pressure and HPNS. In: Brauer RW (ed) Hydrogen as a diving gas. 33rd Undersea and Hyperbaric Medicine Workshop. Undersea and Hyperbaric Medical Society, Bethesda, MD, 125–138

Fructus X, Agarate C, Naquet R, Rostain JC 1976 Postponing the high pressure nervous syndrome to 1640 feet and beyond. In: Lambertsen CJ (ed) Underwater physiology V. FASEB, Bethesda, MD, 21–33

Fry DL 1958 Theoretical considerations of the bronchial pressure-flow-volume relationships with particular reference to the maximum expiratory flow volume curve. Physics in Medicine and Biology 3(2):174–194

Gardette B 1989 Compression procedures for mice and human hydrogen deep diving: COMEX HYDRA program. In: Rostain JC, Martinez E, Lamaire C (eds) High pressure syndrome twenty years later. ARAS-SNHP, Marseilles, 217–231

Goff LG, Frassetto R, Specht H 1956 Oxygen requirements in underwater swimming. Journal of Applied Physiology 9:219–221

Hamilton RW, Schmidt TC, Kenyon DJ, Freitag M, Powell MR 1974 ACCESS: diver performance and physiology in rapid compression to 31 ats. Tech Memo CRL-T-789. Union Carbide, Tarrytown, NY

Hayes PA, Padbury EH, Florio JT, Fyfield TP 1981 Respiratory heat transfer in cold water and during rewarming. Report 80–401, Admiralty Marine Technology Establishment. HMSO, London

Hayward JS, Lisson PA, Collis ML 1978 Survival suits for accidental immersion in cold water: design-concepts and their thermal protection performance. University of Victoria, BC, Canada

Hempleman H, Andrews B, Burgess D, Carlyle R, Collis S, Florio J, Garrard M, Harris D, Hayes P, Herbert M, Lewis V, McKenzie R, Nichols G, Pearson R, Stock M, Torok Z, Towse J, Williams J, Winsborough M 1978 Observations on men at pressures of up to 300 msw (31 bar). Report 78–401, Admiralty Marine Technology Establishment. HMSO, London

Hempleman H, Atherton P, Baddely A, Carlyle R, Castle J, Collis S, Florio J, Garrard M, Habert M, Hall G, Harris D, Hayes P, Hennessy T, Lewis V, McKenzie D, McKenzie R, Nichols G, Paciorek J, Spencer N, Stock M, Torok Z, Towse J, Winsborough 1980 Human physiological studies at 43 bar. Report 80–402, Admiralty Marine Technology Establishment. HMSO, London

Hesser CM, Fagraeus L, Linnarsson D 1968 Cardio-respiratory responses to exercise in hyperbaric environment. Report of the Laboratory of Aviation and Naval Medicine, Karolinska Institutit, Stockholm

Hong SK, Rahn H, Kang DH, Song SH, Kang BS 1963 Diving patterns, lung volumes and alveolar gas of the Korean diving women. Journal of Applied Physiology 18:457–465

Hong SK, Cerretelli P, Cruz JC, Rahn H 1969 Mechanics of respiration during submersion in water. Journal of Applied Physiology 27:535–538

Johnston FH, Flagler EA 1950 Hydrostatic pressure reversal of narcosis in tadpoles. Science 112:91–92

Kerem D, Melamed Y, Moran A 1980 Alveolar PCO_2 during rest and exercise in divers and non-divers breathing O_2 at 1 ATA. Undersea Biomedical Research 7:17–26

Kety SS, Schmidt CF 1948 The effects of altered arterial tensions of carbon dioxide and oxygen on cerebral blood flow and cerebral oxygen consumption of normal young men. Journal of Clinical Investigation 27(4):484–492

Kohshi K, Wong RM, Abe H, Katoh T, Okudera T, Mano Y 2005 Neurological manifestations in Japanese Ama divers. Undersea and Hyperbaric Medicine 32(1):11–20

Lalley DA, Zechman FW, Tracy RA 1974 Ventilatory responses to exercise in divers and non-divers. Respiratory Physiology 20:117–129

Lambertsen CJ, Owen SG, Wendel H Stroud MW, Lurie AA, Lochner W, Clark GF 1959 Respiratory cerebral circulatory control during exercise at 0.21 and 2.0 atmospheres inspired PO_2. Journal of Applied Physiology 14:966–982

Lanphier EH 1954 Oxygen consumption in underwater swimming. Report 14–54, US Navy Experimental Diving Unit, Washington, DC

Lanphier EH 1963 Influence of increased ambient pressure upon alveolar ventilation. In: Lambertsen CJ Greenbaum LJ (eds) Proceedings of the 2nd Symposium on Underwater Physiology. National Academy of Sciences National Research Council, Washington, DC, 124–133

Lanphier EH, Camporesi EM 1982 Respiration and exercise. In: Bennett PB, Elliott DH (eds) The physiology and medicine of diving, 3rd edn. Baillière Tindall, London, 99–156

Lever MJ, Miller KW, Paton WD, Smith EB 1971a Pressure reversal of anaesthesia. Nature 231:368–371

Lever MJ, Miller KW, Paton WDM, Streett WB, Smith EB 1971b Effects of hydrostatic pressure on mammals In: Lambertsen CJ (ed) Proceedings of the 4th Symposium on Underwater Physiology. Academic Press, New York, 101–108

Lindholm P, Gennser M 2005 Aggravated hypoxia during breath-holds after prolonged exercise. European Journal of Applied Physiology 93(5–6):701–707

Lollgen H, Niedling GV, Horres R 1980 Respiratory and hemodynamic adjustment during head out water immersion. International Journal of Sports Medicine 1:25–29

Maio DA, Farhi LE 1967 Effect of gas density on mechanics of breathing. Journal of Applied Physiology 23:687–693

Mass T 2007 The case for a device to manage freediver blackout. BlueWater Freedivers Publishing. Available online at: http://freedive.net/SWB/vest1_hi_rez.pdf

Mead J, Turner JM, Macklem PT, Little JB 1967 Significance of the relationship between lung recoil and maximum expiratory flow. Journal of Applied Physiology 22:95–108

Meduna LJ 1950 Carbon dioxide therapy. A neurophysiological treatment of nervous disorders. Charles C Thomas, Springfield, IL

Mekjavic B, Golden FS, Eglin M, Tipton MJ 2001 Thermal status of saturation divers during operational dives in the North Sea. Undersea and Hyperbaric Medicine 28:149–155

Mekjavic IB, Tipton MJ, Eiken O 2003 Thermal considerations in diving. In: Brubakk AO, Neuman TS (eds) Physiology and medicine of diving, 5th edn. Saunders, New York, 323–357

Milic-Emili J, Tyler JM 1963 Relationship between work output of respiratory muscles and end-tidal CO_2 tension. Journal of Applied Physiology 18:497–504

Miller SL, Cooper C 2000 The Aquarius underwater laboratory: America's 'inner space' station. Marine Technology Society Journal 34(4):69–74

Miller KW, Paton WD, Streett WB, Smith EB 1967 Animals at very high pressures of helium and neon. Science 157:97–98

Morrison JB 1973 Oxygen uptake studies of divers when fin swimming with maximum effort at depths of 6–176 feet. Aerospace Medicine 44:1120–1129

Morrison JB, Butt WS 1972 Effect of underwater breathing apparatus and absolute air pressure on diver's ventilatory capacity. Aerospace Medicine 43:881–886

Morrison JB, Conn ML 1980 Unpublished observations

Morrison JB, Reimers SD 1982 Design principles of underwater breathing apparatus. In: Bennett PB, Elliott DH (eds) The physiology and medicine of diving, 3rd edn. Baillière Tindall, London, 55–98

Morrison JB, Taylor NAS 1990 Measurement of static and dynamic pulmonary work during pressure breathing. Undersea Biomedical Research 17(5):453–467

Morrison JB, Butt WS, Florio JT, Mayo IC 1976 The effect of increased O_2-N_2 pressure and breathing apparatus on respiratory function. Undersea Biomedical Research 3:217–234

Morrison JB, Florio JT, Butt WS 1978 Observations after loss of consciousness underwater. Undersea Biomedical Research 5:(2)179–187

Morrison JB, Voogt SL, Wright WP 1993 Evaluation of underwater breathing apparatus used in British Columbia industries according to international performance and safety standards. Report to Workers' Compensation Board of British Columbia, Richmond, BC, Canada

Morrison JB, Zander JK 2007a The effects of exposure time, pressure and cold on hand skin temperature and manual performance when wearing 3-fingered neoprene gloves. Report CR-2007–164, Defence Research and Development Canada – Toronto

Morrison JB, Zander JK 2007b Factors influencing manual performance in cold water diving. Report CR-2007–165, Defence Research and Development Canada – Toronto

Neuman TS 2003 Arterial gas embolism and pulmonary barotrauma. In: Brubakk AO, Neuman TS (eds) Physiology and medicine of diving, 5th edn. Saunders, New York, 323–357

Overfield EM, Saltzman HA, Kylstra JA, Salzano JV 1969 Respiratory gas exchange in normal men breathing 0.9% oxygen in helium at 31.3 ats. Journal of Applied Physiology 27:471–475

Patterson JL, Heyman H, Battey LL, Ferguson RW 1955 Threshold of response of the cerebral vessels of man to increases in blood carbon dioxide. Journal of Clinical Investigation 34(12):1857–1864

Pendergast DR, Lindholm P, Wylegala J, Warkander D, Lundgren CE 2006 Effects of respiratory muscle training on CO_2 sensitivity in scuba divers. Undersea and Hyperbaric Medicine 33(6):447–453

Pollock NW 2006 Development of the DAN breath-hold incident database. In: Lindholm P, Pollock NW, Lundgren CEG (eds) Breath-hold diving. Proceedings of the Undersea and Hyperbaric Medical Society/Divers Alert Network Workshop. Divers Alert Network, Durham, NC, 46–55

Qvist J, Hurford WE, Park YS, Ferguson RW 1993 Arterial blood gas tensions during breath-hold diving in the Korean Ama. Journal of Applied Physiology 75(1):285–293

Rostain JC, Gardett-Chauffour MC, Naquet R 1980 HPNS during rapid compression of men breathing He-O_2 and He-N_2-O_2 at 300m and 180m. Undersea Biomedical Research 7:77–94

Rostain JC, Gardette-Chauffour MC, Lemaire C, Naquet R 1988 Effects of a N_2-He-O_2 mixture on the HPNS up to 450m. Undersea Biomedical Research 15:257–270

Rostain JC, Gardett-Chauffour MC, Naquet R 1990 Studies of neurophysiological effects of hydrogen-oxygen mixture in man up to 30 bars. Undersea Biomedical Research 17(Suppl):159

Rostain JC, Gardett-Chauffour MC, Gardett B 1999 Hydrogen, a gas for diving: a mini review. Undersea Biomedical Research 26:62

Ryerson GG, Block AJ 1991 Oxygen as a drug: clinical properties, benefits, modes and hazards of administration. In: Respiratory care, 3rd edn. JB Lippincott, Philadelphia, 319–325

Salzano JV, Camporesi EM, Stolp BW, Moon RE 1984 Physiological responses to exercise at 47 and 66 ATA. Journal of Applied Physiology 57:1055–1068

Schaefer KE 1965 Adaptation to breath-hold diving. In: Rahn H, Yokoyama T (eds) Physiology of breath-hold diving in the Ama of Japan. National Academy Sciences National Research Council, Washington, DC, 237–251

Schagatay E, Andersson JP, Hallén M, Pålsson B 2001 Selected contribution: role of spleen emptying in prolonging apneas in humans. Journal of Applied Physiology 90:1623–1629

Seusing J, Drube HC 1960 Die bedeutung der hyperkapnie fur das auftreten des tiefenrausches. Klinische Wochenschrifte 38:1088–1090

Sherman D, Eilender E, Shefer A, Kerem D 1980 Ventilatory and occlusion-pressure responses to hypercapnia in divers and non-divers. Undersea Biomedical Research 7:61–74

Spaur WH, Raymond LW, Knott MM, Crothers JC, Braithwaite WR, Thalmann ED, Uddin DF 1977 Dyspnea in divers at 49.5 ATA: mechanical not chemical in origin. Undersea Biomedical Research 4:183–198

Sterba JA 1990 Hypercapnia during deep air and mixed gas diving. Report 12–90. US Navy Experimental Diving Unit, Panama City, FL

Sterk W 1973 Respiratory mechanics of diver and diving apparatus. PhD thesis, University of Utrecht, Netherlands

Taylor NAS, Morrison JB 1989 Lung centroid pressure in immersed man. Undersea Biomedical Research 16:3–19

Taylor NAS, Morrison JB 1990 Effects of breathing-gas pressure on pulmonary function and work capacity during immersion. Undersea Biomedical Research 17(5):413–428

Taylor NAS, Morrison JB 1991 Lung volume changes in response to altered breathing gas pressure during upright immersion. European Journal of Applied Physiology 62:122–129

Tikuisis P, Gerth WA 2003 Decompression theory. In: Brubakk AO, Neuman TS (eds) Physiology and medicine of diving, 5th edn. Saunders, New York, 419–454

Torok Z 1984a Invited review: behaviour and performance in deep experimental diving with man – a review of recent work. In: Backrach AJ, Matzen MM (eds) Underwater physiology VIII. Undersea Medical Society, Bethesda, MD, 739–760

Torok Z 1984b Deep diving: trimix and heliox compared by EEG and tremor criteria. In: Backrach AJ, Matzen MM (eds) Underwater physiology VIII. Undersea Medical Society, Bethesda, MD, 697–705

US Navy Diving Manual 2005 US Navy diving manual, revision 5, volumes 1–5. Naval Sea Systems Command. US Govt Printing Office, Washington, DC, Available online at: www.supsalv.org/pdf/Diveman.pdf

Vaernes R, Hammerborg D, Ellertsen B, Peterson R, Tønjum S 1985 CNS reaction at 51 ata on trimix and heliox during decompression. Undersea Biomedical Research 12:25–39

Vann RD, Freiberger JJ, Caruso JL, Denoble PJ, Pollock NW, Uguccioni DM, Dovenbarger JA, Nord DA 2006 Annual diving report: 2006 edition. Divers Alert Network, Durham, NC, 59–63

Wood WB 1963 Ventilatory dynamics under hyperbaric states. In: Lambertsen CJ, Greenbaum LJ (eds) Proceedings of the 2nd Symposium on Underwater Physiology. National Academy of Sciences National Research Council, Washington, DC, 108–123

Chapter 24

Altitude physiology: the impact of hypoxia on human performance

Claudio Marconi   Paolo Cerretelli

Maximal aerobic power and glycolytic capacity are affected by various environmental variables, among which barometric pressure plays a major role, setting the oxygen partial pressure in the inspired air. As a consequence of acute or chronic reduction of barometric pressure, oxygen partial pressure decreases in the blood and tissues: hypobaric hypoxia. In the 1860s, Denis Jourdanet (1815–1892), a French physician who spent 19 years in Mexico, hypothesised that the effects of high altitude were caused by reduced arterial oxygen pressure. This was subsequently proved by Paul Bert, the French physiologist who is considered the father of

modern high-altitude physiology and medicine. Bert made measurements in a laboratory provided by Jourdanet, equipped with high- and low-pressure chambers. His studies were summarised in the monumental work *La Pression Barométrique: Recherches de Physiologie Expérimentale*, published in 1878, in which the author established that the harmful effects of high altitude were caused by the low partial pressure of oxygen in the inspired air (i.e. the product of barometric pressure and the fractional concentration of oxygen).

At sea level (normobaric conditions) acute hypoxia may be induced by reducing the fraction of inspired oxygen (acute normobaric hypoxia). In some pathological conditions, such as anaemia and chronic obstructive lung disease, tissue hypoxia may be due to a reduction in the total oxygen content in arterial blood with normal (anaemic hypoxia) or low (hypoxic hypoxia) oxygen partial pressures, respectively. In other conditions (e.g. chronic heart failure, peripheral arterial occlusive disease) arterial oxygen content may be normal, whereas tissue blood flow is inadequate, which leads to a greater reduction of oxygen pressure in the tissues (stagnant or ischaemic hypoxia). Finally, tissue hypoxia may be due to the inability of cells to take up or use oxygen from the bloodstream, despite normal arterial oxygen content and blood flow. This condition (histotoxic hypoxia) results from tissue poisoning, such as that caused by alcohol, narcotics and cyanide. This chapter deals mainly with hypobaric hypoxia, though it is a useful physiological model for other forms of hypoxia.

As a consequence of tissue hypoxia, hypoxia-inducible factor 1, a protein known to undergo rapid degradation in normoxia, becomes stabilised, thereby promoting the transcription of several genes, the expression of which increases oxygen delivery and induces metabolic adaptations limiting the functional impairment associated with hypoxia. Beside barometric pressure, important variables to be considered for the study of exercise at altitude are the density, viscosity and humidity of air, which affect the mechanics of ventilation and tissue dehydration.

1 ENVIRONMENTAL VARIABLES

1.1 Barometric pressure

Barometric pressure arises from the force exerted by the gravitational field of the Earth on the molecules contained within a column of air above a given surface area. This pressure decreases exponentially with the distance above sea level. It can be approximated on the basis of a formula provided by the International Civil Aviation Organisation, but this underestimates the actual pressure, since it assumes a uniform temperature in the atmosphere. By contrast, temperature is not uniform and decreases with altitude. In fact, in the inner part of the atmosphere surrounding the Earth, thermal convection causes a rapid mixing of air and expansion of gases. Such expansion occurs without exchange of heat (adiabatic conditions) and therefore causes a reduction in the air temperature. In addition, due to the shape of the Earth, the gravitational field is not uniform and, at a given altitude, air density (mass per unit volume) and temperature vary according to the latitude and season.

The first measurement of barometric pressure on the summit of Mt Everest (8848 m) was made by Pizzo (24 October 1981) in the course of the American Medical Research Expedition (West et al. 1983). He recorded a pressure of 33.73 kPa (253 mmHg), 2.0 kPa higher than previously predicted. This value was confirmed on 23 May 1997 (33.66 kPa). From over 2000 measurements made during May, June, July and August 1998, the average air pressures

at the South Col (7986 m) were 37.86, 38.00, 38.13 and 38.26 kPa, respectively (West 1999). These data confirm that, at extreme altitudes, air pressure is higher than previously thought and changes according to the season, thus favouring attempts to reach the summit of the highest peaks in the summer. On the basis of these measurements, the model atmosphere equation was developed for altitudes above 4000 m, which allows one to predict barometric pressure of most locations with an accuracy of about 1%:

Equation 1:   Barometric pressure =
$$e^{(6.63268-0.1112h-0.00149 \cdot h^2)} \text{ mmHg } (1 = 0.13 \text{ kPa})$$

where:

h = altitude in km.

1.2 Air density and kinematic viscosity

Air density is the ratio between air mass and the volume it occupies. The density, pressure and temperature of a gas are related to each other through the Van Der Waals equation, in such a way that air density decreases with increasing altitude. On the other hand, viscosity is a measure of the resistance of a fluid to deformation under shear stress. Kinematic viscosity is the ratio of viscosity to density. Due to the large reduction of air density with decreasing air pressure, kinematic viscosity increases progressively with altitude. As is well known, the pressure required for a given flow is considerably greater when air flow is turbulent (or when there are flow eddies) than when flow is laminar (streamlined). At altitude, the increase in pressure due to hyperpnoea-induced airway turbulences is counterbalanced by the decrease in air density, whereas the role of viscosity is negligible.

1.3 Absolute humidity and water loss

The absolute humidity of air is the mass of water vapour present per unit volume of air. Since warmer air can hold a greater number of water molecules, absolute humidity decreases with altitude as a result of the temperature drop. The dryness of cold inspired air, coupled with altitude-induced hyperventilation, increases airways water loss. During a 10-h walk at average speed in a cold environment, respiratory water loss may be ~1.5 L, and in subjects climbing Mt Everest, it may be as high as 3.3 L per day. However, Westerterp (2001) has argued that body water loss at extreme altitude is not greater than at sea level, being related not only to ambient temperature but also to water intake. However, at altitude, water intake may be reduced, mainly due to its limited availability (provided only by melting snow). During a prolonged sojourn in a hypobaric chamber, under constant temperature and relative humidity conditions, total water loss was found to be slightly lower at simulated altitudes >7000 m than between 5000 and 7000 m. This is likely to be the consequence of reduced daily energy expenditure, thus limiting the exercise-induced increase in respiratory water loss.

1.4 Other physical variables

Other physical variables, less relevant for exercise at altitude, are ultraviolet light and cold (Chapter 20). Exercise or work at altitude is usually performed with a minimum of skin exposure, due to the low temperature, but face, arms and hands are often exposed to solar radiation with less protective cloud filter. Ultraviolet radiation has different wavelengths (UVA, UVB, UVC) and energy levels, and these may penetrate and damage the dermis, and even subcutaneous tissues, increasing the production of oxygen free radicals and the level of oxidative stress. The latter induces molecular damage with accelerated skin ageing or increased incidence of cutaneous melanoma. Cold exposure might contribute to oxidative stress (Askew 2002), likely via increased thermogenic activity. On the other hand, free radicals may be involved in the impaired cold-induced vasodilatation response at altitude (Purkayastha et al. 1999).

1.5 Hypoxia–inducible factor

The hypoxia-inducible factor (HIF) comprises the heterodimeric transcription factors HIF-α and HIF-β of the Per-Arnt-Sim (PAS) family of basic helix-loop-helix proteins, which are regulated by cellular oxygen tension. These proteins bind to regulatory promoter regions of hypoxia-responsive genes. HIF-1α is the most ubiquitously expressed and best characterised of the family, and is recognised as a master regulator of hypoxic signalling (Semenza 2004). HIF-2α is similar in regulation to HIF-1α but its expression is restricted mainly to endothelial cells. Genes under the control of HIF-1α include those involved in vasodilatation (e.g. the inducible form of nitric oxide synthase), angiogenesis (e.g. vascular endothelial growth factor), enhanced blood oxygen-carrying capacity (e.g. erythropoietin) and glycolysis (e.g. glucose transporters GLUT1 and GLUT3).

Mitochondria play an important role in regulating HIF activation. In normoxia and under steady-state conditions, mitochondria consume ~90% of the available oxygen, generating ATP via oxidative phosphorylation to meet metabolic requirements. The remaining 10% of the oxygen consumed is used for other cellular processes, including HIF-1α and HIF-2α degradation. In hypoxia, mitochondria act like a sink, consuming most of the available oxygen due to the high affinity of cytochrome c oxidase for oxygen (Gnaiger et al. 1998). Thus, the oxygen availability for the degradation of HIF is reduced and the concentration of the latter increases. In contrast, inhibition of cytochrome c oxidase activity by nitric oxide (Antunes et al. 2004) makes oxygen available for HIF-1α degradation. During hypoxia, a paradoxical increase in the production of reactive oxygen species at the electron transport chain may also lead to a further HIF-1α accumulation with consequent increased protein expression by HIF-1α dependent genes (Brunelle et al. 2005).

1.6 Adaptation to hypoxia

The general concepts of adaptation to unusual environments are discussed in Chapter 21, whereas the effects of chronic adaptation to hypoxia will be described in Chapter 25. Therefore, the next few paragraphs will address the functional changes occurring when lowlanders are exposed acutely to hypoxia or sojourn at high altitude from a few days up to 2–3 months. These changes characterise acclimatisation, as opposed to developmental (after years of stay at altitude) and genetic adaptations (characteristic of altitude natives).

2 PULMONARY FUNCTION DURING REST AND EXERCISE

2.1 Lung volumes

The first assessment of the lung volumes at altitude was made by Angelo Mosso (1897), who found that vital capacity decreased ~11% in individuals moving rapidly from sea level to 4559 m. This has been confirmed at various altitudes, also revealing that acute normoxia does not restore vital capacity in acclimatised lowlanders (Cerretelli 1980). With increasing altitude, forced vital capacity also decreases, whereas peak expiratory flow increases, as a consequence of reduced air density. For instance, Cogo et al. (1997; Ev-K2-CNR Laboratory, 5050 m, Nepal) found that the maximal expiratory flow at 25% of the forced vital capacity of lowlanders decreased to 82% of the value measured at sea level, recovering up to 94% after 7 days of exposure. These data have been interpreted as a consequence of increased pulmonary blood volume or the development of interstitial oedema. In this context, the closing volume was found to be increased at 4559 m, also in subjects with no clinical evidence of high-altitude pulmonary oedema, and was attributed to the accumulation of peribronchial fluid (Cremona et al. 2002).

2.2 Respiratory mechanics

Lung compliance of both acclimatised lowlanders and high-altitude natives is not affected by hypobaric hypoxia. In both groups, airway resistance is lower than at sea level, but not as much as expected on the basis of reduced air density (Cruz 1973). As a consequence, the work of breathing is also expected to be somewhat less. However, at 5050 m the work of breathing of acclimatised lowlanders performing exercise at 75% of maximal mechanical power output was found to be greater than at sea level, due to an increase in pulmonary ventilation, and in particular respiratory rate (Cibella et al. 1996). That is, whilst the work of ventilating a given volume of air may be lower, subjects must increase ventilation at altitude to sustain a fixed workload and oxygen uptake. Consequently, at altitude, the energy cost of breathing for any given workload is greater than at sea level, and during maximal effort it may interfere with energy supply to the locomotor muscles and limit exercise (Chapters 2 and 23).

2.3. Pulmonary ventilation during rest and exercise

2.3.1 Lowlanders

Exposure to acute hypoxia, corresponding to an altitude of 4000 m (alveolar oxygen partial pressure ~6.50–7.80 kPa (50–60 mmHg)), does not affect resting minute ventilation of healthy sea-level dwellers, even though peripheral chemoreceptor (carotid body) activity is enhanced. Likewise, alveolar carbon dioxide partial pressure remains constant, while alveolar oxygen partial pressure declines (Figure 24.1, thicker dashed line; Rahn & Otis 1949). More powerful hypoxic stimuli (<6.50 kPa or 50 mmHg) result in a progressive elevation of resting ventilation, due to carotid body stimulation.

For any given hypoxic stimulus, acclimatised subjects are characterised by higher resting ventilation and alveolar oxygen tension, and correspondingly lower alveolar carbon dioxide partial pressure (Figure 24.1, solid line), relative to that seen during an acute exposure (dashed line). This is a true hyperventilatory response. Even though chemoreceptor drive is somewhat diminished, resting ventilation keeps increasing (ventilatory acclimatisation). In addition, as appears from Figure 24.1, at a given altitude, alveolar air composition varies with the value of the respiratory exchange ratio, according to the alveolar air equation:

$$\text{Equation 2:} \quad P_AO_2 = P_IO_2 - P_ACO_2/R + [P_ACO_2 \cdot F_IO_2 \cdot (1-R)/R]$$

where:

P_AO_2 = alveolar oxygen partial pressure
P_IO_2 = inspired oxygen partial pressure
P_ACO_2 = alveolar carbon dioxide partial pressure
R = respiratory exchange ratio
F_IO_2 = fractional concentration of inspired oxygen.

For example, at 6000 m, when the respiratory exchange ratio rises from 0.8 to 1.0, the alveolar oxygen tension of acclimatised lowlanders increases by about 0.4 kPa (3 mmHg). For this reason, from the respiratory standpoint, at extreme altitudes, the oxidation of carbohydrates is more advantageous than that of lipids.

It is interesting to note that an early application of the alveolar air equation, based on the erroneous assumption that the minimal alveolar carbon dioxide tension would be ~2.7 kPa, led Margaria & De Caro (1950) to calculate that climbers could not go higher than 7500 m without supplementary oxygen. However, actual values of alveolar oxygen and carbon dioxide tensions, as determined by West et al. (1983), are compatible with a ceiling height close to that of Mt Everest, as proven by Messner and Habeler (8 May 1978).

Even though central chemoreceptor drive is somewhat diminished, resting ventilation keeps increasing in hypoxia (ventilatory acclimatisation). The underlying mechanisms are not known. It has been hypothesised, but not proven, that compensation of hypocapnic alkalosis in the brain and restoration of prehypoxia pH may occur close to the central chemoreceptors, thus sustaining hyperventilation. It has also been suggested that the carotid bodies may contribute to this ventilatory acclimatisation by increasing their sensitivity to hypoxia, and establishing a new threshold (Chapter 18) for the hypoxic response (Lahiri et al. 2000). The carotid bodies sense changes in local oxygen tension via reduced oxygen availability for mitochondrial oxidative phosphorylation, at the level of cytochrome a3 in the respiratory transport chain, leading to increased afferent flow to the dorsal and ventral respiratory groups of the medulla oblongata. In addition, carotid bodies may modulate their oxygen sensitivity by changing the conductance of oxygen-sensitive ion channels in the cell membranes. Long-term exposure to high altitude elicits progressive adaptations in the carotid bodies, most likely promoted by HIF-1α. In fact, HIF-1α knockout mice (Kline et al. 2002) are characterised by a blunted ventilatory response to hypoxia, compared to wild animals. The above described changes begin within minutes but progress with chronic exposure, resulting in cellular enlargement and biochemical alterations.

In the chronically adapted carotid body, the response to acute changes in oxygen partial pressure is enhanced, being reversed upon return to low altitude (Wilson et al. 2005). It is noteworthy that erythropoietin, besides its erythroid function, has been recently regarded as a key factor that may modulate neural respiratory control during hypoxia. In particular, during 3 days of severe hypoxia, overexpression of erythropoietin in transgenic mice, or its administration in the wild genotype, enhanced their hypoxic ventilatory response, most probably by acting on both the central nervous system and peripheral chemoreceptors (Soliz et al. 2005).

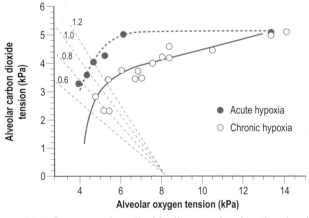

Figure 24.1 Oxygen–carbon dioxide diagram showing the alveolar air composition in acute (closed symbols) and chronic (open symbols) hypoxia. Dotted oblique lines represent the respiratory exchange ratios at about 6000 m. In chronic hypoxia, when the respiratory exchange ratio moves from 0.8 to 1.0, alveolar oxygen partial pressure increases. Modified from Rahn & Otis (1949) with permission.

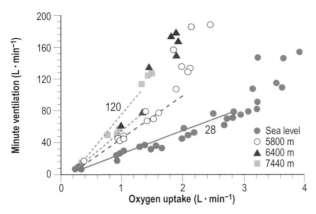

Figure 24.2 Minute ventilation as a function of oxygen uptake (ventilatory equivalent: numbers) in acclimatised lowlanders at sea level and increasing altitudes. Slopes are the ventilatory equivalents. Modified from Pugh et al. (1964) with permission.

The ventilatory responses of acclimatised lowlanders to increased oxygen uptake are shown in Figure 24.2 (ventilatory equivalent). For a given submaximal oxygen uptake, minute ventilation is higher as barometric pressure decreases, as shown by the increased slope of the ventilation-oxygen uptake relationship (ventilatory equivalent). These greater ventilatory responses enhance arterial oxygen saturation, but also induce more pronounced respiratory alkalosis (true hyperventilation). On the other hand, greater ventilation during exercise requires a greater work of breathing, despite reduced air density. Thus, there may be a trade-off between increased arterial blood oxygenation and greater cost of breathing.

2.4 Alveolar–arterial oxygen partial pressure gradient and pulmonary diffusing capacity

Among the various reductions in oxygen partial pressure along the oxygen cascade between inspired air and the mitochondria (Chapters 2 and 10.1), that which occurs between alveolar air and arterial blood, the alveolar–arterial oxygen partial pressure gradient, is considered of great importance in the process of altitude acclimatisation. At sea level, this gradient may be attributable to incomplete oxygen diffusion, an uneven distribution of the ventilation–perfusion ratio and true venous–arterial shunting. Thus, the alveolar–arterial oxygen gradient is ~1.45 kPa (11 mmHg) when resting at sea level, and increases progressively during incremental exercise to ~3.25 kPa (25 mmHg) at exhaustion.

An adaptive reduction of the alveolar-arterial oxygen gradient during acclimatisation represents an effective defence against hypoxia. At 4000 m, the alveolar–arterial oxygen gradient, at rest, is almost identical in lowlanders acutely exposed or acclimatised to hypoxia (0.65–1.04 kPa, 5–8 mmHg). However, at all workloads during exercise in acute hypoxia, this gradient is greater than observed during normoxic exercise, showing a tendency to diminish with acclimatisation. This finding is likely to result from a more

complete alveolar to end-capillary diffusion equilibration (section 3.3). In fact, after 2 weeks at 3800 m, arterial oxygen partial pressure increases during maximal exercise by ~0.65 kPa (5 mmHg). On the other hand, after 8 weeks at 4100 m, Lundby et al. (2004) found similar increases in both maximum exercise alveolar and arterial oxygen tensions in acclimatised lowlanders, and, consequently, the maximal alveolar–arterial oxygen gradient remained unchanged (Chapter 25).

3 EFFECTS OF ALTITUDE ON BLOOD COMPOSITION, ARTERIAL BLOOD GASES, BLOOD–OXYGEN EQUILIBRIUM, BLOOD PH AND FLUID BALANCE

3.1 Regulation of erythropoiesis

Erythropoiesis is generally modulated by oxygen availability, through the stabilisation of HIF-1α which, along with HIF-1β, binds to the hypoxia-response element of the erythropoietin gene and induces production of erythropoietin. In subjects acclimatised to altitude, red blood cell mass increases linearly with decreasing arterial oxygen tension below a threshold of ~8.70 kPa (67 mmHg), or when arterial oxygen saturation is below ~95%. From 2000 to 2600 m, a moderate increase of red cells mass, haemoglobin concentration and haematocrit may be observed following prolonged exposure to hypoxia. However, no effects on red blood cell mass can be observed below 1800 m.

For a single normobaric hypoxic stimulus equivalent to an altitude of 4000 m, the shortest exposure time necessary to elicit a significant increase in erythropoietin production varies from 80 to 120 min. In such conditions, plasma erythropoietin concentration peaks (50% elevation) 4–5 h after the onset of hypoxia. Generally, the altitude-induced increase in erythropoietin production is dose dependent, with 2100–2500 m being the threshold for stimulating sustained erythropoietin release in most subjects (Ge et al. 2002).

Nevertheless, there is marked inter- and intraindividual variability in the erythropoietic response, with some subjects developing stronger responses (high responders). At the molecular level, the kinetics of HIF-1α expression varies among organs. In the kidney and the liver, HIF-1α reaches a peak after about 60 min, and then returns to baseline after ~4 h of continuous hypoxia. In the brain, both expression and subsequent downregulation are delayed 5 and 12 h, respectively. The molecular mechanisms responsible for the decrease of HIF-1α to baseline after a short hypoxic exposure and reduced erythropoietin production after a few days of continuous exposure to hypoxia are still unknown (Schmidt 2002).

3.2 Acid–base balance

As is well known, the hyperventilatory response to hypoxia lowers arterial carbon dioxide partial pressure and elevates blood and tissue pH. This respiratory alkalosis depends also on the capacity of the kidney to excrete enough bicarbonate to provide a full metabolic compensation. As altitude increases, however, such metabolic compensation is progressively less effective and, consequently, respiratory alkalosis is only partially compensated. Whereas the bicarbonate component of blood buffer capacity is reduced, the non-bicarbonate components, mainly haemoglobin and 2,3-diphosphoglyceric acid, are increased (Cerretelli & Samaja 2003). In lowlanders acclimatised to 6450 m, arterial pH may be as high as 7.5. More alkaline values have been measured in individuals who are not fully acclimatised and display abnormal hyperventilation, as may occur on the summit of Mt Everest or in people with acute mountain sickness.

Ventilatory and acid–base balance adjustments are primarily involved in maintaining the homeostasis of oxygen delivery. It has been shown that under conditions of extreme hypoxia, oxygen delivery can be enhanced at the expense of uncompensated respiratory alkalosis. The latter increases the haemoglobin–oxygen affinity and helps to maintain the arterovenous oxygen difference, despite low arterial oxygen tension.

3.3 Oxygen dissociation curve and blood composition

The oxygen dissociation (blood–oxygen equilibrium) curve and the oxygen partial pressure at which 50% saturation occurs (P_{50}) are useful indices of the blood–oxygen affinity. Besides pH and arterial carbon dioxide tension, factors such as temperature, carbon monoxide-bound haemoglobin concentration and the red blood cell concentration of 2,3-diphosphoglyceric acid influence these indices.

Alkalosis increases blood–oxygen affinity and to assess the contribution of alkalosis to the blood oxygen-carrying properties, Samaja et al. (1997) calculated the theoretical arterial oxygen saturation gain at altitude due to blood alkalinisation. It appears that the saturation gain for a given elevation in pH becomes progressively greater as altitude increases. On this basis, respiratory alkalosis is beneficial for oxygen loading in the pulmonary capillary. However, prolonged alkalosis is incompatible with normal body functions, particularly those of the central nervous system, eventually inducing coma. Indeed, one of the effects of acclimatisation is to reduce alkalosis. Therefore, an equilibrium must be attained between the conflicting needs of achieving an adequate oxygen delivery and avoiding perturbations in pH homeostasis. In acclimatised lowlanders, this equilibrium requires high red cell concentrations of 2,3-diphosphoglyceric acid, which decreases the blood–oxygen affinity and counterbalances the effects of alkalosis on the oxygen dissociation curve.

It is of note that this concentration in blood depends, in part, on the age of the red blood cells. Due to the augmented production of erythropoietin, after a 2-week sojourn at 4500 m, red blood cells concentration of Caucasians increases from about 5 to 6.5 million·μL^{-1} of blood. Enhanced erythropoiesis gives rise to a greater fraction of young red cells, in which the intracellular content of 2,3-diphosphoglyceric acid (per unit haemoglobin concentration) is higher than in aged red cells. As a consequence, the oxygen dissociation curve is shifted more rightward for younger red cells. A very similar result on the oxygen dissociation curve is attained by altitude Sherpa natives during acclimatisation from 3000 to 6450 m, but in a different way. At 6450 m, Sherpas hyperventilate less than acclimatised lowlanders and, consequently, their arterial carbon dioxide partial pressure is higher (2.99 and 2.49 kPa, respectively) and pH lower (7.454 and 7.496, respectively) than observed in Caucasians (Samaja et al. 1997). In addition, the blood concentration of 2,3-diphosphoglyceric acid is lower in Sherpas than in Caucasians.

3.4 Pulmonary capillary transit time

According to Fick's Law of Diffusion (Chapters 1 and 10.1), the uptake of oxygen by red blood cells in the lung is determined by the alveolar to mixed venous oxygen partial pressure gradient, and by the thickness and surface area of the membranes separating these compartments.

During rest at sea level, the time spent by red blood cells within the pulmonary capillary (transit time, estimated by the ratio of the pulmonary capillary blood volume to the cardiac output) is ~0.7 s, and is slow enough to allow complete equilibration between alveolar oxygen and capillary blood. This typically occurs within ~0.25 s. However, at high altitude, alveolar oxygen tension is much lower and arterial saturation is kept relatively high by alkalosis. As a result, the oxygen diffusion gradient becomes narrower and the equilibration time increases. Since exercise elevates cardiac output more than pulmonary blood volume, then blood moves more rapidly through the pulmonary capillaries (transit time is reduced). Neither altitude nor exercise is a problem, unless the transit time becomes shorter than the equilibration time.

It has been calculated that, when alveolar oxygen tension is ~6.5 kPa (50 mmHg) transit time is inadequate for complete oxygen loading. On the summit of Mt Everest, the resting partial pressure of oxygen in the pulmonary capillary blood rises slowly from an estimated mixed venous level of 2.73 kPa (21 mmHg), but does not attain equilibrium with alveolar gas, which is ~4.03 kPa (31 mmHg). The situation rapidly worsens when the climber attempts to increase oxygen uptake to 500 mL·min^{-1}. In such conditions, alveolar oxygen tension rises to 4.29 kPa (33 mmHg) whereas the mixed venous blood oxygen tension is only 1.82 kPa (14 mmHg). Due to the increased cardiac output, capillary transit time decreases, resulting in the end-capillary oxygen partial pressure attaining only 2.86 kPa (22 mmHg; West & Wagner 1980).

3.5 Fluid balance in acute hypoxia

Recently, Loeppky et al. (2005) investigated the separate and combined effects of reduced barometric pressure and hypoxia on body fluid balance, and the hormones involved in its regulation, in individuals resident at 1620 m and exposed for 10 h to hypobaric hypoxia (simulating 4800 m), normobaric hypoxia and normoxic hypobaria. Compared to normobaric hypoxia, hypobaric hypoxia favoured a greater fluid retention, as shown by reduced urine volume, while plasma volume was higher. This was mainly due to increased secretion of antidiuretic hormone. When hypoxia was relieved by breathing an oxygen-enriched mixture (normoxic hypobaria), there was an increase in blood aldosterone concentration and plasma renin activity, accompanied by a small reduction in plasma volume. The latter was even greater in normobaric hypoxia. Indeed, numerous studies have shown that normobaric hypoxia results in a diuresis within minutes to hours by way of an inhibition of antidiuretic hormone, a finding that is still under close examination.

4 CARDIAC FUNCTION AND CIRCULATION IN ACUTE AND CHRONIC HYPOXIA

4.1 Rest and acute hypoxia

Acute exposures up to 3500 m do not affect resting heart rate. By contrast, at higher altitudes, with arterial oxygen tensions of 5.85–4.55 kPa (45–35 mmHg), both heart rate and cardiac output increase. The rise of the former has been attributed to changes in the control of sinoatrial node activity by the autonomic nervous system, with increased sympathetic and reduced vagal activity. Mean arterial blood pressure is unchanged during acute hypoxia, whereas mean pulmonary arterial pressure after breathing 10% oxygen for 10 min increases almost twofold.

Unlike skeletal muscle blood vessels, those of the pulmonary vasculature constrict with local hypoxia. This is a short-term adaptive vasomotor response aimed at redistributing blood to highly ventilated alveoli. For instance, in healthy subjects, acute inhalation of 12.5% oxygen reduces arterial oxygen tension to <6.50 kPa (50 mmHg), increasing pulmonary vascular resistance by 100–150%.

Many factors, such as alveolar carbon dioxide tension, mixed venous oxygen tension, cardiac output, the hypoxic stimulus duration and genetic characteristics, affect vasoconstriction (Dorrington & Talbot 2004). However, the functional role of this hypoxic vasoconstriction response in humans remains uncertain. Recently, it has been demonstrated that hypoxic pulmonary vasoconstriction is unevenly distributed within the lung. This finding gives substantial support to the concept of regional pulmonary overperfusion, leading to locally increased capillary pressure that may exceed the capillary dilatation capacity on the venous side. In these circumstances, the Starling forces are disturbed, favouring fluid leakage into the interstitium and the possible development of high-altitude pulmonary oedema.

Such an oedema is therefore a non-cardiogenic pulmonary oedema, with a typical patchy distribution in the lungs. It usually occurs at altitudes >3000 m, and in rapidly ascending non-acclimatised individuals within the first 2–5 days after arrival at altitude. It may also occur in high-altitude Andean dwellers who return from sojourns at low altitudes (Bärtsch et al. 2005).

4.2 Rest and chronic hypoxia

In the course of acclimatisation, the resting heart rate tends to resume sea-level values, despite sympathetic and parasympathetic activity remaining unchanged, compared to acute hypoxia up to at least 5000 m. Therefore, the lower resting heart rate in acclimatised lowlanders may be due to a progressive reduction in adrenergic sensitivity of the heart. Compared to sea level, resting cardiac output increases slightly (+20%) after 2 weeks at 4300 m, thereafter resuming normal values. Cardiac output does not change with duration of exposure, or increases in altitude, at least up to 5350 m.

Arterial blood pressure is usually well regulated within normal limits, at least up to 6000 m. By contrast, and despite acclimatisation, pulmonary arterial pressure remains elevated, with no apparent improvement of the ventilation–perfusion matching. Pulmonary hypertension increases the load on the right ventricle, thereby reducing the cardiac functional reserve. In chronic hypoxia, pulmonary hypertension may be sustained by a remodelling of the pulmonary vascular wall. This is characterised by hypertrophy and hyperplasia, or by a reduction in the rate of apoptosis of smooth muscle cells in the tunica media of the pulmonary artery (Remillard & Yuan 2005). Interestingly, chronic hypoxia results also in increased total pulmonary vessel length, volume, endothelial surface area and number of endothelial cells (Howell et al. 2003). The hypoxia-induced angiogenesis recently found in the lungs of animals may have important beneficial consequences for gas exchange. Should it occur also in humans, it might be responsible for the higher arterial oxygen saturation found in acclimatised lowlanders after years of altitude exposure, and in Tibetan altitude natives (Chapter 25).

4.3 Exercise during acute and chronic hypoxia

In acute hypoxia, at any submaximal exercise intensity, heart rate and cardiac output are elevated, compared to normoxia, as a consequence of a greater sympathetic stimulation. At 4000 m, both heart rate and cardiac output are about 15% higher than at sea level for the same absolute work rate, whereas at exhaustion, maximal values are unaltered. After a few weeks of exposure to high altitude, the heart rate response to submaximal exercise is still slightly elevated, whereas cardiac output resumes normoxic values. At peak exercise, however, the maximal cardiac output is significantly reduced, with the drop varying from 20% (after 2 weeks at 4300 m) to 30% (after 8–12 weeks at 5800 m).

In any case, due to the increase in haemoglobin concentration, maximal oxygen delivery to the tissues is unaffected by chronic hypoxia. Interestingly, both submaximal and maximal cardiac outputs are related to oxygen uptake exactly as they are at sea level.

Wagner (2000) has suggested that neither an increased blood viscosity nor a reduced blood volume, due to dehydration, with a consequent decrease in right ventricular filling pressure, play a significant role in reducing maximal cardiac output. However, it is worth noting that after a 9-week acclimatisation to 5260 m, when haemoglobin concentration was lowered to its sea-level value by haemodilution, both maximal leg blood flow and the vascular conductance of lowlanders were increased (Calbet et al. 2002). Furthermore, it has been shown that, at 5050 m, acclimatised Tibetan lowlanders have lower haemoglobin concentration and higher peak heart rates, when compared to acclimatised Caucasians (Marconi et al. 2004). Moreover, in the latter there is no evidence that the myocardium self-limits its own pumping (Chapter 10.2) by reducing contractility to avoid ischaemia. As is well known, maximal heart rate drops progressively as altitude increases, possibly as a consequence of a slight reduction in the cardiac β-receptors sensitivity, and of hypoxia per se. However, a compensatory partial increase in stroke volume also occurs (Calbet et al. 2003). In conclusion, so far, there is no clear explanation for the altitude-related reduction in maximal cardiac output, and the hypothesis that it may be dictated by the maximal oxygen uptake of skeletal muscles appears attractive, although difficult to test.

The increase in mean arterial blood pressure in the course of heavy exercise is the same in acclimatised lowlanders as in sea-level dwellers. The mean pulmonary arterial pressure during exhausting exercise is 30% higher at 2400 m than at sea level (3.64 versus 2.73 kPa, respectively).

5 EFFECTS OF ACUTE AND CHRONIC HYPOXIA ON AEROBIC METABOLISM

5.1 Maximal mechanical power output

In 1929, Margaria was the first to demonstrate a progressive reduction of maximum mechanical power output during cycle ergometer exercise in a hypobaric chamber with air pressure decreasing to 39 kPa (300 mmHg). At 52 kPa, corresponding to 5400 m, maximum mechanical power was 62% of that measured at sea level. Interestingly, the curve describing the drop of maximal power output with increasing altitude can be almost superimposed on that obtained later describing the relationship between maximal oxygen uptake (aerobic power) reduction and altitude in acute and chronic hypoxia (section 5.3).

5.2 Maximal aerobic power in acute hypoxia

Changes in maximal aerobic power during acute hypoxia have been investigated in hypobaric chambers and whilst breathing hypoxic gas mixtures at sea level (normobaric hypoxia). In general, these experiments yield data identical with those obtained shortly after reaching equivalent altitudes in the mountains (Cerretelli & Hoppeler 1996), and universally demonstrate a progressive reduction in the maximal aerobic power of lowlanders with declines in air pressure and inspired oxygen partial pressure.

It is worth noting that, up to 1500 m, untrained sea-level dwellers undergo little or no apparent decrement in maximal aerobic power. By contrast, well-trained athletes experience a 6–7% reduction in their sea-level maximal aerobic power when acutely exposed to a simulated altitude of 580 m (Gore et al. 1996). However, interindividual variability in the magnitude of these changes upon acute or subacute exposure to hypoxia is considerable. For example, Young et al. (1985) determined maximal aerobic power in 51 soldiers at 50 m, and after 1–8 days at 4300 m, observing an altitude-related reduction of 27%, but with individual changes ranging from 9% to 54%, with the more aerobically fit subjects suffering larger decrements.

5.3 Maximal aerobic power in acclimatised lowlanders

The relationship between maximal oxygen uptake and altitude for acclimatised lowlanders is shown in Figure 24.3. It is evident that, at any given altitude, whilst maximal aerobic power is reduced, the relative reduction varies widely among individuals. Such variability appears to be mainly related to the extent of acclimatisation and endurance fitness.

A prolonged (8–12 weeks) sojourn at ≥5000 m affects maximal aerobic power both positively, by increasing blood oxygen carrying capacity, and negatively, as a consequence of a progressive reduction in muscle mass and, possibly, muscle deterioration (Cerretelli & Hoppeler 1996). As a result, in the above conditions, acclimatised lowlanders can recover only a minor fraction of their initial maximal oxygen uptake. Thus, the decrease accompanying chronic

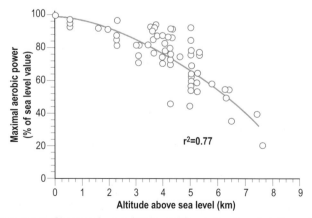

Figure 24.3 Changes in maximal aerobic power as a function of altitude.

exposure is essentially the same as that occurring with acute hypoxia.

However, if the duration of the sojourn is long enough (years) and altitude does not exceed 3500–4000 m, adaptations may occur, allowing improved gas exchange at the lung, as shown by increased arterial oxygen saturation at the end of exhaustive exercise, and almost complete recovery of sea-level maximal heart rates. Consequently, maximal aerobic power may progressively increase, attaining levels only slightly lower than those found at sea level in age-, gender- and fitness-matched individuals. This topic will be addressed in more detail in Chapter 25.

As noted above, preexposure endurance fitness may affect the reduction in maximal oxygen uptake at altitude. A recent project compared four groups of subjects with different sea-level maximal oxygen uptakes, using untrained and trained Caucasians and Tibetans (39 versus 61 mL·kg^{-1}·min^{-1} and 38 versus 49 mL·kg^{-1}·min^{-1}, respectively). All subjects spent 30 days at 5050 m (Ev-K2-CNR Laboratory, Nepal). At the end of the sojourn, all subjects experienced a reduced maximal aerobic power, but these changes were most apparent within the trained subjects (Caucasians: −45% versus −30%; Tibetans: −15% and −8%; Marconi et al. 2004). Thus trained individuals, who are low responders to increments in training stimuli (Chapter 21), appear to be high responders to chronic hypoxia and detraining (Chapter 9). The decrement within the trained individuals was independent of their ethnic background and might be due to greater maximal cardiac output of those subjects, which increases the velocity of pulmonary blood flow. The consequent reduction in red blood cell transit time in the alveolar capillaries may further impair alveolar-blood oxygen equilibration. In fact, the loss of maximal aerobic power appears to be inversely related to arterial oxygen saturation at exhaustion.

This observation may explain, in part, the discrepancy evident within elite Caucasian mountaineers between their climbing performance and sea-level maximal oxygen uptake. Indeed, one of the greatest climbers of the last century, and the first to reach the summit of Mt Everest without supplementary oxygen (Reinhold Messner), was characterised by a sea-level maximal aerobic power of only 49 mL·kg^{-1}·min^{-1}. Indeed, this index has long been known to have relatively poor predictive qualities in elite performers (Chapter 10.2).

5.4 Factors limiting maximal aerobic power in acclimatised lowlanders

The cardiovascular and pulmonary factors limiting maximal aerobic performance at sea level are discussed in detail in Chapters 1, 2, 10.1 and 10.2. At sea level, the maximal convective transport of oxygen to the active tissues is the major determinant of maximal oxygen uptake (di Prampero & Ferretti 1990). However, at altitude, reduced diffusive conductance in the lungs and muscles, along with the efficiency

of oxygen utilisation by the mitochondria, are more important limiting factors.

5.5 Energy cost of locomotion

It was widely recognised that, compared to sea level, chronic hypoxia exposures do not significantly alter the energy cost of physical activity (cycling and stepping), at least when lowlanders are acclimatised up to 5400 m. The energy cost of locomotion in high-altitude natives will be addressed in Chapter 25.

5.6 Energy substrates

Mosso (1897) was the first to realise that, at altitude, the intake of carbohydrates needs to be increased to delay the onset of fatigue. Almost one century later, the question whether the type of substrate utilisation is affected by acute or chronic hypoxia is still open. In fact, Brooks et al. (1991) have shown that, compared to sea level (Chapter 7), exposure to 4300 m increases the use of blood glucose during submaximal exercise. Acclimatisation resulted in greater glucose utilisation also at rest. An increased reliance on glucose metabolism at altitude may be advantageous, because glucose is a more efficient fuel than lipids, and at a given altitude, a shift of the respiratory gas exchange ratio from 0.8 towards 1.0 also increases alveolar oxygen tension.

However, this conclusion concerning substrate use has been challenged by Lundby & Van Hall (2002) who found that, in Caucasians acclimatised to 4100 m, substrate utilisation was unaffected by either acute or chronic hypoxia, when the work rate was matched to the same relative intensity as at sea level. Thus, the principle that relative exercise intensity determines the mixture of fuels oxidised seems to hold true also at altitude. However, in animal models, acclimatisation to hypoxia strongly stimulates lipolysis (McClelland et al. 2001) and there are also hints that native Tibetans have a very active lipid metabolism (Chapter 25). Thus, the role of relative substrate utilisation during exercise at altitude remains unresolved.

6 EFFECTS OF ACUTE AND CHRONIC HYPOXIA ON ANAEROBIC METABOLISM

6.1 Peak power

Chronic hypoxia does not affect the capacity of a given muscle mass to generate short-duration (<10 s) peak force and power. This conclusion is based on the findings that the maximal voluntary contraction (isometric elbow flexion), vertical jump height and the average mechanical power output during a 10-s, all-out cycle sprint are not affected by a 4-week exposure to 5050 m (Grassi et al. 2001). Moreover, compared to sea-level measurements, no differences were found in lowlanders acclimatised to 5050 m regarding α-motoneuron excitability, nerve and muscle fibre conduction velocity, synaptic and muscle end-plate signal transmission, and excitation–contraction coupling of the adductor pollicis and of the quadriceps muscles (Kayser et al. 1993).

From the energetic standpoint, it is well known that ATP and phosphocreatine concentrations in resting muscle are not affected by acute hypoxia, and likely by chronic hypoxia, although this is not yet proven.

6.2 Anaerobic power: revisiting the lactate paradox

During acute hypoxia, blood and muscle lactate concentrations, for any given submaximal exercise level, are greater than during normoxia, but peak lactate values are unchanged. After a prolonged stay at altitude (>3 weeks), resting blood lactate is essentially unchanged. However, during incremental exercise, blood lactate increases at the same fraction of maximal oxygen consumption to a lesser extent and attains lower peak levels at voluntary exhaustion. The latter finding was first described by Dill et al. (1931) and Edwards (1936), and was later confirmed and extended to altitudes up to 7600 m (Marconi et al. 1998), as it appears in Figure 24.4 (Cerretelli & Samaja 2003). This apparently reduced reliance on glycolysis during chronic hypoxia appeared paradoxical (West 1986), particularly in view of the progressive reduction in maximal aerobic power. Indeed, one might predict a greater activation of glycolysis, hence the origin of the term: lactate paradox (Hochachka 1988). It is notable that the lactate paradox is only scarcely affected by inducing acute normoxia. This was shown by Edwards (1936) in an acclimatised Caucasian subject, and later confirmed by Cerretelli et al. (1982) in groups of Caucasians and altitude Sherpas sojourning for 6–8 weeks at Mt Everest base camp (or above), and by other investigators, both in acclimatised Caucasians and Bolivian Mestizos (high-altitude natives) at ~4000 m.

The origin of the lactate paradox was and still is rather controversial (Cerretelli & Samaja 2003). Several hypotheses

have been put forward to explain why it occurs: (1) a down-regulation, during chronic hypoxia, of the enzymes controlling glycolysis; (2) a lower concentration of muscle glycogen at altitude; (3) a progressive preferential recruitment of slow-twitch muscle fibres during acclimatisation; (4) a downregulation of β-adrenergic receptors followed by a reduction of the maximum glycolytic flux; (5) a lowering of tissue bicarbonate and non-bicarbonate buffers; and (6) a decrease in maximum mechanical power generation due to impaired motor control by the central nervous system. However, none of these hypotheses has (individually) gained sufficient experimental support.

An interesting feature of the lactate paradox was the observation of its slow reversal upon restoring normoxia (Grassi et al. 1996). These authors concluded that it takes >5 weeks to deacclimatise Caucasians to the extent that they can achieve their preexposure peak blood lactate concentrations (Figure 24.5). This is also apparently the case for a group of Quechuas (high-altitude natives), transferred from altitude to sea level (Hochachka et al. 1991), in whom the lactate paradox persisted for at least 6 weeks, leading the authors to hypothesise that the lactate paradox is a permanent characteristic of high-altitude natives.

In this context, research by Danish investigators is of particular interest. Lundby et al. (2000) confirmed the occurrence of the lactate paradox in Caucasians after 2–4 weeks exposure to 5400 m, but showed a reversal of the phenomenon after 6 weeks. On the other hand, Van Hall et al. (2001) showed a restoration of preexposure peak blood lactate concentration after 9 weeks of acclimatisation at 5200 m breathing air or oxygen-enriched gas mixtures. Moreover, two recent unpublished observations by the same Danish group would indicate that, in healthy, well-motivated and acclimatised lowlanders, the lactate paradox does not exist. First, they have found equivalent peak muscle (vastus lateralis) lactate concentrations at exhaustion in lowlanders at

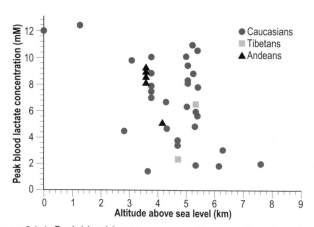

Figure 24.4 Peak blood lactate concentration as a function of altitude in acclimatised subjects from different ethnic groups. Modified from Cerretelli & Samaja (2003) with permission.

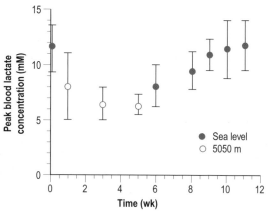

Figure 24.5 Peak blood lactate concentrations of lowlanders, obtained during the first minute of recovery after exhaustive incremental exercises (15–30 min) at sea level, and at different times during a sojourn at 5050 m. Modified from Grassi et al. (1996) with permission.

sea level, during acute hypoxia and after 2–8 weeks exposure to 4100 m. Second, they have observed substantially greater muscle lactate concentrations at exhaustion in high-altitude natives (Bolivians) compared to acclimatised Caucasians.

Furthermore, unpublished measurements by Marconi's group also induce one to reconsider the occurrence and characteristics of the lactate paradox. They have shown that, in Tibetan migrants, after a 1–4 week sojourn at 1300 m, peak blood lactate concentrations were identical with those of age- and exercise-matched Tibetan lowlanders (~12 mM). In addition, they found peak blood lactate concentrations >12 mM in a group of very well-trained and highly motivated high-altitude natives (Lhasa; 3600 m), who were further acclimatised at Shegar (Tibet; 4300 m).

It is apparent that the lactate paradox is a rather elusive and a quantitatively variable phenomenon, the origin of which is multifactorial. Besides the partial role played by one or more of the metabolic mechanisms described above, two other variables seem to be involved. First, there is a subjective factor that relates to the motivation and mental capacity of subjects to carry out heavy and unpleasant physical efforts that result in maximal activation of glycolytic pathways, and thereby prevent the lactate paradox from occurring.

The second factor is related to possible hypoxia-dependent functional changes in lactate, hydrogen ion and electrolyte transporters in the cell membranes. However, acclimatisation to high altitude seems to induce only moderate changes in transporters within the sarcolemma, whereas it has relatively large effects upon the erythrocyte membrane transporters. Indeed, after 8 weeks at 4100 m, the erythrocyte lactate–hydrogen ion co-transporter (MCT1) and the erythrocyte chloride-bicarbonate exchanger were found to be increased three- to fivefold, compared to preexposure conditions (Juel et al. 2003). The increase in MCT1 is expected to enhance the lactate–hydrogen ion transport capacity across the erythrocyte membrane and, during exercise, to reduce the corresponding plasma lactate concentration. It would appear that the size of the lactate paradox, as well as its temporal, training- and ethnic-dependent variability, may underlie a complex gene-based reorganisation of cell metabolism during hypoxia that is likely to be under the control of the hypoxia-inducible factor (HIF-1), and may involve the activity of lactate–hydrogen ion co-transporters.

In conclusion, the reduction in peak blood lactate concentration, which appears to occur in many subjects after prolonged exposure to hypoxia, may not be an indicator of a blunted energy contribution by glycolysis, but rather the consequence of a changed translocation rate of lactate between muscle and blood, and within the blood. In addition, it can also result from an increased rate of lactate use by the muscle and other tissues (turnover; Chapters 6 and 10.3). Thus, from the energetic standpoint, it would be inappropriate to define the phenomenon as a lactate paradox. On the other hand, the changes in blood lactate concentra-

tion found in various experimental conditions may have a different significance, being also a possible marker of the function of the lactate–hydrogen ion transport system, which may impose a different kinetics for lactic acid or lactate washout.

7 MUSCLE ADAPTATION TO HYPOXIA IN ACCLIMATISED LOWLANDERS

7.1 Morphological and biochemical adaptations

Muscle tissue adaptations in lowlanders acclimatised to hypoxia have been described extensively (Hoppeler & Vogt 2001). Briefly, muscle atrophy is a common feature during traditional mountaineering expeditions to the Himalayas. For example, the reduced muscle mass after an extended exposure to altitudes >5000 m is associated with a 20–25% reduction of the cross-sectional area of muscle fibres which is independent of fibre type. This change resembles the sarcopenia seen during ageing (Chapter 16) and depends, at least in part, on an imbalance between energy expenditure and caloric intake, with protein absorption being in the normal range. When optimal nutritional conditions are provided, changes in muscle mass and cross-sectional area are minimised.

There is no evidence for fibre type transformation in response to hypoxia. The distribution of type II fibres in the vastus lateralis muscle appears to be unaffected by altitude or ethnic grouping, being 19% in Bolivian residents of 3600 m, 15.9% in Tibetans and 17.4% in Nepalese born at 1300 m. These distributions are not notably different from values found at sea-level in individuals with similar levels of habitual physical activity. This finding has recently been confirmed by determining the distribution of myosin heavy chain isoforms in lowlanders acclimatised to 4100 m and in native Bolivians (Juel et al. 2003).

As a consequence of fibre size reduction, capillary density in the vastus lateralis of acclimatised lowlanders is increased ~10%. However, the capillary-to-fibre ratio remains unchanged, arguing against increased capillarisation, as confirmed by the finding that the expression of the vascular endothelial growth factor is not enhanced after 8 weeks at 4100 m (Lundby et al. 2004). It is notable that muscle fibre atrophy may improve oxygen diffusion, because the same capillary bed now supplies a smaller muscle volume and the diffusion distance is reduced.

Oxidative enzymes are affected by chronic hypoxia. For example, following a Himalayan expedition (Howald et al. 1990), or an expedition to Mt Everest simulated in a hypobaric chamber (Operation Everest II; Green et al. 1989), the activity of some key enzymes of the citric acid (Krebs) cycle (citrate synthase, succinate dehydrogenase, hexokinase and cytochrome oxidase) was reduced by >20%, as was muscle mitochondrial volume density. It is worth noting that subjects with the highest pre-expedition mitochondrial volume density suffered the greatest reduction in muscle oxidative capacity. This decrease is likely to be the result of an adaptation to hypoxia, since it has also been found in high-altitude natives (Tibetans and Bolivians). However, it is worth noting that despite reduced mitochondrial volume density, Tibetans are characterised by a maximal oxygen uptake to mitochondrial volume ratio higher than that of acclimatised lowlanders (Kayser et al. 1991). This finding suggests that oxidative metabolism is more efficient in Tibetans than acclimatised lowlanders (Marconi et al. 2006).

7.2 Molecular adaptation in acclimatised lowlanders

Lowlanders sojourning at high altitude are paradoxically at an increased risk of reactive oxygen species generation, which may lead to the formation of altered molecules, including DNA, proteins and lipids (Lundby et al. 2003), and to the accumulation of degradation products such as lipofuscin (Martinelli et al. 1990). Interestingly, an accumulation of lipofuscin (age pigment) is also found in ageing tissues and in patients with chronic obstructive pulmonary disease. Hypoxia, and the accumulation of reactive oxygen species, may also play a role in reducing protein synthesis and in downregulating many ATP-dependent processes, like ion pumps. Indeed, decreased sodium-potassium-ATPase activity has often, but not always, been described in lowlanders exposed to hypoxia (Marconi et al. 2006). It is likely that the duration, magnitude and characteristics of the hypoxic exposure, as well as the level of fitness of the subject, may differentially modulate sodium-potassium-

ATPase activity at altitude. However, it is notable that downregulation of the ion pumps may be a short-term adaptive mechanism, allowing cells to save energy, but in the long term, it may be accompanied by further production of reactive oxygen species and the accumulation of mitochondrial nitric oxide.

8 CONCLUSION

Exercise performance of lowlanders exposed to acute and chronic hypoxia is the result of the interaction of multiple factors, affecting oxygen delivery and metabolism, and also through molecular adaptations elicited by hypoxia-inducible factor. The latter may depend on the duration of exposure to hypoxia, training conditions and ethnic characteristics of the subjects. As will be shown in Chapter 25, in the study of acclimatisation to hypoxia, the most appropriate end-point for a comparison is represented by the condition of high-altitude natives (e.g. Tibetans) who have attained an optimal adaptation, and, until recently, have not been in contact with migrating lowlanders.

Altitude investigations, besides their intrinsic interest, are of growing importance for the study of training for performance at sea level and of ageing in healthy subjects. In addition, hypobaric hypoxia may be a useful model for the study of the consequence of normobaric hypoxia (e.g. anaemic, hypoxic, ischaemic) in different pathological conditions, such as chronic obstructive pulmonary disease, chronic heart failure, peripheral obstructive arterial disease, the metabolic syndrome and diabetes.

References

Antunes F, Boveris A, Cadenas E 2004 On the mechanism and biology of cytochrome oxidase inhibition by nitric oxide. Proceedings of the National Academy of Sciences 101: 16774–16779

Askew EW 2002 Work at high altitude and oxidative stress: antioxidant nutrients. Toxicology 180:107–119

Bärtsch P, Mairbäurl H, Maggiorini M, Swenson ER 2005 Physiological aspects of high-altitude pulmonary edema. Journal of Applied Physiology 98:1101–1110

Brooks GA, Butterfield GE, Wolfe RR, Groves BM, Mazzeo RS, Sutton JR, Wolfel EE, Reeves JT 1991 Increased dependence on blood glucose after acclimatization to 4,300 m. Journal of Applied Physiology 70:919–927

Brunelle JK, Bell EL, Quesada NM, Vercauteren K, Tiranti V, Zeviani M, Scarpulla RC, Chandel NS 2005 Oxygen sensing requires mitochondrial ROS but not oxidative phosphorylation. Cell Metabolism 1:409–414

Calbet JAL, Rådegran G, Boushel R, Søndergaard H, Saltin B, Wagner PD 2002 Effect of blood haemoglobin concentration on O₂max and cardiovascular function in lowlanders acclimatised to 5260 m. Journal of Physiology 545:715–728

Calbet JAL, Boushel R, Rådegran G, Søndergaard H, Wagner PD, Saltin B 2003 Why is V$_{O_{2max}}$ after altitude acclimatization reduced despite normalization of arterial O₂ content? American Journal of Physiology. Regulatory, Integrative and Comparative Physiology 284:R304–R316

Cerretelli P 1980 Gas exchange at high altitude. In: West JB (ed) Pulmonary gas exchange. Academic Press, New York, 97–147

Cerretelli P, Hoppeler H 1996 Morphologic and metabolic response to chronic hypoxia: the muscle system. In: Fregly MJ, Blatteis CM (eds) Handbook of physiology. Environmental physiology, vol. 4. Oxford University Press, New York, 1155–1181

Cerretelli P, Samaja M 2003 Acid-base balance at exercise in normoxia and in chronic hypoxia. Revisiting the 'lactate paradox.' European Journal of Applied Physiology 90:431–448

Cerretelli P, Veicsteinas A, Marconi C 1982 Anaerobic metabolism at high altitude: the lactacid mechanism. In: Brendel W, Zink RA (eds) High altitude physiology and medicine. Vol I. Physiology of adaptation. Springer Verlag, New York, 94–102

Cibella F, Cuttitta G, Kayser B, Narici M, Romano S, Saibene F 1996 Respiratory mechanics during exhaustive submaximal exercise at high altitude in healthy humans. Journal of Physiology 494:881–890

Cogo A, Legnani D, Allegra L 1997 Respiratory function at different altitudes. Respiration 64:416–421

Cremona G, Asnaghi R, Baderna P, Brunetto A, Brutsaert T, Cavallaro C, Clark TM, Cogo A, Donis R, Lanfranchi P, Luks A, Novello N, Panzetta S, Perini L, Putnam M, Spagnolatti L, Wagner H, Wagner PD 2002 Pulmonary extravascular fluid accumulation in recreational climbers: a prospective study. Lancet 359:303–309

Cruz JC 1973 Mechanics of breathing in high altitude and sea level subjects. Respiration Physiology 17:146–161

Dill DB, Edwards HT, Folling A, Oberg SA, Pappenheimer AM Jr, Talbott JH 1931 Adaptations of the organism to changes in oxygen pressure. Journal of Physiology (London) 71:47–63

di Prampero PE, Ferretti G 1990 Factors limiting maximal oxygen consumption in humans. Respiration Physiology 80:113–127

Dorrington KL, Talbot NP 2004 Human pulmonary vascular response to hypoxia and hypercapnia. Plügers Archives, European Journal of Physiology 449:1–15

Edwards HT 1936 Lactic acid in rest and work at high altitude. American Journal of Physiology 116:367–375

Ge R-L, Witkowski S, Zhang Y, Alfrey C, Sivieri M, Karlsen T, Resaland GK, Harber M, Stray-Gundersen J, Levine BD 2002 Determinants of erythropoietin release in response to short-term hypobaric hypoxia. Journal of Applied Physiology 92:2361–2367

Gnaiger E, Lassnig B, Kuznetsov AV, Margreiter R 1998 Mitochondrial respiration in the low oxygen environment of the cell. Effect of ADP on oxygen kinetics. Biochimica Biophysica Acta 1365:249–254

Gore CJ, Little SC, Hahn AG, Scroop GC, Watson DB, Norton KI, Wood RJ, Campbell DP, Emonson DL 1996 Increased arterial desaturation in trained cyclists during maximal exercise at 580 m altitude. Journal of Applied Physiology 80:2204–2210

Grassi B, Marzorati M, Kayser B, Bordini M, Colombini A, Conti M, Marconi C, Cerretelli P 1996 Peak blood lactate and blood lactate vs. work load during acclimatization to 5,050 m and in deacclimatization. Journal of Applied Physiology 80:685–692

Grassi B, Mognoni P, Marzorati M, Mattiotti S, Marconi C, Cerretelli P 2001 Power and peak blood lactate at 5050 m with 10 and 30 s 'all out' cycling. Acta Physiologica Scandinavica 172:189–194

Green HJ, Sutton JR, Cymerman A, Young PM, Houston CS 1989 Operation Everest II: adaptations in human skeletal muscle. Journal of Applied Physiology 66:2454–2461

Hochachka PW 1988 The lactate paradox: analysis of underlying mechanisms. Annals of Sports Medicine 4:184–188

Hochachka PW, Stanley C, Matheson GO, McKenzie DC, Allen PS, Parkhouse WS 1991 Metabolic and work efficiencies during exercise in Andean natives. Journal of Applied Physiology 70:1720–1730

Hoppeler H, Vogt M 2001 Muscle tissue adaptations to hypoxia. Journal of Experimental Biology 204:3133–3139

Howald H, Pette D, Simoneau J-A, Uber A, Hoppeler H, Cerretelli P 1990 III. Effects of chronic hypoxia on muscle enzyme activities. International Journal of Sports Medicine 11 (suppl 1):S10–S14

Howell K, Preston RJ, McLoughlin P 2003 Chronic hypoxia causes angiogenesis in addition to remodelling in the adult rat pulmonary circulation. Journal of Physiology 547:133–145

Juel C, Lundby C, Sander M, Calbet JAL, Van Hall G 2003 Human skeletal muscle and erythrocyte proteins involved in acid-base homeostasis: adaptations to chronic hypoxia. Journal of Physiology (London) 548:639–648

Kayser B, Hoppeler H, Claassen H, Cerretelli P 1991 Muscle structure and performance capacity of Himalayan Sherpas. Journal of Applied Physiology 70:1938–1942

Kayser B, Bokenkamp R, Binzoni T 1993 Alpha-motoneuron excitability at high altitude. European Journal of Applied Physiology 66:1–4

Kline DD, Peng Y-J, Manalo DJ, Semenza GL, Prabhakar NR 2002 Defective carotid body function and impaired ventilatory responses to chronic hypoxia in mice partially deficient for hypoxia-inducible factor 1alpha. Proceedings of the National Academy of Sciences 99:821–826

Lahiri S, Rozanov C, Cherniack NS 2000 Altered structure and function of the carotid body at high altitude and associated chemoreflexes. High Altitude Medicine and Biology 1:63–74

Loeppky JA, Roach RC, Maes D, Hinghofer-Szalkay H, Roessler A, Gates L, Fletcher ER, Icenogle MV 2005 Role of hypobaria in fluid balance response to hypoxia. High Altitude Medicine and Biology 6:60–71

Lundby C, Van Hall G 2002 Substrate utilization in sea level residents during exercise in acute hypoxia and after 4 weeks of acclimatization to 4100 m. Acta Physiologica Scandinavica 176:195–201

Lundby C, Saltin B, Van Hall G 2000 The 'lactate paradox,' evidence for a transient change in the course of acclimatization to severe hypoxia in lowlanders. Acta Physiologica Scandinavica 170:265–269

Lundby C, Pilegaard H, Van Hall G, Sander M, Calbet J, Loft S, Moller P 2003 Oxidative DNA damage and repair in skeletal muscle of humans exposed to high-altitude hypoxia. Toxicology 192:229–236

Lundby C, Calbet JAL, Van Hall G, Saltin B, Sander M 2004 Pulmonary gas exchange at maximal exercise in Danish lowlanders during 8 wk of acclimatization to 4,100 m and in high-altitude Aymara natives. American Journal of Physiology. Regulatory, Integrative and Comparative Physiology 287:R1202–R1208

McClelland GB, Grant B, Hochachka PW, Reidy SP, Weber J-M 2001 High-altitude acclimation increases the triacylglycerol/fatty acid cycle at rest and during exercise. American Journal of Physiology. Endocrinology and Metabolism 281:E537–E544

Marconi C, Pogliaghi S, Grassi B, Rasia Dani E, Colombini A, Cerretelli P 1998 Energy metabolism at 7,600 m. FASEB Journal 12:A724

Marconi C, Marzorati M, Grassi B, Basnyat B, Colombini A, Kayser B, Cerretelli P 2004 Second generation Tibetan lowlanders acclimatise to high altitude more quickly than Caucasians. Journal of Physiology (London) 556:661–671

Marconi C, Marzorati M, Cerretelli P 2006 Work capacity of permanent residents of high altitude. High Altitude Medicine and Biology 7:105–115

Margaria R 1929 Die Arbeitsfahigkeit des Menschen bei vermindertem Luftdruck. Arbeitphysiologie 2:261–272

Margaria R, De Caro L 1950 Principi di fisiologia umana. Vol 1, 2nd edn. Vallardi, Milano, 382–383

Martinelli M, Winterhalder R, Cerretelli P, Howald H, Hoppeler H 1990 Muscle lipofuscin content and satellite cell volume is increased after high altitude exposure in humans. Experientia 46:672–676

Mosso A 1897 Fisiologia dell'uomo sulle Alpi. Fratelli Treves Editori, Milano

Pugh LGCE, Gill MB, Lahiri S, Milledge JS, Ward MP, West JB 1964 Muscular exercise at great altitude. Journal of Applied Physiology 19:431–440

Purkayastha SS, Sharma RP, Ilavazhagan G, Sridharan K, Ranganathan S, Selvamurthy W 1999 Effect of vitamin C and E in modulating peripheral vascular response to local cold stimulus in man at high altitude. Japanese Journal of Physiology 49:159–167

Rahn H, Otis AB 1949 Man's respiratory response during and after acclimatization to high altitude. American Journal of Physiology 157:445–462

Remillard CV, Yuan JX-J 2005 High altitude pulmonary hypertension: role of K⁺ and Ca²⁺ channels. High Altitude Medicine and Biology 6:133–146

Samaja M, Mariani C, Prestini A, Cerretelli P 1997 Acid-base balance and O_2 transport at high altitude. Acta Physiologica Scandinavica 159:249–256

Schmidt W 2002 Effects of intermittent exposure to high altitude on blood volume and erythropoietic activity. High Altitude Medicine and Biology 3:167–176

Semenza GL 2004 Hydroxylation of HIF-1: oxygen sensing at the molecular level. Physiology 19:176–182

Soliz J, Joseph V, Soulage C, Becskei C, Vogel J, Pequignot JM, Ogunshola O, Gassmann M 2005 Erythropoietin regulates hypoxic ventilation in mice by interacting with brainstem and carotid bodies. Journal of Physiology 568:559–571

Van Hall G, Calbet JAL, Søndergaard H, Saltin B 2001 The re-establishment of the normal blood lactate response to exercise in humans after prolonged acclimatization to altitude. Journal of Physiology 536:963–975

Wagner PD 2000 Reduced maximal cardiac output at altitude – mechanisms and significance. Respiration Physiology 120:1–11

West JB 1986 Lactate during exercise at extreme altitude. Federation Proceedings (FASEB) 45:2953–2957

West JB 1999 Barometric pressures on Mt. Everest: new data and physiological significance. Journal of Applied Physiology 86:1062–1066

West JB, Wagner PD 1980 Predicted gas exchange on the summit of Mt. Everest. Respiration Physiology 42:1–16

West JB, Lahiri S, Maret KH, Peters RM Jr, Pizzo CJ 1983 Barometric pressure at extreme altitudes on Mt. Everest: physiological significance. Journal of Applied Physiology 54:1188–1194

Westerterp KR 2001 Energy and water balance at high altitude. News in Physiological Sciences 16:134–137

Wilson DF, Roy A, Lahiri S 2005 Immediate and long-term response of the carotid body to high altitude. High Altitude Medicine and Biology 6:97–111

Young AJ, Cymerman A, Burse RL 1985 The influence of cardiorespiratory fitness on the decrement in maximal aerobic power at high altitude. European Journal of Applied Physiology 54:12–15

Chapter 25

Human adaptation to altitude and hypoxia: ethnic differences, chronic adaptation and altitude training

Carsten Lundby Claudio Marconi Paolo Cerretelli
Benjamin D. Levine

1 INTRODUCTION

This chapter addresses the physiological responses accompanying adaptation to hypoxia, such as in native highlanders and long-term or chronic altitude exposure (acclimatisation) in lowlanders. In addition, the various paradigms of altitude training are discussed. For the more acute influence of hypoxia from hours up to 2–3 months on exercise-related physiological responses, see Chapter 24.

2 HIGH-ALTITUDE RESIDENTS

Approximately 140 million people reside permanently at altitudes above 2500 m, mainly in the Himalayas, Andes, Rocky Mountains and the plateaux of east Africa. According to data recently released by the Food and Agricultural Organisation of the United Nations (Huddleston et al. 2003), there are about 17 million individuals living at altitudes higher than 3500 m, with 4 million living permanently above 4500 m. This last group is distributed mainly in the Himalayan and Karakoram areas, and in the Andes. At present, the highest permanently inhabited settlements on the planet are La Riconada, a mining village of over 7000 people in southern Peru, and Wenzhuan, a town founded in 1955 on the Qinghai–Tibet road, north of the Tangla mountain range in Tibet, both at 5100 m altitude (Marconi et al. 2006). Of these, the Tibetan plateau has been inhabited the longest, and humans have resided here for some 50,000 years, as compared to only 4000–6000 years on the Altiplano in the Andes. In addition, in Ecuador, Peru and Bolivia, the estimated European admixture varies from 5% to 30%.

The general concepts of adaptation to extreme environments have been discussed in Chapter 21. As far as chronic hypoxia is concerned, successful adaptation is reflected in the ability of one generation to successfully reproduce the next. Indeed, one of the best documented differences between high-altitude natives and lowlanders is a reduction in birth weight, approximately 100 g per 1000 m of altitude. Growth retardation persists throughout adolescence, and adult stature remains shorter than at sea level. However, at a given altitude, the reduction in birth weight is lower in Tibetans than in other groups of high-altitude natives or acclimatised lowlanders. For the above reasons, compared to acclimatised lowlanders, Tibetans and, to a lesser extent, Andeans are considered well adapted to chronic hypoxia.

3 ACUTE AND CHRONIC RESPONSES TO ALTITUDE EXPOSURE IN SEA-LEVEL RESIDENTS

Although the main proportion of the inhabitants of our world reside at sea level, almost all humans can acclimatise to a reduced oxygen partial pressure. Indeed, most people can successfully tolerate altitudes up to 2000–2500 m without much effort, due to the flat position of the blood–oxygen dissociation curve at this altitude (Chapter 24). At higher elevations, however, anatomical, physiological and biochemical adjustments to the low oxygen partial pressure may be necessary to sustain life. These changes are referred to as acclimatisation and, in the following sections, the most common strategies developed by sea-level residents upon chronic exposure to altitude are discussed.

3.1 Changes in pulmonary ventilation

One of the very first defences against hypoxia is an increase in alveolar ventilation (Table 25.1). Such a ventilatory increase exceeds the metabolic demand for oxygen, resulting in the flushing of carbon dioxide from the blood (true hyperventilation; Chapter 2). With hyperventilation, a greater fraction of the alveolar air is exchanged and therefore the percentage of oxygen in the alveoli will be slightly elevated. As a consequence, arterial oxygen partial pressure, saturation and oxygen content are elevated.

3.1.1 Mechanisms of breathing

More than a century ago, changes in the static lung volumes of sea-level residents exposed to high altitude were first investigated, and these are discussed in Chapter 24 for vital capacity and forced expiratory flows for acclimatised lowlanders. High-altitude natives born in Morococha (4540 m)

had a 38% larger residual volume than individuals of the same ethnicity but born and living at sea level. The vital capacity was approximately the same and, as a result, total lung capacity was higher in high-altitude natives (Hurtado 1964). It appears that the larger lung volumes of the latter are mainly the result of chronic adaptations to hypoxia that occur during growth and development.

Altitude also has direct effects on ventilation due to a decreased density of the surrounding (ambient) air, with barometric pressure halving every 5500 m. The lower density decreases airway resistance and the dynamic work of breathing, together with increased maximal inspiratory and expiratory flows (this is directly opposite that which is seen with increased air pressure; Chapter 23). Cotes (1954) measured maximal voluntary ventilation in subjects exposed acutely to 3050, 5200 and 8200 m, observing respective increases of 13%, 24% and 31% relative to sea level. In most studies, increases in the forced expired volume in 1 second have also been observed at altitude.

3.1.2 Control of pulmonary ventilation at rest and exercise in native highlanders

Resting Himalayan and Andean natives are characterised by a blunted (habituated) or less pronounced hypoxic ventilatory response. In fact, compared to acclimatised lowlanders, Tibetans are characterised by lower resting ventilation and, consequently, by higher arterial carbon dioxide partial pressures (3.8 versus 2.9 kPa at 3400 m and 3.0 versus 2.5 kPa at 6450 m; Samaja et al. 1997). According to Moore (2000), Tibetans ventilate more at rest than do Andeans residing at the same altitude (4200 m), as shown also by a lower average end-tidal carbon dioxide partial pressure (3.9 versus 4.1 kPa).

It is likely that in most native lowlanders studied at altitude, the higher ventilatory response depends, at least in part, on incomplete acclimatisation to the altitude at which the measurements were made. However, after a 7-month sojourn at Lhasa (3680 m), the minute ventilation of Chinese Han lowlanders seemed to approach that of Tibetan natives, both at rest and during graded exercise (Niu et al. 1995). On the other hand, after a 3–4 week exposure to 5350 m, the ventilatory response to graded exercise of Sherpas born at 2500–4000 m was similar to that of acclimatised lowlanders, up to oxygen uptakes of about 2 L·min^{-1} (Cerretelli 1980). In any case, it is noteworthy that at exhaustion, native Tibetans or Sherpas attain a lower maximal minute ventilation than acclimatised lowlanders, when normalised to body mass (mL·kg^{-1}·min^{-1}). No differences in submaximal exercise ventilations were found at 3600 m among acclimatised Europeans, European migrants and lifelong residents at that altitude, or Bolivian Aymara natives at 3850 m (Brutsaert et al. 2004).

As is well known (Chapter 24), the acute (seconds to minutes) ventilatory response to hypoxia results chiefly from hypoxic stimulation of the peripheral chemoreceptors, primarily those of the carotid bodies. Immediately follow-

Table 25.1 Increments in resting ventilation ($\dot{V}$E) with increasing altitude and decreasing partial pressure of inspired oxygen (PIO$_2$) (data obtained from Reeves et al. 1994)

Barometric pressure (kPa)	Altitude (m)	PIO$_2$ (kPa)	$\dot{V}$E (L·min^{-1})
101	0	19.9	11
57	4800	10.7	15
46	6300	8.4	21
37	8100	6.5	37
34	8848	5.6	42

ing this increase, ventilation declines somewhat over the subsequent 10–30 min, although remaining above normoxic levels. This decline in ventilation is somewhat surprising, and the mechanisms are the subject of considerable investigation. It has been concluded, however, that a decreased carotid body sensory feedback (reduced chemoreceptor sensitivity) and hypocapnia are not involved, and that the response is most likely mediated within the central nervous system. After this initial decline, ventilation undergoes a progressive increase in the following hours to days, before reaching a plateau. Since ventilation is increased (or remains elevated), while at the same time arterial oxygen tension is increased and carbon dioxide tension decreased, the elevated ventilation has often been ascribed to increased carotid body sensitivity (over time) to hypoxia. Considerable evidence has accumulated to show that the carotid bodies play a specific role in acclimatisation. In this context, using the vascular isolated–perfused carotid body technique, Bisgard et al. (1986) separated the circulation to the carotid body from the rest of the systemic circulation. When they rendered the carotid body hypoxic for several hours, while maintaining the rest of the body normoxic, they observed essentially normal ventilatory acclimatisation responses.

In some indigenous populations, or migrants resident for many years at high altitude, the ventilatory response to hypoxia may be much lower than that of the acclimatised lowlander. Moreover, specific pharmacological stimulation of the carotid bodies in native highlanders produced a ventilatory response lower than in sojourners at the same altitude. Interestingly, this blunting effect is more pronounced in Andean Aymara and Quechua than in Tibetans.

3.1.3 Gas exchange

High-altitude natives from North America (Dempsey et al. 1971), Tibet (Zhuang et al. 1996) and South America (Schoene et al. 1990, Wagner et al. 2002) have unique pulmonary gas transport characteristics, keeping a low alveolar–arterial oxygen partial pressure difference at maximum exercise, thus better preserving arterial oxygen tension and saturation. This confers a clear advantage to high-altitude natives, compared to the lowlanders, during exercise at altitude. Although pulmonary gas exchange in high-altitude natives has been the focus of several studies, only a few reports exist on pulmonary gas exchange during exercise in lowlanders acclimatised to high altitude.

The classical study by Dempsey et al. (1971) investigated the alveolar–arterial oxygen partial pressure difference in a group of lowlanders acclimatised to 3100 m for 4, 21 and 45 days. The results were then compared to data obtained in first- to third-generation high-altitude residents. Despite the limited number of subjects analysed (four lowlanders), a comparatively lower exercise alveolar–arterial oxygen partial pressure difference was observed in the natives, whereas lowlanders seemed to undergo a reduction of this alveolar–arterial oxygen pressure difference during exer-

cise as altitude exposure was prolonged. More recently, it was shown that pulmonary gas exchange of lowlanders may improve with acclimatisation, even though after 8 weeks of acclimatisation gas exchange did not reach the values found in high-altitude natives (Lundby et al. 2004a). However, there are hints that, after years of exposure to hypoxia, gas exchange of acclimatised lowlanders may attain values close to those found in high-altitude natives. In fact, Sun et al. (1990) found that a group of adult Chinese Han, resident at Lhasa since 8 years of age, had arterial oxygen saturations at exhaustive exercise similar to those of high-altitude Tibetan natives. As hypothesised in Chapter 24, this may be the consequence of a remodelling of the vascular bed in the lungs.

3.2 Changes in blood variables

Oxygen-sensing cells within the kidneys stabilise the transcription factor hypoxia inducible factor 1 (HIF-1) which, in turn, initiates the synthesis of erythropoietin (and several other changes). This erythropoietin release stimulates the production of erythrocytes in the bone marrow. With exposure to high altitude, plasma erythropoietin concentration peaks within the first 2–4 days, and then gradually returns toward sea-level values. However, although erythropoietin concentration reaches a nadir early upon exposure to high altitude, it may take weeks for the maturation and release of new erythrocytes, and to eventually increase the total red cell mass (polycythaemia). Despite this somewhat lengthy process, haematocrit is increased very rapidly with exposure to hypoxia, as a consequence of a reduction in plasma volume. This process is initiated within hours of exposure to hypoxia and persists for several days. Plasma volume may decrease by as much as 20% over 12 days. This change appears to be an aspect of a generalised redistribution of fluids from the extracellular to the intracellular fluid compartment, with no net loss in total body water (Hannon et al. 1969). The mechanisms of this response are partially unknown, but could include increased vasoconstriction, secondary to an augmented sympathetic nervous activity. However, α-adrenergic receptor blockade with propranolol was found not to modify the altitude-induced decrease in plasma volume (Grover et al. 1998). Volume-regulating hormones such as atrial natriuretic peptide, renin and angiotensin could also be involved, and at least atrial natriuretic peptide has been shown to be activated during acute hypoxia (Albert et al. 1997).

As indicated above, true polycythaemia develops when residing at high altitude for several weeks, and varies greatly among individuals. On average, the expansion of the red cell mass may require up to 1 month to become significant and, in some individuals, the increased red cell mass may not prove sufficient to increase blood volume above sea-level values. This may, however, depend upon the severity of hypoxia. In iron-deficient anaemic females, daily supplementation with 200 mg iron has proven effective in increasing red cell mass. Nonetheless, with lifelong residence at high altitude, red cell volume is increased. For instance, Weil et al. (1968) quantified red cell volume in 73 resting individuals living permanently at sea level, at 1600 m and at 3100 m. A linear increase in red cell volume was found, along with a decreasing haemoglobin oxygen saturation.

In sea-level residents, after a few weeks' exposure to high altitude, haematocrit and haemoglobin concentration may increase to levels found in high-altitude Andean indigenes (native Tibetans have haemoglobin concentrations lower than those of Andeans for a given altitude). Prolonged acclimatisation is not followed by further blood changes. Indeed, with just 2 weeks of acclimatisation to 4100 m, the haematocrit of lowlanders was increased from 42.7% to 49.2%, compared to 50.2% observed in natives. With such an haematocrit, arterial oxygen content at about 4000 m is approximately 200 mL·L^{-1}, and is not substantially different from the value observed at sea level. This could be a reason for haematocrit not increasing to higher values (Lundby et al. 2004a). Interestingly, in four mountaineers studied at 5800 m, whose haematocrit had risen to 58%, an isovolaemic haemodilution lowering haematocrit to 50% did not significantly reduce maximal aerobic power (Sarnquist et al. 1986). This implies that with a higher haematocrit (viscosity), blood flow may be impaired. Presumably, lowering haematocrit improved blood flow as a consequence of a lower blood viscosity. Hence, it appears that the optimal haematocrit for gas transport during exercise appears to be about 50%.

The sigmoid shape of the oxygen dissociation (equilibrium) curve facilitates blood oxygenation in the lung capillaries, as virtually all the haemoglobin is loaded (saturated) with oxygen, even at a relative low arterial oxygen tension (Figure 25.1). The capability of haemoglobin to bind with oxygen is expressed as the P_{50} value, which represents the arterial oxygen partial pressure at which oxygen saturation is 50%. While the major determinant of the haemoglobin oxygen saturation is arterial oxygen pressure, the binding of oxygen to haemoglobin can be greatly influenced by many factors, including: plasma pH, carbon dioxide tension, the concentration of 2,3-diphosphoglyceric acid, magnesium, adenosine triphosphate and chloride, blood temperature and the amount of haemoglobin bound to carbon monoxide. It is generally believed that a leftward shift in the oxygen dissociation curve (i.e. a lowering of P_{50}) is advantageous for the uploading of oxygen in the pulmonary capillaries, whereas a rightward shift is supposed to facilitate oxygen unloading at the tissue level (Bencowitz et al. 1982, Winslow 1988). Thus, in theory, if P_{50} is low, pulmonary oxygen uptake is enhanced, whereas tissue oxygen unloading is impaired, and vice versa.

With acclimatisation to altitudes of 4000–5300 m, the blood–oxygen affinity of resting humans is decreased (rightward shift in the dissociation curve), and the stan-

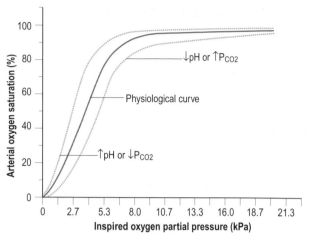

Figure 25.1 The blood–oxygen dissociation (equilibrium) curve. With short-term hypoxic exposure, ventilation increases while the partial pressure of arterial carbon dioxide (P_aCO_2) decreases, and the blood becomes more alkaline. As a result, the curve shifts leftward. In the early part of acclimatisation to hypoxia, the curve is shifted rightward, possibly due to an increase in 2,3-diphosphoglyceric acid concentration.

dard P_{50} is increased by 0.3–0.7 kPa (Lundby et al. 2006, Wagner et al. 2002). This change is probably mediated by increased blood content of 2,3-diphosphoglyceric acid, magnesium, adenosine triphosphate or chloride (Lenfant et al. 1971, Mairbaurl et al. 1993). The result of these changes is a net decrease in blood–oxygen binding capacity. Although an increase in standard P_{50} with altitude exposure may seem paradoxical, since the ability of haemoglobin to bind oxygen in the lung capillaries decreases, the effect of this change on oxygen unloading to the tissues may be beneficial. That is, the favouring of oxygen unloading to the muscles without concomitantly lowering capillary oxygen tension will enhance oxygen delivery.

So far, there is no general agreement concerning whether a decreased or increased blood–oxygen affinity is preferable. Results from animals adapted to live at altitude, the great majority of which have blood P_{50} values lower than their sea-level counterparts, indicate that an increased blood–oxygen affinity is advantageous. In high-altitude Aymaras, however, P_{50} was reported to be higher (3.8 kPa) than in sea-level residents (3.5 kPa). As noted in Chapter 24, Samaja et al. (1997) have suggested that a decreased blood–oxygen affinity is preferable up to altitudes of 5500 m, because a decrease in venous oxygen saturation tends to maximise the change in arterial and venous oxygen saturation, thereby lowering the circulatory load. In contrast, above 5500 m, an increased blood–oxygen affinity is preferred because the preservation of arterial oxygen saturation becomes a priority.

4 THE CARDIOVASCULAR SYSTEM

The major role of the cardiovascular system is to transport oxygen and substrates to support the metabolic demands of the body (Chapter 1). In 1930, it was shown that, at an altitude of 4300 m, the resting cardiac output can increase by approximately 40% (Grollman 1930). Since then, this change has been confirmed on numerous occasions, and it is directly related to the degree of hypoxia, and independent of age and gender. Thus, the cardiac output increases to ensure that oxygen delivery matches metabolic demand, and this is the principal focus of this section (Table 25.2). Subsequently, with acclimatisation to altitude, the drop in plasma volume reduces stroke volume. This, in turn, may cause the resting cardiac output to decrease to levels below that observed at sea level, depending on the degree and duration of hypoxia. In such conditions, oxygen extraction is increased to maintain sufficient oxygenation.

4.1 Heart rate

The initial increase in resting cardiac output with an acute exposure to hypoxia is, for the most part, a function of an increased heart rate (a chronotropic response). This change is sustained by hypoxia-dependent sympathetic activation, directly via stimulation of the peripheral chemoreceptors (Kahler et al. 1962), and vagal withdrawal, indirectly via an increase in ventilation. With acclimatisation to altitudes >3000 m (which corresponds to the commencement of the relatively flat part of the oxygen dissociation curve), the elevation in resting heart rate persists, slightly decreasing toward, sea level after 2–3 weeks.

With acute hypoxic exposure, as indicated in Chapter 24, β-receptor blockade diminishes most of the initial increase in resting heart rate. However, this is not the case with acclimatisation. In the course of such adaptation, heart rate remains somewhat elevated, even when administering supplemental oxygen or β-blockers. The exact mechanisms for these changes remain unknown but it seems to indicate a higher degree of parasympathetic withdrawal with long-term exposure.

4.2 Stroke volume

The initial increase in resting cardiac output is usually not a function of an augmented stroke volume. However, such changes become much more important with acclimatisation. Since heart rate is consistently elevated at altitude, the reduction in cardiac output noted above must be a consequence of a decreased stroke volume, and this has been confirmed in various studies. This reduction is mainly caused by a decrease in plasma volume. Since stroke volume is the difference between end-diastolic and end-systolic volumes, stroke volume can only be reduced if end-systolic volume is increased due to impaired contractile function, or if end-diastolic volume is reduced due to impaired left ventricular filling. Laboratory studies conducted as part of Operation Everest II showed that myocardial contractility is well preserved, even at extreme altitudes (Suarez et al. 1987), and stroke volume is therefore reduced in parallel with changes in left ventricular end-diastolic volume. Such changes are secondary to a hypoxia-induced plasma (blood) volume reduction (Grover et al. 1976).

5 THE AUTONOMIC NERVOUS SYSTEM

Exposure to hypoxia causes sympathetic excitation in humans. This has been determined indirectly from measurements of the hypoxia-induced increases in noradrenaline (Cunningham et al. 1965), and directly from increases in muscle sympathetic nerve activity (Saito et al. 1988). The primary mechanism for this elevated sympathetic activity is the activation of chemoreceptors within the carotid body (Marshall 1994) and the brain stem (Solomon 2000). Thus, during acute exposure to hypoxia, sympathetic nerve activity changes significantly when arterial oxygen saturation decreases to ~85% (Smith et al. 1996).

Recently, it was demonstrated that sea-level residents acclimatising for 4 weeks to an altitude of 5260 m exhibited a surprisingly high level of muscle sympathetic nerve activity (Hansen & Sander 2003). The average muscle sympathetic burst frequency increased to 300% above the sea-level

---

Table 25.2 Resting heart rate, cardiac output, stroke volume, arterial-mixed venous oxygen difference (AV O_2 diff), oxygen delivery and mean arterial pressure (MAP) in healthy, sea-level native men studied at sea level, during acute hypoxia (4 h), and following acclimatisation to 4300 m (21 days; data from Wolfel et al. 1991,1998)

	Sea level	Acute hypoxia	Acclimatised
Heart rate (beats·min⁻¹)	72 ±5	80 ±4[†]	80 ±4[†]
Cardiac output (L·min⁻¹)	6.6 ±0.6	6.7 ±0.6	5.5 ±0.6[†]
Stroke volume (mL)	91 ±6	84 ±6	70 ±7[††]
AV O_2 diff (volume %)	4.4 ±0.5	4.7 ±0.8	6.8 ±0.8[††]
O_2 delivery (L O_2·min⁻¹)	1230 ±120	1010 ±90[†]	1015[†]
MAP (mmHg)	88 ±3	86 ±3	107 ±3[††]

[†]P<0.05 compared to sea level; [†]P <0.05 compared to acute hypoxia.

values, which is considerably more than the 50–100% expected during acute exposure to a corresponding hypoxic gas mixture. The mechanisms underlying this apparent high-altitude sympathetic excitation are unclear. Concurrent breathing of 100% oxygen and intravenous infusion of saline (to restore blood volume) at high altitude only caused a minor decrease in muscle sympathetic nerve activity, indicating that activation of the peripheral chemoreceptors or the cardiopulmonary baroreceptors cannot account for this altered sympathetic excitation. Instead, chronic exposure to hypoxia may cause a resetting of the central nervous pathways involved in the sympathetic excitatory reflexes.

6 MAXIMUM AEROBIC POWER

6.1 Altitude natives

The maximal aerobic power of high-altitude natives, as well as that of acclimatised lowlanders, depends on age, gender, nutritional status, training status, the total muscle mass involved in the exercise (arms, legs, whole body), and, particularly, on altitude and the time spent by the subjects in hypoxia prior to the measurements. On average, the maximal aerobic power (cycle ergometer) of young, physically active but non-athletic Tibetans and Andeans living at around 3600–4000 m varies from 41 to 52 mL·kg^{-1}·min^{-1} (Marconi et al. 2006). These values are in the range of those found at sea level in comparable individuals. It appears therefore that acclimatised highlanders may achieve sea-level values thanks to adaptations involving not only oxygen transport but also muscle energetics, as shown at the molecular level by the analysis of the muscle proteome (Gelfi et al. 2004).

A peculiar feature of altitude adaptation is that both Tibetans and Andeans, despite increased blood convective and diffusive oxygen transport, undergo only a small (8–15%) or even no elevation in peak aerobic power, compared to their reference altitude value, upon migration from 3500–5000 m to ~1000 m (Hochachka et al. 1991, Marconi et al. 2004), or as a consequence of acute hypobaric-normoxic breathing (Favier et al. 1995, Lundby et al. 2004a, Wagner et al. 2002). The above findings may be accounted for, among other factors, by their generally low muscle mitochondrial density and blunted mitochondrial function (Papandreou et al. 2006). Due to the latter, an acute generalised reoxygenation may result in the mitochondrial machinery becoming the bottleneck of the aerobic pathway. In this case, the expected gain in peak aerobic power is not achieved, whereas at altitude, both central (respiratory and cardiovascular) and peripheral (microcirculatory and metabolic) adaptations may still be adequate to optimise and raise peak aerobic power to the levels indicated above.

When Tibetan and Andean lowlanders move from low to high altitudes, the reduction of peak aerobic power appears to be limited, being of the same order of magnitude as the gain seen during descent. This indicates that, unlike Caucasians (Cerretelli & Hoppeler 1996), the maximal aerobic power of altitude populations may be only moderately impaired by lowering barometric pressure, at least below 5000 m. This hypothesis has been strengthened recently, when second-generation Tibetan lowlanders, born at 1300 m and never previously exposed to high altitudes, were studied after 30 days at 5050 m. These individuals were found to recover most (92%) of their pre-exposure peak aerobic power. By contrast, in the same conditions, untrained and trained acclimatised Caucasians were able to recover only 70% and 55% (respectively) of their reference sea-level peak aerobic power (Marconi et al. 2004). Even when prolonging the sojourn at 4100 m for 60 days or more, trained Caucasian lowlanders could not recover their initial peak aerobic power, which attained, on average, only 85% of their sea-level control value (Lundby et al. 2004a).

6.2 Acclimatised lowlanders

For lowlanders wishing to restore a larger fraction of their sea-level peak aerobic power when acclimatising at altitude, the duration of the sojourn must be increased. In fact, this is most likely to require extended acclimatisation, possibly extending to years, during which pulmonary gas exchange improves, and almost normal sea-level peak heart rates are attained. These developmental adaptations may enable acclimatised lowlanders to progressively recover peak aerobic power to values only slightly lower than those prevailing at sea level, and similar to those found in comparable high-altitude natives. For example, upon arrival to 3680 m, the peak aerobic power of a large group of Chinese Han lowlanders was, on average, 23% lower than observed at sea level. After a 7- and a 15-month sojourn, however, the reduction became smaller (i.e. 15% and 8%, respectively) and peak aerobic power attained levels close to those of Tibetan natives (Niu et al. 1995).

A number of investigators have compared maximum aerobic power of high-altitude natives to that of lowlanders born or resident for 1–15 years at the same altitude (Brutsaert et al. 1999, 2003, 2004, Chen et al. 1997, Favier et al. 1995, Frisancho et al. 1973, Ge et al. 1994, Huang et al. 1992, Niu et al. 1995). Figure 25.2 summarises the results of the above studies, showing that peak aerobic power of high-altitude natives (Tibetans: $N = 152$, 42 mL·kg^{-1}·min^{-1}; Andeans: $N = 116$, 47 mL·kg^{-1}·min^{-1}), when normalised to body mass, was only slightly, but not significantly, higher than that of acclimatised lowlanders (Chinese Hans: $N = 116$, 39 mL·kg^{-1}·min^{-1}; Caucasians: $N = 70$, 42 mL·kg^{-1}·min^{-1}; Marconi et al. 2006).

It is notable that these ethnic differences vanish when the degree of genetic admixture between highlanders and lowlanders increases, as is the case for Andean Mestizos. It is therefore unlikely that the anecdotal evidence of superior physical performance of high-altitude natives, compared to acclimatised altitude-resident lowlanders, can be based on differences in maximal aerobic power. Indeed, this conclu-

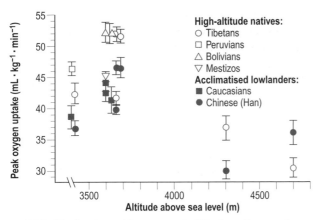

Figure 25.2 Maximal aerobic power of altitude natives and acclimatised lowlanders, both permanent residents of the same altitude for more than 1 year. Data are from: Frisancho et al. (1973), Huang et al. (1992), Ge et al. (1994), Favier et al. (1995), Niu et al. (1995), Chen et al. (1997) and Brutsaert et al. (1999, 2000, 2004). Reproduced from Marconi et al. (2006) with permission.

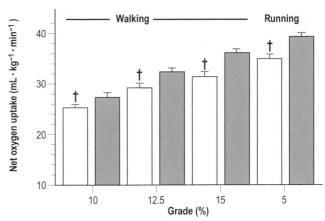

Figure 25.3 Net pulmonary oxygen uptake (steady-state minus resting standing value) assessed at 1300 m of altitude in Tibetans and Nepali lowlanders during treadmill walking at 6 km·h^{-1} on inclines of 10%, 12.5% and 15%, and during running at 10 km·h^{-1} on a 5% incline. Reproduced from Marconi et al. (2006) with permission.

sion led Matheson et al. (1991) to coin the term 'maximal aerobic power paradox' to indicate the higher submaximal work capacity and lower fatigability of Andean Quechuas when rapidly transferred from 3700–4500 m to 700 m, despite a peak aerobic power similar to, or even lower than, that of lowlanders.

6.3 Energy cost of locomotion

There is increasing evidence that, compared to altitude-acclimatised lowlanders, high-altitude Tibetans are characterised by lower energy expenditure during walking and running on a treadmill at a constant speed (Figure 25.3; Marconi et al. 2005). This is consistent with the observation that the metabolic cost of carrying 1 kg of load over a fixed distance at 3500 m is lower for Sherpas than Caucasian mountaineers (Bastien et al. 2005). The mechanisms underlying the greater efficiency of locomotion found in Tibetans are so far not clear, even though there is growing evidence of hypoxia-induced metabolic adaptations in the muscle. Although this observation is valid for Tibetans and Sherpas, it does not seem to be the case for Aymaras (Lundby et al. 2007).

6.4 Muscle structure

During hypoxia, an increase in skeletal muscle capillarisation could be advantageous, since the diffusion distance for oxygen would be reduced. Indeed, after an expedition to Mt Everest (Hoppeler et al. 1990), and following an altitude simulation in which the hypoxic stimulus was equivalent

to that of Mt Everest (MacDougall et al. 1991), muscle biopsies revealed an increase in muscle capillarisation as a consequence of a decrease in muscle fibre cross-sectional area. These results, however, could be affected by reduced physical activity and nutritional status, both of which occur at altitude, and are known causes of muscle atrophy. Recently, it was shown that at the altitude of 4100 m, capillarisation and muscle fibre area were unchanged in physically active and well-nourished subjects (Lundby et al. 2005). This has subsequently been confirmed in subjects exposed for 75 days to 5300 m (B. Saltin, unpublished observation). Thus, in healthy humans, altitude exposure appears not to have an angiogenic effect on the skeletal muscle vascular bed.

For a long time, it was speculated that it would be advantageous during acclimatisation to shift muscle fibres towards the metabolic characteristics of the slow oxidative fibres. However, in lowlanders acclimatised for up to 10 weeks, no changes in the metabolic properties of skeletal muscle fibres could be documented. In addition, no metabolic differences were found between a Danish control group and nine Aymara high-altitude natives (Lundby et al. 2004a).

Although it has been proposed on several occasions that chronic hypoxia is a stimulus for mitochondrial enzymes to be increased, this has not yet been demonstrated. In fact, in the studies performed to date, the observations reveal either no change or a decrease in mitochondrial enzyme concentrations. One of the factors possibly affecting the results is that in some studies, the muscle biopsy was obtained at altitude after 3 weeks' exposure to 4300 m, whereas others were obtained on return to sea level with sampling delays of up to 15 days. In a more recent investigation, muscle biopsies were obtained at 5250 m after 75 days of exposure, and no changes were observed in either citrate synthase or hydroxyacyl-CoA-dehydrogenase activity (B. Saltin, unpublished observation). In this study, muscle buffer capacity was enhanced with altitude exposure, and this was consistent with similar results obtained after high-altitude training. In these studies, however, the altitude was lower (≈2000 to 2700 m) and the exposure duration was only up to 21 days. Thus, the severity of hypoxia and the duration of the stimulus do not appear to be directly linked to the degree of muscle buffer capacity.

Compared to lowlanders, the vastus lateralis muscle of altitude-native Sherpas was found to be characterised by a low lipofuscin content (a biomarker of exposure to reactive oxygen species), which was in the range found in Caucasian mountaineers before high-altitude exposure (Chapter 24). The skeletal muscle of Tibetans who recently migrated to 1300 m is characterised by the greater expression of a number of proteins that influence, directly and indirectly, the metabolic and cellular respiratory function (Gelfi et al. 2004). Among them, enoyl-CoA hydratase concentration (an intra-mitochondrial enzyme involved in β-oxidation of fatty acids) was four times higher than in lowlanders. This indicates enhanced flux of acyl-CoA through the mitochondrial membrane, and is consistent with reports of a 50% decreased intramyocellular fat content in high-altitude Sherpas. In addition, glutathione-S-transpherase P1-1 content was four times higher than that found in lowlanders, thus providing the muscle fibres of Tibetans with a greater protection against reactive oxygen species accumulation, and thus preventing mitochondrial swelling and dysfunction. Moreover, the myoglobin isoform with isoelectric point = 7.29 has been found to be upregulated 100% in high-altitude Tibetans. Besides being an intramuscular oxygen store and transporter, myoglobin seems to be implicated in scavenging reactive oxygen species and tuning nitric oxide concentration at the microvascular and tissue level. In addition, it may play a role in the control of oxidative metabolism. In fact, by binding nitric oxide, myoglobin may relieve the nitric oxide-induced inhibition of cytochrome c oxidase (Brunori 2001), thus optimising the rate of oxygen inflow and consumption by the skeletal muscles.

7   HIGH–ALTITUDE TRAINING

Studies on the various forms of high-altitude training were started in the mid-1960s, in preparation for the Olympic Games in Mexico City (1968). Two reasons exist to undertake such training. First, familiarisation and adaptation are absolutely necessary to enable optimal physical performance within a low-pressure and hypoxic environment. Second, some individuals hope to gain an ergogenic advantage at sea level following hypoxia-induced adaptations. The merits of this are extensively debated within the scientific literature (Genderson et al. 2004, Gore et al. 2005, Julian et al. 2004, Truijens et al. 2003). Today several approaches are used including live high-train high, live high-train low, live low-train high and intermittent hypoxic exposure. In this section, studies focusing on the potential advantages of high-altitude training on sea level performance will be discussed.

7.1   Live high–train high

Live high-train high, a condition where the athlete resides and trains at altitude, was the original altitude training regimen. The initial thought was that an altitude-dependent increase in the total circulating haemoglobin mass, and thus blood oxygen content, would improve exercise performance upon return to sea level. In general, the experimental results of a live high-train high regimen on performance at sea level go in two directions. First, a very limited number of studies show a positive effect on sea-level performance. Second, a large number of studies show no effect on sea-level performance, with a very limited number of them showing even a negative influence. The reason for performance not to be increased in some studies, despite an augmented haemoglobin mass, could be the consequence of a decrease in the training intensity that can be tolerated at altitude (see adaptation theory, Chapter 21). As noted above, maximal aerobic power decreases with increasing altitude, and therefore the ability to maintain high training loads decreases. The live high-train high method has, to a large extent, been replaced by live high-train low regimens, where all training is undertaken as close to sea level as logistically possible, and the remaining time is spent at altitude.

7.2   Live high–train low

The live high-train low method tries to employ the advantages of two environmental conditions: the altitude-associated increase in haemoglobin mass and the ability to maintain high-intensity exercise during sea-level training. The initial live high-train low study conducted by Levine & Stray-Gundersen (1997) was performed with athletes living at 2500 m and training at 1250 m. The hours spent at altitude were approximately 20 per day for 28 days. This allowed an increase in haemoglobin concentration, a concomitant increase in maximal aerobic power and improved 5000 m running performance. The positive effects of this training protocol were maintained for 3 weeks after returning to sea level. Subsequently, the same researchers showed that it was sufficient to descend to sea level for the hard exercise sessions, whereas those sessions characterised by moderate intensities might be conducted at the residing altitude (Stray-Gundersen et al. 2001). Other groups found similar results (Wehrlin et al. 2006), and it was also shown that this approach may be used to increase maximal aerobic power and performance at 2350 m altitude (Schuler et al. 2007).

One obvious drawback of the live high-train low approach is that it may be logistically demanding for the athletes. However, it has been shown that it is sufficient to administer supplemental oxygen while training at the residing altitude (Morris et al. 2000). The latter procedure, however, does not permit the athlete to move freely and sporting disciplines usually performed in the field would now have to be performed in very restricted locations, such as indoor cycle ergometer training sessions for road cyclists. In countries where it is impossible to move to altitudes sufficient to increase erythropoiesis, 'nitrogen houses', developed by Finnish scientists in the early 1990s, have become popular. These chambers are flushed with very high concentrations of nitrogen, thereby lowering the oxygen partial pressure, and simulating altitude (normobaric hypoxia). From live high-train low experiments conducted in 'nitrogen houses', it has become apparent that, in order to increase the circulating haemoglobin mass, the simulated altitude should be around 2500–3000 m, and the daily exposure should be no less than 14–16 hours a day (Brugniaux et al. 2006, Robach et al. 2006). A limited number of investigators have suggested that running and cycling efficiency may be increased with the sleep high-train low paradigm, but a recent study, which included more than 100 subjects, did not confirm such effects (Lundby et al. 2007). Confinement to the limited space in most 'nitrogen houses' for long periods of the day may limit the popularity of these settings among athletes and their families. Furthermore, the use of these facilities has been banned by the World Anti-Doping Agency.

7.3 Intermittent hypoxic exposure at rest and during exercise (live low–train high)

Intermittent hypoxic exposure has been employed both at rest and during exercise. The relative ease of this method has contributed to its popularity. However, convincing evidence for either one of these procedures to increase sea level performance is still lacking.

7.3.1 Intermittent hypoxic exposure at rest

Based on the fact that circulating erythropoietin concentration increases within a few hours of hypoxic exposure (Chapter 24), it has been speculated that repeated, short-term exposures to hypoxia could progressively stimulate an increase in haemoglobin mass. Examples of such protocols include 2–3 hours of daily hypoxic exposure to up to 5000 m equivalent altitude for several weeks. Although early studies found positive effects associated with this hypoxic protocol, more recent observations failed to confirm these observations (Frey et al. 2000, Julian et al. 2005, Lundby et al. 2005).

7.3.2 Intermittent hypoxic exposure during exercise (live low–train high)

The use of intermittent hypoxic exposure in conjunction with training sessions is referred to as live low-train high. One of the early investigations carried out by Terrados et al. (1988) indicated that total work capacity and maximal power output were increased more in subjects training at 2300 m than in control subjects training at sea level. In this study, the total training duration was between 21 and 28 days. This pioneering work was followed by a variety of studies with some controversial results. Recently, however, a randomised double-blind study found no improvement in performance time, maximal aerobic power or maximal power output with this method (Truijens et al. 2003).

In conclusion, so far there are not sufficient data to support the claim that either form of intermittent hypoxic exposure has positive effects on sea-level performance (Wilber 2004).

References

Albert TSE, Tucker VL, Renkin EM 1997 Atrial natriuretic peptides levels and plasma volume contraction in acute alveolar hypoxia. Journal of Applied Physiology 82:102–110.

Bastien GJ, Schepens B, Willems PA, Heglund NC 2005 Energetics of load carrying in Nepalese porters. Science 308:1755

Bencowitz HZ, Wager PD, West JB 1982 Effect of change in P50 on exercise tolerance at high altitude: a theoretical study. Journal of Applied Physiology 53:1487–1495

Bisgard GE, Busch MA, Forster HV 1986 Ventilatory acclimatization to hypoxia is not dependent on cerebral hypocapnic alkalosis. Journal of Applied Physiology 60:1011–1015

Brugniaux JV, Schmitt L, Robach P, Nicolet G, Fouillot JP, Moutereau S, Lasne F, Pialoux V, Saas P, Chorvot MC, Cornolo J, Olsen NV, Richalet JP 2006 Eighteen days of 'living high, training low' stimulate erythropoiesis and enhance aerobic performance in elite middle-distance runners. Journal of Applied Physiology 100:203–211

Brunori M 2001 Nitric oxide, cytochrome-c oxidase and myoglobin. Trends in Biochemical Sciences 26:21–23

Brutsaert TD, Spielvogel H, Soria R, Caceres E, Buzenet G, Haas JD 1999 Effect of developmental and ancestral high-altitude exposure on O₂ peak of Andean and European/North American natives. American Journal of Physical Anthropology 110:435–455

Brutsaert TD, Parra EJ, Shriver MD, Gamboa A, Palacios J-A, Rivera M, Rodriguez I, Leòn-Velarde F 2003 Spanish genetic admixture is associated with larger O₂max decrement from sea level to 4,338 m in Peruvian Quechua. Journal of Applied Physiology 95:519–528

Brutsaert TD, Haas JD, Spielvogel H 2004 Absence of work efficiency differences during cycle ergometry exercise in Bolivian Aymara. High Altitude Medicine and Biology 5:41–59

Cerretelli P 1980 Gas exchange at high altitude. In: West JB (ed) Pulmonary gas exchange. Academic Press, New York, 97–147

Cerretelli P, Hoppeler H 1996. Morphologic and metabolic response to chronic hypoxia : the muscle system. In: Fregly MJ, Blatteis CM (eds) Handbook of physiology, sect 4 : environmental physiology, vol. 4. Oxford University Press, New York, 1155–1181

Chen Q-H, Ge R-L, Wang X-Z, Chen H-X, Wu T-Y, Kobayashi T, Yoshimura K 1997 Exercise performance of Tibetans and Han adolescents at altitude of 3,417 and 4,300 m. Journal of Applied Physiology 83:661–667

Cotes JE 1954 Ventilatory capacity at altitude and its relation to mask design. Proceedings of the Royal Society B 143:32–39

Cunningham WL, Becker EJ, Kreuzer F 1965 Catecholamines in plasma and urine at high altitude. Journal of Applied Physiology 20:607–610

Dempsey JA, Reddan WG, Birnbaum ML, Forster HV, Thodens JS, Grover RF, Rankin J 1971 Effects of acute trough life-long hypoxic exposure on exercise pulmonary gas exchange. Respiration Physiology 13:62–89

Favier R, Spielvogel H, Desplanches D, Ferretti G, Kayser B, Hoppeler H 1995 Maximal exercise performance in chronic hypoxia and acute normoxia in high-altitude natives. Journal of Applied Physiology 78:1868–1874

Frey WO, Zenhausern PC, Colombani PC, Fehr J 2000 Influence of intermittent exposure to normoxic hypoxia on hematological indexes and exercise performance. Medicine and Science in Sport and Exercise 32:65

Frisancho AR, Martinez C, Velasquez T, Sanchez J, Montoye H 1973 Influence of developmental adaptation on aerobic capacity at high altitude. Journal of Applied Physiology 34:176–180

Ge R-L, Chen Q-H, Wang L-H, Gen D, Yang P, Hubo K, Fujimoto K, Matsuzawa Y, Yoshimura K, Takeoka M, Kobayashi T 1994 Higher exercise performance and lower O_2max in Tibetan than Han residents at 4,700 m altitude. Journal of Applied Physiology 77:684–691

Gelfi C, De Palma S, Ripamonti M, Wait R, Eberini I, Bajracharya A, Marconi C, Schneider A, Hoppeler H, Cerretelli P 2004 New aspects of altitude adaptation in Tibetans: a proteomic approach. FASEB Journal 18:612–614

Grollman A 1930 Physiological variations of the cardiac output in man. VII. The effect of high altitude on the cardiac output and its related functions: an account of experiments conducted on the summit of Pikes Peak, Colorado. American Journal of Physiology 93:19–40

Grover RF, Reeves JT, Maher JT, McCullough RE, Cruz JC, Denniston JC, Cymerman A 1976 Maintained stroke volume but impaired arterial oxygenation in man at high altitude with supplemental CO_2. Circulation Research 38:391–396

Grover RF, Selland MA, Mazzeo RS, McCullough R G, Dahms TA, Wolfel EE, Butterfield G E, Reeves JT, Greenleaf J E 1998 Beta-adrenergic blockade does not prevent polycythemia or decrease in plasma volume in men to 4300 m altitude. European Journal of Applied Physiology 77:264–270

Hannon JP, Shields JL, Harris CW 1969 Effects of altitude acclimatization on blood composition of women. Journal of Applied Physiology 26:540–547

Hansen J, Sander M 2003 Sympathetic neural overactivity in healthy humans after prolonged exposure to hypobaric hypoxia. Journal of Physiology 546:921–929

Hochachka PW, Stanley C, Matheson GO, McKenzie DC, Allen PS, Parkhouse WS 1991 Metabolic and work efficiencies during exercise in Andean natives. Journal of Applied Physiology 70:1720–1730

Hoppeler H, Kleinert E, Schlegel C, Claassen H, Howald H, Kayar SW, Cerretelli P 1990 Morphological adaptations of human skeletal muscle to chronic hypoxia. International Journal of Sports Medicine 11:3–9

Huang SY, Sun S, Droma T, Zhuang J, Tao JX, McCullough RG, McCullough RE, Micco AJ, Reeves JT, Moore L 1992 Internal carotid arterial flow velocity during exercise in Tibetan and Han residents of Lhasa (3,658 m). Journal of Applied Physiology 73:2638–2642

Huddleston B, Ataman E, Fe d'Ostiani L 2003 Towards a GIS-based analysis of mountain environments and populations. FAO, Rome

Hurtado A 1964 Animals in high altitudes: resident man. In: Dill DB, Adolph EF, Wilber CG (eds) Handbook of physiology: adaptations to environment. American Physiological Society, Washington, DC, 843–860

Julian CG, Gore CJ, Wilber RL, Daniels JT, Fredericson M, Stray-Gundersen J, Hahn AG, Parisotto R, Levine BD 2004 Intermittent normobaric hypoxia does not alter performance or erythropoietic markers in highly trained distance runners. Journal of Applied Physiology 96:1800–1807

Kahler RL, Goldblatt A, Braunwald E 1962 The effects of acute hypoxia on the systemic venous and arterial systems and on myocardial contractile force. Journal of Clinical Investigations 41:1553–1563

Lenfant C, Torrance JD, Reynafarje C 1971 Shift of the O_2-Hb dissociation curve at altitude: mechanism and effect. Journal of Applied Physiology 30:625–631

Levine BD, Stray-Gundersen J 1997 'Living high-training low': effect of moderate-altitude acclimatization with low-altitude training on performance. Journal of Applied Physiology 83:102–112

Lundby C, Calbet JA, Van Hall G, Saltin B, Sander M 2004a Pulmonary gas exchange at maximal exercise in Danish lowlanders during 8 wk of acclimatization to 4,100 m and in high-altitude Aymara natives. American Journal of Physiology. Regulatory, Integrative and Comparative Physiology 287:R1202–R1208

Lundby C, Pilegaard H, Andersen JL, Van Hall G, Sander M, Calbet JA 2004b Acclimatization to 4100 m does not change capillary density or mRNA expression of potential angiogenesis regulatory factors in human skeletal muscle. Journal of Experimental Biology 207:3865–3871

Lundby C, Nielsen TK, Dela F, Damsgaard R 2005 The influence of intermittent altitude exposure to 4100 m on exercise capacity and blood variables. Scandinavian Journal of Medicine and Science in Sports 15:182–187

Lundby C, Sander M, Van Hall G, Saltin B, Calbet JAL 2006 Maximal exercise and muscle oxygen extraction in acclimatizing lowlanders and high altitude natives. Journal of Physiology 573(2):535–547

Lundby C, Calbet JAL, Sander M, Van Hall G, Mazzeo RS, Stray-Gundersen J, Stager JM, Chapman RF, Saltin B, Levine BD 2007 Exercise economy does not change after acclimatization to moderate to very high altitude. Scandinavian Journal of Medicine and Science in Sports 17(3):281–291

MacDougall JD, Green HJ, Sutton JR, Coates G, Cymerman A, Young P, Houston CS 1991 Operation Everest II: structural adaptations in skeletal muscle in response to extreme simulated altitude. Acta Physiologica Scandinavica 142:421–427

Mairbaurl H, Oelz O, Bartsch P 1993 Interactions between Hb, Mg, DPG, ATP, and Cl determine the change in Hb-O_2 affinity at high altitude. Journal of Applied Physiology 74:40–48

Marconi C, Marzorati M, Grassi B, Basnyat B, Colombini A, Kayser B, Cerretelli P 2004 Second generation Tibetan lowlanders acclimatise to high altitude more quickly than Caucasians. Journal of Physiology (London) 556:661–671

Marconi C, Marzorati M, Sciuto D, Ferri A, Cerretelli P 2005 Economy of locomotion in high-altitude Tibetan migrants exposed to normoxia. Journal of Physiology (London) 569:667–675

Marconi C, Marzorati M, Cerretelli P 2006 Work capacity of permanent residents of high altitude. High Altitude Medicine and Biology 7:105–115

Marshall JM 1994 Peripheral chemoreceptors and cardiovascular regulation. Physiological Reviews 74:543–594

Matheson GO, Allen PS, Ellinger DC, Hanstock CC, Gheorghiu D, McKenzie DC, Stanley C, Parkhouse WS, Hochachka PW 1991 Skeletal muscle metabolism and work capacity: a ^{31}P-NMR study of Andean natives and lowlanders. Journal of Applied Physiology 70:1963–1976

Moore LG 2000 Comparative human ventilatory adaptation to high altitude. Respiration Physiology 121:257–276

Morris DM, Kearney JT, Burke ER 2000 The effects of breathing supplemental oxygen during altitude training on cycling performance. Journal of Science and Medicine in Sports 3:165–175

Niu W, Wu Y, Li B, Chen N, Song S 1995 Effects of long-term acclimatization in lowlanders migrating to high altitude: comparison with high altitude residents. European Journal of Applied Physiology 71:543–548

Papandreou J, Cairns RA, Fontana L, Lim AL, Denko NC 2006 HIF-1 mediated adaptation to hypoxia by actively downregulating mitochondrial oxygen consumption. Cell Metabolism 3:187–197

Robach P, Schmitt L, Brugniaux J, Roels B, Millet GG, Hellard P, Nicolet G, Duvallet A, Fouillot JP, Moutereau SP, Lasne F, Pialoux V, Olsen N, Richalet JP 2006 Living high-training low: effect on erythropoiesis and aerobic performance in highly-trained swimmers. European Journal of Applied Physiology 96:423–433

Saito M, Mano T, Iwase S, Koka K, Abe H, Yamazaki Y 1988 Responses in muscle sympathetic activity to acute hypoxia in humans. Journal of Applied Physiology 66:1736–1743

Samaja M, Mariani C, Prestini A, Cerretelli P 1997 Acid-base balance and O_2 transport at high altitude. Acta Physiologica Scandinavica 159:249–256

Sarnquist FH, Schoene RB, Hacket PH, Townes TB 1986 Hemodilution of polycythemic mountaineers: effects on exercise and mental function. Aviation, Space and Environmental Medicine 57:313–317

Schoene RB, Roach RC, Lahiri S, Peters RM, Hacket PH, Santolaya R 1990 Increased diffusion capacity maintains arterial saturation during exercise in Quechua Indians of Chilenian Altiplano. American Journal of Human Physiology 2:663–668

Schuler B, Thomsen JJ, Gassmann M, Lundby C 2007 Timing the arrival at 2340 m altitude for aerobic performance. Scandinavian Journal of Medicine and Science in Sports 17(5):588–594

Smith ML, Niedermaier ONW, Hardy SM, Decker MJ, Strohl KP 1996 Role of hypoxemia in sleep apnea-induced sympathoexcitation. Journal of the Autonomic Nervous System 56:184–190

Solomon IC 2000 Excitation of phrenic and sympathetic output during acute hypoxia: contribution of medullary oxygen detectors. Respiration Physiology 121:101–117

Stray-Gundersen J, Chapman RF, Levine BD 2001 'Living high-training low' altitude training improves sea level performance in male and female elite runners. Journal of Applied Physiology 91:1113–1120

Suarez J, Alexander JK, Houston CS 1987 Enhanced left ventricular systolic performance at high altitude during operation Everest II. American Journal of Cardiology 60:137–142

Sun SF, Droma TS, Zhang JG, Tao JX, Huang SY, McCullough RG, McCullough RE, Reeves CS, Reeves JT, Moore LG 1990 Greater maximal O_2 uptakes and vital capacities in Tibetan than Han residents of Lhasa. Respiration Physiology 79:151–162

Terrados N, Melichna J, Sylven C, Jansson E, Kaijser L 1988 Effects of training at simulated altitude on performance and muscle metabolic capacity in competitive road cyclists. European Journal of Applied Physiology 57:203–209

Truijens MJ, Toussaint HM, Dow J, Levine BD 2003 Effect of high-intensity hypoxic training on sea-level swimming performances. Journal of Applied Physiology 94:733–743

Wagner PD, Araoz M, Boushel R, Calbet JA, Jessen B, Radegran G, Spielvogel H, Sondegaard H, Wagner H, Saltin B 2002 Pulmonary gas exchange and acid-base state at 5,260 m in high-altitude Bolivians and acclimatized lowlanders. Journal of Applied Physiology 92:1393–1400

Wehrlin JP, Zuest P, Hallen J, Marti B 2006 Live high-train low for 24 days increases hemoglobin mass and red cell volume in elite endurance athletes. Journal of Applied Physiology 100:1938–1945

Weil JV, Jamieson G, Brown DW, Grover RF 1968 The red cell mass–arterial oxygen relationship in normal man. Application to patients with chronic obstructive airway disease. Journal of Clinical Investigations 47:1627–1639

Wilber RL 2004 Altitude training and athletic performance. Human Kinetics, Champaign, IL

Winslow RM 1988 Optimal hematologic variables for oxygen transport, including P50, hemoglobin cooperativity, hematocrit, acid-base status, and cardiac function. Biomaterials Artificial Cell Artificial Organs 16:149–171

Wolfel EE, Groves BM, Brooks GA, Butterfield GE, Mazzeo RS, Moore LG, Sutton JR, Bender PR, Dahms TE, McCullough RE, McCullough RG, Huang S-Y, Sun S-F, Grover RF, Hultgren HN, Reeves JT 1991 Oxygen transport during steady-state submaximal exercise in chronic hypoxia. Journal of Applied Physiology 70:1129–1136

Wolfel EE, Selland MA, Cymerman A, Brooks GA, Butterfield GE, Mazzeo RS, Grover RF, Reeves JT 1998 O_2 extraction maintains O_2 uptake during submaximal exercise with ß-adrenergic blockade at 4,300 m. Journal of Applied Physiology 85:1092–1102

Zhuang J, Droma T, Sutton JR, Groves BM, McCullough RE, McCullough RG, Sun S, Moore LG 1996 Smaller alveolar-arterial O_2 gradients in Tibetan than Han residents of Lhasa (3658 m). Respiration Physiology 103:75–82

Chapter 26

Physiological considerations of human performance in space

Helmut Hinghofer–Szalkay Ronald J. White

1 INTRODUCTION: THE SPECIAL ENVIRONMENT IN A SPACECRAFT

When a person ventures into space, that person enters a realm not visited by humans prior to 1961, and where complex interactions between humans and machines are commonplace. Human performance in space hinges on an operational understanding of these complex events and how they impact upon mission task performance. This chapter will focus on the human physiological changes that occur during a typical space mission, with Figure 26.1 illustrating some of the factors that affect physiology during a mission.

First, because of the harshness of the space environment, the spacecraft itself must provide all the support necessary for the life and health of the astronaut, including control of the internal temperature, air composition, humidity, lighting, noise, etc. (Sulzman & Genin 1994). This is normally handled by a combination of automated and semi-automated systems, with control shared between crew and ground personnel. Second, depending on the mission and its stage, the person either always floats weightless in the air within the spacecraft, or floats between periods of partial weightlessness on a foreign body (e.g. Moon). This weightless (microgravity) state has profound effects on the precise physiological state of the body, a state discussed in detail in this chapter and Chapter 9, whilst Chapter 22 describes the physiological responses associated with head-out (upright) immersion, which is used to simulate microgravity.

The spacecraft is surrounded by a hostile radiation environment (Nelson 1996) and an altered electromagnetic field (Schmitt 2006); the materials used in the construction of the spacecraft are the first line of defence against some of the worst consequences of these environmental threats, but the protection provided by the spacecraft is not sufficient to satisfactorily reduce this risk, particularly for longer missions or missions away from low-Earth orbit. Over time, the physiological effects of some of these environmental components can lead to serious health problems.

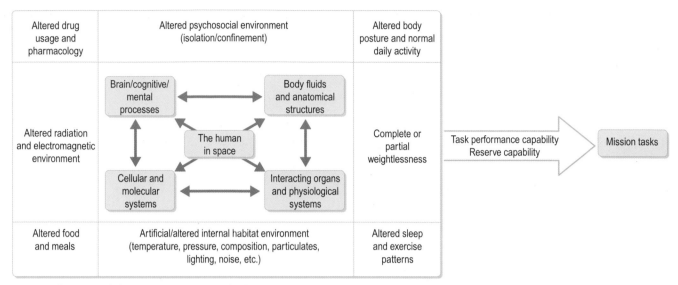

Figure 26.1 Conceptual diagram representing the human during a space mission, and showing some of the many factors influencing both the physiological state of the human in space and the ultimate performance of mission tasks.

In addition, for longer space missions, the unchanging social environment for the crew can lead to stresses that manifest themselves in physiological terms (Kanas & Manzey 2003). Compounding these environmentally related events are an altered set of daily activities, undertaken from a unique postural state with a unique locomotor strategy (Lackner & DiZio 2000) and altered sleep (Czeisler & Khalsa 2000), diet (Lane & Schoeller 2000) and exercise patterns. Furthermore, attempts to deal with minor aches, pains and sleep problems often involve introducing drugs, the effectiveness of which may be altered in space (Cintron & Putcha 1996). All these factors, taken together, lead to a time-dependent physiological state and one that is difficult to model on Earth. In addition, many of the factors are difficult or impossible to control and are likely to vary from person to person, even within the same crew.

So far as the mission itself is concerned, the bottom line for crew members is the performance of certain mission-related tasks, involving either planned activities or unplanned events. From this perspective, overall performance in space involves having the crew members carry out the planned mission activities successfully and appropriately cope with unplanned events. However, from a crew member's personal perspective, performance is more complicated, involving individual physiological capability and health, as well as protection against the long-term health consequences of a mission, even after a mission is complete and the person returns to normal life. To understand a few of these connected personal events, we will examine some of the more important physiological changes and performance issues confronted during a mission.

Several recent books and reviews provide much more detailed information about the weightless state and the other factors that influence the human physiological state in space than is appropriate for this short chapter (Brown & Sawin 1999, Buckey 2006, Buckey & Homick 2003, Churchill 1997, Clément 2003, Dietlein & Pestov 2004, Fregly & Blatteis 1996, Huntoon et al. 1998, Planel 2004, Prisk et al. 2001, Taylor 1993, Watenpaugh 2001, White & Averner 2001).

2 WEIGHTLESSNESS AND HUMAN PHYSIOLOGY: GENERAL CONSIDERATIONS, PHYSICAL EVENTS

Some of the most dramatic physiological events surrounding human spaceflight occur right at the beginning of a mission. As soon as Earth orbit is achieved, everything in the spacecraft, including the people, become weightless, floating if not tied down. Weightlessness instantaneously removes all other physical processes that depend on gravity for their effect. Thus, among other things, fluids do not exert their normal gravitational pressure within the body and normal convection and sedimentation simply cease. The effects of weightlessness are expressed in different ways, but it is convenient to discuss some of the consequences of weightlessness by considering three of the body's components: body fluids, gravity receptors and weight-bearing bones. Eventually, however, either directly or indirectly, weightlessness will affect every part of the body.

2.1 Initial physiological responses

Removal of the normal gravitational (hydrostatic) fluid pressure causes a rapid fluid shift towards the upper body. This is externally manifested in the rounded faces and thin legs of crew members. This immediate, cephalad fluid shift is accompanied by a slightly elevated cardiac output with little or no change in heart rate, similar to that observed during head-out water immersion (Chapter 22). Since central venous pressure drops during the first few seconds to minutes of weightlessness, the implication is that it is likely that atrial transmural pressure increases which, in turn, argues that the local intrathoracic pressure surrounding the heart drops more than central venous pressure. These affect the Starling forces and transmural body fluid shifts. Ultimately, the blood and extracellular fluid volumes are reduced and the body achieves a new state of fluid balance with lower plasma and red cell volumes. This adapted state in space is one of the major contributing factors to the postflight orthostatic intolerance commonly seen when the physiological state must change back to a state appropriate for upright ambulation on Earth.

In weightlessness, the body's many gravity receptors immediately receive information consistent with free fall (zero gravity or microgravity). Thus, afferent signals received by the brain and originating from the vestibular system and tactile sensors, proprioceptors and mechanoreceptors of the joints, muscles and the feet change, yet signals sent from the visual system remain normal. This state is thought to induce a sensory conflict, leading to symptoms of space motion sickness. Once again, returning space travellers must deal with a number of problems in balance and gait associated with the readaptation process.

The onset of weightlessness removes the forces within the musculoskeletal system that are related to supporting the body in a normal posture on Earth, and during normal daily activities. Force removal triggers responses in the muscles and bones that are initiated rapidly, but are manifest only with the passage of days, weeks and months in space. Eventually, muscle mass, strength and endurance generally decrease (Chapter 9) and bone mineral density can decrease significantly in some bones in some people. Although variable, these changes in bone mineral density can be much more rapid and severe than is generally seen in postmenopausal women on Earth (Chapter 12).

2.2 Other challenges

The other challenges of life in a spacecraft, described briefly above (Figure 26.1), act together to precipitate a cascade of time-related responses in each of the body's many cellular and physiological systems. It is hypothesised that the gravity-related changes are appropriate for life in the weightless environment, and are part of the normal adaptation to spaceflight. However, this new physiological state, in which body fluids, muscle function and bone density are reduced, is inappropriate when the space traveller returns to a gravitational environment. Returning to Earth generally requires a significant readaptation period, during which performance of a number of the body's physiological systems is markedly reduced. This reduction in performance could be quite serious in the event of an accident requiring rapid escape from a spacecraft on landing day.

An additional challenge, particularly for researchers studying humans in space, is the fact that, in the current working environment, we will no longer see data from space travellers that come from a uniform population of crew members, with similar initial physiological states, and carrying out similar activities in space. Each crew member also carries out a set of specific activities designed to maintain the body in a healthy state, enabling completion of mission tasks – countermeasures (Nicogossian et al. 1994). Such countermeasures are prescribed in general, but each person has the freedom to modify the prescription to fit their own personal choices. Unfortunately, records of actual individual activities completed during space travel are rarely available. Thus, major determinants of the physiological status are not always clear. Robust state changes in space stand out above the individual variations, but less robust changes are sometimes masked by the differences in the initial physiological state and daily choices of the individual astronauts. This fact should be kept in mind when examining the literature pertaining to human space travel.

3 ADAPTATION AND READAPTATION: DYNAMIC CHANGES AND THE ADAPTED STATE

3.1 Body fluid volumes and distribution

Absence of the downward (gravitational) force that pulls fluids towards the lower parts of the upright body causes body fluids to shift towards the chest, neck and head regions. This cephalad displacement peaks after 1 day and a new steady state is attained within 3–4 day. Leg circumference decreases up to 30% over this time and is sustained for the rest of the flight, even for extended durations. In addition, there are haemodynamic and neurohumoral consequences for the cardiovascular system, as this situation also impinges upon the state of tissues and organs in terms of fluid-holding capacity and volume regulation.

Based on head-down, bed-rest and water immersion simulation studies, weightlessness should promote renal excretion of sodium (natriuresis) and water (diuresis), leading to dehydration. However, it has been observed that, after several days in flight, the diuretic and natriuretic responses to an intravenous isotonic saline load were attenuated, and plasma norepinephrine and renin concentrations increase compared with those observed following an acute (supine) postural change before flight. Renal fluid excretion after an oral water load was also attenuated (Christensen et al. 2001). Sympathoadrenal activity seems to be increased during spaceflight (Eckberg 2003, Eckberg & Fritsch 1991), and the activation of antinatriuretic, as well as sympathoadrenal, activity could be caused by the early reduction in total and central blood volume. A decreased plasma volume may be explained by factors such as redistribution of plasma from the lower to the upper body, reduced food intake and decreased muscle activity. The subsequent increase in sympathetic activity is due, at least in part, to the cessation of activity in large muscle groups during microgravity, which normally counteracts the effects of gravity in the upright posture (Christensen et al. 2001).

This state could lead to the accumulation of fluid and protein in tissue compartments. Whereas the total blood volume comprises approximately 7% of body mass, about twice as much fluid resides in the extravascular–extracellular domain. This interstitial space contains specialised fibres, fibrils and molecules that form an intricate meshwork, and together determine important biophysical features, like tunnel flow with certain hydrodynamic resistances and electrical charges. Such properties are salient for the percolation of extracellular fluid and plasma proteins on their way from the bloodstream towards the lymphatic drainage system (Katz 1980, Aukland & Nicolaysen 1981, Aukland & Reed 1993) and thereby for the nourishment and metabolism of all cells. The interstitial system also conveys a multitude of complex physiological information (Rössler & Hinghofer-Szalkay 2003). For all these reasons, one might think of the interstitium as an organ in its own right.

The extracellular fluid compartment is a key player in the distribution of body fluid volumes and fluid balance. During steady-state conditions, ~10 $g \cdot h^{-1}$ of protein moves from the vascular compartment into the interstitium, and the same volume is shuttled back via the lymphatic system (Renkin 1986). The content of the various protein fractions within the blood and lymph differs, being dependent upon factors such as posture and physical activity (Olszewski et al. 1977, Reichel et al. 1976).

The main barrier for albumin exchange is not the capillary wall but the interstitial compartment, and the major tissues taking up albumin are the skin, muscle, lung and gut (Bent-Hansen 1991). The transcapillary escape rate of albumin, under steady-state conditions, is ~4–5%$\cdot h^{-1}$ of the intravascular pool, whereas immunoglobin-G escapes at 2.6–2.8%$\cdot h^{-1}$ and immunoglobin-M leaves at only 1.9%$\cdot h^{-1}$ (Parving et al. 1974). Besides large regional differences in protein loss, there is a multitude of transport gates, partly receptor mediated, for albumin and various globulins (Schnitzer 1993). The regulation of body fluid volumes during microgravity states is a major element of cardiovascular stability and organ functioning, with unexpected functional states possibly arising during long-term spaceflight.

It is well established that microgravity alters the distribution and composition of body fluids, but little is known concerning its effect on capillary fluid or protein transport changes. Hypotheses concerning the pattern of macromolecular exchange between circulating blood, interstitial space and lymphatics should be tested in future flights. Changes in the hydration of the interstitial gel matrix affect the partition of plasma proteins between intra- and extravascular spaces. Adaptation to microgravity alters the amount and distribution of extravascular fluid distribution along the body axis. These readjustments create a unique pattern when commencing spaceflight (Antonutto & di Prampero 2003, Kirsch et al. 1993).

3.2 Cardiovascular and pulmonary systems

Cardiovascular deconditioning comes about with decreased circulating blood and interstitial fluid volumes, as well as baroreceptor resetting. In parallel, and over time, left ventricular mass and stroke volume are reduced. Postflight orthostatic intolerance and reduced exercise capacity are the logical consequences of these changes (Antonutto & di Prampero 2003, Sides et al. 2005). Orthostatic instability causes trouble when microgravity-adapted astronauts evacuate their vessel in an emergency, with little time for antiorthostatic prevention, particularly if insufficient cooling causes high external thermal loads (Chapter 19).

Resting cardiac output (5–7 L$\cdot min^{-1}$) can increase up to fourfold during strenuous extravehicular exercise. Cardiovascular control mechanisms stabilise (regulate) mean arterial pressure by means of intrinsic, autonomic, central, reflex and humoral elements (Levine et al. 1991). These include minimising blood pooling in the lower limb (dependent) capacitance vessels, an important mechanism because much volume can be stored within lower body veins, thereby diminishing cardiac preload. Leg volume changes are larger in space than with microgravity simulation (Thornton et al. 1992). A reduced vasoconstrictive reserve would explain postflight orthostatic problems because a reduced blood volume increases sympathetic tone, limiting further vasoconstriction while standing (Convertino & Cooke 2005).

Increased whole-body net filtration during orthostasis leads to a partial displacement of the blood volume into the interstitial space (Brown & Hainsworth 1999, Hinghofer-Szalkay & Moser 1986), reducing the effective circulating volume, cardiac output and, ultimately, blood pressure. This is primarily mediated through the systemic circulation, with pulmonary vessels experiencing hydrostatic pressure gradients of approximately the same magnitude, regardless of posture. Spaceflight deconditioning aggravates this problem. Adaptive cardiovascular changes are mediated by concomitant alterations of extracellular fluid volume and its distribution, vascular responsiveness and capacitance, and neurohumoral mechanisms (Christensen et al. 2001).

Inflight resting heart rate and blood pressure stay within normal limits (Bungo et al. 1987, Fritsch et al. 1992) and it is still debated if, and under what circumstances, cardiac function is weakened and myocardial atrophy ensues (Convertino & Cooke 2005, Gisolf et al. 2005). Resting cardiac contractility seems to remain within nominal limits, even with long-duration spaceflight (Atkov et al. 1987). Presently, there is no convincing evidence for the occurrence of space cardiomyopathy (Convertino & Cooke 2005, Sides et al. 2005). However, experimental evidence from simulation studies supports the concept of microgravity-induced diastolic dysfunction, linked to hypovolaemia and reduced ventricular mass (Perhonen et al. 2001, Spaak et al. 2005). Physical and cardiovascular fitness are closely connected, and cardiomyocytes swiftly adapt to the average and peak mechanical load they are experiencing. Spaceflight might reduce maximum cardiac performance to a level that might prove particularly dangerous in emergency situations.

Central venous pressure is increased prior to launching due to a semi-supine position adopted by crew members, with the legs elevated above the chest for at least 2 h (Kirsch et al. 1984, Lathers et al. 1989). It is further increased during launch, where up to +3.5 Gx (anteroposterior) forces compress the thorax, but drops immediately below the supine baseline pressure when microgravity commences (Buckey et al. 1996, Foldager et al. 1996). An inflight thoracic expansion, with a concomitant fall in the local thoracic pressure on the heart, is one explanation of this reduction in central venous pressure (Buckey 2006, White & Blomqvist 1998). Note that even head-down tilt causes a biphasic central venous pressure response (Nixon et al. 1979), but for different reasons.

The pulmonary system is particularly sensitive to the influence of gravity. A change in posture alters chest wall mechanics, the relative displacement of rib cage and abdominal compartments and their compliances, as well as ventilation and perfusion patterns. The latter can have a pronounced effect on gas exchange. Indeed, weightlessness is a unique situation, ideally suited to test hypotheses of gravitational effects on the lung.

It has been argued that the orthostatic reduction in apical pulmonary blood flow is not so much a matter of raising blood against the pull of gravity as it is a consequence of increased vascular resistance in the upper parts of the lung (Badeer 1982). For example, evidence has been presented that pulmonary blood flow distribution is only marginally influenced by gravity in the canine lung (Glenny et al. 1991). In addition to the direct effect of gravity, non-gravitational mechanisms also produce inhomogeneities of ventilation and perfusion.

Microgravity experiments arguably offer the best physiological approach to evaluate the relative role played by some of these gravitational and non-gravitational factors (Chapter 9). Contrary to expectation, perfusion and convective inhomogeneities persist in spaceflight, despite the absence of gravitational influences on pulmonary perfusion patterns (Prisk et al. 1993, 1994, 1998).

Previous observations have shown some inconsistency in the preflight versus postflight pulmonary function comparisons. However, extensive measurements ($N = 10$) during long-duration flights (130–196 days) recently demonstrated unchanged vital capacity and respiratory muscle strength, throughout their exposure to microgravity (Prisk et al. 2006).

Gravity contributes to aerosol deposition within the lungs by deposition on the surface of air passages; this mechanism disappears during weightlessness. Filtering by gravitational settling prevails in the periphery of the lung (terminal alveolar ducts), where air velocities are low, the time spent within a given airway increases and there is no flow turbulence.

The persistence of aerosol droplets in the air is also more prolonged during weightlessness, with only a fraction (<20%) of the total deposition of medium-sized particles being observed after inhalation during weightlessness, than within a 1-G environment (Engel 1991).

There have been no observations suggesting serious dysfunction of the respiratory system during spaceflight, and crew members have not complained of impaired breathing. There is, however, a feeling of fullness in the head, nasal stuffiness and a sensation similar to having a cold. This is most marked during the first few days, but may last for several weeks after launch. Almost certainly the sensation is related to the cephalad shift of blood, resulting in congestion of the facial sinuses by the increase in blood flow. In general, only limited information is available on chemoreceptor reflex changes or regional differences in the lung during weightlessness.

A change from upright to supine posture, or the immersion of seated subjects into water, is associated with an inward displacement of the anterior abdominal wall, a cephalad displacement of the diaphragm and an increased intrathoracic blood volume, all of which combine to reduce the functional residual capacity and modify the mechanics of breathing (Taylor & Morrison 1991, 1999). In the absence of gravity, these changes occur because the weight of the abdominal contents is removed, and respiratory plethysmography has revealed the decrease in functional residual capacity in microgravity to be primarily due to an abdominal chest wall volume decrease (Edyvean et al. 1991, Paiva et al. 1989). End-expiratory rib cage volume was found to be either unchanged (Paiva et al. 1989) or increased during microgravity exposure (Edyvean et al. 1991). Magnetometric determination of changes in rib cage dimensions in seated subjects during parabolic flight, a method that simulates gravitational unloading during the first phase of descent, confirmed that microgravity is associated with a consistent motion of the sternum in the cephalad direction, and an increase in the anteroposterior diameter of the lower rib cage (Estenne et al. 1992).

Electromyographic recordings from the scalene muscles, which inflate the upper portion of the rib cage during quiet inspiration at 1 G (De Troyer 1983, Estenne et al. 1985), have shown a consistent decrease in phasic inspiratory activity during weightlessness (Estenne et al. 1992). This may be part of a reflex referred to as operational length compensation (Green et al. 1978). When the operating length of the diaphragm increases, as it presumably does during microgravity, the whole muscle is placed in a more favourable part of its length–tension curve, enabling greater force generation for a constant neural activation. In this state, the inspiratory activation of all inspiratory muscles is reduced to keep tidal volume constant, thus ensuring the regulation of blood gases and arterial pH. This mechanism has been demonstrated during changes from upright to supine posture, and during water immersion (Druz & Sharp 1981, Reid et al. 1986).

Pulmonary diffusion capacity, pulmonary capillary blood volume and membrane diffusion capacity have been measured in four crew members during a 9-day spaceflight, as well as prior to and following flight in both standing and supine postures. Each function was significantly increased after 1, 4 and 8 days in microgravity. The changes in pulmonary capillary blood volume were of similar magnitude to those seen with a postural change on Earth (standing to supine). Postural changes have no substantial effect on membrane diffusion capacity, but microgravity caused it to rise significantly, suggesting there was a considerably greater surface area available for gas exchange in that state. The increase in diffusion capacity observed in space was almost twice as great as that elicited by the postural transition (standing to supine), and was directly related to an increase in, and a more uniform distribution of capillary blood volume throughout the lung (Prisk et al. 1993).

3.3 Metabolism and endocrine function

Adaptation of metabolic systems to weightlessness is mirrored by corresponding endocrine adjustments, which eventually find a new steady state. Before discussing these changes, it is necessary to highlight some methodological considerations, so that the literature can be more readily interpreted.

Measurements of hormone concentrations in the blood, or other body fluids, can be taken under steady-state (static or chronic) conditions, where the effects of longer term physiological changes become evident. However, the time course of adaptation differs for various physiological systems, with functions needing no more than seconds to hours to adapt, whereas others take weeks, months or even years to do so. Therefore, dynamic investigations of stress-response patterns are necessary to evaluate the magnitude and time course of hormonal changes following the acute application of physiological stresses. The responsiveness of various hormones allows for systematic analysis of the underlying physiology of endocrine function. However, many hormones, particularly the peptides, are subject to decomposition within the sample before measurement can be performed, if insufficient preventive measures are not undertaken. Therefore, equipment for spaceflight research must enable sampling into chilled syringes, centrifuging at low temperature (4°C) and storage at −20°C or lower. Another problem is the pulsatile release of many hormones, requiring frequent sampling and various data-processing strategies. Different subsystems may exhibit specific hypogravity sensitivity curves, so that the maximum response of one subsystem can occur at a different gravity stress than that of others. Close attention to these difficulties makes the difference between good and inadequate science.

It was originally expected that, due to the absence of gravitational pull, energy requirements should be reduced in space, since postural muscles are activated to the same extent. However, the caloric requirements of space travellers may have been unchanged, or even increased, due to exhaustive activities in space (Lane 1992). Metabolic changes associated with muscular adaptation during spaceflight, including a fuel shift toward glycolysis (described below), decrease the capacity for fat oxidation and energy substrate accumulation in the atrophied muscles. Glycolysis is very effective for high-intensity, short-duration acute activities but if sustained output is needed, an energy profile where fat use is favoured rather than compromised is desirable (Chapter 7). The shift toward increased glycolytic activity in muscle that loses mass, particularly the weight-bearing muscles, is accommodated by an increase in hepatic gluconeogenic capacity (Stein & Wade 2005).

Investigations have found changes in insulin and glucose metabolism suggestive of a subclinical, diabetes-like state in prolonged microgravity: decreased glucose tolerance, increased plasma glucose and a relative decrease in circulating insulin for the level of prevailing glucose (Tobin et al. 2002). These changes are diabetogenic, resembling the symptoms associated with subclinical insulin secretory deficiency, insulin resistance, glucose intolerance, compensatory hyperinsulinaemia and altered amino acid metabolism (Chapter 30). Observations of increased C-peptide (Stein et al. 1994) indicate a relative hyperinsulinaemia, induced by peripheral insulin resistance to the stress of spaceflight and the hyperglycaemia that ensues, resulting in an increased insulin secretion by the pancreatic islets. This compensatory increase, however, is insufficient to offset the peripheral resistance to insulin. However, the mechanisms involved in altered regulation of insulin secretion in microgravity are not yet fully understood (Cena et al. 2003).

Ground-based studies have found similar diabetogenic effects when using microgravity simulations. For example, prolonged bed rest has long been used as a paradigm for insulin resistance and glucose intolerance, and it induces metabolic alterations much like those observed in microgravity (Lipman et al. 1970), including a loss in lean body mass and decreased insulin sensitivity. The glucose intolerance of bed rest is believed to be modulated secondary to a decrease in peripheral tissue insulin sensitivity, which results in a decreased ability to mobilise glucose transporters from the cytosolic pool and insert them into the cellular membrane in insulin-sensitive tissues. Thus, observations during and after spaceflight, as well as ground-based experiments, collectively support changes similar to the glucose intolerance of subclinical diabetes, ageing (Chapter 16) and physical inactivity (Chapter 28).

Spaceflight is associated with increased oxidative stress after returning to Earth, which is more pronounced after long-duration spaceflight. The effects last for several weeks after landing. Indeed, recent data provide evidence for oxidative damage with long-duration space travellers. For example, serum iron, ferritin saturation and transferrin were decreased and serum ferritin was increased in 11 crew members after 128–195 days aboard the International Space

Station. Following the flight, urinary 8-hydroxy-2'-deoxyguanosine concentration was greater and erythrocytic superoxide dismutase decreased (Smith et al. 2005b). These changes have been attributed to a combination of the energy deficiency that occurs during flight, and substrate competition for amino acids occurring between repleting muscle and other tissues during the recovery phase (Stein 2002). Decreasing the imbalance between the production of endogenous oxidant defences and oxidant production, by increasing the supply of dietary antioxidants, may reduce the severity of postflight oxidative stress.

3.4 Muscle function

Regular mechanical loading of the muscular system is necessary to maintain the balance of contractile protein synthesis and degradation (catabolism), and consequently muscle mass and power output (Chapter 9). Inactivation of the weight-bearing (antigravity) muscles has an impact on strength, speed and endurance, and results in disuse atrophy and decreased expression of protein isoforms comprising the contractile system (Caiozzo et al. 1992, Diffee et al. 1991, 1993). This remodelling process involves a transition from slow to fast myosin fibre types, which have twice the shortening velocity potential compared to the others (Adams et al. 2003, Haddad et al. 2005, Stein & Wade 2005). The underlying physiological processes and their implications are dealt with in Chapter 9 of this book.

In response to decreased workload, skeletal muscle undergoes an adaptive, reductive remodelling, with the mechanism of this process being largely independent of the reason for disuse. However, crew members need to maintain as much functional capacity as possible during spaceflight for extravehicular activities. In space, there is a profound functional redistribution within the musculoskeletal system, due to altered physical activity and force patterns. Muscles that have an antigravity function, such as the calf and quadriceps muscles, rapidly shrink during spaceflight, while others are barely affected. Exercise is a natural countermeasure for fighting disuse atrophy in space. Alternatively, electrical stimulation could be employed, if the amount of exercise performed is unable to balance the mechanical unloading (Duvoisin et al. 1989). It seems that novel ways should be identified that allow crew members to exercise for an extended time at the desired level (Chapter 9), without causing overly cumbersome side-effects like excessive boredom, skin lesions, etc. The lack of motivation to activate large parts of the musculoskeletal system in microgravity conditions stems from the absence of any immediate need to do so. Paradoxically, this is one of the examples of how humans must fight an adaptation process that makes sense in the given situation (i.e. losing unnecessary muscle mass), but would have dangerous consequences when reentering 1-G conditions, particularly after longer lasting journeys of exploration.

The limited access to microgravity environments to study muscle adaptation and evaluate countermeasure programmes has necessitated the use of ground-based models and simulations to conduct both basic and applied research. The models of muscle unweighting include bed rest, cast immobilisation and unilateral lower limb suspension. Comparisons of changes in muscle strength and size between these models, in the context of the limited results available from spaceflight, suggest that each model may be useful for certain aspects of muscle unweighting during microgravity (Adams et al. 2003).

For instance, it has been shown that unilateral limb suspension induces atrophy and reduced strength of the affected muscle group, and that resistance exercise is effective in ameliorating these deficits. Using this model, it has been determined that alterations in contractile protein gene expression (myosin heavy chain and actin) provide molecular markers concerning the deficits that occur in muscle mass and volume. The data indicated that there are deficits in total RNA, mRNA, actin and myosin heavy chain mRNA expression and these changes can be blunted when resistance exercise was applied (Gallagher et al. 2005, Haddad et al. 2005).

It appears that muscular deconditioning is not a spaceflight-specific effect, but a normal physiological adaptation to a lack of mechanical challenge (disuse atrophy), as seen with any comparable model or simulation. Indeed, the obvious and straightforward solution to all such cases is to increase mechanical loading, using either artificial gravity or resistance exercise. In addition, regular exercise brings considerable cardiovascular benefit, even in ambulatory subjects (Evans et al. 2004). Protein or essential amino acid supplementation may also be employed to mitigate loss of muscle mass and strength during simulated (bed rest, immobilisation) and spaceflight. Most interestingly, however, it seems that such a muscular countermeasure may, at the same time, exacerbate bone metabolism because of an acidifying effect, consequently leading to osseal calcium resorption and excretion. Thus, this potential muscle loss countermeasure has negative effects on bone metabolism (Zwart et al. 2005).

Without direct scientific evidence, head-down bed rest (−6°) has long been hypothesised to mimic the cardiovascular effects of microgravity, and many studies have shown rapid disuse atrophy within muscles and bones, as well as cardio-respiratory deconditioning (Chapter 9). A recent parallel study comparing cardiorespiratory responses to exercise and work by four crew members on a 17-day spaceflight with eight earthbound, bed rest subjects specifically tested this hypothesis (Trappe et al. 2006). Like bed rest, exercise capacity falls almost immediately, apparently reaching a low point at 13 days in flight. Maximal oxygen uptake decreased by 11% and 9%, and oxygen pulse by 18% and 12% for spaceflight and head-down bed rest, respectively. Thus, the direction, magnitude and time course of these cardiorespiratory responses to exercise were similar. The recovery data lend support to the possibility that programmes designed from head-down bed rest to help astronauts once they arrive at the moon may be sufficiently effective.

3.5 Skeletal system

A change in the gravitational environment alters the intensity of mechanical stress on the skeletal system. Lessons learned from spaceflight studies have the potential to find novel treatments and countermeasures for ameliorating or preventing bone loss (Mundy et al. 1999, Vogel 1999). Muscle atrophy and increased bone resorption are observed with body casting, prolonged bed rest without exercise training and spaceflight, with striking similarities (Bikle et al. 1997, Bloomfield 1997, Zerwekh et al. 1998).

Bone mineral loss during prolonged deconditioning may well exceed $10\%\cdot y^{-1}$ (Leblanc et al. 1990; Chapters 13 and 28), with urinary and faecal calcium excretion increased by 20–50% (Arnaud et al. 1992, Van Der Wiel et al. 1991, Zerwekh et al. 1998). Calcium loss begins a few days into bed rest and stays elevated, leading to an ever-increasing negative calcium balance (Greenleaf & Kozlowski 1982, Krasnoff & Painter 1999). Without physical activity, the balance between bone formation and breakdown is disrupted, with resorption predominating, resulting in bone loss and osteoporosis (Bloomfield 1997, Fukuoka et al. 1994, Leblanc et al. 1990, 1995, Nishimura et al. 1994, Vico et al. 1987). Bone loss with spaceflight, however, is a consequence of both elevated bone resorption and decreased intestinal calcium absorption (Smith et al. 2005a).

Osteoporosis is a common metabolic bone disease, and represents a major health-care problem affecting up to 50% of women and 25% of men over age 50 (Chapters 13 and 16), and is associated with a high incidence of hip and vertebral fractures. The disorder is characterised by parallel reductions in bone mineral and bone matrix, so that bone density is decreased but its normal composition remains (Finkelstein et al. 1997). The mechanism of osteoporosis is increased bone resorption, generally with reduced bone formation, and often accompanied by low calcium availability, high calcium loss and hormonal disturbances (Nordin 1997).

Prolonged bed rest, inactivity and spaceflight are all useful models for investigating the mechanisms of, and preventive strategies for skeletal deconditioning and osteoporosis (Cowin 1998, White 1998). The most consistent forces affecting humans are those associated with gravity, which are transmitted to bone as the supportive and power-distributing system. Thus, gravitation governs the trophic stimuli that bone continually receives. Matrix and cell surface proteoglycans control cellular growth factors during chondrogenesis and osteogenesis. Integrins, which transduce signals from the extracellular matrix to the intracellular compartment, mediate adhesion of osteoclasts during bone resorption. Vitamin D upregulates integrin expression in mononucleated osteoclast precursors and also stimulates their differentiation into osteoclasts, suggesting that integrins perform a vital role during osteoclast differentiation (Boissy et al. 1998).

Osteocytes communicate via canaliculi by means of cytoplasmic processes (Figure 26.2), and this network connects periostal and the vast endosteal surfaces (1000–5000 m^2). Due to its sponge-like structure, trabecular bone provides more than 80% of this exchange interface, although its mass is only ~20% of the total skeleton.

Osteocytes are the most abundant cells of the osteoblast lineage, receiving nourishment and signals via their gap junction-equipped cytoplasmic processes. These cells are differentiated osteoblasts that became entrapped in bone matrix during growth or remodelling. Together with osteoblasts and the quiescent lining cells, they comprise the bone membrane. The bone surface is mostly covered by flat (bone-lining) cells. These are also connected to each other and to superficial osteocytes with cell processes extending into canaliculi, equipped with gap junctions, and thus contributing to a syncytium formed by all bone cells except osteoclasts (Moss 1991). This system comprises an information network where each osteocyte has probably up to 80 cytoplasmic processes, approximately 15 mm long, arrayed in a three-dimensional manner and interconnected with up to 12 neighbouring osteocytes (Palumbo et al. 1990). Canalicular extracellular space contains fluid and macromolecular complexes, with a high proportion of large proteoglycans (Sauren et al. 1992). This entire arrangement provides an intracellular (gap junctions) and extracellular route for the rapid passage of electrical and chemical information (Curtis et al. 1985).

Can an osteocyte or an osteoblast sense changes in the gravitational field directly and independently of changes in its environment, or does it detect those changes from its environment indirectly by contact stress? Adhesive forces on osteoblasts or osteocytes are 3–4 orders of magnitude larger than gravitational forces due to cell weight (Cowin 1998). Is the magnitude or the rate of strain the controlling factor for local bone metabolism? Strategies for coping with deterioration of the musculoskeletal system during long-term bed rest, immobilisation or spaceflight are dependent upon the answers to these questions.

It appears that the functional responses during deconditioning involve simultaneous mechanical, bioelectric and biochemical processes. Strain affects both collagen and mineral microarchitecture, and tensile forces are associated with increased tissue anisotropy and associated physical load (Takano et al. 1999). Bone seems to sense only time-varying forces because a constant, non-time varying force applied to bone has the same effect as no force (Rubin & Lanyon 1987). Thus, it would not be the absence of gravity per se that induces bone loss during spaceflight or inactivity, but rather the time-varying force systems acting on the bone that are fundamentally changed due to ambulatory changes (Cowin 1998).

Cytokines in the osseal microenvironment regulate the dynamics of bone metabolism. For instance, bone repre-

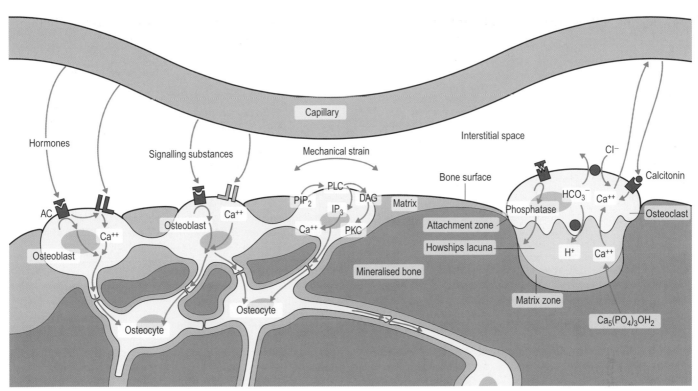

Figure 26.2 Bone formation (left) and resorption (right). Signalling substances and mechanical strain influence calcium influx and G-protein dependent enzyme activity (AC, adenylate cyclase; PLC, phospholipase C). Osteoblast-derived cytokines and prostaglandins activate osteoclasts, which release hydrogen ions, proteases and phosphatases and form a Howship's lacuna. Calcitonin reduces osteoclast motility, Ca^{++} stimulates osteoclast retraction.

sents the largest reservoir for transforming growth factor, a potent osteoblastic mitogen, which is attached to a special binding protein. This growth factor inhibits bone resorption by suppressing osteoclast recruitment and activity. Interleukin-6, produced by osteoblasts and stromal cells, increases resorption and promotes osteoclastogenesis. Some components of the insulin-like growth factor system are also abundantly expressed in human bone (IGF-I and IGF-II). IGF-I and IGF-II are mitogens that enhance differentiation of osteoblasts. The actions of such cytokines provide a target for steroid hormones, most notably oestrogens and androgens (Hofbauer & Khosla 1999).

Bone mineral density accounts for 70–75% of bone strength (Faulkner 2000, Heany 1989, Ott 1993). Several types of bone are routinely measured to represent this skeletal feature. For example, the radius is used to represent cortical bone, cancellous bone is represented by the lumbar spine, mixed bone by the proximal hip or neck of the femur, and the calcaneus is used since it is 90–95% trabecular bone. Bone density changes are used to assess altered mineralisation in the lower extremities with spaceflight; calcaneal mineral density is a good predictor of vertebral and femoral neck fractures (Cheng et al. 1994, Vogel et al. 1988). Absorptiometry appears to be the most sensitive method for monitoring bone mineral content, with ultrasound techniques also providing information concerning bone quality (Brandenburger 1993, Sone et al. 1998) and fragility (Schnitzler 1993).

Bone resorption markers should reflect osteoclast activity or collagen degradation, formation markers, osteoblastic synthetic activity or extracellular metabolism of procollagen.

Changes in bone structure with microgravity deconditioning do not constitute true systemic osteoporosis, since it is only the weight-bearing bones that lose mass during microgravity, whereas those in the upper body remain more or less unaffected, or may even gain substance. Microgravity-induced bone loss in humans, due to direct gravitational sensing, is highly unlikely because constant, non-varying forces applied to bone have the same effect as no force (Rubin & Lanyon 1987). Thus, a change in effective gravity, as with bed rest deconditioning or spaceflight, has essentially no effect on the single bone cell, but it has a major effect on the intact skeleton. Bone cells receive information related to gravitational changes directly from the immediate environment; 1-G strain on an isolated cell level is too weak to be perceived (Cowin 1998). However, several days of exposure to weightlessness can reduce the differentiation of osteoblasts in response to growth-promoting signal substances (Carmeliet et al. 1998).

Recent research has shown that bone resorption starts to predominate from the very beginning of a period with reduced stimulation (Baecker et al. 2003), indicating there is practically no delay in osseal adaptation to a changed mechanical environment. Bone is a plastic tissue, capable of responding to altered stimulation patterns and intensity on a real-time basis.

References

Adams GR, Caiozzo VJ, Baldwin KM 2003 Skeletal muscle unweighting: spaceflight and ground-based models. Journal of Applied Physiology 95:2185–2201

Antonutto G, di Prampero PE 2003 Cardiovascular deconditioning in microgravity: some possible countermeasures. European Journal of Applied Physiology 90:283–291

Arnaud SB, Sherrard DJ, Maloney N, Whalen RT, Fung P 1992 Effects of 1-week head-down tilt bed rest on bone formation and the calcium endocrine system. Aviation, Space and Environmental Medicine 63:14–20

Atkov OY, Bednenko VS, Fomina CA 1987 Ultrasound techniques in space medicine. Aviation, Space and Environmental Medicine 58: A69-A73

Aukland K, Nicolaysen G 1981 Interstitial fluid volume: local regulatory mechanisms. Physiological Reviews 61:556–643

Aukland K, Reed RK 1993 Interstitial-lymphatic mechanisms in the control of extracellular fluid volume. Physiological Reviews 73:1–78

Badeer HS 1982 Gravitational effects on the distribution of pulmonary blood flow: hemodynamic misconceptions. Respiration 43:408–413

Baecker N, Tomic A, Mika C, Gotzmann A, Platen P, Gerzer R, Heer M 2003 Bone resorption is induced on the second day of bed rest: results of a controlled crossover trial. Journal of Applied Physiology 95:977–982

Bent-Hansen L 1991 Whole body capillary exchange of albumin. Acta Physiologica 143(S 603):5–10

Bikle DD, Halloran BP, Morey-Holton E 1997 Spaceflight and the skeleton: lessons for the earthbound. Endocrinologist 7:10–22

Bloomfield SA 1997 Changes in musculoskeletal structure and function with prolonged bed rest. Medicine and Science in Sports and Exercise 29:197–206

Boissy P, Machuca I, Pfaff M, Ficheux D, Jurdic P 1998 Aggregation of mononucleated precursors triggers cell surface expression of alpha v beta 3 integrin, essential to formation of osteoclast-like multinucleated cells. Journal of Cell Science 111:2563–2574

Brandenburger GH 1993 Clinical determination of bone quality: is ultrasound the answer? Calcified Tissue International 53:S151–S156

Brown CN, Hainsworth R 1999 Assessment of capillary fluid shifts during orthostatic stress in normal subjects and subjects with orthostatic intolerance. Clinical Autonomic Research 9:69–73

Brown JT, Sawin CF 1999 Extended duration orbiter medical project final report. NASA SP-1999-534, Houston

Buckey JC 2006 Space physiology. Oxford University Press, New York

Buckey JC, Homick JL 2003 The neurolab Spacelab mission: neuroscience research in space. NASA SP-2003-535, Houston

Buckey JC, Gaffney FA, Lane LD, Levine BD, Watenpaugh DE, Wright SJ, Yancy CW, Meyer DM, Blomqvist CG 1996 Central venous pressure in space. Journal of Applied Physiology 81(1):19–25

Bungo MW, Goldwater DJ, Popp RL, Sandler H 1987 Echocardiographic evaluation of Space Shuttle crewmembers. Journal of Applied Physiology 62:278–283

Caiozzo VJ, Ma E, McCue SA, Herrick RE, Baldwin KM 1992 A new animal model for modulating myosin isoform expression by mechanical activity. Journal of Applied Physiology 73:1432–1440

Carmeliet G, Nys G, Stockmans I, Bouillon R 1998 Gene expression related to the differentiation of osteoblastic cells is altered by microgravity. Bone 22:139S–143S

Cena H, Sculati M, Roggi C 2003 Nutritional concerns and possible countermeasures to nutritional issues related to spaceflight. European Journal of Nutrition 42:99–110

Cheng S, Suominen H, Era P, Heikkinen E 1994 Bone density of the calcaneus and fractures in 75- and 870-year old men and women. Osteoporosis International 4:48–54

Christensen NJ, Drummer C, Norsk P 2001 Renal and sympathoadrenal responses in space. American Journal of Kidney Disease 38:679–683

Churchill S (ed) 1997 Fundamentals of space life sciences, volumes 1 and 2. Krieger, Malabar

Cintrón NM, Putcha L 1996 Pharmacokinetics in flight. In: Huntoon CSL, Antipov VV, Grigoriev AI (eds) Space biology and medicine, volume III, book 2, humans in spaceflight. American Institute of Aeronautics and Astronautics, Washington, DC, 547–557

Clément G 2003 Fundamentals of space medicine. Kluwer, Dordrecht

Convertino VA, Cooke WH 2005 Evaluation of cardiovascular risks of spaceflight does not support the NASA bioastronautics critical path roadmap. Aviation, Space and Environmental Medicine 76:869–876

Cowin SC 1998 On mechanosensation in bone under microgravity. Bone 22:S119–S125

Curtis TA, Ashrafi SH, Weber DF 1985 Canalicular communication in the cortices of human long bones. Anatomical Records 212:336–344

Czeisler CA, Khalsa SB 2000 The human circadian timing system and sleep-wake regulation. In: Kryger MH, Roth T, Dement WC (eds) Principles and practice of sleep medicine, 3rd edn. Saunders, Philadelphia, 353–375

De Troyer A 1983 Mechanical role of the abdominal muscles in relation to posture. Respiratory Physiology and Neurobiology 53:341–353

Dietlein LF, Pestov ID 2004 Health, performance and safety of space crews, volume IV of space biology and medicine. AIAA, Reston

Diffee GM, Haddad F, Herrick RE, Baldwin KM 1991 Control of myosin heavy chain expression: interaction of hypothyroidism and hindlimb suspension. American Journal of Physiology 30: C1099–C1106

Diffee GM, Caiozzo VJ, McCue SA, Herrick SE, Baldwin KM 1993 Activity-induced regulation of myosin isoform distribution: comparison of two contractile activity programs. Journal of Applied Physiology 74:2509–2516

Druz WS, Sharp JT 1981 Activity of respiratory muscles in upright and recumbent humans. Journal of Applied Physiology 51:1552–1561

Duvoisin MR, Convertino VA, Buchanan P, Gollnick PD, Dudley GA 1989 Characteristics and preliminary observations of the influence of electromyostimulation on the size and function of human skeletal muscle during 30 days of simulated microgravity. Aviation, Space and Environmental Medicine 60:671–678

Eckberg DL 2003 Bursting into space: alterations of sympathetic control by space travel. Acta Physiologica 177:299–311

Eckberg DL, Fritsch JM 1991 Human autonomic responses to actual and simulated weightlessness. Journal of Clinical Pharmacology 31:951–955

Edyvean J, Estenne M, Paiva M, Engel LA 1991 Lung and chest wall mechanics in microgravity. Journal of Applied Physiology 71:1956–1966

Engel LA 1991 Effect of microgravity on the respiratory system. Journal of Applied Physiology 70:1907–1911

Estenne M, Yernault JC, De Troyer A 1985 Rib cage and diaphragm abdomen compliance in humans: effects of age and posture. Journal of Applied Physiology 59:1842–1848

Estenne M, Gorini M, Van Muylem A, Ninan, V, Paiva M 1992 Rib cage shape and motion in microgravity. Journal of Applied Physiology 73:946–954

Evans JM, Stenger MB, Moore FB, Hinghofer-Szalkay H, Rössler A, Patwardhan AR, Pelligra R, Brown DR, Zielger MG, Knapp CF 2004 Centrifuge training increases presyncopal orthostatic tolerance in ambulatory men. Aviation, Space and Environmental Medicine 75:850–858

Faulkner KG 2000 Bone matters: are density increases necessary to reduce fracture risk? Journal of Bone and Mineral Research 15:183–187

Finkelstein JS, Mitlak BH, Slovick DM 1997 Osteoporosis. In: Andreoli TE, Bennett JC, Carpenter CCJ, Plum F (eds) Cecil's essentials in medicine. Saunders, Philadelphia

Foldager N, Andersen TA, Jessen FB, Ellegaard P, Stadeager C, Videbaek R, Norsk P 1996 Central venous pressure in humans during microgravity. Journal of Applied Physiology 81:408–412

Fregly MJ, Blatteis CM (eds) 1996 Handbook of physiology section 4: environmental physiology, the gravitational environment, volumes I and II. Oxford University Press, New York

Fritsch JM, Charles JB, Bennett BS, Jones MM, Eckberg DL 1992 Short duration spaceflight impairs human arterial baroreflex function. Journal of Applied Physiology 73:664–671

Fukuoka H, Kiriyama M, Nishimura Y, Higurashi M, Suzuki Y, Gunji A 1994 Metabolic turnover of bone and peripheral monocyte release of cytokines during short-term bed rest. Acta Physiologica 150 (suppl 616):37–41

Gallagher P, Trappe S, Harber M, Creer A, Mazzetti S, Trappe T, Alkner B, Tesch P 2005 Effects of 84-days of bed rest and resistance training on single muscle fibre myosin heavy chain distribution in human vastus lateralis and soleus muscles. Acta Physiologica 185:61–69

Gisolf J, Immink RV, Van Lieshout JJ, Stok WJ, Karemaker JM 2005 Orthostatic blood pressure control before and after spaceflight, determined by time-domain baroreflex method. Journal of Applied Physiology 98:1682–1690

Glenny RW, Lamm WJE, Albert RK, Robertson HT 1991 Gravity is a minor determinant of pulmonary blood flow distribution. Journal of Applied Physiology 71:620–629

Green M, Mead J, Sears TA 1978 Muscle activity during chest wall restriction and positive pressure breathing in man. Respiratory Physiology and Neurobiology 35:283–300

Greenleaf JE, Kozlowski S 1982 Physiological consequences of reduced physical activity during bed rest. Exercise and Sports Sciences Reviews 20:83–119

Haddad F, Baldwin KM, Tesch PA 2005 Pretranslational markers of contractile protein expression in human skeletal muscle: effect of limb unloading plus resistance exercise. Journal of Applied Physiology 98:46–52

Heany RP 1989 Osteoporotic space: an hypothesis. Bone and Mineral 6:1–13

Hinghofer-Szalkay H, Moser M 1986 Fluid and protein shifts after postural changes in humans. American Journal of Physiology. Heart and Circulatory Physiology 250:H68–H75

Hofbauer LC, Khosla S 1999 Androgen effects on bone metabolism: recent progress and controversies. European Journal of Endocrinology 140:271–286

Huntoon CSL, Grigoriev AI, Natochin YV 1998 Fluid and electrolyte regulation in spaceflight. American Astronautical Society, San Diego, CA

Kanas N, Manzey D 2003 Space psychology and psychiatry. Kluwer, Dordrecht

Katz MA 1980 Interstitial space – the forgotten organ. Medical Hypotheses 6:885–898

Kirsch KA, Röcker L, Gauer OH, Krause R 1984 Venous pressure in man during weightlessness. Science 225:218–219

Kirsch KA, Baartz FJ, Gunga HC, Röcker L 1993 Fluid shifts into and out of superficial tissues under microgravity and terrestrial conditions. Clinical Investigator 71:687–689

Krasnoff J, Painter P 1999 The physiological consequences of bed rest and inactivity. Advances in Renal Replacement Therapy 6:124–132

Lackner JR, DiZio P 2000 Human orientation and movement control in weightless and artificial gravity environments. Experimental Brain Research 130:2–26

Lane HW 1992 Energy requirements for spaceflight. Journal of Nutrition 122:13–18

Lane HW, Schoeller DA 2000 Nutrition in spaceflight and weightless models. CRC Press, Boca Raton, FL

Lathers C, Charles JB, Elton KF, Holt TA, Mukai C, Bennett BS, Bungo MW 1989 Acute hemodynamic responses to weightlessness in humans. Journal of Clinical Pharmacology 29:615–627

Leblanc AD, Schneider VS, Evans HJ, Engelbretson DA, Krebs JM 1990 Bone mineral loss and recovery after 17 weeks of bed rest. Journal of Bone and Mineral Research 5:843–850

Leblanc A, Schneider V, Spector E, Evans H, Rowe R, Lane H, Demers L, Lipton A 1995 Calcium absorption, endogenous secretion and endocrine changes during and after long-term bed rest. Bone 16:301S–304S

Levine BD, Buckey JC, Fritsch JM, Yancy CW Jr, Watenpaugh DE, Snell PG, Lane LD, Eckberg DL, Blomqvist CG 1991 Physical fitness and cardiovascular regulation: mechanisms of orthostatic intolerance. Journal of Applied Physiology 70:112–122

Lipman RL, Ulvedal F, Schnure JJ, Bradley EM, Lecocq FR 1970 Gluco-regulatory hormone response to 2-deoxy-d-glucose infusion in normal subjects at bed rest. Metabolism 19:980

Moss ML 1991 Bone as a connected cellular network: modeling and testing. In: Ross G (ed) Topics in biomechanical engineering. Pergamon, New York, 117–119

Mundy G, Garrett R, Harris S, Chan J, Chen D, Rossini G, Boyce B, Zhao M, Gutierrez G 1999 Stimulation of bone formation in vitro and in rodents by statins. Science 286:1946–1949

Nelson GA 1996 Radiation in microgravity. In: Fregly MJ, Blatteis CM (eds) Handbook of physiology, section 4: environmental physiology, the gravitational environment, volume II. Oxford University Press, New York, 785–798

Nicogossian AE, Sawin CF, Grigoriev AI 1994 Countermeasures to space deconditioning. In: Nicogossian AE, Huntoon CL, Pool SL (eds) Space physiology and medicine, 3rd edn. Lea and Febiger, Philadelphia, 447–467

Nishimura Y, Fukuoka H, Kiriyama M, Suzuki Y, Oyama K, Ikawa S, Higurashi M, Gunji A 1994 Bone turnover and calcium metabolism during 20 days bed rest in young healthy males and females. Acta Physiologica 150(suppl 616):27–35

Nixon JV, Murray RG, Bryant C, Johnson RL, Mitchell JH, Holland OB, Gomez-Sanchez C, Vergne-Marini P, Blomqvist CG 1979 Early cardiovascular adaptation to simulated zero gravity. Journal of Applied Physiology 46:541–548

Nordin BEC 1997 Calcium and osteoporosis. Nutrition 13:664–686

Olszewski WL, Engeset A, Sokolowski J 1977 Lymph flow and protein in the normal male leg during lying, getting up and walking. Lymphology 10:178–183

Ott SM 1993 When bone mass fails to predict bone failure. Calcified Tissue International 53:S7–S13

Paiva M, Estenne M, Engel LA 1989 Lung volume, chest wall configuration and pattern of breathing in microgravity. Journal of Applied Physiology 67:1542–1550

Palumbo C, Palazzini S, Marotti G 1990 Morphological study of intercellular functions during osteocyte differentiation. Bone 11:401–406

Parving HH, Rossing N, Nielsen SL, Lassen NA 1974 Increased transcapillary escape rate of albumin, IgG and IgM after plasma volume expansion. American Journal of Physiology 227:245–250

Perhonen MA, Zuckerman JH, Levine BD 2001 Deterioration of left ventricular chamber performance after bed rest. Circulation 103:1851–1857

Planel H 2004 Space and life. CRC Press, Boca Raton, FL

Prisk GK, Guy HJB, Elliott AR, Deutschmann III RA, West JB 1993 Pulmonary diffusing capacity, capillary blood volume and cardiac output during sustained microgravity. Journal of Applied Physiology 75:15–26

Prisk GK, Guy HJB, Elliott AR, West JB 1994 Inhomogeneity of pulmonary perfusion during sustained microgravity on SLS-1. Journal of Applied Physiology 76:1730–1738

Prisk GK, Elliott AR, Guy HJB, Verbanck S, Paiva M, West JB 1998 Multiple-breath washing of helium and sulfur hexafluoride in sustained microgravity. Journal of Applied Physiology 84:244–252

Prisk GK, Paiva M, West JB (eds) 2001 Gravity and the lung. Marcel Dekker, New York

Prisk GK, Finel JM, Cooper TK, West JB 2006 Vital capacity, respiratory muscle strength and pulmonary gas exchange during long-duration exposure to microgravity. Journal of Applied Physiology 101:439–447

Reichel A, Rother U, Werner J, Reichel F 1976 On the transport of various endogenous plasma proteins from blood to peripheral lymph in man. Lymphology 9:118–121

Reid MB, Loring SH, Banzett RB, Mead J 1986 Passive mechanics of upright human chest wall during immersion from hips to neck. Journal of Applied Physiology 60:1561–1570

Renkin EM 1986 Some consequences of capillary permeability to macromolecules: Starling's hypothesis reconsidered. American Journal of Physiology 250:H706–H710

Rössler A, Hinghofer-Szalkay H 2003 Hyaluronan fragments: an information-carrying system? Hormone and Metabolic Research 35:1–3

Rubin CT, Lanyon LE 1987 Osteoregulatory nature of mechanical stimuli: function as a determinant for adaptive bone remodeling. Journal of Orthopedic Research 5:300–310

Sauren YMHF, Mieremet RHP, Groot CG, Scherft JP 1992 An electron microscopic study on the presence of proteoglycans in the mineralized matrix of rat and human compact lamellar bone. Anatomical Record 232:36–44

Schmitt HH 2006 Return to the Moon. Copernicus, New York, 305

Schnitzer JE 1993 Update on the cellular and molecular basis of capillary permeability. Trends in Cardiovascular Medicine 3:124–130

Schnitzler CM 1993 Bone quality: a determinant for certain risk factors for bone fragility. Calcified Tissue International 53:S27–S31

Sides MB, Vernikos J, Convertino VA, Stepanek J, Tripp LD, Draeger J, Hargens AR, Kourtidou-Papadeli C, Pavy-LeTraon A, Russomano T, Wong JY, Buccello RR, Lee PH, Nangalia V, Saary MJ 2005 The Bellagio report. Cardiovascular risks of spaceflight: implications for the future of space travel. Aviation, Space and Environmental Medicine 76:877–895

Smith SM, Wastney ME, O'Brien KO, Morukov BV, Larina IM, Abrams SA, Davis-Street JE, Oganov V, Shackelford LC 2005a Bone markers, calcium metabolism and calcium kinetics during extended-duration spaceflight on the Mir Space Station. Journal of Bone and Mineral Research 20(2):208–218

Smith SM, Zwart SR, Block G, Rice BL, Davis-Street JE 2005b The nutritional status of astronauts is altered after long-term spaceflight aboard the International Space Station. Journal of Nutrition 135:437–443

Sone T, Imai Y, Tomomitsu T, Fukunaga M 1998 Calcaneus as a site for the assessment of bone mass. Bone 22:155S–157S

Spaak J, Montmerle S, Sundblad P, Linnarsson D 2005 Long-term bed rest-induced reductions in stroke volume during rest and exercise: cardiac dysfunction vs. volume depletion. Journal of Applied Physiology 98:648–654

Stein TP 2002 Spaceflight and oxidative stress. Nutrition 8:867–871

Stein TP, Wade CE 2005 Metabolic consequences of muscle disuse atrophy. Journal of Nutrition 135:1824S–1828S

Stein TP, Schulter MD, Boden G 1994 Development of insulin resistance by astronauts during spaceflight. Aviation, Space and Environmental Medicine 65:1091–1096

Sulzman FM, Genin AM (eds) 1994 Space biology and medicine, volume II, life support and habitability. American Institute of Aeronautics and Astronautics, Washington, DC

Takano Y, Turner CH, Owan I, Martin RB, Lau ST, Forwood MR, Burr DB 1999 Elastic anisotropy and collagen orientation of osteonal bone are dependent on the mechanical strain distribution. Journal of Orthopaedic Research 17:59–66

Taylor GR 1993 Overview of spaceflight immunology studies. Journal of Leukocyte Biology 54:179–188

Taylor NAS, Morrison JB 1991 Lung volume changes in response to altered breathing gas pressure during upright immersion. European Journal of Applied Physiology 62:122–129

Taylor NAS, Morrison JB 1999 Static respiratory muscle work during immersion with positive and negative respiratory loading. Journal of Applied Physiology 87:1397–1403

Thornton WE, Hedge V, Coleman E, Uri JJ, Moore TP 1992 Changes in leg volume during microgravity simulation. Aviation, Space and Environmental Medicine 63:789–794

Tobin BW, Uchakin PN, Leeper-Woodford SK 2002 Insulin secretion and sensitivity in spaceflight: diabetogenic effects. Nutrition 18:842–848

Trappe T, Trappe S, Lee G, Widrick J, Fitts R, Costill C 2006 Cardiorespiratory responses to physical work during and following 17 days of bed rest and spaceflight. Journal of Applied Physiology 100:951–957

Van Der Wiel HE, Lips P, Nauta J, Netelenbos JC, Hazenberg GJ 1991 Biochemical parameters of bone turnover during ten days of bed rest and subsequent mobilization. Bone and Mineral 13:123–129

Vico L, Chappard D, Alexandre C, Palle S, Minaire P, Riffat G, Morukov B, Rakhmanov S 1987 Effects of a 120-day period of bed-rest on bone mass and bone cell activities in man: attempts at countermeasure. Bone and Mineral 2:383–394

Vogel G 1999 Capturing the promise of youth. Science 286:2238–2239

Vogel JM, Wasnich RD, Ross PD 1988 The clinical relevance of calcaneus bone mineral measurements: a review. Bone and Mineral 5:35–58

Watenpaugh DE 2001 Fluid volume control during short-term spaceflight and implications for human performance. Journal of Experimental Biology 204:3209–3215

White RJ 1998 Weightlessness and the human body. Scientific American 279:39–43

White RJ, Averner M 2001 Humans in space. Nature 409:1115–1118

White RJ, Blomqvist CG 1998 Central venous pressure and cardiac function during spaceflight. Journal of Applied Physiology 85:738–746

Zerwekh JE, Ruml LA, Gottschalk F, Pak CYC 1998 The effects of twelve weeks of bed rest on bone histology, biochemical markers of bone turnover and calcium homeostasis in eleven normal subjects. Journal of Bone and Mineral Research 13:1594–1601

Zwart SR, Davis-Street JE, Paddon-Jones D, Ferrando AA, Wolfe RR, Smith SM 2005 Amino acid supplementation alters bone metabolism during simulated weightlessness. Journal of Applied Physiology 99:134–140

Chapter **27**

Topical debates

Chapter 27.1

Do humans have selective brain cooling?

Lars Nybo   Matthew D. White

Selective brain cooling is defined as a lowering of the average brain temperature below that of arterial blood (IUPS Thermal Physiology Commission 2001). The case for selective cooling has been demonstrated in animals with a carotid rete (Jessen 2001, Mitchell et al. 2002). Whilst humans lack such an anatomical structure, the basis for cooling arterial blood prior to its reaching the brain may exist (Rubenstein et al. 1960). However, there is a long-standing debate among thermal physiologists on the existence, or non-existence, of this temperature gradient in hyperthermic humans. In this chapter, the scientific evidence from both sides of this debate will be reviewed.

Part A: The case against
Lars Nybo

The idea that humans, like several animal species, are capable of selectively cooling the brain during exercise-induced hyperthermia has arisen from the observation that tympanic membrane temperature may be reduced below that of other body core temperature measurement sites (oesophageal or rectal), if active cooling is applied to the head (Brinnel et al. 1987, Cabanac & Caputa 1979a, Cabanac et al. 1987, Nagasaka et al. 1998). However, it is important to emphasise that, although the tympanic membrane is located close to the surface of the brain, it is neither a true nor reliable index of the global brain temperature.

As demonstrated in Figure 27.1.1, tympanic temperature follows arterial and jugular venous temperatures during exercise with progressive hyperthermia (uncompensable heat stress), when no fanning is applied to the head. However, the deviation between the tympanic and internal jugular blood temperature during facial fanning signifies that the average brain temperature and tympanic temperature are independent in humans (Shiraki et al. 1988). Thus, evidence for selective brain cooling based on measurements of the tympanic membrane temperature should be disre-

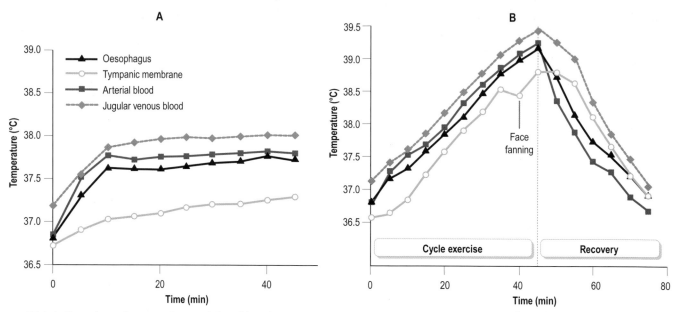

Figure 27.1.1 Oesophageal, tympanic, arterial and jugular venous temperature responses during cycling ($N = 7$) with a normal core temperature response (A: control), and during a similar exercise bout with progressive hyperthermia (B). Standard deviations are omitted for clarity, but were in the range of 0.1–0.3°C. Reprinted from Nybo et al. (2002) with permission.

garded, as membrane temperature is influenced by the skin temperature of the head, while the average brain temperature remains unaffected by such changes.

It should be noted that brain temperatures are not evenly distributed, and that some superficial layers of the brain, especially areas close to the nasal cavities, may be lower than the body core, and affected by pulmonary ventilation (Mariak et al. 1999). However, these subdural temperatures are not representative of the average brain temperature, and, unlike some animal species, it appears that humans are not able to establish a global brain temperature which is lower than that of the trunk and aortic blood.

Selective brain cooling is best achieved in animals with a carotid rete, such as the artiodactyls and felids (Jessen 2001, Mitchell et al. 2002). In humans, aortic blood and the tissue adjacent to the internal carotid artery have similar temperatures at rest when the ventilation is normal. However, we have previously observed that the temperature of connective tissue adjacent to the internal carotid artery may be ~2°C lower than the aortic blood temperature during exercise with hyperthermia, and ~1°C lower during voluntary hyperventilation (Nybo et al. 2002). Therefore, when pulmonary ventilation increases, this temperature gradient makes it physically possible for arterial blood to release heat during its passage from the heart to the brain (Hanson 1974). However, the transit time of blood within the carotid artery is too short, and the blood will not equilibrate with the thermal energy content of the surrounding tissues (Crezee & Lagendijk 1992). According to measures of cerebral heat balance, it appears that blood temperature is lowered by <0.09°C on its passage from the body core to the brain (Nybo et al. 2002).

This loss of thermal energy is not sufficient to lower brain temperature below that of aortic blood (body core). Both at rest and during exercise, the human brain has an average metabolic rate of 3–3.5 mL O_2·100 g cerebral tissue^{-1}·min^{-1} (Lassen 1985, Madsen et al. 1993). This corresponds to a cerebral heat production of ~0.6 J·g^{-1}·min^{-1}, and cerebral heat balance is established with a jugular venous to arterial temperature difference of ~0.3°C and a cerebral blood flow of ~50 mL·100 g cerebral tissue^{-1}·min^{-1} (Nybo et al. 2002, Yablonskiy et al. 2000). This temperature difference, especially that between the jugular vein and aortic arch, may be narrowed to 0.2°C during exercise, due to precooling of arterial blood. But, as seen in Figure 27.1.1, the jugular venous blood, and hence the brain, remains warmer than the body core.

The precooling of arterial blood during its passage through the carotid artery could be considered as a form of brain cooling. However, it is similar during both normothermic and hyperthermic exercise, and it is therefore unlikely that the precooling of arterial blood is a mechanism that can be selectively used during hyperthermic exercise. It has been suggested that selective brain cooling does not take place during normothermia but becomes relevant during hyperthermia (Cabanac 1993). However, in the study represented in Figure 27.1.1, the jugular venous blood temperature was, in all subjects and at all times (including the period with face fanning, which restored head skin temperature to normal levels), higher than the oesophageal and aortic arch temperatures. This was evident even though subjects reached quite high body temperatures; the highest individual core temperature was 40.1°C, with a corresponding jugular venous blood temperature of 40.4°C.

In conclusion, the only direct assessment of the cerebral heat balance in exercising humans demonstrates that the cerebral venous blood temperature, during both normothermia and hyperthermia (with or without facial cooling), is above that of the arterial blood, signifying that the average brain temperature is always higher than that of the body core (Figure 27.1.1; Nybo et al. 2002). Thus, there is no valid scientific evidence for selective brain cooling in humans.

Part B: The supporting position
Matthew White

Following the evidence presented by Baker & Hayward (1967), Magilton & Swift (1968) and Taylor (1966) of selective brain cooling in hyperthermic, non-human mammals, physiologists were intrigued with the possibility that hyperthermic humans might also selectively cool the brain. The potential mechanism(s) for this response, or lack thereof, have previously been reviewed by both the proponents (Cabanac 1986, 1993, Nagasaka et al. 1998) and opponents (Jessen 2001, Mitchell et al. 2002, Nielsen 1988) of human selective brain cooling. The purpose of this contribution is to provide an interpretation and summary of recent results that have either directly demonstrated selective brain cooling in humans, or present evidence that suggests the contrary. In this context, the goal of this counterpoint is to give the reader a balanced integration of these recent results into the existing scientific literature, and to show that such evidence collectively supports the existence of selective brain cooling in hyperthermic humans.

Before discussing the evidence on human selective brain cooling, three background points need to be noted. First, it is exceedingly difficult to obtain direct human intracranial temperature measurements, and this has limited the study of human selective brain cooling. Second, it is difficult to decide which intracranial temperature accurately reflects human brain temperature. This is so because a characteristic of intracranial temperatures for humans (Mariak et al. 1993, Mellergard 1994) and other mammals, including the cat and monkey (Baker et al. 1972), is the presence of pronounced radial temperature gradients from the central cerebral ventricles to the cooler brain surface and meninges. Third, the premise of several human selective brain cooling studies was that tympanic temperature gives an accurate index of intracranial temperature. This index of brain temperature has been validated against intracranial temperatures in humans (Mariak et al. 1994, 2003, Mellergard & Nordstrom 1990) and other mammals (Baker et al. 1972), thus lending credence to studies that have used this measurement site (Cabanac & Caputa 1979a,b). Tympanic temperature gives a global index of intracranial temperatures (Mariak et al. 1994, 2003, Mellergard & Nordstrom 1990), and the criterion for its accurate measurement is that it must be equal to, or greater than, oesophageal temperature during normothermia (Cabanac 1986). This follows from

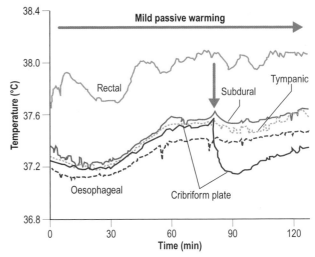

Figure 27.1.2 Time course of intracranial and core temperatures in a patient before and after removal of endotracheal tube (vertical arrow). Restitution of airflow through the upper airways caused intracranial temperature, at the basal aspect of frontal lobes on the cribriform plate, to decrease below that of the core temperature indices (oesophageal, tympanic, rectal) and subdural temperature on the brain convexity. Reproduced from Mariak et al. (1999) with permission.

direct measures of intracranial temperatures in normothermic humans when tympanic and intracranial temperatures exceed oesophageal temperature (Mariak et al. 1999).

The evidence indicates that there are three independent mechanisms that permit humans to selectively cool the brain during hyperthermia: (i) convective and evaporative cooling of the upper airways, leading to cooling of adjacent blood vessels; (ii) cooling venous blood in the scalp, face and head, followed by drainage to the intracranium through valveless emissary and other veins; and (iii) a countercurrent heat exchange in the cavernous sinus between warm arterial blood in the internal carotid arteries supplying the cranium, and the cooled venous blood in the internal jugular veins that has drained from the face, scalp and head.

Some of the first intracranial temperatures measured in conscious, hyperthermic humans were provided by Mariak and colleagues (1999). Figure 27.1.2 gives an example of these data, which were recorded prior to, and following upper airway extubation. During passive warming prior to extubation, there was no evidence of selective brain cooling, with cribriform exceeding oesophageal temperature. However, after extubation, the precipitous drop in cribriform temperature to less than oesophageal temperature is direct evidence of selective brain cooling in humans. In these same volunteers, subsequent volitional hyperventilation elicited repeatable decreases in cribriform temperature (Mariak et al. 1999). Together, these results support the possibility that heat loss from the upper airways is an important avenue of heat loss, and contributes to selective brain cooling in mildly hyperthermic humans.

Selective brain cooling includes surface cooling on the scalp, face and head, followed by the drainage of this cooled blood, including that from the pteryroid plexus, through bidirectional valveless emissary veins to the intracranium, and subsequently to dural venous sinuses, as well as the internal jugular veins. Sweat secretion on the forehead and face is especially pronounced relative to other body surfaces (Hertzman 1957), and surface cooling due to evaporation is a prerequisite for this avenue of selective brain cooling, although sweating and evaporation are not necessarily equivalent (Chapter 19). In humans, the directional nature of blood flow in the emissary veins was demonstrated by Cabanac & Brinnel (1985), and confirmed by Nagasaka et al. (1990) to travel from the scalp to intracranium during hyperthermia, and to be either absent or travel from the intracranium to the scalp during hypothermia. Data from face fanning support this selective brain cooling mechanism (Mariak et al. 2003); however, this brain cooling does not appear to extend to the brainstem (Deklunder 1992, Mekjavic et al. 2002).

Recently, Nybo et al. (2002) measured blood temperatures in exercising humans, at the aortic arch (inflow) and the jugular bulb of the internal jugular vein (outflow). They suggested that, since internal jugular temperatures were greater than aortic arch temperatures during hyperthermic or normothermic exercise, no counter-current heat exchange was possible in the cavernous sinus, and these humans did not display a selective brain cooling. However, an alternative interpretation of these data is possible.

First, the blood temperatures measured were all extracranial. The unspecified location of one thermocouple within the jugular bulb was at the base of the cranium. There are two jugular bulbs in each internal jugular vein, and the bulb used could have been at the level of the clavicles or just inferior to the jugular foramen. Arterial blood temperature was measured at about the level of the clavicles. Thus, both temperatures were measured in either the neck or thoracic regions, and their values should mirror thoracic or oesophageal temperatures more so than cranial temperatures during exercise.

Second, although the ambient conditions were not described, a companion paper (Nybo & Nielsen 2001), with presumably the same conditions and volunteers, described high air temperatures and humidity. Such conditions are likely to impede or block contributions to selective brain cooling from evaporative heat loss in the upper airways, face and scalp (Chapter 19). It is possible that, in these ambient conditions, neither of these two main avenues of cranial heat loss would have been effective enough to allow normal cranial thermoregulation or selective brain cooling.

Third, the authors suggested there was a reduction of ~20% in cerebral blood flow, in both the middle cerebral artery (transcranial Doppler sonometry; $N = 7$) and globally (Kety–Schmidt method; $N = 3$). These decreases were reasoned to be a function of cerebral hypocapnia, induced by the hyperthermia-induced hyperventilation, and resulting in cerebral vasoconstriction (Nybo & Nielsen 2001). This decrease was, in part, suggested to be accounted for by a ~5% decrease in cardiac output (Nybo & Nielsen 2001). These observations collectively indicate that the autoregulation of cerebral blood flow was abandoned in these participants. However, other studies with either submaximal (Thomas et al. 1989) or hyperthermic maximal (González-Alonso et al. 2004) exercise report an increase in cerebral blood flow, as would be expected for any tissue with an elevated metabolic rate. Furthermore, a similar exercise study illustrated that cardiac output was increased or maintained during hyperthermia (MacDougall et al. 1974).

A reduction in cranial blood flow will diminish the convective heat load delivered to the brain (Nybo et al. 2002). However, if mass is conserved, reduced inflow would be coupled with a reduced venous efflux, and this would increase the cranial heat load by lowering the brain-to-blood heat exchange. Figure 27.1.1 demonstrates a relatively constant venous to arterial temperature gradient, despite the lower cranial blood flow and a 7% increase in cerebral metabolic heat production. If convective heat transfer to the intracranial blood is the main mechanism for cranial heat removal, it is not apparent why, with a 20% reduction in cranial blood perfusion, there was no influence on the arterial-to-venous temperature gradient. It was argued that there was cranial heat storage during hyperthermic exercise, but this would need to be reflected by a progressive elevation of the internal jugular above arterial influx temperatures. Their own evidence does not support this view.

An alternative explanation for these results is the possibility of dilation of the middle cerebral artery and possibly other large cerebral arteries during exercise (González-Alonso et al. 2004, Thomas et al. 1989), when core temperatures approached 39°C. Rearranging Poiseuille's Law ($\dot{Q} = \Delta P \cdot \pi r^4 / 8\eta l$) for resistance to blood flow in blood vessels shows that blood flow ($\dot{Q}$) is directly proportional to perfusion pressure (ΔP), blood vessel radius (r) raised to the fourth power, and inversely proportional to blood viscosity (η) for a given straight length (l) of a blood vessel. Accordingly, a 20% decrease in cerebral blood flow could result from a blood vessel radial reduction of only 5%.

Alternatively, such results could be explained in the presence of a constant or elevated blood flow to the cranium via the internal carotid artery (MacDougall et al. 1974). A small degree of middle cerebral artery or global cranial vasodilatation (González-Alonso et al. 2004, Thomas et al. 1989) will increase cranial perfusion, and this is consistent with the reported velocity reduction. This would be coupled with an elevated venous efflux to internal jugular vein. To maintain a constant arterial–venous temperature difference, despite an elevated metabolic heat production, surface cooling would be needed from the face and scalp, with the cooled venous blood directed intracranially through emissary veins (Cabanac & Brinnel 1985). This is evidence of intracranial selective brain cooling, and the explanation is consistent with an autoregulation of cranial blood flow so as to match an elevated cranial heat production.

Finally, in the treatment state, participants were rendered hyperthermic through exercise, whilst wearing an impermeable suit and rubber gloves, with only the head exposed (Nybo et al. 2002). This very stressful exercise might induce a fight-or-flight response, during which selective brain cooling is now suggested to be abandoned (Jessen 2001, Mitchell et al. 2002). However, in the control (normothermic) trials (Nybo et al. 2002), a relatively greater drop of tympanic temperature from thoracic temperatures was evident, supporting selective brain cooling. Figure 27.1.1 shows that, early during normothermic exercise, tympanic temperature was ~0.47°C below aortic blood temperature. This difference increased to ~0.88°C at the mid-exercise point, and it remained ~0.72°C at the end of exercise. Thus, in the control state, there was a lowering of cranial (as reflected by tympanic) temperature below aortic temperature and this closely follows the definition of selective brain cooling. As such, these results support a selective brain cooling during a non-fight-or-flight, exercise-induced hyperthermia, as previously demonstrated (Cabanac & Caputa 1979a,b, White & Cabanac 1996).

In conclusion, the recent and past evidence supports the existence of selective brain cooling in hyperthermic humans. Three main avenues of heat loss for this response have been described. These include heat loss from the airways, that gives a selective brain cooling on the cribriform plate; surface cooling of blood from the face and head, followed by drainage of cooled venous blood to the intracranial space; and counter-current heat exchange between a main arterial supply to cranium (internal carotid) and the internal jugular vein.

Part C: Rebuttal
Lars Nybo

First, it is important to note that a single brain temperature measured in the superficial layers of the brain may not be representative of the average brain temperature, since temperatures in the brain are heterogeneously distributed (Nybo & Secher 2004, Yablonskiy et al. 2000). Second, any conclusion based on tympanic temperature is likely to be unreliable, since this measure can be contaminated by the skin temperature of the head, if these temperatures are different. Therefore, at present, the closest assessment of the average brain temperature in exercising and resting humans is provided from the temperature of the cerebral mixed-venous blood in the internal jugular vein. Since convective heat transfer between the tissue and capillaries is a very fast process (Pennes 1948), the temperature of the blood passing the cerebral capillaries will equilibrate with that of the cerebral tissue (Yablonskiy et al. 2000).

Jugular venous temperature is measured using a catheter inserted retrogradely into the internal jugular vein (Seldinger technique) and advanced toward the brain as far as possible. At the sample site (catheter tip), where the vein leaves the cranium, more than 98% of the blood is of intracranial origin, as verified by >50 years of research studying cerebral metabolism and circulation (Friberg et al. 1986, Ide & Secher 2000, Kety & Schmidt 1948, Madsen et al. 1993). In our hands, the thermocouple probe was always advanced at least 0.5 cm further to measure temperature even closer to the cerebral capillaries and the brain tissue.

The jugular vein–arterial temperature difference remains relatively unchanged and is always positive, because the temperature of blood that enters and leaves the brain rises in parallel. This indicates that heat removal from the brain via the blood remains fairly stable. Dr White states that cerebral heat accumulation (resulting in an increased brain temperature) '. . . would need to be reflected by a progressive elevation of the internal jugular above arterial influx temperatures'. However, the arteriovenous temperature difference does not reflect absolute brain tissue temperature, but the rate of heat release. The same can be observed in exercising muscle, where the arteriovenous temperature difference stabilises at ~0.4°C, while the arterial, femoral vein blood temperature and the temperature of the muscle tissue gradually rises to more than 40°C (González-Alonso et al. 1999). The only way that the venous blood can remain, or become warmer than the arterial blood, is because the perfused tissue has a temperature that is higher than the arterial blood, and equal to or slightly higher than that of the venous blood. This will be the case for both the brain and exercising muscle.

Concerning our previous research (Nybo et al. 2002), the room temperature was 20°C, with the subject heat stressed simply by exercising in impermeable clothing. Thus, the subjects were actually inspiring air that was ~20°C cooler than the arterial blood temperature, and it was much lower than the air temperature normally inhaled when subjects are exposed to environmental heat stress. Furthermore, when we lowered the overall head skin temperature to a level >6°C cooler than the arterial and jugular vein temperatures, the arteriovenous temperature difference remained unchanged, whilst the jugular venous blood temperature kept increasing.

In accordance with the work of Friberg et al. (1986), this confirms that our cerebral venous blood temperatures were not contaminated by the temperature of extracranial blood. In contrast, tympanic temperature was affected by lowering head skin temperature because this measure is not representative of intracranial temperature but was contaminated by skin temperature, since venous blood from the surface of the head passes the ear drum. With our head cooling procedure, we created a condition where all extracranial temperatures (skin, tissues adjacent to the carotid arteries, inhaled air) were much lower than the arterial blood. Yet, we observed that the blood leaving the brain was warmer than the body core and blood entering the brain. This is only possible because the cerebral tissue, due to its metabolic heat production, has a temperature higher than that of the body core (and arterial blood). As noted above, the main route for cranial heat removal is via the blood, since the rate of heat release through the skull is very limited.

It is true that cerebral blood flow is reduced during exercise with hyperthermia; we have measured this with a technique that quantifies arterial inflow, and with the Kety–Schmidt technique, which provides a measure of the global cerebral outflow. However, this reduction is not due to a failure of cerebral autoregulation, but relates to a hyperventilation-induced reduction of the arterial carbon dioxide content and thus a reduction in cerebral perfusion. The regulation of regional and global cerebral blood flow is complex, but under the present conditions, the arterial carbon dioxide tension appears to become the dominant factor determining cerebral blood flow (Ide & Secher 2000, Nybo & Secher 2004). However, since the cerebral circulation removes heat from the brain and not the other way around as stated by Dr White, this actually implies that less heat is removed from the brain tissue.

It is true that our subjects were exposed to stressful conditions, as indicated by increased circulating catecholamine concentrations. However, hyperthermic humans *are* stressed, especially when exercising, and we did not observe noradrenaline or adrenaline concentrations that differed from other studies with combined exercise and heat stress. It is also correct that some animals capable of selective brain cooling rarely utilise this ability when they are stressed by the presence of humans. However, this applies to animals with a carotid rete, where arterial blood destined for the brain loses heat to venous blood returning from evaporative surfaces in the upper respiratory tract. During laboratory experiments, fear-associated activation of the sympathetic nervous system appears to interfere with the animal's ability to utilise selective brain cooling since stress may alter the route for venous drainage of the cool extracranial blood. This does not apply to humans as we do not have a carotid rete, and therefore only a very limited possibility to precool the arterial blood before it reaches the brain. Furthermore, humans have a brain with a high metabolic rate and consequently the cerebral heat production is

of such a magnitude that it is impossible to establish an average brain temperature that is lower than the body core.

Part D: Rebuttal
Matthew White

In the first paragraph of his section, Dr Nybo's dismissal of tympanic temperature as a true and reliable index of global brain temperature is based mainly on hearsay. The only evidence to support his statements was data from a young normothermic patient with elevated intracranial pressure, where selective brain cooling is known not to occur. This pressure elevation impairs venous return from the scalp, and prevents brain cooling. This is demonstrated by tympanic temperature remaining 1.3°C higher in febrile hydrocephalic children than in febrile controls (Chmielowa et al. 1980). Indeed, the evidence of direct intracranial temperature measurements in adult humans that does exist supports that tympanic temperature is a true and reliable index of global brain temperature (Mariak et al. 1999, 2003).

From Figure 27.1.1B, Dr Nybo suggests face fanning influenced tympanic independently from oesophageal or other extra-cranial blood temperatures. However, it is clear at time zero in their exercise trials that tympanic temperature was lower than oesophageal temperature, indicating the temperature probe had not been correctly placed on the tympanic membrane. As such, this was not a correctly measured cranial temperature, and shows that aural canal temperature was influenced by fanning, as one would expect for any other surface skin temperature.

It needs to be emphasised that Dr Nybo follows a 'black box' approach to the study of human cranial heat balance. Blood inflow temperature measurements are made in the thorax at the level of the clavicles, and the outflow temperatures are measured in the internal jugular vein. This approach ignores heat exchange to and from the cranium, and temperatures within the cranium. Surface heat loss from the head during exercise is substantial (Rasch et al. 1991), and needs to be considered to understand cranial heat balance and selective brain cooling in hyperthermic humans.

References

Baker MA, Hayward JN 1967 Carotid rete and brain temperature of cat. Nature 216(111):139–141

Baker MA, Stocking RA, Meehan JP 1972 Thermal relationship between tympanic membrane and hypothalamus in conscious cat and monkey. Journal of Applied Physiology 32(6):739–742

Brinnel H, Nagasaka T, Cabanac M 1987 Enhanced brain protection during passive hyperthermia in humans. European Journal of Applied Physiology 56:540–545

Cabanac M 1986 Keeping a cool head. News in Physiological Sciences 1:41–43

Cabanac M 1993 Selective brain cooling in humans: 'fancy' or fact? FASEB Journal 7(12):1143–1146

Cabanac M, Brinnel H 1985 Blood flow in the emissary veins of the human head during hyperthermia. European Journal of Applied Physiology 54(2):172–176

Cabanac M, Caputa M 1979a Open loop increase in trunk temperature produced by face cooling in working humans. Journal of Physiology (London) 289:163–174

Cabanac M, Caputa M 1979b Natural selective cooling of the human brain: evidence of its occurrence and magnitude. Journal of Physiology (London) 286:255–264

Cabanac M, Germain M, Brinnel H 1987 Tympanic temperatures during hemiface cooling. European Journal of Applied Physiology 56:534–539

Chmielowa M, Kielczewska-Mrozikiewicz D, Skuratowicz A 1980 Temperatura blony bebenkowej w niektorych scherzeniach goraczkowych. Roczn. A. M Jbznan 1:157–160

Crezee J, Lagendijk JJW 1992 Temperature uniformity during hyperthermia: the impact of large vessels. Physics in Medicine and Biology 37:1321–1337

Deklunder G 1992 Influence of ventilation of the face on thermoregulation on man during hyper- and hypothermia. European Journal of Applied Physiology 64:282

Friberg L, Kastrup J, Hansen M, Bulow J 1986 Cerebral effects of scalp cooling and extracerebral contribution to calculated blood flow values using the intravenous 133Xe technique. Scandinavian Journal of Clinical Laboratory Investigation 46(4):375–379

González-Alonso J, Calbet J, Nielsen B 1999 Metabolic and thermodynamic responses to dehydration-induced reductions in muscle blood flow in exercising humans. Journal of Physiology 520(2):577–589

González-Alonso J, Dalsgaard M, Osada T, Volianitis S, Dawson E, Yoshiga C 2004 Brain and central haemodynamics and oxygenation during maximal exercise in humans. Journal of Physiology (London) 557(1):331–342

Hanson RDG 1974 Respiratory heat loss at increased core temperature. Journal of Applied Physiology 37:103–107

Hertzman AB 1957 Individual differences in regional sweating. Journal of Applied Physiology 10(2):242–248

Ide K, Secher N 2000 Cerebral blood flow and metabolism during exercise. Progress in Neurobiology 61:397–414

IUPS Thermal Physiology Commission 2001 Glossary of terms for thermal physiology, 3rd edn. Revised by the Commission for Thermal Physiology of the International Union of Physiological Sciences. Japanese Journal of Physiology 51(2):245–280

Jessen C 2001 Selective brain cooling in mammals and birds. Japanese Journal of Physiology 51(3):291–301

Kety SS, Schmidt CF 1948 The nitrous oxide method for the quantitative determination of cerebral blood flow in man: theory, procedure and normal values. Journal of Clinical Investigation 27:476–483

Lassen NA 1985 Normal average value of CBF in young adults is 50 ml/100 g/min (editorial). Journal of Cerebral Blood Flow and Metabolism 5:347–349

MacDougall JD, Reddan WG, Layton CR, Dempsey JA 1974 Effects of metabolic hyperthermia on performance during heavy prolonged exercise. Journal of Applied Physiology 36(5):538–544

Madsen PL, Sperling BK, Warming T, Schmidt JF, Secher NH, Wildschiødtz G, Holm S, Lassen NA 1993 Middle cerebral artery blood velocity and cerebral blood flow and O$_2$ uptake during dynamic exercise. Journal of Applied Physiology 74:245–250

Magilton J, Swift C 1968 Description of two physiological heat exchange systems for the control of brain temperature. In: IEEE Conference Record: Fifth Annual Rocky Mountain Bioengineering Symposium, pp 24–27

Mariak Z, Bondyra Z, Piekarska M 1993 The temperature within the circle of Willis versus tympanic temperature in resting normothermic humans. European Journal of Applied Physiology 66(6):518–520

Mariak Z, Lewko J, Luczaj J, Polocki B, White MD 1994 The relationship between directly measured human cerebral and tympanic temperatures during changes in brain temperatures. European Journal of Applied Physiology 69(6):545–549

Mariak Z, White MD, Lewko J, Lyson T, Piekarski P 1999 Direct cooling of the human brain by heat loss from the upper respiratory tract. Journal of Applied Physiology 87(5):1609–1613

Mariak Z, White MD, Lyson T, Lewko J 2003 Tympanic temperature reflects intracranial temperature changes in humans. Pflugers Archives 446(2):279–284

Mekjavic IB, Rogelj K, Radobuljac M, Eiken O 2002 Inhalation of warm and cold air does not influence brain stem or core temperature in normothermic humans. Journal of Applied Physiology 93(1):65–69

Mellergard P 1994 Monitoring of rectal, epidural and intraventricular temperature in neurosurgical patients. Acta Neurochirurgica Suppl (Wien) 60:485–487

Mellergard P, Nordstrom CH 1990 Epidural temperature and possible intracerebral temperature gradients in man. British Journal of Neurosurgery 4(1):31–38

Mitchell D, Maloney SK, Jessen C, Laburn HP, Kamerman PR, Mitchell G 2002 Adaptive heterothermy and selective brain cooling in arid-zone mammals. Comparative Biochemistry and Physiology. Part B, Biochemistry and Molecular Biology 131(4):571–585

Nagasaka T, Hirashita M, Tanabe M, Sakurada S, Brinnel H 1990 Role of the veins in the face in brain cooling during body warming in human subjects. Japanese Journal of Biometeorology 27:113–120

Nagasaka T, Brinnel H, Hales JRS, Ogawa T 1998 Selective brain cooling in hyperthermia – the mechanisms and medical implications. Medical Hypotheses 50(3):203–211

Nielsen B 1988 Natural cooling of the brain during outdoor bicycling? Pflugers Archives 411:456–461

Nybo L, Nielsen B 2001 Middle cerebral artery blood velocity is reduced with hyperthermia during prolonged exercise in humans. Journal of Physiology 534(Pt 1):279–286

Nybo L, Secher NH 2004 Cerebral perturbations provoked by prolonged exercise. Progress in Neurobiology 72:223–261

Nybo L, Secher NH, Nielsen B 2002 Inadequate heat release from the human brain during prolonged exercise with hyperthermia. Journal of Physiology 545:697–704

Pennes HH 1948 Analysis of tissue and arterial blood temperatures in the resting human forearm. Journal of Applied Physiology 1:93–122

Rasch W, Samson P, Cote J, Cabanac M 1991 Heat loss from the human head during exercise. Journal of Applied Physiology 71:590–595

Rubenstein E, Meub D, Eldridge F 1960 Common carotid blood temperature. Journal of Applied Physiology 15:603–604

Shiraki K, Sagawa S, Tajima F, Yokota A, Hashimoto M, Brengelmann GL 1988 Independence of brain and tympanic temperatures in an unanesthetized human. Journal of Applied Physiology 65:482–486

Taylor CR 1966 The vascularity and possible thermoregulatory function of horns in goats. Physiological Zoology 39:127–139

Thomas SN, Schroeder T, Secher NH, Mitchell JH 1989 Cerebral blood flow during submaximal and maximal dynamic exercise in humans. Journal of Applied Physiology 67(2):744–748

White MD, Cabanac M 1996 Exercise hyperpnea and hyperthermia in humans. Journal of Applied Physiology 81(3):1249–1254

Yablonskiy DA, Ackerman J, Raichle ME 2000 Coupling between changes in human brain temperature and oxidative metabolism during prolonged visual stimulation. Proceedings of the National Academy of Sciences 97:7603–7608

Chapter **27.2**

A critical core temperature and the significance of absolute work rate

José González–Alonso   Ola Eiken   Igor B. Mekjavic

Body core temperature increases in response to physical exercise (metabolic heat production; Chapter 19). In this chapter, two issues are discussed regarding this exercise-induced rise in core temperature, and these have been the focus of much controversy over the last few decades. First is the manner in which core temperature is regulated during exercise (see Chapter 18), while the second is how this rise in core temperature may influence exercise performance.

1 REGULATION OF CORE TEMPERATURE DURING EXERCISE

In 1938, Marius Nielsen demonstrated that, in response to prolonged leg exercise performed at a steady work rate, core temperature increased and then stabilised at an elevated level. The exercise-induced elevation in core temperature was similar across a wide range of ambient temperatures, suggesting to Nielsen that the increase is a well-regulated response, rather than the result of a failure of heat-dissipating mechanisms to cope with the increased heat production. This finding raised the question as to what determines the level of core temperature increase during exercise.

Two parallel avenues of research emanated from this simple observation. One avenue focused on the manner in which exercise might cause a change in the level at which core temperature was being regulated (Chapter 18), while another investigated the nature of the exercise-induced changes in thermoregulatory effector mechanisms.

1.1 Exercise-induced alterations in temperature regulation

In the resting condition, core temperature is predominantly regulated by input from peripheral and central thermoreceptors. The level at which core temperature is regulated may be altered by a variety of physiological and pathological factors of non-thermal origin. It was once considered that such regulation was analogous to that of a thermostat, and changes in core temperature caused by non-thermal factors were thought to be due to a change in the 'set-point' temperature. Thus, for example, during fever, the set-point core temperature is shifted to a higher temperature, with core temperature being regulated at this new set-point. Although the set-point concept, together with the simple thermostat model of temperature regulation, is no longer considered to be a proper representation of the manner in which body temperature is regulated (Chapter 18), it is apparent that the multitude of non-thermal factors associated with exercise, and its consequences, may impinge upon the thermoregulatory integrators and, hence, affect the regulated level of core temperature (Mekjavic & Eiken 2006). Thus, the transition from rest to exercise leads to neural and humoral alterations capable of affecting thermal homeostasis. Researchers are now documenting these exercise-related, non-thermal factors and are attempting to understand the mechanism of their action.

To understand the manner in which such factors influence core temperature, we need to identify how they affect heat loss and heat production effectors. Dehydration, for example, will induce greater increases in core temperature during exercise than would occur in the euhydrated state. This is not due to increased heat production during exercise, but to reduced sweating and skin blood flow responses. Studies have shown that changes in plasma osmolality affect the rate and onset of sweating by altering the firing rate of central warm-sensitive neurons that contribute to the regulation of sweating (Silva & Boulant 1984).

We must appreciate that exercise induces many changes in the internal environment of the body, and that some of these changes may impact upon a number of physiological systems and not just the thermoregulatory system. Thus, it is tenable that exercise is associated with several other, as yet unidentified, factors impinging on thermoregulation. We must also consider that, during exercise, physiological systems work in concert. Thus, an effect of an exercise-induced factor on one physiological system (i.e. cardiovascular function), may influence the functioning of another (i.e. thermoregulation). This interaction can be nicely illustrated using the dehydration example.

It is well known that dehydration potentiates exercise-induced increments in core temperature (Chapters 19, 33 and 34.2). This is a consequence of its action on both the cardiovascular and the thermoregulatory system. A reduced exercising cardiac output when dehydrated results in a lower skin blood flow. This reduces convective and conductive heat losses at the skin and results in an elevated core temperature. The increase in plasma osmolality, concomitant with dehydration, alters the sweating response and the reduction in evaporative heat loss elicits a greater core temperature rise. Thus, dehydration has affected two physiological systems, resulting in an augmented elevation of the exercise-induced increase in core temperature.

1.2 Is an exercise–induced elevation in core temperature a function of absolute or relative work rate?

The above example illustrates that an alteration in the set-point is not required to explain a change in the regulated core temperature. In this case, a greater increment in core temperature during exercise was due to dehydration. Indeed, it is the ability of a portion of the central neurons in the thermoregulatory centre to act as both warm-sensitive thermoreceptors and osmoreceptors that explains why the neurogenic drive for sweating is attenuated during dehydration. This example can be further extended to help understand why maximal work rate is significantly reduced during dehydration.

For example, if we were to compare the peak (maximal) achievable work rates during incremental exercise trials (cycle ergometry) in the same individuals, during both euhydrated and dehydrated states, we may observe respective peak work rates of 250 and 200 W. Thus, a steady-state work rate of 125 W would represent 63% of the peak work rate when dehydrated, but only 50% of the euhydrated peak. That is, the relative workload (strain) for the same absolute work rate differs between the two conditions. A greater increase in core temperature in the dehydrated condition could then be interpreted as a dependence of the exercise-induced elevation in core temperature on the relative workload since, in both conditions, the absolute work rate is the same.

The question tackled by investigators working in this area has important practical implications, including: is the magnitude of core temperature rise predictable from the intensity and nature of the exercise? It is commonly suggested that the magnitude of the exercise-induced increase in core temperature is related to the relative, rather than to the absolute work intensity (Kenney & Johnson 1992). This might support the concept that the altered core temperature is not merely a consequence of increased heat production. The notion of a close correlation between relative work rate and core temperature is based on findings from cross-sectional studies in which individuals with varying working capacity were compared. These studies have shown that, at a given work intensity, the magnitude of core temperature increases are larger in unfit than in endurance-trained individuals (Davies et al. 1976, Saltin & Hermansen 1966). Likewise, longitudinal studies have shown that the magnitude of the exercise-induced core temperature increase is less following a training regimen that results in increased aerobic power, and hence an increase in the absolute/relative work intensity ratio (Saltin 1970).

On the other hand, it appears that the close correlation between the exercise core temperature response and the relative work does not hold true in conditions where the ratio between relative and absolute work intensity is experimentally manipulated. For example, such changes can be induced by reducing the oxygen content of inspired air or by inducing graded ischaemia in the working leg muscles. Instead, under such conditions, the exercise-induced rise in core temperature seems to be more closely related to the absolute work intensity (Eiken & Mekjavic 2004, Greenleaf et al. 1969, Kacin et al. 2005). The general conclusion from these studies must therefore be that the absolute work rate determines the level of endogenous heat produced, whereas the relative work rate modulates the efficiency with which the body can dissipate this heat. Since endurance training results in physiological adaptations that also enhance heat dissipation, then training lowers the core temperature associated with a given submaximal work rate.

In situations where heat loss is impaired, due to environmental conditions or non-thermal factors, exercise may cause core temperature to rise to levels that may impair physical performance. Core temperature is only one of several factors known to limit exercise performance. However, the attainment of a critically high level of core temperature has been proposed as the main cause of fatigue during exercise in hot environments (Nielsen et al. 1993).

2 LIMITATIONS TO EXERCISE PERFORMANCE IN HOT ENVIRONMENTS

Environmental heat stress depends upon the interaction among the physical variables that determine heat transfer (exchange) from the body shell (subcutaneous and skin) tissues to the environment (Chapter 19). It is well documented that exercise endurance is impaired in environments that have a limited capacity for evaporative heat loss (Hales et al. 1996, Montain et al. 1994, Nielsen et al. 1993, Rowell et al. 1966). Such conditions are typified by hot and humid environments, and are referred to as uncompensable states. An elevated ambient humidity (water vapour partial pressure) reduces evaporation. To an exercising individual, this means that sweat will not completely evaporate and its contribution to cooling is reduced. As a consequence, heat storage will increase during exercise, potentiating the exercise-induced increase in core temperature. In contrast, people exercising in a dry environment at the same temperature can achieve thermal, cardiovascular and metabolic homeostasis, as long as the combination of clothing and exercise intensity is not too heavy (Chapter 19) and normal body fluid status can be maintained (González-Alonso et al. 1995, 1998, 1999b, 2000). This compensable state is due to the fact that drier air optimises the evaporation of sweat. During strenuous work and exercise in such environments, in which hyperthermia and dehydration develop in concert, fatigue may result from their synergistic effects. The focus of the following discussion is on the mechanisms causing fatigue during exercise in environments where core temperature rises, even when maintaining body fluid status.

2.1 The critical core temperature hypothesis

The attainment of a critically high body core temperature has been proposed as the main factor limiting endurance

performance in hot environments (Nielsen et al. 1993). Although there is compelling evidence showing that fatigue in the heat is closely related to high core temperatures (~40°C) in trained and in some untrained subjects (Montain et al. 1994, Nielsen et al. 1993), few studies have systematically manipulated the initial core temperature and its rate of rise in an attempt to isolate the effect of body temperature on performance.

MacDougall et al. (1974) showed that humans always became exhausted during heavy prolonged exercise at a rectal temperature of 39.4°C, even though its rate of rise was deliberately and extensively varied. More recently, González-Alonso et al. (1999a) showed that trained subjects fatigued at remarkably similar levels of tissue temperature (core: ~40°C; exercising muscle: ~41°C), cardiovascular strain (heart rate: 196–198 beats·min^{-1}; cardiac output: ~20 L·min^{-1}) and perceived exertion (19 Borg units), despite differences in the starting core temperature, the rate of heat storage and the final skin temperature. It is notable that cardiac output, and thus peripheral blood flow, declined ~2 L·min^{-1} with increasing thermal strain (González-Alonso et al. 1999a). Thus, the impact of thermal strain on fatigue in individuals exercising in hot environments cannot be dissociated from that of cardiovascular strain, and the metabolic consequences of reduced oxygen delivery to locomotor muscles (González-Alonso & Calbet 2003, González-Alonso et al. 1998, 1999b).

The severity of the effects of heat stress on performance is clearly evident in trained subjects who are capable of cycling intensely for several hours, but become exhausted after only ~30 min when the initial value of core temperature is high or its rate of rise is fast (González-Alonso et al. 1999a). These deleterious effects on performance are also clear during maximal exercise lasting 3–10 min (González-Alonso & Calbet 2003) and during repeated sprint performance (Drust et al. 2005). However, heat stress does not affect supramaximal exercise lasting only a few seconds (Drust et al. 2005). Measures of hypothalamic and jugular venous blood temperatures in rats and humans during exhaustive exercise indicate that the increase in brain temperature closely mirrors the rise in core temperature (Fuller et al. 1998, Nybo et al. 2002). It is therefore reasonable to assume that hypothalamic and other internal organ temperatures reach a similar value at the point of fatigue, and that temperature differences among internal organs and tissues are small. Thus, the possibility arose that a ceiling core temperature may limit exercise.

The concept that an absolute and critical core temperature level may be the primary factor underlying fatigue with heat stress is challenged by studies that have manipulated body temperature during maximal and supramaximal exercise (González-Alonso & Calbet 2003, González-Alonso et al. 2004, Nybo et al. 2001). The maximal exercise reports show that the exhaustion occurring at core temperatures of 39–40°C is preceded by marked reductions in systemic, brain and locomotor skeletal muscle blood flow and oxygen supply, and reduced contracting muscle aerobic metabolism (González-Alonso & Calbet 2003, González-Alonso et al. 2004, Mortensen et al. 2005). Moreover, exercise hyperthermia does not hamper one single 15 s bout of supramaximal exercise but impairs repeated sprint performance (Drust et al. 2005). Although there is evidence that hyperthermia reduces maximal voluntary contraction and interpolated twitch force during both knee extension and grip strength (Nybo & Nielsen 2001), the ability to perform intense whole-body exercise for very short periods is unaltered (Drust et al. 2005). Pointing towards a cardiovascular limitation, repeated sprint performance in the hyperthermic state was associated with a lower whole-body oxygen uptake during bouts 2–4, suggesting that cardiovascular instability became limiting only after the second bout of sprinting (Drust et al. 2005). Together, these findings suggest that the interaction between hyperthermia and cardiovascular strain, rather than an absolute critical level of core temperature, determines fatigue in individuals performing prolonged moderate and short high-intensity exercise in hot environments.

2.2 Mechanisms underlying hyperthermia–induced fatigue

The precise mechanisms underlying heat stress-induced fatigue and the chain of events leading to exhaustion are not well understood. The studies manipulating the rate of rise and initial level of body temperature suggest that the high core temperature and concomitant cardiovascular strain play a major role. There are at least three possibilities by which local and systemic hyperthermia could either directly or indirectly impair exercise capacity. First, high muscle temperature could directly impair active muscle mitochondrial function and overall myocyte metabolism. Second, high brain temperature could suppress central arousal and the voluntary activation of muscles (Nielsen et al. 2001). Third, high myocardial tissue temperature and systemic thermal strain could indirectly impair cardiac output and blood flow to locomotor muscles, brain and splanchnic tissues, leading to a compromised locomotor muscle metabolism (González-Alonso & Calbet 2003, González-Alonso et al. 2004, Mortensen et al. 2005).

While in vitro evidence clearly demonstrates that a tissue temperature of ≥42–45°C is associated with muscle dysfunction, cellular damage and protein degradation (see Hales et al. 1996), it is unlikely that such phenomena are occurring to a significant extent at exhausting core temperatures of 39–40°C. A muscle temperature of 40–41°C is also

unlikely to suppress muscle oxygen uptake at rest or during light exercise when blood flow is not limiting. Thus, reduced oxygen delivery, rather than temperature-mediated mitochondrial dysfunction, is the most likely explanation for the impaired locomotor muscle oxygen uptake seen with hyperthermia during moderate and severe exercise (González-Alonso & Calbet 2003, González-Alonso et al. 1998).

There is some evidence that the hyperthermia-associated, impaired ability to exercise is related to a reduced arousal and central neuromuscular drive (Nielsen & Nybo 2003, Nybo & Secher 2004). For example, Nielsen et al. (2001) measured brain activity during exercise in both hot and cool environments, and showed that hyperthermia was associated with a depression in the high-frequency β waves, such that the ratio of α and β increased. Since the altered encephalographic activity with heat stress is similar to that which normally occurs during sleep, it may indicate that hyperthermia reduces the state of arousal (Nielsen et al. 2001). On the other hand, the intimate correlation between the rise in core temperature, the increase in heart rate and the reduction in stroke volume during constant exercise with altered initial body temperature lends support to the idea that hyperthermia is involved in the reductions in cardiac output, by either reducing diastolic filling time or impairing cardiac contractility (González-Alonso et al. 1997, 1999a, Rubin 1987). Taken together, available evidence suggests that functional alterations in multiple bodily tissues including skeletal muscle, brain and heart are associated with the hyperthermia-induced fatigue. In this construct, exhaustion is preceded by dysfunction of multiple systems in response to thermal, cardiovascular and metabolic strain, rather than the attainment of a critically high level of temperature.

3 CONCLUSION

Following the initial observation by Marius Nielsen (1938) that exercise caused an increase in core temperature, research has focused on the manner in which core temperature is regulated during exercise. In addition, recent studies have emphasised the importance of core temperature in limiting exercise performance. It is now clear that non-thermal factors may alter heat loss responses, some of them in such a manner that they impair heat loss, thereby potentiating exercise-induced hyperthermia and decreasing performance. The mechanisms by which hyperthermia limits exercise performance are not fully understood, but may involve dysfunction of several physiological systems, including the cardiovascular and central nervous systems.

References

Davies CT, Brotherhood JR, Zeidifard E 1976 Temperature regulation during severe exercise with some observations on effects of skin wetting. Journal of Applied Physiology 41:772–776

Drust B, Rasmussen P, Mohr M, Nielsen B, Nybo L 2005 Elevations in core and muscle temperature impairs repeated sprint performance. Acta Physiologica Scandinavica 183:181–190

Eiken O, Mekjavic IB 2004 Ischaemia in working muscles potentiates the exercise induced sweating response in man. Acta Physiologica Scandinavica 181:305–311

Fuller A, Carter RN, Mitchell D 1998 Brain and abdominal temperatures at fatigue in rats exercising in the heat. Journal of Applied Physiology 84:877–883

González-Alonso J, Calbet JAL 2003 Reductions in systemic and skeletal muscle blood flow and oxygen delivery limit maximal aerobic capacity in humans. Circulation 107:824–830

González-Alonso J, Mora-Rodríguez R, Below PR, Coyle EF 1995 Dehydration reduces cardiac output and increases systemic and cutaneous vascular resistance during exercise. Journal of Applied Physiology 79(5):1487–1496

González-Alonso J, Mora-Rodríguez R, Coyle EF 1997 Dehydration markedly impairs cardiovascular function in hyperthermic endurance athletes during exercise. Journal of Applied Physiology 82(4):1229–1236

González-Alonso J, Calbet JAL, Nielsen B 1998 Muscle blood flow is reduced with dehydration during prolonged exercise in humans. Journal of Physiology 513:895–905

González-Alonso J, Teller C, Andersen SL, Jensen FB, Hyldeg T, Nielsen B 1999a Influence of body temperature on the development of fatigue during prolonged exercise in the heat. Journal of Applied Physiology 86(3):1032–1039

González-Alonso J, Calbet JAL, Nielsen B 1999b Metabolic and thermodynamic responses to dehydration-induced reductions in muscle blood flow in exercising humans. Journal of Physiology 520:577–589

González-Alonso J, Mora-Rodríguez R, Coyle EF 2000 Stroke volume during exercise: interaction of environment and hydration. American Journal of Physiology 278:H321–H330

González-Alonso J, Dalsgaard MK, Osada T, Volianitis S, Dawson EA, Yoshiga CC, Secher NH 2004 Brain and central haemodynamics and oxygenation during maximal exercise in humans. Journal of Physiology 557:331–342

Greenleaf JE, Greenleaf CJ, Card DH, Saltin B 1969 Exercise temperature regulation in man during exposure to simulated altitude. Journal of Applied Physiology 26:290–296

Hales JRS, Hubbard RW, Gaffin SL 1996 Limitation of heat tolerance. In: Fregly MJ, Blatteis CM (eds) Handbook of physiology. Environmental physiology. American Physiology Society, Bethesda, MD, 285–355

Kacin A, Golja P, Eiken O, Tipton MJ, Gorjanc J, Mekjavic IB 2005 Human temperature regulation during cycling with moderate leg ischemia. European Journal of Applied Physiology 95:213–220

Kenny WL, Johnson JM 1992 Control of skin blood flow during exercise. Medicine and Science in Sport and Exercise 24:303–312

MacDougall JD, Reddan WG, Layton CR, Dempsey JA 1974 Effects of metabolic hyperthermia on performance during heavy prolonged exercise. Journal of Applied Physiology 36:538–544

Mekjavic IB, Eiken O 2006 Contribution of thermal and nonthermal factors to the regulation of body temperature in humans. Journal of Applied Physiology 100:2065–2072

Montain SL, Sawka MN, Cadarette BS, Quigley MD, McKay JM 1994 Physiological tolerance to uncompensable heat stress: effect of exercise intensity, protective clothing and climate. Journal of Applied Physiology 77:216–222

Mortensen SP, Dawson EA, Yoshiga CC, Dalsgaard MK, Damsgaard R, Secher N, González-Alonso J 2005 Limitations to systemic and locomotor limb muscle oxygen delivery and uptake during maximal exercise in humans. Journal of Physiology 566:273–285

Nielsen M 1938 Die Regulation der Körpertemperatur bei Muskelarbeit. Skandinavisches Archiv der Physiologie 79:193–230

Nielsen B, Nybo L 2003 Cerebral changes during exercise in the heat. Sports Medicine 33(1):1–11

Nielsen B, Hales JRS, Strange S, Christensen NJ, Warberg J, Saltin B 1993 Human circulatory and thermoregulatory adaptations with heat acclimation and exercise in a hot, dry environment. Journal of Physiology 460:467–485

Nielsen B, Hyldig T, Bidstrup F, González-Alonso J, Christoffesen GRJ 2001 Brain activity and fatigue during prolonged exercise in the heat. Pflügers Archive: European Journal of Physiology 442:41–48

Nybo L, Nielsen B 2001 Hyperthermia and central fatigue during prolonged exercise in humans. Journal of Applied Physiology 91:1055–1160

Nybo L, Secher NH 2004 Cerebral perturbations provoked by prolonged exercise. Progress in Neurobiology 72(4):223–261

Nybo L, Jensen T, Nielsen B, González-Alonso J 2001 Effects of marked hyperthermia with and without dehydration on VO_2 kinetics during intense exercise. Journal of Applied Physiology 90:1057–1064

Nybo L, Secher NH, Nielsen B 2002 Inadequate heat release from the human brain during prolonged exercise with hyperthermia. Journal of Physiology 545(2):697–704

Rowell LB, Bruce HJ, Conn RD, Kusumi F 1966 Reductions in cardiac output, central blood volume and stroke volume with thermal stress in normal men during exercise. Journal of Clinical Investigation 45:1801–1816

Rubin SA 1987 Core temperature regulation on heart rate during exercise in humans. Journal of Applied Physiology 62:1997–2002

Saltin B 1970 Circulatory adjustments and body temperature regulation during exercise. In: Hardy JD, Gagge AP, Stolwijk JAJ (eds) Physiological and behavioural temperature regulation. Charles C Thomas, Springfield, IL, 316–323

Saltin B, Hermanssen L 1966 Esophageal, rectal and muscle temperature during exercise. Journal of Applied Physiology 21:1757–1762

Silva LN, Boulant AJ 1984 Effects of osmotic pressure, glucose and temperature on neurons in preoptic tissue slices. American Journal of Physiology. Regulatory, Integrative and Comparative Physiology 247:R335–R345

Chapter 27.3

Do training–induced plasma volume changes improve athletic performance?

Hiroshi Nose   Scott J. Montain

CHAPTER CONTENTS

Part A: Plasma volume expansion improves performance
Hiroshi Nose

Humans are unique in that we exercise in an upright posture and regulate mean body temperature via modulations of skin blood flow and sweat rate. Since the cardiac stroke volume during exercise is largely limited by venous return to the heart according to Starling's Law of the heart (Chapter 1), and in humans 70% of the blood volume is located below heart level in the upright position (Rowell 1986), it is plausible that even a slight decrease in plasma volume through dehydration will decrease stroke volume during exercise (Sawka & Coyle 1999). Conversely, hypervolaemia induced through endurance training is likely to increase stroke volume, cardiac output and peripheral blood flow to the contracting muscles (oxygen delivery) and the skin surface (heat dissipation), leading to improved endurance performance with enhanced resistance to heat and dehydration.

According to Fick's Law, maximal aerobic power is determined by maximal heart rate, maximal stroke volume and the difference in oxygen content between arterial and mixed venous blood (Chapters 10.1 and 10.2). However, when these variables are compared between untrained and trained subjects, noticeably higher values are only observed in maximal stroke volume, while the arteriovenous oxygen difference is minimal, with maximal heart rate possibly even being reduced in trained subjects (McArdle et al. 1991). Experimentally, maximal (peak) aerobic power in individuals is highly correlated with plasma volume (Mack et al. 1988), and also with maximal left atrial pressure (cardiac filling pressure) at maximal exercise intensity (Reeves et al. 1990). Moreover, these variables increase after aerobic training (Nadel 1985). Also, there are several studies indicating that acute plasma volume expansion, following saline infusion, increases aerobic power by elevating stroke volume (Hopper et al. 1988). Furthermore, Kamijo et al. (2000) suggested that the lactate threshold during graded exercise can be elevated when continuous negative pressure breathing is used to increase venous return to the heart (see Chapter 10.3 for a critique of the lactate and anaerobic thresholds). These results tend to support the idea that a training-induced plasma volume expansion improves endurance performance.

There are many studies indicating that an acute reduction in cardiac filling pressure, such as that associated with hypovolaemia (Fortney et al. 1981a, 1983, Nadel et al. 1980), postural change from supine to upright (Brengelman et al. 1977) or lower body negative pressure (Mack et al. 1987), decreases skin vascular conductance and skin blood flow, resulting in an acceleration of hyperthermia during exercise. Conversely, an acute increase in cardiac filling pressure can be induced by manoeuvres such as the intravenous infusion of saline (Nose et al. 1990), head-out water immersion (Nielsen et al. 1984) or continuous negative pressure breathing (Nagashima et al. 1998), and thereby enhancing skin vasodilatation. These results are consistent with plasma volume expansion enhancing cutaneous vasodilatation during exercise.

In contrast to the studies of the effects of acute plasma volume modifications on thermoregulation, there have been a few studies that support the merits of endurance training-induced plasma volume expansion for cutaneous vasodilatation during exercise. Recently, Okazaki et al. (2002) observed that, in older men, the sensitivity of the cutaneous vasodilatory response to increased core temperature (oesophageal) during exercise was enhanced after 18 weeks of endurance or resistance training in the subjects with an elevated plasma volume, while it was reduced in those in whom plasma volume was decreased (Figure 27.3.1A). Moreover, they suggested that the increase in cutaneous vasodilatory response was accelerated when the plasma volume was expanded using carbohydrate-protein supplementation during 8 weeks of endurance training (Okazaki et al. 2004).

These results were recently confirmed in young men (Goto et al. 2007), showing that the increase in cutaneous vasodilatation after 5 days of endurance training was enhanced threefold via carbohydrate and protein supplementation designed to increase the plasma volume. Furthermore, Ichinose et al. (2005a) found that the enhanced sensitivity of cutaneous vasodilatation (in young men) was accompanied by an increased stroke volume with an enlarged plasma volume, following 10 days of endurance training. They also suggested that the suppression of cutaneous vasodilatation that accompanies dehydration-induced hyperosmolality is attenuated when the plasma volume is expanded following endurance training (Ichinose et al. 2005b). These results support the idea that training-induced plasma volume expansion improves thermoregulation during exercise, by enhancing cutaneous vasodilatation.

However, in hot environments (>30°C), an increase in cutaneous vasodilatation does not contribute to heat dissipation as much as in a cool environment, due to a reduced (or reversed) skin–air temperature gradient (Chapter 19). Experimentally, Montain & Coyle (1992) have shown that thermoregulation during exercise at 32.7°C was more powerfully influenced by hyperosmolality than hypovolaemia. Since sweating is not reduced by acute hypovolaemia as much as cutaneous vasodilatation (Fortney et al. 1981b, Kamijo et al. 2001), and sweating is the principal heat dis-

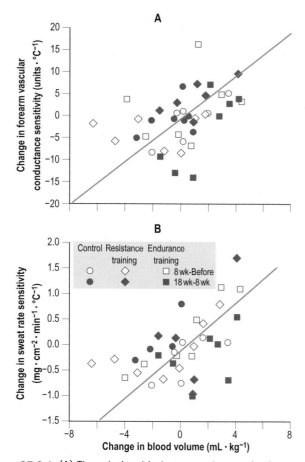

Figure 27.3.1 (A) The relationship between changes in the sensitivity (slope or gain) of forearm skin vascular conductance (relative to core temperature (oesophageal)) and blood volume change following three treatments: no training (control), resistance training and endurance training. Open symbols represent changes from the pretreatment state (no training) to 8 wk; solid symbols are for differences between 8 and 18 wk of training. The blood volume change was significantly correlated with the sensitivity change for forearm skin vascular conductance (r = 0.45, P < 0.01). (B) The relationship between changes in sweat rate sensitivity (relative to oesophageal temperature), and blood volume changes during the same experiment. The blood volume change was significantly correlated with the sweat rate sensitivity change (r = 0.51, P < 0.01). Redrawn from Okazaki et al. (2002) with permission of the American Physiological Society.

sipation mechanism in hot environments, training-induced plasma volume expansion may not contribute significantly to heat dissipation. However, since the increase in sensitivity of the sweating response (Chapter 18) to core temperature change was enhanced in parallel with training-induced plasma volume expansion in both older (Okazaki et al. 2002; Figure 27.3.1B) and young men (Ichinose et al. 2005a, 2005b), then an increased cutaneous vasodilatory response, also accompanying a training-induced plasma volume expansion, may supply a greater blood flow to the sweat glands, thereby supporting an elevated sweat secretion.

Notwithstanding these thermoregulatory benefits, an acute plasma volume expansion has a limited capacity to improve aerobic power during exercise. Hopper et al. (1988)

suggested that, in untrained subjects, stroke volume during submaximal exercise increased 11% in response to a 14% plasma volume expansion, but further expansion did not elicit further changes in stroke volume. Coyle et al. (1990) examined the effects of graded plasma volume expansion on maximal aerobic power, suggesting that a larger plasma volume expansion and the consequent haemodilution resulted in aerobic power and performance changes that were not different from those observed in the control condition, or significantly less than observed with smaller plasma volume expansions. Thus, it appears that plasma volume expansion increases maximal aerobic power more when other cardiac and oxygen delivery functions (cardiac contractility, muscle blood flow, oxygen extraction) are improved (Chapter 10.1).

Similarly, plasma volume expansion also has a limited capacity to improve thermoregulation. For example, Takeno et al. (2001) studied the effects of 10 days endurance training (cycling) in cool (20°C) and warm (30°C) environments, observing that the sensitivity of the cutaneous vasodilatory response to increased core temperature was higher in a warm environment, although the increase in plasma volume was similar between the two conditions. These results imply that plasma volume expansion improves thermoregulation more when central or peripheral thermoregulatory mechanisms are also improved during repeated heat exposure (heat acclimation; Chapter 21).

In conclusion, although plasma volume expansion alone has a limited capacity to increase aerobic power and thermoregulation, it is more effective when other primary aerobic and thermoregulatory functions have acquired endurance training- or heat-induced adaptations.

Part B: Plasma volume expansion is not critical to exercise performance
Scott Montain

Whether or not plasma volume expansion is beneficial to performance is largely dependent on how the expansion affects oxygen delivery to the tissues. For example, if the haemodilution produced by plasma volume expansion reduces oxygen delivery to the working muscle, it can be expected that such expansion would be detrimental rather than beneficial to performance (Chapter 10.1). Therefore, if there is any advantage to be gained from an expansion of the plasma volume, it must overcome the accompanying reduction in the volume-specific oxygen content, resulting from haemoglobin dilution (haemodilution).

Modest reductions in oxygen content are associated with altered central and peripheral modifications to preserve oxygen delivery to the working muscles. Isovolaemic haemodilution, producing a lowering of haemoglobin concentration by >30 g·L^{-1}, is accompanied by an elevated cardiac output and increased leg blood flow during submaximal exercise; thereby preserving oxygen delivery (González-Alonso et al. 2006, Roach et al. 1999). Similarly, an acute removal of ~300 mL of blood is accompanied by greater heat storage during subsequent exercise-heat stress and

reduced skin blood flow sensitivity. However, there is an upper limit for compensating for this reduced oxygen content. Beyond this limit, maximal power will be compromised (Koskolou et al. 1997).

While there is supportive evidence that plasma volume expansions of 300–400 mL can increase stroke volume, maximal oxygen uptake and endurance time in untrained and recreational athletes (Coyle et al. 1990, Hopper et al. 1988), further expansion produces reductions in oxygen content that cannot be compensated, and there is a reversal of these physiological and performance gains (Hopper et al. 1988). Thus, while some expansion of plasma volume is ergogenic in nature in untrained individuals, too much expansion can be disadvantageous.

Endurance training is typically associated with ~10% expansion of plasma volume and exercise stroke volume. Experimentally inducing further expansion of the plasma volume in this population does not further increase stroke volume (Coyle et al. 1986, Kanstrup & Ekblom 1982). Thus, endurance training per se appears to maximise cardiac filling. When Coyle et al. (1986) expanded plasma volume expansion ~429 mL using a dextran infusion, the plasma volume expansion was accompanied by a non-significant reduction in maximal oxygen uptake (4.42 to 4.37 L·min^{-1}) and an 8% reduction in exercise time to exhaustion (9.13 to 8.38 min). Similarly, Kanstrup & Ekblom (1982) reported that acute plasma volume expansion by 700 mL lowered haemoglobin 8–10%, and the time to exhaustion declined from 5.45 to 5.02 min. Thus, it can be expected that experimental interventions to selectively expand plasma volume will produce no physiological advantage in already plasma volume-expanded athletes, and rather than being ergogenic, will more likely be detrimental to performance.

It might be argued that athletes would benefit from plasma volume expansion during exercise-heat stress, as a means of reducing cardiovascular strain and facilitating heat transfer. However, the available evidence again indicates that plasma volume expansion per se in endurance-trained and heat-acclimated individuals is not beneficial. Montain & Coyle (1992) found there was no advantage for the preservation of skin blood flow and heat loss when the plasma volume was selectively preserved, independently of the interstitial and intracellular body water compartments, during 2 h of exercise-heat stress. In their experiment, infusion of ~390 mL of dextran maintained plasma and blood volumes equal to, or higher than that observed when the subjects drank copious amounts of fluid during exercise. Despite this intervention, the core temperature response was similar to that observed when drinking was not permitted. While no performance measures were made, the observation that perceived exertion rose similarly during the plasma volume expansion and no fluid trials argues against performance advantages. Even in less fit volunteers, where acute plasma volume expansion does increase stroke volume (Fortney et al. 1981a, b), core temperatures and skin blood flow responses were not improved. Thus, selective expansion of the plasma volume does not seem to offer either thermoregulatory or performance advantages during exercise-heat stress for heat-acclimatised endurance-trained athletes.

When viewed comprehensively, it appears that much of the confusion regarding the advantages of plasma volume expansion stems from the subject populations being tested. Whereas acute plasma volume expansion can produce cardiovascular and performance advantages for sedentary to recreationally active individuals, these ergogenic responses are less apparent or absent in individuals accustomed to endurance exercise or adapted to exertional heat stress (heat acclimatised). Therefore, it is important to consider training as well as heat acclimation status when determining the potential of plasma volume expansion to alter physiological function.

In summary, the plasma volume expansion accompanying endurance training provides the necessary volume expansion to optimise cardiac filling. Any benefit of artificially expanding plasma volume will dilute oxygen content, making it more difficult to provide adequate oxygen delivery to working muscles. In situations where the aerobic requirements of the task produce maximal stroke volumes, the selective expansion of plasma volume would be likely to compromise performance.

References

Brengelmann GL, Johnson JM, Hermansen L, Rowell LB 1977 Altered control of skin blood flow during exercise at high internal temperature. Journal of Applied Physiology 43:790–794

Coyle EF, Hemmert MK, Coggan AR 1986 Effects of detraining on cardiovascular responses to exercise: role of blood volume. Journal of Applied Physiology 60:95–99

Coyle EF, Hopper MK, Coggan AR 1990 Maximal oxygen uptake relative to plasma volume expansion. International Journal of Sports Medicine 11:116–119

Fortney SM, Nadel ER, Wenger CB, Bove JR 1981a Effect of acute alterations of blood volume on circulatory performance in humans. Journal of Applied Physiology 50:292–298

Fortney SM, Nadel ER, Wenger CB, Bove JR 1981b Effect of blood volume on sweating rate and body fluids in exercising humans. Journal of Applied Physiology 51:1594–1600

Fortney SM, Wenger CB, Bove JR, Nadel ER 1983 Effects of plasma volume on forearm venous and cardiac stroke volume during exercise. Journal of Applied Physiology 55:884–890

González-Alonso J, Mortensen SP, Dawson EA, Secher NH 2006 Erythrocytes and the regulation of human skeletal muscle blood flow and oxygen delivery: role of erythrocyte count and oxygenation state of haemoglobin. Journal of Physiology 572:295–305

Goto M, Kamijo Y, Okazaki K, Okazaki K, Masuki S, Miyagawa K, Nose H 2007 Protein and carbohydrate supplementation during 5-day aerobic training enhanced improvement of thermoregulation in young men. FASEB Journal 21:A1296

Hopper MK, Coggan AR, Coyle EF 1988 Exercise stroke volume relative to plasma volume expansion. Journal of Applied Physiology 64:404–408

Ichinose T, Okazaki K, Masuki S, Mitono H, Chen M, Endoh H, Nose H 2005a Enhanced sensitivity of cutaneous vasodilation and cardiac stroke volume after 10-day exercise training in humans. FASEB Journal 19:A1193

Ichinose T, Okazaki K, Masuki S, Mitono H, Chen M, Endoh H, Nose H 2005b Ten-day endurance training attenuates the hyperosmotic suppression of cutaneous vasodilation during exercise but not sweating. Journal of Applied Physiology 99:237–243

Kamijo Y, Takeno Y, Sakai A, Inaki M, Okumoto T, Itoh J, Yanagidaira Y, Masuki S, Nose H 2000 Plasma lactate concentration and muscle blood flow during dynamic exercise with negative pressure breathing. Journal of Applied Physiology 89:2196–2205

Kamijo Y, Okumoto T, Takeno Y, Okazaki K, Itoh J, Masuki S, Nose H 2001 The interactive effects of hypovolemia and hyperosmolality on cutaneous vasodilation and sweating during exercise in a hot environment. Japanese Journal of Physiology 51:S266

Kanstrup I-L, Ekblom B 1982 Acute hypervolemia, cardiac performance and aerobic power during exercise. Journal of Applied Physiology 52:1186–1191

Koskolou MD, Roach RC, Calbet JAL, Rådegran G, Saltin B 1997 Cardiovascular responses to dynamic exercise with acute anemia in humans. American Journal of Physiology 42:H1787–H1793

McArdle WD, Katch FI, Katch VL 1991 Exercise physiology, 3rd edn. Lea and Febiger, Malvern, PA, 428

Mack GW, Shi X, Nose H, Tripathi A, Nadel ER 1987 Diminished baroreflex control of forearm vascular resistance in physically fit humans. Journal of Applied Physiology 63:105–110

Mack GW, Nose H, Nadel ER 1988 Role of cardiopulmonary baroreflexes during dynamic exercise. Journal of Applied Physiology 65:1827–1832

Montain SJ, Coyle EF 1992 The influence of graded dehydration on hyperthermia and cardiovascular drift during exercise. Journal of Applied Physiology 73:1340–1350

Nadel ER 1985 Physiological adaptation to aerobic training. American Scientist 73:334–343

Nadel ER, Fortney SM, Wenger CB 1980 Effect of hydration state on circulation and thermal regulations. Journal of Applied Physiology 49:715–721

Nagashima K, Nose H, Takamata A, Morimoto T 1998 Effect of continuous negative pressure breathing on skin blood flow during exercise in a hot environment. Journal of Applied Physiology 84:1854–1851

Nielsen B, Rowell LB, Bonde-Pedersen F 1984 Cardiovascular responses to heat stress and blood volume displacement during exercise in man. European Journal of Applied Physiology and Occupational Physiology 52:370–374

Nose H, Mack GW, Shi X, Morimoto K, Nadel ER 1990 Effect of saline infusion during exercise on thermal and circulatory regulations. Journal of Applied Physiology 69:609–616

Okazaki K, Kamijo Y, Takeno Y, Okumoto T, Masuki S, Nose H 2002 Effects of exercise training on thermoregulatory reponses and blood volume in older men. Journal of Applied Physiology 93:1630–1637

Okazaki K, Ichinose T, Mitono H, Masuki S, Endoh H, Chen M, Hayase H, Doi T, Nose H 2004 Protein and CHO supplementation during aerobic training increased plasma volume and thermoregulatory capacity in older men. FASEB Journal 18:A1099

Reeves JT, Groves BM, Cymerman A, Sutton RJ, Wagner PD, Turkevich D, Houston CS 1990 Operation Everest II: cardiac filling pressure during cycle exercise at sea level. Respiratory Physiology 80:147–154

Roach RC, Koskolou MD, Calbet JAL, Saltin B 1999 Arterial O$_2$ content and tension in regulation of cardiac output and leg blood flow during exercise in humans. American Journal of Physiology 276: H438–H445

Rowell LB 1986 Adjustments to upright posture and blood loss. In: Human circulation regulation during physical stress. Oxford University Press, New York, 137–173

Sawka MN, Coyle EF 1999 Influence of body water and blood volume on thermoregulation and exercise performance in the heat. In: Holloszy JO (ed) Exercise and sport sciences reviews, vol 27. Lippincott, Williams and Wilkins, Philadelphia, PA, 167–218

Takeno Y, Kamijo Y, Nose H 2001 Thermoregulatory and aerobic changes after endurance training in a hypobaric hypoxic and warm environment. Journal of Applied Physiology 91:1520–1528

SECTION 5

Exercise interactions

Section introduction: Does exercise have a role in the treatment of chronic disease?

Herbert Groeller

Unquestionably yes, and probably no.

However, to both open and close a section introduction with such a statement, although succinct, would be far too brief and ambiguous to provide any meaningfully consideration of the question.

Chronic diseases typically develop over an extended time, during which the normal structure or function of tissues, organs or physiological systems gradually experience adverse changes (e.g. osteoporosis, some cancers, coronary heart disease, type 2 diabetes). Thus, the manifestation of a chronic disease can take considerable time to be fully expressed. For example, a chronically sedentary person would be unlikely to be aware of the progressive development of coronary artery disease, until it impacted upon daily activities. Yet, intravascular ultrasound assessment of 262 heart transplant recipients, one month after transplant from asymptomatic donors, revealed that one in six donor teenage hearts had evidence of atherosclerotic lesions (Tuzcu et al. 2001). Due to the largely, and habitually sedentary behaviour of such individuals, a significant attenuation of coronary blood flow will be required for the person to be impeded during their typical daily physical tasks.

In this example, the individual has acquired a subclinical state of a developing chronic disease. The signs of this disease may be revealed in a thorough medical examination, although the individual is largely asymptomatic, except when stressed physically. Indeed, this state is ubiquitous in contemporary, sedentary humans and the dramatic rise in the incidence of chronic disease has prompted some scientists to suggest that a war must be waged against such diseases, to impede their inexorable progression (Booth et al. 2000). It is clearly apparent that one of the primary fronts of this battle is to arrest the significant and relatively recent decline in the level of habitual physical activity (Chapters 17.1 and 28).

One must consider the potential of physical exercise (short versus prolonged, infrequent versus frequent, low versus high intensity) to act as a means for correcting the debilitating impact of chronic disease on the body, and to have a positive impact upon physiological function. Thus, in a manner similar to the use of drugs to treat disease, we should consider the therapeutic index of exercise: the ratio of a beneficial dose to that of a toxic dose. Let us first consider the responses associated with the latter.

Concerns regarding the effect of excessive physical activity on health were present in early Greek times.

Festivals were regularly held that displayed athletic prowess, with valuable prizes awarded for superior performance, thus providing the impetus for the genesis of the full-time, professional athlete (MacAuley 1994). The Greek physician Hippocrates (c 460–370 BC), universally considered the father of medicine, was uneasy about some of the practices of these athletes and the benefits of conducting such intense physical activity: 'In athletes a perfect condition that is at its highest pitch is treacherous. Such conditions cannot remain the same or be at rest, and, change for the better being impossible, the only possible change is for the worse' (Jones 1967, p. 99). Indeed, the view that vigorous exercise was detrimental endured into the 19th century (MacAuley 1994).

Excessive, sustained levels of training stress can evoke a broad range of systemic physiological responses, resulting in a prolonged period of depressed physical function (Chapter 29). In contrast, more moderate exercise stimuli may fail to provoke the attainment of the highest performance goals. Athletes must therefore navigate along a slim and lengthy path of progressive exercise, to successfully arrive at maximal physical performance, while avoiding the negative effects of a prolonged excessive dose of physical training.

In contrast, relative moderation of the exercise dose was also recognised in ancient Greece to provide significant health and therapeutic benefits. Hippocrates stated: 'In a word, all parts of the body which were made for active use, if moderately used and exercised at the labour to which they are habituated, become healthy, increase in bulk, and bear their age well, but when not used, and when left without exercise, they become diseased, their growth arrested, and they soon become old' (Adams 1849, p. 629).

Despite this remarkable insight from almost 2500 years ago, it is an extraordinary paradox that we still debate the notion of the beneficial effects of exercise, while simultaneously observing a world community that has failed to embrace habitual vigorous physical activity. The evidence is clear and unequivocal: increased habitual physical exercise affords its participants extensive health benefits. For example, regular exercise provides significant protection against coronary heart disease (Sesso et al. 2000). Indeed, the scientific literature is replete with evidence supporting both the benefits that accrue from an adequate dose (Chapters 17.1 and 17.2), as well as the adverse effect of the sedentary lifestyle (Chapters 28 and 30). Yet, despite this evidence, considerable challenges lie ahead for scientists, policy makers, town planners and employers to bolster routine exercise participation within the daily activities of all individuals (Booth et al. 2000; Chapter 31.1).

One of those challenges is to attain significant compliance to a minimum of 30 min of moderate-intensity exercise each day (Chapters 17.1 and 28). For it is when exercise is of a sufficient dose, with respect to its intensity, duration and frequency, that the health benefits are optimised (Blair et al. 2001). Indeed, exercise of insufficient stimulus, although marginally better than no exercise at all, provides the participant with limited health benefits, particularly when exercise adherence is transient. However, when the exercise stimulus is sufficient, significant therapeutic benefits have been observed for many common chronic diseases (Chapters 28 and 30). Indeed, for some chronic conditions, such as sarcopenia, exercise is the only current means of arresting disease progression (Doherty 2003). Therefore, appropriately prescribed exercise unquestionably has a substantial role in the treatment of chronic disease.

References

Adams F 1849 The genuine works of Hippocrates. Volume II: translated from the Greek with preliminary discourse and annotations by Francis Adams. Sydenham Society, London

Blair SN, Cheng Y, Holder SJ 2001 Is physical activity or physical fitness more important in defining health benefits? Medicine and Science in Sports and Exercise 33(6):S379–S399

Booth FW, Gordon SE, Carlson CJ, Hamilton MT 2000 Waging war on modern chronic diseases: primary prevention through exercise biology. Journal of Applied Physiology 88(2):774–787

Doherty TJ 2003 Invited review: aging and sarcopenia. Journal of Applied Physiology 95:1717–1727

Jones WHS (trans) 1967 Hippocrates, Vol. IV. Harvard University Press, Cambridge, MA

MacAuley D 1994 A history of physical activity, health and medicine. Journal of the Royal Society of Medicine 87(January):32–35

Sesso HD, Paffenbarger RS, Lee IM 2000 Physical activity and coronary heart disease in men: the Harvard Alumni Health Study. Circulation 102:975–980

Tuzcu ME, Kapadia SR, Tutar E, Ziada KM, Hobbs RE, McCarthy PM, Young JB, Nissen SE 2001 High prevalence of coronary atherosclerosis in asymptomatic teenagers and young adults. Circulation 103:2705–2710

Chapter 28

Physiological penalties of the sedentary lifestyle

Manu V. Chakravarthy

CHAPTER CONTENTS

1 DEFINITION OF A SEDENTARY LIFESTYLE AND SCOPE OF THE PROBLEM

While much of this textbook is focused on the physiology of exercise, this Chapter, along with Chapters 17.1, 30 and 31.1, deals with sedentary behaviour. However, as will become apparent, most of the world is in fact sedentary, and a relatively small proportion of people are engaged in habitual, moderate-intensity physical activities. Therefore, an aim of this chapter is to highlight the physiological penalties of physical inactivity and through that, to introduce the notion of an inherently programmed evolutionary basis for physical activity in humans.

The definition of a sedentary lifestyle is based on the concept of a health-related exercise threshold: the Expert Panel of the Centers for Disease Control and Prevention (CDC) and the American College of Sports Medicine (ACSM) recommended that adults who engage in moderate-intensity physical activity, resulting in a daily energy expenditure of ~900 $kJ \cdot d^{-1}$ (~200 $kcal \cdot d^{-1}$), can expect many health benefits. Such an energy expenditure would require the accumulation of ~30 $min \cdot d^{-1}$ of moderate-intensity physical activity (Pate et al. 1995). Based on this definition, those without at least 30 $min \cdot d^{-1}$ of brisk walking are termed sedentary for the purposes of this chapter. Other reports indicate that <30 $min \cdot d^{-1}$ of moderate-intensity physical activity offered no significant risk reduction from coronary artery disease, stroke or type 2 diabetes (Hu et al. 1999, 2000; see also Chapters 13 and 17.1). Therefore, from this health perspective, the definition of sedentary includes those who undertake no leisure time physical activity and those who undertake <30 $min \cdot d^{-1}$ of physical activity.

Our highly mechanised lifestyle in the 21st century has encouraged sedentary living, since there is little impetus for us to be active. Indeed, we have to make conscious efforts to actually schedule time for physical activity as part of our daily life, akin to the way that we schedule a meeting or an important engagement. Ready-prepared food can be obtained 24 hours a day, requiring no major physical effort on the part of the consumer. Contrast this to the inextricable relationship between caloric acquisition (gathering of food) and caloric expenditure (physical activity) that was necessary for the survival of our species throughout the long course of human and prehuman evolution, during which the genes regulating the metabolism of our progenitors were selected.

Thus, circumstances of human existence in the 21st century have made it exceedingly difficult to engage in the natural dependence of physical activity, as was the habit of our ancestors. Physical activity is no longer obligatory for daily living, and the relationship between eating and physical work has been altered. However, genetic evolution has been unable to match the rapidity of our modern lifestyle changes and consequently, our genes remain adapted for conditions that existed during their selection over tens of thousands of years ago. Simply stated, it is this discordance between the circumstances of our modern life and our genetic make-up that has contributed to the burgeoning of many of our current health problems.

2 SEDENTARY LIVING IS A DIRECT CAUSE OF MANY CHRONIC HEALTH CONDITIONS AND MORTALITY

Epidemiological evidence shows that sedentary lifestyle is an independent risk factor for at least 20 chronic diseases (Table 28.1).

Compared to the number of deaths from microbial agents, firearms, illicit usage of drugs, sexually transmitted diseases and motor vehicle accidents, deaths from sedentary living are three times greater (McGinnis & Foege 1993). Such research may form the basis for the CDC decision to

Table 28.1 Chronic health conditions associated with sedentary living

Coronary heart disease
Breast cancer
Colon cancer
Congestive heart failure
Cognitive dysfunction
Depression
Dyslipidaemia
Gallstone disease
Hypertension
Obesity
Osteoarthritis
Osteoporosis
Pancreatic cancer
Peripheral vascular disease
Physical frailty
Premature mortality
Prostate cancer
Sleep apnoea
Stroke
Type 2 diabetes

designate sedentary living as an actual cause of death (defined as lifestyle and behavioural factors that directly contribute to the leading causes of deaths from heart disease, cancer, stroke, etc.). Thus, in 2000, sedentary lifestyle accounted for 334,000 premature deaths in the US from these diseases, trailing tobacco use (430,000 deaths), making it the second most dangerous lifestyle choice (Chakravarthy & Booth 2003). In other words, within the last 100 years, the major causes of death have largely shifted from infectious agents in the early 20th century to those resulting from sedentary lifestyle in the 21st century, thereby constituting a new scourge for humanity.

Hence, the obvious question must be raised: how exactly does sedentary living produce such devastating effects on the population's health? An answer to this question requires us to consider the evolutionary origins of how our genome was moulded during an era of obligatory physical activity, and the resultant discordance between our ancient genotype and the modern phenotype.

3 WHY IS A SEDENTARY LIFESTYLE NON-PHYSIOLOGICAL? AN EVOLUTIONARY PERSPECTIVE

Through nearly all of human evolutionary history, physical exercise and food procurement were irrevocably linked to the survival of our ancestors. Much of human biology, and presumably some of human behaviours are thought to have been naturally selected during the Late Palaeolithic era. During this period (50,000–10,000 BC, the Old Stone Age), humans mainly existed as hunter-gatherers and consequently, it was not unusual for our ancestors to undergo cycles of feast and famine, as food was never guaranteed. Famines commonly occurred through drought conditions, an unsuccessful hunt or an inability to hunt due to incapacitation or illness.

Besides cycles of feast and famine, cycles of physical activity and rest were also present. Archaeological records suggest that men undertook a hunt usually on 1–4 non-consecutive days a week, whereas women gathered food every 2–3 days (Cordain et al. 1998). The major adaptations for human survival therefore had to evolve to support cycles of habitual physical activity–rest and feast–famine. Such circumstances most likely demanded a metabolic framework in which homeostasis was maintained by an oscillating enzymatic regulation of fuel storage and usage (Figure 28.1).

3.1 Concept of the 'thrifty genes'

In a cyclical environment where food was not assured, individuals highly efficient in caloric intake and utilisation would have had a survival advantage during famines, using their larger, previously stored energy to maintain homeostasis, while those without such ability would be at a disadvantage, and less likely to survive. Stated another way, the former individuals could be said to be more thrifty

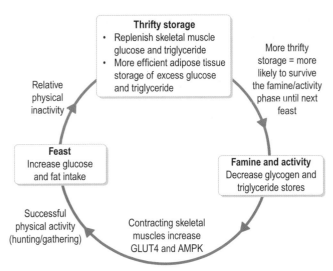

Figure 28.1 The normal feast–famine and physical activity cycle. In the Late Palaeolithic era, during periods of feast, thrifty mechanisms were used to ensure adequate storage of fuel for periods of impending famine/fast. Such efficient storage and utilisation of fuel (for example, via glucose transporter 4 (GLUT4) and adenosine monophosphate–activated protein kinase (AMPK) mechanisms allowing for greater fuel extraction in working skeletal muscles) permitted our ancestors to continue intense physical labour to hunt for food despite a prolonged fasted state. Once the hunt was completed, feast once again ensued and the exhausted fuel stores were replenished for another cycle. The highly conserved thrifty mechanisms of our hunter-gatherer ancestors continue to be in operation today. Although there have been no true famines in developed countries in the 21st century, the presence of a certain threshold of physical activity ensures that this cycling of metabolic processes continues. Illustration reproduced with permission from Chakravarthy & Booth (2004).

with regard to their fuel (energy) balance. These notions are formalised by the so-called thrifty gene hypothesis, initially proposed by Neel (1962), in which he argued that certain genes were incorporated into our genome because of their selective advantage over less thrifty genes. It was under the environmental pressures of the physically active, hunter-gatherer environment that existed over tens of thousands of years that most of the current human genome evolved and was selected. Remarkably, the portion of the human genome that determines basic anatomy and physiology has remained relatively unchanged to this day.

However, the physical environment, especially with regard to physical activity and food availability, has dramatically changed compared to 10,000 years ago. Though the absolute caloric intake of humans in the 21st century is thought to be lower compared to our Late Paleolithic ancestors, it is nevertheless high compared to the corresponding decrease in caloric expenditure by physical activity. Hence, those thrifty genes that evolved for a selective advantage and survival 10,000 years ago are now being exposed to a constant food supply and physical inactivity, resulting in homeostatic disruption, and a disadvantage with respect to

chronic diseases and longevity. The genes of our ancestors were not likely to be selected for a sedentary existence; those whose genes only supported sedentary living were probably eliminated from the gene pool due to their incompatibility with hunting and gathering. Accordingly, natural selection has decreed that contemporary humans have the genotype of hunter-gatherers.

Thus, the modern sedentary environment, on the background of our palaeolithically programmed genome, leads to a mismatch in gene–environmental interactions, with dysregulated gene expression in multiple organ systems ultimately resulting in a wide range of pathological states. The contention is that the absence of both famine and physical activity in modern life eliminates the obligate metabolic cycling of fuel stores that is normally induced by the feast–famine and activity–rest cycles needed to maintain homeostasis.

3.2 Cyclical utilisation and storage of fuels

The major fuel sources are glycogen and triglyceride. In the fed state, storage of glycogen, triglyceride synthesis and carbohydrate oxidation would take priority. In the fasted state, preservation of glycogen, gluconeogenesis and fatty acid oxidation predominate (Chapter 7). While after physical activity, resynthesis of glycogen and triglyceride dominate, during exercise (especially in endurance-trained skeletal muscle), fatty acid oxidation and glycogen sparing occurs, similar to that seen in the fasted state. Although the duration of physical activity–rest cycling is shorter (hours) than feast–famine cycling (days), similar biochemical events are observed in both exercising and fasted individuals, for the conservation of skeletal muscle glycogen and fatty acids, compared with the sedentary and food-abundant state (see Table 28.2).

These speculations are corroborated by established physiological principles. For example, the human body only stores ~3.8 MJ (~900 kcal) of glycogen, but can store ~500 MJ (~120,000 kcal) of triglyceride. Why would evolution select for such a small storage of carbohydrate for periods of famine, since 3.8 MJ is hardly sufficient to supply even one day of total caloric output? One answer could be that the liver evolved to store glycogen to ensure the provision of a constant supply of glucose for the brain and red blood cells, since they depend exclusively on glucose for their fuel supply. In contrast, skeletal muscle glycogen provides the primary fuel source for high-intensity activities, and could therefore be related to survival during evolution. This idea is supported by empirical observations. Following an exercise bout that depleted muscle and liver glycogen, there was a complete repletion of skeletal muscle glycogen stores that occurred 1–2 hours before that of the liver, which had less than 50% repletion at four hours postexercise (Terjung et al. 1974). These data suggest that the small storage of glycogen in skeletal muscle, relative to demand during physical activity, may establish a cycle of glycogen

Table 28.2 Directional changes in key regulatory processes during feast, famine, exercise, and that expected after recovery from exercise. Note the similarities in the directional changes of arrows in feast and recovery from exercise columns (2 and 3) and in the famine, and during exercise columns (4 and 5) for all parameters, except insulin sensitivity. ↑, increased; ↓, decreased (reproduced with permission from Chakravarthy & Booth 2004)

1 Parameter	2 Feast	3 Recovery from exercise	4 Famine	5 During exercise
Blood glucose	↑	↑ (if decreased by exercise)	↓	↓ (>3 h)
Blood insulin	↑	↑ (from decreased level by exercise)	↓	↓
Insulin sensitivity	↓	↓	↓	↑
Skeletal muscle glycogen level	↑	↑ (from decreased level by exercise)	↓	↓
Skeletal muscle fatty acid oxidation	↓	↓ (from increased level by exercise)	↑	↑ (goes up significantly to preserve glycogen stores)

depletion and repletion. It is possible that evolution may have selected for those genes that would be the most efficient to conserve and utilise muscle glycogen.

An example of such a gene is pyruvate dehydrogenase kinase 4. Exercising when muscle glycogen concentration is low markedly induces gene expression for this enzyme, compared to when muscle glycogen concentration is high at the start of exercise (Furuyama et al. 2003). Pyruvate dehydrogenase kinase 4 inhibits the reaction that allows the products of glycolysis to enter the mitochondria, thereby limiting the amount of energy gained from carbohydrates, allowing glycolytic products to go to the liver for gluconeogenesis. Thus, induction of pyruvate dehydrogenase kinase 4 in skeletal muscle at the end of a long exercise bout, appears not only to be a defensive mechanism, reflecting priority given to the metabolic needs of the brain, but also to ensure the replenishment of glycogen stores as quickly as possible, preparing the body for the next challenge. It is conceivable that those hunter-gatherers who had a survival advantage during famines may have had genes that were more efficient in conserving glycogen during and after an unsuccessful hunt for food.

Taken together, the glycogen-cycling regulatory mechanisms for these hunter-gatherer activities could be a common product of natural selection. It appears that evolution placed a high selective priority on the storage and use of skeletal muscle glycogen to provide rapid energy for immediate tasks related to muscle work and survival. However, when both famine and physical activity are removed from the genetically selected expectation of metabolic cycling, as is the case in our modern society, the feast–famine and physical activity–rest cycles stall in feast and inactivity. Consequently, the cycling that certain metabolic genes were programmed to expect also stalls. As a result, there is an even greater and unhealthy storage of fuel (triglyceride), ultimately resulting in adverse metabolic outcomes (Figure 28.2).

4 WHY IS A SEDENTARY LIFESTYLE NON-PHYSIOLOGICAL? EVIDENCE FOR THE EVOLUTIONARY PERSPECTIVE

The evolutionary concepts described above are supported by both epidemiological and basic physiological data.

4.1 Epidemiological studies

Studies in current hunter-gatherer societies support the notion of the discordance between our genetically controlled biology and the circumstances of our current environment, including changes in habitual exercise and nutrition. For example, current hunter-gatherer societies rarely develop hypertension, obesity, sarcopenia, hypercholesterolaemia, non-occlusive atheromata or insulin resistance, compared with their prevalence in similarly aged, sedentary populations (Eaton et al. 2002). Even modern humans, if engaged in routine habitual physical activity, can stave off many chronic ills. Compared with cohorts who had >2.5 h·wk^{-1} of moderate-intensity physical activity, participants in the Harvard Nurses Health Study who undertook less than this level of physical activity had a 41% higher prevalence of mortality, 22% increase in breast cancer, 43% increase in coronary heart disease, 85% increase in type 2 diabetes and colon cancer, 92% increase in diabetic cardiomyopathy and 117% increase in ischaemic stroke (Hu et al. 1999, 2000, Rockhill et al. 2001).

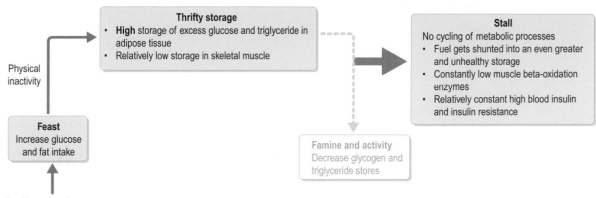

Figure 28.2 Stalling of the feast–famine and physical activity cycle in modern Western society: thrifty storage exists, but famine and physical activity are not utilised. When neither a famine nor an adequate physical activity threshold is present because of abundant food and sedentary living, normal metabolic cycles stall. The result is an unabated storage of fuel without the stimulus for its utilisation. As a consequence of this unhealthy accumulation of fuel stores, in concert with misexpression of thrifty genes, metabolic derangements ensue. Illustration reproduced with permission from Chakravarthy & Booth (2004).

Estimates of physical activity in the Late Palaeolithic era and contemporary physically active societies are both much greater than in the current sedentary population. Hominid energy expenditure declined from ~206 kJ·kg^{-1}·d^{-1} (49 kcal·kg^{-1}·d^{-1}), a value present for much of the past 3.5 million years, to ~134 kJ·kg^{-1}·d^{-1} (32 kcal·kg^{-1}·d^{-1}) for contemporary humans, a reduction of 35% (Cordain et al. 1998). Such reductions, when factored over time, translate to deleterious clinical consequences. For example, the prevalence of type 2 diabetes is six times greater for Arizona Pima Indians than for Mexican Pimas. This dramatic difference between two geographically separate, but genetically similar populations can be explained by lifestyle and behaviour patterns. The Arizona Pimas had <5 h·wk^{-1} of work-related physical activity, yet they consumed a typical US diet, whereas the Mexican Pimas had 23 h·wk^{-1} of physical activity and ate mainly vegetable staples. These findings clearly underscore the importance of environmental interactions with the genome.

Similarly, in the Pacific island of Naura, where diabetes was virtually unknown 50 years ago, it is now present in approximately 40% of adults. In general, the estimated prevalence of type 2 diabetes is 1.1% in present-day hunter-gatherer societies, while it is 6% in developed countries. The CDC estimate that 33% of those born in 2000 in the US will develop diabetes in their lifetime. As genes and gene polymorphisms have not changed in the past 40 years, 100% of this epidemic increase must therefore be due to environmental modulation of existing diabetes susceptibility genes. Taken together, these observations further support the notion that contemporary physical ills are related to the incompatibility between lifestyles and the environments in which humans currently live, and the conditions under which human biology evolved.

4.2 Physiological studies

Adverse health risk factors of sedentary living manifest in a relatively short period of time. Prediabetic conditions in healthy humans (decreased oral glucose tolerance with increased fasting plasma glucose and insulin concentration) occur within 3 days of commencing continuous bed rest when trained individuals stop exercising (Heath et al. 1983; see also Chapter 9). Similarly, when endurance-trained subjects refrained from physical training for several days, the metabolic clearance rate of glucose (measured using the euglycaemic clamp technique) decreased by ~46% 7 days after detraining commenced, compared to the clearance rate observed just 12 h after the last bout of exercise (Burstein et al. 1985). These data suggest that physical inactivity plays a key role in the rapid development of insulin resistance (Chapter 30).

Dysregulation in glucose homeostasis is also present in animal models of physical inactivity. Abrupt cessation of physical activity following 3 weeks of voluntary running in rats resulted in a rapid and synchronous decline in submaximal, insulin-stimulated glucose uptake, and decreased insulin binding to its receptor. Several components of the insulin signal transduction pathway were affected just 53 h after ceasing physical activity, including decreased insulin receptor β-tyrosine phosphorylation, decreased Akt phosphorylation and decreased glucose transporter 4 concentrations from the muscles of these rats (Kump & Booth 2005).

Remarkably, in the same animal model, there was a 25% and 48% increase in the epididymal (testicular) and omental (visceral) fat masses, respectively, just 53 h after the cessation of physical activity. This was due to increased triglyceride synthesis rates, indicating that triglyceride synthesis cycles with daily physical activity. CCAAT/enhancer binding protein α, a marker of adipose differentiation, was 41% higher in sedentary rats as compared to the group that ran for 3 weeks before becoming sedentary (Kump et al. 2006). Triglyceride synthesis was suppressed during and for 5 h after an exercise bout, which was mediated in part by an increase in adenosine monophosphate-activated protein kinase, a critical sensor of cellular energy status (Kahn et al. 2005). However, triglyceride levels subsequently overshot sedentary values due to increased protein abundance and activity of mitochondrial glycerol 3 phosphate acyltransferase-1, the rate-controlling enzyme in glycerolipid synthesis that aids in partitioning acyl-CoAs toward triacylglycerol synthesis and away from degradative pathways, by 3.5-fold from the 10th to the 53rd h (Kump et al. 2006).

The above data provide two critical insights. First, they provide experimental evidence for the previously conjectured metabolic cycling of fuels (Figure 28.1), as daily physical activity cycles triglyceride synthesis in the fat pads of rats, and is abrogated when physical activity ceases for only a few days, stalling triacylglycerol synthesis at its apparent zenith. Second, the adaptive and maladaptive changes occur relatively rapidly (2 days) following the cessation of physical activity, such as the disruption in glucose handling (insulin signalling) and changes in proteins controlling triglyceride metabolism. This latter point further provides the scientific rationale for the recommendation that physical activity be performed routinely (daily and habitual) to obtain health benefits.

5 PATHOPHYSIOLOGICAL CONSEQUENCES OF A SEDENTARY LIFESTYLE

The remainder of this chapter will provide a brief overview highlighting the multisystem dysfunction resulting from chronic, sedentary living. Readers interested in more information on primary research material and detailed references to these and other related topics should consult Booth et al. (2002) and Chakravarthy & Booth (2003).

5.1 Cardiovascular

5.1.1 Vasculature

Endothelial cells are an important cell type for detecting preclinical cardiovascular disease. Accumulative evidence indicates that physical inactivity produces endothelial dysfunction, in part by diminishing the number of pulsatile increases in blood flow through coronary blood vessels. As a result of an absence of exercise-induced, pulsatile increases in coronary blood flow, the corresponding lack of vascular shear stresses removes the stimulus for vasodilatory (acute) and structural enlargement (chronic) adaptations. The prevalence of some clinical conditions that depress endothelial function is enhanced by sedentary behaviour. For example, obesity and insulin resistance are associated with blunted endothelium-dependent but not endothelium-independent vasodilatation; patients with type 1 or type 2 diabetes have significant abnormalities in endothelial function, and reduced high-density lipoprotein is associated with endothelial vasomotor dysfunction.

A major factor contributing to endothelial dysfunction is the loss of nitric oxide, a potent antiatherogenic agent mediating its actions via vasodilatation, inhibition of platelet aggregation, smooth muscle cell proliferation and leucocyte adhesion in the vessel wall. Hypercholesterolaemia, diabetes and hypertension are all associated with reduced synthesis or increased degradation of vascular nitric oxide.

Physical inactivity decreases nitric oxide production by lowering endothelial nitric oxide synthase expression, consequently producing vasoconstriction. All nitric oxide synthase isoforms catalyse reactive oxygen species such as superoxide anion formation, which in turn reduces oxidative stress in endothelial cells. Oxidative stress is a condition implicated in the pathogenesis of diabetes and atherosclerosis. The sedentary state further decreases the elimination of these reactive intermediates as the concentration of extracellular superoxide dismutase, the enzyme that converts superoxide anion into hydrogen peroxide, is reduced, thereby enhancing the potential of superoxide anion to degrade the exercise-induced increases in nitric oxide, resulting in vasoconstriction and further endothelial damage (Kingwell 2000).

Clinical and postmortem investigations of recent hunter-gatherer societies reveal little or no heart disease, with low serum cholesterol concentrations, despite consuming 65% of their energy from animal food (see also Eaton et al. 2002). However, when individuals from these societies became westernised, their incidence of coronary heart disease rose significantly. Therefore, the qualitative differences in the intake of fats, salt, antioxidants, fibre, vitamins and phytochemicals may have operated synergistically with habitual exercise, less stress and no smoking to suppress cardiovascular disease in the hunter-gatherers.

5.1.2 Myocardium

Common convention recognises two major categories of cardiac hypertrophy: one in which cardiac reserve and contractility are enhanced (physiological hypertrophy associated with endurance-trained individuals), and the other in which contractility diminishes (pathological hypertrophy produced by pressure overload, such as hypertension leading to congestive heart failure). While the former improves cardiac function by decreasing oxygen demand and increasing filling time, venous return and maximal cardiac output, the latter decreases ejection fraction, filling time and increases myocardial oxygen demand.

Physiological hypertrophy of cardiac myocytes cannot be explained solely by an inherited and fixed genome, but rather, it is attributable to the plastic nature of cardiac tissue, which in turn is influenced by a dynamic and changing microenvironment. For example, cardiac dimensions of sedentary young men rapidly increase with swim training and decrease with deconditioning. As palaeolithic humans laboured for their survival, they possibly exhibited physiological left ventricular hypertrophy and high cardiac reserves.

Pathological hypertrophy results in cardiac dysfunction, ultimately leading to congestive heart failure. A sedentary lifestyle is considered an independent risk factor for the development of congestive heart failure, accounting for 9.2% of all cases. To put this number in perspective, compare this to the contributions from hypertension (10.2%), diabetes (3.2%) and obesity (8.0%; He et al. 2001). Therefore, habitual physical inactivity can directly (via a lack of physiological hypertrophy) or indirectly (by prevention of hypertension, diabetes, obesity) account for the development of a significant percentage of cases of pathological cardiac hypertrophy.

The two forms of cardiac hypertrophy are distinguishable by unique molecular signatures. While physiological hypertrophy in rats is associated with specific increases in the messenger ribonucleic acid (mRNA) of transforming growth factor-1, calcineurin, insulin-like growth factor I and noradrenaline, pathological hypertrophy is associated with selective increases in the mRNA of transforming growth factor-3, fibronectin and preprocollagen (Calderone et al. 2001). Also, a greater accumulation of total collagen was noted in pressure-overloaded rat hearts compared to hearts from voluntarily running rats.

Taken together, these data show that habitual physical activity produces a distinct cardiac phenotype, with superior function (physiological cardiac hypertrophy), and possibly represented the norm in 10,000 BC, thereby facilitating survival. In contrast, the prevalent form of cardiac enlargement in the current sedentary environment is pathological cardiac hypertrophy, which predisposes to increased mortality. Ironically, despite the fact that the inheritance of our genome was shaped by a physically active environment, the current dogma defines the heart of a sedentary human as normal or the control state, while physiological hypertrophy (i.e. athlete's heart) is defined as an adaptation. In much the same manner, we hear some in the exercise sciences refer to exercise as a health intervention strategy. Instead, it may be argued that habitual exercise is the normal state, whereas habitual physical inactivity is the intervention, the result of which has serious health consequences. In short, as physically active individuals are healthier than sedentary individuals, then physically active subjects should compose the control group in exercise studies (Booth & Lees 2006).

5.2 Metabolic

5.2.1 Insulin resistance and type 2 diabetes

Sedentary living elevates the risk of type 2 diabetes, even in normal-weight individuals, underscoring the fact that habitual physical inactivity is an independent risk factor for

this disease (Chapter 30). There is a strong inverse association between walking score and the risk of type 2 diabetes. Compared with women who were consistently sedentary (metabolic equivalent (MET) score of ≤0.5), women who were consistently active (median MET score of 20, which is at least 2.5 h·wk^{-1} of brisk walking) had a lower risk of developing diabetes (relative risk = 0.74), even after additional adjustment for body mass index (Hu et al. 1999). The MET value is the energy need per kilogram of body weight per hour of activity, divided by the energy need per kilogram of body mass per hour at rest. Because sedentary individuals are likely to have a higher body fat content, physical inactivity also contributes to an increased prevalence of type 2 diabetes by its direct effect on increasing adiposity in certain individuals, as the prevalence of type 2 diabetes increases in individuals with a body mass index >25 kg·m^{-2}.

Skeletal muscle is the predominant site of insulin and non-insulin dependent glucose disposal in humans. Habitual physical activity increases insulin sensitivity because of an increased number and activity of glucose transporters (GLUT4) in both muscle and adipose tissue. During hyperinsulinaemia, insulin-mediated glucose uptake in skeletal muscle represents 75% and 95% of total body rate of glucose disappearance at euglycaemia and hyperglycaemia, respectively. But, in patients with type 2 diabetes, skeletal muscles have impaired glucose response, even to normal levels of circulating insulin.

The molecular mechanisms leading to insulin- and exercise-induced stimulation of glucose uptake in skeletal muscle are distinct. Although contracting skeletal muscles increase their glucose uptake, proximal insulin signalling steps are not components of the signalling mechanism by which physical activity stimulates glucose uptake. For example, contractile activity does not stimulate autophosphorylation of insulin receptors, insulin receptor substrate tyrosine phosphorylation or phosphatidylinositol 3' kinase activity (Goodyear & Kahn 1998). However, muscle contraction is thought to stimulate adenosine monophosphate-activated protein kinase activity, which in turn stimulates the expression of glucose transporter 4 and hexokinase (both of which increase glucose uptake), and mitochondrial enzymes (which increase oxidative phosphorylation). However, recent findings suggest that the increase in glucose transporter 4 expression, in response to exercise and denervation, does not require adenosine monophosphate-activated protein kinase (Holmes et al. 2004), but is obligatory for insulin- and exercise-stimulated glucose uptake in skeletal muscle, and its transcription and protein levels are markedly decreased in inactive muscles.

Besides activation of adenosine monophosphate-activated protein kinase, muscle contraction also induces additional signalling pathways, including calcium, protein kinase C, nitric oxide and glycogen, all of which are hypothesised to enhance glucose uptake into moderately contracting skeletal muscles (Richter et al. 2001). A rise in the intracellular calcium concentration is a contributing factor to enhanced glucose uptake during muscle contractions, as increased calcium not only enhances glucose transporter 4 translocation to the sarcolemma directly through protein kinase C, but also indirectly via the induction of myocyte enhancer factors 2A and 2D, transcription factors that activate the promoter of the glucose transporter 4 gene, enhancing its transcription (Mora & Pessin 2000). While the role of nitric oxide in exercise-stimulated glucose uptake remains controversial, lower muscle glycogen content appears to induce adenosine monophosphate-activated protein kinase activity (Barnes et al. 2005).

5.2.2 Obesity and dyslipidaemia

Sedentary subjects tend to have larger adipose tissue stores and decreased fat oxidation. Habitual physical activity increases the activation efficiency of the lipolytic β-adrenergic pathway in subcutaneous abdominal adipose tissue. As noted in section 4.2, abrupt cessation of voluntary running activity in rats resulted in a rapid accumulation of epididymal and omental fat mass, caused by an increase in triglyceride synthesis rates, mediated by the induction of mitochondrial glycerol-3-phosphate acyltransferase activity.

Sedentary lifestyle in the absence of simultaneous dietary interventions results in mean increases in triglycerides, low-density lipoprotein cholesterol and total cholesterol of 3.8%, 5.3% and 1.0%, respectively (Leon & Sanchez 2001). Though it remains unknown whether repeated elevations in postprandial lipoproteins directly lead to the development of atherosclerosis (i.e. after food consumption), it is well established that the sedentary state markedly increases fasting and postprandial triglyceride-rich lipoprotein levels, which in turn are strongly linked with coronary heart disease. Several studies have documented a significant attenuation of the postprandial rise in total triglyceride concentration and triglycerides associated with very low-density lipoproteins and chylomicrons, through physical activity performed 12–16 h prior to eating a fatty meal. Increased high-density lipoprotein cholesterol concentrations are also seen in the venous blood obtained from exercising muscles, with higher levels seen if the exercise bout had been performed 12 h prior to the meal. Physical inactivity decreases plasma high-density lipoprotein cholesterol levels by 4.4%, which translates to an approximate increase in risk for coronary heart disease by 4% in men and 6% in women (Leon & Sanchez 2001).

The mechanism by which the sedentary state increases postprandial lipaemia involves a suppressed lipoprotein lipase-mediated process that reduces clearance of triglyceride-rich lipoproteins. Lipoprotein lipase activity in plasma and muscle peaks about 4–18 h after exercise. Subjects who had the lowest skeletal muscle lipoprotein lipase activity after exercise also had the most noticeable increases in postprandial lipaemia. Detraining in athletes (Chapter 9) results

in a differential response in lipoprotein lipase activity: decreased muscle and increased adipose tissue (both of which occur through posttranslational mechanisms), such that the adipose to muscle lipoprotein lipase ratio rises from 0.51 before detraining to 4.45 after detraining (Simsolo et al. 1993). Therefore, the sedentary state results in a preferential uptake of fatty acids or glucose into adipose tissue. In contrast, lipoprotein lipase activity is decreased in skeletal muscles, which in turn minimises the lipolytic effect in the capillaries supplying muscle.

It is important to bear in mind that the effect of a single bout of physical activity in decreasing postprandial lipaemia is short-lived, again underscoring the fact that persistent, habitual (daily) physical activity is needed to obtain and maintain the lipid-lowering effects.

5.3 Skeletal muscle

5.3.1 Skeletal muscle mass and hypertrophy

Sedentary behaviour accelerates the loss of skeletal muscle strength and consequently, the onset of physical frailty during ageing (Chapters 13 and 16). Individuals who have lost more than 10% of their body mass after age 50 have a relatively high death rate. A comprehensive review of the scientific literature by Spirduso & Cronin (2001) further corroborates the inverse relationship between regular physical activity and physical disability. For example, 60-year-old women gained strength in three muscle groups after 12 months of resistance exercise, and these gains occurred throughout the year. Such training also improved their gait and balance, leading to fewer falls and fractures, ultimately decreasing nursing home admissions (Chapter 31.1).

Skeletal muscle hypertrophy is mediated by the complex interplay of several factors. Actin promoter activity, messenger ribonucleic acid and protein synthesis have all been shown to increase in an animal overload model of muscle hypertrophy and serum response element 1 was identified as the specific hypertrophy regulatory site on the actin promoter (Carson et al. 1995). Serum response element 1 activates specific contractile protein genes to produce more messenger ribonucleic acid in response to overload conditions by homodimerising to a transcription factor called serum response factor. In addition, early adaptive changes in skeletal muscle during increased loading are also due to enhanced translation of existing mRNAs to increase protein production after a few days of overloading.

The type of physical activity stimulus governs the intricate balance by which signalling pathways are turned on or off, providing for a regulation of phenotypic outcomes. For example, aerobic exercise does not affect phosphorylation of p70S6 kinase, whereas high-resistance exercise does. The stimulus for muscle hypertrophy is also dictated by the extrinsic microenvironment, which in turn regulates intracellular mediators of hypertrophy such as Akt. For instance, increasing extracellular concentrations of insulin-like growth factor I resulted in the recovery of skeletal muscle from atrophy. Akt is critical for the induction of skeletal muscle hypertrophy, as overexpression of a constitutively active form of Akt alone was sufficient to produce marked hypertrophy (Bodine et al. 2001).

5.3.2 Aerobic fitness and oxidation of fuels

A direct association between the duration of contractile activity and mitochondrial density of the contracting skeletal muscle has long been established. Cytochrome c is a marker of mitochondrial density and of the ability to oxidise fuels. Increases and decreases in cytochrome c mRNA abundance occur with habitual exercise and physical inactivity, respectively. Inactive skeletal muscles have lower adenosine monophosphate-activated protein kinase activity that decreases nuclear regulatory factor 1 protein, a transcription factor that binds to promoters for aminolaevulinic acid synthase and mitochondrial transcription factor A genes, in turn leading to decreased cytochrome c protein concentration and mitochondrial density (Hood 2001). Because not all promoters of genes transcribing mitochondrial proteins have nuclear regulatory factor 1 binding sites, other transcription factors would also be involved in contractile activity-modulated mitochondrial biogenesis. Though surprisingly, inactivation of adenosine monophosphate-activated protein kinase in skeletal muscle was shown not to have a significant effect on contraction-induced muscle glucose uptake (Jorgensen et al. 2004), earlier studies have shown adenosine monophosphate-activated protein kinase to be involved in the adaptations to aerobic exercise training (increasing hexokinase, uncoupling protein 3, mitochondrial oxidative enzymes and mitochondrial biogenesis; Winder 2001). Clearly, the underlying mechanisms are complex and continue to be an area of intense investigation (Kahn et al. 2005).

Overall, the existing data suggest that sedentary behaviour decreases skeletal muscle mitochondria concentration. The physiological significance of decreased mitochondrial content is the absence of protective homeostasis during disruption, which occurs within contracting skeletal muscles. As demonstrated by the classical work of Saltin & Karlsson (1971), when the same human is tested at the same submaximal oxygen uptake before and after endurance training, glycogen depletion and lactate concentrations in the quadriceps muscle are lower. Endurance-trained muscles have increased concentrations of enzymes for β-oxidation and oxidise more fatty acids (sparing the limited stores of glycogen) at the same absolute workload. This has a resultant protection against hypoglycaemia-induced fatigue and increases exercise time to exhaustion. Creatine phosphate concentrations are higher and inorganic phosphate, adenosine diphosphate, adenosine monophosphate and lactate concentrations are lower in muscles of endurance-trained rats with higher mitochondrial concentrations, as compared with untrained rats during the same contractile activity

(Constable et al. 1987; see also Chapter 6). Thus, exercise-deficient skeletal muscles, as seen in sedentary conditions, undergo a greater homeostatic disruption at the same absolute work intensity. This translates to a decreased aerobic potential (i.e. diminished endurance fitness or aerobic power) that is ultimately associated with increased mortality.

5.4 Brain

5.4.1 Cognitive dysfunction

Sedentary lifestyle is associated with lower cognitive skills and is accompanied by structural and physiological changes in the brain. A recent report of 2300 women aged 65 years or older showed that habitual physical activity was associated with 37–50% reduced risk of cognitive impairment, Alzheimer's disease and dementia of any type, compared with those who were habitually sedentary (Laurin et al. 2001). A sedentary lifestyle may be a risk factor in neurodegenerative diseases because it is associated with higher risk of cerebrovascular accidents, and is more pronounced in the elderly.

Conversely, physical activity enhances spatial learning, attenuates motor deficits and impedes age-related neuronal loss. Mice undergoing voluntary running learned to negotiate a water maze test better and exhibited an enhanced long-term potentiation in the dentate gyrus. Compared with the sedentary group, voluntary running led to distinct changes in gene expression patterns within the rat hippocampus, known to be associated with neuronal activity, synaptic structure and neuronal plasticity. Exercised aged rats not only had 11% more Purkinje cells and 9% larger Purkinje cell volumes compared to sedentary aged rats, but also had the same number of Purkinje cells as young rats (Larsen et al. 2000). These protective processes are akin to physiologically successful ageing (Chapter 16).

Physical activity also ameliorates neurological impairments in different neurodegenerative processes. For example, exercise improved the recovery from brain damage caused by stroke or multiple sclerosis (Eldar & Marincek 2000). These neuroprotective effects could be mediated by enhancement of cerebral blood flow, lowering lipid levels, inhibiting platelet aggregability and increasing cerebral nutrient supply. Physical activity induces a mild stress response, resulting in the expression of genes that encode neurotrophic factors and heat shock proteins that serve to suppress oxyradical production and stabilise cellular calcium homeostasis.

Sedentary behaviour decreases neural cell proliferation and survival by lowering many growth factors, such as insulin-like growth factor I, fibroblast growth factor-2, brain-derived neurotrophic factor and glial cell-derived neurotrophic factor in the brain, compared with physically active rats (see Dishman et al. 2006 for more references). The fibroblast growth factor family and brain-derived neurotrophic factor increase neurogenesis, thereby playing a key role in learning and synaptic plasticity. Consistent with this notion, lumbar spinal cords of sedentary rats had decreased brain-derived neurotrophic factor mRNA expression with lower neurotrophic factor protein levels in the motor neuron cell bodies and axons of the ventral horns of their spinal cords. Sedentary animals also have reduced brain uptake of serum insulin-like growth factor I compared with exercising animals. When uptake of insulin-like growth factor I by brain cells was blocked in rats undergoing exercise training, the exercise-induced increase on c-fos expression was also blocked, suggesting that increased brain levels are caused by increased uptake of insulin-like growth factor I from serum during exercise. Because peripheral administration of insulin-like growth factor I also resulted in increases in the number of new neurons in the hippocampus of hypophysectomised rats, circulating insulin-like growth factor I might be mediating the stimulatory effects of exercise on the number of new hippocampal neurons in normal adult rats (Trejo et al. 2001). Taken together, these data imply that being sedentary increases the susceptibility to neurodegenerative processes attributable to insufficient brain uptake of serum insulin-like growth factor I.

5.5 Bone

5.5.1 Osteoporosis

Osteoporosis is a systemic skeletal disease characterised by low bone mass and microarchitectural deterioration of bone tissue, with a consequent increase in bone fragility and susceptibility to fracture (Chapter 13). It is defined as a bone density at, or more than 2.5 standard deviations below the normal peak values for young adults. Osteoporosis occurs when bone reabsorption exceeds bone formation. Current evidence indicates that three environmental factors accelerate bone loss: habitual physical inactivity, insufficient nutrient and calcium intake, and reduced reproductive hormones. Bone loss is continual with ageing in the sedentary individual and inactivity speeds the onset of osteoporosis. The results from the National Osteoporosis Risk Assessment (Siris et al. 2001) indicated that people who habitually exercised had a significantly reduced risk of developing osteoporosis.

Low bone mineral density is the single best predictor of fracture risk, with hip fractures being associated with a 20% increase in overall mortality. Epidemiological data show that bed rest markedly accelerates bone loss. Significant quantities of bone mineral were lost in healthy subjects after 17 weeks of bed rest (Chapter 9). Immobilised patients can lose up to 40% of their bone mineral density in 1 year, whereas simply standing upright for as little as 30 $min \cdot d^{-1}$ can prevent this loss, at least within load-bearing bones.

Although not fully understood, it is thought that formation of new bone through increased loading may be regulated through complex interactions of increases in insulin-like growth factor I, prostaglandins and nitric oxide (Chow 2000). These adaptive changes may be disrupted by sedentary behaviour. During the early phases of mechanical loading, the expression of insulin-like growth factor I is increased in osteocytes. This increased expression is consistent with the model in which insulin-like growth factor I, generated by osteocytes in response to mechanical loading, participates in the induction of bone formation. In addition, the increase in insulin-like growth factor I is thought to play a significant role in the regulation of bone formation, by its ability to induce proliferation and differentiation of osteoblastic cells in culture. Prostaglandins are produced soon after the administration of mechanical strain in osteoblastic cells. Furthermore, it is known that new bone formation, induced by mechanical strain, can be inhibited by drugs that inhibit prostaglandin formation (e.g. indometacin). Interestingly, prostaglandins have been shown to increase insulin-like growth factor I in osteoblastic cells. This suggests that prostaglandins can be elevated by mechanical strain, thereby activating insulin-like growth factor I and inducing the net formation of new bone.

Finally, nitric oxide was also shown to be involved in the formation of new bone, using both agonists and antagonists of nitric oxide production that affected the induction and inhibition of new bone formation under mechanical strain, respectively (Chow 2000). Expression of the endothelial nitric oxide synthase isoform recently detected in osteoblasts and osteocytes was shown to be sufficient to stimulate proliferation of osteoblasts in cell culture.

6 CONCLUSION

Sedentary behaviour is extremely common. Indeed, it can be considered a clinical condition in much the same way as any other chronic health condition, as a sedentary lifestyle directly leads to pathophysiological changes, affecting the structural and functional regulation of multiple organ systems (Figure 28.3).

The modern deleterious consequences of habitual physical inactivity have their origins in evolution based on the natural selection of the human genome, under conditions of obligate physical activity. In this sense, sedentary living is an unnatural condition, and the body's physiological response to this condition is an adaptation to reset homeostasis towards levels to which the selected genes were programmed: obligate and habitual physical activity. Consequently, these adaptations (phenotypes) turn out to be maladaptations in the modern era, manifesting themselves as pathological conditions, ranging from weaker bones to heart disease. Therefore, the reintroduction of habitual physical activity into the fabric of our daily life is vital to help restore this homeostasis, thereby allowing for healthier living and physiologically successful ageing.

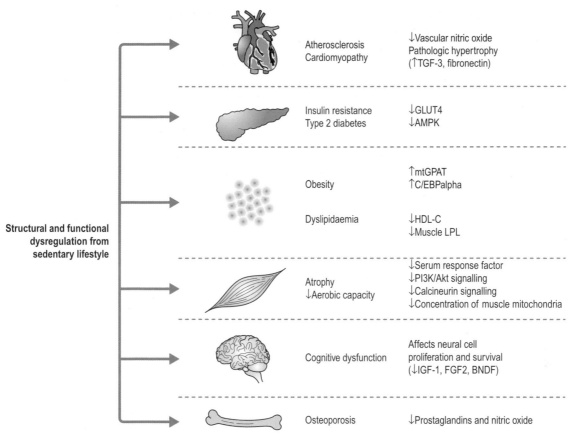

Figure 28.3 A schematic overview of the protean adverse organ system manifestations of sedentary living. Some of the potential mechanisms described for the respective diseases are highlighted in the far right column. Abbreviations: TGF, transforming growth factor; GLUT4, glucose transporter 4; AMPK, adenosine monophosphate-activated protein kinase; TNF, tumour necrosis factor; mtGPAT, mitochondrial glycerol-3-phosphate acyltransferase; C/EBP, CCAAT enhancer binding protein; HDL-C, high-density lipoprotein cholesterol; LPL, lipoprotein lipase; PI3K, phosphatidylinositol 3' kinase; IGF-I, insulin-like growth factor I; FGF; fibroblast growth factor; BNDF, brain-derived neurotrophic factor.

References

Barnes BR, Glund S, Long YC, Hjalm G, Andersson L, Zierath JR 2005 5'-AMP-activated protein kinase regulates skeletal muscle glycogen content and ergogenics. FASEB Journal 19(7):773–779

Bodine SC, Stitt TN, Gonzalez M, Kline WO, Stover GL, Bauerlein R, Zlotchenko E, Scrimgeour A, Lawrence JC, Glass DJ, Yancopoulos GD 2001 Akt/mTOR pathway is a crucial regulator of skeletal muscle hypertrophy and can prevent muscle atrophy in vivo. Nature Cell Biology 3(11):1014–1019

Booth FW, Lees SJ 2006 Physically active subjects should be the control group. Medicine and Science in Sports and Exercise 38(3):405–406

Booth FW, Chakravarthy MV, Gordon SE, Spangenburg EE 2002 Waging war on physical inactivity: using modern molecular ammunition against an ancient enemy. Journal of Applied Physiology 93(1):3–30

Burstein R, Polychronakos C, Toews CJ, MacDougall JD, Guyda HJ, Posner BI 1985 Acute reversal of the enhanced insulin action in trained athletes. Association with insulin receptor changes. Diabetes 34(8):756–60

Calderone A, Murphy RJ, Lavoie J, Colombo F, Beliveau L 2001 TGF beta and prepro ANP mRNAs are differentially regulated in exercise induced cardiac hypertrophy. Journal of Applied Physiology 91(2):771–776

Carson JA, Yan Z, Booth FW, Coleman ME, Schwartz RJ, Stump CS 1995 Regulation of skeletal alpha actin promoter in young chickens during hypertrophy caused by stretch overload. American Journal of Physiology 268(4 Pt 1):C918–C924

Chakravarthy MV, Booth FW 2003 Exercise – hot topics. Elsevier, Philadelphia

Chakravarthy MV, Booth FW 2004 Eating, exercise and 'thrifty' genotypes: connecting the dots toward an evolutionary understanding of modern chronic diseases. Journal of Applied Physiology 96(1):3–10

Chow JW 2000 Role of nitric oxide and prostaglandins in the bone formation response to mechanical loading. Exercise and Sport Science Reviews 28(4):185–188

Constable SH, Favier RJ, McLane JA, Fell RD, Chen M, Holloszy JO 1987 Energy metabolism in contracting rat skeletal muscle: adaptation to exercise training. American Journal of Physiology 253(2 Pt 1):C316–C322

Cordain L, Gotshall RW, Eaton SB, Eaton SB 3rd 1998 Physical activity, energy expenditure and fitness: an evolutionary perspective. International Journal of Sports Medicine 19(5):328–335

Dishman RK, Berthoud HR, Booth FW, Cotman CW, Edgerton VR, Fleshner MR, Gandevia SC, Gomez-Pinilla F, Greenwood BN, Hillman CH, Kramer AF, Levin BE, Moran TH, Russo-Neustadt

AA, Salamone JD, Van Hoomissen JD, Wade CE, York DA, Zigmond MJ 2006 Neurobiology of exercise. Obesity 14(3):345–356

Eaton SB, Strassman BI, Nesse RM, Neel JV, Ewald PW, Williams GC, Weder AB, Eaton SB 3rd, Lindeberg S, Konner MJ, Mysterud I, Cordain L 2002 Evolutionary health promotion. Preventive Medicine 34(2):109–118

Eldar R, Marincek C 2000 Physical activity for elderly persons with neurological impairment: a review. Scandinavian Journal of Rehabilitation Medicine 32(3):99–103

Furuyama T, Kitayama K, Yamashita H, Mori N 2003 Forkhead transcription factor FOXO1 (FKHR)-dependent induction of PDK4 gene expression in skeletal muscle during energy deprivation. Biochemical Journal 375(Pt 2):365–371

Goodyear LJ, Kahn BB 1998 Exercise, glucose transport and insulin sensitivity. Annual Reviews in Medicine 49:235–261

He J, Ogden LG, Bazzano LA, Vupputuri S, Loria C, Whelton PK 2001 Risk factors for congestive heart failure in US men and women: NHANES I epidemiologic follow-up study. Archives of Internal Medicine 161(7):996–1002

Heath GW, Gavin JR 3rd, Hinderliter JM, Hagberg JM, Bloomfield SA, Holloszy JO 1983 Effects of exercise and lack of exercise on glucose tolerance and insulin sensitivity. Journal of Applied Physiology 55(2):512–517

Holmes BF, Lang DB, Birnbaum MJ, Mu J, Dohm GL 2004 AMP kinase is not required for the GLUT4 response to exercise and denervation in skeletal muscle. American Journal of Physiology. Endocrinology and Metabolism 287(4):E739–E743

Hood DA 2001 Invited review: contractile activity-induced mitochondrial biogenesis in skeletal muscle. Journal of Applied Physiology 90(3):1137–1157

Hu FB, Sigal RJ, Rich-Edwards JW, Colditz GA, Solomon CG, Willett WC, Speizer FE, Manson JE 1999 Walking compared with vigorous physical activity and risk of type 2 diabetes in women: a prospective study. Journal of the American Medical Association 282(15):1433–1439

Hu FB, Stampfer MJ, Colditz GA, Ascherio A, Rexrode KM, Willett WC, Manson JE 2000 Physical activity and risk of stroke in women. Journal of the American Medical Association 283(22):2961–2967

Jorgensen SB, Viollet B, Andreelli F, Frosig C, Birk JB, Schjerling P, Vaulont S, Richter EA, Wojtaszewski JF 2004 Knockout of the alpha2 but not alpha1 5′-AMP-activated protein kinase isoform abolishes 5-aminoimidazole-4-carboxamide-1-beta-4-ribofuranosidebut not contraction-induced glucose uptake in skeletal muscle. Journal of Biological Chemistry 279(2):1070–1079

Kahn BB, Alquier T, Carling D, Hardie DG 2005 AMP-activated protein kinase: ancient energy gauge provides clues to modern understanding of metabolism. Cell Metabolism 1(1):15–25

Kingwell BA 2000 Nitric oxide-mediated metabolic regulation during exercise: effects of training in health and cardiovascular disease. FASEB Journal 14(12):1685–1696

Kump DS, Booth FW 2005 Alterations in insulin receptor signalling in the rat epitrochlearis muscle upon cessation of voluntary exercise. Journal of Physiology 562(Pt 3):829–838

Kump DS, Laye MJ, Booth FW 2006 Increased mitochondrial glycerol-3-phosphate acyltransferase protein and enzyme activity in rat epididymal fat upon cessation of wheel running. American Journal of Physiology. Endocrinology and Metabolism 290(3):E480–E489

Larsen JO, Skalicky M, Viidik A 2000 Does long-term physical exercise counteract age-related Purkinje cell loss? A stereological study of rat cerebellum. Journal of Comparative Neurology 428(2):213–222

Laurin D, Verreault R, Lindsay J, MacPherson K, Rockwood K 2001 Physical activity and risk of cognitive impairment and dementia in elderly persons. Archives of Neurology 58(3):498–504

Leon AS, Sanchez OA 2001 Response of blood lipids to exercise training alone or combined with dietary intervention. Medicine and Science in Sports and Exercise 33(6):S502–S515

McGinnis JM, Foege WH 1993 Actual causes of death in the United States. Journal of the American Medical Association 270(18):2207–2212

Mora S, Pessin JE 2000 The MEF2A isoform is required for striated muscle-specific expression of the insulin-responsive GLUT4 glucose transporter. Journal of Biological Chemistry 275(21):16323–16328

Neel JV 1962 Diabetes mellitus: a 'thrifty' genotype rendered detrimental by 'progress'? American Journal of Human Genetics 14:352–353

Pate RR, Pratt M, Blair SN, Haskell WL, Macera CA, Bouchard C, Buchner D, Ettinger W, Heath GW, King AC 1995 Physical activity and public health. A recommendation from the Centers for Disease Control and Prevention and the American College of Sports Medicine. Journal of the American Medical Association 273(5):402–407

Richter EA, Derave W, Wojtaszewski JF 2001 Glucose, exercise and insulin: emerging concepts. Journal of Physiology 535(Pt 2):313–322

Rockhill B, Willett WC, Manson JE, Leitzmann MF, Stampfer MJ, Hunter DJ, Colditz GA 2001 Physical activity and mortality: a prospective study among women. American Journal of Public Health 91(4):578–583

Saltin B, Karlsson J 1971 Muscle ATP, CP and lactate during exercise after physical conditioning. In: Pernow B, Saltin B (eds) Muscle metabolism during exercise. Plenum Press, New York, 395–399

Simsolo RB, Ong JM, Kern PA 1993 The regulation of adipose tissue and muscle lipoprotein lipase in runners by detraining. Journal of Clinical Investigation 92(5):2124–2130

Siris ES, Miller PD, Barrett-Connor E, Faulkner KG, Wehren LE, Abbott TA, Berger ML, Santora AC, Sherwood LM 2001 Identification and fracture outcomes of undiagnosed low bone mineral density in postmenopausal women: results from the National Osteoporosis Risk Assessment. Journal of the American Medical Association 286(22):2815–2822

Spirduso WW, Cronin DL 2001 Exercise dose-response effects on quality of life and independent living in older adults. Medicine and Science in Sports and Exercise 33(6):S598–S610

Terjung RL, Baldwin KM, Winder WW, Holloszy JO 1974 Glycogen repletion in different types of muscle and in liver after exhausting exercise. American Journal of Physiology 226(6):1387–1391

Trejo JL, Carro E, Torres-Aleman I 2001 Circulating insulin-like growth factor I mediates exercise-induced increases in the number of new neurons in the adult hippocampus. Journal of Neuroscience 21(5):1628–1634

Winder WW 2001 Energy-sensing and signaling by AMP-activated protein kinase in skeletal muscle. Journal of Applied Physiology 91(3):1017–1028

Chapter 29

Overreaching and overtraining

Laurel T. Mackinnon Shona L. Halson Sue L. Hooper
Asker E. Jeukendrup

1 INTRODUCTION

Overtraining is the process of excessive exercise training that, if left unchecked, may lead to overtraining syndrome, which is characterised by persistent fatigue, performance decrements, mood state changes and an altered hormonal profile. Athletes also associate overtraining with susceptibility to mild illness, such as upper respiratory tract infection. Overtraining syndrome is thought to reflect the body's inability to adapt to the cumulative fatigue caused by daily intense exercise that is not balanced by the right type and amount of rest or recovery.

Overtraining is important from a practical perspective. An overtrained athlete cannot perform to the level expected and may then train even harder, exacerbating the symptoms and causing performance to decline even further. Studying the physiological dysfunction that accompanies overtraining also contributes to our understanding of the limits of physiological adaptations to exercise stress.

2 DEFINITION AND OVERVIEW OF OVERTRAINING

Overtraining has been called by several terms and defined differently by various groups. Terms frequently used include staleness, underperformance syndrome, overtraining syndrome, burnout, overstrain and overfatigue. There is no single accepted diagnostic tool to identify overtraining. At present, the working definition of overtraining is also used as the diagnostic tool.

2.1 Definitions of fatigue, overreaching and overtraining

Fatigue is a complex and multifaceted phenomenon that has been defined in a variety of ways. This chapter uses the definition of fatigue presented by Gandevia (2001) because it reflects both peripheral and central fatigue, and it focuses on the reduction in force that occurs as fatigue progresses. Muscle fatigue is defined as any exercise-induced reduction in the ability of a muscle to generate force or power; it has both central and peripheral causes (Chapters 5, 6, 7).

Peripheral fatigue is produced by changes at, or distal to the neuromuscular junction, whereas central fatigue is a progressive reduction in voluntary activation of muscle during exercise.

For overreaching and overtraining, we have used the definitions of Kreider et al. (1998), which underline the importance of a decrease in performance as a prerequisite to indicating the state of overreaching or overtraining. These definitions also differentiate between overreaching and overtraining according to the time required for performance to recover. Overreaching is defined as an accumulation of training or non-training stress, resulting in a short-term decrement in performance capacity with or without related physiological and psychological signs and symptoms of overtraining, in which restoration of performance capacity may take several days to several weeks (Kreider et al. 1998). Overtraining is defined similarly but it has an extended timeframe because the restoration of performance may take several weeks or months (Kreider et al. 1998).

2.1.1 Signs and symptoms of overtraining and overreaching

Athletes and coaches associate overtraining with many signs and symptoms, although not all of these have been substantiated by empirical research. Those that have been substantiated are contained in Table 29.1. The symptoms of overreaching, and overtraining are generally similar and only a few symptoms are specific for one outcome or the other. For example, resting heart rate usually increases in overreaching but may be normal in overtraining (Halson & Jeukendrup 2004). The responses to intense training are also highly individual. For example, athletes undertaking similar training may present with different symptoms. This explains why there are, at present, no clear diagnostic markers of overreaching and overtraining besides the operational definitions of Kreider et al. (1998).

2.1.2 Differences between fatigue, overreaching and overtraining

The process by which intense training, in combination with limited recovery leads to overreaching or overtraining is often viewed as a continuum (Fry et al. 1991, Halson & Jeukendrup 2004). This continuum begins with the acute fatigue associated with a single training session, progresses to overreaching when there is an imbalance between training and recovery, and terminates with overtraining if intense training is continued with inadequate recovery (Figure 29.1).

Frequent endurance and resistance exercise stimulates positive physiological and morphological adaptations (Chapter 21), and performance generally improves. However, an imbalance between training and recovery can induce overreaching or a short-term decrement in performance resulting from cumulative fatigue. Continuing to train intensely, with limited or inadequate recovery (cause),

Table 29.1 Signs and symptoms of overtraining and overreaching

Physiological signs and symptoms:
Impaired or unexpected poor performance
Decreased muscular strength and power
Decreased aerobic capacity and power
Increased difference between lying and standing heart rate
Decreased maximal heart rate
Decreased plasma lactate concentration during maximal exercise
Decreased ratio of plasma lactate concentration to effort sense

Psychological signs and symptoms:
Depression-like symptoms
Mood state disturbances: anxiety, apathy, loss of vigour
Disturbed sleep
Difficulty in concentrating at work and training
Decreased ability to narrow concentration
Restlessness and irritability

Biochemical and hormonal signs and symptoms:
Hypothalamic dysfunction
Decreased ratio of free testosterone to cortisol by >30%
Decreased intrinsic sympathetic activity
Decreased β-adrenoreceptor density
Increased plasma norepinephrine concentration
Decreased urinary excretion of norepinephrine

Immunological signs and symptoms:
Increased susceptibility to and severity of upper respiratory tract infection
Frequent mild flu-like illness
Decreased functional activity of neutrophils
Decreased total lymphocyte count
Shift from T helper cell 1 to T helper cell 2 lymphocytes
Decreased interferon-γ production by lymphocytes
Viral reactivation
Decreased mucosal immunoglobulin A concentration

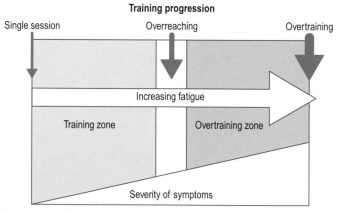

Figure 29.1 The overtraining continuum during continued intense training, but with inadequate recovery. Modified from Halson & Jeukendrup (2004) with permission.

moves the athlete along the overtraining continuum to the more serious state of overtraining (outcome).

2.1.3 Fatigue and overreaching in elite athletes

In the elite athlete, fatigue is a normal part of the training process and can be an important indicator that an athlete is training at the level needed to improve. Many athletes intentionally train intensely over a period of a few days to weeks, with limited recovery, and then follow this with a period of recovery (reduced intensity or volume) to induce supercompensation. According to the overtraining continuum model (see Figure 29.1), fatigue that approaches overreaching is considered a normal part of training at the elite level (Halson & Jeukendrup 2004). However, overreaching may lead to overtraining if an appropriate recovery period (or taper) is not incorporated into the training programme after the period of intense training. The taper is a 1–4-week period of decreased training load (usually volume) that athletes use to peak for major competition.

2.1.4 Diagnosis of overreaching and overtraining

Because fatigue, even to the point of overreaching, is considered a normal part of training, the elite athlete might regularly experience periods of reduced performance during an intense training cycle (before recovery or taper). Therefore, other diagnostic criteria are needed to classify an athlete as overreached or overtrained. Any of the signs and symptoms listed in Table 29.1 may accompany overtraining or overreaching. For example, an increase in mood disturbance occurs frequently in overreached and overtrained athletes, and may help differentiate between normal training fatigue and the fatigue caused by overreaching or overtraining (Halson & Jeukendrup 2004, Hooper et al. 1997, Martin et al. 2000, Morgan et al. 1988). However, as discussed later in this chapter, athletes can show clear signs of overtraining such as poor performance and persistent fatigue without mood disturbances (Hooper et al. 1997, Martin et al. 2000). By definition, both overreaching and overtraining are characterised by a decrement in performance, and neither can be diagnosed if performance remains unchanged despite the level of fatigue or other symptoms (Kreider et al. 1998).

2.1.5 Overreaching and overtraining have similar symptoms

Overreaching and overtraining cause similar symptoms and the same degree of performance decrement, and cannot be distinguished by performance or symptoms alone. There is only limited evidence to indicate that an overtrained athlete experiences a greater decrement in performance than an overreached athlete (Halson & Jeukendrup 2004). The best way to distinguish overreaching from overtraining is the time needed for performance to return to the original or expected values. Recovery of performance to the expected level may take as little as one week or perhaps a few weeks in an overreached athlete, but much longer (months and sometimes years) in an overtrained athlete (Kreider et al. 1998). Unfortunately, for the overtrained athlete, differentiating between overreaching and overtraining is often retrospective.

2.2 Prevalence of and susceptibility to overreaching and overtraining

The incidence of overreaching and overtraining has not been clearly established because it is very difficult to survey a large number of athletes across a range of sports, and because athletes and coaches are often reluctant to label an athlete as overtrained. However, given sufficiently rigorous training, most elite athletes will experience overreaching for short periods (up to 4 weeks; Lehmann et al. 1992, Mackinnon et al. 1997).

Researchers have estimated that, at any given time, 5–20% of elite athletes exhibit symptoms of overtraining. For example, Naessens et al. (2000) followed 10 semi-professional soccer players over a competitive season, and found that two players demonstrated clinical symptoms of overtraining syndrome. Hooper et al. (1993) followed 14 elite swimmers over a 6-month season, and diagnosed three (21%) as overtrained. In a sample of 272 Swedish athletes from 16 sports (48% from individual sports and 30% from team sports), 37% reported experiencing 'staleness' at least once (Kentta et al. 2001). In 257 athletes on British national teams, 15% were classified as overtrained (Koutedakis & Sharp 1998). The latter study reported a similar incidence of overtrained athletes in aerobic and anaerobic sports, with a slightly higher percentage of males (17%) than females (11%) showing symptoms.

Although overtraining occurs in athletes from many sports, it is thought that highly motivated athletes (Hooper et al. 1995) and individuals showing anxiety traits (Kentta & Hassmen 1998) are more susceptible to overtraining.

2.3 Models to study overreaching and overtraining

Overtraining has been studied using two basic models. In one model, athletes are assessed over several months, and performance and physiological or psychological responses are compared at different times in the training cycle, or between athletes classified as overtrained and not overtrained. Athletes are studied in their natural training environment, but the effects of other factors (e.g. competition stress, travel, illness) cannot be controlled.

In the second model, training is intensified by increasing the duration or intensity of exercise for a defined period, usually no more than 4 weeks, for ethical reasons. Performance and physiological or psychological variables are compared before and after intensified training, or between athletes who adapt to the training and those who show symptoms of overreaching. This model allows one to control training and possibly eliminate confounding variables, but the sudden increase in training volume or intensity is greater than that usually experienced by athletes during their normal training cycle. Each model has limitations, but together they provide insight into the outcomes and mechanisms responsible for overtraining syndrome.

3 CHANGES IN PHYSIOLOGICAL RESPONSES AND PERFORMANCE WITH OVERREACHING AND OVERTRAINING

To understand both the underlying causes of overtraining and markers to diagnose overtraining, researchers have measured a number of variables. However, the lack of definitive diagnostic criteria for overtraining poses one challenge to research on this topic.

3.1 Performance testing

Assessing performance is critical to diagnosis. It is likely that changes in the physiological responses to exercise underlie at least part of the decrement in performance. Any changes in physiological responses should be considered along with the type of performance test. For example, the overreached or overtrained athlete may reach volitional fatigue earlier than when not overreached or overtrained. This would give lower than expected test results in maximal tests, but not necessarily in submaximal tests.

3.1.1 Time trial

Time trial protocols are highly reproducible and often closely reflect the demands of competition, and several studies have shown that overreaching or overtraining can cause a time trial performance decrement of 2–10%. For example, Jeukendrup et al. (1992) reported a 5% increase in time to complete a 15-min time trial in overreached cyclists. Hooper et al. (1993) observed a 2.4% increase in time trial performance in overtrained swimmers and Halson et al. (2002) reported a 10% increase in time to complete a 40 km cycling time trial (~60 min duration) after overreaching. In runners, the time to complete an 8 km treadmill time trial increased by 155 s (8%) after 11 days of intensified running training (Achten et al. 2004).

3.1.2 Time to fatigue

Large decreases in endurance capacity, as determined in a time-to-fatigue protocol, occur in overreached athletes and several studies have shown 20–30% decreases in performance (Fry et al. 1992, Halson et al. 2004, Urhausen et al. 1998b). Meeusen et al. (2004) used a two-bout exercise protocol to detect changes in performance in overreached and overtrained athletes. The test involved two graded incremental cycle tests to exhaustion separated by 4 hours. In non-fatigued athletes, the time to exhaustion was 3% lower after the second bout than the first. In athletes diagnosed as overreached, the time to exhaustion was an average of 6% lower and 11% lower in a single overtrained athlete. Thus,

the ability to reproduce repeat maximal efforts may be reduced in overreached and overtrained athletes. These studies show that the time to fatigue decreases more than time trial performance.

3.1.3 Maximal work output

Although few studies have measured maximal power generated by overtrained athletes, incremental cycle tests to exhaustion reveal 3–8% decreases in peak power after intensified training (Halson et al. 2002, Jeukendrup et al. 1992, Snyder et al. 1995). These changes result from a decrease in both total exercise time and average power, probably as a consequence of fatigue.

3.2 Physiological measures

A variety of physiological measures have been used to assess and help explain the impaired performance and fatigue that accompany overtraining syndrome.

3.2.1 Maximal aerobic power

Peak (maximal) oxygen uptake may remain unchanged (Fry et al. 1991, Hooper et al. 1995, Urhausen et al. 1998b) or may decrease by 5–8% in overreached or overtrained athletes (Halson et al. 2002, Jeukendrup et al. 1992, Snyder et al. 1995). When observed, decreases probably result from the shorter exercise duration, when the athlete ends the test before true exhaustion because of greater perceived fatigue (Jeukendrup et al. 1992). Thus, decreased performance does not necessarily reflect abnormal physiological or metabolic function.

3.2.2 Blood lactate variables

Submaximal and maximal blood lactate concentrations, and the work rate at the lactate threshold may decrease during overreaching and overtraining. Jeukendrup et al. (1992) noted a shift to the right in the lactate–work rate curve in cyclists who underwent 2 weeks of intensified training, and a decrease in maximal blood lactate concentration. Similarly, Lehmann et al. (1996) reported a decrease in submaximal and maximal lactate concentrations in overtrained runners. Urhausen et al. (1998b) found lower lactate concentration at maximal work rate and lower power output at exhaustion. Achten et al. (2004) observed decreased blood lactate concentration during treadmill running after 11 days of intensified training. Halson et al. (2004) found that lactate concentration at a fixed exercise intensity and duration decreased after 8 days of intensified training in subjects on both low- or high-carbohydrate diets. However, other studies have reported non-significantly lower blood lactate concentrations after significant increases in training load (Fry et al. 1992, Lehmann et al. 1991, Snyder et al. 1995, Urhausen et al. 1998b).

The shift to the right of the lactate curve reported by Jeukendrup et al. (1992) is generally considered a positive adaptation to training. The shift may indicate that less lactate is being produced at a given power output. However, this shift may also indicate chronic muscle glycogen depletion, which would limit lactate production. This also highlights the need to combine measures of performance together with measures of physiological, metabolic or hormonal function.

However, the interpretation of blood lactate (turnover) measures in the absence of indices of production or removal can be difficult to interpret. Recall that blood lactate concentration is not necessarily an index of metabolic fatigue, but may instead reflect the redistribution of energy among tissues as part of the energy shuttle (Chapters 6, 7 and 10.3). Blood lactate concentration may also reflect blood flow redistribution between sites of production and removal. Thus, the physiological significance of this measure is debated (Chapter 6), and caution must be exercised in its interpretation.

3.2.3 Heart rate

Although coaches and athletes often monitor resting or early morning heart rate, most research indicates that neither measure changes significantly with overtraining (Hooper et al. 1993, 1995, Lehmann et al. 1992, Snyder et al. 1995; Urhausen et al. 1998b). In contrast, decreases in submaximal and maximal heart rates have been noted consistently during overreaching and overtraining (Costill et al. 1988, Jeukendrup et al. 1992, Lehmann et al. 1992, 1996, Urhausen et al. 1998b). Heart rate during moderate-intensity submaximal exercise decreased in overreached runners (Achten et al. 2004) and during constant-load exercise (Halson et al. 2004) in overreached athletes. However, in another study, heart rate at a fixed work rate remained unchanged following intensified training in cyclists (Halson et al. 2002).

It is unclear whether a lower maximal heart rate in overreached athletes results from a lower exercise intensity or duration during the assessment (i.e. athletes reach volitional fatigue earlier during assessment), or whether overreaching alters cardiac function. The lower submaximal heart rate observed in some studies is consistent with an underlying physiological impairment, although the exact nature of this is unknown. However, Israel (1976) suggested that overtrained athletes experienced an increase in the parasympathetic activity relative to that of the sympathetic nervous system. An increase in parasympathetic activity or decrease in sympathetic nervous system activity is consistent with reduced maximal heart rate.

3.2.4 Glycogen depletion

Muscle glycogen depletion causes fatigue and impairs performance (Karlsson & Saltin 1971; Chapter 7) and repeated bouts of high-intensity exercise will deplete muscle glycogen stores (Costill et al. 1971). Accordingly, a high-carbohydrate diet is needed for optimal adaptations to training (Jacobs & Sherman 1999), and the carbohydrate content of a diet may play a critical role in performance ability during intense training.

Simonsen et al. (1991) intensified training in rowers (4 weeks) and examined the effects of consuming moderate- ($5 \, \mathrm{g \cdot kg^{-1} \cdot d^{-1}}$) and high-carbohydrate diets ($10 \, \mathrm{g \cdot kg^{-1} \cdot d^{-1}}$). Athletes on the moderate diet maintained muscle glycogen content and increased rowing power output (2%), whereas the high-carbohydrate diet increased muscle glycogen content by 65% and performance by 11%. This study indicates that high carbohydrate intake may enhance adaptation to intensified training. However, athletes in this study did not demonstrate signs of overreaching despite intensified training (i.e. performance improved in both groups), and these data may not be directly relevant to overtraining, although they are consistent with the observation that low muscle glycogen stores may contribute to reduced exercise capacity and fatigue in some overreached or overtrained athletes.

Because intense training with limited recovery causes overreaching and overtraining, it is conceivable that the fatigue and underperformance accompanying these conditions are related to low muscle glycogen concentration. Costill et al. (1988) examined the effects of 10 days of increased training volume on performance and muscle glycogen content in collegiate swimmers. Four of the 12 swimmers were unable to tolerate the increase from 4000 to 9000 $\mathrm{m \cdot d^{-1}}$ and were classified as non-responders. This group consumed ~4186 $\mathrm{kJ \cdot d^{-1}}$ (1000 $\mathrm{kcal \cdot d^{-1}}$) less than their estimated energy requirement, and less carbohydrate ($5.3 \, \mathrm{g \cdot kg^{-1} \cdot d^{-1}}$) than the responders ($8.2 \, \mathrm{g \cdot kg^{-1} \cdot d^{-1}}$). However, muscular power, sprint swimming ability and swimming endurance ability were not affected in either group. Costill et al. (1988) concluded that the muscle glycogen content of the non-responders was sufficient to maintain performance, but inadequate to support the higher training volume.

These observations prompted Snyder et al. (1995) to examine the responses to intensified training in athletes given sufficient dietary carbohydrate to determine whether overreaching can occur in the presence of normal muscle glycogen content. Subjects consumed 160 g of carbohydrate in the 2 h after each training session; they completed 7 days of normal training, 15 days of intensified training and 6 days of recovery training. Resting muscle glycogen content did not change significantly but all athletes showed self-reported symptoms of overreaching and a decreased ratio of blood lactate to the rating of perceived exertion. This study shows that athletes can have some symptoms of overreaching despite having a normal muscle glycogen concentration.

3.2.5 Haematological measures

Blood variables, such as red blood cell count, haematocrit and the concentrations of iron, ferritin, haemoglobin, urea and ammonia are usually normal in overreached or overtrained athletes. Studies using clear criteria of overreaching or overtraining have shown that, except for blood lactate concentration, these variables do not change with overreaching or overtraining (Hooper et al. 1993, Mackinnon et al. 1997, Rowbottom et al. 1995). For example, in a 7-month study of elite swimmers, Hooper et al. (1993) found no differences in haematocrit and the concentrations of haemoglobin, creatine phosphokinase and ferritin between swimmers showing clear symptoms of overtraining (poor performance, persistent fatigue, sleep disturbances) and swimmers from the same teams who were not overtrained. Rowbottom et al. (1995) reported clinically normal blood concentrations of urea, creatinine, albumin, electrolytes, creatine phosphokinase, haemoglobin and ferritin, and red blood cell count and red blood cell volume in 10 athletes with clear symptoms of overtraining syndrome. Mackinnon et al. (1997) found no adverse changes in red blood cell count and mean cell volume, haematocrit and concentrations of ferritin and haemoglobin in swimmers during 4 weeks of intensified training; these variables did not differ between overreached and non-overreached athletes.

We note that anaemia or other iron-related blood disorders can cause fatigue, mimicking that caused by overtraining syndrome. It is important that blood disorders are excluded by a physician before diagnosing a tired, under-performing athlete as overtrained.

3.3 Valid markers of overtraining

Many studies have attempted to determine valid and reliable indicators of overreaching and overtraining, and several reviews have been published recently (e.g. Halson & Jeukendrup 2004, Urhausen & Kindermann 2002). Coaches are interested in using markers to titrate training and recovery, and any marker must be both valid and practical in the training environment. Effective overtraining markers must be readily available, inexpensive, not require sophisticated equipment or expertise, and be consistently related to the only universally accepted objective indicator of overreaching and overtraining: performance decrement (McKenzie 1999). Performance by itself cannot be the only, or main, marker because other factors (e.g. nutritional and hydration states, muscle fatigue, lack of sleep, jet lag, psychological factors) can affect performance independently of overtraining. Athletes are also reluctant to perform maximally often enough for performance to be the main marker of overtraining or overreaching, and the lack of motivation makes regular maximal efforts, such as time trials, impractical. In addition, significant impairment of performance often occurs too late in the process to be effective for monitoring and adjusting training to prevent overreaching or overtraining.

Most research conducted to date has assessed markers based on their response to short-duration (<4 weeks) increases in training, rather than to overtraining, because it is unethical to induce overtraining intentionally.

Many markers have been suggested as valid indicators of overtraining including ratings of perceived exertion (Kentta & Hassmen 1998), plasma concentration and urinary excretion of norepinephrine (Hooper et al. 1993, Lehmann et al. 1992, Mackinnon et al. 1997, Naessens et al. 2000), self-ratings of well-being (Hooper et al. 1995, Lehmann et al. 1991) and reaction time (Rietjens et al. 2005). Physiological, immunological and biochemical variables have not received widespread support in providing useful markers. In contrast, psychological testing or rating of well-being seem to be useful early-warning markers (Hooper et al. 1993, Kentta & Hassmen 1998, Lehmann et al. 1991, McKenzie 1999, Mackinnon & Hooper 1996, Urhausen et al. 1995). Changes in mood state (Halson & Jeukendrup 2004, Kentta & Hassmen 1998, Morgan et al. 1988) and self-rated measures of well-being (e.g. fatigue, quality of sleep, stress) seem to be particularly useful. For example, in distance runners, subjective ratings in a 'complaints index' (self-ratings by the athletes of their well-being and physical complaints) reflected the overreached state after 4 weeks of increased training volume (Lehmann et al. 1991). Similarly, daily ratings of well-being (stress, quality of sleep, fatigue, muscle soreness) predicted overtraining in elite swimmers several weeks before performance declined (Hooper et al. 1995). Self-ratings were also able to predict, by 1–2 weeks, declining performance in swimmers showing signs of overreaching after 4 weeks of intensified training (Mackinnon & Hooper 1996).

Although mood state or self-ratings of well-being seem to identify overreached or overtrained athletes, some have questioned whether these measures are useful in all individuals, or as a way to differentiate between overreached and overtrained athletes (Hooper et al. 1997, Martin et al. 2000). Although changes in mood are good indicators of psychological distress, mood on its own has not yet been established as a valid and reliable marker of overreaching and overtraining.

Because these states occur on a continuum of severity, valid and reliable markers must also change in relation to this continuum and it is possible that no single marker will consistently identify overreached or overtrained athletes. Table 29.2 includes the most valid indicators of overtraining syndrome.

4 MECHANISMS UNDERLYING OVERTRAINING SYNDROME

Although the mechanisms underlying overtraining syndrome have not been identified clearly, it is thought that overtraining syndrome represents the final stages of a stress response resulting from an imbalance between excessive stress and the body's ability to recover. This section discusses the various mechanisms proposed to explain the physiological and psychological responses to excessive training leading to overtraining syndrome. Although we discuss each separately, we note that they are not mutually exclusive and that a complex phenomenon, such as over-

Table 29.2 Indicators of overtraining syndrome

Useful indicators:
Performance on standard exercise test (time trial, time to fatigue)
Self-analysis of well-being (fatigue, vigour, stress)

Potentially useful indicators:
Changes in mood state (anxiety, depression, tension)
Response to standardised exercise (maximum heart rate, perceived exertion, blood lactate, lactate:exertion ratio)
Stress hormones (blood cortisol, urinary catecholamine excretion)
Sleep disturbances

Not useful as indicators:
Body mass
Early morning or resting heart rate
Haematological measures (red blood cell count, blood concentrations of ferritin or creatine phosphokinase)
Immunological measures (immunoglobulin A concentration)

training syndrome, is likely to result from dysfunction within more than one system.

4.1 Stress adaptation models and central fatigue

The numerous and multifaceted symptoms of overtrained athletes suggest the involvement of higher brain centres. Changes in mood state, fatigue and performance may be considered as consequences of dysfunction of the neuro-endocrine system and this may occur at any of several sites within the central nervous system.

4.1.1 Selye's theory of stress adaptation

Selye examined the concept and characteristics of homeo-stasis (maintenance of a dynamic equilibrium; Chapter 18), and developed the general adaptation syndrome model (Selye 1976). Selye believed the adaptation syndrome to be triphasic, beginning with the alarm phase, followed by a stage of resistance and ending with exhaustion. Selye's theory was the first to examine the effects of stress on the hypothalamus, pituitary, adrenal and other systems. Selye's work also gave rise to the notion of 'diseases of adaptation', in which he suggested that many diseases did not necessarily result from some external agent (e.g. infection), but were a consequence of an inability to adequately adapt to external stress (Selye 1976).

It is possible that, under extreme physiological and psychological stress, the mechanisms responsible for maintaining homeostasis fail to adapt. The recently named 'disorders of the stress system' may result from inappropriate or insufficient adaptation to stress (Chrousos & Gold 1992). The concept that overtraining syndrome represents an accumulation of physical and psychological stress caused by intense training with inadequate recovery fits Selye's model. The alarm phase of the model may correspond to fatigue, the

resistance phase to overreaching, and the exhaustion phase to overtraining.

4.1.2 Serotonergic system

The serotonergic system is the most active modulator of behaviour in the brain, and influences fatigue and mood state (Struder & Weicker 2001). Increased activation of the serotonergic system affects arousal, lethargy, the sleep–wake cycle and mood (Davis & Bailey 1997). This may be caused through inhibition of dopamine or through the reduction of arousal and elevated perception of effort (Davis & Bailey 1997). The neurotransmitter 5-hydroxytryptamine is released during exercise, and drugs that manipulate its activity affect physical performance, possibly by changing the perception of effort. Because of its central role regulating arousal, fatigue, sleep and mood state, the serotonergic system may be involved in overtraining. However, few studies have investigated the role of the serotonergic system in the fatigue associated with overtraining.

Lehmann et al. (1996) subjected experienced runners to a progressive increase in training volume (distance) over 4 weeks, which was followed 12 months later by a progressive increase in training intensity, again over 4 weeks. Total distance run in an incremental treadmill test decreased after the increased volume protocol, but increased following the increase in training intensity. The volume increase caused symptoms of overreaching (e.g. fatigue, poor performance, muscle soreness and decreased lactate threshold) in most athletes, whereas performance improved after the increase in training intensity protocol. However, both protocols induced a similar increase in the ratio of free tryptophan to branched-chain amino acids. Thus, this ratio does not change during a period of intensified training that causes a performance decrement, and this ratio does not explain the mechanisms responsible for overtraining syndrome.

Weicker & Struder (2001) examined the effects of 4 weeks of increased training duration on basal prolactin concentration and 5-hydroxytryptamine transporters and receptors in isolated blood platelets. Although performance was not assessed, athletes reported increased self-perceived fatigue after intensified training. Maximal receptor binding decreased, but the number of 5-hydroxytryptamine transporters did not change after intensified training. Weicker & Struder (2001) suggested that intensified training disturbs central 5-hydroxytryptamine neurotransmission, resulting in reduced performance capacity, altered mood state and sleep disturbance.

The 5-hydroxytryptamine receptors may play a role in fatigue during exercise but may be adaptable, such that receptor sensitivity may decrease after endurance training. It is possible that the availability of 5-hydroxytryptamine is more important in causing fatigue during overtraining than altered receptor sensitivity. This is consistent with the lack of change in the ratio of free tryptophan to branched-chain amino acids during overtraining. However, although theoretically possible, no study has examined whether the sensitivity of these receptors changes during overtraining.

Recently, Uusitalo (2004) used single-photon emission computed tomography to examine serotonin reuptake in an athlete diagnosed with overtraining syndrome. The athlete had a low number of 5-hydroxytryptamine transporters in a left frontal lobe and was also diagnosed with major depression. Thus, it is impossible to tell whether the low number of 5-hydroxytryptamine transporters was related to depression or overtraining or both. Indeed, it is impossible to attribute these changes only to overtraining.

4.1.3 Altered effort sense

The rating of perceived exertion is a perceptual and subjective method of quantifying effort sense (Borg 1973). The rating of perceived exertion tends to be higher in athletes showing symptoms of overreaching than when they are training normally and not overreached (Urhausen et al. 1998b). However, only recently have researchers examined effort sense at submaximal exercise intensities in relation to overreaching or overtraining (Achten et al. 2004, Halson et al. 2004).

Elevations in effort sense may indicate that overreaching and overtraining are accompanied by changes in the athlete's perception of effort. This altered perception may be protective. However, the mechanism responsible for altered perception has not been identified, and it is not clear whether it relates to changes in brain or neurotransmitter function, peripheral factors (e.g. local fatigue), psychological factors or some combination of these processes.

4.2 Hormonal imbalance

The physiological and psychological changes that occur during overtraining may arise from the central nervous system and might involve changes in hormones released during exercise. Several hormones are released in response to physical and psychological stress (cortisol, testosterone, growth hormone, adrenocorticotrophic hormone and catecholamines), and these have far-reaching effects on physiological function. Hormonal changes are thought to underlie at least some of the symptoms associated with overtraining.

4.2.1 Cortisol

Cortisol, a steroid and primary stress hormone, is catabolic in action and is released in response to high-intensity (>60% maximum) exercise (Stone et al. 1991). The cortisol response to exercise and other stresses appears to be blunted during overreaching. For example, Barron et al. (1985) reported lower serum cortisol responses to insulin-induced hypoglycaemia in overtrained athletes than in asymptomatic runners, despite higher basal cortisol concentrations. Lehmann et al. (1991) found that 24-h urinary cortisol excre-

tion decreased after 21 days of intensified training that resulted in underperformance.

However, Urhausen et al. (1998a) reported no significant changes in resting cortisol concentration after intensified training. Similar observations were noted by Flynn et al. (1994) and Rowbottom et al. (1995), and also between athletes showing symptoms of overtraining or overreaching and those who were healthy (Hooper et al. 1995, Mackinnon et al. 1997).

The cortisol response to maximal exercise appears to be blunted during overreaching. Snyder et al. (1995) found a 25% lower plasma cortisol concentration after a period of intensified training that resulted in overtraining. Urhausen et al. (1998a) and Halson et al. (2004) reported similar reductions in maximal cortisol levels.

The assessment of serum cortisol concentration during submaximal exercise can be an important indictor of the cortisol responsiveness to exercise. Under such conditions, exercise intensity and duration are kept constant, and the concentration of cortisol can be compared in athletes when they are, and are not, showing symptoms of overreaching. Halson et al. (2004) found that submaximal plasma cortisol concentration decreased significantly after 60 min of cycling at a fixed workload, following 8 days of intensified training that resulted in overreaching. It was suggested that this decline resulted from reduced adrenocorticotrophic hormone secretion, inhibition of negative feedback inhibition or decreased sensitivity of target cells.

Cortisol mobilises and redistributes metabolic fuels and enhances the responsiveness of the cardiovascular system (Armstrong & VanHeest 2002). A decline in cortisol concentration after intensified training that results in overreaching may induce metabolic changes sufficient to adversely affect performance. Cortisol also has significant effects on emotion and mood state (Young 2004), and changes in cortisol release during maximal and submaximal exercise may underlie some of the symptoms of overtraining such as the inability to train and perform at the expected level.

4.2.2 Testosterone

Testosterone is a gonadal hormone with primarily androgenic–anabolic effects. Its release is stimulated by exercise, particularly at intensities >60% of maximum (Stone et al. 1991), and, depending on the intensity and duration of exercise, testosterone can have anabolic effects (Urhausen et al. 1995). Testosterone may be important during recovery because of its role in protein synthesis and its possible effect on increasing glycogen storage through increased muscle glycogen synthetase activity (Urhausen et al. 1995).

The response of total and free testosterone concentrations in the blood of overtrained athletes is confusing and offers little insight into the physiological mechanisms. For instance, Flynn et al. (1994) observed decreased serum total and free testosterone concentrations coincident with a decrease in performance after intense training in swimmers and runners. Vervoorn et al. (1991) also reported lower testosterone concentration in rowers after intense training but performance did not change, and these athletes were not considered overreached. In contrast, Urhausen et al. (1998a) found that resting testosterone concentration did not differ significantly between normal training and when athletes were overtrained.

4.2.3 Testosterone:cortisol ratio

The testosterone:cortisol ratio has been suggested as an indicator of the balance between the anabolic activity (testosterone) and catabolic (cortisol) activities of these two hormones (Stone et al. 1991). A 30% decrease in the testosterone:cortisol ratio, or a ratio of their blood concentrations below 0.35×10^{-3}, has been suggested to indicate overtraining (Adlercreutz et al. 1986). However, the ratio can remain unchanged in underperforming, overtrained (Hooper et al. 1993, Urhausen et al. 1998a) and overreached (Mackinnon et al. 1997) athletes. A decreased ratio has been reported in athletes whose performance was normal (not impaired) after intense training (Vervoorn et al. 1991). Thus, this ratio does not seem helpful in explaining the mechanisms underlying overtraining syndrome.

4.2.4 Growth hormone

Growth hormone or somatotrophic hormone has anabolic activity, stimulates lipolysis and has insulin-like effects (Keizer 1998). Growth hormone is under the control of the hypothalamic-pituitary axis and is partly responsible for the anabolic effects of exercise training. The limited research suggests that the growth hormone response to exercise is similar to the response of other hormones under control of the hypothalamic–pituitary axis. During endurance exercise, plasma growth hormone concentration peaks before the end of exercise and returns to resting levels normally within 1–2 h. Growth hormone release in response to both insulin-induced hypoglycaemia (Barron et al. 1985) and exercise (Urhausen et al. 1998a) appears to be blunted in overreached athletes.

4.2.5 Adrenocorticotrophic hormone

Adrenocorticotrophic hormone controls the function of the adrenal cortex and the release of cortisol. However, despite this relationship, little research has been conducted on the role of this hormone in overtraining. The exceptions are a study by Barron et al. (1985), who reported decreased adrenocorticotrophic responses to insulin-induced hypoglycaemia, and a study by Urhausen et al. (1998a), who observed lower resting serum concentration and less release in response to exercise.

4.2.6 Catecholamines

Israel (1976) attempted to distinguish between a parasympathetic (vagal) form of overtraining and a sympathetic form. The parasympathetic form is characterised by increased fatigue, apathy and changes in mood state and immune function. Lehmann et al. (1998) suggested this form is observed more frequently, and may be the contemporary form of overtraining. This form of overtraining is said to be the consequence of an imbalance between prolonged, intense endurance training and adequate recovery, possibly in combination with other non-training stress factors such as travel, poor diet and stress (Lehmann et al. 1998). Catecholamine concentration in urine and plasma reflects the activity of the sympathetic nervous system, and can be used to examine the possible role of parasympathetic–sympathetic imbalance or autonomic dysfunction (Urhausen et al. 1995).

In a 6-month prospective study of elite swimmers, resting plasma norepinephrine concentration was higher in overtrained swimmers than in non-overtrained swimmers (Hooper et al. 1993). Norepinephrine concentration was highest late in the season and during the taper before major competition. Lehmann et al. (1992) also observed increased resting norepinephrine concentration after a period of increased training volume that resulted in performance incompetence. In contrast, Urhausen et al. (1998a) found no significant differences in submaximal and maximal plasma catecholamine concentrations in overreached athletes compared with values obtained earlier in the season when they were not overreached. However, Achten et al. (2004) reported unchanged norepinephrine and epinephrine concentrations at rest and after 30 and 60 min of steady-state exercise, after a period of intensified running training that resulted in overreaching. It is possible that plasma norepinephrine concentration changes only with overtraining and not with shorter-term overreaching.

Urinary catecholamine excretion declines significantly in overreached athletes (Lehmann et al. 1992, 1996, 1998, Mackinnon et al. 1997). For example, urinary norepinephrine excretion declined progressively over a 4-week period of intensified training in male runners (Lehmann et al. 1992, 1996), was negatively correlated with fatigue ratings in overtrained athletes and returned to baseline values after recovery (Lehmann et al. 1998). In swimmers undergoing 4 weeks of intensified training, urinary norepinephrine excretion was significantly lower at the start of the study in swimmers who were asymptomatic but later developed symptoms of overreaching (Mackinnon et al. 1997). The authors speculated that the swimmers who developed overreaching might have been predisposed toward the syndrome by their training or other factors before the start of the study. Urinary catecholamine excretion is a better indicator of sympathetic function than is its plasma concentration, and the low values associated with overreaching and overtraining suggest impairment of sympathetic function.

4.3 Immune function and possible role of cytokines

Athletes and coaches associate overtraining with an increased susceptibility to mild illness, such as upper respiratory tract infection (common cold, sore throat, flu-like symptoms), and much attention has focused on whether overtraining is associated with impaired immune system function. Only a handful of studies have assessed immune function in athletes diagnosed with, or showing signs of, overtraining or overreaching. Because so little is known, we must also consider the immune system response to intense exercise training, which may evoke symptoms of overtraining or overreaching.

4.3.1 Illness and overreaching and overtraining

Endurance athletes experience a high incidence of symptoms of upper respiratory tract infection during periods of intense training (Mackinnon et al. 1993, Novas et al. 2002), after major competition (Nieman et al. 2006, Peters & Bateman 1983), and at other times in their training cycles (Nieman et al. 1990). For example, in the 2 weeks after an ultramarathon, 33% of runners reported symptoms of upper respiratory tract infection, more than twice the percentage of age-matched non-runners, and there was a correlation between pre-race training volume or race pace and the incidence of such infections (Peters and Bateman 1983). Similarly, Novas et al. (2002) found the incidence of upper respiratory tract infection in tennis players was correlated with training energy expenditure over a 12-week period. In contrast, some studies have failed to find a higher incidence of these infections in athletes (Gleeson et al. 1995, Pyne et al. 1995). These divergent observations may relate to differences in athlete populations (e.g. elite versus non-elite), sport and the time frame.

Few studies have reported the incidence of upper respiratory tract infection in overtrained athletes. In 24 swimmers who undertook intensified training for 4 weeks, eight (33%) showed symptoms of overreaching and 10 (42%) had symptoms of respiratory tract infection (Mackinnon & Hooper 1996). However, fewer athletes classified as overreached (8) reported these symptoms than the well-trained (but not overreached) swimmers (16). These data imply that athletes who experienced illness may have been protected from developing the symptoms of overreaching by consciously or subconsciously reducing their training loads (i.e. before symptoms were noticeable, the athletes sensed, either consciously or subconsciously, the impeding illness and eased their training (Mackinnon & Hooper 1996)).

In a study of well-trained athletes, those experiencing persistent fatigue and impaired performance had a higher incidence (and duration) of upper respiratory tract infection symptoms than healthy, non-fatigued athletes (Clancy et al. 2006). However, these athletes had presented to a medical clinic because of fatigue and persistent illness, and it is unclear whether they are representative of all athletes. At this point, we do not know whether fatigue or overtraining contributes to illness or vice versa. It is possible that both are concomitant outcomes of prolonged periods of intense training with inadequate recovery. Athletes seem to be more susceptible to illness when training exceeds an individual threshold of combined volume and lack of variety (Foster 1998).

Overtraining is associated with reactivation of the Epstein–Barr virus, a common virus that most adults are exposed to, which causes symptoms of upper respiratory tract infection (Clancy et al. 2006, Gleeson et al. 2002, Reid et al. 2004). In a study of elite swimmers, 11 of 14 swimmers had antibodies to Epstein–Barr virus in their blood (seropositive), indicating previous exposure to the virus (Gleeson et al. 2002). During 30 days of intensified training, seven of the 11 seropositive swimmers had Epstein–Barr virus DNA in their blood, a sign of viral reactivation, and six of these developed symptoms of upper respiratory tract infection. However, no seronegative swimmers developed symptoms.

Similarly, in a study of 41 athletes presenting to a medical clinic because of persistent fatigue or poor performance, 22% exhibited evidence of Epstein–Barr virus reactivation (Reid et al. 2004). In a double-blind, placebo-controlled study from the same laboratory, an antiviral agent (Valtrex™) decreased the Epstein–Barr virus load but did not decrease the incidence of upper respiratory tract infection, when given to elite distance runners over a 4-month period (Cox et al. 2004). Thus, it is unclear whether the symptoms of respiratory tract infection, associated with overtraining and prolonged periods of intense training, are caused by an infectious agent. It is possible that the localised symptoms of the infection may have an inflammatory rather than an infectious origin.

4.3.2 Changes in immune function

Researchers have focused on immune function to try to explain this apparent increased susceptibility to upper respiratory tract infection and viral reactivation during prolonged periods of intense training and overtraining.

4.3.2.1 Leucocyte number

The resting concentration of blood leucocytes is generally normal in athletes, even during periods of intense or high-volume training and overtraining (Gabriel et al. 1998, Halson et al. 2003). However, leucocyte concentration may decline to the low end of the clinically normal range during heavy training. In a study of middle-distance runners, doubling training volume over 4 weeks resulted in a progressive decline in resting leucocyte concentration (Lehmann et al. 1996); increasing training intensity had no effect on cell counts. Overtraining or overreaching has little effect on the relative numbers of most types of leucocytes in the blood (Halson et al. 2003, Hooper et al. 1993, Rowbottom et al. 1995, Mackinnon 2000).

Although immune cell number is relatively unaffected by overtraining, certain aspects of immune function, and the overall regulation of the immune system, may change during overtraining and prolonged periods of intense training.

4.3.2.2 Neutrophil function

Neutrophils are the most prevalent immune cell, comprising 60–70% of immune cells in the blood. Neutrophils are important to the body's early defence against microorganisms and are integral to inflammation. Lower resting and postexercise neutrophil activity has been reported in athletes from a variety of sports (Peake 2002, Pyne et al. 1995, Smith et al. 1990).

Pyne et al. (1995) found that neutrophil activity in elite swimmers declined progressively as training was intensified over 12 weeks, and was lowest in the weeks with the most intense training. However, the change in neutrophil activity was not related to upper respiratory tract infection. It has been suggested that downregulation of neutrophil function reflects an adaptive response to chronic inflammation caused by tissue microtrauma resulting from intense daily training (Smith 1994).

4.3.2.3 Immunoglobulin

Immunoglobulin is a glycoprotein found in serum, various body fluids (saliva, tears) and within the gastrointestinal, urinary and respiratory tracts. Antibodies are immunoglobulin molecules that react with specific antigens (foreign protein, microorganisms) and are important in recognising and initiating the immune response.

Serum immunoglobulin concentrations may be normal or low during periods of intense training (Gleeson et al. 1995, Reid et al. 2004). Deficiency of the immunoglobulin subclass associated with susceptibility to upper respiratory tract infection (IgG3) was noted in 28% of 41 athletes attending a medical clinic because of persistent fatigue or recurrent infections (Reid et al. 2004). Immunoglobulin A, contained in respiratory tract fluid, is an important first line of defence against viral infection, and has been investigated thoroughly to try to explain the link between intense training, overtraining and respiratory infections.

Salivary immunoglobulin A concentration declines acutely after intense exercise (Gleeson et al. 2004a, Mackinnon 1999). Elite athletes exhibit low resting salivary IgA concentration (Gleeson et al. 1999), and IgA concentration is lower in overtrained than in non-overtrained athletes (Mackinnon & Hooper 1994). A decrease in salivary immunoglobulin A concentration precedes and predicts the subsequent appearance of an upper respiratory tract infection (Gleeson et al. 1999, Mackinnon et al. 1993, Nieman et al. 2006, Pyne & Gleeson 1998). These changes might reflect dysfunction of immune responses to infectious agents.

4.3.2.4 Cell-mediated immunity and cytokines

Cell-mediated immunity is an immune response that does not involve antibodies, but instead involves several types of immune cells, in particular T lymphocytes and the release of soluble mediators (cytokines). Cytokines are intercellular signalling molecules that mediate the immune response, inflammation, haematopoiesis, metabolism and tissue repair. Several cytokines are released during and after exercise and their release is generally proportional to exercise intensity and duration (Petersen & Pedersen 2005).

Cytokines can be classified according to their role in inflammation. Proinflammatory cytokines promote inflammation and are released early in the inflammatory process; anti-inflammatory cytokines function to limit inflammation and restore homeostasis and are released later. T helper1 lymphocytes are associated with cell-mediated immunity and release proinflammatory cytokines; T helper 2 lymphocytes are associated with humoral immunity (involving antibodies). Both T helper 1 and T helper 2 cells are needed for a competent immune system and the two cell types normally exist in balance with each other. Physical stress or infection can shift this balance.

Intense prolonged exercise may alter cell-mediated immunity (Bruunsgaard et al. 1997), leading to a shift toward T helper 2 cells (Lancaster et al. 2004, Suzuki et al. 2003). For example, in cyclists, the number of cells producing interferon-γ, an antiviral cytokine produced by T helper1 cells, decreased after 6 days of intensified training, but returned to baseline after 2 weeks of recovery training (Lancaster et al. 2004). Downregulation of cell-mediated immunity and the shift toward a T helper 2 response can compromise resistance to viral infection, and is considered one possible mechanism for the higher incidence of upper respiratory tract infection experienced by athletes training intensely or when overtrained (Lancaster et al. 2004, Smith 2000, 2004). However, Gleeson et al. (2004b) found no difference in cell-mediated immunity between elite swimmers and non-athletes, and no evidence of decreased cell-mediated immunity measured at different stages of the training cycle in swimmers, even during high-intensity training.

Fatigued athletes show some evidence of a shift away from T helper 1 toward T helper 2 immunity. For example, Clancy et al. (2006) found that immune cells from fatigued athletes produced less interferon-γ, which plays a vital role in the body's defence against viral infection and reactivation. This might explain the Epstein–Barr virus reactivation observed in the fatigued athletes. Cortisol and catecholamines suppress the T helper 1 response and cell-mediated immunity, and increased concentrations of these hormones may be involved in these changes in cell-mediated immunity and viral reactivation (Smith 2004). However, it is unclear whether viral reactivation is a cause or consequence of fatigue associated with intense training in athletes.

4.3.3 Glutamine and branched–chain amino acids

Glutamine is the most abundant amino acid in the body and is required by immune cells for normal function and replication. Plasma glutamine concentration declines acutely after endurance exercise (Hiscock & Pedersen 2002) and during intense training (Keast et al. 1995, Krieger et al. 2004), and is lower in overtrained or overreached athletes (Mackinnon & Hooper 1996, Rowbottom et al. 1995). Low glutamine levels are associated with immunosuppression associated with major trauma, such as burns or surgery (Hiscock & Pedersen 2002). When first studied in the context of exercise, it was thought that low plasma glutamine concentration might impair the ability of immune cells to proliferate, a key step in the immune response. However, exercise-induced decreases in plasma glutamine concentration are not associated with impaired lymphocyte proliferation and even the lowest concentration in plasma is sufficient to support lymphocyte proliferation (Hiscock & Pedersen 2002). Low plasma glutamine concentration is not related to the appearance of upper respiratory tract infection in overtrained athletes (Mackinnon & Hooper 1996).

Glutamine supplementation may alter some of the exercise-induced changes in immune function. For instance, glutamine supplementation enhances the release of interleukin-6 from skeletal muscle after endurance exercise (Hiscock et al. 2003). Glutamine supplementation increased nasal immunoglobulin A, but not the salivary concentration, after 9 days of intensified training (Krieger et al. 2004). Supplementation with branched-chain amino acids (precursors in glutamine synthesis) restores the ability of immune cells to proliferate after intense exercise and shifts the balance of the immune response more toward the T helper 1 profile (Bassit et al. 2002). These data indicate that, although glutamine concentration does not affect immune cell function directly, adequate glutamine availability may help maintain cell-mediated immunity (the T helper 1 response) through its effects on cytokines, in particular interleukin-6.

4.3.4 Cytokines as mediators of immune system changes

The cytokine hypothesis proposes that cytokines are mediators of overtraining syndrome (Smith 2000, 2004). The hypothesis holds that frequent intense exercise induces microtrauma to joints, muscles and connective tissue, which activates immune cells to release proinflammatory cytokines. These initiate a whole-body response involving changes in the T helper 1/T helper 2 balance, mild systemic inflammation (sickness behaviour) and changes in mood state, and fit within the third stage of Seyle's general adaptation model.

Regular, moderate exercise has overall anti-inflammatory effects. That is, it promotes the increase of anti-inflammatory cytokines and inhibits the release of proinflammatory cytokines, changes now thought responsible for many of the health benefits of moderate exercise (Petersen & Pedersen 2005). The predominant anti-inflammatory response is thought to protect against chronic, systemic (low-grade) inflammation and is a positive adaptation to exercise training. The cytokine hypothesis proposes that excessive exercise, or a sudden increase in training volume, disrupts the balance between anti-inflammatory and proinflammatory responses, leading to increased release of proinflammatory mediators and chronic inflammation. This change in cyto-

kine patterns is consistent with the downregulation of T helper 1 cells and viral reactivation associated with overtraining. Proinflammatory cytokines also active the hypothalamic–pituitary-adrenal axis, possibly modulating hormone release (Smith 2000, 2004).

Robson (2003) hypothesised that overtraining syndrome is caused by excessive production of, or intolerance to, the cytokine interleukin-6. Interleukin-6 is produced by and released from skeletal muscle during and after intense prolonged exercise, and has both proinflammatory and anti-inflammatory activities. Acute experimental administration of low doses of interleukin-6 and chronically elevated levels causes fatigue, changes in mood state and disturbed sleep–symptoms associated with depression, posttraumatic stress disorder and overtraining syndrome. Robson (2003) proposed that sensitisation to repeatedly elevated interleukin-6 levels causes either excessive production or intolerance to its subsequent increase. Some people seem to be genetically predisposed toward an elevated interleukin-6 response to various stressors. Robson also proposed that interventions to limit its release after exercise (carbohydrate ingestion, adequate rest between sessions, adequate recovery after infection) might help prevent overtraining syndrome.

Although the cytokine hypothesis and the proposed role of interleukin-6 might explain the complex symptoms of overtraining syndrome, few have studied the cytokine profile in overtrained or overreached athletes. Recently, Halson et al. (2003) found no changes in the concentrations of interleukin-6 or tumour necrosis factor-α in the blood of cyclists who showed symptoms of overreaching. However, cycling has no eccentric component and causes only limited microtrauma to muscle, and it is unlikely that this type of training greatly increases the production or release of cytokines. Moreover, serum cytokine concentration (turnover) may not directly reflect its production or activity, because cytokines act locally and are cleared rapidly from the blood. The expression of a cytokine's gene, as measured by its mRNA level, may give a better indication of cytokine production or regulation. Such studies have shown that interleukin-6 is produced within skeletal muscle during and after exercise (Steensberg 2003). Obviously, further studies are needed to document the cytokine profile in well-trained and overtrained athletes, and to determine whether cytokines play a causal or contributory role in overtraining.

5 PRACTICAL ASPECTS: PREVENTING AND TREATING OVERTRAINING

Overtraining syndrome may adversely affect an athlete's career for several months to years, undoing months and often years of hard work, and in some cases causing premature retirement (Hooper & Mackinnon 1995). Therefore, preventing overtraining by monitoring athletes and adjusting their training appropriately is vital to the management of elite athletes.

5.1 Preventing overtraining

Preventing overtraining requires a multifaceted approach based on scientific training principles such as periodisation and individualisation of training (Table 29.3). This is most effective when the coach uses experience and intuition to carefully consider the diverse and complex information available about each athlete. Although the physical loading and regeneration of the athlete is the coach's priority, coaches may also need to consider the importance of helping the athlete manage life stresses and recovery.

Many consider that overtraining reflects a fundamental mismatch between training and recovery (Kentta & Hassmen 1998). Coaches have a vast array of tools to alter programming by manipulating the frequency, intensity, volume and type of training and regeneration. The number of factors, and their interaction, can make it difficult to modify these systematically and doing so may require adequate resources. For example, individualising training requires the coach to consider each athlete's training programme in the context of susceptibility to overtraining, and the ability to cope with different types of stresses, which are unpredictable and may change frequently (Hooper & Mackinnon 1995).

Further complicating the process are the different types of regeneration techniques available. These include, but are

---

Table 29.3 Strategies for preventing overtraining

Follow scientific principles to design training programmes:
Periodise training
Individualise training
Programme recovery sessions into training

Identify susceptible athletes and monitor for warning signs:
Unexpected and unexplained persistent fatigue
Changes in mood state
Life stresses not directly related to training

Minimise known causes of overtraining:
Sudden or large increases in training volume
Heavy competition schedules with inadequate recovery
Inadequate recovery between seasons or after illness

Monitor diet:
To ensure adequate total energy and carbohydrate intake, especially in the first few hours after training or competition

Reinforce the use of regenerative techniques:
Relaxation
Psychological practices
Recovery sessions
Massage

Seek medical advice to exclude:
Anaemia
Depression
Acute infection
Immune deficiency

---

not limited to, nutrition, hydration, sleep, massage, active and passive rest, saunas and baths, psychological practices such as visualisation and meditation, and emotional support from family and friends (Barnett 2006). For example, inadequate carbohydrate intake and muscle glycogen depletion are considered contributing factors to overreaching or overtraining (Urhausen et al. 1998b). Low carbohydrate intake is associated with poor race performance and symptoms of overtraining in competitive cyclists (Manetta et al. 2002). Although overreaching or overtraining may occur without muscle glycogen depletion (Snyder et al. 1995), sufficient dietary carbohydrate is needed for athletes to adapt positively to intense training and to prevent overreaching and overtraining.

There is little scientific information about the time course of recovery from overreaching and overtraining. Many coaches believe that performance may return to the expected level within 2–4 weeks in overreached athletes, given adequate rest and recovery. However, an overtrained athlete may need months to years to recover fully. When recovering from overreaching, many athletes are tempted to return to training earlier or at a higher intensity than is appropriate. For this reason, training should be structured and supervised to ensure a full recovery without pushing the athlete towards overtraining syndrome.

Self-assessment by the athlete may be beneficial in preventing poor performance. This can be ad hoc and informal, but is likely to be more effective if documented daily and reviewed regularly, even weekly. Self-report tools are potentially useful for monitoring training and identifying overtraining (Hooper et al. 1995, Lehmann et al. 1991), although their efficacy for successfully preventing overtraining is yet to be determined. These tools aim to efficiently present relevant information about factors that influence the athlete's ability to cope, and are a well-established practice among many elite athletes. These tools can help coaches understand how athletes are coping with training and may help predict overtraining (Hooper et al. 1995) and overreaching (Mackinnon & Hooper 1996). Training diaries may include self-ratings of fatigue, muscle soreness, quality of sleep, injury, illness and general well-being, as well as training details.

The total quality recovery tool also uses the athlete's self-assessment of training and recovery, and was developed to measure psychophysiological recovery (Kentta & Hassmen 1998). The recovery-stress questionnaire (Kallus 1995) is another tool developed to simultaneously assess general stress and recovery in athletes, and it is useful in evaluating the impact of training schedules (Kellmann et al. 2001). It contains items related to psychological affect, sleep, physical complaints and recovery, fitness, injury, performance and coping. The daily analyses of life demands for athletes questionnaire (Rushall 1990) highlights the sources and symptoms of stress, and was designed to indicate when an athlete is not coping with life. It has been used to monitor athletes undertaking intensified training (Halson et al.

2002). Although self-reports can be manipulated by athletes to portray themselves in a positive light, judicious checking and encouragement by the coach help athletes to complete these accurately.

Using objective markers overcomes the possibility that athletes might manipulate self-assessment tools. Further guidance of practically viable, valid, reliable and objective markers would help prevent overtraining. These objective and subjective markers need to be readily available and sensitive if training and recovery are to be altered quickly enough to prevent declining performance. Markers intended to predict future performance (outcomes in training) that have the level of accuracy to confidently alter training programmes for elite athletes require individualised monitoring (Kinugasa et al. 2004).

5.2 Treating overtraining

When overtraining is suspected, the athlete should undergo clinical diagnosis from an experienced sports physician to identify and treat any illness, infection or other medical condition that may be contributing to the fatigue, poor performance and other symptoms. Part of this diagnostic process will consider causal and contributing factors, which should be documented and used to plan an effective recovery strategy. This is likely to be holistic in nature, and a central feature will be rest and a greatly reduced training load. Other important considerations should include preventing monotony or lack of variety in the athlete's training and competition (Foster 1998), regeneration techniques such as massage and hydrotherapy, and the support of family and friends in reducing sources of stress.

6 CONCLUSION

Overtraining is the process of excessive exercise training that, if left unchecked, may lead to overtraining syndrome, which is characterised by persistent fatigue and a decrement in performance. Performance can decline by 2–25% in an overtrained athlete, depending on the test used. Other physiological and psychological changes accompanying overtraining syndrome should be monitored. Overtrained athletes exhibit signs of hormonal dysfunction, especially of the hypothalamic–pituitary–adrenal axis. Such athletes may also exhibit signs of viral reactivation, which may indicate a shift in the regulation of immune cell function and might explain altered susceptibility to illness. However, the mechanism responsible for overtraining syndrome is not known at present but may involve an altered cytokine profile that favours proinflammatory processes.

References

Achten J, Halson SL, Moseley L, Rayson MP, Casey A, Jeukendrup AE 2004 Higher dietary carbohydrate content during intensified running training results in better maintenance of performance and mood state. Journal of Applied Physiology 96(4):1331–1340

Adlercreutz H, Härkönen M, Kuoppasalmi K, Näveri H, Huhtaniemi I, Tikkanen H, Remes K, Dessypris A, Karvonen J 1986 Effect of training on plasma anabolic and catabolic steroid hormones and their response during physical exercise. International Journal of Sports Medicine 7(Suppl 1):27–28

Armstrong LE, VanHeest JL 2002 The unknown mechanism of the overtraining syndrome: clues from depression and psychoneuroimmunology. Sports Medicine 32(3):185–209

Barnett A 2006 Recovery modalities and between-training session recovery in elite athletes. Sports Medicine 36(9):781–796

Barron JL, Noakes TD, Levy W, Smith C, Millar RP 1985 Hypothalamic dysfunction in overtrained athletes. Journal of Clinical Endocrinology and Metabolism 60(4):803–806

Bassit RA, Sawada LA, Bacurau RF, Navarro F, Martins E Jr, Santos RV, Caperuto EC, Rogeri P, Costa Rosa LF 2002 Branched-chain amino acid supplementation and the immune response in long-distance runners. Nutrition 18:376–379

Borg G 1973 Perceived exertion: a note on 'history' and methods. Medicine and Science in Sports and Exercise 5:90–93

Bruunsgaard H, Hartkopp A, Mohr T, Konradsen H, Heron I, Mordhorst CH, Pedersen BK 1997 In vivo cell-mediated immunity and vaccination response following prolonged, intense exercise. Medicine and Science in Sports and Exercise 29:1176–1181

Chrousos GP, Gold P W 1992 The concepts of stress and stress system disorders. Overview of physical and behavioral homeostasis. Journal of the American Medical Association 267(9):1244–1252

Clancy RL, Gleeson M, Cox A, Callister R, Dorrington M, D'Este C, Pang G, Pyne D, Fricker P, Henriksson A 2006 Reversal in fatigued athletes of a defect in interferon gamma secretion after administration of Lactobacillus acidophilus. British Journal of Sports Medicine 2006 40(4):351–354

Costill DL, Bowers R, Branam G, Sparks K 1971 Muscle glycogen utilization during prolonged exercise on successive days. Journal of Applied Physiology 31:834–838

Costill DL, Flynn MG, Kirwan JP, Houmard JA, Mitchell JB, Thomas R, Park SH 1988 Effects of repeated days of intensified training on muscle glycogen and swimming performance. Medicine and Science in Sports and Exercise 20:249–254

Cox AJ, Gleeson M, Pyne DB, Saunders PU, Clancy RL, Fricker PA 2004 Valtrex® therapy for Epstein–Barr virus reactivation and upper respiratory symptoms in elite runners. Medicine and Science in Sports and Exercise 36(7):1104–1110

Davis JM, Bailey SP 1997 Possible mechanisms of central nervous system fatigue during exercise. Medicine and Science in Sports and Exercise 29(1):45–57

Flynn MG, Pizza FX, Boone JB Jr, Andres FF, Michaud TA, Rodriguez-Zayas JR 1994 Indices of training stress during competitive running and swimming seasons. International Journal of Sports Medicine 15(1):21–26

Foster C 1998 Monitoring training in athletes with reference to overtraining syndrome. Medicine and Science in Sports and Exercise 30(7):1164–1168

Fry RW, Morton AR, Keast D 1991 Overtraining in athletes. An update. Sports Medicine 12(1):32–65

Fry RW, Morton AR, Garcia-Webb P, Crawford GP, Keast D 1992 Biological responses to overload training in endurance sports. European Journal of Applied Physiology 64(4):335–344

Gabriel HH, Urhausen A, Valet G, Heidelbach U, Kindermann W 1998 Overtraining and immune system: a prospective longitudinal study in endurance athletes. Medicine and Science in Sports and Exercise 30(7):1151–1157

Gandevia SC 2001 Spinal and supraspinal factors in human muscle fatigue. Physiological Reviews 81(4):1725–1789

Gleeson M, McDonald WA, Cripps AW, Pyne DB, Clancy RL, Fricker PA 1995 The effect on immunity of long-term intensive training in elite swimmers. Clinical and Experimental Immunology 102:210–216

Gleeson M, McDonald WA, Pyne DB, Cripps AW, Francis JL, Fricker PA, Clancy RL 1999 Salivary IgA levels and infection risk in elite swimmers. Medicine and Science in Sports and Exercise 31(1):67–73

Gleeson M, Pyne DB, Austin JP, Lynn Francis J, Clancy RL, McDonald WA, Fricker PA 2002 Epstein–Barr virus reactivation and upper-respiratory illness in elite swimmers. Medicine and Science in Sports and Exercise 34(3):411–417

Gleeson M, Pyne DB, Callister R 2004a The missing links in exercise effects on mucosal immunity. Exercise Immunology Review 10:107–128

Gleeson M, Pyne DB, McDonald WA, Bowe SJ, Clancy RL, Fricker PA 2004b In-vivo cell mediated immunity in elite swimmers. Journal of Science and Medicine in Sport 7(1):38–46

Halson SL, Jeukendrup AE 2004 Does overtraining exist: an analysis of overreaching and overtraining research. Sports Medicine 34:967–981

Halson SL, Bridge MW, Meeusen R, Busschaert B, Gleeson M, Jones DA, Jeukendrup AE 2002 Time course of performance changes and fatigue markers during intensified training in trained cyclists. Journal of Applied Physiology 93(3):947–956

Halson SL, Lancaster GI, Jeukendrup AE, Gleeson M 2003 Immunological responses to overreaching in cyclists. Medicine and Science in Sports and Exercise 35(5):854–861

Halson SL, Lancaster GI, Achten J, Gleeson M, Jeukendrup AE 2004 Effects of carbohydrate supplementation on performance and carbohydrate oxidation after intensified cycling training. Journal of Applied Physiology 97(4):1245–1253

Hiscock N, Pedersen BK 2002 Exercise-induced immunosuppression – plasma glutamine is not the link. Journal of Applied Physiology 93:813–822

Hiscock N, Petersen EW, Krzywkowski K, Boza J, Halkjaer-Kristensen J, Pedersen BK 2003 Glutamine supplementation further enhances exercise-induced plasma IL-6. Journal of Applied Physiology 95:145–148

Hooper S, Mackinnon LT 1995 Monitoring overtraining in athletes: recommendations. Sports Medicine 20:321–327

Hooper SL, Mackinnon LT, Gordon RD, Bachmann AW 1993 Hormonal responses of elite swimmers to overtraining. Medicine and Science in Sports and Exercise 25(6):741–747

Hooper SL, Mackinnon LT, Howard A, Gordon RD, Bachmann AW 1995 Markers for monitoring overtraining and recovery. Medicine and Science in Sports and Exercise 27(1):106–112

Hooper S, Mackinnon L, Hanrahan S 1997 Mood states as an indication of staleness and recovery. International Journal of Sports Psychology 28(1):1–12

Israel S 1976 Problems of overtraining from an internal medical and performance physiological standpoint. Medizine Sport 16:1–12

Jacobs KA, Sherman WM 1999 The efficacy of carbohydrate supplementation and chronic high-carbohydrate diets for improving endurance performance. International Journal of Sport Nutrition 9:92–115

Jeukendrup AE, Hesselink MK, Snyder AC, Kuipers H, Keizer HA 1992 Physiological changes in male competitive cyclists after two weeks of intensified training. International Journal of Sports Medicine 13(7):534–541

Kallus KW 1995 Recovery-stress questionnaire manual. University of Wurzburg, Wurzburg, Germany

Karlsson J, Saltin B 1971 Diet, muscle glycogen and endurance performance. Journal of Applied Physiology 31:203–206

Keast D, Arstein D, Harper W, Fry RW, Morton AR 1995 Depression of plasma glutamine concentration after exercise stress and its possible influence on the immune system. Medical Journal of Australia 162:15–18

Keizer H 1998 Neuroendocrine aspects of overtraining. In: Kreider RB, Fry AC, O'Toole ML (eds) Overtraining in sport. Human Kinetics, Champaign, IL, 145–167

Kellmann M, Altenburg D, Lormes W, Steinacker JM 2001 Assessing stress and recovery during preparation for the World Championships in rowing. Sport Psychologist 15:151–167

Kentta G, Hassmen P 1998 Overtraining and recovery: a conceptual model. Sports Medicine 26(1):1–16

Kentta G Hassmen P, Raglin JS 2001 Training practices and overtraining syndrome in Swedish age-group athletes. International Journal of Sports Medicine 22 (6):460–465

Kinugasa, T Cerin E, Hooper S 2004 Single-subject research designs and data analyses for assessing elite athletes' conditioning. Sports Medicine 34(15):1035–1050

Koutedakis Y, Sharp NC 1998 Seasonal variation of injury and overtraining in elite athletes. Clinical Journal of Sports Medicine 8(1):18–21

Kreider R, Fry AC, O'Toole M 1998 Overtraining in sport: terms, definitions and prevalence. In Kreider R, Fry AC, O'Toole M (eds) Overtraining in sport. Human Kinetics, Champaign, IL, vii–ix

Krieger JW, Crowe M, Blank SE 2004 Chronic glutamine supplementation increases nasal but not salivary IgA during 9 days of interval training. Journal of Applied Physiology 97:585–591

Lancaster GI, Halson SL, Khan Q, Drysdale P, Wallace F, Jeukendrup AE, Drayson MT, Gleeson M 2004 Effects of acute exhaustive exercise and chronic exercise training on type 1 and type 2 T lymphocytes. Exercise Immunology Review 10:91–107

Lehmann M, Dickhuth HH, Gendrisch G, Lazar W, Thum M, Kaminski R, Aramendi JF, Peterke E, Wieland W, Keul J 1991 Training-overtraining. A prospective, experimental study with experienced middle- and long-distance runners. International Journal of Sports Medicine 12(5):444–452

Lehmann M, Schnee W, Scheu R, Stockhausen W, Bachl N 1992 Decreased nocturnal catecholamine excretion: parameter for an overtraining syndrome in athletes? International Journal of Sports Medicine 13(3):236–242

Lehmann M, Mann H, Gastmann U, Keul J, Vetter D, Steinacker JM, Häussinger D 1996 Unaccustomed high-mileage vs intensity training-related changes in performance and serum amino acid levels. International Journal of Sports Medicine 17(3):187–192

Lehmann M, Foster C, Dickhuth HH, Gastmann U 1998 Autonomic imbalance hypothesis and overtraining syndrome. Medicine and Science in Sports and Exercise 30(7):1140–1145

McKenzie DC 1999 Markers of excessive exercise. Canadian Journal of Applied Physiology 24(1):66–73

Mackinnon LT 1999 Advances in exercise immunology, Human Kinetics, Champaign IL, 178–198

Mackinnon LT 2000 Overtraining effects on immunity and performance in athletes. Immunology and Cell Biology 79:502–509

Mackinnon LT, Hooper SL 1994 Mucosal (secretory) immune system responses to exercise of varying intensity and during overtraining. International Journal of Sports Medicine 15:S179–S183

Mackinnon LT, Hooper SL 1996 Plasma glutamine concentration and upper respiratory tract infection during overtraining in elite swimmers. Medicine and Science in Sports and Exercise 28(4):285–290

Mackinnon LT, Ginn E, Seymour GJ 1993 Temporal relationship between exercise-induced decreases in salivary IgA and subsequent appearance of upper respiratory tract infection in elite athletes. Australian Journal of Science and Medicine in Sport 25:94–99

Mackinnon LT, Hooper SL, Jones S, Gordon RD, Bachmann AW 1997 Hormonal, immunological and hematological responses to intensified training in elite swimmers. Medicine and Science in Sports and Exercise 29(12):1637–1645

Manetta J, Brun JF, Maimoun L, Galy O, Coste O, Maso F, Raibaut JL, Benezis C, Lac G, Mercier J 2002 Carbohydrate dependence during hard-intensity exercise in trained cyclists in the competitive season: importance of training status. International Journal of Sports Medicine 23:516–523

Martin D, Andersen M, Gates W 2000 Using profile of mood states (POMS) to monitor high-intensity training in cyclists: group versus case studies. Sport Psychologist 14:138–156

Meeusen R, Piacentini MF, Busschaert B, Buyse L, De Schutter G, Stray-Gundersen J 2004 Hormonal responses in athletes: the use of a two bout exercise protocol to detect subtle differences in (over)training status. European Journal of Applied Physiology 91(2–3):140–146

Morgan WP, Costill DL, Flynn MG, Raglin JS, O'Connor PJ 1988 Mood disturbance following increased training in swimmers. Medicine and Science in Sports and Exercise 20:401–414

Naessens G, Chandler J, Kibler WB, Driessens M 2000 Clinical usefulness of nocturnal urinary noradrenaline excretion patterns in the follow-up of training processes in high-level soccer players. Journal of Strength and Conditioning Research 14(2):125–131

Nieman DC, Johanssen LM, Lee JW, Arabatzis K 1990 Infectious episodes in runners before and after the Los Angeles Marathon. Journal of Sports Medicine and Physical Fitness 29:289–296

Nieman DC, Henson DA, Dumke CL, Lind RH, Shooter LR, Gross SJ 2006 Relationship between salivary IgA secretion and upper respiratory tract infection following a 160-km race. Journal of Sports Medicine and Physical Fitness 46(1):158–162

Novas A, Rowbottom D, Jenkins D 2002 Total daily energy expenditure and incidence of upper respiratory tract infection symptoms in young females. International Journal of Sports Medicine 23:465–470

Peake JM 2002 Exercise-induced alterations in neutrophil degranulation and respiratory burst activity: possible mechanisms of action. Exercise Immunology Review 8:49–100

Peters EM, Bateman ED 1983 Ultramarathon running and upper respiratory tract infections. South African Medical Journal 64:582–584

Petersen AMW, Pedersen BK 2005 The anti-inflammatory effect of exercise. Journal of Applied Physiology 98:1154–1162

Pyne DB, Gleeson M 1998 Effects of intensive exercise training on immunity in athletes. International Journal of Sports Medicine 19: S183–S194

Pyne DB, Baker MS, Fricker PA, McDonald WA, Telford RD, Weidemann MJ 1995 Effects of an intensive 12-wk training program by elite swimmers on neutrophil oxidative activity. Medicine and Science in Sports and Exercise 27(3):536–542

Reid VL, Gleeson M, Williams N, Clancy RL 2004 Clinical investigation of athletes with persistent fatigue and/or recurrent infections. British Journal of Sports Medicine 38:42–45

Rietjens GJ, Kuipers H, Adam JJ, Saris WH, van Breda E, van Hamont D, Keizer HA 2005 Physiological, biochemical and psychological markers of strenuous training-induced fatigue. International Journal of Sports Medicine 26:16–26

Robson PJ 2003 Elucidating the unexplained underperformance syndrome in endurance athletes: the interleukin-6 hypothesis. Sports Medicine 33(10):771–781

Rowbottom DG, Keast D, Goodman C, Morton AR 1995 The haematological, biochemical and immunological profile of athletes suffering from the overtraining syndrome. European Journal of Applied Physiology and Occupational Physiology 70(6):502–509

Rushall BS 1990 A tool for measuring stress tolerance in elite athletes. Applied Sport Psychology 2:51–66

Selye H 1976 The stress of life. New York, McGraw Hill, 5–45

Simonsen JC, Sherman WM, Lamb DR, Dernbach AR, Doyle JA, Strauss R 1991 Dietary carbohydrate, muscle glycogen and power output during rowing training. Journal of Applied Physiology 70:1500–1505

Smith JA 1994 Neutrophils, host defense and inflammation: a double-edged sword. Journal of Leucocyte Biology 56:672–686

Smith LL 2000 Cytokine hypothesis of overtraining: a physiological adaptation to excessive stress? Medicine and Science in Sports and Exercise 32(2):317–331

Smith LL 2004 Overtraining, excessive training and altered immunity: is this a T helper-1 versus T helper-2 lymphocyte response? Sports Medicine 33(5):347–364

Smith JA, Telford RD, Mason IB, Weidemann MJ 1990 Exercise, training and neutrophil microbicidal activity. International Journal of Sport Medicine 11:179–187

Snyder AC, Kuipers H, Cheng B, Servais R, Fransen E 1995 Overtraining following intensified training with normal muscle glycogen. Medicine and Science in Sports and Exercise 27(7):1063–1070

Steensberg A 2003 The role of IL-6 in exercise-induced immune changes and metabolism. Exercise Immunology Review 9:40–47

Stone MH, Keith RE, Kearney JT, Fleck SJ, Wilson GD, Triplett NT 1991 Overtraining: a review of the signs, symptoms and possible causes. Journal of Applied Sport Science Research 5:35–50

Struder HK, Weicker H 2001 Physiology and pathophysiology of the serotonergic system and its implications on mental and physical performance. Part II. International Journal of Sports Medicine 22:482–497

Suzuki K, Nakaji S, Kurakake S, Totsuka M, Sato K, Kuriyama T, Fujimoto H, Shibusawa K, Machida K, Sugawara 2003 Exhaustive exercise and type-1/type-2 cytokine balance with special focus on interleukin-12 p40/p70. Exercise Immunology Review 9:48–57

Urhausen A, Kindermann W 2002 Diagnosis of overtraining: what tools do we have? Sports Medicine 32:95–102

Urhausen A, Gabriel H, Kindermann W 1995 Blood hormones as markers of training stress and overtraining. Sports Medicine 20(4):251–276

Urhausen A, Gabriel HH, Kindermann W 1998a Impaired pituitary hormonal response to exhaustive exercise in overtrained endurance athletes. Medicine and Science in Sports and Exercise 30(3):407–414

Urhausen A, Gabriel HH, Weiler B, Kindermann W 1998b Ergometric and psychological findings during overtraining: a long-term follow-up study in endurance athletes. International Journal of Sports Medicine 19(2):114–120

Uusitalo AL 2004 Abnormal serotonin reuptake in an overtrained, insomniac and depressed team athlete. International Journal of Sports Medicine 25(2):150–153

Vervoorn C, Quist AM, Vermulst LJ, Erich WB, de Vries WR, Thijssen JH 1991 The behaviour of the plasma free testosterone/cortisol ratio during a season of elite rowing training. International Journal of Sports Medicine 12(3):257–263

Weicker H, Struder HK 2001 Influence of exercise on serotonergic neuromodulation in the brain. Amino Acids 20(1):35–47

Young AH 2004 Cortisol in mood disorders. Stress 7(4):205–208

Chapter 30

Exercise and disease states

Arthur B. Jenkins Guy Plasqui

CHAPTER CONTENTS

1 INTRODUCTION

Chapter 28 presents a strong case that the absence of habitual physical activity (sedentary lifestyles), as a behavioural consequence of breaking the link in consumer societies between physical activity and food gathering, is a primary cause of much morbidity and mortality in those societies. Some of the consequences of physical inactivity relate specifically to the physiology of those systems directly involved in muscular activity. Others are a consequence of the positive energy balance, which generally accompanies a sedentary lifestyle, and the resulting overweight or obesity. Many, but not all, of the diseases or conditions covered in this chapter are strongly associated with sedentary behaviour and the resulting changes in metabolism and body composition.

Benefits of regular physical activity may therefore be expected in these diseases of affluence, especially when combined with dietary restriction leading to weight loss (Chapter 32), and there is considerable evidence supporting these expectations. Other diseases discussed have a pathophysiology independent of physical activity. Here, sedentary behaviour, and the concurrent metabolic complications, are a consequence rather than a cause of the disease. For these diseases, exercise can have some therapeutic effect on the progression of the disease itself or help to reduce long-term metabolic complications. A theme that will arise often in this chapter relates to the practical difficulties encountered in realising these potential benefits, due to the often low levels of compliance with recommendations for lifestyle change. This low compliance may be related to specific features of the diseases that make physical activities more difficult, or to increased risks of physical activity due to concurrent pathologies (cardiovascular disease, hypertension, musculoskeletal or circulatory pathologies), or to motivational or other personal factors. The main challenges in rational applications of physical therapy to the diseases and conditions covered in this chapter are to find ways of promoting general exercise compliance or to target those individuals most likely to benefit from exercise programmes.

Much of the background to this chapter has been very well covered in a recent review by Pedersen & Saltin (2006), and the reader is referred to that article for more specific details regarding evidence for the benefits of physical activity and guidelines for the prescription and delivery of exercise programmes.

2 INSULIN RESISTANCE AND THE METABOLIC SYNDROME

Almost 20 years ago, Reaven (1988) put forward the idea that insulin resistance was an underlying and perhaps causative feature of a cluster of common diseases including type 2 diabetes, dyslipidaemias, certain forms of hypertension and cardiovascular disease, all of which are associated with overweight or obesity. Insulin resistance is defined as reduced ability of insulin to lower blood glucose concentration and has two major components: (1) reduced glucose uptake into and storage within skeletal muscle, and (2) reduced ability of insulin to lower glucose output from the liver. Insulin resistance is correlated with high concentrations of insulin in the blood, for reasons which are disputed and to an extent that insulin concentration is often used as a surrogate measure of insulin resistance. Subsequently, much evidence has accumulated in support of the concept of insulin resistance or the metabolic syndrome but the concept has proved less useful therapeutically than was initially hoped.

Recently, the metabolic syndrome has come to be seen primarily as a clustering of cardiovascular disease risk factors with an underlying pathology related to insulin resistance. As emphasised in a recent review, there is very little evidence to support this view (Kahn et al. 2005), and in the current state of knowledge, the treatment of individuals with diseases and conditions included under the metabolic syndrome should target primarily the symptoms that they exhibit (e.g. diabetes, hypertension, dyslipidaemias), rather than the insulin resistance presumed to underlie those conditions. However, since the recommended treatments for all of these conditions include lifestyle modification (diet and exercise) aimed at reducing body weight and improving cardiovascular fitness (Kahn et al. 2005), it is encouraging to note that increased physical activity can reduce insulin resistance through effects on skeletal muscle and cardiovascular physiology (Hawley 2004).

2.1 Measurement of insulin resistance in humans

Any consideration of the effects of physical activity on insulin resistance must first address the problem of measurement of insulin action in vivo. The widely accepted gold standard method is the hyperinsulinaemic euglycaemic clamp in which circulating insulin concentration is raised by intravenous infusion of insulin, while an intravenous glucose infusion is varied to maintain a constant blood glucose concentration. The rate of glucose infusion required to maintain euglycaemia provides a direct measure of the ability of insulin to lower the blood glucose concentration. While some studies have used this method to investigate the effects of physical activity, many have not for logistical or other reasons. These studies rely instead on either mathematical models of insulin–glucose relationships or on direct measures of circulating insulin concentrations. However, interpretation of plasma insulin concentrations as an index of insulin resistance is often ambiguous. More generally, the diversity of methods used to measure insulin resistance complicates and confuses the study of effects of interventions in humans. This problem with the interpretation of measures of insulin resistance in humans, and the partly related problems of measurement of insulin secretion, were well described by Groop et al. (1993), but the methods used in this area are still essentially unchanged and the problems of data interpretation remain.

2.2 Effects of physical activity on insulin resistance

Despite the measurement problems noted above, it is clear that increased physical activity can decrease insulin resistance in humans in at least two ways (Plasqui & Westerterp 2007). Immediately after a bout of either aerobic or resistance activity, skeletal muscle shows increased insulin sensitivity, which persists for up to 24 h. In the longer term, physical activity programmes produce an additional improvement in insulin sensitivity, which reverses with detraining. In part, the confidence in this conclusion is due to the demonstration of very clear benefits of training on directly measured insulin sensitivity in animal models (Kim et al. 2000, Kraegen et al. 1989). However, uncertainties, due in part to measurement problems, arise when considering the types, intensities and duration of exercise training programmes that are necessary for producing such benefits in humans, their mechanisms and their benefits in producing improvements in associated conditions. With regard to mechanisms, the animal data indicate that physical training compensates for, rather than corrects, the insulin resistance induced by high-fat feeding (Kim et al. 2000, Kraegen et al. 1989). At least some studies in humans are consistent with this observation. Dengel et al. (1996) showed that aerobic exercise training and weight loss produced separate and additive effects on glucose tolerance in sedentary older men. The potential benefits of physical activity programmes for individuals with insulin resistance may therefore be additional to any benefits associated with diet-induced weight loss.

The optimal exercise prescription (type, intensity, frequency, duration) to achieve significant benefits in people with insulin resistance can still be debated, but is that really the most important question? From the studies reviewed by Plasqui & Westerterp (2007), three outcomes are clear. First, a single bout of exercise improves insulin sensitivity, whether it is aerobic or resistance exercise. Second, both aerobic and resistance training have a prolonged positive effect on insulin sensitivity. Third, higher levels of habitual physical activity are associated with improved insulin action and a risk reduction for the development of type 2 diabetes (see section 4.3). So, as for many of the diseases and conditions covered in this chapter, the question is not whether or not physical activity can be useful, but rather how it can be implemented. Obviously, one is more likely to see the anticipated positive physiological adaptations if the dose of physical activity is maximised, but it has to be taken into account that a sedentary individual will most likely not continue to undergo a high-intensity activity exercise regimen (Kriska 2000). Given the rapid (days) decrements in insulin sensitivity after physical activity has ceased (Houmard et al. 1993, Vukovich et al. 1996), long-term compliance is more essential and beneficial than short-term improvements. In that regard, a moderate level of physical activity seems more feasible to incorporate into one's lifestyle, and is less likely to result in overuse injury.

3 OVERWEIGHT AND OBESITY

3.1 Aetiology

Overweight and obesity, which have reached epidemic proportions in many Western countries, are key risk indicators of preventable morbidity and mortality due to many diseases, particularly hypertension, cardiovascular disease and type 2 diabetes mellitus. The literature on the treatment of these conditions is vast and complex, and there is much misleading information present in both the lay and scientific literature. It would be impossible to summarise the evidence and the rational approaches to these problems within just part of a chapter, so the approach taken here is to refer the reader to a comprehensive governmental report designed to assist clinicians in managing the problems of overweight and obesity (Commonwealth of Australia 2003). Much of what follows is extracted from that report and so citations to this source also include section numbers.

Overweight and obesity are the result of excessive stores of body fat (adiposity) and are usually defined on the basis of the body mass index (BMI), which is calculated as body mass (kg) divided by height (m) squared. Overweight is defined as $25 <$ BMI ≤ 30 and obesity as BMI > 30. It is important to note that body mass index is not a measure of body composition or fatness, and it can be misleading when applied to individuals or particular populations, but under many circumstances it can provide a useful surrogate measure (Commonwealth of Australia 2003; 3.2.1). There is evidence that intra-abdominal obesity may have additional deleterious effects on insulin resistance and cardiovascular disease risk, and this is usually indexed in clinical situations by waist circumference measurements (Commonwealth of Australia 2003; 3.2.2).

At one level, the causes of obesity are simple and obvious, based on the Second Law of Thermodynamics (Chapter 19). Excessive body fat stores must be the result of an imbalance between energy intake (diet) and energy expenditure (resting metabolism plus the energy costs of physical and other activities). However, it is now clear that this simple equation, while valid, is of limited use by itself in devising strategies for sustained weight reduction at the individual or population levels (Commonwealth of Australia 2003; 1.7). So while it is true that weight loss can only be achieved and maintained by some combination of dietary restriction and physical activity, there are many biological, psychological and societal barriers to implementing and maintaining the necessary behavioural changes.

3.2 Physical activity in the treatment of obesity and overweight

An increase in physical activity is an important component of weight loss therapy, although at moderate levels, it will not lead to substantially greater weight loss over 12 months (Commonwealth of Australia 2003; 6.2.1). Sustained physical activity is most helpful in the prevention of weight regain (Commonwealth of Australia 2003; 6.2.5). In addition, it has a benefit in reducing cardiovascular and diabetes risks beyond that produced by weight reduction alone (Commonwealth of Australia 2003; 6.2.1). Exercise should generally be initiated slowly and the intensity should be increased gradually. An additional expenditure of 400–800 kJ per day should be achievable. The Australian guidelines recommend that adults should set a long-term goal to accumulate at least 30 min or more of moderate-intensity physical activity on most, and preferably all, days of the week. However, the consistent misconception is that one can adequately achieve this target merely by accumulating incidental exercise. This is clearly erroneous (Chapter 17.1). Indeed, there is now growing evidence that a minimum of 60 min activity per day may be necessary to maintain reduced body weight (Westerterp & Plasqui 2004; Chapter 28). These regimens can be adapted to many forms of physical activity, but walking is particularly attractive because of its safety and accessibility. Reducing sedentary time is another strategy to increase activity by undertaking frequent, less strenuous activities (Expert Panel on the Identification, Evaluation and Treatment of Overweight in Adults 1998).

Adherence to these or similar recommendations, coupled with appropriate dietary restriction, will lead to significant weight loss and reductions in abdominal adiposity in the medium term (3–6 months) in most overweight or obese people, and will generally result in improved cardiovascular fitness and general well-being (Commonwealth of Australia 2003; 6). Improvement in the insulin resistance, often associated with overweight and obesity, could also be expected (see section 30.2.2).

It is widely acknowledged that the initial success in weight loss programmes, which can be quite high over 3–6 months, is followed by weight regain to the initial or higher levels after 1–2 years; most estimates of failure by this criterion cluster around 80% of participants. It is in this area of reduced weight maintenance that increases in physical activity may be particularly important. Observational studies indicate that successful maintenance of reduced weight is accompanied in 90% of cases by regular physical activity at levels above those recommended for the general population (Wing & Hill 2001).

4 TYPE 2 DIABETES MELLITUS

4.1 Aetiology, pathophysiology and treatment

Diabetes mellitus is a disease group characterised by a high blood glucose concentration. Diagnosis is based on the concentration of glucose in the blood after an overnight fast or the blood glucose response to ingestion of a standard amount of glucose (oral glucose tolerance test), using diagnostic cut-offs that are continually under review in relation to therapeutic, preventative and economic goals (American Diabetes Association 2004a).

Type 2 diabetes, which accounts for approximately 90% of cases of diabetes mellitus, is a disorder characterised by both insulin resistance and insulin secretory failure (American Diabetes Association 2004a). The failure of insulin secretion is usually not absolute but relative to the high concentration of glucose in the blood, and many people with type 2 diabetes have normal or even high concentrations of insulin in the blood. Insulin resistance and insulin secretion may influence each other and both are influenced by genetic and environmental factors. The interactions among these physiological processes and the factors influencing them is not well understood (Jenkins & Campbell 2004). Except in extremely rare monogenetic forms of the disease, it is not clear what the primary causes of the disease are, but excess body fat is clearly a factor in most aetiologies.

The main goals of treatment of type 2 diabetes are to reduce the high blood glucose levels (hyperglycaemia) and to reduce adiposity. People with type 2 diabetes are at increased risk of many common, chronic, serious and potentially fatal so-called secondary complications, including various forms of cardiovascular and peripheral vascular disease, kidney disease, neuropathies and retinopathy. Chronic hyperglycaemia is associated with many of these complications, and their occurrence and progression can be reduced by aggressive control of the blood glucose concentration (Prospective Diabetes Study Group UK 1998a,b). These complications may constitute significant barriers to the use of physical exercise as treatment in people with type 2 diabetes. Treatment usually commences with attempts at weight reduction through diet and exercise programmes, but these are ineffective in most patients (see below), who then progress to treatment with one or more of a rapidly growing arsenal of blood glucose-lowering drugs. Many ultimately progress to insulin injections, even though they may have quite high endogenous plasma insulin concentrations.

There were estimated to be 150 million people with diabetes in the world in 2001 (80–90% type 2 diabetes) and this was predicted to rise to 300 million by 2025 (Zimmet et al. 2001). The impact of this tidal wave is beginning to be felt at a time when, in the USA, diabetes is already responsible for one in 10 dollars of health-care costs. The most recent Australian data indicate that approximately 7% of the adult population have diabetes (80–90% type 2) (Commonwealth Department of Health and Aged Care and Australian Institute of Health and Welfare 1998). While type 2 diabetes used to be seen as a disease of middle age (mature-onset diabetes), there is a striking trend towards increased incidence of the disease in younger age groups, including adolescents and children (Zimmet et al. 2001). This trend parallels the trends in sedentary lifestyles and obesity associated with globalisation and industrialisation (Zimmet et al. 2001).

4.2 Physical activity in the treatment of type 2 diabetes

Exercise and dietary interventions have long been described as the cornerstones of therapy of type 2 diabetes. In theory, habitual physical activity should offer many benefits, including acute reduction of glycaemia due to increased utilisation of circulating glucose, reduction in insulin resistance, reduced requirements for glucose-lowering drugs and counteraction of the effects of sedentary lifestyles on many of the risk factors (adiposity, blood lipid concentration, cardiovascular fitness) associated with the complications of type 2 diabetes (Pedersen & Saltin 2006).

Care must be taken to screen individuals with type 2 diabetes for cardiovascular and other circulatory, retinal, sensory, kidney and autonomic nervous system complications before recommending appropriate exercise programmes (American Diabetes Association 2004b). Individuals being treated with insulin do not appear to be at any greater risk of acute hypoglycaemia (low blood glucose concentration) during exercise (Turner & Holman 1990), unlike insulin-treated type 1 diabetics (see section 5.1).

The evidence for the therapeutic effectiveness of exercise interventions has been limited. Many of the studies of exercise-based interventions have been in relatively small samples of patients and results have been variable. Epidemiological studies suffer from confounding by other lifestyle factors, and from the inadequacy of survey-based estimates of physical activity levels. A meta-analysis (Boule et al. 2001) of controlled clinical trials of aerobic or resistance training interventions of ≥ 8 weeks duration ($N = 14$) did find a clinically and statistically significant reduction in haemoglobin A_{1c} (a standard measure of long-term blood glucose control). However, no significant effect on body mass was demonstrated. Most of the studies reviewed by

Boule et al. (2001) included a dietary intervention with the exercise intervention and in a separate analysis, exercise was shown to have an additional effect over dietary interventions alone. However, it is important to note that this meta-analysis was restricted to those controlled studies that demonstrated compliance with the exercise prescription, either by direct supervision or self-report. Because of this, the results obtained provide support for potential benefits, rather than a demonstration of what can be achieved in clinical practice or by self-management.

The implications of this are highlighted by one study excluded from the analysis on the grounds that no effect of the exercise intervention on estimates of physical activity was obtained. Samaras et al. (1997) delivered an exercise intervention programme designed using a health promotion model and compared it with standard treatment, including dietary advice, in a group of 40–70-year-old individuals with type 2 diabetes. The aim was to evaluate a more intensive but still logistically feasible approach to behaviour modification in a group clinical setting. While the results showed that individuals who did increase their level of physical activity (irrespective of the group they were randomised to) showed improvements in blood glucose control and body composition, there was no sustained effect of the exercise intervention. This result is consistent with the experience of most clinical practices, and emphasises the crucial importance of patient compliance in realising the potential of exercise interventions in type 2 diabetes. The barriers to compliance are many (see Samaras et al. 1997) and include motivational difficulties, pathophysiological factors which are secondary or predisposing to the disease, as well as other factors such as age and inflexible social obligations.

In summary, it seems clear that the potential benefits of habitual physical activity are significant, but their full achievement is a difficult, perhaps impossible challenge for the majority of people with this disease. Efforts to promote and prescribe physical activity in patients with type 2 diabetes will no doubt continue and will continue to have beneficial effects in a minority of patients. However, it may be that similar efforts applied to those at high risk of developing the disease will offer more benefits in the long run.

4.3 Physical activity and the onset of type 2 diabetes

In the last decade, there has been a growing international recognition that efforts designed to prevent or delay the onset of the disease may be justified at the individual and population levels (American Diabetes Association and National Institute of Diabetes and Digestive and Kidney Diseases 2004, National Health and Medical Research Council of Australia 2005, Task Force on Diabetes and Cardiovascular Diseases of the European Society of Cardiology and of the European Association for the Study of Diabetes 2007). Type 2 diabetes meets many criteria that would justify such an approach, including the magnitude of the personal and societal burdens of the disease, the presence of reliable indicators of disease risk and progression, the availability of effective preventive measures and the affordability of identifying individuals at risk and of delivering preventive programmes (American Diabetes Association and National Institute of Diabetes and Digestive and Kidney Diseases 2004). The last of these is the least clear, due to uncertainties about how best to identify individuals and the early stage of development of preventive programmes, but there are some grounds for optimism.

The most powerful single predictor of increased risk of developing type 2 diabetes is the presence of a higher than normal fasting blood glucose concentration or a higher than normal response to an oral glucose tolerance test, which are below the diagnostic threshold for diabetes: impaired fasting glucose or impaired glucose tolerance. However, other factors, such as mature age, high body mass index, family history of diabetes, elevated blood pressure and blood lipid levels, contribute significantly to the risk (American Diabetes Association and National Institute of Diabetes and Digestive and Kidney Diseases 2004). All of these additional factors, except perhaps family history, are associated with sedentary lifestyles and can potentially be modified by moderate physical activity programmes, particularly when combined with dietary restriction (Chapters 17.1 and 28).

The evidence that interventions incorporating physical activity programmes can prevent or delay the progression to type 2 diabetes in individuals at high risk is very strong. The Swedish Malmo Study (Eriksson & Lindgarde 1991) used increased physical exercise and weight loss as major intervention strategies to prevent or delay type 2 diabetes. High-risk subjects had less than half the risk of developing type 2 diabetes during 5 years of follow-up, compared with those who did not take part in the lifestyle modification programme. Similar results were obtained subsequently in large-scale Finnish (Tuomilehto et al. 2001) and US (Knowler et al. 2002) studies.

Less is known about the type of exercise that is most protective. Indeed, some forms of exercise may be contraindicated; for example, resistance training and high-intensity exercise may be inappropriate for hypertensive individuals (Pedersen & Saltin 2006, Wallberg-Henriksson et al. 1998). Nevertheless, vigorous sports activity (expending at least 42 kJ·min^{-1}) appears protective against type 2 diabetes (Helmrich et al. 1994). Due to the greater glucose utilisation that results from the use of large muscle groups, activities such as walking, swimming, rowing or cycling appear to be preferable to exercises isolating small muscle groups, such as some calisthenics or some forms of weight lifting (National Health and Medical Research Council of Australia 2005).

Compliance with an exercise programme is also important. Therefore, flexible programmes, based on accumulated lifestyle-oriented activities, may be more conducive to improvements in long-term exercise adherence, and to improvements in metabolic health, than more structured programmes (Jakicic et al. 1995). Clearly, individuals at high risk of developing type 2 diabetes will share many characteristics with those diagnosed with the disease, and will therefore exhibit some of the same barriers and contraindications to habitual physical activity. However, it could be expected that, because of their age and less developed pathologies on average, better compliance with programmes may be obtained in younger individuals. In support of this, the investigators of one of the large-scale intervention programmes commented that 'The reasonably low dropout rate in our study . . . indicates that subjects with impaired glucose tolerance are willing and able to participate in a demanding intervention programme if it is made available to them' (Tuomilehto et al. 2001).

5 TYPE 1 DIABETES MELLITUS

5.1 Aetiology, pathophysiology and treatment

Most cases of type 1 diabetes, which accounts for 5–10% of all cases of diabetes mellitus, are caused by autoimmune destruction of the pancreatic β cells, resulting in a complete deficiency of insulin. Affected individuals require insulin treatment for survival, usually administered by subcutaneous injection, often three times daily. Age of onset is usually before or around puberty, but can be later in life, even in the eighth or ninth decades. Onset is often rapid, with complete destruction of β cells occurring within days, but may be more gradual in some individuals. The disease has multiple genetic predispositions and is also related to environmental factors, but these are poorly defined (American Diabetes Association 2004a).

The consequences of untreated type 1 diabetes for energy metabolism are extreme, reflecting the crucial role of insulin in metabolic regulation. Hepatic glucose output is unrestrained and peripheral glucose utilisation is low. Together, these result in extremely high blood glucose concentrations. Similarly, the breakdown of fats stored in adipose tissue is unrestrained, resulting in very high concentrations of fatty acids and ketone bodies in the blood. Many patients present initially with ketoacidosis, which would rapidly become fatal if not reversed by insulin injection.

The therapeutic problem in type 1 diabetes is to control blood glucose concentration within or near the normal range by appropriate injections of insulin. In normal physiology, the concentration of insulin in the blood is under rapid and tight regulation (Chapter 18) by many signals, including blood glucose concentration, sympathetic and parasympathetic outflows and hormones released by the gastrointestinal tract. While there are now many types of insulin preparation available, with different absorption rates and other pharmacokinetic properties, it is not possible to replicate (by insulin injection) the normal relationships between metabolic requirements and the concentration of insulin in the blood. Patients with type 1 diabetes are constantly at risk of either hyperglycaemia, due to underinsulinisation, or hypoglycaemia due to overinsulinisation.

Hyperglycaemia, while rarely as severe now as it was before the use of insulin, nevertheless results, over time, in the same severe secondary complications that are a feature of type 2 diabetes (section 4.1). It is clear that tight control of blood glucose in type 1 diabetes has a marked beneficial effect on the occurrence and progression of those complications (Diabetes Control and Complications Trial Research Group 1993).

On the other hand, hypoglycaemia carries severe acute risks; if the blood glucose concentration falls below a critical threshold (approximately $1.5 \, mmol \cdot L^{-1}$), the brain and central nervous system are unable to extract sufficient glucose from the blood to meet their energy requirements. The resulting hypoglycaemic coma results in permanent brain damage or death, if not reversed, within minutes. For this reason, many patients and their clinicians tend to target a blood glucose concentration on the high side of normal.

5.2 Exercise in type 1 diabetes

Exercise is not thought at present to provide substantial improvements in the underlying pathology of type 1 diabetes, although there is presumed to be some small benefit from the acute reduction in blood glucose concentration in well-managed patients, caused by the increased utilisation of glucose by active skeletal muscles. However, there is a recognition that patients with type 1 diabetes should be able to perform any form of physical activity they desire, for their chosen lifestyle or profession, for the beneficial effects on some of the secondary complications and for general health benefits (American Diabetes Association 2004b). Patients should be screened in the same way recommended for type 2 diabetic patients (American Diabetes Association 2004b), but there is the additional risk of exercise-induced hypoglycaemia to be considered. Hypoglycaemia can occur during, immediately after or many hours after physical activity. Avoiding this complication requires that the patient has an adequate knowledge of the metabolic and hormonal consequences of physical activity, as well as good self-management skills. Insulin doses can be adjusted and carbohydrates can be consumed in relation to the patient's responses to particular types of exercise.

Self-monitoring of blood glucose concentrations is an important component of this process (American Diabetes Association 2004b). These skills can be difficult to master, particularly for the majority of new cases of type 1 diabetes who are children or adolescents. However, it is believed that with careful instruction, the majority are able to incorporate physical activities into their lives, and individuals with type 1 diabetes have reached the highest levels of competitive sports.

6 RHEUMATOID ARTHRITIS

6.1 Aetiology

Rheumatoid arthritis is a systemic inflammatory, autoimmune disease that produces a progressive degeneration of the musculoskeletal system. It affects approximately 1% of the adult population and is most prevalent among those aged 40–60 years. The risk of developing rheumatoid arthritis is about five times higher in women (Ottawa Panel 2004). Rheumatoid arthritis is characterised by chronic, symmetric polyarthritis and erosive synovitis, which may lead to several degrees of articular destruction, loss of function and increased energy expenditure (De Carvalho et al. 2004). Even with appropriate drug therapy, up to 7% of patients are disabled to some extent 5 years after disease onset, and 50% are too disabled to work 10 years after onset (Yelin et al. 1980). Rheumatoid arthritis is also accompanied by a loss of body cell mass, mainly muscle mass, known as rheumatoid cachexia, which contributes to a 2–5 times higher all-cause mortality and reduced life expectancy of 3–18 years (Walsmith & Roubenoff 2002). The loss of body cell mass is linked to an excess of inflammatory cytokines and increased protein catabolism, although the exact mechanism is still unknown (Roubenoff et al. 1994).

6.2 Functional classification

Patients with rheumatoid arthritis can be classified according to their functional capacity into the following classes: (1) complete functional capacity, with ability to carry out all usual duties without handicap; (2) functional capacity adequate to conduct normal activities, despite the handicap of discomfort or limited mobility of one or more joints; (3) functional capacity adequate to perform only a few or none of the duties of usual occupation or of self-care; or (4) largely or wholly incapacitated, with the patient bedridden or wheelchair bound, permitting little or no self-care (Helewa & Walker 2004).

6.3 The role of physical activity

6.3.1 Physical inactivity

Patients with rheumatoid arthritis have restricted mobility, considerably reduced muscle strength, ranging from 30–70% of that seen in people of similar age, and reduced endurance, typically 50% of healthy controls (Ekdahl & Broman 1992, Hakkinen et al. 1995, Pedersen & Saltin 2006). Reduced habitual physical activity may be caused by joint pain, restricted mobility and fatigue, and will result in decreased physical fitness. Since total body cell mass is the main determinant of functional capacity, the lower body cell mass observed in cachectic patients might be both a consequence and a cause of lower physical activity. Furthermore, the metabolic cost of performing a specific activity might be higher in patients compared to healthy subjects (De Carvalho et al. 2004), and may be an additional cause

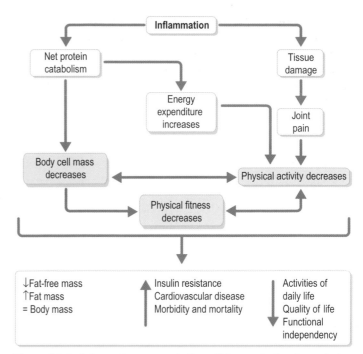

Figure 30.1 Schematic representation of the cascade of events in rheumatoid cachexia leading to decreases in body cell mass, physical fitness and physical activity.

of decreased physical activity. The end result is a vicious circle (Figure 30.1), where inflammation leads to pain, joint destruction and muscle wasting, resulting in decreased physical activity and physical fitness. Decreased physical fitness will lead to a lower functional capacity and ability to exercise which, in turn, will decrease physical activity and fitness even further.

In the long term, this cascade of events has consequences on morbidity and mortality. The result of the loss of body cell mass and decreased physical activity is an unfavourable body composition. For example, patients have a lower fat-free mass and a relatively high fat mass, while body mass often remains unchanged (Rall & Roubenoff 2004, Roubenoff et al. 1994). This is also referred to as cachectic obesity, and may lead to insulin resistance and a higher risk for cardiovascular disease. A schematic representation is given in Figure 30.1.

6.3.2 Exercise therapy: beneficial or prejudicial?

Unlike the metabolic disorders of diabetes or obesity, where a sedentary lifestyle can lead to the development of the disorder, rheumatoid arthritis is never the consequence, but always the cause of a low activity level. Rheumatoid arthritis acts directly on the movement apparatus, causing joint pain and inflammation. Therefore the question arises whether or not exercise, which puts extra strain on joints and muscles, is beneficial. Indeed, exercise may aggravate the disease activity. In an attempt to answer this question, one has to weigh up the risks versus the benefits in both the short and long term.

6.3.2.1 Evidence for the benefits of exercise

The ultimate goal of prescribing exercise in rheumatoid arthritis is to prevent or minimise functional loss in the long run. A reduced function will result in decreased ability to perform activities of daily life, decreased independence and the adoption of a sedentary lifestyle, with a negative psychosocial impact and increased risk for cardiovascular disease. With respect to the musculoskeletal system, the three most essential elements for optimal functioning are range of motion (flexibility), strength and aerobic power (endurance). Most exercise intervention trials are based on resistance or aerobic training.

A large number of trials have been published with respect to the effect of exercise training on disease progress, pain, quality of life, range of motion, strength and aerobic fitness. Studies differ with respect to the duration and frequency of exercise, the types of patients studied, the specifics of the exercise regimen and the end points used. Recently, the Ottawa Panel reviewed published evidence with regard to the role of therapeutic exercise in the management of rheumatoid arthritis in adults (Ottawa Panel 2004). They identified 90 relevant publications, of which 16 met the selection criteria and were included in the analysis. The Panel concluded there was sufficient evidence to support the use of therapeutic exercises, especially knee functional strengthening, general physical activity and whole-body, low-intensity exercises for the management of rheumatoid arthritis. Conversely, evidence was lacking at present as to whether the use of shoulder- and hand-strengthening exercises and whole-body, high-intensity exercises should be included or excluded in the daily practice of physical rehabilitation for rheumatoid arthritis management (Ottawa Panel 2004).

Another recent review assessed the positive effect of training on pathogenesis (Pedersen & Saltin 2006), symptoms specific to rheumatoid arthritis, physical fitness or strength, and quality of life, and rated the available evidence as strong, moderate, limited or absent. They concluded there was considerable agreement between the studies that dynamic physical activity improves physical fitness and muscle strength, but has no, or only a moderate effect on disease activity and pain. However, the majority of studies involved patients in functional classes one and two, and only a very few used patients from classes three and four (Pedersen & Saltin 2006). Stenström & Minor (2003) concluded, after reviewing 15 randomised controlled trials, that evidence was growing for the beneficial effect of aerobic or strengthening exercise on aerobic power and muscle function in patients with rheumatoid arthritis. Most studies, however, found no effect on pain, range of motion, the ability to perform activities of daily life or health-related quality of life. Furthermore, these authors concluded that neither positive nor negative evidence existed for the effects of exercise on disease activity or joint destruction.

With regard to rheumatoid cachexia, a lack of exercise exacerbates the cytokine-driven loss of muscle mass. Resistance training increases muscle strength and physical function, and has a direct positive effect on the maintenance of muscle and body cell masses. Aerobic training will positively affect insulin resistance and cardiovascular risk, and may prevent fat accumulation. Therefore, with respect to muscle wasting or cachectic obesity, any type of physical activity could be considered to be beneficial.

6.3.2.2 Contraindications

The contraindications of exercise are often assessed by outcome measures such as pain, changes in range of motion and disease activity measured by inflammatory markers. An overview of randomised controlled studies assessing these variables is provided by Stenström & Minor (2003). The conclusion of these studies was that pain, and the ability to perform activities of daily life, remained unchanged in most studies, and that disease activity was either reduced or unchanged. These variables provide an indication of disease progress but the ultimate index of interest in rheumatoid arthritis is joint damage. Unfortunately, radiographic evidence of the effect of exercise on joint damage is scarce.

Nordemar et al. (1981) investigated the effectiveness and safety of a supervised, long-term (4–6 years) exercise programme, performed once every other week, compared with the standard patient care. Radiological progression of clinically affected joints was less pronounced in the exercise than in the control group. In a study by Stenström et al. (1991), patients with rheumatoid arthritis performed intensive dynamic, water-based exercises once a week, and radiographic evaluation was compared with data from a control (care) group. After 4 years, there were no differences in radiological progression between the groups. It has to be noted, however, that although exercise intensity in both these trials was sufficiently high, the frequency was low: once every second week (Nordemar et al. 1981) and once a week (Stenstrom et al. 1991).

Results of other studies investigating the effect of exercise on radiographic progression showed no differences between intervention and control groups (de Jong et al. 2003, Hakkinen et al. 2001, 2004, Hansen et al. 1993), or were slightly in favour of the exercise group (de Jong et al. 2004). Long-term, high-intensity exercise in a patient training trial showed no statistically significant differences in radiographic progression of the large joints between exercise and control groups (de Jong et al. 2003). A subgroup analysis, however, showed that the association between long-term, high-intensity weight-bearing exercise and joint damage was influenced by baseline damage (Munneke et al. 2005).

6.3.3 Conclusions

The consensus of systematic reviews is that persons with rheumatoid arthritis demonstrate improved aerobic fitness and muscle strength. As a consequence, patients' ability to perform activities of daily life and health-related quality of life should improve as well, although not all studies have found these effects. It is possible that questionnaires designed to assess these variables, such as the Stanford Health Assessment Questionnaire (Fries et al. 1980), are not sensitive enough to capture and tease out the exercise effects relative to those associated with medication (Stenstrom & Minor 2003).

With regard to pain, disease activity and joint damage, there is insufficient evidence that exercise has detrimental effects on disease progression (de Jong & Vlieland 2005, Pedersen & Saltin 2006, Stenstrom & Minor 2003). Furthermore, evidence is lacking for either positive or negative effects of exercise in patients from functional classes three and four (Pedersen & Saltin 2006). Training is contraindicated in cases of severe inflammation and care should be taken with the prescription of high-intensity exercises, especially weight-bearing activities. Nevertheless, patients will benefit most from an overall increase in physical activity, to improve cardiovascular and muscular fitness, which can be maintained throughout life.

Despite a growing body of evidence that exercise and increased physical activity are beneficial in terms of physical functioning, and the lack of evidence for the detrimental effects on disease activity, clinicians still have reservations about prescribing exercise for patients with rheumatoid arthritis. Approximately 58% of rheumatologists in one arthritis centre believed aerobic exercises were not useful for rheumatoid arthritis patients (Finckh et al. 2003). There is no doubt that care should be taken with high-intensity exercises that apply high loads on the joints, and more research is needed for the effect of such exercises on long-term radiological damage. However, in the absence of acute severe inflammation, an overall increase in daily physical activity can only be beneficial. As with the general population, exercise programmes are often hard to sustain over longer periods. In fact, patients should be encouraged to be as physically active as possible, have a variety of activity options, build activities into their daily routines and to develop an active lifestyle, rather than just following a regimented exercise prescription (Finckh et al. 2003).

7 OSTEOARTHRITIS

7.1 Aetiology

Osteoarthritis is the most common joint disease and is strongly related to age and overweight, but can also be the result of joint injury. Virtually everyone over 60 years shows signs of osteoarthritis in at least one joint (Pedersen & Saltin 2006). It most frequently affects the hands, spine, knees and hips while involvement of the wrists, elbows and shoulders is uncommon (Sarzi-Puttini et al. 2005). Osteoarthritis is a progressive joint disease, characterised by varying degrees of pain and degeneration. It affects the structural and functional integrity of articular cartilage, as well as the adjacent bone and joint tissues (Griffin & Guilak 2005). Loss of artic-

ular cartilage is one of the dominant factors in the pathogenesis of osteoarthritis and this is accompanied by joint deformation, bone sclerosis, capsule shrinkage, muscle atrophy and varying degrees of synovitis (Pedersen & Saltin 2006). The aetiology of osteoarthritis is multifactorial, with inflammatory, metabolic and mechanical causes (Sarzi-Puttini et al. 2005).

Patients with symptomatic osteoarthritis of the hip or knee will complain of deep, aching pain. In the early stages of the disease, pain will be intermittent and mostly associated with joint use. When the disease progresses, pain becomes more chronic and may also be present during rest and at night (Fransen et al. 2003). Crepitus, a crackling or grating sound when the joint is moved, may be due to cartilage loss and joint surface irregularity (Sarzi-Puttini et al. 2005). The joint feels stiff, resulting in pain and difficulty when initiating movement after a period of rest (Fransen et al. 2003). Short-lasting morning stiffness is a common complaint (Sarzi-Puttini et al. 2005).

7.2 Physical activity and obesity in osteoarthritis

Increasing age is the most important risk factor for this disease. Given the scope of this chapter, the focus here will be on the biomechanical factors related to the disease, with the most important issues being habitual physical activity and obesity.

7.2.1 Obesity

Obesity is very relevant to osteoarthritis because it is an important risk factor for its development (Sarzi-Puttini et al. 2005), and because of its relationship with habitual exercise. Recent studies have established that being overweight antedates the development of osteoarthritis and increases the risk of radiographic progression (Lievense et al. 2002). Weight loss can reduce the risk of osteoarthritis (Felson et al. 1992), and a higher body mass index is positively correlated with an increased risk of knee osteoarthritis (Coggon et al. 2001). Continuous high loads placed on the joints, as a consequence of obesity, accelerate joint wear. Thus, habitual exercise could positively affect osteoarthritis via superior weight management.

7.2.2 Physical activity
7.2.2.1 Physical activity as a cause of osteoarthritis
The risk of osteoarthritis is increased by some factors related to physical activity such as occupation, type and level of sports participation and exercise intensity levels (Griffin & Guilak 2005). Occupations involving heavy loading (Felson et al. 2000) or repetitive tasks overloading the joints and muscles increase the risk for osteoarthritis (Sarzi-Puttini et al. 2005). Some sports of high intensity, those involving heavy loading and twisting of the knee or those with repeated and direct impact on the joints also increase the risk of osteoarthritis (Felson et al. 2000, Griffin & Guilak 2005, Sarzi-Puttini et al. 2005). Sports such as soccer, rugby,

racket sports and other track and field sports, practised at a high level, can contribute to the development of osteoarthritis at a relatively early age (Lequesne et al. 1997). However, elevated daily physical activity levels are not a risk factor for osteoarthritis (Arokoski et al. 2000). On the contrary, physical activity has a fundamental role in the treatment of osteoarthritis.

7.2.2.2 Physical activity in the treatment of osteoarthritis

Several authors have reviewed the available literature on the effect of exercise on the treatment of osteoarthritis. Van Baar et al. (1999) summarised the results of 11 randomised clinical trials on exercise therapy for osteoarthritis of the hip or knee. The outcome measures used were pain, self-reported disability, observed disability or patient's global assessment of effect. There was a small to moderate effect of exercise therapy on pain, small beneficial effects on both disability outcome measures and moderate to pronounced beneficial effects according to patient's global assessment of effect. The conclusion was that exercise was effective in patients with osteoarthritis of the hip or knee but that those conclusions were based on only a small number of good studies (Van Baar et al. 1999).

Fransen et al. (2003) reviewed randomised, controlled trials comparing some form of land-based therapeutic exercise with a non-exercise control group. Insufficient data existed to draw any conclusions about subjects with osteoarthritis of the hip, but for osteoarthritis of the knee, the results of 17 studies indicated a positive treatment effect on pain and self-reported physical function. There were also no significant differences found between group programmes or treatments provided on a one-to-one basis (Fransen et al. 2003).

Two recent meta-analyses focused specifically on the efficacy of strengthening (Pelland et al. 2004) and aerobic exercise (Brosseau et al. 2004) for osteoarthritis. Twenty-two trials of strengthening exercise were identified and included isometric, isotonic, isokinetic, concentric, concentric-eccentric and dynamic modalities. Improvements in strength, pain, function and quality of life were noted with muscle strengthening, but there was no evidence that the type of exercise influences the outcome. Aerobic exercises included walking programmes, aquatic exercises, jogging in water, yoga and tai chi. Results indicated that aerobic exercise alleviated pain and joint tenderness, and promoted functional status and respiratory capacity (Bennell & Hinman 2005, Brosseau et al. 2004, Pelland et al. 2004).

7.2.2.3 Mechanism

There are no grounds for believing that training works through a direct effect on the disease pathogenesis. The primary aim of physical training in the treatment of osteoarthritis is to enhance muscle strength around the affected joints (Pedersen & Saltin 2006). Where strengthening exercises have a direct effect on stabilising the joint, and hence pain and function, endurance exercises have a more long-term effect on functional capacity, and are relevant in the prevention of other diseases and weight loss.

7.2.2.4 Contraindications

As was the case with rheumatoid arthritis, affected joints should be rested when acute inflammation occurs. If pain worsens after exercise, exercise should be temporarily discontinued and the exercise programme should be modified (Pedersen & Saltin 2006). As indicated above, sports or exercises that place a high workload on joints, in the form of both axial compression and twisting, should be avoided, as should running on hard surfaces (Pedersen & Saltin 2006).

7.2.3 Conclusions

The overall consensus of the studies reviewed is that strengthening exercises reduce pain and enhance joint function and thereby generally improve the quality of life. Most of the studies, however, were based on osteoarthritis of the knee and more evidence is needed to verify whether or not these conclusions also apply to other joints. Endurance training has additional beneficial effects on physical functioning and is highly relevant with regards to obesity and the related co-morbidities, such as cardiovascular disease. Again, long-term compliance is a key factor, since a higher habitual exercise level has to be a life-long effort for the beneficial effects to be sustained.

8 CANCER

8.1 Aetiology

Cancer can be defined as a group of diseases characterised by uncontrolled growth and spread of abnormal cells, resulting in the compression, invasion and degradation of adjacent fresh tissue. When malignant cells are transported through the blood or lymph to other locations in the body, secondary tumours or metastases can be formed. Breast cancer is the most common cancer in women, followed by lung and colorectal cancers. In men, prostate cancer is the most common, followed by cancers of the lung and colon. For both genders combined, lung cancer is the leading killer of all cancers (American Cancer Society 2006). Environmental factors such as smoking, radiation, diet and physical inactivity (Chapter 28) increase the risk of developing cancer.

The symptoms related to cancer are numerous, and depend on the type and localisation of the tumour and progress of the disease. The demanding nature of cancer treatment (chemotherapy, radiotherapy, surgery) contributes to common symptoms such as fatigue, sickness, poor appetite and weight loss. Often, not only weight loss but a specific loss of muscle mass is observed (cancer cachexia). It is a significant cause of morbidity and mortality, occurring in up to 80% of patients with advanced cancer and responsible for death in up to 20% of all cancer cases (Tisdale 2002). Cachexia causes muscle loss, leading to decreased physical fitness and function. Co-existing physical inactivity exacerbates this muscle wasting.

8.2 The role of physical activity

8.2.1 Physical activity and cancer prevention

There is increasing evidence from observational studies that physical activity protects against the development of cancer (Chapter 28). Thune & Furberg (2001) reviewed the available literature for a dose–response association between physical activity and overall and site-specific cancer risk. The evidence indicated a protective effect of both leisure time and occupational physical activity on overall and site-specific cancer risk. A crude graded inverse dose–response relationship was observed between physical activity and cancers of the colon and of the breast (Thune & Furberg 2001). Further research is needed concerning cancer of other organs and to reveal the biological mechanism behind this protective effect.

8.2.2 Exercise therapy during and after cancer treatment

Stevinson et al. (2004) summarised the results of 33 controlled trials involving exercise therapy and including several types of cancer, but with the majority being breast cancer. The two main outcomes studied were physical functioning and fatigue. Significant improvements were observed in tests of aerobic power or timed walk distances following aerobic exercise programmes (13 trials). In one study, the typical loss of physical performance was attenuated among inpatients receiving high-dose chemotherapy who exercised during hospitalisation. Increases in muscular strength were recorded after resistive training (three trials), and no improvements in fitness parameters or muscle strength were recorded in six trials. The pooled standardised mean difference between exercisers and controls showed significantly greater physical function for the exercisers, with the strongest effect observed in patients with breast cancer. However, the authors noted that the largest study, which was also the only study using intention-to-treat analysis, found no effect of exercise on physical function

(Stevinson et al. 2004). Pooling the data from 12 trials that assessed fatigue indicated there was no overall effect of exercise on symptoms of fatigue. For outcomes such as quality of life and psychological symptoms, there was no clear or consistent evidence that exercise was beneficial (Stevinson et al. 2004).

Knols et al. (2005) reviewed 34 randomised clinical trials and controlled clinical trials. Results were presented separately for exercise during and after breast cancer treatment, during high-dose chemotherapy following bone marrow and peripheral bone stem cell transplantation, and during and after treatment in a mixed solid tumour population. The overall results demonstrated that cancer patients in specific populations may benefit from physical exercise, both during and after cancer treatment. Positive results have been observed for a diverse set of outcomes, including physiological measures, objective performance indicators, self-reported functioning and symptoms (particularly fatigue), psychological well-being and overall health-related quality of life (Knols et al. 2005).

8.2.3 Conclusions

Some controversy still exists concerning the efficacy of physical therapy during cancer treatment. However, when these results are reviewed collectively, the overall evidence indicates that patients can benefit from increased physical exercise. Variability in study outcomes may be due to differences in study design, sample size and the specific outcome measures used. Positive effects of exercise may vary significantly as a function of the type of cancer, the stage of the disease, the medical treatment, the nature, intensity and duration of the exercise programme, and the lifestyle of the patient (Knols et al. 2005). It is important to note that there are no known adverse effects of exercise on the disease or its symptoms (Stevinson et al. 2004). At present, however, there is insufficient evidence concerning the impact of exercise on either survival or the recurrence of cancer (Stevinson et al. 2004).

References

American Cancer Society 2006 Cancer facts and figures 2006. Available online: www.cancer.org/docroot/home/index.asp

American Diabetes Association 2004a Diagnosis and classification of diabetes mellitus. Diabetes Care 27 (Suppl 1):S5–S10

American Diabetes Association 2004b Physical activity/exercise and diabetes. Diabetes Care 27 (Suppl 1):S58–S62

American Diabetes Association and National Institute of Diabetes and Digestive and Kidney Diseases 2004 Prevention or delay of type 2 diabetes. Diabetes Care 27 (Suppl 1):S47–S54

Arokoski JP, Jurvelin JS, Vaatainen U, Helminen HJ 2000 Normal and pathological adaptations of articular cartilage to joint loading. Scandinavian Journal of Medicine and Science in Sport 10:186–198

Bennell K, Hinman R 2005 Exercise as a treatment for osteoarthritis. Current Opinion in Rheumatology 17:634–640

Boule NG, Haddad E, Kenny GP, Wells GA, Sigal RJ 2001 Effects of exercise on glycemic control and body mass in type 2 diabetes mellitus: a meta-analysis of controlled clinical trials. Journal of the American Medical Association 286:1218–1227

Brosseau L, Pelland L, Wells G, Macleay L, Lamothe C, Michaud G, Lambert J, Robinson V, Tugwell P 2004 Efficacy of aerobic exercises for osteoarthritis (part II): a meta-analysis. Physical Therapy Reviews 9:125–145

Coggon D, Reading I, Croft P, McLaren M, Barrett D, Cooper C 2001 Knee osteoarthritis and obesity. International Journal of Obesity and Related Metabolic Disorders 25:622–627

Commonwealth Department of Health and Aged Care and Australian Institute of Health and Welfare 1998 National Health Priority Areas Report: Diabetes Mellitus. Canberra, Commonwealth Department of Health and Aged Care. Available online: www.aihw.gov.au/publications/index.cfm/title/4463

Commonwealth of Australia 2003 Clinical practice guidelines for the management of overweight and obesity in adults. Available online: www.obesityguidelines.gov.au

De Carvalho MR, Tebexreni AS, Salles CA, Barros Neto T, Natour J 2004 Oxygen uptake during walking in patients with rheumatoid arthritis – a controlled study. Journal of Rheumatology 31:655–662

de Jong Z, Vlieland TP 2005 Safety of exercise in patients with rheumatoid arthritis. Current Opinion in Rheumatology 17:177–182

de Jong Z, Munneke M, Zwinderman A, Kroon H, Jansen A, Ronday K, Van Schaardenburg D, Dijkmans B, Ven Den Ende C, Breedveld F, Vliet Vlieland T, Hazes J 2003 Is a long-term high-intensity exercise program effective and safe in patients with rheumatoid arthritis? Results of a randomized controlled trial. Arthritis and Rheumatism 48:2415–2424

de Jong Z, Munneke M, Zwinderman A, Kroon H, Ronday K, Lems W, Dijkmans B, Breedveld F, Vliet Vlieland T, Hazes J, Huizinga T 2004 Long term high intensity exercise and damage of small joints in rheumatoid arthritis. Annals of the Rheumatic Diseases 63:1399–1405

Dengel DR, Pratley RE, Hagberg J, Rogus E, Goldberg A 1996 Distinct effects of aerobic exercise training and weight loss on glucose homeostasis in obese sedentary men. Journal of Applied Physiology 81:318–325

Diabetes Control and Complications Trial Research Group 1993 The effect of intensive treatment of diabetes on the development and progression of long-term complications in insulin-dependent diabetes mellitus. New England Journal of Medicine 329:977–986

Ekdahl C, Broman G 1992 Muscle strength, endurance and aerobic capacity in rheumatoid arthritis: a comparative study with healthy subjects. Annals of the Rheumatic Diseases 51:35–40

Eriksson KF, Lindgarde F 1991 Prevention of type 2 (non-insulin-dependent) diabetes mellitus by diet and physical exercise. The 6-year Malmo feasibility study. Diabetologia 34:891–898

Expert Panel on the Identification, Evaluation and Treatment of Overweight in Adults 1998 Clinical guidelines on the identification, evaluation and treatment of overweight and obesity in adults: executive summary. American Journal of Clinical Nutrition 68:899–917

Felson DT, Zhang Y, Anthony J, Naimark A, Anderson J 1992 Weight loss reduces the risk for symptomatic knee osteoarthritis in women. The Framingham Study. Annals of Internal Medicine 116:535–539

Felson DT, Lawrence R, Dieppe P, Hirsch R, Helmick C, Jordan J, Kington R, Lane N, Nevitt M, Zhang Y, Sowers M, McAlindon T, Spector T, Poole A, Yanovski S, Ateshian G, Sharma L, Buckwalter J, Brandt K, Fries J 2000 Osteoarthritis: new insights. Part 1: the disease and its risk factors. Annals of Internal Medicine 133:635–646

Finckh A, Iversen M, Liang MH 2003 The exercise prescription in rheumatoid arthritis: primum non nocere. Arthritis and Rheumatism 48:2393–2395

Fransen M, McConnell S, Bell M 2003 Exercise for osteoarthritis of the hip or knee. Cochrane Database Syst Rev: CD004286

Fries JF, Spitz P, Kraines R, Holman H 1980 Measurement of patient outcome in arthritis. Arthritis and Rheumatism 23:137–145

Griffin TM, Guilak F 2005 The role of mechanical loading in the onset and progression of osteoarthritis. Exercise and Sport Science Review 33:195–200

Groop LC, Widen E, Ferrannini E 1993 Insulin resistance and insulin deficiency in the pathogenesis of type 2 (non-insulin-dependent) diabetes mellitus: errors of metabolism or methods. Diabetologia 36:1326–1331

Hakkinen A, Hannonen P, Hakkinen K 1995 Muscle strength in healthy people and in patients suffering from recent-onset inflammatory arthritis. British Journal of Rheumatology 34:355–360

Hakkinen A, Sokka T, Kotaniemi A, Hannonen P 2001 A randomized two-year study of the effects of dynamic strength training on muscle strength, disease activity, functional capacity and bone mineral density in early rheumatoid arthritis. Arthritis and Rheumatism 44:515–522

Hakkinen A, Kokka T, Kautiainen H, Kotaniemi A, Hannonen P 2004 Sustained maintenance of exercise induced muscle strength gains and normal bone mineral density in patients with early rheumatoid arthritis: a 5 year follow up. Annals of the Rheumatic Diseases 63:910–916

Hansen TM, Hansen G, Langgaard A, Rasmussen J 1993 Longterm physical training in rheumatoid arthritis. A randomized trial with different training programs and blinded observers. Scandinavian Journal of Rheumatology 22:107–112

Hawley JA 2004 Exercise as a therapeutic intervention for the prevention and treatment of insulin resistance. Diabetes/Metabolism Research Reviews 20:383–393

Helewa A, Walker JM 2004 Epidemiology and economics of arthritis. In: Physical therapy in rheumatoid arthritis. WB Saunders, Toronto, 9–18

Helmrich SP, Ragland DR, Paffenbarger RS 1994 Prevention of non-insulin-dependent diabetes mellitus with physical activity. Medicine and Science in Sports and Exercise 26:824–830

Houmard JA, Hortobagyi T, Neufer P, Johns R, Fraser D, Israel G, Dohm G 1993 Training cessation does not alter GLUT-4 protein levels in human skeletal muscle. Journal of Applied Physiology 74:776–781

Jakicic JM, Wing R, Butler B, Robertson R 1995 Prescribing exercise in multiple short bouts versus one continuous bout: effects on adherence, cardiorespiratory fitness and weight loss in overweight women. International Journal of Obesity 19:893–901

Jenkins AB, Campbell LV 2004 The genetics and pathophysiology of diabetes mellitus type II. Journal of Inherited Metabolic Disease 27:331–347

Kahn R, Buse J, Ferrannini E, Stern M 2005 The metabolic syndrome: time for a critical appraisal: joint statement from the American Diabetes Association and the European Association for the Study of Diabetes. Diabetes Care 28:2289–2304

Kim CH, Youn JH, Park JY, Hong SK, Park KS, Park SW, Suh KI, Lee KU 2000 Effects of high-fat diet and exercise training on intracellular glucose metabolism in rats. American Journal of Physiology. Endocrinology and Metabolism 278:977–984

Knols R, Aaronson N, Uebelhart D, Fransen J, Aufdemkampe G 2005 Physical exercise in cancer patients during and after medical treatment: a systematic review of randomized and controlled clinical trials. Journal of Clinical Oncology 23:3830–3842

Knowler WC, Barrett-Connor E, Fowler S, Hamman R, Lachin J, Walker E, Nathan D 2002 Reduction in the incidence of type 2 diabetes with lifestyle intervention or metformin. New England Journal of Medicine 346:393–403

Kraegen EW, Storlien L, Jenkins A, James D 1989 Chronic exercise compensates for insulin resistance induced by a high fat diet in rats. American Journal of Physiology 256:E242–E249

Kriska A 2000 Physical activity and the prevention of type 2 diabetes mellitus: how much for how long? Sports Medicine 29:147–151

Lequesne MG, Dang N, Lane NE 1997 Sport practice and osteoarthritis of the limbs. Osteoarthritis and Cartilage 5:75–86

Lievense AM, Bierma-Zeinstra S, Verhagen A, Van Baar M, Verhaar J, Koes B 2002 Influence of obesity on the development of osteoarthritis of the hip: a systematic review. Rheumatology (Oxford) 41:1155–1162

Munneke M, de John Z, Zwinderman A, Ronday H, Van Schaardenburg D, Dijkmans B, Kroon H, Vliet Vlieland T, Hazes J 2005 Effect of a high-intensity weight-bearing exercise program on radiologic damage progression of the large joints in subgroups of patients with rheumatoid arthritis. Arthritis and Rheumatism 53:410–417

National Health and Medical Research Council of Australia 2005 National evidence based guidelines for the management of type 2 diabetes mellitus. Available online: www.nhmrc.gov.au

Nordemar R, Ekblom B, Zachrisson L, Lundqvist K 1981 Physical training in rheumatoid arthritis: a controlled long-term study. I. Scandinavian Journal of Rheumatology 10:17–23

Ottawa Panel 2004 Ottawa Panel evidence-based clinical practice guidelines for therapeutic exercises in the management of rheumatoid arthritis in adults. Physical Therapy 84:934–972

Pedersen BK, Saltin B 2006 Evidence for prescribing exercise as therapy in chronic disease. Scandinavian Journal of Medicine and Science in Sports 16(Suppl 1):3–63

Pelland L, Brosseau L, Wells G, MacLeay L, Lambert J, Lamothe C, Robinson V, Tugwell P 2004 Efficacy of strengthening exercises for osteoarthritis (Part I): a meta-analysis. Physical Therapy Review 9:77–108

Plasqui G, Westerterp K 2007 Physical activity and insulin resistance. Current Nutrition and Food Science 3:157–160

Prospective Diabetes Study (UKPDS) Group UK 1998a Effect of intensive blood-glucose control with metformin on complications in overweight patients with type 2 diabetes (UKPDS 34). Lancet 352:854–865

Prospective Diabetes Study (UKPDS) Group UK 1998b Intensive blood-glucose control with sulphonylureas or insulin compared with conventional treatment and risk of complications in patients with type 2 diabetes (UKPDS 33). Lancet 352:837–853

Rall LC, Roubenoff R 2004 Rheumatoid cachexia: metabolic abnormalities, mechanisms and interventions. Rheumatology (Oxford) 43:1219–1223

Reaven GM 1988 Role of insulin resistance in human disease. Diabetes 37:1595–1607

Roubenoff R, Roubenoff RA, Cannon J, Kehayias J, Zhuang H, Dawson-Hughes B, Dinarello C, Rosenberg I 1994 Rheumatoid cachexia: cytokine-driven hypermetabolism accompanying reduced body cell mass in chronic inflammation. Journal of Clinical Investigation 93:2379–2386

Samaras K, Ashwell S, Mackintosh A, Fleury A, Campbell L, Chisholm D 1997 Will older sedentary people with non-insulin-dependent diabetes mellitus start exercising? A health promotion model. Diabetes Research and Clinical Practice 37:121–128

Sarzi-Puttini P, Cimmino M, Scarpa R, Caporali R, Parazzini F, Zaninelli A, Atzeni F, Canesi B 2005 Osteoarthritis: an overview of the disease and its treatment strategies. Seminars in Arthritis and Rheumatism 35:1–10

Stenstrom CH, Minor MA 2003 Evidence for the benefit of aerobic and strengthening exercise in rheumatoid arthritis. Arthritis and Rheumatism 49:428–434

Stenstrom CH, Lindell B, Swanberg E, Swanberg P, Harms-Ringdahl K, Nordemar R 1991 Intensive dynamic training in water for rheumatoid arthritis functional class II – a long-term study of effects. Scandinavian Journal of Rheumatology 20:358–365

Stevinson C, Lawlor DA, Fox KR 2004 Exercise interventions for cancer patients: systematic review of controlled trials. Cancer Causes and Control 15:1035–1056

Task Force on Diabetes and Cardiovascular Diseases of the European Society of Cardiology (ESC) and of the European Association for the Study of Diabetes (EASD) 2007 Guidelines on diabetes, pre-diabetes and cardiovascular diseases. European Heart Journal 28:88–136

Thune I, Furberg AS 2001 Physical activity and cancer risk: dose-response and cancer, all sites and site-specific. Medicine and Science in Sports and Exercise 33:S530–550; discussion S609–S610

Tisdale MJ 2002 Cachexia in cancer patients. Nature Reviews. Cancer 2:862–871

Tuomilehto J, Lindstrom J, Eriksson J, Valle T, Hamalainen H, Ilanne-Parikka P, Keinanen-Kiukaanniemi S, Laakso M, Louheranta A, Rastas M, Salminen V, Uusitupa M, Aunola S, Cepaitis Z, Moltchanov V, Hakumaki M, Mannelin M, Martikkala V, Sundvall J 2001 Prevention of type 2 diabetes mellitus by changes in lifestyle among subjects with impaired glucose tolerance. New England Journal of Medicine 344:1343–1350

Turner RC, Holman RR 1990 Insulin use in NIDDM. Rationale based on pathophysiology of disease. Diabetes Care 13:1011–1020

Van Baar ME, Assendelft W, Dekker J, Oostendorp R, Bijlsma J 1999 Effectiveness of exercise therapy in patients with osteoarthritis of the hip or knee: a systematic review of randomized clinical trials. Arthritis and Rheumatism 42:1361–1369

Vukovich MD, Arciero P, Kohrt W, Racette S, Hansen P, Holloszy J 1996 Changes in insulin action and GLUT-4 with 6 days of inactivity in endurance runners. Journal of Applied Physiology 80:240–244

Wallberg-Henriksson H, Rincon J, Zierath JR 1998 Exercise in the management of non-insulin-dependent diabetes mellitus. Sports Medicine 25:25–30

Walsmith J, Roubenoff R 2002 Cachexia in rheumatoid arthritis. International Journal of Cardiology 85:89–99

Westerterp KR, Plasqui G 2004 Physical activity and human energy expenditure. Current Opinion in Clinical Nutrition and Metabolic Care 7:607–613

Wing RR, Hill JO 2001 Successful weight loss maintenance. Annual Review of Nutrition 21:323–341

Yelin E, Meenan R, Nevitt M, Epstein W 1980 Work disability in rheumatoid arthritis: effects of disease, social and work factors. Annals of Internal Medicine 93:551–556

Zimmet P, Alberti KG, Shaw J 2001 Global and societal implications of the diabetes epidemic. Nature 414:782–787

Chapter **31**

Topical debate

Chapter **31.1**

It is not economically viable to address the penalties of sedentary behaviour through primary prevention strategies

Roy J. Shephard

Chair: The motion before us is that 'It is not economically viable to address the penalties of sedentary behaviour through primary prevention strategies'. This will be proposed by **Cassandra**, with **Asclepius** sustaining the opposing viewpoint.

Cassandra: Given the many health problems which have been attributed to a sedentary lifestyle (Bouchard et al. 1992; Chapters 17.1, 28, 30), I would be delighted if personal behaviour could be appropriately corrected by some primary prevention strategy. However, the disappointing fact is that widely publicised public health interventions have failed to change even immediate exercise behaviour, let alone modify future health. Look, for example, at the lack of response to intensive exercise promotion programmes of up to 6 months duration in the Canadian cities of Saskatoon and Lindsay, Ontario (Jackson 1975). Likewise, extensive primary prevention campaigns in California have struggled hard to demonstrate any gains in habitual physical activity, energy expenditure or health status (see Calfas et al. 2000).

Asclepius: Surely, you ignore the very successful fitness and lifestyle programmes that have been established in many commercial enterprises (Shephard 1986, 1992a)?

Cassandra: The supposed success of many of these programmes is anecdotal; very few studies have used the experimental or quasiexperimental design necessary to facilitate appropriate scientific scrutiny of the primary observations (Shephard 1991a). Furthermore, I would question the actual success of such programmes. Look at perhaps the simplest criterion: attendance or adherence. Even given the enthusiasm associated with a demonstration project, only a third to half of employees are initially recruited. Furthermore, some of this group were previously active elsewhere, and as many as a half of the initial participants will no longer be attending the programme after 6 months (Shephard 1991a). And these are people who volunteer to exercise! If you were to look at a randomised sample of the general population, as is required when assessing a public health intervention, I am convinced that the marginal costs of recruitment would be much higher, and adherence would be even poorer. Currently, we lack the data to predict the cost of either short- or long-term campaigns to enhance the lifestyle of the general population; most studies have been based on volunteers and almost nothing is known concerning lifelong exercise adherence (habitual physical activity).

Asclepius: I agree that current adherence figures are disappointing, and that we need more data on the responses of the general population. However, if I may draw an analogy with the problem of discouraging cigarette smoking, adherence in many early smoking withdrawal trials was very disappointing. Nevertheless, a dramatic decrease in the proportion of smokers has been achieved in developed countries over a span of 50 years; this reflects, in part, persistent health education and, in part, a restructuring of society (for instance, the progressive prohibition of smoking in public places and court challenges to cigarette manufacturers). Other contributing factors have included the increasing fraction of non-smokers, and identification of the smoker with undesirable personal characteristics (antisocial, low intelligence, low social class; Shephard, 1982, US Department of Health and Human Services 2000). Interestingly in the context of our debate, these advances in population health have been achieved with only a small fraction of the budget spent by those advertising cigarettes. Those engaged in the advocacy of greater physical activity do not face such powerful adversaries as the cigarette manufacturers. So, I think that with modest but persistent health promotional efforts, we shall find a much more positive attitude towards physical activity in 40 or 50 years' time.

Cassandra: Surely, you are not advocating Orwellian legislation that will compel people to exercise?

Asclepius: There have been informal suggestions that health insurance premiums should be reduced for those who exercise or (perhaps more acceptably) that tax incentives should be offered to encourage membership in exercise clubs. But I think our main focus should be not on external rewards associated with exercising, but rather on such internal rewards as personal satisfaction, greater self-esteem, enhanced mood state, and ability to undertake the physical tasks needed in daily life. Furthermore, I do not think membership of an expensive sports club or the purchase of expensive athletic equipment is necessary to achieve the health benefits of exercise; indeed, such purchases can become obstacles to participation (Shephard 1991b). The emphasis on exotic activities, supported by the latest fads in equipment, may contribute to our limited success as yet. Rather, the emphasis should be on restructuring the urban environment; we should be gracing our cities with attractive walkways, cycle paths and pedestrian precincts that make it attractive for people to exercise. Population efforts must adopt a very long-term perspective, concentrating on environmental changes that make active commuting and recreation normative and pleasant forms of social behaviour (Atkinson et al. 2005, Owen et al. 2004).

Cassandra: It is difficult for either of us to predict whether an active lifestyle will be acceptable to a substantial proportion of the general population in 50 years' time. But, even if this does happen, I think the economic dividends from an increase of physical activity (Klarman 1981) will remain greatly overstated. For a start, there is much double counting. One instance of this is that the same health benefits are claimed by those interested in cardiovascular disease and by those concerned with obesity and the metabolic syndrome. Furthermore, some of the intangible attributed benefits of exercise, such as a reduction in the need for physical and emotional support from other family members, are, at best, wild guesses and little thought has been given to the discounting of long-distant health benefits.

Asclepius: There may be some truth in this, but for many Western countries the economic benefits associated with a habitually active lifestyle are likely to remain large, even after making allowance for weaknesses in the estimates, some double counting and the effects of discounting, For example, direct medical costs in Canada amount to more than US $20 billion per year and some 30% of these costs are attributable to conditions (cardiovascular disease and cancer) that are much less prevalent in the active part of the population. Likewise, it has been estimated that encouragement of physical activity in the labour force yields savings of around $500 per worker per year, due to greater productivity and worker satisfaction, less absenteeism, reduced employee turnover, fewer industrial injuries and reduced health insurance premiums. Finally, in the elderly segment of the population, enhanced personal fitness is likely to defer by as much as 10 years the age at which expensive institutional care is required (Shephard 1986).

Cassandra: You speak of huge benefits, but do not forget that these rather dubious estimates are often based on the response of small samples, tested under ideal experimental conditions. When extrapolated to the general population, the possible magnitude of benefit shrinks dramatically. Less than 50% of people are attracted to a typical fitness programme, many fail to show the lifelong adherence and compliance needed for enhanced health outcomes, and even some of those who do adhere may, for various reasons, be non-respondent to exercise (low responders; Shephard 1991a). For instance, there is little evidence that the costs associated with prostate cancer will be averted by exercise. Likewise, regular physical activity is unlikely to bring about any substantial reduction in the need for institutional support associated with geriatric blindness or Alzheimer's disease.

Asclepius: Some categories of disease show little response to primary prevention programmes. For other conditions such as obesity, most people respond to exercise, but there are a few conditions where reduction of body fat is hampered by an adverse genotype. But, if we take the specific example of obesity, one of the big concerns of health promotion at the present time, there can be little argument that the problem has arisen largely from a small discrepancy between the individual's energy intake and energy expenditure, continued over many years (Chapter 30). If overweight members of society can be persuaded to spend just a few hundred kilojoules more than they ingest as food each day, and any compensatory reduction in resting metabolism is countered by a moderate exercise programme, then the obesity and its attendant health risks will progressively disappear (Shephard 1994).

Cassandra: Another problem with your calculations of fiscal benefit is that too often no account is taken of exercise-induced heart attacks (Vuori 1995) and injuries (Kallinen & Markku 1995). Several studies have shown that the risk of a heart attack is increased five or more fold during and following a bout of vigorous exercise. Other reports chronicle a horrendous toll of injuries associated with both team and individual sports.

Asclepius: The issue of exercise-induced heart attacks is answered fairly easily. Although the risks of myocardial infarction and sudden cardiac death are increased in any individual, sedentary or fit during, and immediately following a period of exercise, this apparent hazard is more than compensated in the fit individuals by a substantial reduction of risk during intervening periods of rest (Siscovick et al. 1984). Taking account of both the exercise bout and subsequent rest, the net risk of a cardiac incident in those who exercise vigorously is thus about a third to a half of that seen in sedentary individuals. At any given absolute intensity of physical effort, it is also likely that the risk that this will provoke a heart attack is less in a fit than in a sedentary person. I agree that the dangers of physical injury during high-level competition and extreme forms of sport are well documented. However, the impact of such injury on the economic balance sheet is less easily assessed. Many of the injured are attracted to their sport by the associated risks. If this source of excitement were denied to them, I believe that they would engage in other forms of hazardous behaviour, such as fast driving. Furthermore, I am not advocating that the general population engage in extreme sport. I am encouraging such pursuits as fast walking, which have extremely low injury rates. Studies from the Johnson & Johnson foundation and the Canada Life Assurance Company, among others, have shown equally that those who engage in the moderate activities of an employee fitness programme incur less immediate medical expense than sedentary controls. Moreover, habitually active workers incur fewer orthopaedic problems (Shephard 1992a). Any decrease in the incidence of most chronic diseases would be a relatively long-term benefit (Chapter 28). So, the immediate decrease in medical consultations and hospitalisation, seen in the work-site studies, is presumably due to an enhancement of mood state, a response akin to that yielding dividends of lesser absenteeism and greater productivity (Shephard 1992a).

Cassandra: Well, let us suppose that your primary prevention programme is effective in enhancing health. Is the end-result not going to be that the population will live longer? Already, the pension plans of governments in developed societies are compromised, and health costs are becoming unsustainable because of increased longevity. If the benefits that you claim are realised, health-care programmes and pension plans will quickly become bankrupt (Russell 1986, Warner et al. 1988)!

Asclepius: Perhaps you are becoming Orwellian now, forbidding exercise in order to increase the fiscal stability of health and pension plans? Surely, if costs rise because people are living longer, then the government has a responsibility to adjust health and pension premiums accordingly. But in any event, such actuarial criticism is based on several important misunderstandings. Let us deal first with the issue of health-care costs. Expenditures are indeed rising rapidly, but this reflects largely heroic efforts at treatment during the final years of life (Fries 1980). Such terminal costs are similar whether a person dies at the age of 80 or 90 years of age. Furthermore, the active person is likely to die suddenly rather than from a chronic disease, so that the final expensive year of treatment is often avoided (Linsted et al. 1991). A second major source of expense is institutional care; because an habitually active person retains a larger muscle strength and aerobic power, he or she has much less need of institutional support than someone who has allowed their muscles to waste from disuse (Shephard 1997; Chapters 16 and 28).

Now let me address the question of pension payments. First, I presume that you have assumed a fixed age of retirement. However, let me stress that the fit person suffers less from chronic disease, and thus remains capable of gainful employment, for a period of 5 or even 10 years beyond when a sedentary person has become dependent on society. Second, many investigators have focused on average life expectancy, rather than the dis-

tribution of ages at death (Chapter 16). The average length of life differs little between habitually active and sedentary individuals. What exercise does is to reduce premature mortality (Chapter 28). Deaths are avoided during working life when a person is contributing to, rather than calling upon, societal wealth (Shephard 1992b, 1997). After the age of 80 years, there is some evidence that the habitually active person has a shorter life expectancy than someone who is sedentary (Linsted et al. 1991). Thus, the promotion of habitual physical activity helps to control numbers in that segment of the population that is of the greatest concern to those administering health care and pension plans.

Cassandra: I would still maintain that you lack the hard data needed to sustain the argument that primary prevention is an economically viable strategy.

Asclepius: I agree that we need much more data on random population samples, collected over very long periods. Furthermore, there are many items that should be included in an ultimate balance sheet which are very hard to quantify. For the individual citizen, it is relatively easy to focus upon morbidity and mortality, but what value should we set upon equally important items such as the quality-adjusted lifespan (Shephard 1997)? Life quality can be approximated by techniques such as a 'standard gamble', where a person is asked to imagine trading 10 years of their current quality of life for a shorter period in perfect health. This is a very important consideration for the elderly; a sedentary person may have a similar calendar survival to an active individual, but 10 years spent in a wheelchair or an institution should be heavily discounted, relative to 10 years in normal good health. The industrialist may ask, what is the fiscal benefit of developing the image of a company that cares about the health of its employees? And in society, a full balance sheet must discuss the many costs of not exercising, including such items as our tremendous current expenditures on the construction and maintenance of highways, bridges and ferries, the many adverse effects of air pollution/greenhouse gas emissions, and the carnage incurred on modern highways.

Chair: Thank you both for presenting these opposing viewpoints so fairly. I shall leave readers to decide whether the proponent or the opponent has carried the day, but perhaps I may express my personal prejudices. I support Asclepius in criticising the purely utilitarian assessment of human life; governmental decisions should not be based strictly upon supposed fiscal dividends. Consideration must be given rather to maximising the happiness of the general population. I agree with Cassandra that we need longer studies with better epidemiological designs before we can be clear how to achieve this. But my current impression is that we shall ultimately conclude that primary prevention has a favourable impact not only on the health and happiness of humankind, but also on the economic balance sheet of society.

References

Atkinson JL, Sallis JF, Saelens BE, Cain KL, Black JB 2005 The association of neighborhood design and recreational environments with physical activity. American Journal of Health Promotion 19:304–309

Bouchard C, Shephard RJ, Stephens T 1992 Physical activity, fitness and health. Human Kinetics, Champaign, IL

Calfas CJ, Sallis JF, Nichols JF, Sarkin JA, Johnson MF, Caparosa S, Thompson S, Gehrman CA, Alcaraz JE 2000 Project GRAD: two year outcomes of a randomized controlled physical activity intervention among young adults. Graduate Ready for Activity Daily. American Journal of Preventive Medicine 18:28–37

Fries JF 1980 Aging well. Addison-Wesley, Reading, MA

Jackson JJ 1975 Diffusion of an innovation. An exploratory study of the consequences of Sport Participation Canada's campaign at Saskatoon. Doctoral dissertation, University of Alberta, Edmonton, AL

Kallinen M, Markku A 1995 Aging, physical activity and sports injuries: an overview. Sports Medicine 20:41–52

Klarman HE 1981 Economics of health. In: Clark DW, MacMahon B (eds) Preventive and community medicine, 2nd edn. Little, Brown, Boston, 603–615

Linsted KD, Tonstad K, Kuzma J 1991 Self-reports of physical activity and patterns of mortality in Seventh-day Adventist men. Journal of Clinical Epidemiology 44:355–364

Owen N, Humpel N, Leslie E, Baumann A, Sallis JF 2004 Understanding environmental influences on walking: review and research agenda. American Journal of Preventive Medicine 27:67–76

Russell LB 1986 Is prevention better than cure? Brookings Institute, Washington, DC

Shephard RJ 1982 The risks of passive smoking. Croom Helm, London

Shephard RJ 1986 The economic benefits of enhanced fitness. Human Kinetics, Champaign, IL

Shephard RJ 1991a Considerations in the cost-benefit evaluation of exercise programs. Sports Medicine, Training and Rehabilitation 3:65–77

Shephard RJ 1991b Evolution of occupational health and exercise promotion concept. In: Oja P, Telama R (eds) Sport for all. Elsevier, Amsterdam, 217–223

Shephard RJ 1992a A critical analysis of work-site fitness programs and their postulated economic benefits. Medicine and Science in Sports and Exercise 24:354–370

Shephard RJ 1992b Economic benefits of secondary and tertiary cardiac rehabilitation. Annals of the Academy of Medicine (Singapore) 21:57–62

Shephard RJ 1994 Aerobic fitness and health. Human Kinetics, Champaign, IL

Shephard RJ 1997 Aging, physical activity and health. Human Kinetics, Champaign, IL

Siscovick DS, Weiss NS, Fletcher RH, Lasky T 1984 The incidence of primary cardiac arrest during vigorous exercise. New England Journal of Medicine 311:874–877

US Department of Health and Human Services 2000 Population based smoking cessation. National Institutes of Health, National Cancer Institute, Bethesda, MD

Vuori V 1995 Sudden death and exercise: effects of age and type of activity. Sport Science Review 4(2):46–84

Warner KE, Wickizer TM, Wolfe RA, Schildroth JE, Samuelson MH 1988 Economic implications of workplace health promotion programs. Journal of Occupational Medicine 30:106–112

SECTION 6

Optimising performance through supplementation

Section introduction: Ethical considerations of human performance optimisation

Andy Miah

At the beginning of the 21st century, the ethics of human performance are being pulled in two directions. The first of these embodies the spirit of the amateur athlete – itself an account of the broader social values ascribed to physical culture – which arose in the late 19th century, and flourished in the early 20th century (Hoberman 1992). The other beckons humanity towards a less familiar era, which is rooted in the democratisation of technology and where the human condition is treated as an unfinished biological entity.

These two eras are united by their mutual appreciation of performative excellence; the difficulty is that they differ in how they define and evaluate this term. For the former, technology compromises and overshadows the natural achievements of individuals though, at times, allows for a more representative appraisal of ability. In this case, we might think of a shoe as a technology that eliminates the relative fragility of the ankle joint and foot structure, that has the effect of revealing which people can cover a given distance in the fastest time. However, even in this simple category, distinctions must be made about how different types of shoe optimise performance

for quite different activities. Thus, a climber's crampon also reveals specific kinds of skills that are deemed to be valuable to climbers. Without the technology, it would not be possible to test such specific skills. For the latter category, technology constitutes the natural athlete, and it becomes all the more necessary to utilise such technological advances as people approach their natural limits. On this view, one might consider what should be done to improve upon the relative strength of the ankle, as other physiological capacities are strengthened within an individual.

It is common within debates about the ethics of human performance optimisation to isolate specific social groupings, through which to explore the problems it raises. Indeed, most notable in undertaking such isolationism is within elite sport. Yet, crucial to understanding these debates is the consideration of how the values that are deemed to be at stake with regard to doping extend beyond sport or, more generally, how the values of sport are also constituted by broader social values. While it is convenient to discuss sport as separate from society, and even identify examples that support this claim – for example, the legitimisation of violence – there are broader elements that cannot be so neatly described. These include the legitimate use of biomedical technology. The ethics of scientific research and medical practice is particularly complicated today, as a wider range of enhancement technologies is made available to people outside sport, for use in either work or leisure (US President's Council on Bioethics 2003). In this context, one might ask whether the rules of anti-doping will still be relevant in an era where non-athletes are modifying themselves through numerous forms of technology (Kayser et al. 2005, Savulescu 2004).

Over the last 10 years, human enhancement technologies have begun to compromise the boundaries of health care. Moreover, the use of body modifications to fit lifestyle choices, rather than to resolve specific health needs, has grown considerably as a commercial market. One might include cosmetic dental work, surgical procedures, the ambiguous prescription of mind-altering pharmaceuticals, nanotechnology and even the development of science that promises the extension of life, such as biogerontology, as indications of this shift towards a biocultural model for understanding health (Morris 2000). Indeed, current parlance is to discuss the implications of 'NBIC' technologies, which comprise nanotechnology, biotechnology, information technology and cognitive science (Roco & Bainbridge 2002). One of the principal questions that confronts the ethics and administration of such technologies is not simply whether it is possible to make a conceptual distinction between therapy, non-therapy (which would seem to accommodate the notion of optimisation) and enhancement, but whether the moral distinctions between these terms will continue to matter, for they are already being transgressed.

A useful indication of how the performance cultures of work and exercise collide is the recent emergence of a genetic test for performance capacity (Genetic Technologies 2004). This test has been criticised by a number of scientists but, nevertheless, has been made available despite the absence of certainty over its reliability and meaningfulness. While policy makers will undoubtedly offer formal guidance over the appropriate use of this technology, it is necessary to take into account the fact that regulative frameworks do not determine the social significance of artefacts or the range of social meanings that might be ascribed to them. Indeed, Nelkin & Lindee (1995) offer this argument most eloquently when observing that the cultural significance and meanings attached to the concept of genes extend far beyond that which responsible scientists would advocate.

The blurred boundaries between the two value systems outlined above are made even more apparent by discussions about optimisation through nutrition (Chapters 32 and 34.1). Indeed, the prospect of functional foods, that are engineered to optimise the performative capacities of nutritional substances, begs the question as to whether it will remain possible to make a meaningful distinction between doping technologies and technologies that optimise performance. The chapters in this section, and others throughout this volume (e.g. Chapter 8), imply a number of ethical questions that concern the distinction between optimisation and enhancement. For example, the authors of Chapter 8 undertake the familiar scientific gesture of characterising the application of medical, therapeutic technologies to enhancement practices as a 'threat' to the meaning of sport and health care. Yet, they also recognise the difficulty of characterising therapy in the context of elite sport where, for instance, much of the scientific knowledge aims to enhance the recovery process when injured. In their case study on gene transfer, the authors note that it will be very difficult to isolate a specific intervention as exclusively therapeutic. Once introduced, it might not be therapeutically sound (or possible) to switch off the genetic intervention that enabled the therapeutic effect. To this extent, while the World Anti-Doping Agency (2003) indicates that gene therapy will not be denied to athletes, it is difficult to foresee how this policy will be applied in any meaningful way. Indeed, it is likely that any therapeutic intervention using either genetic or nanotechnology would need to take place at the presymptomatic stage. Thus, even the therapeutic use of such technology involves the need to rethink such concepts as health (Chapters 17.1 and 28), ageing (Chapters 16 and 17.2) and disease (Chapter 30).

So understood, the supposed threat from technologies that enhance performance is multifaceted, but perhaps indistinguishable from the effects of technologies that optimise performance. It encompasses the possibly dehumanising effects of too much technology, the possibility of maintaining social justice, the prospect of harm, but also the value of preserving a competitive environment where individuals can expect minimal medical interference. It also involves concern that the commercial model of medicine does not compromise the care of professionals. A worry that is often advanced in relation to elite sport occurs when the decision of team physicians is compromised by coaches, who are under pressure to make decisions that will optimise the likelihood of competitive success (Murray 1984).

A number of the chapters in this volume also draw attention to the complexity of engineering biology. They also remind us that characterising technology as distinct from biology is difficult. For instance, Chapters 33 and 34.2 describe what is known about the performance effects of hydration and thereby explain how one might consider water as a technological artefact that is no less complex than, say, the science of performance genetics. Indeed, the salient point seems to involve our appreciation of the interrelatedness of biological systems. While a systems-based theory of biological processes might not apply equally to all kinds of modifications (not all forms of performance modification are equally complex), the claim of complexity from which ethical concerns about safety derive, seems central to the ethical resistance to performance enhancement.

These chapters also reinforce the need for ethical analyses to take into account the non-functional elements of performative culture. For instance, Chapter 32 indicates how some athletes use prohibited substances and methods to improve aesthetic appearance, which most likely has no performance benefit. Indeed, recognising the athlete as a body located within a visual culture, rather than merely a performing body, is crucial to understanding the value system underpinning enhancement practices in work and exercise. They also raise a question about which people should be culpable for ethical transgressions in sport. Often, it seems there is little sympathy for athletes who test positive for a prohibited substance. However, Chapter 34.1 indicates that the regulatory structure for nutritional supplements is inadequate, which limits an athlete's capacity to ensure compliance with existing rules. This requires that responsibility for enabling an ethical culture is shared across a number of stakeholders.

Finally, one might suggest that one of the central values of elite performance practices, such as sport, music or dance, is the demonstrable capacity to extend what is previously assumed concerning the limits of humanity. As such, if society expects individuals to break world records or extend creative genius, then technologies that transcend mere optimisation will become a necessity. In the near future, we might not see the engineering of pianists with six fingers on each hand, as depicted in the science fiction film *Gataca* (Nicol 1997) who are able to play divine new compositions. Nevertheless, it is pertinent to scrutinise the moral concern that arises from such a prospect as conceptually similar achievements are already undertaken via body modification.

References

Genetic Technologies Limited 2004 Your Genetic Sports Advantage™. Available online: www.genetictechnologies.com.au

Hoberman JM 1992 Mortal engines: the science of performance and the dehumanization of sport. Free Press, New York (Reprinted 2001, Blackburn Press)

Kayser BA, Mauron A, Miah A 2005 Legalisation of performance-enhancing drugs. Lancet 366 (Supplement on Medicine and Sport):21

Morris DB 2000 How to speak postmodern: medicine, illness, and cultural change. Hastings Center Report 30(6):7–16

Murray TH 1984 Divided loyalties in sports medicine. Physician and Sportsmedicine 13(8):134–140

Nelkin D, Lindee MS 1995 The DNA mystique: the gene as a cultural icon. WH Freeman, New York

Niccol A (Writer and Director) 1997 Gattaca

Roco MC, Bainbridge WS (eds) 2002 Converging technologies for improving human performance: nanotechnology, biotechnology, information technology and cognitive science. National Science Foundation, Arlington, VA

Savulescu J, Foddy B, Clayton M 2004 Why we should allow performance enhancing drugs in sport. British Journal of Sports Medicine 38:666–670

US President's Council on Bioethics 2003 Beyond therapy: biotechnology and the pursuit of happiness. US Government, Washington, DC. Available online: http://bioethics.gov/reports/beyondtherapy/index.html

World Anti-Doping Agency 2003 International standard for the prohibited list 2004. Available online: www.wada-ama.org/docs/web/standards_harmonization/code/list_standard_2004.pdf

Chapter 32

Optimising and enhancing human performance through nutrition

Louise M. Burke   Bente Kiens   Kevin D. Tipton

1 INTRODUCTION

Good nutrition plays an important role in allowing athletes to achieve training and competition goals. A well-chosen eating plan is needed to maximise the success of the training programme and prepare the athlete for competition. Strategies for fluid and fuel intake before, during and after exercise can reduce fatigue and promote optimal performance. These strategies are particularly important in the competition arena. Despite the degree of expertise that underpins the majority of guidelines for sports nutrition, many athletes do not appear to follow good nutrition practices. The aim of this chapter is to provide an overview of the different ways in which nutrition can contribute to sporting success.

2 EATING TO OPTIMISE TRAINING

The major role of the everyday diet is to supply the athlete with fuel and nutrients needed to optimise the adaptations achieved during training, and to recover quickly between workouts. The athlete must also eat appropriately to stay in good health and to achieve and maintain an optimal physique.

2.1 Energy needs for training and the ideal physique

The body continuously expends energy to maintain physiological functions, for the biosynthesis of macromolecules such as proteins, glycogen and triacylglycerols, and for muscular work. However, most of this energy is lost as heat (~80%; Chapter 19), due to the inefficiency of the metabolic pathways. This relationship means that energy expenditure can be assessed from the direct measurement of heat production (calorimetry). Since there is a close relation between energy metabolism and oxygen uptake, steady-state oxygen uptake can also be used to estimate energy expenditure (indirect calorimetry).

Total daily energy expenditure is composed of three components: the basal (or resting) metabolic rate, the thermic effect of food and physical activity (Figure 32.1).

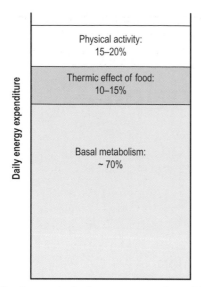

Figure 32.1 The three principal components of total daily energy expenditure in an inactive individual. PA, physical activity; TEF, postprandial thermogenic effect of food; BMR, basal metabolic rate.

A certain amount of energy is required to support life, and the rate at which a resting organism oxidises its own stored fuels is called the basal metabolic rate which is measured under standardised conditions (awake, supine rest (at least 30 min), comfortably warm environment, after 10–12 h fast). A distinction exists between the basal and resting metabolic rates. However, these may be considered similar if measurements are performed in the postabsorptive state.

Basal metabolic rate appears to vary with age when normalised to body mass, height or surface area, since muscle mass declines beyond ~50 years. However, when normalised to the summed mass of the most metabolically active tissues (heart, kidney, brain, liver), which retain mass, basal metabolic rate is stable with ageing (Chapter 16). Fat cells are metabolically active but contain a substantial amount of inert fat, making adipose one of the least active tissues. Thus, the larger fat mass of an average woman results in a lower basal metabolic rate, when normalised to body mass but not when normalised to the fat-free mass.

Basal metabolic rate is also dependent on body size, physiological status (growth, pregnancy) and hormonal status. Most women show cyclic variations in basal metabolic rate (±5%), which is lowest in the late follicular phase of the menstrual cycle, increasing at ovulation and peaking in the late luteal phase.

Besides the basal metabolic requirements, energy is also required for processing food (eating, digestion, absorption, transportation, storing) – the thermic effect of food or dietary-induced thermogenesis (Figure 32.1). The remaining energy expenditure is accounted for by daily physical activity, over and above the resting state.

Due to the often huge training volume (intensity and frequency) of many athletes, energy expenditure can be several fold higher compared to a sedentary person, resulting in a large increase in energy needs. Since athletes also vary in size (female gymnast versus heavy male rower), and body size influences energy expenditure, then body mass influences the energy requirement.

Growth is another important factor to consider. An individual is in a state of energy balance if energy intake equals energy expenditure. For growth to occur, intake must exceed output (energy turnover). This does not only apply to young athletes, since an increased body mass may also be of importance to athletes in sports where a high power output is desired. However, whenever energy intake and expenditure are not equal, a change in body mass will occur; a negative energy balance results in the use of stored energy (protein, glycogen, fat), while a positive energy balance results in energy storage (primarily as fat). If performance is to be maintained during periods of intense training, high energy expenditures must be matched by equivalent energy intakes.

Experimental data indicate that most athletes are in energy balance. Despite this, numerous cross-sectional observation studies have repeatedly reported a negative energy balance, primarily in female, but also in male athletes. In male athletes, this is often related to weight classification sports. Furthermore, most but not all studies have reported that amenorrhoeic athletes consume even less energy than eumenorrhoeic athletes (Chapter 11), when matched for training level, size and body mass (Loucks 2004). Of interest, however, is that despite apparent negative energy balance, body mass often remains stable. Although these studies collectively imply that female athletes, in particular amenorrhoeic athletes, are chronically exposed to a state of low-energy availability, many studies have been questioned due to the under-reporting of energy intake, undereating during the registration period and methodological difficulties in measuring energy intake and expenditure.

However, low energy intake in female athletes is reported from various laboratories, especially in aesthetic sports and in those where low body mass is desired. This may suggest that, in some situations, energy balance is not maintained on a daily basis, and that many athletes might be energy deficient during their heavy exercise training programmes. Repeatedly low energy intake may indicate an adaptation to a lower energy balance in these individuals.

There is considerable evidence that a low energy availability can have serious consequences for the hormonal, immunological and health status of athletes. This is exemplified in females who develop the female athlete triad: low energy availability, impaired menstrual function and reduced bone mineral density (Loucks 2004). Many female athletes develop metabolic, reproductive and bone disruptions because they excessively restrict energy intake. Among these is an increased plasma cortisol concentration, a catabolic hormone that accelerates protein degradation during states of energy deprivation and especially carbohydrate deprivation. Furthermore, plasma growth hormone concentrations will increase, while plasma insulin, insulin growth factor type I, triiodothyronine, leptin and glucose concentrations decrease with energy deficiency (Loucks et al. 1998).

In a non-human primate model, Williams et al. (2001) demonstrated that the induction of amenorrhoea was a product of the volume of calories consumed during training, which decreased the energy availability for reproductive and other necessary metabolic functions. Furthermore, prospective studies in a primate model, examining the short-term effect of low energy availability on circulating reproductive hormone levels, provide evidence that the energy cost of exercise can result in a suppression of reproductive hormone secretion, when exercise-induced increase in energy expenditure is not offset by supplemental caloric intake.

When young lean men were exposed to an average energy deficiency of $4\,MJ \cdot d^{-1}$ for 8 weeks in multi-stress environments (heat, cold, sleep deprivation; Friedl et al. 2000), they reduced fat mass by 51% and fat free mass by 6%. Reductions in metabolic substrates and hormones were similar to those reported by Loucks et al. (1998) for women. But interestingly, Friedl et al. (2000) demonstrated that, after 1 week of refeeding, the plasma concentrations of growth hormone, insulin growth factor type I and triiodothyronine were restored, despite the continuation of exercise and other stresses (Friedl et al. 2000). In accordance with this, Williams et al. (2001) found that induced amenorrhoea in primates was reversed by supplementing energy intake, but without modifying training volume. Thus, these data indicate that it is the decreased energy availability, resulting from a failure to increase energy intake to match expenditure (and carbohydrate utilisation), and not exercise per se that leads to a disruption of metabolic and reproductive functions.

When energy availability was restricted for exercising women and men to $<126\,kJ \cdot kg^{-1}$ fat-free mass per day (over 5 days), the pulsatile secretion of luteinising hormone was depressed in both genders, especially with low carbohydrate availability (Loucks et al. 1998). In exercising women, glucoregulatory hormones do not maintain normal plasma glucose concentrations below an energy availability of $126\,kJ \cdot kg^{-1}$ fat-free mass per day (Loucks & Nattiv 2005). It is noteworthy that energy balance normally occurs in young adults at an energy availability of about $190\,kJ \cdot kg^{-1}$ fat-free mass per day. Some athletes, especially amenorrhoeic athletes, have caloric intakes of only $67\,kJ \cdot kg^{-1}$ fat-free mass per day, even when training (Loucks & Nattiv 2005).

In summary, while the measurement of low dietary energy intake in athletes, especially in female athletes, has been questioned, evidence is accumulating that some

athletes restrict, whilst others in endurance sports fail to modify, caloric intake to compensate for increased energy expenditure. Such caloric deficits increase the risk of hormonal dysfunctions, impaired menstrual status, poor bone health, immune function and growth. For those athletes who are on fat loss programmes, it is recommended that caloric intake should not fall below $126\,kJ \cdot kg^{-1}$ fat-free mass per day.

2.2 Strategies to reduce mass and body fat

An adequate energy intake is critical for optimal physical performance. However, some athletes want to reduce body mass to improve their aesthetic appearance, while others want to lose body fat (increase fat-free mass) to optimise performance. In addition, athletes involved in weight category sports must achieve fixed mass targets prior to competition. The similarity between these athletes is that they often try to reduce body mass well below that considered normal for their stature. For example, athletes engaged in weight category sports often compete in a class 5–10% below their usual body mass, but competition is often followed with periods of unrestricted food intake and mass gains. This often leads to unhealthy nutritional practices including deliberate vomiting, overexercising, voluntary dehydration and the use of diet pills and diuretics. These practices may result in severe health consequences, such as delayed maturation, impaired growth, menstrual irregularities, increased rate of infections, eating disorders and depression. However, is there an optimal strategy for reducing body mass without experiencing adverse health implications or reducing performance?

To lose weight a negative energy balance must be elicited, and to maintain lost body weight, a lower energy balance must be maintained. Negative energy balance can be achieved by restricting energy intake, increasing energy expenditure by additional training or through simultaneously modifying both sides of the equation.

When body mass is reduced through energy restriction alone, a large percentage of this loss can be accounted for by reductions in lean body mass and total body water. To what extent lean mass is lost depends on the extent of the energy restriction and the duration of that restriction. For instance, caloric restriction with rowers reduced body mass by 2–8 kg over 2–4 months but muscle mass loss accounted for 32–87% of the mass change (Koutedakis et al. 1994, Slater et al. 2006a).

There is some evidence that resting metabolic rate is largely related to the lean body mass, since, in adults <50 years, muscle mass accounts for about 40% of the body mass. Thus, whilst the resting metabolic rate of muscle ($54\,kJ \cdot kg^{-1} \cdot d^{-1}$) is only a small fraction of that of the heart ($1842\,kJ \cdot kg^{-1} \cdot d^{-1}$), its mass-specific energy consumption is more than twofold greater. Reduced thyroid function most certainly contributes to this metabolic reduction. Repeated episodes of mass loss and gain (weight cycling) have also been associated with reduced resting metabolic rate, altered patterns of body fat distribution and increased rates of mass gain. These changes will make subsequent mass loss more difficult, since a greater energy restriction is required to achieve a negative energy balance. Most knowledge on this aspect, as it relates to athletes, has been obtained from studies of wrestlers. The data indicate that, during the season, when body mass was lowest, resting metabolic rate was significantly reduced (Melby et al. 1990).

The effect of rapid mass loss on performance appears to depend on how the loss is achieved, its magnitude and the type of exercise performed. Absolute maximal oxygen uptake may decrease after mass losses. Some would suggest this may affect endurance performance (Fogelholm 1994). However, this needs to be viewed cautiously, particularly in weight-bearing activities, where a mass reduction equates with a reduced energy expenditure to move at a constant velocity. That is, a reduction in the size or number of cells is only detrimental if it impinges upon one's ability to perform, which, at elite levels, is often unrelated to slight changes in aerobic power (Chapter 10.2).

Burge et al. (1993) observed that a 5.2% decrease in body mass over 24 h resulted in a 22 s increase in a simulated 2000 m ergometer performance in competitive rowers. However, this cannot be due to the loss of metabolically active cells, but to dehydration and perhaps some muscle glycogen depletion. Such performance decrements are entirely predictable (Viitasalo et al. 1987). The effect of such acute mass losses is reduced or eliminated when repeated over several days (Slater et al. 2006b). In a study of three heavyweight rowers, who were prepared to compete as lightweight rowers (16 weeks), body mass decreased 2.0–8.0 kg, with muscle mass accounting for a large proportion of this change (32–85%). Two athletes maintained performance. However, performance was compromised in the athlete who experienced the greatest mass loss (Slater et al. 2006a).

Can dietary strategies modify physiological adaptation to energy restrictions and prevent a decrease in performance? Horswill et al. (1990) found that performance was unimpaired after a mass loss of 6% over 4 days, if a relatively high carbohydrate (energy) consumption was achieved. In addition, low carbohydrate intake was suggested to explain impaired performance obtained in judo athletes after energy restriction in combination with intense training that caused mass losses (Degoutte et al. 2006).

A high carbohydrate diet during energy restriction seems mandatory for maintaining physical performance, probably because it may prevent glycogen depletion that might otherwise compromise performance (Chapter 7). Moreover, for athletes who are on fat loss programmes, energy availability should not be below 126 kJ·kg^{-1} fat-free mass per day (Loucks & Thuma 2003). Thus, to avoid performance and training decrements and also health complications, mass losses should not exceed ~0.5–1.0 kg·wk^{-1} or an energy deficit of 2–4 MJ. Hence, acute mass losses should be avoided and weight loss should slowly be achieved over several weeks, and be planned well in advance.

Evidence from wrestlers has shown that while resting metabolic rate was significantly reduced during the season, their off-season body masses returned to normal, as did resting metabolic rate (Melby et al. 1990). Thus, participating in numerous cycles of mass loss and gain did not permanently lower resting metabolic rate in these athletes. On the other hand, a recent study from a cohort of 1838 male athletes engaged in international competitions from 1929 to 1965, including 370 males engaged in boxing, weight lifting and wrestling, indicated that repeated cycles of mass loss and gain appeared to enhance subsequent mass gains and may predispose to obesity later in life (Saarni et al. 2006).

Thus, when mass or fat reductions are required, these should be achieved by a programme of eating and exercise that allows the athlete to perform well, stay healthy and remain free of unreasonable stress, in both the short and long term. Many athletes need assistance to plan dietary programmes that meet goals for adequate energy intake, and sufficient protein and micronutrients consumption. Although it is difficult to get reliable figures on the prevalence of eating disorders among athletes, there appears to be a higher risk of problems among female athletes and athletes in sports that require specific mass targets or lower body fat levels than in the general population (Beals & Manore 1994, Sundgot-Borgen 2000).

2.3 Requirements for growth and gaining lean body mass

Lean body mass represents several tissues but for athletes, the focus is muscle mass. The metabolic foundation for changes in muscle mass is the difference between muscle protein synthesis and breakdown (net muscle protein balance, nitrogen balance or protein turnover), which occur continually and concurrently.

Accretion of muscle proteins results when protein turnover, particularly the balance of myofibrillar proteins, is positive (net muscle protein synthesis). Exercise and nutrition have an immense influence on protein turnover which, on a daily basis, can be either positive or negative, depending on feeding and exercise situations. The length and duration of these periods of positive and negative balance determine the net loss or gain of muscle mass. Consequently, in healthy, mass-stable adults, periods of positive and negative turnover will be equal and no growth occurs. Muscle growth only results when a cumulative positive protein turnover prevails.

A clear relationship between energy intake and muscle growth should not be surprising. Nevertheless, athletes most often focus on protein intake when muscle growth is desired. However, it is not clear that increasing protein intake above habitual levels should be the primary objective. First and foremost, the athlete must at least maintain energy balance, and most likely a positive energy turnover.

After all, protein accretion is an energetically expensive process; the deposition of 1 g of protein consumes ~100 kJ of energy.

It has been estimated that ~30% of the variation in protein turnover may be attributed to differences in energy balance (Pellet & Young 1992). As much as 100 years ago, Chittenden (1907) demonstrated that athletes gain strength and maintain muscle mass even during periods of low protein intake, provided energy intake is sufficient. In a series of classical studies, Butterfield & Calloway (1984) and Todd et al. (1984) established that maintenance of a balanced protein turnover during training is not possible if energy balance is negative, regardless of protein intake. More recently, studies have shown that additional energy intake results in greater gains in lean body mass than additional protein intake during resistance training (Gater et al. 1992, Rozenek et al. 2002). Clearly, energy intake is critical for protein accretion and muscle growth.

3 PROTEIN NEEDS FOR MUSCLE GAIN, TRAINING ENHANCEMENT AND REPAIR

Most athletes feel that high protein intake is critical for muscle growth, repair and enhancement of training adaptations, and a huge supplement industry has been built upon this assumption (Chapter 34.1). The scientific evidence for high protein intakes in athletes is, at best, equivocal and is extensively debated in the scientific community (Phillips 2004, Rennie & Tipton 2000, Tarnopolsky 2004, Tipton & Wolfe 2004).

Generally, there is much disagreement as to the protein needs for athletes and exercising relative to sedentary individuals. Well-controlled studies have demonstrated that nitrogen balance is generally greater for athletes than in sedentary controls (Lemon et al. 1992, Tarnopolsky et al. 1988, 1992). Increased protein needs are likely to stem from increased amino acid oxidation during exercise (McKenzie et al. 2000, Phillips et al. 1993), and the growth and repair of muscle. During recovery from both endurance (Carraro et al. 1990, Tipton et al. 1996) and resistance training (Biolo et al. 1995, Phillips et al. 1997), muscle protein synthesis is elevated. Thus, increased protein intake may provide amino acids for the elevated synthesis for repairing damaged protein, muscle growth and mitochondrial biogenesis.

On the other hand, many authors maintain that protein needs for active individuals, even those involved in heavy training, are not increased (Rennie & Tipton 2000, Tipton & Wolfe 2004). This argument is supported by the fact that the efficiency of amino acid utilisation is increased by exercise (Todd et al. 1984), perhaps due to increased efficiency of reutilisation of amino acids from muscle protein breakdown (Phillips et al. 1999). Whole-body protein balance decreases following training, indicating that protein requirements would actually be less with regular training (Hartman et al. 2006).

The disagreement possibly originates from two sources: methodological limitations (nitrogen balance and leucine oxidation) and, perhaps more fundamentally, a lack of consideration for the primary reason why athletes need protein. Rather than the attainment of nitrogen balance, the amount of protein that optimises training and maximises performance is the important consideration. Each athlete will have a unique protein intake that optimises adaptations to training and performance. Thus, a single numerical value indicating the protein requirement for all athletes, or even relatively arbitrary divisions for endurance and strength athletes, seems illogical.

For many, if not most, athletes, the point may be inconsequential. Most athletes ingest enough protein to cover even the higher estimates of ~1.2–1.5 $g \cdot kg^{-1} \cdot d^{-1}$ (Phillips 2004, Tarnopolsky 2004). Thus, recommending increased protein intake would not be necessary for the majority of athletes consuming a well-chosen diet that meets energy needs. In fact, for some athletes, extra protein may be detrimental. For example, if carbohydrate intake is reduced to make room for protein, given a limited energy intake, performance may be impaired (Macdermid & Stannard 2006).

On the other hand, there are undoubtedly athletes for whom increased protein intake may be beneficial. If increased muscle mass and strength is the primary goal, there seems little reason to limit protein intake, provided the requirements for other nutrients are satisfied. However, given the high energy intakes necessary to support increased muscle mass, habitual protein consumption is likely to assure maximum muscle accretion. Certainly, no evidence exists to suggest the anabolic response to protein from food sources is inferior to that from commercially available supplements (Elliot et al. 2006, Phillips et al. 2005).

Athletes desiring mass reduction, and who are in negative energy balance, may benefit from higher protein consumption (Layman & Walker 2006). Use of a risk/benefit approach may offer some insights. If risk is minimal and there is a rationale for potential benefit, then there is no reason to recommend against increasing protein intake. Health problems have often been touted as reasons for avoiding protein intake, particularly kidney damage. While the relationship between high protein intake and chronic diseases has not been established, it should be noted that individuals with pre-existing problems, particularly kidney disease, should not consume high-protein diets (Zello 2006).

A further complication to assigning specific amounts of daily dietary protein to all athletes, or even groups of athletes, is that amino acids utilisation and the metabolic response to ingested protein are variable among individuals, depending on the circumstances in which the protein was ingested (Tipton & Wolfe 2004). For instance, Phillips and colleagues (2005) reported that amino acid uptake from proteins into muscle is greater for milk than soy proteins, following resistance training. However, unlike whole-body amino acid uptake at rest (Dangin et al. 2001), the use of individual milk proteins by muscle following exercise cannot be distinguished (Tipton et al. 2004).

Similarly, the anabolic response to protein ingestion will vary with other concurrently ingested nutrients. Following exercise, ingestion of carbohydrates increases amino acid use by muscle (Borsheim et al. 2004, Miller et al. 2003), an effect likely to be mediated by the insulin response (Biolo et al. 1999). Interestingly, recent evidence implies that amino acids from protein ingestion may be used to a greater extent when fat is simultaneously ingested (Elliot et al. 2006). However, the mechanism for increased amino acid use with fat ingestion is unclear, and these observations require more systematic investigation before firm conclusions may be drawn. Nonetheless, taken together, it is clear that ingesting a given amount of protein results in differential muscle use (Figure 32.2), and thus training adaptations may depend less on the amount of protein ingested and more on the type of proteins ingested, and other nutrients ingested in the same meal.

The anabolic response of muscle is determined not only by nutrients but also by timing the ingestion of protein in relation to the exercise bout (Roy et al. 1997, 2000, Tipton et al. 2001). It seems there is an interaction between the type of amino acid source, nutrients ingested concurrently and timing in relation to exercise (Tipton et al. 2001, 2007), and the complexities of assessing the relationship of the anabolic response should be readily apparent. Indeed, muscle mass may be maintained, and even increased, on a wide range of protein intakes. The anabolic response is not determined solely by protein ingested, but varies depending on

other nutritional factors associated with consuming the protein. Undoubtedly, future work will uncover more regarding these interactions.

4 FUEL NEEDS FOR TRAINING AND RECOVERY

An important goal of the athlete's diet is the provision of adequate fuel to the muscles to support the training programme. The major fuels for exercise are body fat and carbohydrate stores. Sources of fat, including plasma free fatty acids derived from adipose tissue and intramuscular triglycerides, are relatively plentiful. In contrast, carbohydrate supplies, such as plasma glucose (derived from the liver or carbohydrate intake) and muscle glycogen stores, are limited. In fact, the availability of carbohydrate as a substrate for muscle and the central nervous system becomes a limiting factor in endurance exercise of submaximal or intermittent high-intensity exercise (>90 min; Chapter 7), and plays a permissive role in the performance of brief, high-intensity work (Coyle 1995). As a result, sports nutrition guidelines have focused on strategies to enhance carbohydrate availability. The present section will focus on refuelling from day to day and the challenge of recovering between daily training sessions or multiple workouts, where fuel requirements are likely to challenge or exceed normal body carbohydrate stores.

Muscle glycogen synthesis follows a biphasic response, consisting of a rapid early phase for the first 30–60 min (non-insulin dependent) followed by a slower phase (insulin dependent), lasting up to several days (Ivy & Kuo 1998). Maximal rates of muscle glycogen storage reported during the first 12 h of recovery are within the range of 5–10 mmol·kg wet weight^{-1}·h^{-1} (Jentjens & Jeukendrup 2003) and 20–24 h of recovery are required to normalise muscle glycogen levels (100–120 mmol·kg wet weight^{-1}) after depletion through prolonged or intense exercise (Coyle 1991). However, since the training and competition schedules of many athletes often provide considerably less time than this, many athletes commence a training session with some degree of muscle glycogen depletion.

Data from a recent study show that training with low glycogen concentrations might be advantageous for training adaptation (Hansen et al. 2005). In this study, untrained subjects achieved greater increases in muscle enzyme content and endurance in the leg that trained with a protocol promoting glycogen depletion than the contralateral leg that undertook the same volume of training in a glycogen-recovered state. However, other chronic studies of diet and training interventions in well-trained athletes show that higher carbohydrate intakes that allow greater glycogen recovery are associated with fewer symptoms of overtraining during high-volume periods (Achten et al. 2004; Chapter 29) and greater training adaptations (Simonsen et al. 1991). It is likely that elite athletes optimise training outcomes by periodising training and diet, so that some sessions are undertaken with relative glycogen depletion, while high-

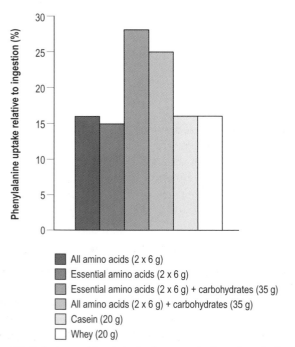

Figure 32.2 Amino acid uptake by leg muscle from ingested amino acids or proteins following exercise.

Legend:
- All amino acids (2 × 6 g)
- Essential amino acids (2 × 6 g)
- Essential amino acids (2 × 6 g) + carbohydrates (35 g)
- All amino acids (2 × 6 g) + carbohydrates (35 g)
- Casein (20 g)
- Whey (20 g)

Y-axis: Phenylalanine uptake relative to ingestion (%)

quality performance sessions occur following complete refuelling.

The major dietary factor involved in postexercise refuelling is the amount of carbohydrate consumed. As long as total energy intake as adequate (Tarnopolsky et al. 2001), increased carbohydrate intake promotes increased muscle glycogen storage, until the threshold for glycogen synthesis is reached. A recent update of the guidelines for sports nutrition of the International Olympic Committee recommended two changes in the recommended carbohydrate intake of athletes (Burke et al. 2004). The first change recognised that guidelines should be scaled according to the training load undertaken by athletes, while the second recommended that guidelines be expressed as grams of carbohydrate relative to the size of the athlete, rather than an arbitrary percentage of the athlete's total energy intake. A summary of some of these revised guidelines is presented in Table 32.1.

Athletes have been advised to enhance recovery by consuming carbohydrates as soon as possible after training. The highest rates of muscle glycogen storage occur during the first hour after exercise, and the intake of carbohydrate immediately after exercise potentiates this effect (Ivy et al. 1988). However, the most important consideration is that an absence of carbohydrate intake leads to very low rates of glycogen restoration. Therefore, an early carbohydrate intake following strenuous exercise is most valuable because it provides an immediate source of substrate to the muscle cell and maximises effective recovery. Although early feeding may be important when there is only 4–8 h between sessions (Ivy et al. 1988), it may have less impact over a longer recovery period (Parkin et al. 1997). Overall it appears that, when the interval between exercise sessions is short,

the athlete should begin to consume carbohydrate as soon as possible to maximise the effective recovery time. In addition, there may be some advantages in the first couple of hours of recovery to achieving a target of $1 \, g \cdot kg^{-1}$ body mass each hour, spread into a series of small snacks (Burke et al. 2004). However, when longer recovery periods are available, the athlete can choose their preferred meal schedule as long as total carbohydrate intake goals are achieved.

The type of carbohydrate consumed may have some effect on glycogen restoration rate. For instance, moderate and high glycaemic index, carbohydrate-rich foods and drinks appear to promote greater glycogen storage than meals based on low glycaemic index carbohydrates (Burke et al. 1993). However, the mechanisms may include factors such as the malabsorption of low glycaemic index carbohydrate, rather than differences in the glycaemic and insulinaemic responses (Burke et al. 1996).

Early research indicated that glycogen synthesis was enhanced by adding protein to carbohydrate snacks consumed after exercise, an observation that was explained by the protein-stimulated enhancement of the insulin response (Zawadzki et al. 1992). However, this has been refuted by other studies (Burke et al. 2004), and the current consensus is that the co-ingestion of protein or amino acids with carbohydrate does not clearly enhance glycogen synthesis (Burke et al. 2004). Benefits to glycogen storage are limited to the first hour of recovery (Ivy et al. 2002) or to situations where protein is added to carbohydrate intakes below the threshold for maximal glycogen synthesis. Of course, the intake of protein within carbohydrate-rich recovery meals may allow the athlete to meet other nutritional goals including the enhancement of net protein balance after exercise.

Table 32.1 Revised guidelines for the carbohydrate intake of athletes (adapted from Burke et al. 2004)

- Aim to achieve carbohydrate intakes that meet fuel requirements of training while optimising muscle glycogen between workouts. Recommendations should be fine-tuned with consideration of total energy needs, specific training needs and performance feedback:
  - Immediate recovery (0–4 h): 1–$1.2 \, g \cdot kg^{-1} \cdot h^{-1}$ consumed at frequent intervals
  - Daily recovery: moderate-duration, low-intensity training: 5–$7 \, g \cdot kg^{-1} \cdot h^{-1}$
  - Daily recovery: moderate-heavy endurance training: 7–$12 \, g \cdot kg^{-1} \cdot h^{-1}$
  - Daily recovery: extreme programme (4–6 h+ per day): 10–$12 \, g \cdot kg^{-1} \cdot h^{-1}$
- Adequate energy intake is important for optimal glycogen recovery.
- Guidelines for carbohydrate (or other macronutrients) should not be provided in terms of percentage contributions to total dietary energy intake.

---

5 EATING TO MINIMISE ILLNESS AND INJURY

Athletes must be able to train hard and compete without the interruptions of illness and injury. Eating well to achieve nutrient needs is also important for general health and wellbeing. However, there are several health challenges that are specific to sport and exercise. These include the risk of iron depletion, immunosuppression that is known to accompany prolonged and strenuous training, and the disturbances of the athlete's endocrine function, with potential implications for illness and bone integrity.

5.1 Calcium, bones and the female athlete triad

Since exercise provides a major stimulus for bone formation and bone health, it seems ironic that many female athletes are reported to suffer from compromised bone health, from frank osteopenia to a failure to achieve an optimal peak bone density. Poor bone health can reduce an athlete's potential by increasing the risk of injury, including stress fractures. Long-term problems include an increased risk of osteoporosis (Chapter 13). Initially, an awareness of poor bone health was identified as the female athlete triad syndrome (Otis et al. 1997), and is a disorder cluster involving disordered eating, amenorrhoea and osteopenia. The focus was directed to the prevalence of menstrual disturbances in females, with the recognition that disruptions to reproductive hormone have a negative effect on bone formation and remodelling. Much debate centred on the cause of the menstrual dysfunction, with theories including low body fat and high training volumes. We now know that the common thread to impairment of menstrual status and other hormonal systems is low energy availability (Loucks 2004).

This syndrome has now been updated (American College of Sports Medicine 2007) to target energy availability, menstrual health and bone density. The new message is that each of these issues involves a continuum between optimal health and frank disorder, and the athlete must be alert to changes in her status of any issue. Athletes must be educated about the benefits of early diagnosis and treatment of problems and the likelihood that negative outcomes occur at a much earlier stage than previously considered. Recent research has shown that low energy availability directly impairs bone formation and resorption (Ihle & Loucks 2004), and problems may also be seen in male athletes.

The detection, prevention and management of this triad, or individual elements within it, require expertise and, ideally, the teamwork of sports physicians, dieticians, psychologists, physiologists and coaches (Beals & Manore 2002). Dietary intervention is important to correct factors that underpin menstrual dysfunction, as well as those that contribute to suboptimal bone density. Prevention or early intervention is clearly the preferred option, since it is not always certain that damage to bone strength can be overturned, particularly when it is long term (Drinkwater et al. 1996). Dietary goals include adequate energy and calcium intakes. In the latter case, daily calcium requirements may be increased to 1200–1500 mg·d^{-1} in athletes with impaired menstrual function. Where adequate calcium intake cannot be met through dietary means (e.g. low-fat dairy foods or calcium-enriched soy alternatives), a calcium supplement may be considered (Kerr et al. 2006).

5.2 Iron depletion

An inadequate iron status is the most likely micronutrient deficiency among athletes and the general community. Exercise affects many measures of iron status, due to changes in the plasma volume or the acute-phase response to stress. Therefore, conventional haematological standards are often inappropriate for diagnosing the true prevalence of problematic iron deficiency in athletics.

Inadequate iron status can reduce performance via suboptimal haemoglobin concentrations and oxygen delivery (Chapters 1 and 10.1), and perhaps also via reduced myoglobin and iron-related enzymes (Hood et al. 1992). However, it is often difficult to detect the stage of iron defi-

ciency at which impairments to exercise performance are observed. Despite initial conflict in the literature, it now appears that iron depletion, in the absence of anaemia (reduced serum ferritin concentrations), may impair exercise performance (Deakin 2006). In addition, athletes with reduced iron stores complain of feeling fatigued and failing to recover between training sessions (Chapter 29). Since low ferritin concentrations may become progressively lower and eventually lead to iron deficiency anaemia, it makes sense to monitor athletes who are at high risk of iron depletion, and to intervene as soon as iron status appears to decline substantially or to symptomatic levels.

The evaluation and management of iron status in athletes should be undertaken by a sports physician. It is tempting for fatigued athletes to self-diagnose iron deficiency and to self-medicate with iron supplements. However, there are dangers in self-prescription or long-term supplementation in the absence of medical follow-up. Iron supplementation is not a replacement for medical and dietary assessment and therapy, since it typically fails to correct underlying problems that have caused iron drain (i.e. factors causing iron requirements and losses to exceed iron intake). Chronic supplementation with high doses of iron carries a risk of iron overload, especially in males for whom the genetic traits for haemochromatosis are more prevalent.

A diagnosis of iron deficiency requires multiple sources of information which assess the presence of risk factors for low iron status and determine whether this has lead to a functional outcome. These include clinical signs and symptoms suggestive of iron deficiency or anaemia (e.g. unexplained fatigue, reduced recovery, recurrent infections, pallor), a dietary assessment which indicates an inadequate intake of bioavailable iron and the presence of other factors that may predict an increase in iron requirements or loss. Haematological evidence of iron deficiency is the presence of pale (hypochromic) and small (microcytic) red blood cells on a blood film, and a plasma haemoglobin concentration below the laboratory reference range (12 g·100 mL^{-1} (females); 14 g·100 mL^{-1} (males)). These parameters will remain normal with iron deficiency without anaemia. Although iron deficiency in the general population is normally denoted by reduced serum ferritin concentrations below the reference range (12 ng·mL^{-1}), in athlete populations thresholds of 20 ng·mL^{-1} (Nielsen & Nachtigall 1998) or 30 ng·mL^{-1} (Fallon 2004) are often applied. Plasma measurements of soluble transferrin receptors have been described as a new marker of iron status, but this needs to be confirmed in athletic populations (Pitsis et al. 2004).

Changes to iron status parameters that occur with acute or chronic training include haemodilution, due to increased plasma volume that accompanies endurance training (Chapter 27.3), and heat adaptation (Chapter 21). These changes do not impair exercise capacity. Alternatively, an increase in serum ferritin (an acute-phase reactant) can be expected in response to a single strenuous bout of exercise, inflammation or infection, without any true change in iron status. Therefore, haematological and biochemical tests undertaken in athletes should be administered in a way that standardises these effects. For example, all tests should be completed in the same laboratory, after a light training day and before any exercise is undertaken for that day (Deakin 2006). Serial monitoring of athletes may help establish normal ranges over which such parameters vary for each athlete over the training and competition year, thereby helping to identify changes that may impair health, function or performance.

Although iron supplementation may play a role in the prevention and treatment of iron deficiency, the management plan should be based on long-term interventions to reverse iron drain, reducing excessive iron losses and increasing dietary iron. Dietary interventions should increase total iron intake and increase the bioavailability of this iron. The haem form of iron found in meat, fish and poultry is better absorbed than the organic (non-haem) iron found in plant foods such as fortified and wholegrain cereals, legumes and green leafy vegetables (Hallberg 1981, Monsen 1988). However, iron bioavailability can be manipulated by matching iron-rich foods with dietary factors promoting iron absorption (e.g. vitamin C and other food acids, 'meat factor' found in animal flesh) and reducing the interaction with inhibitory factors for iron absorption (e.g. phytates in fibre-rich cereals, tannins in tea; Hallberg 1981, Monsen 1988). Finally, changes to iron intake should be achieved with eating patterns that are compatible with the athlete's other nutritional goals.

5.3 Nutrition for the immune system

Nutrition is an important component of proper immune function (Gleeson 2006, Gleeson et al. 2004; Chapter 29). High-intensity exercise is associated with an increased incidence of infection (Nieman et al 1990) and immunosuppression (Gleeson 2006, Gleeson et al. 2004). The prevailing notion is that exercise of sufficient intensity and duration results in high plasma concentrations of stress hormones (cortisol, catecholamines), and immunosuppression ensues. Immune system depression for several hours following strenuous exercise increases the opportunity for infection (the open window hypothesis). However, despite ample evidence of the acute and chronic impact on immune function, there is little direct evidence of a link with increased illnesses (Gleeson 2006).

Nutritional deficiencies can have a profound impact on immune function, with immune dysfunction linked with severe energy restriction, which is quickly corrected with refeeding (Walrand et al. 2001). Severe energy restriction is not common among athletic populations, but subclinical eating disorders in athletes are associated with increased infection rates (Beals & Manore 1994). It is clear that insufficient protein intake (Daly et al. 1990) and deficiencies of micronutrients may lead to immunosuppression (Gleeson 2006). However, athletes who consume sufficient energy to support training demands should not be in danger of deficiencies leading to immune impairment.

Since the exercise-induced depression of the immune system is linked to increased stress hormones, nutritional manipulations that ameliorate this rise should effectively limit immune dysfunction. Carbohydrate intake may be used to minimise the immune impairments associated with prolonged exercise (Nieman 1998) and glutamine, vitamin C and zinc have also been implicated in the immune response. However, evidence for the efficacy of these supplements is equivocal, and excesses of several nutrients result in depression of immune responses (Gleeson 2006). Thus, it is clear that modulation of the immune system results from heavy exercise but there is much to be investigated about these interactions and nutrition.

5.4 Vitamins, minerals and the antioxidant system

Vitamins, minerals and the antioxidant system, as regulators of metabolism, are integral parts of nutritional considerations for all involved in regular exercise. Deficiencies of these nutrients clearly impair performance, but scientific evidence does not necessarily support vitamin and mineral supplementation to improve performance.

The main issues concerning vitamins and minerals for athletes seem to be whether regular, rigorous exercise increases their requirements and whether supplementation increases performance. Since vitamins and minerals are integral for many metabolic processes, there is ample rationale to expect exercise to impact upon nutrient requirements. Certainly, deficiencies will impair performance (Lukaski 2004, Manore 2000). However, most athletes consume ample vitamins and minerals to support training and performance, but observations are often complicated by the uncertainty of assessing vitamin and mineral status (Lukaski 2004). An obvious point of concern is for athletes with restricted energy intakes (e.g. making weight or those in body image sports) in whom low vitamin and mineral intakes would not be surprising.

Several vitamins and minerals, including vitamins C, E, A (as β-carotene), selenium, zinc, iron, copper and manganese, as well as other dietary components (e.g. flavonoids), play a role as part of antioxidant defences. Muscles produce free radicals and other reactive oxygen species during exercise (Davies et al. 1982, Jackson et al 1998), and the type of activity is likely to determine the pattern and magnitude of free radical production (Patwell & Jackson 2004). These radicals may contribute to oxidative damage and perhaps fatigue (Powers et al. 2004, Urso & Clarkson 2003). However, cells are protected by a complex antioxidant defence mechanism, to which dietary components contribute, thereby providing the rationale for antioxidant supplementation for athletes during heavy training loads (Powers et al. 2004, Urso & Clarkson 2003).

However, it is not clear at this time that supplemental antioxidants are beneficial for performance, but supplementation may play a role in scavenging free radicals and possibly preserving cell structure and function (Powers et al. 2004). Nevertheless, it is not certain that performance is impacted, and the interpretation that athletes need antioxidants to protect against oxidative damage is based primarily on studies that measure cellular and extracellular damage (Alessio 1993, Mastaloudis et al. 2001), leaving the question open. Ingestion of antioxidants may reduce markers of damage, but due primarily to a lack of well-designed studies, there is no consensus on the efficacy of antioxidants for exercise performance. On the contrary, there is clear evidence that reactive oxygen species regulate gene expression through stimulation of signalling pathways (Jackson et al. 2002). Thus, it is conceivable that antioxidant supplementation may interfere with the adaptive process to training.

6 EATING FOR COMPETITION PERFORMANCE

To achieve optimal performance, the athlete should identify nutritional factors that are likely to cause fatigue during their event, and undertake strategies before, during and after the event that minimise or delay the onset of this fatigue. Potential factors include dehydration (Chapters 19, 33 and 34.2), depletion of glycogen stores (Chapter 7), low blood glucose concentrations and other disturbances of the central nervous system (Chapter 5), gastrointestinal distress and hyponatraemia (Chapters 33 and 34.2). These nutritional challenges present according to the length and intensity of the event, the environment and factors that influence opportunities to eat and drink during the event or recovery. Of course, practical considerations are important, including the availability of suitable foods or drinks, gastrointestinal challenges to eating or drinking while exercising, and finding access to food supplies when competition takes place away from home.

6.1 Making weight to meet competition weight targets

In weight class sports, it is common practice for athletes to train at a higher body mass, before rapidly reducing mass to qualify at a lower class division against smaller, weaker opponents. There are many different practices used to achieve this reduction, but most involve severe restriction of food intake and dehydration (Steen & Brownell 2000). However, the use of diuretics and other pharmacological agents, as well as dehydration, should be avoided.

Rapid mass losses reduce lean body mass as well as fat mass, and may decrease performance (Horswill 1993) and result in health problems and even death (CDCP, 1998). A more reasonable approach may be to select the weight class that optimises each athlete's performance. In other sports where weight loss is prevalent, an optimal mass/fat level

must be determined and appropriate dietary strategies should be used to achieve and maintain these goals. These strategies should maximise the opportunity to meet all nutrition goals, but without undue food-related stress.

6.2 Fuelling for competition

A key part of the preparation for competition is to ensure that muscle fuel stores are adequate for the demands of the event. Resting muscle glycogen concentrations of trained athletes (100–120 mmol·kg wet weight^{-1}) appear adequate for events lasting up to 60–90 min (Hawley et al. 1997). Such stores can be achieved by 24 h of rest and an adequate carbohydrate intake (7–10 g·kg^{-1}·d^{-1}; Costill et al. 1981), unless there is severe muscle damage. For some athletes, glycogen restoration can be achieved with everyday eating plans. However, athletes following restricted diets may need to increase carbohydrate (and energy) intake over the day before competition, and make fuelling up a higher priority than body mass concerns.

Carbohydrate loading describes practices that aim to maximise muscle glycogen stores prior to longer events and loading protocols evolved in the 1960s. These typically involved a 6-day strategy, starting with glycogen depletion (3 days on low carbohydrate diet and training) followed by glycogen supercompensation (3 days with tapered training and high carbohydrate intake; Bergstrom & Hultman 1966). This strategy was shown to boost muscle glycogen stores to ~150–250 mmol·kg wet weight^{-1}.

In the 1980s, it was found that well-trained athletes did not need to include the depletion or glycogen-stripping phase (Sherman et al. 1981). More recent studies show that maximal glycogen storage can be achieved by well-trained athletes in as little as 36–48 h following the last exercise session, proving the athlete rests and consumes an adequate carbohydrate intake (Bussau et al. 2002).

Theoretically, carbohydrate loading could enhance the performance in sports that would otherwise be limited by glycogen depletion (e.g. >90 min; Hawley et al. 1997). Increased pre-event glycogen stores prolong the duration for which moderate-intensity exercise can be undertaken before fatiguing, and may enhance the performance of steady state by ~20% and time-trial performance or the completion of a set amount of work by 2–3%, by preventing the decline in work output (pace) that would otherwise occur (Hawley et al. 1997).

Such preparation of fuel stores may enhance performance in prolonged distance events, but may also be useful for athletes in prolonged intermittent sports, who may otherwise incur fatigue from depleted glycogen reserves. The benefits of carbohydrate loading may be specific not only to the sport but also to the athlete, depending on the requirements of their position or style of play. Of course, the logistics of competition in many sports, where games may be played every day or every second day, might prevent pre-event optimisation of glycogen stores. Indeed, a recent study showed that it is not possible to supercompensate muscle glycogen stores several times within a short time period, although performance can be restored between several bouts of prolonged exercise by high carbohydrate eating (McInerney et al. 2005). An example of an eating plan for carbohydrate loading is provided in Table 32.2.

6.3 Fat adaptation and glycogen restoration strategies

Different dietary strategies have been used to improve endurance performance and especially focusing on optimising muscle glycogen stores. In the classical studies of Christensen & Hansen (1939) and Bergstrom and co-workers (1967), it was shown that a 3–5 day diet consisting primarily of carbohydrates was superior to a fat-rich diet for improving endurance time during exhaustive exercise.

On the other hand, endurance-trained athletes have a high capacity for fat oxidation, and it has been hypothesised that if fat availability to muscle cells was enhanced through the diet, it would increase fat oxidation during exercise, thereby sparing muscle glycogen. Several studies have tested this hypothesis, using both pharmacological and dietary interventions to acutely increase plasma fat availability (Hawley 2002, Kiens & Helge 2000). In most of these studies, plasma fatty acid concentration was only increased slightly relative to baseline, but in studies where the fatty acid concentration was successfully elevated, no clear enhancement of exercise performance was observed. In addition, it is evident from studies including brief high-fat diets lasting less than 7 days that endurance performance was impaired (Bergstrom et al. 1967, Galbo et al. 1979). Longer-term adaptations to a high-fat diet in combination with exercise training might, on the other hand, induce metabolic and morphological skeletal muscle adaptations, which could influence performance and the capacity for fat oxidation during exercise. Training-induced skeletal muscle adaptations include increased capillarisation and enhanced activity of the oxidative enzymes (Henriksson 1977, Kiens et al. 1993), and these all play a significant role in elevating the fat oxidative capacity of muscle. Accordingly, there has been interest in the impact of the combined adaptations to a high-fat diet and endurance training on performance.

In those studies where the dietary period lasted between 1 and 4 weeks, the aerobic fitness level of subjects used

Table 32.2 A carbohydrate loading menu providing carbohydrate intakes of ~10 g·kg^{-1}·d^{-1} for a 65 kg male runner; scale this intake up or down according to body mass

Day	Diet plan (~650 g·d^{-1} carbohydrate)
Day 1 Focuses on carbohydrate-rich foods; other foods can be added to balance the meal. An exercise taper should accompany this menu to optimise glycogen storage. Glycogen supercompensation can be achieved in 2 days with this diet in well-trained runners who can arrange a suitable taper	Breakfast: 2 cups flake cereal + cup milk + banana 250 mL sweetened fruit juice Snack: 500 mL bottle soft drink 2 slices thick toast + jam Lunch: 2 large bread rolls with fillings 200 g carton flavoured yoghurt Snack: Coffee scroll or muffin 250 mL sweetened fruit juice Dinner: 3 cups cooked pasta + ¾ cup sauce and 2 cups jelly Snack: 2 crumpets and honey 250 mL sweetened fruit juice
Day 2	Breakfast: 2 cups flake cereal + cup milk + cup sweetened canned fruit 250 mL sweetened fruit juice Snack: 500 mL fruit smoothie Lunch: 3 stack pancake + syrup + 2 scoops ice-cream 500 mL soft drink Snack: 100 g dried fruit 250 mL sweetened fruit juice Dinner: 3 cups rice dish (fried rice, risotto) Snack: 2 cups fruit salad + 2 scoops ice-cream
Day 3 Many like to increase the focus on low-fibre/low-residue eating on day before competition, thus reaching the line feeling light, rather than with gastrointestinal fullness	Breakfast: 2 cups cereal (low fibre) + cup milk + banana 250 mL sweetened fruit juice Lunch: 4 white crumpets + jam Dinner: 2 cups white pasta + small amount of sauce Over day: 1 L liquid meal drink or 1 L sports drink + 3 sports gels 200 g jelly confectionery

varied from untrained subjects to endurance-trained athletes. Furthermore, the fat content of diets varied from 35 to 80 energy-% and the methods to measure performance varied across studies (Helge et al. 1998, Lambert et al. 1994, Muoio et al. 1994, Phinney et al. 1983). Nevertheless, the effect of these dietary strategies on performance was negligible (Helge et al. 1998, Lambert et al. 1994, Phinney et al. 1983), and improved endurance was only obtained in endurance athletes after 7 days on a semi-high fat diet (Muoio et al. 1994), relative to a carbohydrate-rich diet. In untrained subjects following supervised training through a 4-week intervention while on a high-fat diet, time to exhaustion was increased to a similar extent as when subjects consumed a high-carbohydrate diet (Helge et al. 1998). However, when a fat-rich diet was consumed beyond 4 weeks, impaired performance was evident compared to a carbohydrate-rich diet (Figure 32.3; Helge et al. 1996).

These studies clearly demonstrate that a habitual fat-rich diet used for a short period (up to 4 weeks), and consumed in association with regular endurance training, is not superior to a carbohydrate-rich diet for improving performance. However, when high-fat, low-carbohydrate eating continues beyond 4 weeks, an impairment of training adaptation is evident, relative to the consumption of high-carbohydrate, low-fat diets (Helge et al. 1996).

Other combinations of dietary strategies have been suggested. Such strategies include a short-term high-fat, low-carbohydrate diet, followed by a high-carbohydrate diet to restore muscle glycogen. Such a combination of dietary strategies would seem the perfect preparation for the athlete, simultaneously restoring carbohydrate stores while maximising the capacity for fat oxidation during exercise. Consistent and robust findings are available that a higher total

fat oxidation during prolonged exercise is achieved in as little as 5 days training, when using a high-fat diet (65–69 energy-%; Burke et al. 2000, 2002, Carey et al. 2001, Goedecke et al. 1999). A reduction in muscle glycogen stores was also achieved after 5 days on the high-fat diet, and consuming a high-carbohydrate diet for 1 day of rest restored muscle glycogen content but only to its initial levels (Burke et al. 2002, Carey et al. 2001).

To test performance following such dietary strategies, most experiments include a prolonged exercise trial (2–4 h), followed by a time trial. Despite higher fat oxidation during the prolonged exercise trial after the high fat-diet, relative to the high-carbohydrate diet, time-trial performance was not significantly different, and was even slower in some investigations (Havemann et al. 2006). Moreover, after 6 days on a high-fat diet followed by 1 day carbohydrate loading, 1 km sprint power output was significantly lower compared with a high-carbohydrate (only) diet (Havemann et al. 2006).

Interestingly, when carbohydrate loading was extended to 1 week, after high-fat adaptation for 7 weeks, muscle glycogen content was not only restored but was supercompensated, and significantly larger than resulting from a high-carbohydrate (only) diet (Helge et al. 2002). Following the high-fat, low-carbohydrate diet for 7 weeks, an impaired response to training was observed, despite supercompensation of the muscle glycogen stores. In addition, endurance performance only increased slightly and was still impaired compared to the high-carbohydrate, low-fat diet which was consumed during the entire 8 weeks of exercise training (Figure 32.3; Helge et al. 1996).

Thus, what was initially viewed as glycogen sparing after adaptation to a high-fat diet may be a downregulation of carbohydrate metabolism. Accordingly, after long-term fat adaptation followed by 1 week carbohydrate loading, skeletal muscle glucose uptake was impaired, despite a high plasma glucose concentration (Helge et al. 2002). Moreover, despite supercompensation of muscle glycogen, exhaustion occurred when only 37% of the muscle glycogen had been used (Helge et al. 2002). It has also been shown that fat adaptation/carbohydrate restoration strategies were associated with a reduced pyruvate dehydrogenase activity during 20 min of steady-state cycling (Stellingwerff et al. 2006).

Therefore, there is now evidence that such dietary strategies may result in a downregulation of carbohydrate metabolism or glycogen impairment during exercise. Moreover, adaptations to high-fat diets also increase heart rate (Havemann et al. 2006, Helge et al. 1996) and sympathetic activation, as measured by plasma epinephrine concentration (Helge et al. 1996, Sasaki et al. 1991) during submaximal exercise, and these trends persisted despite restoring muscle glycogen to supercompensated levels (Helge et al. 1996). Accordingly, it seems that fat adaptation and fat-loading strategies cannot be considered as valuable methods (Burke & Kiens 2006).

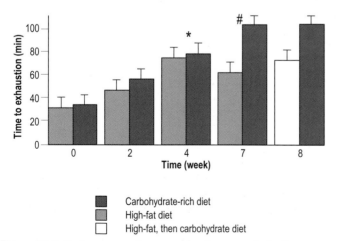

Figure 32.3 Endurance performance (cycle ergometer) after 2–7 weeks on a high-fat diet (65 energy-%) and a carbohydrate-rich diet. After 7 weeks on the high-fat diet, these subjects switched to a high-carbohydrate diet*, significantly different from week 0, significantly different between carbohydrate diet (week 4) and fat plus carbohydrate diet (week 7). Adapted from Kiens & Helge (2000) with permission.

6.4 Pre-event eating (1–4 h)

It is well known that exercise metabolism and performance are influenced by the composition and amount of energy in the diet. The pre-event meal provides the athlete with a final opportunity to address fluid and carbohydrate needs for competition, whilst avoiding gastrointestinal problems during competition (balancing feelings of hunger against gastrointestinal discomfort, vomiting or diarrhoea). Therefore, much emphasis has been on the timing, the dietary composition, the types of carbohydrates and the total energy of the pre-exercise meal, either before training or competition.

The ingestion of a carbohydrate-rich meal can result in a rapid and large increase in plasma glucose and insulin concentrations. The plasma insulin elevation facilitates glucose uptake and decreases lipolysis, possibly resulting in increased glucose and glycogen use during exercise. These metabolic perturbations can persist for up to 6 h after carbohydrate ingestion (Montain et al. 1991).

With regard to timing of the pre-exercise meal, when comparing the effect between a meal ingested 3–4 h before exercise and an overnight fast on endurance performance, no differences in a 10 km time trial were found when participants had breakfast containing 250 g of carbohydrates, 4 h before, when compared with no meal (Whitley et al. 1998). On the other hand, endurance was significantly greater after breakfast (100 g of carbohydrates and milk) ingested 3 h before steady-state exercise (70% maximal oxygen uptake) to exhaustion, when compared with an overnight fast (Schabort et al. 1999). Similarly, Casey et al. (2000) found that a meal 3–4 h before exercise improved performance, relative to exercise in the fasting state. This is mainly due to an optimisation of liver glycogen stores, as these are substantially reduced after an overnight fast. Based on this, a carbohydrate meal 3–4 h before exercise is better than exercising in the overnight fasting state.

The amount of carbohydrates ingested 3–4 h before exercise seems also to play a role. For instance, while endurance can be improved (Sherman et al. 1989), eating large amounts of carbohydrate 3–4 h before exercise may cause gastrointestinal discomfort in some individuals. Thus, drinking carbohydrate solutions 3–4 h before exercise has been suggested.

Furthermore, not all carbohydrates elicit similar metabolic effects. Thus, when foods with a low-glycaemic index are ingested 3 h before prolonged exercise, increases in plasma glucose and insulin concentrations during the postprandial period and during exercise are smaller. The reduction in fatty acid mobilisation is less and carbohydrate oxidation during exercise is lower, as compared to ingestion of food items of a high glycaemic index (Wee et al. 1999). However, neither high- nor low-glycaemic carbohydrate ingestion (3 h before exercise) appeared to be either detrimental or advantageous to performance (Wee et al. 1999).

Carbohydrates ingested in the hour before exercise will induce a rapid fall in blood glucose concentration during the first period of exercise due to the enhanced plasma glucose and insulin concentrations at onset of exercise, and in some cases hypoglycaemia will last for a considerable time. The degree of metabolic perturbation seems also in this situation to be related to the glycaemic index of the carbohydrates. When a pre-exercise meal consisting of carbohydrates with a low-to-moderate glycaemic index was ingested 30–60 min before exercise, a lower plasma glucose and insulin response was observed before exercise start and hypoglycaemia did not occur compared to when carbohydrates of high glycaemic index were ingested (DeMarco et al. 1999, Kirwan et al. 2001, Thomas et al. 1991) During the following exercise session, the plasma glucose concentration was increased when the low-to-moderate glycaemic index meal was consumed, compared to when the high-glycaemic index carbohydrate meal was consumed (DeMarco et al 1999, Thomas et al. 1991).

Exercise performance (time to exhaustion) is markedly increased after consuming low and moderate glycaemic index pre-exercise meals, compared to high glycaemic index meals (DeMarco et al. 1999, Kirwan et al. 2001, Thomas et al. 1991). However, other studies show no performance change, despite metabolic alterations before and during exercise (Febbraio et al. 2000, Wee et al. 1999). This disparity could be explained by differences in study design, exercise intensities and the training status of subjects, but it may also be due to the extent of the metabolic perturbation caused by the ingested carbohydrates which, in turn, may be related to meal timing, the amount of carbohydrates ingested and the glycaemic index of those carbohydrates. However, data also indicate improved performance after ingesting a low-to-moderate glycaemic index pre-exercise meal, if the meal can maintain euglycaemia during exercise (Burke 2006).

An aspect to consider regarding the composition and timing of the pre-exercise meal is the rapid fall in plasma glucose during exercise, especially after ingesting high glycaemic index carbohydrates <1 h before exercise. This phenomenon is more likely to occur when the exercise intensity is low. Achten & Jeukendrup (2003) showed that when exercising (55%, 77%, 90% maximal oxygen uptake) after the ingestion of a 75 g carbohydrate solution, glucose concentration decreased within the first 5 min, and to a similar extent at all intensities. On average, no evidence of hypoglycaemia was evident. However, on an individual basis, several of the subjects developed hypoglycaemia at each of the three intensities. When the 75 g carbohydrate solution was ingested 15, 45 or 75 min before 20 min of submaximal exercise (65% maximal), followed by a time trial, subjects became hypoglycaemic during the first 10 min of exercise in all situations, but this did not affect performance in the subsequent exercise bout. Thus, some athletes are more prone to developing hypoglycaemia when exercise is performed <1 h after high glycaemic carbohydrate ingestion, and some individuals are also more sensitive to low plasma glucose concentrations, which is important to consider when planning a pre-exercise meal for <1 h before competition.

The athlete should also be conscious of fluid needs and consume enough fluid to ensure that adequate hydration is achieved before competition. This includes restoring losses from previous training or competition, and from intentional dehydration strategies to fine tune body mass (Chapter 33).

6.5 Fuelling during events

When food and fluid consumption can occur during competition, it is important to consider the interaction of strategies undertaken before and during exercise, particularly in relation to fuel metabolism and performance. Carbohydrate consumed during exercise changes the metabolic impact of carbohydrates eaten prior to exercise (Burke et al. 1998). There is also some evidence that the benefits of combining these two strategies to enhance carbohydrate availability for endurance exercise are additive (Chryssanthopoulos & Williams 1997, Wright et al. 1991). However, another study found that ingesting carbohydrates before exercise is only beneficial to time-trial performance late during exercise, when there is further intake of carbohydrate during the session (Febbraio et al. 2000). This deserves further study.

6.6 Postevent recovery

Following a competitive event, the nutrition needs are similar to, if perhaps sometimes more exaggerated than, those following heavy training sessions. The more rapidly an athlete must return to competition or training, the more important it will be to rehydrate, refuel and repair from the first session. Thus, athletes who compete in tournaments, stage races or events involving heats and finals should be directed to follow the prescribed recovery eating strategies described above. Some consideration of the practical issues involved in achieving these nutritional goals may be needed, since many athletes are required to travel interstate or internationally for their most important competitions (Table 32.3).

Table 32.3 Challenges and solution for the travelling athlete

Challenges of travelling	Strategies to cope with the challenges of travelling

• Disruptions to normal training routine and lifestyle
• Changes in climate and environment that modify nutritional needs
• Jet lag
• Changes in the availability of familiar foods
• Reliance on hotel, restaurant and takeaway foods instead of home cooking
• Exposure to new foods and eating cultures
• Temptations of an 'all you can eat' dining hall in an athletes' village
• Risk of gastrointestinal illnesses due to exposure to food and water with poor hygiene standards
• Excitement and distraction of a new environment
	1. **Planning ahead**
	  ○ Investigate food issues on travel routes (e.g. airlines) and at the destination before leaving home. Caterers and food organisers should be contacted well ahead of the trip to let them know meal timing and menu needs.
	2. **Taking supplies to supplement the local fare**
	  ○ A supply of portable and non-perishable foods should be taken to the destination to replace important items that may be missing.
	3. **Eating and drinking well en route**
	  ○ Many will turn to boredom eating when confined. They should eat according to real needs, taking into account the forced rest while travelling
	  ○ When moving to a new time zone, the athlete should adopt eating patterns that suit their destination as soon as the trip starts. This will help the body clock to adapt.
	  ○ Unseen fluid losses in air-conditioned vehicles and pressurised plane cabins should be recognised, and a drinking plan should be organised to keep athletes well hydrated.
	4. **Taking care with food/water hygiene**
	  ○ If the local water supply is unsafe to drink, then drink from sealed bottles, or hot drinks made from well-boiled water. Ice added to drinks is often made from tap water and may be a problem.
	  ○ In high-risk environments, eat only at good hotels or restaurants. Food from local stalls and markets should be avoided.
	  ○ Food that has been well cooked is the safest; it is best to avoid salads or unpeeled fruit that has been in contact with local water or soil.
	5. **Adhering to the food plan**
	  ○ Choose the best of the local cuisine to meet nutritional needs, supplementing with your own supplies where needed.
	  ○ Be assertive in asking for what is needed at catering outlets (e.g. low-fat cooking styles or an extra carbohydrate choice).
	  ○ The challenge of 'all you can eat' dining should be recognised. Resist the temptation to eat 'what is there' or 'what everyone else is eating'. Follow your own meal plan.

7 CONCLUSION

Various nutrition strategies assist the athlete to train hard in preparation for an event, providing the energy, fuel and nutrient requirements set by their workouts and allowing the athlete to recover between sessions. In some cases, dietary manipulations can assist the athlete to achieve the physique that promotes good performance. For competition, athletes should consider the factors that limit performance or cause fatigue in their event. In many cases, nutritional strategies can be undertaken to reduce or delay the onset of fatigue. Dietary strategies for optimal performance will vary among sports and in some cases, even among athletes in the same sport. Therefore, the athlete should seek professional advice from a sports dietician to determine the strategies that may be of benefit, then experiment to find a nutritional plan that allows optimal training and competition.

References

Achten J, Jeukendrup AE 2003 Effect of pre-exercise ingestion of carbohydrates on glycemic and insulinaemic responses during subsequent exercise at different intensities. European Journal of Applied Physiology 88:466–471

Achten J, Halson SL, Moseley L, Rayson MP, Casey A, Jeukendrup AE 2004 Higher dietary carbohydrate content during intensified running training results in better maintenance of performance and mood state. Journal of Applied Physiology 96:1331–1340

Alessio HM 1993 Exercise-induced oxidative stress. Medicine and Science in Sports and Exercise 25:218–224

Beals KA, Manore MM 1994 The prevalence and consequences of subclinical eating disorders in female athletes. International Journal of Sport Nutrition 4:175–195

Bergstrom J, Hultman E 1966 Muscle glycogen synthesis after exercise: an enhancing factor localized to the muscle cells in man. Nature 210:309–310

Bergstrom J, Hermansen L, Hultman E, Saltin B 1967 Diet, muscle glycogen and physical performance. Acta Physiologica Scandinavica 71:140–150

Biolo G, Maggi SP, Williams BD, Tipton KD, Wolfe RR 1995 Increased rates of muscle protein turnover and amino acid transport after resistance exercise in humans. American Journal of Physiology 268: E514–E520

Biolo G, Williams BD, Fleming RY, Wolfe RR 1999 Insulin action on muscle protein kinetics and amino acid transport during recovery after resistance exercise. Diabetes 48:949–957

Børsheim E, Cree MG, Tipton KD, Elliott TA, Aarsland A, Wolfe RR 2004 Effect of carbohydrate intake on net muscle protein synthesis during recovery from resistance exercise. Journal of Applied Physiology 96:674–678

Burke L 2006 Preparation for competition. In: Burke L, Deakin V (eds) Clinical sports nutrition, 3rd edn. McGraw-Hill, Sydney, 355–384

Burke L 2007 Practical sports nutrition. Human Kinetics, Champaign, IL

Burke LM, Hawley JA 2002 Effects of short-term fat adaptation on metabolism and performance of prolonged exercise. Medicine and Science in Sports and Exercise 34:1492–1498

Burke LM, Kiens B 2006 'Fat adaptation' for athletic performance – the nail in the coffin? Journal of Applied Physiology 100:7–8

Burke LM, Collier GR, Hargreaves M 1993 Muscle glycogen storage after prolonged exercise: the effect of the glycemic index of carbohydrate feedings. Journal of Applied Physiology 75:1019–1023

Burke LM, Collier GR, Davis PG, Fricker PA, Sanigorski AJ, Hargreaves M 1996 Muscle glycogen storage after prolonged exercise: effect of the frequency of carbohydrate feedings. American Journal of Clinical Nutrition 64:115–119

Burke LM, Claassen A, Hawley JA, Noakes TD 1998 Carbohydrate intake during prolonged cycling minimizes effect of glycemic index of preexercise meal. Journal of Applied Physiology 85:2220–2226

Burke LM, Angus DJ, Cox GR, Cummings NK, Febbraio MA, Gawthorn K, Hawley JA, Minehan M, Martin DT, Hargreaves M 2000 Effect of fat adaptation and carbohydrate restoration in metabolism and performance during prolonged cycling. Journal of Applied Physiology 89:2413–2421

Burke LM, Kiens B, Ivy JL 2004 Carbohydrates and fat for training and recovery. Journal of Sports Sciences 22:15–30

Bussau VA, Fairchild TJ, Rao A, Steele P, Fournier PA 2002 Carbohydrate loading in human muscle: an improved 1 day protocol. European Journal of Applied Physiology and Occupational Physiology 87:290–295

Butterfield GE, Calloway DH 1984 Physical activity improves protein utilization in young men. British Journal of Nutrition 51:171–84

Carey AL, Staudacher HM, Cummings NK, Stepto NK, Nikolopoulos V, Burke LM, Hawley JA 2001 Effect of fat adaptation and carbohydrate restoration on prolonged endurance exercise. Journal of Applied Physiology 91:115–122

Carraro F, Stuart CA, Hartl WH, Rosenblatt J, Wolfe RR 1990 Effect of exercise and recovery on muscle protein synthesis in human subjects. American Journal of Physiology 259:E470–E476

Casey A, Mann R, Banister K, Fox J, Morris PG, Macdonald IA, Greenhaff PL 2000 Effect of carbohydrate ingestion on glycogen resynthesis in human liver and skeletal muscle, measured by 13C. MRS. American Journal of Physiology 278:E65–E75

Chittenden RH 1907 The nutrition of man. Heinemann, London

Christensen EH, Hansen O 1939 Arbejdsfähigkeit und ernärung. Skandinavisches Archiv für Physiologie 81:160–171

Chryssanthopoulos C, Williams C 1997 Pre-exercise carbohydrate meal and endurance running capacity when carbohydrates are ingested during exercise. International Journal of Sports Medicine 18:543–548

Costill DL, Sherman WM, Fink WJ, Maresh C, Witten M, Miller JM 1981 The role of dietary carbohydrates in muscle glycogen resynthesis after strenuous running. American Journal of Clinical Nutrition 34:1831–1836

Coyle EF 1991 Timing and method of increased carbohydrate intake to cope with heavy training, competition and recovery. Journal of Sports Sciences 9:29–52

Coyle EF 1995 Substrate utilization during exercise in active people. American Journal of Clinical Nutrition 61(suppl):968S–979S

Daly JM, Reynolds J, Sigal RK, Shou J, Liberman MD 1990 Effect of dietary protein and amino acids on immune function. Critical Care Medicine 18:S86–S93

Dangin M, Boirie Y, Garcia-Rodenas C, Gachon P, Fauquant J, Callier P, Ballèvre O, Beaufrère B 2001The digestion rate of protein is an independent regulating factor of postprandial protein retention. American Journal of Physiology. Endocrinology and Metabolism 280:E340–E348

Davies KJ, Quintanilha AT, Brooks GA, Packer L 1982 Free radicals and tissue damage produced by exercise. Biochemistry and Biophysics Research Communications 107:1198–1205

Deakin V 2006 Iron depletion in athletes. In: Burke L, Deakin V (eds) Clinical sports nutrition, 3rd edn. McGraw-Hill, Sydney, 263–312

Degoutte F, Jouanel P, Bègue RJ, Colombier M, Lac G, Pequignot JM, Filaire E 2006 Food restriction, performance, biochemical, physiological and endocrine changes in judo athletes. International Journal of Sports Medicine 27(1):9–18

DeMarco HM, Sucher KP, Cisar CJ, Butterfield GE 1999 Pre-exercise carbohydrate meals: application of glycemic index. Medicine and Science in Sports and Exercise 31:164–170

Drinkwater BL, Nilson K, Ott S, Chesnut CH 3rd 1986 Bone mineral density after resumption of menses in amenorrheic athletes. Journal of the American Medical Association 256:380–382

Elliot TA, Cree MG, Sanford AP, Wolfe RR, Tipton KD 2006 Milk ingestion stimulates net muscle protein synthesis following resistance exercise. Medicine and Science in Sports and Exercise 38:667–674

Fallon KE 2004 Utility of hematological and iron-related screening in elite athletes. Clinical Journal of Sports Medicine 14:145–152

Febbraio MA, Chiu A, Angus DJ, Arkinstall MJ, Hawley JA 2000 Effects of carbohydrate ingestion before and during exercise on glucose kinetics and performance. Journal of Applied Physiology 89:2220–2226

Fogelholm M 1994 Effect of bodyweight reduction on sports performance. Sports Medicine 18:249–267

Friedl KE, Moore RJ, Hoyt RW, Marchitelli LJ, Martinez-Lopez LE, Askew EW 2000 Endocrine markers in semistarvation in healthy lean men in a mutistressor enviroment. Journal of Applied Physiology 88:1820–1830

Galbo H, Holst JJ Christensen NJ 1979 The effect of different diets and of insulin on the hormonal response to prolonged exercise. Acta Physiologica Scandinavica 107:19–32

Gater DR, Gater DA, Uribe JM, Bunt JC 1992 Impact of nutritional supplements and resistance training on body composition, strength and insulin-like growth factor-1. Journal of Applied Sport Science Research 6:66–76

Gleeson M 2006 Can nutrition limit exercise-induced immunodepression? Nutrition Reviews 64:119–131

Gleeson M, Nieman DC, Pedersen BK 2004 Exercise, nutrition and immune function. Journal of Sports Science 22:115–125

Goedecke JH, Christie C, Wilson G, Dennis SC, Noakes TD, Hopkins WG, Lambert EV 1999 Metabolic adaptations to a high-fat diet in endurance cyclists. Metabolism 48:1509–1517

Hallberg L 1981 Bioavailability of dietary iron in man. Annual Review of Nutrition 1:123–147

Hansen AK, Fischer CP, Plomgaard P, Andersen JL, Saltin B, Pedersen BK 2005 Skeletal muscle adaptation: training twice every second day vs. training once daily. Journal of Applied Physiology 98:93–99

Hartman JW, Moore DR, Phillips SM 2006 Resistance training reduces whole body protein turnover and improves net protein retention in untrained young males. Applied Physiology. Nutrition and Metabolism 31:1–8

Havemann L, West SJ, Goedecke JH, Macdonald IA, St Clair Gibson A, Noakes TD, Lambert EV 2006 Fat adaptation followed by carbohydrate-loading compromises high-intensity sprint performance. Journal of Applied Physiology 100:194–202

Hawley J 2002 Effect of increased fat availability on metabolism and exercise capacity. Medicine and Science in Sports and Exercise 34:1485–1491

Hawley JA, Schabort EJ, Noakes TD, Dennis SC 1997 Carbohydrate-loading and exercise performance: an update. Sports Medicine 24:73–81

Helge J, Richter EA, Kiens B 1996 Interaction of training and diet on metabolism and endurance in man. Journal of Physiology 292:293–306

Helge J, Wulff B, Kiens B 1998 Impact of a fat-rich diet on endurance performance in man: role of the dietary period. Medicine and Science in Sports and Exercise 30:456–461

Helge JW, Watt PW, Richter EA, Kiens B 2002 Partial restoration of dietary fat induced metabolic adaptation to training by 7 days of carbohydrate diet. Journal of Applied Physiology 93:1797–1805

Henriksson J 1977 Training induced adaptation of skeletal muscle and metabolism during submaximal exercise. Journal of Physiology 270:661–675

Hood DA, Kelton R, Nishio ML 1992 Mitochondrial adaptations to chronic muscle use: effect of iron deficiency. Comparative Biochemistry and Physiology 101A:597–605

Horswill CA, Hickner RC, Scott JR, Costill DL, Gould D 1990 Weight loss, dietary carbohydrate modifications and high intensity physical performance. Medicine and Science in Sports and Exercise 22:470–476

Ihle R, Loucks AB 2004 Dose-response relationships between energy availability and bone turnover in young exercising women. Journal of Bone and Mineral Research 19:1231–1240

Ivy JL, Kuo CH 1998 Regulation of GLUT4 protein and glycogen synthase during muscle glycogen synthesis after exercise. Acta Physiologica Scandinavica 162:295–304

Ivy JL, Katz AL, Cutler CL, Sherman WM, Coyle EF 1988 Muscle glycogen synthesis after exercise: effect of time of carbohydrate ingestion. Journal of Applied Physiology 64:1480–1485

Ivy JL, Goforth HW Jr, Damon BM, McCauley TR, Parsons EC, Price TB 2002 Early post-exercise muscle glycogen recovery is enhanced with a carbohydrate-protein supplement. Journal of Applied Physiology 93:1337–1344

Jackson MJ, McArdle A, McArdle F 1998 Antioxidant micronutrients and gene expression. Proceedings of the Nutrition Society 57:301–305

Jackson MJ, Papa S, Bolaños J, Bruckdorfer R, Carlsen H, Elliott RM, Flier J, Griffiths HR, Heales S, Holst B, Lorusso M, Lund E, Øivind Moskaug J, Moser U, Di Paola M, Polidori MC, Signorile A, Stahl W, Viña-Ribes J, Astley SB 2002 Antioxidants, reactive oxygen and nitrogen species, gene induction and mitochondrial function. Molecular Aspects of Medicine 23:209–285

Jentjens R, Jeukendrup AE 2003 Determinants of post-exercise glycogen synthesis during short-term recovery. Sports Medicine 33:117–144

Kerr D, Khan K, Bennell K 2006 Bone, exercise, nutrition and menstrual disturbances. In: Burke L, Deakin V (eds) Clinical sports nutrition, 3rd edn. McGraw-Hill, Sydney

Kiens B, Helge J 2000 Adaptations to a high fat diet. In: Maughan R (ed) Nutrition in sport. Blackwell Science, Oxford, 192–204

Kiens B, Essen-Gustavsson B, Christensen NJ, Saltin B 1993 Skeletal muscle substrate utilization during submaximal exercise in man: effect of endurance training. Journal of Physiology (London) 469:459–478

Kirwan JP, Cyr-Campbell D, Campbell WW, Scheiber J, Evans WJ 2001 Effects of moderate and high glycemic index meals on metabolism on exercise performance. Metabolism 50:849–855

Koutedakis Y, Pacy PJ, Quevedo RM, Millward DJ, Hesp R, Boreham C, Sharp NC 1994 The effect of two different periods of weight-reduction on selected performance parameters in elite lightweight oarsmen. International Journal of Sports Medicine 15:472–477

Lambert EV, Speechly DP, Dennis SC, Noakes TD 1994 Enhanced endurance in trained cyclists during moderate intensity exercise following 2 weeks adaptation to a high fat diet. European Journal of Applied Physiology 69:287–293

Layman DK, Walker DA 2006 Potential importance of leucine in treatment of obesity and the metabolic syndrome. Journal of Nutrition 136:319S–323S

Lemon PW, Tarnopolsky MA, MacDougall JD, Atkinson SA 1992 Protein requirements and muscle mass/strength changes during intensive training in novice bodybuilders. Journal of Applied Physiology 73:767–775

Loucks AB 2004 Energy balance and body composition in sports and exercise. Journal of Sports Sciences 22:1–14

Loucks AB, Nattiv A 2005 The female athlete triad. Lancet 366:S49–S50

Loucks AB, Thuma JR 2003 Luteinizing hormone pulsatility is disrupted at a threshold of energy availability in regularly menstruating women. Journal of Clinical Endocrinology and Metabolism 88:297–311

Loucks AB, Verdun M, Heath EM 1998 Low energy availability, not stress of exercise, alters LH pulsatility in exercising women. Journal of Applied Physiology 84:37–46

Lukaski HC 2004 Vitamin and mineral status: effects on physical performance. Nutrition 20:632–644

Macdermid PW, Stannard SR 2006 A whey-supplemented, high-protein diet versus a high-carbohydrate diet: effects on endurance cycling performance. International Journal of Sport Nutrition and Exercise Metabolism 16:65–77

McInerney P, Lessard SJ, Burke LM, Coffey VG, Lo Giudice SL, Southgate RJ, Hawley JA 2005 Failure to repeatedly supercompensate muscle glycogen stores in highly trained men. Medicine and Science in Sports and Exercise 37:404–411

McKenzie S, Phillips SM, Carter SL, Lowther S, Gibala MJ, Tarnopolsky MA 2000 Endurance exercise training attenuates leucine oxidation and BCOAD activation during exercise in humans. American Journal of Physiology. Endocrinology and Metabolism 278:E580–E587

Manore MM 2000 Effect of physical activity on thiamine, riboflavin and vitamin B-6 requirements. American Journal of Clinical Nutrition 72:598S–606S

Mastaloudis A, Leonard SW, Traber MG 2001 Oxidative stress in athletes during extreme endurance exercise. Free Radical Biology Medicine 31:911–922

Melby CL, Schmidt WD, Corrigan D 1990 Resting metabolic rate in weight-cycling collegiate wrestlers compared with physically active, noncycling control subjects. American Journal of Clinical Nutrition 52:409–414

Miller SL, Tipton KD, Chinkes DL, Wolf SE, Wolfe RR 2003 Independent and combined effects of amino acids and glucose after resistance exercise. Medicine and Science in Sports and Exercise 35:449–455

Monsen ER 1988 Iron nutrition and absorption: dietary factors which impact iron bioavailability. Journal of the American Dietetic Association 88:786–790

Montain SJ, Hopper MK, Coggan AR, Coyle EF 1991 Exercise metabolism at different time intervals after a meal. Journal of Applied Physiology 70:882–888

Muoio DM, Leddy JJ, Horvath PJ, Awad AB, Pendergast DR 1994 Effects of dietary fat on metabolic adjustment to maximal VO2 and endurance in runners. Medicine and Science in Sports and Exercise 26:81–88

Nielsen P, Nachtigall D 1998 Iron supplementation in athletes: current recommendations. Sports Medicine 26:207–216

Nieman DC 1998 Influence of carbohydrate on the immune response to intensive, prolonged exercise. Exercise and Immunology Reviews 4:64–76

Nieman DC, Johanssen LM, Lee JW, Arabatzis K 1990 Infectious episodes in runners before and after the Los Angeles Marathon. Journal of Sports Medicine and Physical Fitness 30:316–328

Otis CL, Drinkwater B, Johnson M, Loucks A, Wilmore J 1997 American College of Sports Medicine position stand. The female athlete triad. Medicine and Science in Sports and Exercise 29:i–ix

Parkin JA, Carey MF, Martin IK, Stojanovska L, Febbraio MA 1997 Muscle glycogen storage following prolonged exercise: effect of timing of ingestion of high glycemic index food. Medicine and Science in Sports and Exercise 29:220–224

Pattwell DM, Jackson MJ 2004 Contraction-induced oxidants as mediators of adaptation and damage in skeletal muscle. Exercise and Sport Science Reviews 32:14–18

Pellett PL, Young VR 1992 The effects of different levels of energy intake on protein metabolism and of different levels of protein intake on energy metabolism: a statistical evaluation from the published literature. In: Scrimshaw NS, Schurch B (eds) Protein-energy interactions. Nestle Foundation, Lausanne, Switzerland, 81–121

Phillips SM 2004 Protein requirements and supplementation in strength sports. Nutrition 20:689–695

Phillips SM, Tipton KD, Ferrando AA, Wolfe RR 1983 The human metabolic response to chronic ketosis without caloric restriction: prevention of submaximal exercise capability with reduced carbohydrate oxidation. Metabolism 32:769–776

Phillips SM, Atkinson SA, Tarnopolsky MA, MacDougall JD 1993 Gender differences in leucine kinetics and nitrogen balance in endurance athletes. Journal of Applied Physiology 75:2134–2141

Phillips SM, Tipton KD, Aarsland A, Wolf SE, Wolfe RR 1997 Mixed muscle protein synthesis and breakdown following resistance exercise in humans. American Journal of Physiology. Endocrinology and Metabolism 273:E99–E107

Phillips SM, Tipton KD, Ferrando AA, Wolfe RR 1999 Resistance training reduces the acute exercise-induced increase in muscle protein turnover. American Journal of Physiology. Endocrinology and Metabolism 76:E118–E124

Phillips SM, Hartman JW, Wilkinson SB 2005 Dietary protein to support anabolism with resistance exercise in young men. Journal of the Americal College of Nutrition 24:134S–139S

Pitsis GC, Fallon KE, Fallon SK, Fazakerley R 2004 Response of soluble transferrin receptor and iron-related parameters to iron supplementation in elite, iron-depleted, nonanemic female athletes. Clinical Journal of Sports Medicine 14:300–304

Powers SK, DeRuisseau KC, Quindry J, Hamilton KL 2004 Dietary antioxidants and exercise. Journal of Sports Science 22:81–94

Rennie MJ, Tipton KD 2000 Protein and amino acid metabolism during and after exercise and the effects of nutrition. Annual Review of Nutrition 20:457–483

Roy BD, Tarnopolsky MA, MacDougall JD, Fowles J, Yarasheski KE 1997 Effect of glucose supplement timing on protein metabolism after resistance training. Journal of Applied Physiology 82:1882–1888

Roy BD, Fowles JR, Hill R, Tarnopolsky M 2000 Macronutrient intake and whole body protein metabolism following resistance exercise. Medicine and Science in Sports and Exercise 32:1412–1418

Rozenek R, Ward P, Long S, Garhammer J 2002 Effects of high-calorie supplements on body composition and muscular strength following resistance training. Journal of Sports Medicine and Physical Fitness 42:340–347

Saarni SE, Rissanen A, Sarna S, Koskenvuo M, Kaprio J 2006 Weight cycling of athletes and subsequent weight gain in middle age. International Journal of Obesity 30(11):1639–1644

Sasaki H, Hotta N, Ishiko T 1991 Comparison of sympatho-adrenal activity during endurance exercise performance under high – and low-carbohydrate diet conditions. Journal of Sports Medicine and Physical Fitness 31:407–412

Schabort EJ, Bosch AN, Weltan SM, Noakes TD 1999 The effect of pre-exercise meal on time to fatigue during prolonged cycling exercise. Medicine and Science in Sports and Exercise 31:464–471

Sherman WM, Costill DL, Fink WJ, Miller JM 1981 Effect of exercise-diet manipulation on muscle glycogen and its subsequent utilisation during performance. International Journal of Sports Medicine 2:114–118

Sherman WM, Brodowicz G, Wright DA, Allen WK, Simonsen J, Dernbach A 1989 Effect of 4 hour pre exercise carbohydrate feeding on cycling performance. Medicine and Science in Sports and Exercise 21:598–604

Simonsen JC, Sherman WM, Lamb DR, Dernbach AR, Doyle JA, Strauss R 1991 Dietary carbohydrate, muscle glycogen and power output during rowing training. Journal of Applied Physiology 70:1500–1505

Slater GJ, Rice AJ, Jenkins D, Gulbin J, Hahn AG 2006 Preparation of former heavyweight oarsmen to compete as leightweight rowers over 16 weeks. Three case studies. International Journal of Nutrition and Exercise Metabolism 16:108–121

Slater GJ, Rice AJ, Tanner R, Sharpe K, Jemkins D, Hahn A 2006 Impact of two different body mass management strategies on repeated rowing performance. Medicine and Science in Sports and Exercise 38:138–146

Sundgot-Borgen J 2000 Eating disorders in athletes. In: Maughan R (ed) Nutrition in sport. Blackwell Science, Oxford, 510–522

Tarnopolsky M 2004 Protein requirements for endurance athletes. Nutrition 20:662–668

Tarnopolsky MA, Atkinson SA, MacDougall JD, Chesley A, Phillips S, Schwarcz HP 1992 Evaluation of protein requirements for trained strength athletes. Journal of Applied Physiology 73:1986–1995

Tarnopolsky MA, MacDougall JD, Atkinson SA 1988 Influence of protein intake and training status on nitrogen balance and lean body mass. Journal of Applied Physiology 64:187–193

Tarnopolsky MA, Zawada C, Richmond LB, Carter S, Shearer J, Graham T, Phillips SM 2001 Gender differences in carbohydrate loading are related to energy intake. Journal of Applied Physiology 91:225–230

Thomas DE, Brotherhood JR, Brand JC 1991 Carbohydrate feeding before exercise: effect of glycemic index. International Journal of Sports Medicine 12:180–186

Tipton KD, Wolfe RR 2004 Protein and amino acids for athletes. Journal of Sports Science 22:65–79

Tipton KD, Ferrando AA, Williams BD, Wolfe RR 1996 Muscle protein metabolism in female swimmers after a combination of resistance and endurance exercise. Journal of Applied Physiology 81:2034–2038

Tipton KD, Rasmussen BB, Miller SL, Wolf SE, Owens-Stovall SK, Petrini BE, Wolfe RR 2001 Timing of amino acid-carbohydrate ingestion alters anabolic response of muscle to resistance exercise. American Journal of Physiology. Endocrinology and Metabolism 281:E197–E206

Tipton KD, Elliott TA, Cree MG, Wolf SE, Sanford AP, Wolfe RR 2004 Ingestion of casein and whey proteins result in muscle anabolism after resistance exercise. Medicine and Science in Sports and Exercise 36:2073–2081

Tipton KD, Elliott TA, Cree MG, Aarsland AA, Sanford AP, Wolfe RR 2007 Stimulation of net muscle protein synthesis by whey protein ingestion before and after exercise. American Journal of Physiology. Endocrinology and Metabolism 292:E71–E76

Todd KS, Butterfield GE, Calloway DH 1984 Nitrogen balance in men with adequate and deficient energy intake at three levels of work. Journal of Nutrition 114:2107–2118

Urso ML, Clarkson PM 2003 Oxidative stress, exercise and antioxidant supplementation. Toxicology 189:41–54

Viitasalo JT, Kyrolainen H, Bosco C, Alen M 1987 Effects of rapid weight reduction on force production and vertical jumping height. International Journal of Sports Medicine 8:281–285

Walrand S, Moreau K, Caldefie F, Tridon A, Chassagne J, Portefaix G, Cynober L, Beaufrère B, Vasson MP, Boirie Y 2001 Specific and nonspecific immune responses to fasting and refeeding differ in healthy young adult and elderly persons. American Journal of Clinical Nutrition 74:670–678

Wcc SL, Williams C, Gray S, Horabin J 1999 Influence of high and low glycemic index meals on endurance running capacity. Medicine and Science in Sports and Exercise 31:393–399

Whitley HA, Humphreys SM, Campbell IT, Keegan MA, Jayanetti TD, Sperry DA, MacLaren DP, Reilly T, Frayn KN 1998 Metabolic and performance responses during endurance exercise after high fat and high carbohydrate meals. Journal of Applied Physiology 85:418–424

Williams NI, Helmreich DL, Parfitt DB, Caston-Balderrama A, Cameron JL 2001 Evidence for a causal role of low energy availability in the induction of menstrual cycle disturbances during strenuous exercise training. Journal of Clinical Endocrinology and Metabolism 86:5184–5193

Wright DA, Sherman WM, Dernbach AR 1991 Carbohydrate feedings before, during or in combination improve cycling endurance performance. Journal of Applied Physiology 71:1082–1088

Zawadzki KM, Yaspelkis BB, Ivy JL 1992 Carbohydrate-protein complex increases the rate of muscle glycogen storage after exercise. Journal of Applied Physiology 72:1854–1859

Zello GA 2006 Dietary reference intakes for the macronutrients and energy: considerations for physical activity. Applied Physiology Nutrition and Metabolism 31:74–79

Chapter 33

Fluid, electrolyte and carbohydrate requirements for exercise

Scott J. Montain Samuel N. Cheuvront

1 INTRODUCTION

The combination of exercise and environmental stress can severely challenge body fluid balance (homeostasis), as sweating is the primary avenue for dissipating heat produced during work. As a consequence, large water deficits can rapidly accrue if fluids are not consumed to compensate. If sufficient dehydration occurs, the ability to perform endurance tasks will be compromised. Conversely, overzealous fluid intake, relative to water turnover and salt losses, can produce, in a matter of hours, physiological changes that will also compromise health status. Persistent overdrinking, or drinking aggressively without replacing the salt lost in sweat, can produce a medical syndrome known as hyponatraemia (water intoxication), which has afflicted marathon runners as well as individuals participating in other longer-duration physical activities. This condition can lead to mental status changes, seizures and in rare instances, death.

This chapter discusses the fluid, electrolyte and carbohydrate requirements for exercise, and the physiological and performance implications of imbalances in their loss and replacement. Throughout the chapter, euhydration refers to the normal body water content, hypohydration refers to a body water deficit and hyperhydration refers to increased body water content.

2 PHYSIOLOGY OF WATER AND ELECTROLYTE BALANCE

Water is the principal chemical constituent of the human body. For an average adult, total body water is relatively constant, representing 50–70% of body mass (Food and Nutrition Board of the Institute of Medicine 2005, Sawka & Coyle 1999). This range, in addition to the differences often attributed to age, gender and endurance fitness, is primarily accounted for by differences in body composition, with adipose tissue containing <10% water. Total body water is distributed among the intracellular fluid (~65%) and extracellular fluid compartments (~35%), with the latter being further divided into the interstitial (~25% of the total body

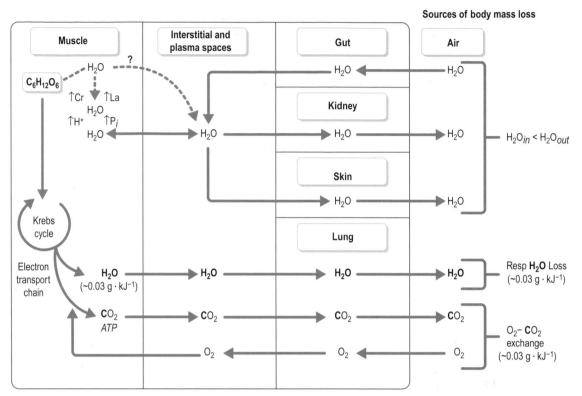

Figure 33.1 Sources of body mass loss during exercise, and associated with the metabolic exchange of oxygen and carbon dioxide and total body water turnover. Abbreviations: ECF, extracellular fluid; ETS, electron transport system.

water) and plasma spaces (<10%). Each fluid compartment experiences dynamic exchange across vascular and cellular membranes.

Independent of exercise-induced water turnover, ~5–10% of total body water is turned over daily. Most of this turnover is the result of fluid intake and urine production, but metabolism and ventilation also contribute. As illustrated in Figure 33.1, the process of metabolism continuously produces water, and at the same time there is continuous loss of water from the lungs. Interestingly, the water produced during metabolism (~0.03 g·kJ^{-1} or 0.13 g·kcal^{-1}) generally approximates respiratory water loss (~0.03 g·kJ^{-1} or 0.12 g·kcal^{-1}), resulting in water turnover, but no net change in total body water volume (Consolazio et al. 1963, Mitchell et al. 1972). In addition, Figure 33.1 illustrates that the combination of respiratory water and carbon exchange contributes independently as a source of body mass loss and therefore requires correction when estimating sweat loses from changes in body mass.

Urine output represents the primary avenue for regulating net body water balance across a broad range of fluid intake volumes and losses from other avenues (Food and Nutrition Board of the Institute of Medicine 2005). As such, any overshoot in oral fluid intake is offset by urine production (1–2 L·d^{-1}), resulting in day-to-day water stability. Sweat losses vary widely and depend upon the physical activity level and environmental conditions. Yet even athletes sweating profusely have remarkably stable total body water as thirst and hunger drives, coupled with ad libitum access to

food and fluid, generally meet energy and fluid needs (Food and Nutrition Board of the Institute of Medicine 2005). Physiologically, hormonal and renal responses (Andreoli et al. 2000) to body water volume and tonicity changes, as well as non-regulatory social-behavioural factors (Rolls 1994), play a large role in this process.

When a body water deficit occurs, as with exercise, plasma volume decreases and plasma osmotic pressure increases in proportion to the decrease in total body water. Plasma volume decreases because it replaces the interstitial fluid lost as sweat, and osmolality increases because sweat is hypotonic relative to plasma (Chapter 19). The increase in plasma osmotic pressure is primarily due to increased plasma sodium and chloride, with no consistent effect on potassium concentrations (Kubica et al. 1983, Montain & Coyle 1992).

3 WATER, ELECTROLYTE AND CARBOHYDRATE REQUIREMENTS FOR EXERCISE

3.1 Water

Normal water and electrolyte needs range widely due to numerous factors (metabolic rate, diet, climate, clothing) and therefore normal hydration is compatible with a wide range of fluid and electrolyte intakes (Food and Nutrition Board of the Institute of Medicine 2005). For example, the daily water requirement of a 70 kg adult male is ~2.5 L if sedentary, and it can increase to ~3.2 L when performing

Table 33.1 Variations in sweat rates across sports (data compiled from Rehrer & Burke 1996)

Sport	Mean (L·h⁻¹)	Range (L·h⁻¹)
Waterpolo	0.55	0.30–0.80
Cycling	0.80	0.29–1.25
Running	1.10	0.54–1.83
Basketball	1.11	0.70–1.60
Soccer	1.17	0.70–2.10

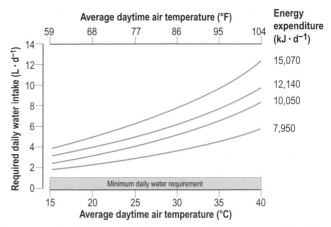

Figure 33.2 Predictions of daily water requirements as a function of daily energy expenditure and air temperature. Adapted from Food and Nutrition Board of the Institute of Medicine 2005.

~60 min of modest-intensity physical activity. More active adults living in warm environments have daily water needs of ~6 L, and water turnover studies show that the daily water turnover is approximately 3.3 L and 4.5 L for sedentary and active men, respectively. Regular physical activity increases water requirements that parallel sweat losses for evaporative heat exchange. For instance, higher volumes of daily (50 km cycling) or weekly (100 km running) activity in a temperate environment increase water flux by an additional 1.2–1.4 L·d⁻¹, owing primarily to sweat loss (Leiper et al. 1996, 2001). The same activities conducted in warmer environments increase water turnover further.

Table 33.1 (Rehrer & Burke 1996) illustrates the wide variability in hourly sweat losses, both within and among sports. Depending upon the duration of physical activity and the nature of the environmental exposure, the impact of these elevated hourly sweat rates on daily water requirements will vary. Figure 33.2 depicts generalised modelling approximations for daily water requirements, based upon calculated sweating rates as a function of daily energy expenditure (activity level) and air temperature (Food and Nutrition Board of the Institute of Medicine 2005). Applying this prediction model, it is clear that daily water requirements can increase 2–6-fold from baseline by simple manipulation of either variable. As a consequence, prolonged strenuous work in hot climates may require fluid replacement of 10–15 L·d⁻¹ (Chapters 19, 21 and 34.2). In addition to air temperature, other environmental factors also modify sweat loss and evaporative cooling, including relative humidity (water vapour pressure), air motion, solar radiation and the use of clothing (Chapters 19, 21), in particular thermal and chemical protective ensembles. Therefore, it is expected that water losses and water needs will vary considerably among moderately active people, based on changing extraneous influences.

3.2 Electrolytes

Sweat is hypotonic to extracellular fluid but contains electrolytes including, but not limited to, sodium, chloride and potassium. Sweat sodium concentration averages ~35 mEq·L⁻¹ (range: 10–70 mEq·L⁻¹) and varies depending upon diet, sweat rate, hydration state and heat acclimation (Allan & Wilson 1971, Costill 1977, Shirreffs & Maughan

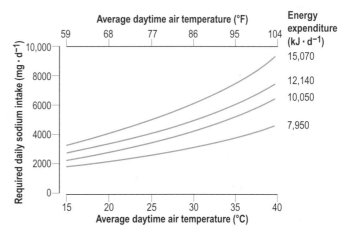

Figure 33.3 Predictions of daily sodium requirements as a function of daily energy expenditure and air temperature. Adapted from Food and Nutrition Board of the Institute of Medicine 2005.

1997). Sweat chloride averages ~30 mEq·L⁻¹ (range: 5–60 mEq·L⁻¹), whilst potassium concentration averages only ~5 mEq·L⁻¹ (range: 3–15 mEq·L⁻¹). Sweat glands reabsorb sodium by active transport across the duct walls, but the ability to reabsorb sodium is inversely related to sweat transit time. As a result, total sodium content and the sodium concentration of sweat increase at high sweating rates (Allan & Wilson 1971, Costill 1977). Heat acclimation improves the ability of the sweat gland to reabsorb sodium (Chapter 21). Thus, heat-acclimated persons typically have lower sweat sodium concentrations (>50% reduction) for a given sweat rate (Allan & Wilson 1971), but will secrete more sweat.

Figure 33.3 depicts generalised (modelling) approximations for daily sodium needs, based upon calculated sweat rates, which were derived as a function of daily energy expenditure (activity level) and air temperature (Food and Nutrition Board of the Institute of Medicine 2005). This analysis assumes that persons are heat acclimated and have a sweat sodium concentration of 25 mEq·L^{-1} (about 0.6 g·L^{-1}). The average daily sodium intake varies greatly around the world, depending upon ethnic-based food preferences (e.g. Australia: ~2 g·d^{-1}; U.S.A.: ~4 g·d^{-1}).

Increases or decreases in sodium stores are usually corrected by adjustments in a person's salt appetite. Additional food intake associated with increased physical activity usually covers the additional sodium requirement. Therefore, sodium supplementation is generally not necessary, as normal dietary sodium intake appears adequate to compensate for sweat sodium losses in all but the most extreme cases.

If individuals need additional sodium, this can readily be obtained by salting food to taste. Another strategy is to rehydrate with fluids containing ~20 mEq·L^{-1} of sodium. Most commercial sports drinks approximate this concentration. However, the addition of common table salt (sodium chloride) to tap water, at the rate of ~1 g·L^{-1}, will also satisfy this requirement. Recently, electrolyte pills (salt tablets) have returned to the marketplace and provide another option for replacing electrolytes. These are a viable option for replacing electrolytes when food containing electrolytes is unavailable. Nevertheless, in most circumstances their use is not necessary, particularly when an adequate and balanced diet is consumed. Indeed, Chapter 34.2 explores the scientific evidence supporting the use of commercial sports drinks.

3.3 Carbohydrates

The rate of carbohydrate oxidation is primarily determined by metabolic rate (see Figure 33.1), but is influenced by other factors, such as diet, heat stress and dehydration. Carbohydrate oxidation rates in excess of 1.5 g·min^{-1} can be sustained for over 2 h, whilst rates >3 g·min^{-1} can only be sustained for ~1 h (Coyle 2005). As resting muscle contains only 21–27 g of glycogen per kg of muscle (wet mass), and gluconeogenesis generates glucose at a rate of only ~1 g·min^{-1}, there are many exercise scenarios where exogenous carbohydrate intake would be likely to prove beneficial for preserving carbohydrate oxidation and the ability to sustain exercise intensity (Chapter 7). Indeed, many studies have demonstrated that carbohydrate feeding can delay fatigue during prolonged cycling and running (Coyle 2005). Carbohydrate feeding can also improve muscle power when people try to complete a specified task as quickly as possible (Coyle 2005). More recently, carbohydrate feeding has proven beneficial during incremental exercise (e.g. shuttle-running; Nicholas et al. 1996).

Classically, the ergogenic effects of carbohydrate feeding were attributed to the provision of a carbohydrate source when muscle glycogen concentration was low. Carbohydrate feeding did not appear to slow (spare) muscle glycogen use, at least during constant-intensity exercise performed at ≥60% of maximal intensity (Coyle et al. 1991). Experiments conducted in the 1980s established that ingested carbohydrate and blood glucose can be oxidised at rates of approximately 1 g·min^{-1}, and this form of glucose becomes the predominant form of carbohydrate oxidised late in a bout of prolonged continuous exercise (Coyle 2005). More recently, it has been shown that regular carbohydrate feeding not only provides an energy source for oxidation but during sustained light-intensity exercise or bouts of intermittent intense exercise or variable intensity exercise, the exogenous carbohydrate appears to be used to sustain muscle glycogen. For example, Nicholas et al. (1999) reported less muscle glycogen use when individuals were fed carbohydrate during an incremental exercise test, compared with tests when a non-carbohydrate placebo beverage was provided. Regardless of the fate of the carbohydrate, regular intake of carbohydrate can be beneficial for sustaining exercise intensity during prolonged exercise.

Carbohydrate supplementation is currently recommended during vigorous work lasting in excess of 60–90 min (American College of Sports Medicine 1996). Typically, 30–60 g·h^{-1} are recommended, but recommendations for up to 60–70 g·h^{-1} exist (Jeukendrup et al. 2005). Pre-exercise carbohydrate meals reduce the effectiveness of, or the requirement for carbohydrate feeding during exercise, particularly for tasks producing fatigue in the 60–90 min timeframe. For tasks lasting longer than 90 min, regular carbohydrate intake is beneficial for sustaining exercise intensity.

Commercial sports drinks are a common method for providing carbohydrate. However, since such drinks are attempting to achieve two goals, adequate fluid replacement and adequate carbohydrate provision, one might wonder whether attempting to accomplish one objective may result in a failure to satisfy the other, by providing either too much or too little. Figure 33.4 illustrates the interaction between fluid (with electrolyte) replacement and carbohydrate delivery. For this comparison, it was assumed that a 70 kg athlete was running a 42 km marathon under two different weather conditions (cool and warm), and that the drink provided contained 7% carbohydrate, a typical concentration for commercial sports drinks. The rate of fluid intake was derived from the predicted sweat rate (Montain et al. 2006), with drinking rate set so that the athlete finished the race with ~2% reduction in body mass due to dehydration (1.4 L water deficit). In the cool conditions, when the race pace is expected to be ≥10 km·h^{-1} (4 h 12 min and faster), drinking a carbohydrate-electrolyte beverage would adequately provide both fluid requirement and the recommended 30–60 g·h^{-1} of carbohydrate (shaded area). In contrast, runners whose pace was slower than 10 km·h^{-1} would have fluid replacement needs insufficient to meet the 30–60 g·h^{-1} carbohydrate objective. In warmer weather, where sweating and therefore drinking rates are higher, both fluid and 30–60 g·h^{-1} of carbohydrate delivery

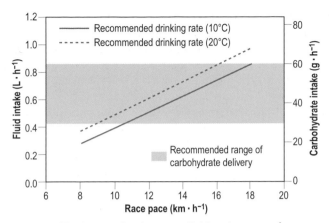

Figure 33.4 The interaction between fluid replacement (to prevent dehydration >2% body mass loss) and carbohydrate provision (30–60 g·h⁻¹) during distance running, when drinking a 7% carbohydrate beverage in two weather conditions: cool (10°C; solid line) and warm (20°C; broken line).

are achieved. However, if there is a need to provide carbohydrate at rates closer to 60 g·h⁻¹, supplementation with more concentrated carbohydrate drinks or items such as carbohydrate gels will be necessary.

The combination of glucose with common mono- or disaccharides (e.g. fructose or sucrose) enhances carbohydrate absorption and carbohydrate oxidation compared to drinks containing glucose alone (Jentjens & Jeukendrup 2005, Jentjens et al. 2006). As glucose and fructose are absorbed via unique intestinal transport proteins, the faster rate of intestinal absorption when the two sugars are consumed simultaneously compared with separately is not altogether surprising. The accompanying higher rates of carbohydrate oxidation, however, imply that the rate of intestinal absorption is a limiting factor in oxidising exogenous carbohydrate.

The inclusion of carbohydrate in a beverage slows the rate of fluid replacement. Gastric emptying and intestinal absorption are appreciatively slower when the beverage carbohydrate concentration is >8% (Coyle & Montain 1992). Whether the slowing compromises fluid replacement will depend on the factors determining sweating rate. However, multiple laboratory experiments have been unable to resolve differences in thermoregulatory and cardiovascular responses when individuals drank water only or beverages containing <8% carbohydrate during prolonged exercise (Coyle & Montain 1992, Lambert et al. 1992). Furthermore, a slowing of gastric emptying due to more concentrated beverages or gels may be an acceptable trade-off when the provision of energy remains high but sweat losses are low, such as during prolonged exercise in very cool weather. Thus, under most circumstances the addition of carbohydrate to a fluid replacement beverage will not compromise the ability to rehydrate.

4 FLUID AND ELECTROLYTE IMBALANCES

It is sometimes difficult to match fluid consumption to sweat losses during exercise, and water losses of 2–6% of body mass have frequently been observed (Sawka et al. 2005), a phenomenon termed voluntary dehydration. Although this is more common in hot environments, similar losses can occur in cold climates when working in heavy clothing (O'Brien et al. 1996). When such a mismatch occurs, the effects on exercise performance are variable, and are likely to depend upon endurance fitness, mode of exercise and the environment (Cheuvront et al. 2003).

4.1 Hypohydration

It is well documented that hypohydration >2% of body mass is associated with impaired endurance exercise performance (Cheuvront et al. 2003, Food and Nutrition Board of the Institute of Medicine 2005). There is some indication that this conclusion may be slightly biased by unrealistic or inadequate convective heat transfer in laboratory studies (Cheuvront et al. 2004, Saunders et al. 2005), but experimental field evidence in hot (Adolph 1947) and more temperate (Armstrong et al. 1985, Wästerlund et al. 2004) environments supports a detrimental impact of dehydration on performance. Whether or not hypohydration impacts upon exercise without an aerobic component (strength, power) remains questionable despite more than 30 studies. A sample of these are reviewed and presented elsewhere (Food and Nutrition Board of the Institute of Medicine 2005). It is also reported that hypohydration by >2% adversely influences cognitive function in the heat (Cian et al. 2001, Gopinathan et al. 1988), but this area also requires more research. Physiological factors that contribute to hypohydration-mediated performance decrements include hyperthermia (Gonzalez-Alonso et al. 1999a, Nielsen et al. 2001), increased cardiovascular strain (Gonzalez-Alonso et al. 1995, Montain & Coyle 1992), altered metabolic function (Febbraio et al. 1994) or perhaps alterations in central nervous system function independent of temperature (Montain et al. 1998).

Hyperthermia associated with exercise is exacerbated by hypohydration in temperate and hot climates, due to alterations in thermal and cardiovascular regulation. A 0.1–0.2°C elevation in exercising core temperature, and 3–5 beats· min⁻¹ greater heart rate, is observed for every percent of body mass loss attributable to water deficit, when the same exercise task is performed with and without fluid replacement (Sawka 1992). The relative hyperthermia associated with dehydration is a result of reduced skin blood flow and altered sweating control (Gonzalez-Alonso et al. 2000, Montain et al. 1995, Sawka 1992). When exercise commences with a water deficit, it takes longer for sweating and skin vasodilatation to occur, and the sensitivity (slope) of the relationship between either variable relative to core temperature is reduced (see Chapter 18). Thus, less vasodilatation and sweating occur with each increment in core temperature when dehydrated. An elevated body core temperature also reduces the capacity for heat storage (Gonzalez-Alonso et al. 1999b). Both the singular and combined effects of plasma hyperosmolality and hypovolaemia are implicated in mediating the reduced heat loss response during exercise-heat stress.

Although higher body temperatures raise circulating catecholamine concentrations, which increase heart rate independently of changes in hydration (Fritzsche et al. 1999), hypohydration increases cardiovascular strain, primarily as a result of a decrease in the central blood volume (Sawka & Coyle 1999). This lowers central venous pressure which decreases cardiac filling (preloading), resulting in a lower stroke volume and greater heart rate. In warm-hot environments, the higher heart rate is not sufficient to offset the fall in stroke volume, resulting in reduced cardiac output and a lower mean arterial pressure. Under these conditions, there is evidence that moderate hypohydration can also compromise muscle blood flow (Gonzalez-Alonso et al. 1998).

In the laboratory, >2% dehydration shortens time to fatigue at any given workload or reduces self-paced exercise intensity (Cheuvront et al. 2003). Maximal oxygen uptake may be maintained or modestly lowered at this level of water deficit, but exercise time at maximal aerobic power is consistently compromised (Sawka & Coyle 1999).

In contrast, cooler climates (4–8°C) produce noticeably smaller alterations in cardiovascular function and heat strain (Gonzalez-Alonso et al. 2000, Kenefick et al. 2004), and cool weather attenuates the performance decrements associated with modest water deficits (2–3% body mass) in temperate and warmer weather (Cheuvront et al. 2005). Other mechanisms, such as diminished psychological drive to exercise (Chapter 5), metabolite accumulation (Chapter 6) or more rapid glycogen depletion (Chapter 7), may also contribute to or help to explain the negative consequences of hypohydration on performance in other circumstances (Brück & Olschewski 1987, Febbraio 2000, Montain et al. 1998).

Acute body water deficits of the order of 9–10% are considered severe and should be avoided. Deficits of this magnitude are typically associated with poor blood pressure regulation and mental status changes. Medically, dehydration of >9% can lead to hypovolaemic shock, seizures, kidney failure, coma and, if left untreated, death. Early indicators of moderate to severe dehydration include thirst, dry mouth, little or no urine production over multiple hours, dizziness or lightheadedness, decreased ability to concentrate, confusion, general lethargy, muscle weakness and headache (Shirreffs et al. 2004b). Physical signs include limited tearing, shrunken eyes and shrivelled skin. Effective treatment is to replace the fluids lost.

4.2 Hyperhydration

A state of hyperhydration is difficult to sustain. Overdrinking of water or carbohydrate-electrolyte solutions produces a fluid overload that is normally excreted rapidly by the kidneys. Greater fluid retention can be achieved by drinking an aqueous solution containing glycerol (Freund et al. 1995, Riedesel et al. 1987), which increases fluid retention by reducing free water clearance. Hyperhydration with glycerol can increase total body water by ~1.5 L for several hours, but glycerol consumption provides no cardiovascular or thermoregulatory advantages over water ingestion alone, when taken during exercise-heat stress (Latzka et al. 1997, Magal et al. 2003, Marino et al. 2003). This is probably because both exercise and heat stress already decrease renal blood flow and free water clearance, which negate glycerol's effectiveness when ingested during exercise, relative to conventional beverages. Glycerol hyperhydration may (Anderson et al. 2001, Coutts et al. 2002, Hitchins et al. 1999) or may not (Magal et al. 2003, Marino et al. 2003) improve exercise performance, but differences in performance measures, climate and study designs make comparisons across the literature difficult. Nevertheless, it appears that glycerol-induced hyperhydration offers minimal benefit, and is probably of no greater benefit than that afforded by maintaining proper hydration.

4.3 Exercise–associated hyponatraemia

Hyponatraemia describes a state of lower than normal blood sodium concentration; typically <135 mEq·L^{-1}. It is also used to describe a clinical syndrome that can occur when there is rapid lowering of blood sodium usually to levels below 130 mEq·L^{-1} and accompanied by altered cognitive status. This clinical syndrome is a serious medical condition that has resulted in death, and is discussed here and in Chapter 34.2.

Exercise-associated hyponatraemia has occurred as a consequence of prolonged work (typically >5 h), where sweating is the primary means of heat dissipation. As sweat contains not only water but small quantities of electrolytes, there is a progressive loss of water, sodium, chloride and potassium. Hyponatraemia most often occurs when individuals consume low sodium drinks or sodium-free water, in excess of sweat losses (typified by mass gains), either during or shortly after completing exercise. However, drinking sodium-free water at rates near to or slightly less than the sweat rate can theoretically produce biochemical hyponatraemia when coupled with a progressive loss of electrolytes. Reductions in the solute concentration of the extracellular fluid promote water movement from the extracellular space into the cells. If this fluid shift is of sufficient magnitude and occurs rapidly, it can congest the lungs, result in brain swelling and alter central nervous system function. Signs and symptoms of hyponatraemia include confusion, disorientation, mental obtundation (loss of faculties), headache, nausea, vomiting, aphasia, loss of coordination and muscle weakness. Complications of severe and rapidly evolving hyponatraemia include seizures, coma, pulmonary oedema and cardiorespiratory arrest.

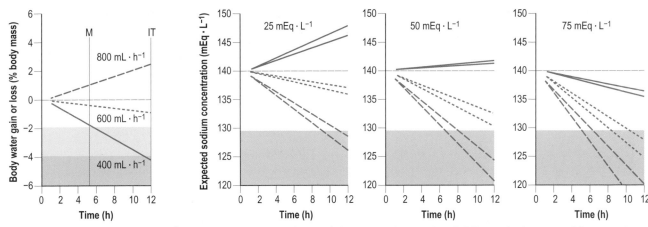

Figure 33.5 Predicted body mass loss (due to water deficit; left panel) for two 70 kg people of different body composition, running at 8.5 km·h⁻¹ in temperate weather (18°C) and drinking water at three rates (400 mL·h⁻¹ (solid line), 600 mL·h⁻¹ (broken line), 800 mL·h⁻¹ (broken dotted line)). The solid shaded areas indicate when water loss would be sufficient to modestly degrade performance (upper) and when water loss would substantially degrade performance (lower). M marks the finishing time for a 42 km marathon, whereas IT marks the approximate finishing time for an Ironman-distance triathlon, based on literature values for participants running the marathon portion at 8.5 km·h⁻¹. Also predicted are plasma sodium concentrations for three rates of sweat sodium loss. Two lines sharing the same line style are the predicted outcomes for people of two different body compositions, with total body water accounting for 50% and 63% (leaner) of body mass. The hatched shaded areas denote the presence of hyponatraemia (plasma sodium concentration <130 mEq·L⁻¹).

The interaction between drinking rate (water only) and plasma sodium concentration is illustrated in Figure 33.5. Since hyponatremia is more common in long-duration activities and slower competitors, a slow running time (8.5 km·h⁻¹) is modelled. Three drinking rates are illustrated, the slowest of which does not elicit hyponatraemia, regardless of the rate of sweat sodium loss. The fastest drinking rate is invariably predicted to produce hyponatraemia because the drinking rate is well in excess of sweating rate; whereas the intermediate drinking rate is predicted to produce hyponatraemia not because the rate of fluid intake exceeded sweating rate, but because of progressive salt deficit. The principal lesson from this interaction is that overdrinking, both in its absolute (volume related) and relative forms (relative to sodium loss), is the mechanism that leads to exercise-associated hyponatraemia.

Exercise-associated hyponatraemia has been observed during marathon and ultramarathon competition (Davis et al. 2001, Hew et al. 2003, Speedy et al. 2001), military training (Garigan & Ristedt 1999, O'Brien et al. 2001) and recreational activities (Backer et al. 1999). In athletic events, the condition is more likely to occur in females and slower competitors, both of which gain weight (due to drinking) during the event. The severity of the symptoms is related to the magnitude by which serum sodium concentration falls, and the rapidity with which it develops (Knochel 1996). If hyponatraemia develops over many hours it might cause less brain swelling and less adverse symptoms (Knochel 1996). As illustrated in Figure 33.5, unreplaced sodium losses contribute to the rate and magnitude of sodium dilution, and may, in certain situations (e.g. salty sweaters), be

the primary reason for development of exercise-associated hyponatraemia (Montain et al. 2001, 2006). Nausea, which increases vasopressin (antidiuretic hormone) secretion, and exercise-heat stress, which reduces renal blood flow and urine output, can negatively affect the ability of the kidney to rapidly correct the fluid–electrolyte imbalance (Zambraski 1996). The syndrome can be prevented by not drinking in excess of sweat rate, and by consuming salt-containing fluids or foods when participating in exercise events that result in many hours of continuous or near-continuous sweating.

The theoretical benefit of consuming electrolyte-containing beverages during endurance exercise, for attenuating the risk of hyponatraemia, is illustrated in Figure 33.6 using a slightly faster running time (10 km·h⁻¹). One drinking rate was modelled, but with two different fluids being consumed (water and a beverage containing 17 mEq·L⁻¹ sodium and 5 mEq·L⁻¹ potassium). Only a mid-range sweat sodium concentration was used. The consumption of water alone may precipitate hyponatraemia. However, the electrolyte drink should not produce this outcome.

5 POSTEXERCISE REHYDRATION

The complete restoration of fluid balance following exercise-induced hypohydration is important for optimal recovery and performance of subsequent work or competition. This is normally not a challenge, since typical fluid losses can be fully replaced with ad libitum drinking and eating from day to day, even when daily water losses are significant.

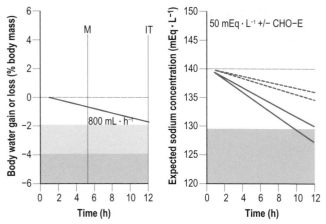

Figure 33.6 The predicted effects of drinking either water or a carbohydrate-electrolyte drink, for attenuating the decline in plasma sodium concentration for a 70 kg person drinking 800 mL·h⁻¹ when running at 10 km·h⁻¹ in warm weather (28°C). Only one sweat sodium concentration is modelled. Shaded areas and finishing time identifiers are the same as in Figure 33.5, except for the slower running speed. For the right panel, the solid lines reflect the effect of drinking water alone, while the broken lines illustrate the effect of consuming the same volume of a drink containing 17 mEq·L⁻¹ sodium and 5 mEq·L⁻¹ potassium. Paired lines represent the predicted outcomes for people of two different body compositions, with total body water accounting for 50% and 63% (leaner) of body mass.

Large acute fluid losses, where there is a need or desire to rehydrate rapidly, require more aggressive rehydration strategies, with particular attention to both volume and solute consumption (Shirreffs et al. 2004a). Drinking water alone or other electrolyte-poor fluid will produce a drop in plasma osmolality, that in turn reduces thirst and stimulates diuresis before euhydration is achieved (Nose et al. 1988a,b). Shirreffs et al. (1996) were the first to systematically characterise the important interaction between fluid volume and electrolyte content during rehydration. Their work demonstrated that rapid full fluid balance restoration requires the replacement of sweat sodium losses and the volume of drink must exceed sweat losses by ~50% (Shirreffs & Maughan 1998). Because the voluntary consumption of drinks containing electrolytes and other flavouring agents is often greater than that of water, such drinks help promote the consumption of larger fluid volumes. They also provide carbohydrates for immediate energy requirements, and the restoration of muscle glycogen stores and can attenuate the risk of developing hyponatraemia (Baker et al. 2005, Montain et al. 2006). However, such drinks are not enough to restore fluid balance in the absence of additional electrolytes (Shirreffs et al. 2004a). This underscores the importance of both food (electrolytes) consumption and fluid intake for the complete restoration of fluid balance follow-ing hypohydration (Maughan et al. 1996). Day-to-day rehydration practices can be considered adequate when the first morning nude body mass varies narrowly day to day (±1%), when urine colour is pale yellow or clear, and when thirst is absent. More details for practical hydration assessment are reviewed elsewhere (Cheuvront & Sawka 2005).

6 HYDRATION SCIENCE IN PRACTICE

This chapter has summarised the science surrounding fluid, electrolyte and carbohydrate requirements for exercise (see also Chapter 34.2). From this information, three simple and practical strategies are provided for optimising body fluid (hydration) and energy (glycogen) balances.

6.1 Drinking rate

During exercise, drink enough fluid to prevent excessive mass loss (>2% of body mass), but never drink so much that body mass increases. The easiest way to track acute hydration changes is to measure nude body mass before and after exercise. If you lose more than 2%, you are drinking too little; if you gain mass, you are drinking too much. This recommendation aims to optimise performance while reducing the risk of hyponatraemia. If the combination of environment, exercise intensity and duration results in fluid losses <2% of body mass without drinking, then fluid intake can be ignored during exercise, but be sure to rehydrate properly before the next exercise bout. Importantly, as illustrated in Figure 33.1, body mass is lost during exercise independently of sweat losses, due to the exchange of oxygen and carbon dioxide and respiratory water loss. When estimates of sweat rate are made during exercise durations of ≤60 min, errors in prediction are fairly small, but since metabolic gas exchanges and respiratory water loss account for 5–15% of mass loss during physical activity (depending on metabolic rate and weather), sweat losses will be overestimated during multiple hour events, if these contributors to mass loss are ignored.

Discussions of fluid replacement requirements often suggest that the liberation of water associated with muscle glycogen storage (~3 mL water per g glycogen) reduces the need for fluid replacement. However, as illustrated in Figure 33.1, water bound to glycogen represents part of the starting total body water pool. Thus, it should not be viewed as appearing de novo, although it could be viewed as a surplus relative to ordinary total body water stores. The precise fate of any water liberated during glycogen utilisation is unknown. Best estimates of liberated water volumes, ubiquitously distributed relative to total body water volume, are small (≤500 mL). It is also possible that this water remains inside the muscle until exercise ceases, due to intracellular osmotic and hydrostatic forces. Either way, the importance of glycogen-bound water to fluid balance and fluid intake recommendations seems minor.

Under conditions that stimulate profuse sweating, drinking sufficient fluid to prevent excessive dehydration from accruing during competition can be a challenge. For example, the elite 42 km marathon runner will need to weigh the advantages of drinking sufficient fluid to prevent slowing caused by excessive dehydration against the time lost when slowing to pick up a water bottle and drinking from it. Similar challenges face athletes in team sports where game rules limit access to fluids (e.g. football, basketball). In addition, the existing literature suggests that in the average-sized adult, gastric emptying and intestinal absorption limit fluid delivery to ~750–1000 L·h^{-1}. Similarly, gastric-emptying rates slow when exercise intensities exceed ~75% of maximal aerobic power (Murray 1987), and are slower during high-intensity, intermittent exercise such as football (Leiper et al. 2005). Thus, under certain competitive situations, sweating rate may be much higher than the rate at which the fluids can be physically replaced. Thus, each athlete must determine their expected fluid losses during competition and devise strategies to drink enough to meet their performance objectives.

The organoleptic properties of the beverage can also impact rehydration. Cool temperature drinks promote greater voluntary intake than warmer drinks. The most pleasurable drink temperature during recovery is relatively cool (~5°C) whereas during exercise, drink temperatures of 15–21°C are generally preferred (American College of Sports Medicine 1996). Similarly, sweetened (artificially or with sugars) flavoured beverages are generally consumed at higher ad libitum rates than plain water.

6.2 Water versus a carbohydrate–electrolyte drink

If exercise duration will exceed 1 h, a carbohydrate-electrolyte (sports) drink is a better choice than water for optimising performance. Prolonged exercise can drain energy reserves and sports drinks provide a steady, useable fuel source. As exercise becomes very prolonged, the electrolytes provided in sports drinks also attenuate the risk of developing hyponatraemia (Baker et al. 2005, Montain et al. 2006).

6.3 Postexercise replacement

The complete restoration of fluid balance requires the replacement of both a fluid volume and its electrolyte content. This is normally achieved by consuming food and beverages ad libitum over a 24 h period, but complete restoration of fluid balance may be more difficult over shorter time frames. Voluntary fluid intake volumes are generally larger when consuming a sports drink, which also provides a small amount of electrolytes and carbohydrates for recovery.

7 CONCLUSION

Water and electrolyte needs increase as a result of exercise. When exercise is prolonged, the addition of carbohydrate to the beverage should be considered. Hypohydration results when sweat losses exceed fluid intakes, and this increases heat storage, by reducing sweat rate and skin blood flow responses for a given core temperature. Endurance exercise is adversely affected when hypohydration is >2% of normal body mass. The magnitude of this effect is dependent largely on the environment, exercise intensity and the duration of exercise. Excessive consumption of hypotonic fluids, over many hours, can lead to hyponatraemia. Marked electrolyte losses can accelerate the dilution of plasma sodium and exacerbate the problem. Hyperhydration provides little or no advantages, and may exacerbate symptomatic hyponatraemia risk. Both hypohydration and hyponatraemia can be avoided with proper fluid intake practices. Proper postexercise rehydration should be considered essential for optimising performance in subsequent work bouts. Although restoration of fluid balance in the short term can be difficult, physiological and behavioural adaptations allow for the maintenance of daily body water and electrolyte balance so long as food and fluid are readily available.

Acknowledgements

The views, opinions and/or findings contained in this report are those of the authors and should not be construed as an official Department of the Army position or decision, unless so designated by other official documentation. Approved for public release; distribution unlimited.

References

Adolph EF 1947 Physiology of man in the desert. Interscience Publishers, New York

Allan JR, Wilson CG 1971 Influence of acclimatization on sweat sodium concentration. Journal of Applied Physiology 30:708–712

American College of Sports Medicine 1996 Position stand on exercise and fluid replacement. Medicine and Science in Sports and Exercise 28:i–vii

Anderson MJ, Cotter JD, Garnham AP, Casley DJ, Febbraio MA 2001 Effect of glycerol-induced hyperhydration on thermoregulation and metabolism during exercise in the heat. International Journal of Sport Nutrition and Exercise Metabolism 11:315–333

Andreoli T, Reeves W, Bichet D 2000 Endocrine control of water balance. In: Fray J, Goodman H (eds) Handbook of physiology, section 7, volume III: endocrine regulation of water and electrolyte balance. Oxford University Press, New York, 530–569

Armstrong LE, Costill DL, Fink WJ 1985 Influence of diuretic-induced dehydration on competitive running performance. Medicine and Science in Sports and Exercise 17:456–461

Backer HD, Shopes E, Collins SL 1999 Exertional heat illness and hyponatremia in hikers. American Journal of Emergency Medicine 17:532–539

Baker LB, Munce TA, Kenney WL 2005 Sex differences in voluntary fluid intake by older adults during exercise. Medicine and Science in Sports and Exercise 37:789–796

Brück K, Olschewski H 1987 Body temperature related factors diminishing the drive to exercise. Canadian Journal of Physiology and Pharmacology 65:1274–1280

Cheuvront SN, Sawka MN 2005 Hydration assessment of athletes. Sports Science Exchange 18:1–6

Cheuvront SN, Carter R III, Sawka MN 2003 Fluid balance and endurance exercise performance. Current Sports Medicine Reports 2:202–208

Cheuvront SN, Carter R III, Montain SJ, Sawka MN 2004 Influence of hydration and airflow on thermoregulatory control in the heat. Journal of Thermal Biology 29:471–477

Cheuvront SN, Carter R III, Castellani JW, Sawka MN 2005 Hypohydration impairs endurance exercise performance in temperate but not cold air. Journal of Applied Physiology 99:1972–1976

Cian C, Barraud PA, Melin B, Raphel C 2001 Effects of fluid ingestion on cognitive function after heat stress or exercise-induced dehydration. International Journal of Psychophysiology 42:243–251

Consolazio FC, Johnson RE, Pecora LJ 1963 The computation of metabolic balances. In: Physiological measurements of metabolic functions in man. McGraw-Hill, New York, 313–339

Costill DL 1977 Sweating: its composition and effects on body fluids. Annals of New York Academy of Sciences 301:160–174

Coutts A, Reaburn P, Mummery K, Holmes M 2002 The effect of glycerol hyperhydration on Olympic distance triathlon performance in high ambient temperatures. International Journal of Sport Nutrition and Exercise Metabolism 12:105–119

Coyle EF 2005 Fluid and fuel intake during exercise. Journal of Sports Sciences 22:39–55

Coyle EF, Montain SJ 1992 Carbohydrate and fluid ingestion during exercise: are there tradeoffs? Medicine and Science in Sports and Exercise 24:671–678

Coyle EF, Hamilton MT, Gonzalez-Alonso J, Montain SJ, Ivy JL 1991 Carbohydrate metabolism during intense exercise when hyperglycemic. Journal of Applied Physiology 70:834–840

Davis DP, Videen JS, Marino A, Vilke GM, Dunford JV, Van Camp SP, Maharam LG 2001 Exercise-associated hyponatremia in marathon runners: a two-year experience. Journal of Emergency Medicine 21:47–57

Febbraio MA 2000 Does muscle function and metabolism affect exercise performance in the heat? Exercise and Sport Science Reviews 28:171–176

Febbraio MA, Snow RJ, Stathis CG, Hargreaves M, Carey MF 1994 Effect of heat stress on muscle energy metabolism during exercise. Journal of Applied Physiology 77:2827–2831

Food and Nutrition Board of the Institute of Medicine 2005 Dietary reference intakes for water, potassium, sodium, chloride and sulfate. National Academies Press, Washington, DC

Freund BJ, Montain SJ, Young AJ, Sawka MN, DeLuca JP, Pandolf KB, Valeri CR 1995 Glycerol hyperhydration: hormonal, renal and vascular fluid responses. Journal of Applied Physiology 79:2069–2077

Fritzsche R, Switzer TW, Hodgkinson BJ, Coyle EF 1999 Stroke volume decline during prolonged exercise is influenced by the increase in heart rate. Journal of Applied Physiology 86:799–805

Garigan T, Ristedt DE 1999 Death from hyponatremia as a result of acute water intoxication in an army basic trainee. Military Medicine 164:234–237

Gonzalez-Alonso J, Mora-Rodríguez R, Below PR, Coyle E 1995 Dehydration reduces cardiac output and increases systemic and cutaneous vascular resistance during exercise. Journal of Applied Physiology 79:1487–1496

Gonzalez-Alonso J, Calbet JAL, Nielsen B 1998 Muscle blood flow is reduced with dehydration during prolonged exercise in humans. Journal of Physiology (London) 513:895–905

Gonzalez-Alonso J, Teller C, Andersen SL, Jensen FB, Hyldig T, Nielsen B 1999a Influence of body temperature on the development of fatigue during prolonged exercise in the heat. Journal of Applied Physiology 86:1032–1039

Gonzalez-Alonso J, Calbet JAL, Nielsen B 1999b Metabolic and thermodynamic responses to dehydration-induced reductions in muscle blood flow in exercising humans. Journal of Physiology (London) 520:577–589

Gonzalez-Alonso J, Mora-Rodriguez R, Coyle EF 2000 Stroke volume during exercise: interaction of environment and hydration. American Journal of Physiology 278:H321–H330

Gopinathan PM, Pichan G, Sharma VM 1988 Role of dehydration in heat stress-induced variations in mental performance. Archives of Environmental Health 43:15–17

Hew TD, Chorley JN, Cianca JC, Divine JG 2003 The incidence, risk factors and clinical manifestations of hyponatremia in marathon runners. Clinical Journal of Sport Medicine 13:41–47

Hitchins S, Martin DT, Burke L, Yates K, Fallon K, Dobson GP 1999 Glycerol hyperhydration improves cycle time trial performance in hot humid conditions. European Journal of Applied Physiology 80:494–501

Jentjens RL, Jeukendrup AE 2005 High rates of exogenous carbohydrate oxidation from a mixture of glucose and fructose ingested during prolonged cycling exercise. British Journal of Nutrition 93:485–492

Jentjens RL, Underwood K, Achten J, Currell K, Mann CH, Jeukendrup AE 2006 Exogenous carbohydrate oxidation rates are elevated after combined ingestion of glucose and fructose during exercise in the heat. Journal of Applied Physiology 100:807–816

Jeukendrup AE, Jentjens RLPG, Moseley L 2005 Nutritional considerations in triathlon. Sports Medicine 35:163–181

Kenefick RW, Mahood NV, Hazzard MP, Quinn TJ, Castellani JW 2004 Hypohydration effects on thermoregulation during moderate exercise in the cold. European Journal of Applied Physiology 92:565–570

Knochel JP 1996 Clinical complications of body fluid and electrolyte balance. In: Buskirk ER, Puhl SM (eds) Body fluid balance: exercise and sport. CRC Press, Boca Raton, FL, 297–317

Kubica R, Neilsen B, Bonnesen A, Rasmussen IB, Stoklosa J, Wilk B 1983 Relationship between plasma volume reduction and plasma electrolyte changes after prolonged bicycle exercise, passive heating and diuretic dehydration. Acta Physiology Poland 34:569–580

Lambert CP, Costill DL, McConell GK, Benedict MA, Lambert GP, Robergs RA, Fink WJ 1992 Fluid replacement after dehydration: influence of beverage carbonation and carbohydrate content. International Journal of Sports Medicine 13:285–292

Latzka WA, Sawka MN, Montain SJ, Skrinar GS, Fielding RA, Matott RP, Pandolf KB 1997 Hyperhydration: thermoregulatory effects during compensable exercise-heat stress. Journal of Applied Physiology 83:860–866

Leiper J, Carnie A, Maughan R 1996 Water turnover rates in sedentary and exercising middle aged men. British Journal of Sports Medicine 30:24–26

Leiper J, Pitsiladis Y, Maughan R 2001 Comparison of water turnover rates in men undertaking prolonged cycling exercise and sedentary men. International Journal of Sports Medicine 22:181–185

Leiper JB, Nicholas CW, Ali A, Williams C, Maughan RJ 2005 The effect of intermittent high-intensity running on gastric emptying of fluids in man. Medicine and Science in Sports and Exercise 37:240–247

Magal M, Webster MJ, Sistrunk LE, Whitehead M, Boyd JC 2003 Comparison of glycerol and water hydration regimens on tennis related performance. Medicine and Science in Sports and Exercise 35:150–156

Marino FE, Kay D, Cannon J 2003 Glycerol hyperhydration fails to improve endurance performance and thermoregulation in humans in a warm environment. Pflügers Archives: European Journal of Physiology 446:455–462

Maughan RJ, Leiper JB, Shirreffs SM 1996 Restoration of fluid balance after exercise-induced dehydration: effects of food and fluid intake. European Journal of Applied Physiology 73:317–325

Mitchell JW, Nadel ER, Stolwijk JAJ 1972 Respiratory weight losses during exercise. Journal of Applied Physiology 32:474–476

Montain SJ, Coyle EF 1992 Influence of graded dehydration on hyperthermia and cardiovascular drift during exercise. Journal of Applied Physiology 73:1340–1350

Montain SJ, Latzka WA, Sawka MN 1995 Control of thermoregulatory sweating is altered by hydration level and exercise intensity. Journal of Applied Physiology 79:1434–1439

Montain SJ, Smith SA, Matott RP, Zientara GP, Jolesz FA, Sawka MN 1998 Hypohydration effects on skeletal muscle performance and metabolism: a ^{31}P-MRS study. Journal of Applied Physiology 84:1889–1894

Montain SJ, Sawka MN, Wenger CB 2001 Hyponatremia associated with exercise: risk factors and pathogenesis. Exercise and Sports Science Review 29:113–117

Montain SJ, Cheuvront SN, Sawka MN 2006 Exertional hyponatremia: quantitative analyses for understanding etiology. British Journal of Sports Medicine 40:98–105

Murray R 1987 The effects of consuming carbohydrate-electrolyte beverages on gastric emptying and fluid absorption during and following exercise. Sports Medicine 4:322–351

Nicholas CW, Williams C, Phillips MI, Nowitz A 1996 Influence of ingesting a carbohydrate-electrolyte solution on endurance capacity during intermittent high intensity shuttle running. Journal of Sports Science 13:283–290

Nicholas CW, Tsintzas K, Boobis L, Williams C 1999 Carbohydrate-electrolyte ingestion during intermittent high-intensity running. Medicine and Science in Sports and Exercise 31:1280–1286

Nielsen B, Hyldig T, Bidstrup F, González-Alonso J, Christoffersen GRJ 2001 Brain activity and fatigue during prolonged exercise in the heat. Pflügers Archives 442:41–48

Nose H, Mack GW, Shi X, Nadel ER 1988a Involvement of sodium retention hormones during rehydration in humans. Journal of Applied Physiology 65:332–336

Nose H, Mack GW, Shi X, Nadel ER 1988b Role of osmolality and plasma volume during rehydration in humans. Journal of Applied Physiology 65:325–331

O'Brien C, Freund BJ, Sawka MN 1996 Hydration assessment during cold-weather military field training exercises. Arctic Medicine Research 55:20–26

O'Brien KK, Montain SJ, Corr WP, Sawka MN, Knapik J, Craig SC 2001 Overhydration hyponatremia in army trainees. Military Medicine 166:405–410

Rehrer N, Burke L 1996 Sweat losses during various sports. Australian Journal of Nutrition and Dietetics 53:S13–S16

Riedesel ML, Allen DY, Peake GT, Al-Qattan K 1987 Hyperhydration with glycerol solutions. Journal of Applied Physiology 63:2262–2268

Rolls BJ 1994 Palatability and fluid intake. In: Marriott BM (ed) Fluid replacement and heat stress. National Academy Press, Washington, DC, 161–168

Saunders AG, Dugas JP, Tucker R, Lambert MI, Noakes TD 2005 The effects of different air velocities on heat storage and body temperature in humans cycling in a hot, humid environment. Acta Physiologica Scandinavica 183:241–255

Sawka MN 1992 Physiological consequences of hypohydration: exercise performance and thermoregulation. Medicine and Science in Sports and Exercise 24:657–670

Sawka MN, Coyle EF 1999 Influence of body water and blood volume on thermoregulation and exercise performance in the heat. Exercise and Sport Science Reviews 27:167–218

Sawka MN, Cheuvront SN, Carter R III 2005 Human water needs. Nutrition Reviews 63:S30–S39

Shirreffs SM, Maughan RJ 1997 Whole body sweat collection in humans: an improved method with preliminary data on electrolyte content. Journal of Applied Physiology 82:336–341

Shirreffs SM, Maughan RJ 1998 Volume repletion following exercise-induced volume depletion in man: replacement of water and sodium losses. American Journal of Physiology 274:F868–F875

Shirreffs SM, Taylor AJ, Leiper JB, Maughan RJ 1996 Post-exercise rehydration in man: effects of volume consumed and drink sodium content. Medicine and Science in Sports and Exercise 28:1260–1271

Shirreffs SM, Armstrong LE, Cheuvront SN 2004a Fluid and electrolyte needs for preparation and recovery from training and competition. Journal of Sports Science 22:57–63

Shirreffs SM, Merson SJ, Fraser SM, Archer DT 2004b The effects of fluid restriction on hydration status and subjective feelings in man. British Journal of Nutrition 91:951–958

Speedy DB, Noakes TD, Kimber NE, Rogers IR, Thompson JMD, Boswell DR, Ross JJ, Campbell RGD, Gallagher PG 2001 Fluid balance during and after an Ironman triathlon. Clinical Journal of Sport Medicine 11:44–50

Wästerlund DS, Chaseling J, Burström L 2004 The effect of fluid consumption on the forest workers' performance strategy. Applied Ergonomics 35:29–36

Zambraski EJ 1996 The kidney and body fluid balance during exercise. In: Buskirk ER, Puhl SM (eds) Body fluid balance: exercise and sport. CRC Press, Boca Raton, FL, 75–95

Chapter **34**

Topical debates

Chapter 34.1

Sports supplements debate: a risky practice that produces expensive urine or legitimate performance boosts that can be found in a packet or bottle?

Louise M. Burke

CHAPTER CONTENTS

Part 1: Supplement use is a risky practice that produces expensive urine

1 INTRODUCTION

Around the world, people spend billions of dollars annually on supplements. The sports world represents a niche market of this industry, with athletes being targeted with products that claim to increase muscle mass, reduce body fat, enhance recovery, keep them healthy or directly improve performance. The marketing and word-of-mouth publicity involving sports foods and supplements are obviously effective, since many surveys have found that their use by athletes is a widespread and accepted practice. Typical outcomes of such studies are a high prevalence of use and a large range of different types and brands of products. For example, a study of 77 elite Australian swimmers (Baylis et al. 2001) found that 94% of the group reported the use of supplements in pill and powder form. When the use of specialised sports foods, such as sports drinks, was also taken into account, 99% of swimmers reported supplement use, and a total of 207 different products was identified. Supplement use, is also widespread among high school and collegiate athletes (Froiland et al. 2004, Massad et al. 1995), and other non-elite and recreational sportspeople.

There are many motives and incentives underpinning supplement use by athletes. Some products are used to address poor eating practices, or because of the belief that everyday foods are unable to provide the required amounts of nutrients or other food chemicals. Other supplements are chosen because of claims to directly enhance performance or physiological components that affect performance. Unfortunately, few of these claims are supported by rigorous scientific research (Chapter 34.2). Furthermore, not all athletes who use supplements and sports foods follow protocols that are known to be safe and effective. So, what is the downside of the use of these products?

Table 34.1.1 Problems identified by the Australian Institute of Sport with current supplement practices by athletes (modified from Burke 2003 with permission)

- Strategies that genuinely enhance performance (e.g. specialised training, sound nutrition practice, good equipment, adequate rest/sleep, mental preparation) are overlooked in favour of supplements.
- Athletes are drawn to new supplements with marketing hype rather than supplements and sports foods that might have true value in achieving nutrition goals.
- Ad hoc use of supplements often means that valuable supplements are not used in a manner that achieves optimal outcomes.
- Products with little value are a drain on limited resources (i.e. money, time, interest).
- Use of unproven supplements by well-known or successful athletes (and institutions) provides endorsement in the eyes of other athletes, and continues false expectations.
- Risk of side-effects.
- Risk of inadvertent positive doping outcomes.

The Australian Institute of Sport has identified a number of concerns regarding the use of supplements by its athletes (Table 34.1.1). Before these issues are explored, there is value in understanding the scene in which supplements and sports foods operate, since the lack of regulation, or the minimisation of its enforcement, is the source of many of these concerns.

2 REGULATION OF THE MANUFACTURE AND SALE OF SUPPLEMENTS AND SPORTS FOODS

There is no universal system for the regulation of the manufacture, labelling and marketing of sports foods and supplements. Countries differ in their approach and practice, with some involving a single government body (e.g. the Food and Drug Administration, USA), while others fall under several government agencies (e.g. Food Standards Australia and New Zealand for food-based products; Therapeutic Goods Administration for pill-based products in Australia). Athletes need to have a global appreciation of the regulation of dietary supplements, since regular travel and modern conveniences, such as mail order and the Internet, provide them with easy access to products that fall outside the scrutiny of their own country's system.

Although it is beyond the scope of this review to discuss the various regulatory issues in different countries, important changes that can be attributed to the Dietary Supplement Health and Education Act of 1994 in the US are worthy of special mention. This Act reduced the regulation of supplements and broadened the category to include new ingredients, such as herbal and botanical products, and constituents or metabolites of other dietary supplements. As a result, the last decade has seen an exponential rise in the number of dietary supplements and the introduction of

a new group of products, including pro-hormones such as androstenedione, dehydroepiandrosterone (DHEA), 19-norandrostenedione and other metabolites found in the steroid pathways that can be converted in the body to testosterone or the anabolic steroid nandrolone (Blue & Lombardo 1999). These products will be discussed later in the context of inadvertent doping outcomes.

The other important outcome of the Dietary Supplement Health and Education Act was to shift responsibility for enforcing safety and claim guidelines from the supplement manufacturer to the Food and Drug Administration. The sophistication of packaging and marketing often suggests that supplements are subjected to the same medical or scientific rigor as pharmaceutical agents. This is not the case. Instead, at most they are meant to comply with simple statutory standards; for example, to exclude ingredients banned by Customs laws within a country, to follow good manufacturing practice and to make limited therapeutic claims. In practice, these products receive little investigation of quality and advertising claims unless they are the subject of serious complaints regarding health and safety issues. Large companies that produce conventional supplements, such as vitamins and minerals, particularly to manufacturing standards used in the preparation of pharmaceutical products, are likely to achieve good quality control. This includes precision with ingredient levels and labelling, and avoidance of undeclared ingredients or contaminants. However, this does not appear to be true for all supplement types or manufacturers, with many examples of poor compliance with labelling laws (Gurley et al. 1998, Hahm et al. 1999, Parasrampuria et al. 1998) and the presence of contaminants and undeclared ingredients.

In addition, although manufacturers are not meant to make unsupported claims about health or performance benefits elicited by supplements, product advertisements and testimonials show ample evidence that this aspect of supplement marketing is unregulated and exploited. It is easy to see how enthusiastic and emotive claims provide a false sense of confidence about the products. Most consumers are unaware that the regulation of such advertising is generally not enforced. Therefore, athletes are likely to believe that claims about supplements are medically and scientifically supported, simply because they believe that untrue claims would not be allowed to exist.

3 POTENTIAL DISADVANTAGES OF SUPPLEMENTS AND SPORTS FOODS

3.1 Expense

An obvious issue with supplement use is the expense which, in extreme cases, can equal or exceed the athlete's weekly food budget. Such extremes include the small number of athletes identified in testimonials and surveys who report a polypharmacy approach to supplements, identifying long lists of products that often overlap in ingredients and claimed functions. However, even an interest in a small number of supplements can be expensive: the cost of some products, such as ribose or colostrum, can exceed AUD50 per week to achieve the manufacturer's recommended dose, or the amounts found to have a true ergogenic outcome in scientific studies. The issue of expense is compounded for teams and sports programmes that have to supply the needs of a group of athletes.

Expense must be carefully considered when there is little scientific evidence to support a product's claims of direct or indirect benefits to athletic performance. But even where benefits do exist, cost is an issue that athletes must acknowledge and prioritise appropriately within their total budget. Supplements or sports foods generally provide nutrients or food constituents at a price that is considerably higher than that of everyday foods. There are often lower-cost alternatives to some supplements and sports foods that the budget-conscious athlete can use. For example, a fruit drink fortified with milk powder is a less expensive choice to supplement energy and protein intake than most protein-rich products marketed to body builders.

3.2 Distraction from the real priorities

The displacement of an athlete's true priorities and distraction of attention from sound strategies to enhance performance are more subtle outcomes of reliance on supplements. Athletes can sometimes be side-tracked from the true elements of success in the search for short-cuts from bottles and packets. Successful sports performance is the product of superior genetics, long-term training, optimal nutrition, state-of-the-art equipment and a committed attitude. These factors cannot be replaced by the use of supplements, but often appear less exciting or more demanding than the enthusiastic and emotive claims made for many supplements and sports foods. Even among supplements, there is often an inverse relationship between the hype associated with the product and the scientific support for the use of the product. Many sports dieticians will attest that athletes are more interested in the latest fad supplement than long-term and scientifically supported products.

The focus on short-cuts at the expense of a commitment to sound practices is a particular concern when it involves younger athletes. The young athlete can expect to see substantial improvements in performance as a result of their growth and maturation, and experience in their sport. Compared with this potential, most people consider the use of supplements to be of minor value. In fact, various expert groups, such as the American Academy of Pediatrics, have condemned the use of ergogenic aids, including various dietary supplements, by children and adolescents (Gomez 2005). The American College of Sports Medicine (2000) recommends that creatine not be used by people under 18 years. These policies are based not only on the unknown health consequences of some supplements, but also the implications of supplement use on the ethics of sport and the morals of a young athlete (see Section 6 Introduction). Some people consider supplements as an entry point to the decision to take more serious compounds, including prohibited drugs, although the evidence to support this claim is not clear.

3.3 Side-effects

Because most supplements are considered by regulatory bodies to be relatively safe, many countries do not have mandatory reporting processes to document adverse side-effects arising from the use of these products. Nevertheless, information from medical registers shows that the risk to public health from the use of supplements and herbal products includes problems of toxicity, allergic reactions, overexposure as a result of self-medication and poisoning due to contaminants (Kozyrskyj 1997, Perharic et al. 1994, Shaw et al. 1997). Tryptophan supplements were associated with deaths and medical problems during the 1980 and 1990s (Roufs 1992), with the suggested cause being contamination of the tryptophan during its manufacture by a microbial process. More recently, products containing the stimulants ephedrine and caffeine have raised health concerns, and have been linked to deaths from heart arrhythmias or heat illnesses in susceptible individuals (Charatan 2003). Many reports call for better regulation and surveillance of supplements and herbal products and increased awareness of potential hazards (Kozyrskyj 1997, Perharic et al. 1994, Shaw et al. 1997).

3.4 Inadvertent doping outcomes

Some supplements contain ingredients that are considered prohibited substances by the codes of the World Anti-Doping Agency, the National Collegiate Athletics Associations and other sports bodies. These include pro-hormones and stimulants, such as ephedrine or related substances. Drug education programmes in sport highlight the need for athletes to read the labels of supplements and sports foods very carefully, to ensure that they do not contain banned substances. This is a responsibility that athletes must master to prevent inadvertent doping outcomes.

Even when athletes take such precautions, inadvertent intake of banned substances from supplement products can still occur. This is because some supplements contain banned products without declaring them as ingredients. This has generally been considered a result of inadvertent contamination or poor labelling within lax manufacturing processes. However, there are some recent examples where the presence of steroid compounds in therapeutic doses in supplements seems a more deliberate activity (Geyer et al. 2003). The pro-hormone compounds seem to be at greatest risk of being found as undeclared contaminants in supplements, and a positive test for the steroid nandrolone is one of the possible outcomes of their intake. The most cited evidence of these problems is a study carried out by a laboratory accredited by the International Olympic Committee (Geyer et al. 2004). This laboratory analysed 634 supplements from 215 suppliers across 13 countries, with products coming from retail outlets (91%), the Internet (8%) and telephone sales. None of these supplements declared pro-hormones as ingredients, yet 94 products (15%) were found to contain hormones or prohormones. A further 10% of samples provided technical difficulties in analysis, such that the absence of hormones could not be guaranteed. Of the positive supplements, 68% contained pro-hormones of testosterone, 7% contained pro-hormones of nandrolone and 25% contained compounds related to both. Forty-nine of the supplements contained only one steroid, but 45 contained more than one, with eight products containing five or more different steroid products. The positive supplements contained steroid concentrations ranging from 0.01 to 190 $\mu g \cdot g^{-1}$ of product. It was noted that a positive urinary test for nandrolone metabolites occurs in the hours following uptake of as little as 1 μg of nandrolone pro-hormones.

Other findings of this study make it difficult to make recommendations to athletes about how to avoid the type and source of supplements that are most at risk of causing a positive doping outcome. According to product labels, the countries of manufacture of all supplements containing steroids were the USA, the Netherlands, the UK, Italy and Germany. However, these products were purchased in other countries. In fact, 10–20% of products purchased in Spain and Austria were found to be contaminated. Just over 20% of the products made by companies which also made other products containing pro-hormones were positive for undeclared pro-hormones, but 10% of products from companies that did not sell steroid-containing supplements were also positive. The brand names of the positive products were not provided in the study, but included amino acid supplements, protein powders and products containing creatine, carnitine, ribose, guarana, zinc, pyruvate, hydroxyl-methyl butyrate, *Tribulus terristris*, herbal extracts and vitamins/minerals.

This is a major area of concern for serious athletes who compete under anti-doping codes, since most codes place strict liability with the athlete for ingestion of banned substances, regardless of the circumstances and the source of ingestion. There are a number of examples where an athlete has received a full or substantial penalty, despite evidence that the source of the banned substance found in their urine was a contaminated or poorly labelled supplement. Further information on contamination of supplements can be found in reviews by Maughan (2005) and Burke (2007). Athletes should make enquiries at the anti-doping agencies within their countries for advice on the specific risks identified with supplement use and any initiatives to reduce this risk.

Part 2: Legitimate performance boosts can be found in a packet or bottle – how can an athlete resist?

1 INTRODUCTION

The margins between the winners in an event and the rest of the field are tantalisingly small (Chapters 10.1 and 10.2).

Table 34.1.2 Potentially valuable characteristics of a sports foods or supplement (modified from Burke 2003 with permission)

- Packages a precise or compact dose of nutrient(s), especially to meet nutrient recommendations for a specialised situation (e.g. pre-event, during event, postevent nutrition).
- Provides a good source of nutrient(s) at risk in the diets of athletes or subgroups of athletes.
- Has simple preparation/storage needs, with a long shelf-life.
- Is portable and conveniently packaged.
- Communicates an educational message related to sports nutrition goals.
- Is easily consumed with a low risk of gastrointestinal upsets or discomfort.
- Contains ergogenic compounds known to enhance sports performance in specific situations.

This helps to explain the motivation of top athletes to search for strategies or products that may enhance performance by even a small amount. But even when the stakes do not involve fame and fortune, athletes are fascinated by the promise of a personal best. Sound eating practices are recognised as an important factor in the achievement of optimal performance. However, there are times when an athlete could benefit from the use of more than everyday foods. Thus, an industry that produces sports foods and supplements has arisen to meet the specialised nutritional needs of athletes. Although many products may not meet the scrutiny of rigorous scientific research, there are a number of legitimate products that may assist the athlete to achieve their sporting goals. The characteristics of useful sports foods and supplements are summarised in Table 34.1.2.

2 DIETARY SUPPLEMENTS THAT ASSIST IN ACHIEVING NUTRITION GOALS

Over the past decades, the science of sports nutrition has become well defined and supported by rigorous research (Chapters 32, 33 and 34.2). In many cases, the guidelines for sports nutrition recommend that an athlete consume energy and nutrients in amounts that are beyond appetite or gastrointestinal comfort or at times when it is difficult to find or consume everyday foods. Under such circumstances, a sports food that allows the athlete to meet these specific goals may directly or indirectly enhance performance. Table 34.1.3 summarises the major classes of sports foods, together with the situations or goals of sports nutrition that these products might address. The substantiation for many of these nutrition goals is well accepted and includes situations where a measurable enhancement of performance can be detected as a result of the correct use of the sports food.

Some specialised sports products (e.g. sports drinks) have crossed successfully into the general market. As long as general consumers are prepared to pay an increased

Table 34.1.3 Sports foods and dietary supplements used to meet nutritional goals (modified from Burke et al. 2006 with permission)

Product	Form	Composition	Sports-related use
Sports drink	Powder or liquid	5–8% carbohydrate 10–35 mmol·L^{-1} sodium 3–5 mmol·L^{-1} potassium	• Optimum delivery of fluid + carbohydrate during exercise • Postexercise rehydration • Postexercise refuelling
Sports gel	Gel 30–40 g sachets or larger tubes	60–70% carbohydrate (~25 g per sachet) Some contain caffeine or electrolytes	• Supplement high-carbohydrate training diet • Carbohydrate loading • Postexercise carbohydrate recovery • May be used during exercise when carbohydrate needs exceed fluid requirements
Electrolyte replacement supplements 1. Oral rehydration solutions 2. Electrolyte-only supplements	1. Powder sachets or tablets to make drink 2. Tablets or sachets of salts to be added to other drinks	1. ≤2% carbohydrate 50–60 mmol·L^{-1} sodium 10–20 mmol·L^{-1} potassium 2. 50–60 mmol·L^{-1} sodium 10–20 mmol·L^{-1} potassium	• Rapid and effective rehydration following dehydration undertaken for weight-making • Replacement of large sodium losses during ultra-endurance activities • Rapid and effective rehydration following moderate to large fluid and sodium deficits
Liquid meal supplement	Powder (mixed with water or milk)	4–6 kJ·mL^{-1} 15–20% protein 50–70% carbohydrate Low to moderate fat Vitamins/minerals: 500–1000 mL supplies RDI/RDAs	• Supplement high energy/carbohydrate/nutrient diet (especially during heavy training/competition or weight gain) • Low-bulk meal replacement (especially pre-event) • Postexercise recovery: provides carbohydrate, protein and micronutrients • Portable nutrition for travelling athlete
Sports bar	Bar (50–60 g)	40–50 g carbohydrate 5–10 g protein Usually low in fat and fibre Vitamins/minerals: 50–100% of RDA/RDIs May contain creatine, amino acids	• Carbohydrate source during exercise • Postexercise recovery: provides carbohydrate, protein and micronutrients • Supplements high energy/carbohydrate/nutrient diet • Portable nutrition

price for specialised products, and sports nutrition messages are left intact, most nutrition experts are not unduly concerned by this outcome. In fact, the use of sports drinks by weekend warriors and recreational exercisers can often be defended, but is vigorously challenged by others (Chapter 34.2). After all, the benefits of fluid intake and carbohydrate replacement during a workout are determined by the physiology of exercise, rather than the calibre of the person who is exercising. It should also be noted that most studies of supplements such as sports drinks have been undertaken on moderate- to well-trained performers rather than elite athletes. Therefore, where evidence of performance benefit does exist, it is directly relevant to these subelite populations.

Dietary supplements that can assist the athlete to achieve their nutrition goals include products supplying micronutrients that are used to correct or prevent a micronutrient deficiency. As with sports foods, these uses are specialised and individualised to a specific athlete or situation. When used according to the situations summarised in Table 34.1.3, these dietary supplements may directly or indirectly enhance performance.

2.1 Substances that are proven to achieve an ergogenic effect

The marketing hype that surrounds the claims for many ingredients in sports supplements sometimes hides the fact that a few products do enjoy sound scientific support for their ability to enhance sports performance. The most credible ergogenic aids are reviewed below. However, it is important that athletes recognise that it is the correct use of the product in the appropriate scenario in sport that achieves the outcome, rather than the product per se. In addition, there is some evidence that some individuals are responders while others are non-responders to these effects. This creates an important role for sports scientists to work with athletes and coaches to find the individuals and situations in which true value from the use of an ergogenic aid is achieved.

As well as the ergogenic aids reviewed below, there are other products that offer promise of benefits via preliminary data or sound hypotheses. Products such as glycerol for hyperhydration (Chapter 33), colostrum, antioxidants and hydroxyl-methyl butyrate possibly merit further investigation and, in future, may be considered to be proven aids for athletic performance. Of course, the limitations of research into performance enhancement must be considered. It is possible that these and other products may produce improvements in performance that are too small to be detected using traditional research design and analytical methods, but are still worthwhile in changing the outcomes of the close competition in sport. Hopkins and colleagues (1999) produced guidelines to improve the ability of research to detect performance changes, as well as new paradigms to interpret the results in light of what is meaningful to sport (Batterham & Hopkins 2006).

2.1.1 Caffeine

Caffeine is a drug that enjoys social acceptance and widespread use around the world because of its entrenched position in daily life. It has been used by athletes for over a century to reduce fatigue and enhance performance, although its use has been restricted or banned by some antidoping codes; it was removed from the World Anti-Doping Agency list of prohibited substances in January 2004. Caffeine exerts a complex range of actions on body organs and it is sometimes difficult to pinpoint the exact mechanism by which it achieves performance enhancements. Nevertheless, caffeine's impact on the central nervous system to mask the perception of fatigue is likely to be an important effect. This may help to explain why caffeine has been shown to enhance endurance and performance of a large range of exercise protocols, particularly with events of prolonged sustained or intermittent activity. The effects on sprint and power events are less clear.

Traditional protocols for the use of caffeine involve the intake of caffeine 1 h before an exercise bout, in doses equivalent to ~6 mg·kg^{-1} body mass (300–500 mg for a typical athlete). However, there is new evidence, at least from studies involving prolonged exercise lasting 60 min or longer, that beneficial effects from caffeine occur at small to moderate levels of intake (1–3 mg·g^{-1} or 50–200 mg of caffeine). In fact, several studies fail to show evidence of a dose–response relationship to caffeine; that is, performance benefits do not increase with increases in the caffeine dose (Cox et al. 2002, Pasman et al. 1995). Finally, it appears that caffeine can be beneficial when consumed at a variety of times during exercise: before or throughout the activity, or towards the end of exercise, when the athlete is becoming fatigued. For more information about caffeine and exercise performance, the reader is directed to Graham (2001).

2.1.2 Creatine

Creatine is a naturally occurring compound found in large amounts in skeletal muscle, as a result of dietary intake and endogenous synthesis from amino acids. Creatine monohydrate is the most common of creatine supplements and a major industry has exploded since reports in the early 1990s that muscle creatine and creatine phosphate content could be increased by protocols of rapid (5 days at 20 g·d^{-1} in split doses) or slow (3–5 g·d^{-1} for 28 d) loading (Hultman et al. 1996). There are individual responses to creatine loading, and it is believed that athletes with the lowest resting muscle content show the greatest response, while those with pre-existing stores of creatine close to the muscle threshold are unlikely to show additional benefits from creatine supplementation (non-responders). Creatine plays a number of roles in cell metabolism, including the provision of phosphocreatine as a rapidly acting but short-lived fuel source for high-intensity exercise. An increase in muscle stores of phosphocreatine would be potentially valuable for exercise in which this fuel source was important but limited in supply.

There are now more than 100 studies of creatine supplementation and exercise, and the consensus is that creatine loading can enhance the performance of exercise involving repeated sprints, or bouts of high-intensity exercise, separated by short recovery intervals. Such an exercise protocol may be limited by the resynthesis of phosphocreatine stores between bouts (Chapter 6). Therefore, creatine supplementation may be of value in resistance training programmes to further increase lean body mass and strength, in interval and sprint training programmes, and to aid training and competition in sports involving intermittent work patterns (e.g. team and racket sports). Recent studies show that creatine can enhance the effectiveness of carbohydrate-loading programme for endurance exercise. One caveat to the current literature is that more studies are needed using highly trained and elite athletes and sports-specific protocols.

Although concerns regarding the long-term use of creatine have been aired, there is currently no evidence of important side-effects or health concerns when athletes use creatine at the doses previously outlined. Further information on creatine supplementation can be found in the following reviews (Branch 2003, Greenhaff 2000, Hespel et al. 2001).

2.1.3 Bicarbonate and citrate for buffering

High rates of anaerobic glycolysis by muscle during high-intensity exercise are associated with a build-up of lactate and hydrogen ions. When intracellular buffering capacity is exceeded, lactate and hydrogen ions diffuse into the extracellular space, aided by a positive pH gradient. Extracellular buffering capacity can be increased by loading with bicarbonate or citrate. These supplements may be taken in the form of specialised sports supplements, as household products (e.g. bicarbonate of soda) or as pharmaceutical urinary alkalinisers (McNaughton 2000). Typical doses for acute loading are 0.3 g·kg^{-1} bicarbonate and 0.3–0.5 g·kg^{-1} citrate, taken 60–90 min before exercise. Buffering agents should be consumed with 1–2 L of water to reduce gastrointestinal problems attributable to osmotic diarrhoea. A longer (chronic) loading protocol with bicarbonate (e.g. 0.5 mg·kg^{-1}·d^{-1} spread over the day) may provide a more sustained increase in blood pH, with benefits being maintained for at least 1 day following the last bicarbonate dose (McNaughton et al. 2000). This protocol may be suited to athletes who compete in a series of events spread over a couple of days, replacing the need to undertake multiple acute dose protocols.

An increase in extracellular buffering capacity may aid an athlete's capacity to produce power during sports or events limited by excessive build-up of hydrogen ions, although readers should carefully consider the discussions in Chapters 6 and 10.3 that challenge some aspects of this fatigue mechanism. There is research support for performance enhancement with bicarbonate loading in high-intensity events lasting 1–7 min, sports involving repeated high-intensity sprints and prolonged high-intensity events lasting 30–60 min (Burke 2007). Recent research indicates that chronic or repeated use of acute bicarbonate supplementation before interval training sessions can enhance training adaptations and subsequent performance of sustained high-intensity exercise (Edge et al. 2006).

2.2 The value of the placebo effect

Even when a supplement or sports food does not produce a true physiological or ergogenic benefit, an athlete might perform better because of a psychological boost or placebo effect associated with supplement use. The placebo effect describes a favourable outcome arising simply from an individual's belief that they have received a beneficial treatment. In a clinical environment, a patient's belief that they need to receive therapy is often addressed in the form of a harmless but inactive (placebo) substance or treatment. This is sometimes associated with a perception of, or even measurable, improvement in the patient's symptoms. In a sports setting, an athlete who receives enthusiastic marketing material about a new supplement or hears glowing testimonials from other athletes who have used it is more likely to report a positive experience.

Despite our belief that the placebo effect is real and potentially substantial, only a few studies have tried to document this effect in relation to sport. In one investigation, weightlifters who received saline injections that they believed to be anabolic steroids increased their gains in lean body mass

(Ariel & Saville 1972). Another investigation involving the use of a sports drink or a sweetened placebo during a 1 h cycling time trial found that performance was affected by the information provided to the subjects (Clark et al. 2000). Subjects who believed they were receiving a carbohydrate drink increased the distance achieved during the time trial by ~4%. Being unsure of which treatment was being received increased the variability of performance, illustrating that the greatest benefits from supplement use occur when athletes are confident they are receiving a useful product.

In this regard, one must also consider this effect within the context of the scientific literature. For example, when an experiment, either through design weaknesses or limitations beyond the control of the researchers, is unable to limit the impact of the placebo effect on the primary dependent variables, then data interpretation may be difficult, and become skewed in favour of the treatment under investigation. Thus, it is possible that some research is also affected by the subjects believing they were being exposed to a substance that may improve physiological performance.

Additional, well-controlled studies are needed to better describe the potential size and duration of the placebo effect, and whether it applies equally to all athletes and across all types of performance. In the meantime, we can accept that the placebo effect exists and may explain, at least partially, why athletes report performance benefits after trying a new supplement or dietary treatment. The placebo effect is probably best used when added to a direct physiological or ergogenic effect achieved by a supplement or sports foods. However, many practitioners are happy to accept that in the absence of side-effects, and when the athlete is prepared to bear the cost of a supplement, the potential for a small confidence boost can be of value to the athlete.

Part 3: Concluding commentary

Athletes, coaches and parents want a single and simple answer to the question 'do I need to take supplements and sports foods to perform at my best?'. In fact, the answer can be either 'yes' or 'no', depending on the strict definition applied to each of the words in this question. The issues involved in the use of supplements and sports foods are complex. There are certainly examples of the beneficial uses of sports foods and supplements – where an athlete has used a product according to evidence-based protocols to achieve his or her nutrition goals, or to gain a real physiological advantage. In these cases, the use of the product may assist the athlete to train or compete at an optimal level, whether it be during an Olympic final or in the pursuit of a personal best by a recreational exerciser. However, there are also many examples where athletes consume products that are unsupported by science, at risk of being contaminated or an unnecessary expense. The decision to use supplements and sports foods must be made on an individual basis with full knowledge of the issues involved.

References

American College of Sports Medicine 2000 Roundtable: the physiological and health effects of oral creatine supplementation. Medicine and Science in Sports and Exercise 32:706–717

Ariel G, Saville W 1972 Anabolic steroids: the physiological effects of placebos. Medicine and Science in Sports and Exercise 4:124–126

Batterham AM, Hopkins WG 2006 Making meaningful inferences about magnitudes. International Journal of Sports Physiology and Performance 1:50–57

Baylis A, Cameron-Smith D, Burke LM 2001 Inadvertent doping though supplement use by athletes: assessment and management of the risk in Australia. International Journal of Sport Nutrition and Exercise Metabolism 11:365–383

Blue JG, Lombardo JA 1999 Steroids and steroid-like compounds. Clinics in Sports Medicine 18:667–689

Branch JD 2003 Effect of creatine supplementation on body composition and performance: a meta-analysis. International Journal of Sport Nutrition and Exercise Metabolism 13:198–226

Burke L 2003 Sports supplements and sports foods. In: Hargreaves M, Hawley J (eds) Physiological bases of sports performance. McGraw-Hill, Sydney, 183–253

Burke L 2007 Supplements and sports foods. In: Practical sports nutrition. Human Kinetics, Champaign, IL

Burke L, Cort M, Cox GR, Crawford R, Minehan M, Wood C 2006 Supplements and sports foods. In: Burke L, Deakin V (eds) Clinical sports nutrition. McGraw-Hill, Sydney, 485–579

Charatan F 2003 Ephedra supplement may have contributed to sportsman's death. British Medical Journal 326:464

Clark VR, Hopkins WG, Hawley JA, Burke LM 2000 Placebo effect of carbohydrate feedings during a 40-km cycling time trial. Medicine and Science in Sports and Exercise 32:1642–1647

Cox GR, Desbrow B, Montgomery PG, Anderson ME, Bruce CR, Macrides TA, Martin DT, Moquin A, Roberts A, Hawley JA, Burke LM 2002 Effect of different protocols of caffeine intake on metabolism and endurance performance. Journal of Applied Physiology 93:990–999

Edge J, Bishop D, Goodman C 2006 Effects of chronic bicarbonate ingestion during interval training on changes to muscle buffering capacity and short term endurance performance. Journal of Applied Physiology 101:918–925

Froiland K, Koszewski W, Hingst J, Kopecky L 2004 Nutritional supplement use among college athletes and their sources of information. International Journal of Sport Nutrition and Exercise Metabolism 14:104–120

Geyer H, Bredehoft M, Mareck U, Parr M, Schänzer W 2003 High doses of the anabolic steroid metandienone found in dietary supplements. European Journal of Sport Science 3:1–5

Geyer H, Parr MK, Mareck U, Reinhart U, Schrader Y, Schänzer W 2004 Analysis of non-hormonal nutritional supplements for anabolic-androgenic steroids – results of an international study. International Journal of Sports Medicine 25:124–129

Gomez J 2005 American Academy of Pediatrics Committee on Sports Medicine and Fitness: use of performance-enhancing substances. Pediatrics 115:1103–1106

Graham TE 2001 Caffeine and exercise: metabolism, endurance and performance. Sports Medicine 31:765–785

Greenhaff PL 2000 Creatine. In: Maughan R (ed) Nutrition in sport. Blackwell Science, Oxford, 367–378

Gurley BJ, Wang P, Gardner SF 1998 Ephedrine-type alkaloid content of nutritional supplements containing Ephedra sinica (Ma-huang) as determined by high performance liquid chromatography. Journal of Pharmaceutical Sciences 87:1547–1553

Hahm H, Kujawa J, Ausberger L 1999 Comparison of melatonin products against USP's nutritional supplements standards and other criteria. Journal of the American Pharmaceutical Association 39:27–31

Hespel P, Eijnde BO, Derave W, Richter EA 2001 Creatine supplementation: exploring the role of the creatine kinase/ phosphocreatine system in the human muscle. Canadian Journal of Applied Physiology 26:S79–S102

Hopkins WG, Hawley JA, Burke LM 1999 Design and analysis of research on sport performance enhancement. Medicine and Science in Sports and Exercise 31:472–485

Hultman E, Söderlund K, Timmons JA, Cederblad G, Greenhaff PL 1996 Muscle creatine loading in men. Journal of Applied Physiology 81:232–237

Kozyrskyj A 1997 Herbal products in Canada. How safe are they? Canadian Family Physician 43:697–702

McNaughton L 2000 Bicarbonate and citrate. In: Maughan R (ed) Nutrition in sport. Blackwell Science, Oxford, 393–404

McNaughton L, Strange N, Backx K 2000 The effects of chronic sodium bicarbonate ingestion on multiple bouts of anaerobic work and power output. Journal of Human Movement Studies 38:307–322

Massad SJ, Shier NW, Koceja DM, Ellis NT 1995 High school athletes and nutritional supplements: a study of knowledge and use. International Journal of Sport Nutrition 5:232–245

Maughan RJ 2005 Contamination of dietary supplements and positive drug tests in sport. Journal of Sports Sciences 23:883–889

Parasrampuria J, Schwartz K, Petesch R 1998 Quality control of dehydroepiandrosterone dietary supplement products. Journal of the American Medical Association 280:1565

Pasman WJ, van Baak MA, Jeukendrup AE, de Haan A 1995 The effect of different dosages of caffeine on endurance performance time. International Journal of Sports Medicine 16:225–230

Perharic L, Shaw D, Colbridge M, House I, Leon C, Murray V 1994 Toxicological problems resulting from exposure to traditional remedies and food supplements. Drug Safety 11:284–294

Roufs JB 1992 Review of L-tryptophan and eosinophilia-myalgia syndrome. Journal of the American Dietetic Association 92:844–850

Shaw D, Leon C, Kolev S, Murray V 1997 Traditional remedies and food supplements. A 5-year toxicological study (1991–1995). Drug Safety 17:342–356

Chapter **34.2**

Current drinking guidelines are not evidence based

Timothy D. Noakes

1 INTRODUCTION

Some current drinking guidelines propose that athletes should drink as much as tolerable during exercise or replace all mass lost during exercise, since thirst is not an accurate guide to fluid replacement requirements during exercise. Since some individuals can tolerate water ingestion that exceeds free water loss during exercise, this advice has caused some to overdrink, leading to water retention, body mass gains and, in a few, death from exercise-associated hyponatraemic encephalopathy (Noakes & Speedy 2006). Fatalities from this preventable condition have been reported in military personnel and female marathoners, uniquely in the USA. Such fatalities are often associated with the inappropriate treatment of affected individuals with intravenous infusions of isotonic or hypotonic saline solutions.

In this chapter, it is argued that contemporary drinking guidelines lack an adequate scientifically proven evidence base, and that they have not been properly evaluated in appropriately controlled clinical trials (also see Noakes 2007a). It is further argued that the evidence of how much to drink during exercise is well established in the published literature, but appears to have been ignored. These guidelines lack an adequate evidence base in several specific areas.

2 DRINKING GUIDELINES

Since 1976, the American College of Sports Medicine has produced four position statements on fluid ingestion. Other organisations, including the US military, the National Athletic Trainers Association, the American Dietetic Association and Dieticians of Canada and, more recently, the International Olympic Committee (Coyle 2004), have produced similar guidelines (Noakes 2007a).

2.1 The ACSM drinking guidelines

The current guidelines include the recommendation that one should attempt to replace all water lost as sweat, consuming the maximal volume tolerable. It is also suggested that carbohydrates can be supplied, without compromising fluid delivery, by drinking a 4–8% carbohydrate solution at rates of 600–1200 mL·h^{-1}.

The goal of these recommendations is to simultaneously optimise performance and reduce the risk of heat illness. However, it is apparent that such guidelines are based on a model of exercise that includes five principal assumptions. The veracity of these assumptions will now be explored.

1. There is no published evidence proving that drinking is necessary to preserve health, or to provide any unique physiological benefit, during exercise lasting <60–90 min, although it does reduce thirst.

2. There is no evidence from realistic (real-world) laboratory studies that drinking according to thirst (ad libitum) produces a less desirable outcome.

3. Whilst there is evidence that dehydration is associated with impaired performance, its relevance to competitive sports is not yet established. No study has yet established the cross-over point at which the performance-enhancing effects of body mass reduction are negated by the established performance-diminishing effects of dehydration.

4. There is no published evidence proving that sodium replacement in excess of that present in the typical Western diet is ever required during any form of exercise, regardless of its intensity or duration.

5. There is proof that the avoidance of overdrinking is necessary to prevent hyponatraemia. This is caused by inadequate renal free water clearance, with an expansion of the total body water and a failure to suppress vasopressin (antidiuretic hormone) secretion in some susceptible individuals.

2.1.1 Assumption 1: mass loss is detrimental to health and performance

This has not been established. As will be argued subsequently, there is no evidence that mass losses (2–4%), incurred when fluid is readily available and when athletes drink according to thirst, place athletes at increased risk of illness or impaired performance.

2.1.2 Assumption 2: fluid ingestion alone can prevent heat illness

This is improbable since there is no evidence that either heatstroke or heat syncope is linked to the degree of sweat loss (Noakes 1995). Furthermore, most athletes treated for heat illness experience difficulties after the completion of exercise (Noakes 2007b). Since cardiovascular strain, caused by fluid loss, must cause collapse during exercise, that is, when the demands on the cardiovascular system are the greatest, this finding shows that dehydration cannot be the cause of the immediate postexercise collapse. Rather, the cause must be linked to the sudden cessation of exercise and the development of postural hypotension (Noakes 2007b).

2.1.3 Assumption 3: thirst is an inadequate guide to fluid replacement

This is a natural consequence of the argument that athletes should drink to prevent mass loss. The logic for this argument is that, since athletes who drink to the dictates of thirst always lose body mass (voluntary dehydration), then clearly the body is unable to accurately determine its fluid requirements during exercise.

But the reality is that the human physiology did not evolve to defend body mass. Rather, the regulated variables of relevance to fluid balance are serum osmolality and blood pressure (mean arterial and central venous: Chapters 18 and 19). Thus, thirst is stimulated by a rising serum osmolality, even whilst it remains within the normal physiological range of 280–295 mOsm·kg H$_2$O^{-1} (Hew-Butler et al. 2006).

In contrast, were the body designed to protect (regulate) its mass (increased drive to drink), then serum osmolality would fall progressively as fuel is used and water stored with glycogen is released, leading to hypotonic hyponatraemia, intracellular fluid overload with cerebral oedema (Noakes et al. 2005).

2.1.4 Assumption 4: it is safe to drink 'as much as tolerable'

Drinking in excess of sweat and urine losses can produce exercise-associated hyponatraemia and may lead to the potentially fatal condition of hyponatraemic encephalopathy. These conditions cannot occur without excessive fluid consumption (Hew-Butler et al. 2005, Noakes et al. 2005). Hence, it is not safe for all people to drink as much as tolerable.

2.1.5 Assumption 5: all people have identical fluid replacement requirements under all conditions

Since sweat rates are influenced by metabolic rate during exercise and, to a lesser extent, environmental conditions, it is most unlikely that all people will have the same fluid replacement requirements. Sweat rates can vary widely: ~200 mL·h^{-1} in ultramarathoners competing in the Alaskan cold (Stuempfle et al. 2002, 2003); ~500 mL·h^{-1} in slow women marathoners (Twerenbold et al. 2003); 1800 mL·h^{-1} in cross-country runners; >2100 mL·h^{-1} in American football players training in the heat (Fowkes Godek et al. 2005). Hence, fluid guidelines for any one of these groups will be hopelessly inappropriate for the others.

2.2 Opposing guidelines

The International Marathon Medical Directors Association and the USA Track and Field have now accepted a different set of guidelines (Noakes 2003), and these differ in a number of ways from those described above. In this section, it is argued that the former guidelines lack an adequate evidence base to support an apparent consensus (Noakes 2004, 2007a). In addition, prior to adoption, these guidelines were not evaluated in properly designed clinical trials. Rather, the drafters of these guidelines appear to have ignored a body of evidence that might support alternative conclusions (Noakes1995, 2003).

Herein, the validity of some of the conclusions that are presented as the singular truth is interrogated. But instead of exhaustively investigating the appropriateness of the evidence base that supports their conclusions, it is perhaps more appropriate to examine the scientific evidence that supports the guidelines in four specific areas where the two groups of guidelines appear to be in greatest disagreement.

2.2.1 Issue 1: dehydration and performance decrement

The consensus guidelines are based on the belief that full replacement of fluid lost during exercise can optimise performance and minimise health risks.

What is the evidence from appropriately controlled, prospective clinical trials that shows that athletes who compete in out-of-doors events benefit by full mass replacement during exercise? Since these guidelines are mostly applied to out-of-doors exercise, it is important that this question is answered. Definitive outcome measures would presumably include proof that this drinking regimen improves exercise performance and reduces the incidence of heatstroke more than does any other drinking behaviour.

Comparison with studies in which no fluid is ingested during exercise would obviously not be appropriate, since no one claims that not drinking is the most appropriate behaviour for athletes. Rather, the control condition needs to be drinking ad libitum, as this is the more natural behaviour.

Experimental variables that need to be considered include the exercise intensity and duration, environmental conditions and exercise mode, in particular whether exercise involves body mass bearing. This is important since some mass loss is advantageous, since it reduces the energy cost of movement. The magnitude of this potential effect needs to be determined.

Answers to these questions would need also to be balanced against evidence that people who attempt to fully replace sweat loses might develop adverse consequences such as impaired performance, gastrointestinal symptoms and an increased probability for a reduced serum sodium concentration (Baker et al. 2005, Glace et al. 2002, Robinson et al. 1995, Stuempfle et al. 2002, 2003, Twerenbold et al. 2003).

If it is crucial to replace all fluid lost during exercise, then why is it that the best athletes in the world seem to religiously avoid this advice? It must be clear, even to the most unobservant, that the world's best marathoners and cyclists, in events lasting 1–3 h, do not ingest 1.2 L·h⁻¹ during international competition.

Indeed, low fluid intakes in competitive athletes are well described in the literature (Buskirk & Beetham1960, Muir et al. 1970, Noakes 1995, Pugh et al. 1967, Wyndham & Strydom 1969), particularly prior to 1969, when athletes were advised not to drink during exercise, regardless of duration, intensity or environmental conditions (Noakes 1993). One must question how these athletes were able to survive this practice prior to adoption of the first ACSM guidelines in 1975, let alone produce remarkable athletic performances, and without any apparent risk to their health. Indeed, the evidence is that world record performances in the marathon improved most between 1930 and 1960 (Nevill & Whyte 2005, Noakes 1993).

One paper used to support the current drinking guidelines reported a linear relationship between average marathon running speed and mass loss, such that athletes who were the most dehydrated ran the fastest (Cheuvront et al. 2003). The authors caution against interpreting such evidence as supporting an ergogenic effect of dehydration. However, the authors provide no explanation of why it is wrong to draw this conclusion, particularly in weight-bearing activities, yet they acknowledge, as many before, that the paradox of elite performance when dehydrated remains unresolved (Buskirk & Beetham1960, Byrne et al. 2006, Laursen et al. 2006, Muir et al. 1970, Pugh et al. 1967, Sharwood et al. 2002, 2004, Wharam et al. 2006). Perhaps humans evolved to run long distances in the heat without drinking, with evolution selecting in favour of this ability (Heinrich 2001).

What is the published evidence showing that replacing all the water lost through sweating improves performance more and reduces the risk of heatstroke more effectively than does drinking ad libitum (according to thirst)? We were unable to trace such evidence. Rather, separate studies show that ad libitum drinking is at least as effective as the current ACSM guideline (Cheuvront & Haymes 2001, Daries et al. 2000, McConell et al. 1997). Drinking ad libitum substantially reduces, but does not absolutely negate, the risk of voluntary overdrinking.

One of the foundation studies of the current ACSM guidelines (Costill et al. 1970) reported that athletes attempting to drink 1.0 L·h⁻¹, for as little as 2 h, developed disabling gastrointestinal symptoms, such that drinking became intolerable. These symptoms were caused by unabsorbed fluid (~300 mL) in the stomach at the end of exercise.

The IOC consensus correctly places the appropriate emphasis on the review of Cheuvront et al. (2003) of the important studies that establish the effects of dehydration on exercise performance. Its authors list 13 studies in which there was a reasonable measure of exercise performance in subjects who completed different exercise bouts, with varying levels of dehydration. Athletes drank either nothing or varying fluid volumes during exercise, thereby developing different levels of dehydration. Such an experimental design is the only one from which it is possible to draw conclusions about the effects of different levels of exercise-induced dehydration on exercise performance. For example, studies in which dehydration is induced before exercise, either by prior exposure to exercise and heat (Armstrong et al. 1997, Sawka et al. 1985) or the use of diuretics (Armstrong et al. 1985), cannot exclude the possibility that the dehydration-inducing intervention, and not the resulting dehydration, was the real cause of the impaired exercise performance, since the experiments did not control for this possibility. Unfortunately, these studies are frequently quoted as the primary evidence that dehydration impairs exercise performance (Gisolfi 1996, Sawka & Montain 2000).

In 10 of the studies reviewed by Cheuvront et al. (2003), exercise performance was impaired in subjects who drank nothing during exercise, and was improved by drinking; in three, however, fluid ingestion was without effect. Notably, studies that failed to show a beneficial effect of drinking were of relatively short duration and were performed in cool conditions. Thus, those data clearly support the conclusion that not drinking during exercise is likely to impair performance, especially during more prolonged exercise in the heat. This is accepted and does not require further argument (Noakes 2003, 2007a). Rather, the relevant question is: 'How much fluid needs to be ingested to enhance performance during exercise; is there an additional performance benefit from drinking "as much as tolerable" compared to drinking some fluid or drinking ad libitum during exercise?'.

Three studies can now be added to those identified by Cheuvront et al. (2003) concerning this question (Dugas et al. 2006, Kay & Marino 2003, Strydom et al. 1966), so that a total of 15 studies have compared the effects of either drinking or not drinking during exercise. In nine studies, there was a clear benefit of fluid ingestion, and in only one was performance impaired by (full) fluid replacement (Robinson et al. 1995), due to the development of gastrointestinal symptoms resulting from excessive fluid consumption. It is also clear that the benefits of fluid ingestion increase with the duration of the exercise bout and are less likely in exercise of short duration.

There are six studies in which the effect of some fluid replacement on exercise performance was compared to full fluid replacement (Backx et al. 2003, Below et al. 1995, Daries et al. 2000, Dugas et al. 2006, McConell et al. 1997, 1998). No study found full fluid replacement to be superior to ad libitum drinking. However, Daries et al. (2000) found that ad libitum drinking, relative to full fluid replacement, was associated with superior performance during a 30-min time trial, but small numbers militated against a significant finding. Dugas et al. (2006) compared the effects on performance during an 80 km cycle time trial in subjects who followed six different fluid replacement regimens, on separate occasions: (i) no fluid; (ii) mouth washing without fluid ingestion; (iii) replacing 33% of fluid loss; (iv) ad libitum drinking (replacing ~55%); (v) replacing 66% of fluid loss; (vi) replacing 100% of fluid loss. There was no significant advantage of drinking more than ad libitum, but drinking less was associated with impaired performance. These studies reinforce the conclusion that no published evidence exists to suggest that drinking in excess of ad libitum is advantageous to exercise performance.

However, the finding that ad libitum fluid ingestion during exercise appears to be at least as good as 'drinking as much as tolerable' has one important intellectual conse-

quence. It implies that it is not the level of dehydration that determines the extent to which performance will be affected by fluid ingestion. Rather, it may be that performance will be optimised regardless of the degree of dehydration that develops, provided that sufficient fluid is ingested to prevent the development of thirst during exercise. This hypothesis indeed invites scientific scrutiny.

If true, this would explain why it is possible for elite athletes to perform well whilst drinking sparingly. For example, the fastest marathon runners are often amongst the most dehydrated (Cheuvront et al. 2003), and athletes who have lost >10% body mass weight are amongst the top finishers in Ironman triathlons (Sharwood et al. 2002, 2004).

2.2.2 Issue 2: dehydration and hyperthermia and heatstroke

Those who argue for drinking to replace mass loss usually equate dehydration and hyperthermia as if dehydration cannot occur without hyperthermia and vice versa.

What is the evidence showing that dehydration is the most important determinant of core temperature, as well as the risk of collapse, in out-of-doors, self-paced exercise? Almost all evidence for this relationship comes from laboratory studies that were not designed to provide adequate convective cooling (Saunders et al. 2005), and in which a constant exercise intensity was used. When adequate convective cooling is provided, the small and biologically insignificant core temperature difference (~0.2°C), produced as a result of drinking to replace all the weight lost during exercise (Montain & Coyle 1992), compared to ad libitum drinking, disappears (Saunders et al. 2005).

What is the evidence from appropriately controlled clinical trials that dehydration increases the risk of heatstroke? There are no such clinical trials in the scientific or medical literature. Thus, it is no longer defensible to argue that dehydration causes heatstroke, or that drinking more during exercise will prevent heatstroke, or indeed the symptom-defined conditions often termed the heat illness. This is especially important if those conclusions affect behaviour in a way that could be detrimental and if those conclusions carry the backing of influential international organisations.

It is interesting that these ideas are based on a novel paradigm: the cardiovascular model of thermoregulation (Noakes 2007a, Noakes & Speedy 2006). This model proposes that dehydration impairs cardiovascular function, reducing skin blood flow and the ability to lose heat via sweating (Cheuvront et al. 2003, Sawka et al. 1985, Stover et al. 2006). It seems to have arisen from early studies which showed that subjects who did not drink during exercise developed elevated heart rates (Brown 1947) and low stroke volumes (Nadel et al. 1980). The danger of this model is that it can be used to justify claims for the value of fluid ingestion that prevents dehydration.

Yet many classical studies (for example, Adolph 1947a,b, Eichna et al. 1945) have not shown that subjects who abstained from drinking during exercise had lower sweat rates than when they ingested fluid at high rates. Thus, Ladell (1955) concluded that dehydration had no effect on sweat rate, until a water deficit >2.5 L occurred: 3.6% mass loss for a 70 kg person. Indeed, Costill et al. (1970) reported that even when not drinking during 2 h of exercise in the heat, the skin was sufficiently wet to permit maximal evaporation. Montain & Coyle (1992) similarly reported that sweat rates were the same in subjects who drank either nothing or 2.4 L of fluid during 2 h of exercise in moderately severe heat. The authors concluded that the higher end-exercise core temperatures in the 'no drink' condition was due to a reduced skin blood flow. But this seems somewhat unlikely if sweat rates were not different, and could presumably have been increased to offset any effect on heat balance of the marginally reduced skin blood flow.

Another explanation may be that the higher core temperature reflects an acute response to optimise the core–air thermal gradient (heat loss) in the absence of drinking (Dugas et al. 2006). Certain hunting mammals like the African hunting dog use this technique to conserve water when hunting (Schmidt-Nielsen 1964). Furthermore, Nielsen et al. (1971) showed that the higher core temperatures during exercise in the dehydrated state are not associated with changes in cardiac output or central circulatory failure. More to the point, the sweating response is regulated by neural mechanisms that are not dependent on the cardiovascular response to exercise (Shibasaki et al. 2003), a point apparently forgotten by those who propose this novel theory. Thus, the principal determinant of the sweating response to exercise is the neural and not the cardiovascular reaction to hyperthermia, so that those without sweat glands are at the greatest risk of heatstroke during exercise.

2.2.3 Issue 3: performance decays linearly with dehydration

It has been argued that dehydration impairs exercise performance as a linear function of dehydration, and this is influenced by environmental temperature (Coyle 2004). This conclusion is, however, based on studies which were not adequately controlled (Noakes 2007a).

What is the evidence from appropriately controlled clinical trials which shows that performance deteriorates linearly with increasing dehydration, and that this relationship becomes steeper as environmental conditions become more severe? The IOC consensus document illustrates this linear relationship (Coyle 2004), which is reproduced in Figure 34.2.1. However, since it lacks units of measure and a description of how data were derived, one must ask whether this diagram is simply a teaching concept for which data are still in the process of being collected.

The second reason for this question is the consistent finding that athletes who win (Buskirk & Beetham1960, Muir et al. 1970, Pugh et al. 1967, Wyndham & Strydom 1969) or finish near the top of competitive endurance events are frequently quite markedly dehydrated, and by up to 8–10% in the case of some Ironman triathletes (Sharwood et al. 2004, Wharam et al. 2006). If dehydration does cause a

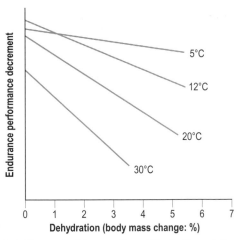

Figure 34.2.1 Theoretical interaction of hydration state and endurance performance. Redrawn from Coyle (2004) with permission.

linear reduction in performance, then these athletes could have finished faster, in some events hours faster, had they simply drunk to prevent mass changes during exercise. Such performances are impossible. Thus, the extent to which performance is impaired by 'dehydration' must be erroneous.

2.2.4 Issue 4: sodium and hyponatraemia

Many fluid replacement guidelines promote sodium ingestion during exercise despite contrary evidence showing that sodium intake in some countries (e.g. USA, Canada) greatly exceeds both the adequate index (1.5 g·d^{-1} or 65 mmol·d^{-1}) and the tolerable upper intake level (2.3 g·d^{-1} or 100 mmol·d^{-1}; Institute of Medicine for the National Academies 2004).

The Institute of Medicine states that a daily sodium intake of 1.5 g·d^{-1} is adequate for moderately active individuals in temperate climates. However, they caution that, for high-intensity exercise in stressful climates, increased water is needed and additional sodium may be required, but experimental data are lacking to support the level of sodium intake that is required. Thus, there is no scientific evidence showing that a sodium intake of 1.5 g·d^{-1} is inadequate for those who are physically active.

This is compatible with the conclusion of the 2005 International Consensus Conference on exercise-associated hyponatraemia (Hew-Butler et al. 2005), which found that only in very prolonged exercise (e.g. Ironman triathlon), undertaken in more extreme environmental conditions, might an acute sodium deficit contribute to exertional hyponatraemia. Thus, only under those unique conditions might an increased sodium intake be beneficial. However, there are no studies to support this hypothesis, yet two actively contradict it (Hew et al. 2006, Speedy et al. 2002).

The finding that the osmotically inactive, but exchangeable sodium stores in the body are likely to play a major role in maintaining serum sodium concentrations during exercise, regardless of the nature or volume of fluids ingested during exercise (Noakes et al. 2005), suggests that it is not the sodium ingested during exercise that is the key determinant of serum sodium concentration during exercise. Rather, it appears to be the individual's ability to mobilise osmotically inactive sodium, or to resist osmotic inactivation of circulating sodium, that may be more important (Noakes et al. 2005).

What is the evidence from appropriately controlled clinical trials that it is important to include sodium in drinks to minimise hyponatraemia? It is this author's opinion that all existing evidence proves this to be wrong.

The evidence shows that exercise-associated hyponatraemia results from inadequate renal free water clearance, in the face of high drinking rates, leading to fluid overload, with acute sodium deficiency playing a minor role (Hew-Butler et al. 2005, Noakes et al. 2005, Weschler 2005). Thus, it is not clear how ingesting low-sodium drinks can minimise hyponatraemia. Rather, since the condition is essentially one of inappropriate antidiuretic hormone secretion, in which sodium excretion is unimpaired, whereas water clearance is inhibited (Schwartz et al. 1957, Zerbe et al. 1980), then the ingestion or intravenous infusion of excessive volumes of any saline solutions, other than those that are markedly hypertonic, will compound the hyponatraemia (Weschler 2005). In fact, hypotonic or isotonic saline treatments are absolutely contraindicated for persons suffering from exercise-associated hyponatraemia (Ayus et al. 2005), whereas the infusion of hypertonic solutions may rapidly reverse symptoms (Hew-Butler et al. 2007).

Furthermore, it has been established that the avoidance of overdrinking can absolutely prevent the development of hyponatraemia (Almond et al. 2005, Noakes et al. 2005), and whilst sodium plays an integral part in its development (Noakes et al. 2005), the real determinant of the serum sodium concentration during exercise is not likely to be the amount lost in sweat and urine, or the amount ingested. Rather, it is more likely to be a result of the extent to which the osmotically inactive, exchangeable sodium stores are mobilised in response to excessive fluid consumption, or the magnitude of the reverse reaction – the conversion of osmotically active circulating sodium into osmotically inactive, intracellular sodium.

Indeed, the ingestion of electrolyte-containing drinks, instead of water, does not prevent the development of hyponatraemia in psychiatric patients with polydypsia (Goldman et al. 1994, Reeves 2004). Similarly, Cade and colleagues (1992) showed that serum sodium concentrations were maintained at or above resting values in marathon runners, whether they drank water or half- or full-strength sports drinks, despite acute sodium losses (400 mmol) that exceed those measured in most subjects with hyponatraemic encephalopathy (Dugas & Noakes 2005, Irving et al. 1991, Noakes et al. 2005). Barr et al. (1991) showed that unreplaced sodium losses of 200–260 mmol did not present a risk of hyponatraemia during exercise ≥6 h, even though sodium losses were substantial. Finally,

the inquest into the cause of the death (hyponatraemic encephalopathy) of a runner in the 2002 Boston Marathon concluded that it was caused by ingesting large volumes of sports drink (Smith 2002).

It is suggested that the inferences of the Gatorade Sports Science Institute (Murray & Eichner 2004), the ACSM (Convertino et al. 1996), the US Army Research Institute of Environmental Medicine (Montain et al. 2006) and now the IOC consensus document favour the promotion of sports drinks over water for all who participate in physical activity. However, there is no scientific evidence that recreational athletes who exercise for <60 min derive any unique physiological benefit by ingesting any fluids (water or sports drinks) during exercise, although they will likely feel less thirsty.

What is the evidence from appropriately controlled clinical trials showing that the excessive sodium loss might cause fatigue due to muscle weakness or cramps? Our understanding is that sodium deficiency has never been linked to muscle cramps or muscle weakness (Maughan 1986, Schwellnus et al. 2004, Sulzer et al. 2005). Indeed, the question may be asked: 'What is the evidence that muscle cramping is a disease of sodium deficiency?'. Are there any other credible explanations for the aetiology of this condition (Schwellnus et al. 1997)?

3 CONCLUSION

It is concluded that:

1. there is no evidence proving that drinking is necessary to preserve health or provide a physiological benefit during exercise <60–90 min

2. there is no evidence from realistic laboratory studies that drinking ad libitum produces a less desirable outcome

3. no study has established the cross-over point at which the performance-enhancing effects of mass reduction are negated by the performance-diminishing effects of dehydration

4. there is no evidence proving that sodium replacement is ever required during exercise, regardless of its intensity or duration

5. there is proof that avoiding overdrinking is necessary to prevent hyponatraemia

6. future guidelines for drinking during exercise should be based on the findings from randomised, appropriately controlled prospective clinical trials conducted under environmental and other conditions that match those found in out-of-doors exercise.

Acknowledgements

The authors' research, on which this review is based, is funded by the Medical Research Council of South Africa, the Harry Crossley and Nellie Atkinson Staff Research Funds of the University of Cape Town, Discovery Health, Bromor Foods and the National Research Foundation of South Africa through its THRIP initiative. T. Noakes's research group has received an annual financial research grant from Bromor (Pty) Ltd, manufacturers of the sports drink Energade. This funding terminated in June 2007. The Sports Science Institute of South Africa also receives financial support from Bromor (Pty) Ltd for its endorsement of that product. However T. Noakes receives no personal benefits, either at present or promised in the future, from this relationship.

References

Adolph EF (ed) 1947a Physiology of man in the desert. Interscience Publishers, New York

Adolph EF 1947b Water metabolism. Annual Review of Physiology 9:381–408

Almond C, Shin A, Fortescue EB, Mannix RC, Wypij D, Binstadt BA, Duncan CN, Olson DP, Salerno AE, Newburger JW, Greenes DS 2005 Hyponatremia among runners in the Boston Marathon. New England Journal of Medicine 352:1550–1556

Armstrong LE, Costill DL, Fink WJ 1985 Influence of diuretic-induced dehydration on competitive running performance. Medicine and Science in Sports and Exercise 17:456–461

Armstrong LE, Maresh CM, Gabaree CV, Hoffman JR, Kavouras SA, Kenefick RW, Castellani JW, Ahlquist LE 1997 Thermal and circulatory responses during exercise: effects of hypohydration, dehydration and water intake. Journal of Applied Physiology 82:2028–2035

Ayus JC, Arieff A, Moritz ML 2005 Hyponatremia in marathon runners. New England Journal of Medicine 353:427–428

Backx K, Van Someren KA, Palmer GS 2003 1H cycling perfomance is not affected by ingested fluid volume. Journal of Sports Science 13:333–342

Baker LB, Munce TA, Kenney WL 2005 Sex differences in voluntary fluid intake by older adults during exercise. Medicine and Science in Sports and Exercise 37:789–796

Barr SI, Costill DL, Fink WJ 1991 Fluid replacement during prolonged exercise: effects of water, saline or no fluid. Medicine and Science in Sports and Exercise 23:811–817

Below PR, Mora-Rodriguez R, Gonzalez-Alonso J, Coyle EF 1995 Fluid and carbohydrate ingestion independently improve performance during 1 h of intense exercise. Medicine and Science in Sports and Exercise 27:200–210

Brown AH 1947 Dehydration exhaustion. In: Adolph EF (ed) Physiology of man in the desert. Interscience Publishers, New York, 208–225

Buskirk ER, Beetham WPJ 1960 Dehydration and body temperature as a result of marathon running. Medicina Sportiva XIV:493–506

Byrne C, Lee JK, Chew SA, Lim CL, Tan EY 2006 Continuous thermoregulatory responses to mass-participation distance running in heat. Medicine and Science in Sports and Exercise 38:803–810

Cade R, Packer D, Zauner C, Kaufmann D, Peterson J, Mars D, Privette M, Hommen M, Fregly MJ, Rogers J 1992 Marathon running: physiological and chemical changes accompanying late-race functional deterioration. European Journal of Applied Physiology. Occupational Physiology 65:485–491

Cheuvront SN, Haymes EM 2001 Ad libitum fluid intakes and thermoregulatory responses of female distance runners in three environments. Journal of Sports Sciences 19:845–854

Cheuvront SN, Carter R III, Sawka MN 2003 Fluid balance and endurance exercise performance. Current Sports Medicine Report 2:202–208

Convertino VA, Armstrong LE, Coyle EF, Mack GW, Sawka MN, Senay LC Jr, Sherman WM 1996 American College of Sports Medicine position stand. Exercise and fluid replacement. Medicine and Science in Sports and Exercise 28:i–vii

Costill DL, Kammer WF, Fisher A 1970 Fluid ingestion during distance running. Archives of Environmental Health 21:520–525

Coyle EF 2004 Fluid and fuel intake during exercise. Journal of Sports Sciences 22:39–55 (www.informaworld.com)

Daries HN, Noakes TD, Dennis SC 2000 Effect of fluid intake volume on 2-h running performances in a 25 degrees C environment. Medicine and Science in Sports and Exercise 32:1783–1789

Dugas JP, Noakes TD 2005 Hyponatraemic encephalopathy despite a modest rate of fluid intake during a 109 km cycle race. British Journal of Sports Medicine 39:e38

Dugas JP, Oosthuizen V, Tucker R, Noakes TD 2006 Drinking 'ad libitum' optimises performance and physiological function during 80 km indoor cycling trials in hot and humid conditions with appropriate convective cooling. Medicine and Science in Sports and Exercise 38:S176

Eichna LW, Bean WB, Ashe WF, Nelson N 1945 Performance in relation to environmental temperature. Bulletin of Johns Hopkins Hospital 76:25–58

Fowkes Godek S, Bartolozzi AR, Godek JJ 2005 Sweat rate and fluid turnover in American football players compared with runners in a hot and humid environment. British Journal of Sports Medicine 39:205–211

Gisolfi CV 1996 Fluid balance for optimal performance. Nutrition Review 54:S159–S168

Glace B, Murphy C, McHugh M 2002 Food and fluid intake and disturbances in gastrointestinal and mental function during an ultramarathon. International Journal of Sport Nutrition and Exercise Metabolism 12:414–427

Goldman MB, Nash M, Blake L, Petkovic MS 1994 Do electrolyte-containing beverages improve water imbalance in hyponatremic schizophrenics? Journal of Clinical Psychiatry 55:151–153

Heinrich B 2001 Racing the antelope. Harper Collins, New York

Hew TD, Sharwood KA, Speedy DB, Noakes TD 2006 Ad libitum sodium ingestion does not influence serum sodium concentrations during an Ironman triathlon. British Journal of Sports Medicine 40:255–259

Hew-Butler TD, Almond CS, Ayus JC, Dugas JP, Meeuwisse WH, Noakes TD, Reid SA, Siegel AJ, Speedy DB, Stuempfle KJ, Verbalis JG, Weschler LB 2005 Consensus Document of the 1st International Exercise-Associated Hyponatremia (EAH) Consensus Symposium, Cape Town, South Africa 2005. Clinical Journal of Sport Medicine 15:207–213

Hew-Butler T, Verbalis JG, Noakes TD 2006 Updated fluid recommendation: position statement from the International Marathon Medical Directors Association (IMMDA). Clinical Journal of Sport Medicine 16:283–292

Hew-Butler T, Anley C, Schwartz P, Noakes T 2007 The treatment of symptomatic hyponatremia with hypertonic saline in an Ironman triathlete. Clinical Journal of Sport Medicine 17:68–69

Institute of Medicine for the National Academies 2004 Dietary reference intakes for water, potassium, sodium, chloride and sulphate. National Academies Press, Washington, DC

Irving RA, Noakes TD, Buck R, Van Zyl SR, Raine E, Godlonton J, Norman RJ 1991 Evaluation of renal function and fluid homeostasis during recovery from exercise-induced hyponatremia. Journal of Applied Physiology 70:342–348

Kay D, Marino FE 2003 Failure of fluid ingestion to improve self-paced exercise performance in moderate-to-warm humid environments. Journal of Thermal Biology 28:29–34

Ladell WS 1955 The effects of water and salt intake upon the performance of men working in hot and humid environments. Journal of Physiology 127:11–46

Laursen PB, Suriano R, Quod MJ, Lee H, Abbiss CR, Nosaka K, Martin DT, Bishop D 2006 Core temperature and hydration status during an Ironman triathlon. British Journal of Sports Medicine 40:320–325

McConell GK, Burge CM, Skinner SL, Hargreaves M 1997 Influence of ingested fluid volume on physiological responses during prolonged exercise. Acta Physiologica Scandinavica 160:149–156

McConell GK, Stephens TJ, Canny BJ 1999 Fluid ingestion does not influence intense 1-h exercise performance in a mild environment. Medicine and Science in Sports and Exercise 31(3):386–392

Maughan RJ 1986 Exercise-induced muscle cramp: a prospective biochemical study in marathon runners. Journal of Sports Science 4:31–34

Montain SJ, Coyle EF 1992 Influence of graded dehydration on hyperthermia and cardiovascular drift during exercise. Journal of Applied Physiology 73:1340–1350

Montain SJ, Cheuvront SN, Sawka MN 2006 Exercise associated hyponatraemia: quantitative analysis to understand the aetiology. British Journal of Sports Medicine 40:98–105

Muir AL, Percy-Robb IW, Davidson IA, Walsh EG, Passmore R 1970 Physiological aspects of the Edinburgh Commonwealth Games. Lancet 2:1125–1128

Murray B, Eichner ER 2004 Hyponatremia of exercise. Current Sports Medicine Reports 3:117–118

Nadel ER, Fortney SM, Wenger CB 1980 Effect of hydration state on circulatory and thermal regulations. Journal of Applied Physiology 49:715–721

Nevill AM, Whyte G 2005 Are there limits to running world records? Medicine and Science in Sports and Exercise 37:1785–1788

Nielsen B, Hansen G, Jorgensen SO, Nielsen E 1971 Thermoregulation in exercising man during dehydration and hyperhydration with water and saline. International Journal of Biometeorology 15:195–200

Noakes TD 1993 Fluid replacement during exercise. Exercise and Sport Sciences Reviews 21:297–330

Noakes TD 1995 Dehydration during exercise: what are the real dangers? Clinical Journal of Sport Medicine 5:123–128

Noakes TD 2003 Fluid replacement during marathon running. Clinical Journal of Sport Medicine 13:309–318

Noakes TD 2004 Can we trust rehydration research? In: McNamee M (ed) Philosophy and the sciences of exercise, health and sport. Taylor and Francis, Abingdon, 144–168

Noakes TD 2007a Drinking guidelines for exercise: what is the evidence that athletes should either drink 'as much as tolerable' or 'to replace all the weight lost during exercise' or 'ad libitum'? Journal of Sports Science 25:781–796

Noakes TD 2007b Reduced peripheral resistance and other factors in marathon collapse. Sports Medicine 37(4–5):382–385

Noakes TD, Sharwood K, Speedy D, Hew T, Reid S, Dugas J, Almond C, Wharam P, Weschler L 2005 Three independent biological mechanisms cause exercise-associated hyponatremia: evidence from 2,135 weighed competitive athletic performances. Proceedings of the National Academy of Sciences 102:18550–18555

Noakes TD, Speedy DB 2006 Case proven: exercise associated hyponatraemia is due to overdrinking. So why did it take 20 years before the original evidence was accepted? British Journal of Sports Medicine 40:567–572

Pugh LG, Corbett JL, Johnson RH 1967 Rectal temperatures, weight losses and sweat rates in marathon running. Journal of Applied Physiology 23:347–352

Reeves RR 2004 Worsening of hyponatremia with electrolyte-containing beverage. American Journal of Psychiatry 161:374–375

Robinson TA, Hawley JA, Palmer GS, Wilson GR, Gray DA, Noakes TD, Dennis SC 1995 Water ingestion does not improve 1-h cycling performance in moderate ambient temperatures. European Journal of Applied Physiology. Occupational Physiology 71:153–160

Saunders A, Dugas JP, Tucker R, Lambert MI, Noakes TD 2005 The effects of different air velocities on heat storage and body temperature in humans cycling in a hot, humid environment. Acta Physiologica Scandinavica 183:241–255

Sawka MN, Montain SJ 2000 Fluid and electrolyte supplementation for exercise heat stress. American Journal of Clinical Nutrition 72:564S–572S

Sawka MN, Young AJ, Francesconi RP, Muza SR, Pandolf KB 1985 Thermoregulatory and blood responses during exercise at graded hypohydration levels. Journal of Applied Physiology 59:1394–1401

Schmidt-Nielsen K 1964 Desert animals. Oxford University Press, London

Schwartz WB, Bennett W, Curelop S, Bartter FC 1957 A syndrome of renal sodium loss and hyponatremia probably resulting from inappropriate secretion of antidiuretic hormone. American Journal of Medicine 23:529–542

Schwellnus MP, Derman EW, Noakes TD 1997 Aetiology of skeletal muscle 'cramps' during exercise: a novel hypothesis. Journal of Sports Science 15:277–285

Schwellnus MP, Nicol J, Laubscher R, Noakes TD 2004 Serum electrolyte concentrations and hydration status are not associated with exercise associated muscle cramping (EAMC) in distance runners. British Journal of Sports Medicine 38:488–492

Sharwood K, Collins M, Goedecke J, Wilson G, Noakes T 2002 Weight changes, sodium levels and performance in the South African Ironman triathlon. Clinical Journal of Sport Medicine 12:391–399

Sharwood KA, Collins M, Goedecke JH, Wilson G, Noakes TD 2004 Weight changes, medical complications and performance during an Ironman triathlon. British Journal of Sports Medicine 38:718–724

Shibasaki M, Kondo N, Crandall CG 2003 Non-thermoregulatory modulation of sweating in humans. Exercise and Sports Science Review 31:34–39

Smith S 2002 Marathon runner's death linked to excessive fluid intake. Boston Globe, August 13, A1

Speedy DB, Thompson JM, Rodgers I, Collins M, Sharwood K, Noakes TD 2002 Oral salt supplementation during ultradistance exercise. Clinical Journal of Sport Medicine 12:279–284

Stover EA, Zachwieja J, Stofan J, Murray R, Horswill CA 2006 Consistently high urine specific gravity in adolescent American football players and the impact of an acute drinking strategy. International Journal of Sports Medicine 27:330–335

Strydom NB, Wyndham CH, Van Graan CH, Holdsworth LD, Morrison JF 1966 The influence of water restriction on the performance of men during a prolonged march. South African Medical Journal 40:539–544

Stuempfle KJ, Lehmann DR, Case HS, Bailey S, Hughes SL, McKenzie J, Evans D 2002 Hyponatremia in a cold weather ultraendurance race. Alaska Medicine 44:51–55

Stuempfle KJ, Lehmann DR, Case HS, Hughes SL, Evans D 2003 Change in serum sodium concentration during a cold weather ultradistance race. Clinical Journal of Sport Medicine 13:171–175

Sulzer NU, Schwellnus MP, Noakes TD 2005 Serum electrolytes in Ironman triathletes with exercise-associated muscle cramping. Medicine and Science in Sports and Exercise 37:1081–1085

Twerenbold R, Knechtle B, Kakebeeke TH, Eser P, Muller G, Von Arx P, Knecht H 2003 Effects of different sodium concentrations in replacement fluids during prolonged exercise in women. British Journal of Sports Medicine 37:300–303

Weschler LB 2005 Exercise-associated hyponatraemia: a mathematical review. Sports Medicine 35:899–922

Wharam PC, Speedy DB, Noakes TD, Thompson JM, Reid SA, Holtzhausen LM 2006 NSAID use increases the risk of developing hyponatremia during an Ironman triathlon. Medicine and Science in Sports and Exercise 38:618–622

Wyndham CH, Strydom NB 1969 The danger of an inadequate water intake during marathon running. South African Medical Journal 43:893–896

Zerbe R, Stropes L, Robertson G 1980 Vasopressin function in the syndrome of inappropriate antidiuresis. Annual Review of Medicine 31:315–327

Index

P